Heart Failure in the Child and Young Adul[t]

Heart Failure in the Child and Young Adult

From Bench to Bedside

Edited by

John L. Jefferies
Anthony C. Chang
Joseph W. Rossano
Robert E. Shaddy
Jeffrey A. Towbin

ELSEVIER
ACADEMIC PRESS
An imprint of Elsevier

Academic Press is an imprint of Elsevier
125 London Wall, London EC2Y 5AS, United Kingdom
525 B Street, Suite 1800, San Diego, CA 92101-4495, United States
50 Hampshire Street, 5th Floor, Cambridge, MA 02139, United States
The Boulevard, Langford Lane, Kidlington, Oxford OX5 1GB, United Kingdom

Notices
Knowledge and best practice in this field are constantly changing. As new research and experience broaden our understanding, changes in research methods, professional practices, or medical treatment may become necessary.

Practitioners and researchers must always rely on their own experience and knowledge in evaluating and using any information, methods, compounds, or experiments described herein. In using such information or methods they should be mindful of their own safety and the safety of others, including parties for whom they have a professional responsibility.

To the fullest extent of the law, neither the Publisher nor the authors, contributors, or editors, assume any liability for any injury and/or damage to persons or property as a matter of products liability, negligence or otherwise, or from any use or operation of any methods, products, instructions, or ideas contained in the material herein.

Library of Congress Cataloging-in-Publication Data
A catalog record for this book is available from the Library of Congress

British Library Cataloguing-in-Publication Data
A catalogue record for this book is available from the British Library

ISBN: 978-0-12-802393-8

For information on all Academic Press publications visit our website at https://www.elsevier.com/books-and-journals

Publisher: Mica Haley
Acquisition Editor: Stacy Masucci
Editorial Project Manager: Samuel Young
Production Project Manager: Anusha Sambamoorthy
Cover Designer: Victoria Pearson

Typeset by TNQ Books and Journals

Jefferies—Heart Failure Dedications

"I would like to dedicate this textbook to my mentors and colleagues who have taught me through the years as well as all those patients and families who have shown me their absolute fortitude in their struggles. I am also extremely grateful to my adopted children Emma and Olivia as they have taught me how to be patient and compassionate as a parent with children who have medical conditions."

—Anthony C. Chang

"This is dedicated to my wife Patti and daughters Jennifer and Sara for all their support over the years and during this project. In addition, to all those who have taught me from my mentors, colleague, trainees, and, most importantly, the patients and their families, I thank you. I hope this book provides others with the wisdom that you all have tried to instill in me."

—Jeffrey A. Towbin

"This book is dedicated to the patients and families that are entrusted in our care, and to my wife and children for their enduring support."

—Joseph W. Rossano

"To family and friends for their support and patience."

—Robert E. Shaddy

"I would like to dedicate this book to my wife Shari and my children John Parker and Caroline for all of their support and encouragement. I am also very grateful to my mentors, colleagues, and, most importantly, the patients and families that have taught me so much over the years."

—John L. Jefferies

Contents

List of Contributors

Iki Adachi Texas Children's Hospital, Houston, TX, United States

Jyothsna Akam-Venkata Wayne State University School of Medicine and Children's Hospital of Michigan, Detroit, MI, United States

Christopher S. Almond Stanford University, Palo Alto, CA, United States

Jeffrey B. Anderson Cincinnati Children's Hospital Medical Center, Cincinnati, OH, United States

Jean Ballweg Le Bonheur Children's Hospital, Memphis, TN, United States

Neha Bansal Wayne State University School of Medicine and Children's Hospital of Michigan, Detroit, MI, United States

Christine Benhase Xavier University, Cincinnati, OH, United States

Daniel Bernstein Stanford University, Stanford, CA, United States

Elizabeth D. Blume Boston Children's Hospital, Boston, MA, United States

Luke J. Burchill Oregon Health and Science University, Portland, OR, United States

Michael Burch Great Ormond Street Hospital, London, Great Britain

Sarah Burki Texas Children's Hospital, Houston, TX, United States

Jonathan W. Byrnes The Heart Institute at Cincinnati Children's Hospital, Cincinnati, OH, United States

Antonio G. Cabrera Baylor College of Medicine/Texas Children's Hospital, Houston, TX, United States

Bryan Cannon Mayo Clinic, Rochester, MN, United States

Charles E. Canter Washington University School of Medicine, St. Louis Children's Hospital, St Louis, MO, United States

Anthony C. Chang Children's Hospital of Orange County, Orange, CA, United States

Steven D. Colan Boston Children's Hospital, Boston, MA, United States

Jennifer L. Conway University of Alberta, Edmonton, AB, Canada

Weining David Xu University of Utah School of Medicine, Salt Lake City, UT, United States

Ryan R. Davies Nemours/A.I. duPont Hospital for Children, Wilmington, DE, United States; Thomas Jefferson University, Philadelphia, PA, United States

Susan W. Denfield Texas Children's Hospital, Houston, TX, United States

Anne I. Dipchand The Hospital for Sick Children and the University of Toronto, Toronto, ON, Canada

Mary T. Donofrio National Children's Health System, Washington, DC, United States

William J. Dreyer Texas Children's Hospital, Houston, TX, United States

David J. Driscoll Mayo Clinic, Rochester, MN, United States

Lucas Eastaugh The Royal Children's Hospital, Melbourne, VIC, Australia; Murdoch Children's Research Institute, Melbourne, VIC, Australia

Melanie D. Everitt University of Colorado, Aurora, CO, United States

James C. Fang University of Utah School of Medicine, Salt Lake City, UT, United States

Theresa J. Faulkner UC Health University Cincinnati Medical Center (UCMS), Cincinnati, OH, United States

Alejandro A. Floh The Hospital for Sick Children and the University of Toronto, Toronto, ON, Canada

Vivian I. Franco Wayne State University School of Medicine and Children's Hospital of Michigan, Detroit, MI, United States

Charles D. Fraser Texas Children's Hospital, Houston, TX, United States

Mark K. Friedberg The Hospital for Sick Children and the University of Toronto, Toronto, ON, Canada

Francis Fynn-Thompson Boston Children's Hospital, Boston, MA, United States

Kristen George The Hospital for Sick Children and the University of Toronto, Toronto, ON, Canada

Matthew J. Gillespie Children's Hospital of Philadelphia, Philadelphia, PA, United States

Andrew C. Glatz Children's Hospital of Philadelphia, Philadelphia, PA, United States

David J. Goldberg The Perelman School of Medicine at the University of Pennsylvania, Philadelphia, PA, United States

Stuart L. Goldstein Cincinnati Children's Hospital Medical Center (CCHMC), Cincinnati, OH, United States

Samuel Hanke Cincinnati Children's Hospital Medical Center, Cincinnati, OH, United States

Karen Hendricks Nursing Informatics at Chamberlain College of Nursing, Chicago, IL, United States

Ray Hershberger Internal Medicine, Division of Human Genetics, Columbus, OH, United States; Wexner Medical Center at the Ohio State University, Columbus, OH, United States

Ziyad M. Hijazi NewYork-Presbyterian Hospital – Weill Cornell Medical Center, New York, NY, United States; Weill Cornell Medical College, New York, NY, United States

Timothy M. Hoffman University of North Carolina, Chapel Hill, NC, United States

Ralf J. Holzer NewYork-Presbyterian Hospital – Weill Cornell Medical Center, New York, NY, United States; Weill Cornell Medical College, New York, NY, United States

Alexander Hussey The Royal Children's Hospital, Melbourne, VIC, Australia

Julia H. Indik The University of Arizona, Tucson, AZ, United States

Frank Ing Children's Hospital Los Angeles, Los Angeles, CA, United States; University of Southern California, Los Angeles, CA, United States

Dunbar Ivy University of Colorado School of Medicine, Aurora, CO, United States

Robert D.B. Jacquiss University of Texas Southwestern Medical Center, Dallas, TX, United States

Edgar T. Jaeggi University of Toronto, Toronto, ON, Canada

Emily Jean-St.-Michel The Hospital for Sick Children and the University of Toronto, Toronto, ON, Canada

Aamir Jeewa The Hospital for Sick Children and the University of Toronto, Toronto, ON, Canada

John L. Jefferies Cincinnati Children's Hosptial Medical Center, Cincinnati, OH, United States

Jason Johnson Le Bonheur Children's Hospital, Memphis, TN, United States

Jonathan N. Johnson Mayo Clinic, Rochester, MN, United States

Ahmad Kaddourah Sidra Medical and Research Center, Doha, Qatar; Cincinnati Children's Hospital Medical Center (CCHMC), Cincinnati, OH, United States

Paul F. Kantor University of Alberta, Edmonton, AB, Canada

Jeffrey J. Kim Texas Children's Hospital, Houston, TX, United States

Steven J. Kindel Children's Hospital of Wisconsin, Milwaukee, WI, United States

James K. Kirklin University of Alabama at Birmingham, Birmingham, AL, United States

Bernhard Kuhn Children's Hospital of Pittsburgh of UPMC, Pittsburgh, PA, United States

Jennifer Lail Cincinnati Children's Hospital Medical Center, Cincinnati, OH, United States

Kory J. Lavine Washington University School of Medicine, St. Louis, MO, United States

Kimberly Y. Lin The Perelman School of Medicine at the University of Pennsylvania, Children's Hospital of Philadelphia, Philadelphia, PA, United States

Steven E. Lipshultz Wayne State University School of Medicine and Children's Hospital of Michigan, Detroit, MI, United States; Karmanos Cancer Institute, Detroit, MI, United States

Angela Lorts Cincinnati Children's Hospital Medical Center, Cincinnati, OH, United States

Kevin O. Maher Emory University School of Medicine, Children's Healthcare of Atlanta, Atlanta, GA, United States

Douglas L. Mann Washington University School of Medicine, St. Louis, MO, United States

Frank I. Marcus The University of Arizona, Tucson, AZ, United States

Renee Margossian Boston Children's Hospital, Boston, MA, United States

Bradley S. Marino Ann & Robert Lurie Children's Hospital of Chicago, Northwestern University Feinberg School of Medicine, Chicago, IL, United States

Jacob Mathew The Royal Children's Hospital, Melbourne, VIC, Australia

Tim Maul Nemours Children's Hospital, Orlando, FL, United States

Luisa Mestroni University of Colorado Anschutz Medical Campus, Aurora, CO, United States

Shelley D. Miyamoto University of Colorado School of Medicine, Children's Hospital Colorado, Aurora, CO, United States

Ana Morales Internal Medicine, Division of Human Genetics, Columbus, OH, United States; Wexner Medical Center at the Ohio State University, Columbus, OH, United States

David L.S. Morales The University of Cincinnati, Cincinnati, OH, United States

Maryam Y. Naim Children's Hospital of Philadelphia, Philadelphia, PA, United States; The University of Pennsylvania Perelman School of Medicine, Philadelphia, PA, United States

Stephanie J. Nakano University of Colorado, Aurora, CO, United States

Deipanjan Nandi Perelman School of Medicine at the University of Pennsylvania, Philadelphia, PA, United States

David P. Nelson The Heart Institute at Cincinnati Children's Hospital, Cincinnati, OH, United States

Michael L. O'Byrne Division of Cardiology, The Children's Hospital of Philadelphia and Perelman School of Medicine University of Pennsylvania, Philadelphia, PA, United States

Matthew J. O'Connor Children's Hospital of Philadelphia, Philadelphia, PA, United States

Alexander R. Opotowsky Boston Children's Hospital, Boston, MA, United States; Brigham and Women's Hospital, Boston, MA, United States

Francis D. Pagani University of Michigan, Ann Arbor, MI, United States

Elfriede Pahl Northwestern University Feinberg School of Medicine, Chicago, IL, United States

Daniel J. Penny Texas Children's Hospital, Houston, TX, United States

Jack F. Price Texas Children's Hospital, Houston, TX, United States

Ilaria Puggia University of Colorado Anschutz Medical Campus, Aurora, CO, United States; Hospital and University of Trieste, Trieste, Italy

Chitra Ravishankar Children's Hospital of Philadelphia, Philadelphia, PA, United States

Andrew N. Redington Cincinnati Children's Hospital Medical Center, Cincinnati, OH, United States

Jonathan J. Rome Division of Cardiology, The Children's Hospital of Philadelphia and Perelman School of Medicine University of Pennsylvania, Philadelphia, PA, United States

David N. Rosenthal Stanford University, Palo Alto, CA, United States

Joseph W. Rossano Perelman School of Medicine at the University of Pennsylvania, Philadelphia, PA, United States

Heather J. Ross University Health Network, Toronto, ON, Canada

Robert D. Ross Children's Hospital of Michigan, Cardiology Division, Wayne State University School of Medicine, Detroit, MI, United States

Teisha J. Rowland University of Colorado Anschutz Medical Campus, Aurora, CO, United States

Thomas D. Ryan Cincinnati Children's Hospital Medical Center, Cincinnati, OH, United States

Kurt R. Schumacher University of Michigan Medical School, C.S. Mott Children's Hospital, Ann Arbor, MI, United States

Matthew C. Schwartz Arnold Palmer Hospital for Children, Orlando, FL, United States

Steven M. Schwartz The Hospital for Sick Children and the University of Toronto, Toronto, ON, Canada

Robert E. Shaddy Children's Hospital Los Angeles and the Keck School of Medicine of the University of Southern California

Maully J. Shah Children's Hospital of Philadelphia, Philadelphia, PA, United States

Jacob Simmonds Great Ormond Street Hospital, London, Great Britain

Kathleen E. Simpson Washington University School of Medicine, St. Louis Children's Hospital, St Louis, MO, United States

Gianfranco Sinagra Hospital and University of Trieste, Trieste, Italy

Juli Sublett Miami University, Oxford, OH, United States; The University of Cincinnati College of Nursing, Cincinnati, OH, United States

Patrick Sullivan Children's Hospital Los Angeles, Los Angeles, CA, United States; University of Southern California, Los Angeles, CA, United States

Hussam Suradi St. Mary Medical Center/Community Healthcare System, Hobart, IN, United States; Rush University Medical Center, Chicago, IL, United States

David L. Sutcliffe University of Texas Southwestern Medical Center, Dallas, TX, United States

Cheryl Takao Children's Hospital Los Angeles, Los Angeles, CA, United States; University of Southern California, Los Angeles, CA, United States

Michael Taylor Cincinnati Children's Medical Center, Cincinnati, OH, United States

Timothy Thiruchelvam Great Ormond Street Hospital, London, Great Britain

Philip T. Thrush Northwestern University Feinberg School of Medicine, Chicago, IL, United States

Jeffrey A. Towbin Le Bonheur Children's Hospital, Memphis, TN, United States

James S. Tweddell Cincinnati Children's Hospital Medical Center; University of Cincinnati, Cincinnati, OH, United States

Simon Urschel University of Alberta, Edmonton, AB, Canada

Christina J. VanderPluym Boston Children's Hospital, Boston, MA, United States

Philip Wackel Mayo Clinic, Rochester, MN, United States

Jack Wallen Cincinnati Children's Hospital Medical Center, Cincinnati, OH, United States

Peter Wearden Nemours Children's Hospital, Orlando, FL, United States

Robert G. Weintraub The Royal Children's Hospital, Melbourne, VIC, Australia; Murdoch Children's Research Institute, Melbourne, VIC, Australia; University of Melbourne, Melbourne, VIC, Australia

Scott L. Weiss Children's Hospital of Philadelphia, Philadelphia, PA, United States; The University of Pennsylvania Perelman School of Medicine, Philadelphia, PA, United States

Shawn West Children's Hospital of Pittsburgh of UPMC, Pittsburgh, PA, United States

James T. Willerson The Texas Heart Institute, Houston, TX, United States

Ivan Wilmot Cincinnati Children's Hospital Medical Center, Cincinnati Children's Hospital Medical Center, Cincinnati, OH, United States

Judith Wilson The Hospital for Sick Children and the University of Toronto, Toronto, ON, Canada

Mahsun Yuerek Children's Hospital of Philadelphia, Philadelphia, PA, United States

Matthew Zinn Children's Hospital of Pittsburgh of UPMC, Pittsburgh, PA, United States

Foreword

In 1941, the subspecialty of Cardiovascular Disease was one of the first four subspecialties of Internal Medicine in which an examination was administered and certificates awarded. (The other three subspecialties were in Allergy, Gastroenterology, and Tuberculosis.) In the late 1940s, Helen Taussig began training pediatricians in the emerging discipline of pediatric cardiology; by 1961, pediatric cardiology became the first subspecialty board in pediatrics [1]. In 2008, the American Board of Internal Medicine approved the third secondary subspecialty of cardiology, Advanced Heart Failure and Transplant Cardiology, a recognition of the unique skills and knowledge required to manage specific and growing number of profoundly ill patients with heart failure, who might undergo heart transplant or ventricular assist device implantation. Likewise, by the mid-1990s, a number of pediatric training programs offered fellowships in pediatric advanced heart failure.

For both pediatric and adult patients, the specter of the heart failure syndrome has not been diminished, despite the spectacular successes of modern medicine and surgery. Indeed, many have argued that with each gain in knowledge and skill—a child once lost in infancy to congenital heart disease or to childhood malignancy, now saved—comes a companion price of the child with chronic cardiac dysfunction. A vigorous and sustained investigation into the genetics of inherited cardiomyopathies has spawned the clinical necessity of genetic counseling, and a widening pool of young people who are potentially at risk for phenotypical disease because of their genotype. Heart failure drug development and testing in children have traditionally faced significant regulatory hurdles; life-prolonging therapy in adults with heart failure and reduced ejection fraction is infrequently tested in clinical trials for children.

Accordingly, the pediatric heart failure community has responded to these many challenges with scientific inquiry and vigor, enthusiastic unity of purpose, and an effective, multipronged approach, attested to by this textbook, Heart Failure in the Child and Young Adult: *From Bench to Bedside*. One such effort deserves special mention. In 1994, the National Heart, Lung, and Blood Institute (NHLBI) funded the Pediatric Cardiomyopathy Registry (PCMR), a large, multicenter observational study of primary and idiopathic cardiomyopathies in children [2]. The PCMR was designed to study the epidemiology and clinical course of selected cardiomyopathies in children and adolescents as well as to promote the development of cause-specific prevention and treatment strategies. Two decades later, this registry has been an invaluable resource for basic scientists, translational studies, and the clinicians who care for these patients. Similar registries for children who have undergone heart transplantation or mechanical circulatory support device implantation have also been organized; a decade long project has followed children who are treated for cancer by a team of multidisciplinary clinicians, including cardiologists. The community partnered again with the NHLBI more recently in a workshop to identify new mechanistic and therapeutic targets for pediatric heart failure [3]. In 2017, pediatric heart failure has devoted space on the American Heart Association's patient education website, (http://www.heart.org/HEARTORG/Conditions/HeartFailure/AboutHeartFailure/Heart-Failure-in-Children-and-Adolescents_UCM_311919_Article.jsp#.WVKlO1PyugQ), and several pages on a popular software system used as a point-of-care medical resource (http://www.uptodate.com/contents/heart-failure-in-children-management). The study and treatment of pediatric heart failure is now mainstream.

In summary, the profound impact of heart failure on the life of a child demands a response from scientists, clinicians, government, industry, and parents alike. The following chapters detail a remarkable progress in this field and define the work yet to be done.

Mariell Jessup, MD

Emeritus Professor of Medicine, University of Pennsylvania, Boston, MA, United States

REFERENCES

[1] J.A. Noonan, A history of pediatric specialties: the development of pediatric cardiology, Pediatr. Res. 56 (2004) 298–306.

[2] J.D. Wilkinson, D.C. Landy, S.D. Colan, et al., The pediatric cardiomyopathy registry and heart failure: key results from the first 15 years, Heart Fail. Clin. 6 (2010) 401–413 vii.

[3] K.M. Burns, B.J. Byrne, B.D. Gelb, et al., New mechanistic and therapeutic targets for pediatric heart failure: report from a National Heart, Lung, and Blood Institute working group, Circulation 130 (2014) 79–86.

Preface

Pediatric Cardiology is, and has always been, a specialty focused on diagnosing and treating all forms of congenital heart disease and the symptoms that occur. Over the past three decades, we have seen dramatic improvements in diagnostic methods, diagnostic accuracy, congenital heart surgery, and outcomes, such that there are now more adults with congenital heart disease than children with congenital heart disease. Many of these patients develop heart failure. Today, suddenly heart failure is becoming one of the major signs and symptoms to be managed by Pediatric Cardiologists and Adult Congenital Heart Disease clinicians but little has been written or learned regarding the care of this population. Recently, the focus on heart failure has been further boosted by a new interest in primary heart muscle disorders in babies, children, adolescents, and young adults. The use of imaging modalities such as cardiac MRI, diagnostic biomarkers, newer heart failure therapeutic approaches, and molecular genetic data has led to the desire to better understand the cardiomyopathies that are prominent in this pediatric population, the similarities and differences seen in this population compared to adults with these same clinical phenotypes, as well as pushing forward the development of advanced fellowship training programs specifically focused on these disorders. In fact, we have witnessed the dawn of what is a new subspecialty in Pediatric Cardiology that of the Pediatric Cardiomyopathy and Heart Failure Cardiologist. It is the development of this burgeoning new area and the need for education that spurred on the editors to create this text. The authors are authorities on the field and topic experts. The reader should come away with increased knowledge of the current state of diagnostic and therapeutic approaches and the pathophysiologic and mechanistic aspects of the disorders causing **Heart Failure in the Child and Young Adult**.

John L. Jefferies, MD
Anthony C. Chang, MD
Joseph W. Rossano, MD
Robert E. Shaddy, MD
Jeffrey A. Towbin, MD

Section I

Basic Science of Heart Failure

Chapter 1

Molecular and Cellular Mechanisms in Heart Failure

Ilaria Puggia[1,2], Teisha J. Rowland[1], Shelley D. Miyamoto[3], Gianfranco Sinagra[2], Luisa Mestroni[1]
[1]University of Colorado Anschutz Medical Campus, Aurora, CO, United States; [2]Hospital and University of Trieste, Trieste, Italy; [3]University of Colorado School of Medicine, Children's Hospital Colorado, Aurora, CO, United States

INTRODUCTION

Heart failure (HF) is classically defined as a "clinical syndrome caused by the inability of the heart to supply blood to the tissues commensurate to the metabolic needs of that tissue" [1,2]. HF results from ventricular dysfunction and volume or pressure overload, alone or in combination, and involves circulatory, neurohormonal, and molecular abnormalities [3]. Clinical presentation and etiology of HF is widely heterogeneous in the pediatric population and also differs greatly between children and adults [4]. Generally, in the pediatric population, the main causes of HF are congenital heart diseases (CHD) and cardiomyopathies. Although CHD is the most common cause of severe HF in the infant population, cardiomyopathies are the most common cause of HF and indication for heart transplantation in older children and adolescents [4], and will be the focus of our discussion in this chapter.

While the etiology of many cardiomyopathies remains unknown (idiopathic), genetic defects (primary forms) or other pathogenic conditions have been implicated. In the primary forms of cardiomyopathy, mutations of genes encoding a variety of structural and functional cellular proteins are involved. In particular, genetic abnormalities of the sarcomere, cytoskeleton, cell membrane proteins, and ion channels have been extensively investigated as causes of cardiomyopathies. Moreover, genetic mutations involving sarcomeric and cytoskeletal proteins may promote the progression of HF through ventricular remodeling, a process resulting from complex and numerous molecular mechanisms including inflammation, oxidative stress, mitochondrial dysfunction, loss of cardiomyocytes, and eventually the fibrotic replacement of myocardial tissue. Understanding the molecular and cellular mechanisms of HF could be exploited in prognostic stratification and clinical management of pediatric patients through identification of biomarkers such as inflammatory mediators or microRNAs (miRNAs). In particular, the expression of specific miRNAs seems to have a role in HF progression in adult populations, and thus miRNAs are currently being investigated as potential therapeutic targets.

Finally, due to a paucity of evidence specific to the pediatric population, treatment of HF in children is primarily based on adult HF guidelines [4]. However, therapies that are known to be effective in adults do not seem to have the same benefit in the pediatric population, and HF outcomes in children have been slow to improve [5]. There are likely many reasons for this differential response to therapy, including the heterogeneous etiologies of HF in children as well as distinctive, age-related molecular and cellular mechanisms of HF. Accordingly, processes involving tissue regeneration and repair after myocardial injury may be different between the young and old. In fact, cardiomyocyte proliferation rate seems to be higher in children than in adults, in whom it is low or absent [6]. This could have important implications in myocardial regenerative therapeutic strategies that are currently under evaluation, which are explored in the final section of this chapter.

GENETICS OF CARDIAC DYSFUNCTION AND HEART FAILURE

Dilated Cardiomyopathy

Dilated cardiomyopathy (DCM) is a myocardial disease characterized by dilation and systolic dysfunction of the left ventricle. Right ventricular dilation and dysfunction may also be present [7]. DCM is the most common cause of HF and indication for transplantation in children. According to the North American Pediatric Cardiomyopathy Registry (PCMR), 71% of children with DCM present with congestive HF at diagnosis and the 1- and 5-year rates of death or heart transplantation are 31% and 46%, respectively [8]. There are 0.58 cases of DCM per 100,000 pediatric patients (<18 years old) per year [8], with

Heart Failure in the Child and Young Adult. http://dx.doi.org/10.1016/B978-0-12-802393-8.00001-6

more boys being affected than girls (0.66 vs. 0.47 per 100,000) and more infants (<1 year old) affected than older children (>1 year old; 4.40 vs. 0.34 cases per 100,000) [9].

DCM is a complex multifactorial disorder that can derive from genetic causes or could be secondary to myocarditis, valvular disease, tachyarrhythmias, cardiotoxic drugs such as chemotherapy, or vascular or immunologic diseases [10]. Unfortunately there is no known cause for the majority of children with DCM (idiopathic), with only about a third of young DCM patients with an identified cause, 5% of them having a familial form [8]. However, many of the idiopathic cases of DCM may also be due to genetic causes. These DCM cases can be mislabeled as idiopathic due to various factors that make identifying the genetic cause difficult, such as a small family size, poor familial history, high genetic heterogeneity of the disease, and low penetrance of the particular genetic variant [11]. De novo genetic variants, while not "familial," may result in a diagnosis of idiopathic DCM, but ultimately may be disease causing [11].

Pediatric and adult DCM share mutations in genes encoding a variety of proteins of the sarcomere, cytoskeleton, nuclear envelope, sarcolemma, ion channels, and intercellular junctions. While it may seem counterintuitive that mutations in such apparently diverse proteins can result in a similar clinical phenotype (i.e., DCM), this similarity is due to these proteins having shared functions or participating in overlapping or related molecular pathways [12]. Overall, genetic mutations are thought to generate DCM phenotypes through impairment of myocardial cell function in terms of contractility and electrical conduction (the latter of which typically results in arrhythmias). For many relevant genes, a single gene mutation that alters the expression of a relevant contractile protein and modifies myocyte structure has been shown to be sufficient to cause DCM and myocardial failure in human and animal models [13,14].

According to recent studies, the most frequent mutations in DCM are thought to be ones that cause truncations of the titin protein (responsible for 18% and 25% of all idiopathic and familial DCM cases, respectively). Titin is the largest-know human protein and functions as a molecular spring by connecting the Z line and the M line in the sarcomere, providing passive force and elasticity in the contraction process [15]. Sarcomeres consist of long, fibrous proteins that contract and relax, and repeated sections of sarcomeres make up the tubular myofibrils (Fig. 1.1). While truncation mutations of the titin gene (TTN) are thought to cause DCM, the pathogenic role of TTN missense mutations is less clear, although they are likely primarily benign [16].

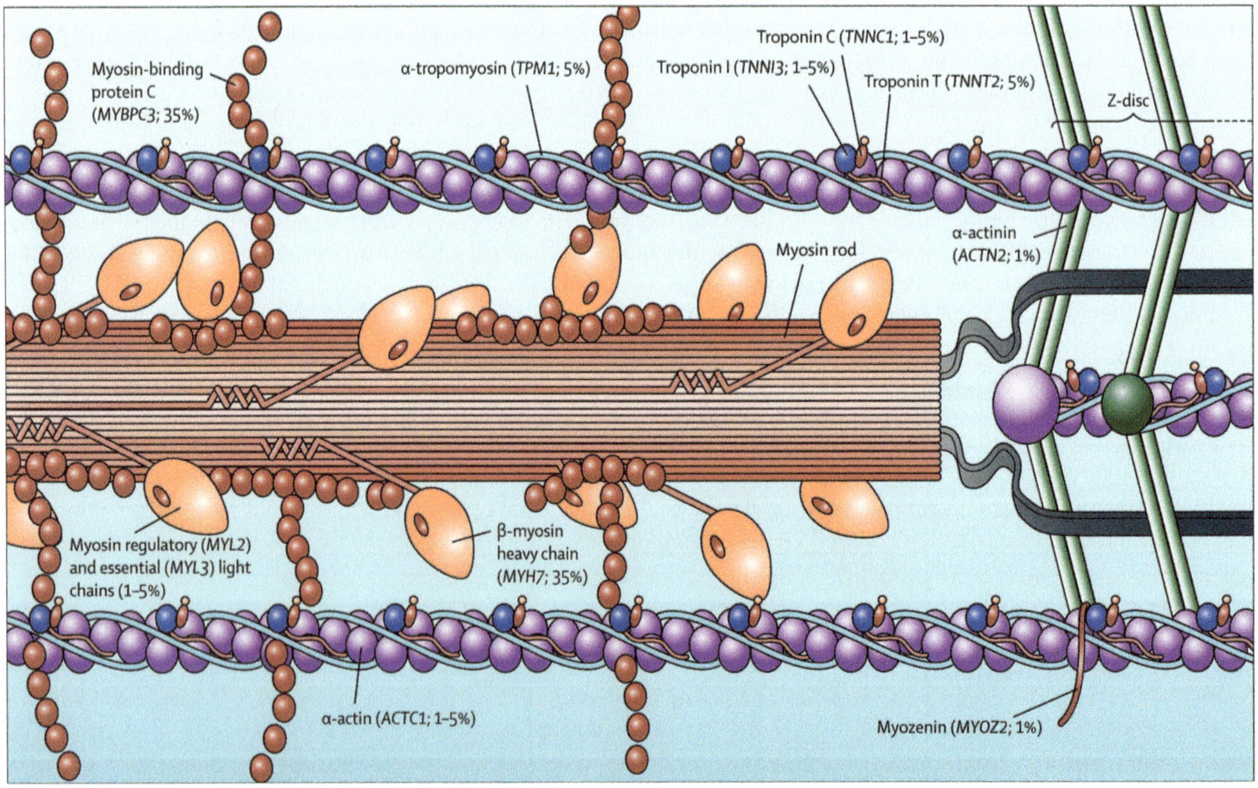

FIGURE 1.1 **Structure of a sarcomere.** Sarcomeres consist of long, fibrous proteins that contract and relax. Mutations in genes encoding the different components of the sarcomere are a frequent cause of dilated cardiomyopathy. *(Reprinted from B.J. Maron, M.S. Maron, Hypertrophic cardiomyopathy, Lancet 381 (9862) (January 19, 2013) 242–255, with permission.)*

Mutations of other genes encoding sarcomeric proteins comprise the next largest group of DCM cases with an identified genetic cause, accounting for 5%–10% of all DCM cases. These sarcomeric genes include the myosin heavy chain 6 (MYH6) and 7 (MYH7), myosin-binding protein C (MYBPC3), α-actin cardiac muscle 1 (ACTC1) and 2 (ACTC2), and α-tropomyosin (TPM1) [11]. DCM-causing sarcomeric mutations typically result in the disruption of a coupling–uncoupling mechanism of the sarcomere that results in a reduction of sarcomere contractility and produces systolic ventricular dysfunction. Recently, studies have shown that mutations in the gene encoding the BCL2-associated athanogene 3 protein (BAG3) are linked to DCM; the BAG3 protein is a cochaperone with antiapoptotic function that is localized to the Z-disc of the striated muscle, and mutations of this gene seem to induce cell apoptosis under metabolic stress. It is estimated that BAG3 mutations are present in 2.8% of Japanese families affected by DCM [17].

Another gene in which mutations can cause DCM is the gene encoding the protein lamin A/C (LMNA); mutations in LMNA are thought to account for 8% of DCM cases and are typically inherited in an autosomal dominant manner [18]. The clinical phenotype of individuals with DCM due to a LMNA variant is characterized by fast or slow arrhythmias, conduction disease, and in some cases variable degrees of skeletal muscle involvement (such as Limb-Girdle Muscular Dystrophy and Emery–Dreifuss Muscular Dystrophy). Association with Familial Partial Lipodystrophy has also been described. Lamins are intermediate filaments that provide strength and stability to the nuclear envelope, which can control the traffic into, and out of, the nucleus, and in this way may regulate the expression of specific genes.

Mutations in genes encoding the cytoskeleton are also known to result in DCM, and in these cases the disease is frequently associated with skeletal myopathy. Specifically, mutations in DES, the gene that encodes the protein desmin, can cause DCM associated with a conduction disorder and myopathy [19]. Mutations in the gene encoding dystrophin (DMD), which connects the cytoskeleton to the extracellular matrix (ECM), can result in an X-linked form of DCM and a skeletal myopathy, specifically Duchenne and Becker muscular dystrophy [20].

Ion channel mutations are associated with DCM frequently with an arrhythmogenic phenotype. Mutations in the gene encoding the sodium channel, voltage-gated, type V α subunit (SCN5A) account for 1.7% of DCM cases and are characterized by an early onset, the presence of conduction disease, and arrhythmias (atrial and ventricular) [21]. Mutations of the phospholamban protein (encoded by the PLN gene), which is involved in regulating the activity of calcium ion pumps (specifically SERCA2a) in cardiac tissue, can lead to DCM through inhibition of these pumps. SERCA2a is an isoform of the cardiac sarcoplasmic reticulum Ca^{2+}-ATPase (SERCA) protein (Fig. 1.2). SERCA2 is the SERCA isoform mainly expressed in cardiomyocytes, and it uses ATP to transport Ca^{2+} released during excitation–contraction coupling against the electrochemical gradient [22]. A PLN founder mutation (R14del) is associated with a high risk of ventricular arrhythmias and end-stage HF in late adolescence [23] and can present as an arrhythmogenic right ventricular cardiomyopathy (ARVC) phenotype.

Hypertrophic Cardiomyopathy

Hypertrophic cardiomyopathy (HCM) is a disease characterized by left ventricular (LV) or septal hypertrophy associated with normal to hyperdynamic systolic function, no dilation of ventricular chambers, and the absence of another cardiac or systemic disease that would cause the hypertrophy [24]. HCM can be classified as being symmetric (involving the LV and septum) or asymmetric (with only septal hypertrophy and normal LV posterior wall thickness). Most individuals who inherit a disease-causing HCM mutation typically present with LV or septal hypertrophy during adolescence, with disease completely manifesting at physical maturity (age ≥17 years). According to the PCMR, the annual incidence of the disease is 0.47 per 100,000 children, making it slightly less common than DCM in the pediatric population [8]. However, HCM is still one of the most frequent causes of life-threatening arrhythmias or sudden death (SD) in young individuals, with an annual mortality rate of 1% [25]. HCM rarely progresses to HF in the pediatric population (with only 13% of pediatric HCM patients developing HF, according to registry data). 8%–9% of infants with HCM have a malformation syndrome (e.g., Noonan, Costello, or Multiple-Lentigines syndrome), a metabolism disorder (e.g., Pompe disease or Danon disease), or a neuromuscular disease [8], which causes additional complications.

Most HCM cases are idiopathic or have an underlying genetic cause (the latter of which comprises almost 50% of cases) [26]. The genetic transmission of the disease is usually autosomal dominant, but maternally inherited mitochondrial patterns of transmission have also been reported [26]. As in DCM, sarcomeric gene mutations are a significant cause of HCM, consisting of 60% of HCM cases with a genetic etiology [27]. They include mutations in MYH6, MYH7, MYBPC3, TPM1, ACTC1, ACTC2, TTN, myosin essential light chain (MLC17), myosin light chain kinase (MYLK), and troponin T type 2 (TNNT2). Mutations in genes encoding nonsarcomeric proteins within the z-disc (e.g., LBD3) and calcium handling control mechanisms (e.g., PLN) can result in a similar HCM phenotype [28]. It is possible particularly for a young individual in an affected family who is positive for an HCM-causing variant to have a normal phenotype, demonstrating a lack of full penetrance.

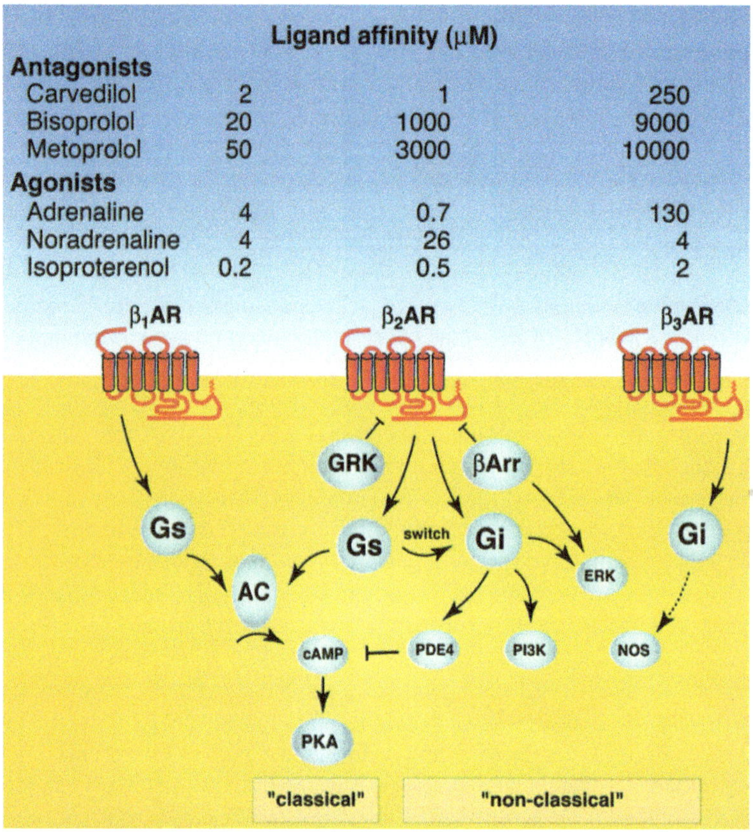

FIGURE 1.2 **β-adrenergic activation.** β1-adrenergic receptors (AR) are the main contributors to the cardiac contractility, β2 are the predominant subtype in most vascular and bronchial smooth cells, while β3 are present in adipose tissue. In the heart, adrenergic agonists bind β1-AR, stimulating the production of cAMP thought G stimulatory protein, and activating PKA. *AC*, adenylyl cyclase; *β Arr*, β-arrestin; *cAMP*, cyclic adenosine monophosphate; *ERK*, extracellular-signal receptor kinase; *Gi*, G inhibitory protein; *GRK*; G protein-coupled receptor kinase; *GS*, G stimulatory protein; *NOS*, nitric oxide synthase; *PDE*, phosphodiesterase; *PI3K*, phosphatidylinositol 3-kinase; *PKA*, protein kinase A. *(Reprinted from M.J. Lohse,* S. Engelhardt, T. Eschenhagen. *What is the role of β-adrenergic signaling in heart failure? Circ. Res. 93 (10) (October 23, 2003) 896–906, with permission.)*

Notably, HCM can be characterized by an obstructive or a nonobstructive phenotype. It is well known that the presence of LV obstruction increases the risk of HF progression by fourfold (compared to patients without obstruction). The likely underlying mechanism of HF in these patients is the chronic elevation of LV pressure secondary to the obstruction, which progressively leads to increased wall stress, myocardial ischemia, and consequent fibrosis. In this case, stiffness of the LV produces a variable degree of diastolic dysfunction, which causes congestive HF symptoms [29]. In nonobstructive HCM disease with a small ventricular cavity, diastolic dysfunction can also occur with even mild or moderate hypertrophy and preserved LV systolic function. Uncontrolled atrial fibrillation can result in progression of HF, especially in presence of obstructive disease. Finally, in the end stage of HCM disease, systolic LV dysfunction may develop and the ventricular chamber can remodel and dilate over time. Mice expressing mutant myosin heavy chains are characterized by a development of hypertrophy and then a late ventricular dilation and decompensation [30]. In human HCM-end-stage hearts, LV dilation and wall thinning are often seen. This is thought to be due to fibrosis that replaces myocardial tissue, especially in the LV septum and free wall [31,32]. A recurrent and silent myocardial ischemia may lead to this scarring and a consequent loss of contractile function [32] (this is further explored later in this chapter in the section "Inflammatory Signaling and Fibrosis").

Left Ventricular Noncompaction

Left ventricular noncompaction (LVNC) is a cardiomyopathy characterized by hypertrabeculation of the LV. According to PCMR registry data, 4.8% of children with a cardiomyopathy specifically have LVNC [33]. LVNC is thought to represent an arrest in the normal process of myocardial compaction, at the end of myocardial morphogenensis [7]. In particular, the NOTCH signaling pathway (a crucial pathway involved in several differentiation processes including cardiac embryonic development) seems to be affected. This results in a persistence of deep trabeculations and intratrabecular recesses resembling the right ventricular morphology [34].

LVNC can be associated with a normal LV size and normal systolic and diastolic function [35]. However, in some cases, underlying arrhythmias are present. LVNC can also occur in association with LV systolic dilation and dysfunction, and when this happens the cardiomyopathy mimics DCM in terms of signs and symptoms, but in young children the outcome is worse than for those with DCM [7]. LVNC can be associated with LV thickening, usually with asymmetric septal hypertrophy, diastolic dysfunction, and hypercontractile systolic function [36]. Other forms of LVNC, such as those with a restrictive phenotype, are rare. LVNC can also be associated with CHD. Similarly to other cardiomyopathy forms, LVNC is known to have genetic causes; several mutations have been identified that are associated with this disease. The first mutation described was in the X-linked gene TAZ (which encodes for tafazzin) and resulted in Barth syndrome (see also "Mitochondrial Dysfunction" section) [37]. Mutations in the Z-line protein-encoding gene LDB3, in the sarcomere genes (MYH7, ACTC, TNNT2, MYBPC3, TPM1, and TNNI3), in LMNA, in dystrophin, in SCN5A, and in DSP have all been reported to have associations with LVNC [38–44].

Arrhythmogenic Right Ventricular Cardiomyopathy

ARVC is a rare cardiomyopathy, with prevalence in the general population estimated to range from 1 in 1000 to 1 in 5000 [45]. In the PCMR, 5% of pediatric patients are affected by ARVC [8]. This cardiomyopathy is usually diagnosed between 20 and 40 years of age, and rarely in individuals younger than 10 years old. Criteria for ARVC diagnosis are well established [46], with it being characterized by a fibro-fatty replacement progressing from the right ventricular epicardium to ultimately becoming transmural. This gradual fibro-fatty replacement interferes with electric impulse conduction, leading to ventricular arrhythmias that often have LV involvement [45]. Among children and young adults it is important to suspect this disease in the presence of recurrent ventricular arrhythmias and a suggestive family history of ARVC or SD. While SD in young asymptomatic ARVC gene carriers may be the first sign of disease, HF mimicking DCM is a less common presentation in the pediatric population [45].

On a molecular and cellular level, ARVC is thought to be caused by defects in cellular adhesion due to mutations in desmosomal genes, including plakophilin-2 (PKP2), desmoplakin (DSP), desmoglein-2 (DSG2), desmocollin-2 (DSC2), and plakoglobin (JUP). Recently, mutations in TTN have also been identified in some ARVC families [47]. In this particular case, a recent study demonstrated that carriers of TTN mutations have a greater risk for supraventricular arrhythmias and conduction disease but a better prognosis than ARVC patients who are desmosomal gene mutation carriers [48]. Mutations in genes that do not encode for demosomal proteins, such as RYR2 and TGFB, have additionally been found to be associated with ARVC [49,50]. Interestingly, PLN (also associated with DCM, as discussed above) and TMEM43 gene variants have also been found to be associated with ARVC, with a TMEM43 missense mutation having been identified as a "founder" ARVC variant observed in populations of the Newfoundland islands and affecting both adults and children [51].

Restrictive Cardiomyopathy

Restrictive cardiomyopathy (RCM) is very rare in childhood, with typically only 5% of pediatric cardiomyopathy patients being affected, based on data from the PCMR [8]. Prognosis for these pediatric patients is often poor, and heart transplantation is usually required. In the adult population, etiologies of RCM can include amyloidosis, sarcoidosis, hemosiderosis, glycogenoses, endomyocardial fibroelastosis, scleroderma, and therapeutic radiation. In children, this disease is often idiopathic, but can also be familial. An important cause of pediatric cases of RCM is mutations in sarcomeric genes [52]. Rarely RCM is caused by an accumulation of mutated desmin proteins in the cardiomyocytes and, in these cases, it is associated with atrioventricular block [53]. Recently, it was demonstrated that mutations in TTN can also cause this disease [54]. HF develops due to a restrictive ventricular physiology and increased filling pressure. The affected heart is characterized by marked atrial enlargement, normal or reduced ventricular diastolic volumes, normal ventricular wall thickness, and (usually) preserved LV ejection fraction [10].

MOLECULAR MECHANISMS OF HEART FAILURE

Ventricular Remodeling

Ventricular remodeling is the process resulting in a modification of structure and function of the heart after an injury of the myocardium that can lead to HF (Table 1.1). This condition is promoted by changes in energetic metabolism,

TABLE 1.1 Some of the Most Important Mechanisms of Ventricular Remodeling in Heart Failure

Mechanisms	Mediators
Genetic mechanism	Cytoskeletal gene mutations
	Sarcomeric gene mutations
	Signaling gene mutations
	Reactivation of "fetal program"
	Posttranslational mRNA modifications
Compensatory mechanisms	β-adrenergic pathway
	Renin–angiotensin–aldosterone system
Inflammatory signaling	Oxidative stress
	Fibrosis
Mitochondrial dysfunction	Reduced energy supply

excitation–contraction coupling, Ca^{2+} handling, contractile proteins or their regulatory elements, or cytoskeleton components [55]. Potentially, changes in the expression of the genes responsible for all of these functions are present in the failing heart and promote the remodeling process [56].

In HF, typically, the primary response is hypertrophic growth of the myocytes in an effort to reduce wall stress of the ventricle in the presence of a pressure or volume overload [55]. A pressure overload could be the consequence of left-sided obstruction, such as in obstructive HCM, severe congenital aortic or subaortic stenosis, aortic coarctation, or hypertensive disorders [4]. In cases with pressure overload, an increase in LV wall thickness due to the parallel assembly of sarcomeres and the growth of the cross-sectional area of cardiomyocytes with a normal chamber volume (i.e., concentric remodeling) occurs [57].

A ventricular volume overload is due to left–right ventricular shunting and atrioventricular or semilunar valve regurgitations [4]. Ventricular volume overload is specifically characterized by the in series array of sarcomeres and longitudinal cardiomyocyte growth. This provokes eccentric hypertrophy with an increase in chamber volume. If stress is prolonged, this leads to a decompensation phase of the failing heart. According to La Place law, the increase of ventricular volume associated with a reduction of thickness promotes wall stress, one of the major determinants of myocardial oxygen consumption. This leads to a shift toward anaerobic glycolytic metabolism, which alters the subcellular ion flux, and contributes to cardiomyocyte dysfunction and consequently to the development of HF [56].

Pathophysiological changes are accompanied by reactivation of fetal gene expression programs (which are normally postnatally downregulated) and repression of the expression of several adult genes. The induction of fetal genes provokes an increase in expression of MYH7, ACTA1, B-type natriuretic peptide, and atrial natriuretic peptide and a decrease in MYH6 and SERCA2. While this gene expression pattern is most well described in adult HF, the decrease of MYH6 was demonstrated to occur in pediatric DCM as well [58]. As a consequence of these gene expression alterations, the quality and bioenergetic yield of contractile proteins and their functions becomes reduced [56,59].

Lastly, cardiomyocyte function is modulated by the β-adrenergic pathway with its inotropic and chromotropic effects. In HF, β-adrenergic stimulation is attenuated because of multiple changes at the signaling level, specifically of G proteins and adenylyl cyclase; this is discussed in further detail in the following section. Finally, at the same time, reduction in parasympathetic drive occurs [60].

Compensatory Mechanisms of Heart Failure

In the development of HF, the role of compensatory mechanisms is crucial. It is well known that the activation of the adrenergic nervous system and renin–angiotensin–aldosterone system (RAAS) contributes to, or is responsible for, the progression of HF. Based on this fact, clinical HF trials in adults have demonstrated the usefulness of angiotensin converting enzyme inhibitors [61–65], angiotensin receptor blockers [66,67], aldosterone receptor antagonist [68,69], and beta blockers [70–73].

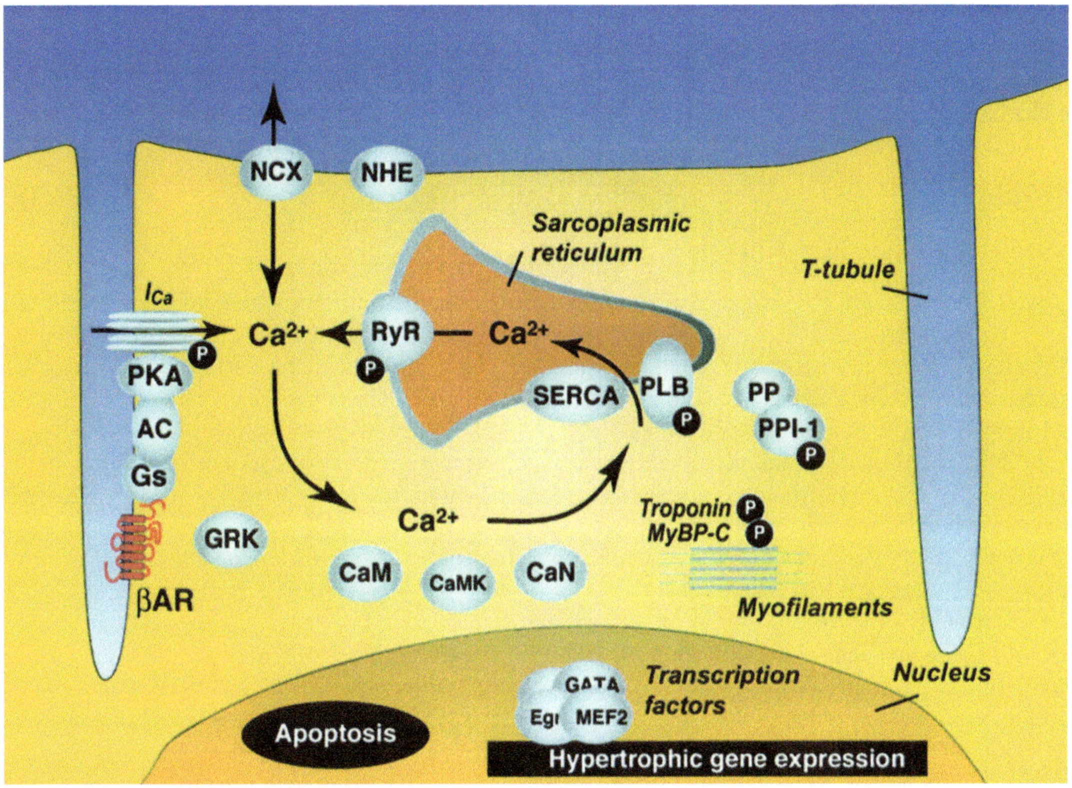

FIGURE 1.3 **Ca^{2+} cycling in cardiomyocytes.** PKA activity affects the cardiac excitation–contraction coupling thought phosphorylation, by increasing intracellular Ca^{2+}, its reuptake in sarcoplasmic reticulum, and the Ca^{+} sensitivity of myofilaments. *AC*, adenylyl cyclase; *AR*, adrenergic receptor; *CaM*, calmodulin; *CaMK*, calmodulin-dependent kinase; *CaN*, calcineurin; *GRK*, G protein-coupled receptor kinase; *GS*, G stimulatory protein; *NCX*, sodium–calcium exchanger; *NHE*, sodium–proton exchanger; *PKA*, protein kinase A; *PLB*, phospholamban; *PP*, protein phosphatase; *RyR*, ryanodine receptor; *SERCA*, sarcoplasmic reticulum calcium ATPase. *(Reprinted from M.J. Lohse, What is the role of β-adrenergic signaling in heart failure? Circ. Res. 93 (10) (October 23, 2003) 896–906, with permission.)*

When a myocardial insult causes systolic dysfunction, β-adrenergic activation (through the β-1 and β-2 receptors) increases heart rate and contractility acutely. The Frank–Starling mechanism is activated in a few hours (by a volume expansion that increases the stroke volume), and cardiac myocyte hypertrophy increases the number of contractile elements in days to 1 week [56]. At the cellular level, the β-adrenergic signaling pathway initially results in increased levels of cyclic adenosine monophosphate (cAMP) through the activation of adenylyl cyclases via stimulatory G proteins. Increased cAMP levels lead to activation of protein kinase A, which phosphorylate several proteins, such as L-type calcium channels, PLN, troponin I, ryanodine receptors, MYBPC3, and protein phosphatase inhibitor-1. This results in impacted myocardial contractility: the phosphorylation of L-type calcium channels increases the Ca^{2+} flux, while the phosphorylation of PLN and SERCA increases the reuptake of Ca^{2+} into the sarcoplasmic reticulum, and MYBPC3 and troponin I phosphorylation modulates the myofilament Ca^{2+} sensitivity. These compensatory adjustments can lead to a stable condition for some days or even months, but they create damage over the long term; chronic stimulation of the β-adrenergic system results in downregulation and desensitization of the β1-adrenergic receptor, resulting in decreased cAMP, dephosphorylation of phospholamban, and repression of SERCA2A activity (Fig. 1.3) [56].

Many differences between adult and pediatric HF populations in terms of myocellular mechanisms (on examination of explanted hearts) have been reported (for a recent review, see Miyamoto et al.) [58]. As one such example [74,75], in adult HF the PLN protein is dephosphorylated, likely through elevated phosphatase activity, resulting in decreased Ca^{2+} reuptake in the sarcoplasmic reticulum. However, PLN phosphorylation has been demonstrated to be unchanged in pediatric HF. The pediatric population is also characterized by downregulation of both the β-1 and β-2 adrenergic receptors, whereas in adult HF the β-2 adrenergic receptor maintains its expression. Therefore, age-related differences in these compensatory mechanisms likely contribute to the different responses to HF therapy between adults and children. For example, a recent randomized controlled trial of carvedilol in pediatric HF patients showed an absence of improvement in long-term mortality, even though this therapy has been shown to be effective in adult patients [76]. While there likely are subsets of pediatric patients that respond to adult-based therapies such as carvedilol, the heterogeneity of pediatric HF and differential age-related adaptations make direct extrapolation of adult HF data challenging. On the other hand, the use of phosphodiesterase 3 inhibitors (PDE3i) in pediatric DCM patients with HF demonstrates an improvement of HF symptoms without an increase in SD and life-threatening arrhythmias, both of which are seen in adults treated with PDE3i [77]. This beneficial treatment response in children may be due to augmented cAMP expression with PDE3i treatment and preserved phospholamban phosphorylation unique to the pediatric failing heart [78]. The unique myocellular changes in pediatric HF continue to be under investigation.

Inflammatory Signaling and Fibrosis

Fibrosis is a determinant of HF outcome, and addressing it using effective antifibrotic therapies in adult HF is crucial for improving patient prognosis. There is a knowledge gap regarding the pathogenesis of fibrosis in children with HF, but pathways of stress-induced fibrosis are thought to be similar in pediatric and adult hearts [79]. Cardiac fibrosis is caused by an irregular deposition of ECM proteins in the cardiac interstitium. The fibroblasts that are central to this process are derived from the differentiation of epicardial cells through endothelial–mesenchymal transformation, which is a process that can be reactivated in adult hearts during stress (e.g., pressure overload) [80] or similarly in pediatric hearts with HCM [81]. Other cells contribute to cardiac fibrosis, including monocytes/macrophages, lymphocytes, mast cells, vascular cells, and cardiomyocytes.

Inflammatory cytokines and chemokines, reactive oxygen species (ROS), matrix metalloproteinases (MMPs), and growth factors (e.g., TGFβ and PDGF) are some of the main fibrosis mediators [82]. Fibrosis can be stimulated by long-term activation of the RAAS. Specifically in the RAAS, angiotensin II (AT II) induces increased levels of aldosterone, which promotes LV remodeling and dysfunction [83,84]. Fibrosis can also be caused by an imbalance between MMPs (which are a family of zinc-dependent enzymes involved in the degradation of the ECM) and their inhibitors, with irregular upregulation of the inhibitors, which can occur during pressure overload. On the other hand, in volume overload (i.e., valvular regurgitation), an overexpression of MMPs occurs [85].

Fibrosis contributes to both diastolic and systolic LV dysfunction, interfering with myocardial excitation–contraction coupling [86]. Initially, fibrosis is associated with an increase in stiffness and a consequent diastolic dysfunction. Over time, the prolonged degradation of the ECM caused by increased levels of MMPs leads to ventricular dilation and an impairment of the systolic function [87]. The generation of fibrotic tissue is also known to alter the electrical conduction of that tissue and creates reentry circuits that promote arrhythmogenesis [88]. Several cardiac diseases are characterized by fibrotic ventricular remodeling. Typically, loss of cell is followed by fibrosis that replaces myocardium with a collagen-based scar [89].

A cardiac condition in which fibrosis plays an important role is HCM. Related to the fibrotic process, elevated collagen accumulation is a hallmark of diastolic impairment in HCM [90]. Moreover, a high level of MMP-2 seems to be related to LV remodeling and a worse prognosis in HCM [91]. Collagen breakdown products and collagen turnover enzymes have also been found to be elevated in HCM patients' family members with pathogenic sarcomere mutations, even in the absence of septal hypertrophy and fibrosis, on clinical examination and MRI imaging. This suggests that increased degradation of collagen, indicating a prefibrotic state, could be present before clinical evidence reveals the presence of pathogenesis [92]. The trigger for increased myocardial fibrosis in this disease is unclear, but it seems to be related to sarcomere mutations and other pathological alterations, such as ischemia secondary to small vessel coronary disease. In fact, hypoxia is another stimuli of the fibrotic process. Studies have shown that increased expression levels of hypoxia-inducible factor 1-α in children with a positive HCM genotype is related to a more severe LV hypertrophy and diastolic dysfunction, and less freedom from surgical myectomy [81]. Finally, a lower oxygen supply in terms of fewer capillaries has been observed in many forms of human adaptive cardiomyopathies, including end-stage DCM. Oxygen deficiency provokes a degeneration of cardiomyocytes, a metabolic imbalance, and interstitial fibrosis [93].

Inflammation and Oxidative Stress in Heart Failure

Inflammation is not well studied in pediatric HF; here we will primarily explore what is known about inflammation in HF in adults, since the process is significantly better characterized.

Inflammation has a primary role in response to cardiac injuries (i.e., ischemia, virus) and secondarily in ventricular remodeling. Notably, tissue damage (e.g., a cardiac injury) can induce an innate immune system response through toll-like receptors, which activate nuclear factor kappa B (NF-κB) transcription factors. Whereas NF-κB activation is known to serve a cardioprotective role in the relatively short-term events of acute hypoxia and reperfusion (i.e., myocardial infarction (MI)) [94], long-term activation (such as caused by long-term cardiac damage) can promote HF through a chronic release of proinflammatory cytokines (i.e., cell signaling proteins) and chemokines (i.e., small cytokines) [95].

The RAAS and sympathetic nervous system are thought to also contribute to the production of cytokines in HF through catecholamines and neurohormonal activation of NF-κB [96]. Chemokines recruit leukocytes to the damaged myocardium; neutrophils and macrophages not only remove the dead cells but also produce other cytokines that promote a local inflammatory response. Cytokines such as tumor necrosis factor-alpha (TNFα) and interleukin 6 (IL-6) are known to directly cause decreases in myocardial contractility and induce myocyte hypertrophy, collagen deposition, and fibrosis [97]. In the same way, IL-1β promotes inflammation, myocardial collagen deposition, and cardiomyocyte apoptosis [98]. Moreover, a high level of circulating inflammatory biomarkers are found in adult HF patients and are associated with a negative prognosis; these include TNFα, the soluble TNFα receptor, and IL-6 [99–101]. On the other hand, high circulating levels of neutrophil gelatinase-associated lipocalin (NGAL) (which is upregulated via various proinflammatory stimuli, including TNFs) [102] are associated with a high negative prognostic value in patients with HF. NGAL levels are also known to be increased in young HF patients [103]. Therefore, stimuli that lead to chronic inflammation are important to analyze when determining if ventricular remodeling is occurring and remain an intriguing therapeutic target.

HF progression is promoted by the loss of cardiomyocytes through apoptosis (i.e., programmed cell death), which can involve regulation of downstream inflammation pathways. Studies have shown that apoptosis rates in patients with end-stage DCM are higher than in nonfailing control hearts. Classically, the apoptosis process is initiated by the activation of cell surface death receptors (i.e., Fas/FasL) that promote the caspase cascade, the latter of which can be critically important for regulating inflammation [104].

Another mechanism involved in ventricular dysfunction is oxidative stress. ROS have been reported to be present in myocardial tissues undergoing HF [105–107]. Aldosterone, produced by the RAAS, stimulates ROS production [108]. Nicotinamide adenine dinucleotide phosphate (NADPH) oxidase is an enzymatic complex that is also known to be a major source of ROS and is thought to have increased enzymatic activity in failing hearts (compared to nonfailing controls) [109] and plays a role in cardiac hypertrophy [110]. NADPH oxidase is activated by AT II, noradrenaline, TNFα, and increased mechanical forces. All these factors are involved in pathophysiology of HF as mentioned above. Finally, increased ROS production contributes to endothelial dysfunction [111] and LV remodeling and dysfunction [112], likely due to a reduction of endothelial nitric oxide synthase-derived nitric oxide (NO). Overall, there are multiple ways in which increased ROS production negatively impacts cardiac remodeling and HF, and a better understanding of these molecular mechanisms, especially in the pediatric population, may improve therapeutic approaches.

Mitochondrial Dysfunction

Augmentation of cardiac output required under times of increased metabolic demand requires mitochondria to be able to rapidly supply energy when needed [113]. The amount of energy, or cellular ATP, demanded by the cardiac tissue varies depending on the effort expended, but, for example, during times of high workload, turnover rate of the cardiac ATP pool can be as fast as 2 s [114,115], making the efficient function of the mitochondria essential for cardiac function. Because of the crucial role of mitochondria, cardiomyopathy is present in an estimated 20%–40% of these individuals [116], and consequently screening for cardiomyopathy has become a standard part of management for people with mitochondrial diseases (which may consist of at least 1 in 5000 live births [117]). Estimated frequencies of mitochondrial cardiomyopathies in pediatric patients are similar, affecting approximately 17%–40% of those with a mitochondrial disease [117–119], and mortality has been reported to be significantly higher in these children than in ones with mitochondrial disease but without cardiomyopathy (71% vs. 26%) [118]. While mitochondrial cardiomyopathies are genetically and phenotypically heterogeneous, in both pediatric and adult patients, HCM has been reported to be the most common cardiomyopathy form, although DCM and LVNC have also been found (comprising 58%, 29%, and 13%, respectively, of the cardiac group in one study of 113 pediatric patients) [116,119]. Some studies suggest that if candidates are selected carefully (i.e., mitochondrial disease isolated primarily to the heart), cardiac transplantation is a feasible treatment strategy [117]. The rest of this section will discuss the more common attributes of pediatric mitochondrial cardiomyopathies; for a recent and thorough review discussing mitochondrial cardiomyopathies in both children and adults see Brunel-Guitton et al. [116].

Barth syndrome is a rare X-linked genetic mitochondrial disease caused by mutations in the gene TAZ, which encodes Tafazzin, a mitochondrial enzyme involved in remodeling cardiolipin. Cardiolipin is a phospholipid primarily found in the inner mitochondrial membrane and is essential for ideal mitochondrial function by maintaining electron flux of the mitochondrial electron transport chain [116,120]. Cardiomyopathy in individuals with Barth syndrome nearly always appears before age 5, and the majority of Barth syndrome patients (73%) present with cardiomyopathy [121]. LVNC and DCM are the cardiomyopathies most commonly associated with this syndrome, while HCM is less common but has been reported [116,121].

Patients also have an increased risk of ventricular arrhythmia and sudden cardiac death. While there is often a significant cardiac component, part of the challenge of diagnosing Barth syndrome is its multisystem and variable nature; in addition to being characterized by cardiomyopathy, affected individuals can also possess skeletal myopathy, neutropenia, growth delay, and increased urinary excretion of 3-methylglutaconic acid [116,121]. Similar to Barth syndrome, a small number of other mitochondrial disorders have characteristic 3-methylglutaconic aciduria, with significant and consistent increases in excretion of 3-methylglutaconic acid in urine (40 to >1000 mmol/mol creatinine) [116,122]. This group includes cardiomyopathies (specifically early onset DCM or LVNC) caused by mutations in the gene encoding the DNAJC19 protein, which resides in the inner mitochondrial membrane, where it is a chaperone protein likely involved in protein import [116,123]. Additionally, it has been reported that pediatric patients with idiopathic DCM have significantly lower expression levels of cardiolipin and dysregulation of enzymes involved in cardiolipin biosynthesis and remodeling [120].

Other mitochondrial diseases that have characteristic cardiomyopathy in the pediatric population include mitochondrial fatty acid β-oxidation defects (FAODs) [116]. Fatty acids are an essential energy source for myocardium, and FAODs can cause a substantial decrease in fatty acid utilization that leads to cardiomyopathy by disrupting different, but interrelated, molecular mechanisms in ways that are not yet fully understood [116]. Clinical presentations of FAODs are variable, with the most severe forms being highly associated with neonatal death [124]. Neonatal presentations most frequently are characterized by cardiac features (22%–47% of cases; specifically cardiomyopathy or arrhythmias associated with SD) [125,126] or liver defects (92%; specifically hepatomegaly) [125], among other symptoms. FAOD presentations can be later-onset, although these are more likely to be myopathic in nature [116].

MicroRNAs

miRNAs (miRs) are relatively short (approximately 22 nucleotides long), single-stranded noncoding RNAs that can bind the complementary 3′ untranslated regions of target messenger RNA (mRNA) to repress gene translation [127]. Changes in the expression of specific miRNAs have been found to take place during heart disease progression; for example, decreased expression of miR-133 has been found to correlate with cardiac hypertrophy [128]. Significant similarities have also been found between the miRNA expression pattern in human failing hearts and fetal cardiac tissue, suggesting that reactivation of fetal miRNAs may contribute to altered gene expression in HF [129]. Such findings have implicated the involvement of miRNAs in heart disease progression, and consequently cardiac-related miRNA applications being pursued include both their use as biomarkers and as therapeutics [127,130,131]. However, while such a therapeutic approach may be advantageous compared to conventional drug molecules because there may be lessened or absent target desensitization (which is a problem with many classical drugs), therapeutic miRNAs potentially have many off-target effects as miRNAs target several mRNAs simultaneously [132]. That said, preclinical animal models are being tested for miRNA-based heart disease therapies, although no therapies have yet begun testing in human clinical trials [127].

Investigations into the potential role of miRNAs in pediatric cardiomyopathies have been limited and warrant more attention due to differences in clinical manifestations and treatment responses between adult and pediatric patients. Our investigations in a pediatric population found that the myocardial miRNA expression profiles of pediatric HF patients (with DCM) share little overlap with the profiles of adult patients with DCM, and such differences may contribute to age-specific differences in response to HF therapies such as PDE3i [133]. We later investigated the circulating miRNA expression profile of pediatric DCM patients to determine if circulating miRNAs could be used as biomarkers to predict patient outcomes [131]; while the 5-year rate of death or transplantation for children with DCM is devastatingly high (40%–60%), a small percentage of pediatric DCM patients recover ventricular function (15%–35%) [9,134,135]. While larger prospective investigations are needed, this study demonstrated that the expression of certain circulating miRNAs could predict recovery of heart function in pediatric subjects with severe DCM. Our study revealed a limited number of miRNAs that were significantly differentially expressed in patients who recovered compared to ones who were transplanted or died (specifically, two miRNAs were upregulated [miR-155 and miR-636] and two were downregulated [miR-646 and miR-639]) [131]. It is unclear whether any of these miRNAs contribute to ventricular function recovery; indeed, an area requiring much further investigation is correlating such descriptive studies of miRNA expression differences with miRNA regulatory mechanisms and outcomes on a molecular level.

MYOCARDIAL REGENERATIVE STRATEGIES

The field of cardiac regenerative medicine has been rapidly growing but has also frequently become an area of considerable controversy, primarily due to lack of reproducibility of findings and methodological heterogeneity. Because HF progression involves a loss of cardiomyocytes thought to be the underlying cause of the HF itself, and no current therapy targets this loss, there is great interest in improving the human heart's limited regenerative abilities [136–138]. (MI also results in a loss of cardiomyocytes, with estimations of more than a billion cells lost from a single MI event [138].) Such interest has led to thousands of patients being enrolled in various clinical trials using stem cells to treat cardiac diseases over the past two decades [139]. Here we will discuss relevant studies investigating cardiomyocytes, cardiac progenitor cells (CPCs), bone marrow-derived stem cells (BMSCs), and pluripotent stem cells, while highlighting relevant pediatric findings.

While studies in neonatal mice and lower vertebrates, such as newts and zebrafish, have revealed these other organisms to have clear regenerative abilities [140–143], the situation has been more uncertain in humans due to the great difficulty of accurately assessing the regenerative capabilities of the human heart and isolating specific cell populations for study. Cardiomyocytes themselves, although they have relatively low renewal rates (estimated to be less than 1%–2% per year), are thought to be the major endogenous cardiac source of new cardiomyocytes in the adult human heart [136,144]. Children may have higher renewal rates, with potentially a 3.5-fold increase in cardiomyocyte numbers between birth and age 20 [6,79]. However, these renewal rates are still much debated, and many questions surrounding these cells remain to be answered before they could be efficiently utilized in regenerative therapies, including whether new cardiomyocytes are in fact generated from existing ones or CPCs, how injury may alter renewal rates, and how to promote cardiomyocyte cytokinesis (the cytoplasmic division of the cell; a process these cells resist undergoing) [136,138].

CPCs, which are Lin^- $c\text{-}kit^+$ cells residing in the heart itself, have been pursued for their regenerative abilities since their discovery in 2003 but are controversial due to mixed findings of their regenerative abilities, making it currently unclear whether these cells are true stem cells that can replenish lost cardiomyocyte populations or they only have regenerative abilities in rare situations (the latter seems more likely based on murine studies) [136]. Other endogenous cell types have also been explored for their cardiac regenerative potential, but due to challenges in isolating these cells in significant numbers, they are difficult to study. CPCs have been used in two small-scale clinical trials that demonstrated safety but were not large enough to prove potential benefits or functional improvement [136]. For a thorough, recent review on cardiac progenitors and early heart development, including signaling pathways and transcription factors involved, see Bulatovic et al. [138].

Although endogenous cardiomyocytes and CPCs likely have some regenerative properties, current cardiac regenerative strategies primarily utilize exogenously added cells—mostly BMSCs—or the addition of molecular factors. BMSCs (which are a type of multipotent, mesenchymal stem cell) originally captured much interest and promise due to a 2001 study showing significant cardiac regeneration in rodents using these cell types [145]. Specifically, this study reported that at 9 days post infarction an injection of Lin^- $c\text{-}kit^+$ BMSCs into the injured myocardial site resulted in regeneration of 68% of the injured area [145]. However, several studies following this one failed to reproduce such positive findings [136,146–148]. Many clinical trials have utilized cellular injections (of autologous or allogeneic BMSCs cells or autologous myocardial tissues [139,149–151]) with similarly mixed results and discrepancies, some retractions of data, and a shared problem being that survival has not been clearly assessed as a primary end point [136,139,152,153]. For a thorough review of 47 recent clinical trials using BMSCs, see Ikebe and Suzuki [154], and for a detailed methodological comparison between a few select clinical trials, see Rosen et al. Such studies and trials have also not utilized standard stratification schemes for age, making it difficult to determine the effect of age on outcomes [139]. However, it is still thought that BMSCs donated from younger patients may be more effective than cells donated from older patients, and younger patients undergoing cellular therapies (and other strategies aimed at stimulating myocardial regeneration) may receive greater benefit than older patients [79,139,149,155–158]. Improved, evidence-based international and regulated standards, following good medical practice code, for the isolation, expansion, and application of donor BMSCs is needed before such therapies can become widely adopted practices [154].

The exact mechanism underlying any potential beneficial effects of injecting BMSCs is unclear; low cell retention rate is a frequent problem, with the injected cells not appearing to substantially remain in the cardiac tissue, nor do these cells appear to significantly transdifferentiate into cardiomyocytes [139]. Currently, it is thought that potential benefits may be caused by the release of paracrine factors and/or recruitment of CPCs, but this effect may not be BMSC-specific, as injections of other cell types have been shown to have similar beneficial effects [139]. If endogenous CPCs are recruited, these cellular therapies may be more effective in younger recipients than older ones, as it is thought younger individuals may have CPCs more capable of healing and repairing tissue [139]. Small improvements in cardiomyocyte production in adult animal models have also been caused by modifying certain transcription factors, altering miRNA expression, and administering recombinant proteins, such as neuregulin1 [79]. Neuregulin1 has undergone clinical testing and so far demonstrated safety in adult patients with chronic HF [159]; if successful at demonstrating functional improvement, it may be possible to use this approach in pediatric HF patients.

While there are multiple ongoing clinical trials using human pluripotent stem cells (both embryonic stem cells [hESCs] and induced pluripotent stem cells [iPSCs]), none yet are aimed at treating a cardiovascular-related disease [139], although robust protocols have been recently developed to differentiate hESCs and iPSCs into cardiomyocytes and other cardiac-related cell types [79,160]. These protocols have been used with patient-derived iPSCs to generate patient-based models of cardiomyopathies and other cardiac conditions, such as long QT syndrome and Danon disease [161–165]. Such models hold great potential for screening of therapeutic drugs, development of treatment strategies, and correction of disease-causing genetic variants, although many hurdles remain to be overcome before such cells can be therapeutically used; for a recent thorough review of these challenges, see Martins et al. [166].

CONCLUSION

The molecular and cellular mechanisms of HF in the pediatric population are still poorly understood, and there is an evolving body of literature demonstrating important differences compared to the adult. Understanding the specific mechanisms involved in the pediatric failing heart is essential for the development of novel targeted therapeutic strategies. Therefore, ongoing focused study specific to children is essential to improve outcomes for this challenging population of patients.

REFERENCES

[1] E. Braunwald, Comment by E. Braunwald, Eur. Heart J. 4 (1983) 447.

[2] E. Braunwald, in: W.B. Saunders (Ed.), Heart Disease. A Textbook of Cardiovascular Medicine, 1997. Philadelphia.

[3] R. Kirk, A.I. Dipchand, D.N. Rosenthal, L. Addonizio, M. Burch, M. Chrisant, et al., The International Society for Heart and Lung Transplantation Guidelines for the management of pediatric heart failure: executive summary, J. Heart Lung Transplant. 33 (9) (September 2014) 888–909.

[4] D.T. Hsu, G.D. Pearson, Heart failure in children: part I: history, etiology, and pathophysiology, Circ. Heart Fail. 2 (1) (January 1, 2009) 63–70.

[5] P.F. Kantor, J.R. Abraham, A.I. Dipchand, L.N. Benson, A.N. Redington, The impact of changing medical therapy on transplantation-free survival in pediatric dilated cardiomyopathy, J. Am. Coll. Cardiol. 55 (13) (March 30, 2010) 1377–1384.

[6] M. Mollova, K. Bersell, S. Walsh, J. Savla, L.T. Das, S.-Y. Park, et al., Cardiomyocyte proliferation contributes to heart growth in young humans, Proc. Natl. Acad. Sci. U.S.A. 110 (4) (January 22, 2013) 1446–1451.

[7] J.L. Jefferies, J.A. Towbin, Dilated cardiomyopathy, Lancet (Lond. Engl.) 375 (9716) (February 27, 2010) 752–762.

[8] J.D. Wilkinson, D.C. Landy, S.D. Colan, J.A. Towbin, L.A. Sleeper, E.J. Orav, et al., The pediatric cardiomyopathy registry and heart failure: key results from the first 15 years, Heart Fail. Clin. 6 (4) (October 2010) 401–413 vii.

[9] J.A. Towbin, A.M. Lowe, S.D. Colan, L.A. Sleeper, E.J. Orav, S. Clunie, et al., Incidence, causes, and outcomes of dilated cardiomyopathy in children, JAMA 296 (15) (October 18, 2006) 1867.

[10] P. Elliott, B. Andersson, E. Arbustini, Z. Bilinska, F. Cecchi, P. Charron, et al., Classification of the cardiomyopathies: a position statement from the European Society of Cardiology Working Group on myocardial and pericardial diseases, Eur. Heart J. 29 (2) (January 4, 2008) 270–276.

[11] L. Mestroni, F. Brun, A. Spezzacatene, G. Sinagra, M.R. Taylor, Genetic causes of dilated cardiomyopathy, Prog. Pediatr. Cardiol. 37 (1–2) (December 2014) 13–18.

[12] N.E. Bowles, K.R. Bowles, J.A. Towbin, The "final common pathway" hypothesis and inherited cardiovascular disease, Herz 25 (3) (June 1, 2000) 168–175.

[13] S. Arber, J. Hunter, J. Ross, M. Hongo, G. Sansig, MLP-deficient mice exhibit a disruption of cardiac cytoarchitectural organization, dilated cardiomyopathy, and heart failure, Cell 88 (February 7, 1997) 393–403.

[14] J.G. Edwards, G.E. Lyons, B.K. Micales, A. Malhotra, S. Factor, L.A. Leinwand, Cardiomyopathy in transgenic myf5 mice, Circ. Res. 78 (3) (March 1, 1996) 379–387.

[15] D.S. Herman, L. Lam, M.R.G. Taylor, L. Wang, P. Teekakirikul, D. Christodoulou, et al., Truncations of titin causing dilated cardiomyopathy, N. Engl. J. Med. 366 (2012) 619–628.

[16] R.L. Begay, S. Graw, G. Sinagra, M. Merlo, D. Slavov, K. Gowan, et al., Role of titin missense variants in dilated cardiomyopathy, J. Am. Heart Assoc. 4 (11) (January 13, 2015) e002645.

[17] T. Arimura, T. Ishikawa, S. Nunoda, S. Kawai, A. Kimura, Dilated cardiomyopathy-associated BAG3 mutations impair Z-disc assembly and enhance sensitivity to apoptosis in cardiomyocytes, Hum. Mutat. 32 (12) (December 2011) 1481–1491.

[18] M.R. Taylor, P.R. Fain, G. Sinagra, M.L. Robinson, A.D. Robertson, E. Carniel, et al., Natural history of dilated cardiomyopathy due to lamin A/C gene mutations, J. Am. Coll. Cardiol. 41 (5) (March 5, 2003) 771–780.

[19] M.R.G. Taylor, L. Ku, D. Slavov, J. Cavanaugh, M. Boucek, X. Zhu, et al., Danon disease presenting with dilated cardiomyopathy and a complex phenotype, J. Hum. Genet. 52 (10) (January 2007) 830–835.

[20] J.A. Towbin, J.F. Hejtmancik, P. Brink, B. Gelb, X.M. Zhu, J.S. Chamberlain, et al., X-linked dilated cardiomyopathy. Molecular genetic evidence of linkage to the Duchenne muscular dystrophy (dystrophin) gene at the Xp21 locus, Circulation 87 (6) (1993) 1854–1865.

[21] W.P. McNair, G. Sinagra, M.R.G. Taylor, A. Di Lenarda, D.A. Ferguson, E.E. Salcedo, et al., SCN5A mutations associate with arrhythmic dilated cardiomyopathy and commonly localize to the voltage-sensing mechanism, J. Am. Coll. Cardiol. 57 (21) (May 24, 2011) 2160–2168.

[22] M.B. Sikkel, C. Hayward, K.T. MacLeod, S.E. Harding, A.R. Lyon, SERCA2a gene therapy in heart failure: an anti-arrhythmic positive inotrope, Br. J. Pharmacol. 171 (1) (January 2014) 38–54.

[23] I.A.W. Van Rijsingen, P.A. van der Zwaag, J.A. Groeneweg, E.A. Nannenberg, J.D.H. Jongbloed, A.H. Zwinderman, et al., Outcome in phospholamban R14del carriers: results of a large multicentre cohort study, Circ. Cardiovasc. Genet. 7 (4) (August 8, 2014) 455–465.

[24] B.J. Gersh, B.J. Maron, R.O. Bonow, J.A. Dearani, M.A. Fifer, M.S. Link, et al., 2011 ACCF/AHA guideline for the diagnosis and treatment of hypertrophic cardiomyopathy: a report of the American College of Cardiology Foundation/American Heart Association Task Force on Practice Guidelines. Developed in collaboration with the American Association for Thoracic Surgery, American Society of Echocardiography, American Society of Nuclear Cardiology, Heart Failure Society of America, Heart Rhythm Society, Society for Cardiovascular Angiography and Interventions, and Society of Thoracic Surgeons, J. Am. Coll. Cardiol. 58 (25) (December 13, 2011) e212–e260.

[25] S.D. Colan, S.E. Lipshultz, A.M. Lowe, L.A. Sleeper, J. Messere, G.F. Cox, et al., Epidemiology and cause-specific outcome of hypertrophic cardiomyopathy in children: findings from the Pediatric Cardiomyopathy Registry, Circulation 115 (6) (February 13, 2007) 773–781.

[26] S.D. Colan, Hypertrophic cardiomyopathy in childhood, Heart Fail. Clin. 6 (4) (October 2010) 433–444 vii – iii.

[27] H. Morita, R. Nagai, J.G. Seidman, C.E. Seidman, Sarcomere gene mutations in hypertrophy and heart failure, J. Cardiovasc. Transl. Res. 3 (4) (August 2010) 297–303.

[28] J.M. Bos, J.A. Towbin, M.J. Ackerman, Diagnostic, prognostic, and therapeutic implications of genetic testing for hypertrophic cardiomyopathy, J. Am. Coll. Cardiol. 54 (3) (July 14, 2009) 201–211.

[29] M.S. Maron, I. Olivotto, S. Betocchi, S.A. Casey, J.R. Lesser, M.A. Losi, et al., Effect of left ventricular outflow tract obstruction on clinical outcome in hypertrophic cardiomyopathy, N. Engl. J. Med. 348 (2003) 295–303.

[30] K.L. Vikstrom, S.M. Factor, L.A. Leinwand, Mice expressing mutant myosin heavy chains are a model for familial hypertrophic cardiomyopathy, Mol. Med. 2 (5) (September 1996) 556–567.

[31] P. Melacini, C. Basso, A. Angelini, C. Calore, F. Bobbo, B. Tokajuk, et al., Clinicopathological profiles of progressive heart failure in hypertrophic cardiomyopathy, Eur. Heart J. 31 (17) (September 31, 2010) 2111–2123.

[32] K.M. Harris, P. Spirito, M.S. Maron, A.G. Zenovich, F. Formisano, J.R. Lesser, et al., Prevalence, clinical profile, and significance of left ventricular remodeling in the end-stage phase of hypertrophic cardiomyopathy, Circulation 114 (3) (July 18, 2006) 216–225.

[33] J.L. Jefferies, J.D. Wilkinson, L.A. Sleeper, S.D. Colan, M. Lu, E. Pahl, et al., Cardiomyopathy phenotypes and outcomes for children with left ventricular myocardial noncompaction: results from the Pediatric Cardiomyopathy Registry, J. Card. Fail. 21 (11) (November 2015) 877–884.

[34] J.A. Towbin, A. Lorts, J.L. Jefferies, Left ventricular non-compaction cardiomyopathy, Lancet 386 (9995) (April 9, 2015) 813–825.

[35] S. Sen-Chowdhry, W.J. McKenna, Left ventricular noncompaction and cardiomyopathy: cause, contributor, or epiphenomenon? Curr. Opin. Cardiol. 23 (3) (May 2008) 171–175.

[36] S.T. Brescia, J.W. Rossano, R. Pignatelli, J.L. Jefferies, J.F. Price, J.A. Decker, et al., Mortality and sudden death in pediatric left ventricular noncompaction in a tertiary referral center, Circulation 127 (22) (June 4, 2013) 2202–2208.

[37] F. Ichida, S. Tsubata, K.R. Bowles, N. Haneda, K. Uese, T. Miyawaki, et al., Novel gene mutations in patients with left ventricular noncompaction or Barth syndrome, Circulation 103 (9) (March 6, 2001) 1256–1263.

[38] S. Klaassen, S. Probst, E. Oechslin, B. Gerull, G. Krings, P. Schuler, et al., Mutations in sarcomere protein genes in left ventricular noncompaction, Circulation 117 (22) (June 3, 2008) 2893–2901.

[39] Y.M. Hoedemaekers, K. Caliskan, M. Michels, I. Frohn-Mulder, J.J. van der Smagt, J.E. Phefferkorn, et al., The importance of genetic counseling, DNA diagnostics, and cardiologic family screening in left ventricular noncompaction cardiomyopathy, Circ. Cardiovasc. Genet. 3 (3) (June 1, 2010) 232–239.

[40] S. Probst, E. Oechslin, P. Schuler, M. Greutmann, P. Boyé, W. Knirsch, et al., Sarcomere gene mutations in isolated left ventricular noncompaction cardiomyopathy do not predict clinical phenotype, Circ. Cardiovasc. Genet. 4 (4) (August 1, 2011) 367–374.

[41] L.M. Dellefave, P. Pytel, S. Mewborn, B. Mora, D.L. Guris, S. Fedson, et al., Sarcomere mutations in cardiomyopathy with left ventricular hypertrabeculation, Circ. Cardiovasc. Genet. 2 (5) (October 1, 2009) 442–449.

[42] L. Shan, N. Makita, Y. Xing, S. Watanabe, T. Futatani, F. Ye, et al., SCN5A variants in Japanese patients with left ventricular noncompaction and arrhythmia, Mol. Genet. Metab. 93 (4) (April 2008) 468–474.

[43] T. Williams, W. Machann, L. Kühler, H. Hamm, J. Müller-Höcker, M. Zimmer, et al., Novel desmoplakin mutation: juvenile biventricular cardiomyopathy with left ventricular non-compaction and acantholytic palmoplantar keratoderma, Clin. Res. Cardiol. 100 (12) (December 2011) 1087–1093.

[44] J. Finsterer, C. Stöllberger, Primary myopathies and the heart, Scand. Cardiovasc. J. 42 (1) (February 12, 2008) 9–24 Taylor & Francis.

[45] C. Basso, D. Corrado, F.I. Marcus, A. Nava, G. Thiene, Arrhythmogenic right ventricular cardiomyopathy, Lancet (Lond. Engl.) 373 (9671) (April 11, 2009) 1289–1300.

[46] F.I. Marcus, W.J. McKenna, D. Sherrill, C. Basso, B. Bauce, D.A. Bluemke, et al., Diagnosis of arrhythmogenic right ventricular cardiomyopathy/dysplasia: proposed modification of the task force criteria, Eur. Heart J. 31 (7) (April 19, 2010) 806–814.

[47] M. Taylor, S. Graw, G. Sinagra, C. Barnes, D. Slavov, F. Brun, et al., Genetic variation in titin in arrhythmogenic right ventricular cardiomyopathy-overlap syndromes, Circulation 124 (8) (August 23, 2011) 876–885.

[48] F. Brun, C.V. Barnes, G. Sinagra, D. Slavov, G. Barbati, X. Zhu, et al., Titin and desmosomal genes in the natural history of arrhythmogenic right ventricular cardiomyopathy, J. Med. Genet. 51 (10) (October 1, 2014) 669–676.

[49] N. Tiso, Identification of mutations in the cardiac ryanodine receptor gene in families affected with arrhythmogenic right ventricular cardiomyopathy type 2 (ARVD2), Hum. Mol. Genet. 10 (3) (February 1, 2001) 189–194.

[50] G. Beffagna, G. Occhi, A. Nava, L. Vitiello, A. Ditadi, C. Basso, et al., Regulatory mutations in transforming growth factor-beta3 gene cause arrhythmogenic right ventricular cardiomyopathy type 1, Cardiovasc. Res. 65 (2) (February 1, 2005) 366–373.

[51] N.D. Merner, K.A. Hodgkinson, A.F.M. Haywood, S. Connors, V.M. French, J.-D. Drenckhahn, et al., Arrhythmogenic right ventricular cardiomyopathy type 5 is a fully penetrant, lethal arrhythmic disorder caused by a missense mutation in the TMEM43 gene, Am. J. Hum. Genet. 82 (4) (April 2008) 809–821.

[52] J.P. Kaski, P. Syrris, M. Burch, M.-T. Tomé-Esteban, M. Fenton, M. Christiansen, et al., Idiopathic restrictive cardiomyopathy in children is caused by mutations in cardiac sarcomere protein genes, Heart 94 (11) (November 1, 2008) 1478–1484.

[53] E. Arbustini, M. Pasotti, A. Pilotto, C. Pellegrini, M. Grasso, S. Previtali, et al., Desmin accumulation restrictive cardiomyopathy and atrioventricular block associated with desmin gene defects, Eur. J. Heart Fail. 8 (5) (August 2006) 477–483.

[54] Y. Peled, M. Gramlich, G. Yoskovitz, M.S. Feinberg, A. Afek, S. Polak-Charcon, et al., Titin mutation in familial restrictive cardiomyopathy, Int. J. Cardiol. 171 (1) (January 15, 2014) 24–30.

[55] J.A. Hill, E.N. Olson, Cardiac plasticity, N. Engl. J. Med. 358 (2008) 1370–1380.

[56] V. Fuster, R.A. Walsh, R.A. Harrington, Hurst's the Heart, 13th Edition: Two Volume Set, 13th ed., McGraw-Hill Education/Medical, 2011.

[57] G.W. Dorn, J. Robbins, P.H. Sugden, Phenotyping hypertrophy: eschew obfuscation, Circ. Res. 92 (11) (June 13, 2003) 1171–1175.
[58] S.D. Miyamoto, B.L. Stauffer, S. Nakano, R. Sobus, K. Nunley, P. Nelson, et al., Beta-adrenergic adaptation in paediatric idiopathic dilated cardiomyopathy, Eur. Heart J. 35 (1) (January 1, 2014) 33–41.
[59] A.-M. Lompre, K. Schwartz, A. d'Albis, G. Lacombe, N. Van Thiem, B. Swynghedauw, Myosin isoenzyme redistribution in chronic heart overload, Nature 282 (5734) (November 1, 1979) 105–107.
[60] P.F. Binkley, E. Nunziata, G.J. Haas, S.D. Nelson, R.J. Cody, Parasympathetic withdrawal is an integral component of autonomic imbalance in congestive heart failure: demonstration in human subjects and verification in a paced canine model of ventricular failure, J. Am. Coll. Cardiol. 18 (2) (August 1, 1991) 464–472.
[61] K. Swedberg, J. Kjekshus, Effects of enalapril on mortality in severe congestive heart failure. Results of the cooperative North Scandinavian Enalapril survival study (CONSENSUS). The Consensus trial study group, N. Engl. J. Med. 316 (23) (1987) 1429–1435.
[62] M. Packer, P.A. Poole-Wilson, P.W. Armstrong, J.G.F. Cleland, J.D. Horowitz, B.M. Massie, et al., Comparative effects of low and high doses of the angiotensin-converting enzyme inhibitor, lisinopril, on morbidity and mortality in chronic heart failure, Circulation 100 (23) (December 7, 1999) 2312–2318.
[63] S. Investigators, Effect of Enalapril on mortality and the development of heart failure in asymptomatic patients with reduced left ventricular ejection fractions, N. Engl. J. Med. 327 (10) (1992) 685–691.
[64] S. Investigators, Effect of enalapril on survival in patients with reduced left ventricular ejection fractions and congestive heart failure, N. Engl. J. Med. 325 (5) (1991) 293–302.
[65] M.A. Pfeffer, E. Braunwald, L.A. Moye, L. Basta, E. Brown, T.E. Cuddy, Effect of Captopril on mortality and morbidity in patients with left ventricular dysfunction after myocardial infarction, N. Engl. J. Med. 327 (10) (1992) 669–677.
[66] J.J.V. McMurray, J. Ostergren, K. Swedberg, C.B. Granger, P. Held, E.L. Michelson, et al., Effects of candesartan in patients with chronic heart failure and reduced left-ventricular systolic function taking angiotensin-converting-enzyme inhibitors: the CHARM-Added trial, Lancet (Lond. Engl.) 362 (9386) (September 6, 2003) 767–771.
[67] J.N. Cohn, G. Tognoni, A randomized trial of the angiotensin-receptor blocker Valsartan in chronic heart failure, N. Engl. J. Med. 345 (23) (2001) 1667–1675.
[68] F. Zannad, J.J. McMurray, H. Krum, D.J. van Veldhuisen, K. Swedberg, H. Shi, J. Vincent, S.J. Pocock, B. Pitt, EMPHASIS-HF Study Group, Eplerenone in patients with systolic heart failure and mild symptoms, N. Engl. J. Med. 364 (1) (January 6, 2011) 11–21.
[69] B. Pitt, F. Zannad, W.J. Remme, R. Cody, A. Castaigne, A. Perez, et al., The effect of spironolactone on morbidity and mortality in patients with severe heart failure, N. Engl. J. Med. 341 (10) (1999) 709–717.
[70] M. Packer, Effect of carvedilol on the morbidity of patients with severe chronic heart failure: results of the carvedilol prospective randomized cumulative survival (COPERNICUS) study, Circulation 106 (17) (October 7, 2002) 2194–2199.
[71] M.D. Flather, S. Yusuf, L. Køber, M. Pfeffer, A. Hall, G. Murray, et al., Long-term ACE-inhibitor therapy in patients with heart failure or left-ventricular dysfunction: a systematic overview of data from individual patients, Lancet 355 (9215) (May 2000) 1575–1581.
[72] Beta-Blocker Evaluation of Survival Trial Investigators, E.J. Eichhorn, M.J. Domanski, H. Krause-Steinrauf, M.R. Bristow, P.W. Lavori, A trial of the beta-blocker bucindolol in patients with advanced chronic heart failure, N. Engl. J. Med. 344 (22) (May 31, 2001) 1659–1667.
[73] P.A. Poole-Wilson, K. Swedberg, J.G.F. Cleland, A. Di Lenarda, P. Hanrath, M. Komajda, et al., Comparison of carvedilol and metoprolol on clinical outcomes in patients with chronic heart failure in the Carvedilol or Metoprolol European Trial (COMET): randomised controlled trial, Lancet 362 (9377) (July 5, 2003) 7–13.
[74] P. Boknik, M. Fockenbrock, S. Herzig, J. Knapp, B. Linck, H. Lüss, et al., Protein phosphatase activity is increased in a rat model of long-term β-adrenergic stimulation, Naunyn Schmiedebergs Arch. Pharmacol. 362 (3) (August 18, 2000) 222–231.
[75] H. Aoyama, Y. Ikeda, Y. Miyazaki, K. Yoshimura, S. Nishino, T. Yamamoto, et al., Isoform-specific roles of protein phosphatase 1 catalytic subunits in sarcoplasmic reticulum-mediated Ca(2+) cycling, Cardiovasc. Res. 89 (1) (January 1, 2011) 79–88.
[76] M. Huang, X. Zhang, S. Chen, Y. Sun, Y. Xiao, J. Sun, et al., The effect of carvedilol treatment on chronic heart failure in pediatric patients with dilated cardiomyopathy: a prospective, randomized-controlled study, Pediatr. Cardiol. 34 (3) (March 2013) 680–685.
[77] J.M. Aranda, R.S. Schofield, D.F. Pauly, T.S. Cleeton, T.C. Walker, V.S. Monroe, et al., Comparison of dobutamine versus milrinone therapy in hospitalized patients awaiting cardiac transplantation: a prospective, randomized trial, Am. Heart J. 145 (2) (February 2003) 324–329.
[78] S.J. Nakano, S.D. Miyamoto, M. Movsesian, P. Nelson, B.L. Stauffer, C.C. Sucharov, Age-related differences in phosphodiesterase activity and effects of chronic phosphodiesterase inhibition in idiopathic dilated cardiomyopathy, Circ. Heart Fail. 8 (1) (January 1, 2015) 57–63.
[79] K.M. Burns, B.J. Byrne, B.D. Gelb, B. Kuhn, L.A. Leinwand, S. Mital, G.D. Pearson, M. Rodefeld, J.W. Rossano, B.L. Stauffer, M.D. Taylor, J.A. Towbin, A.N. Redington, New mechanistic and therapeutic targets for pediatric heart failure: report from a National Heart, Lung, and Blood Institute Working Group, Circulation 130 (1) (2014) 79–86.
[80] E.M. Zeisberg, O. Tarnavski, M. Zeisberg, A.L. Dorfman, J.R. McMullen, E. Gustafsson, et al., Endothelial-to-mesenchymal transition contributes to cardiac fibrosis, Nat. Med. 13 (8) (August 2007) 952–961 Nat. Publishing Group.
[81] J. Alkon, M.K. Friedberg, C. Manlhiot, A.K. Manickaraj, C. Kinnear, B.W. McCrindle, et al., Genetic variations in hypoxia response genes influence hypertrophic cardiomyopathy phenotype, Pediatr. Res 72 (6) (December 2012) 583–592 International Pediatric Research Foundation, Inc.
[82] P. Kong, P. Christia, N.G. Frangogiannis, The pathogenesis of cardiac fibrosis, Cell Mol. Life Sci. 71 (4) (February 2014) 549–574.
[83] E.E. Creemers, Y.M. Pinto, Molecular mechanisms that control interstitial fibrosis in the pressure-overloaded heart, Cardiovasc. Res. 89 (2) (February 1, 2011) 265–272.
[84] J. Katada, T. Meguro, H. Saito, A. Ohashi, T. Anzai, S. Ogawa, et al., Persistent cardiac aldosterone synthesis in angiotensin II type 1A receptor-knockout mice after myocardial infarction, Circulation 111 (17) (May 3, 2005) 2157–2164.

[85] D.L. Mann, G.M. Felker, Heart Failure: A Companion to Braunwald's Heart Disease, Elsevier Health Sciences, 2014. 832 p.
[86] J.S. Janicki, G.L. Brower, The role of myocardial fibrillar collagen in ventricular remodeling and function, J. Card. Fail. 8 (6 Suppl.) (December 2002) S319–S325.
[87] Y. Iwanaga, T. Aoyama, Y. Kihara, Y. Onozawa, T. Yoneda, S. Sasayama, Excessive activation of matrix metalloproteinases coincides with left ventricular remodeling during transition from hypertrophy to heart failure in hypertensive rats, J. Am. Coll. Cardiol. 39 (8) (April 17, 2002) 1384–1391.
[88] R. Khan, R. Sheppard, Fibrosis in heart disease: understanding the role of transforming growth factor-beta in cardiomyopathy, valvular disease and arrhythmia, Immunology 118 (1) (May 2006) 10–24.
[89] N.G. Frangogiannis, Regulation of the inflammatory response in cardiac repair, Circ. Res. 110 (1) (January 6, 2012) 159–173.
[90] R. Lombardi, S. Betocchi, M.A. Losi, C.G. Tocchetti, M. Aversa, M. Miranda, et al., Myocardial collagen turnover in hypertrophic cardiomyopathy, Circulation 108 (12) (September 23, 2003) 1455–1460.
[91] H. Kitaoka, T. Kubo, M. Okawa, K. Hayato, N. Yamasaki, Y. Matsumura, et al., Impact of metalloproteinases on left ventricular remodeling and heart failure events in patients with hypertrophic cardiomyopathy, Circ. J. 74 (6) (May 25, 2010) 1191–1196.
[92] C.Y. Ho, B. Lopez, O.R. Coelho-Filho, N.K. Lakdawala, A.L. Cirino, C.G.C. Petr Jarolim, et al., Myocardial fibrosis as an early manifestation of hypertrophic cardiomyopathy, N. Engl. J. Med. 363 (2010) 552–563.
[93] D. Hilfiker-Kleiner, U. Landmesser, H. Drexler, Molecular mechanisms in heart failure, J. Am. Coll. Cardiol. 48 (9) (November 7, 2006) A56–A66.
[94] A. Misra, S.B. Haudek, P. Knuefermann, J.G. Vallejo, Z.J. Chen, L.H. Michael, et al., Nuclear factor-kappaB protects the adult cardiac myocyte against ischemia-induced apoptosis in a murine model of acute myocardial infarction, Circulation 108 (25) (December 23, 2003) 3075–3078.
[95] J.W. Gordon, J.A. Shaw, L.A. Kirshenbaum, Multiple facets of NF-κB in the heart: to be or not to NF-κB, Circ. Res. 108 (9) (April 29, 2011) 1122–1132.
[96] E.T. Askevold, L. Gullestad, C.P. Dahl, A. Yndestad, T. Ueland, P. Aukrust, Interleukin-6 signaling, soluble glycoprotein 130, and inflammation in heart failure, Curr. Heart Fail. Rep. 11 (2) (June 2014) 146–155.
[97] M. Nian, P. Lee, N. Khaper, P. Liu, Inflammatory cytokines and postmyocardial infarction remodeling, Circ. Res. 94 (12) (June 25, 2004) 1543–1553.
[98] L. Gullestad, P. Aukrust, Review of trials in chronic heart failure showing broad-spectrum anti-inflammatory approaches, Am. J. Cardiol. 95 (11A) (June 6, 2005) 17C–23C discussion 38C – 40C.
[99] G. Torre-Amione, Immune activation in chronic heart failure, Am. J. Cardiol 95 (11A) (June 6, 2005) 3C–8C (Internet) discussion 38C – 40C.
[100] T. Tsutamoto, T. Hisanaga, A. Wada, K. Maeda, M. Ohnishi, D. Fukai, et al., Interleukin-6 spillover in the peripheral circulation increases with the severity of heart failure, and the high plasma level of Interleukin-6 is an important prognostic predictor in patients with congestive heart failure, J. Am. Coll. Cardiol. 31 (2) (February 1, 1998) 391–398.
[101] K.H. Miettinen, J. Lassus, V.-P. Harjola, K. Siirilä-Waris, J. Melin, K.R. Punnonen, et al., Prognostic role of pro- and anti-inflammatory cytokines and their polymorphisms in acute decompensated heart failure, Eur. J. Heart Fail. 10 (4) (April 2008) 396–403.
[102] V.M. Van Deursen, K. Damman, A.A. Voors, M.H. van der Wal, T. Jaarsma, D.J. van Veldhuisen, et al., Prognostic value of plasma neutrophil gelatinase-associated lipocalin for mortality in patients with heart failure, Circ. Heart Fail. 7 (1) (January 1, 2014) 35–42.
[103] S. Sayed, N.K. Idriss, A. Blann, H.G. Sayyed, D.M. Raafat, D. Fouad, et al., The number of GT(n) repeats in the Hemeoxygenase-1 gene promoter is increased in pediatric heart failure but is unrelated to renal, antioxidant and anti-inflammatory markers, Pediatr. Cardiol. 36 (6) (August 2015) 1204–1211.
[104] R.S.-Y. Foo, K. Mani, R.N. Kitsis, Death begets failure in the heart, J. Clin. Investig. 115 (3) (March 2005) 565–571.
[105] Z. Mallat, I. Philip, M. Lebret, D. Chatel, J. Maclouf, A. Tedgui, Elevated levels of 8-iso-prostaglandin F2 in pericardial fluid of patients with heart Failure: a potential role for in vivo oxidant stress in ventricular dilatation and progression to heart failure, Circulation 97 (16) (April 28, 1998) 1536–1539.
[106] S. Kinugawa, H. Tsutsui, S. Hayashidani, T. Ide, N. Suematsu, S. Satoh, et al., Treatment with dimethylthiourea prevents left ventricular remodeling and failure after experimental myocardial infarction in mice: role of oxidative stress, Circ. Res. 87 (5) (September 1, 2000) 392–398.
[107] F. Sam, D.L. Kerstetter, D.R. Pimental, S. Mulukutla, A. Tabaee, M.R. Bristow, et al., Increased reactive oxygen species production and functional alterations in antioxidant enzymes in human failing myocardium, J. Card. Fail. 11 (6) (August 2005) 473–480.
[108] G.M. Kuster, E. Kotlyar, M.K. Rude, D.A. Siwik, R. Liao, W.S. Colucci, et al., Mineralocorticoid receptor inhibition ameliorates the transition to myocardial failure and decreases oxidative stress and inflammation in mice with chronic pressure overload, Circulation 111 (4) (February 1, 2005) 420–427.
[109] C. Heymes, J.K. Bendall, P. Ratajczak, A.C. Cave, J.-L. Samuel, G. Hasenfuss, et al., Increased myocardial NADPH oxidase activity in human heart failure, J. Am. Coll. Cardiol. 41 (12) (June 18, 2003) 2164–2171.
[110] J.K. Bendall, Pivotal role of a gp91phox-containing NADPH oxidase in angiotensin II-induced cardiac hypertrophy in mice, Circulation 105 (3) (January 22, 2002) 293–296.
[111] J. Bauersachs, A. Bouloumie, D. Fraccarollo, K. Hu, R. Busse, G. Ertl, Endothelial dysfunction in chronic myocardial infarction despite increased vascular endothelial nitric oxide synthase and soluble guanylate cyclase Expression: role of enhanced vascular superoxide production, Circulation 100 (3) (July 20, 1999) 292–298.
[112] M. Scherrer-Crosbie, R. Ullrich, K.D. Bloch, H. Nakajima, B. Nasseri, H.T. Aretz, et al., Endothelial nitric oxide synthase limits left ventricular remodeling after myocardial infarction in mice, Circulation 104 (11) (September 11, 2001) 1286–1291.
[113] A.N. Carley, H. Taegtmeyer, E.D. Lewandowski, Matrix revisited: mechanisms linking energy substrate metabolism to the function of the heart, Circ. Res. 114 (4) (February 14, 2014) 717–729.
[114] R.S. Balaban, Cardiac energy metabolism homeostasis: role of cytosolic calcium, J. Mol. Cell. Cardiol. 34 (10) (October 2002) 1259–1271.
[115] V.K. Mootha, A.E. Arai, R.S. Balaban, Maximum oxidative phosphorylation capacity of the mammalian heart, Am. J. Physiol. 272 (2 Pt 2) (February 1997) H769–H775.
[116] C. Brunel-Guitton, A. Levtova, F. Sasarman, Mitochondrial diseases and cardiomyopathies, Can. J. Cardiol. 31 (11) (2015) 1360–1376.

[117] A.S. Golden, Y.M. Law, H. Shurtleff, M. Warner, R.P. Saneto, Mitochondrial electron transport chain deficiency, cardiomyopathy, and long-term cardiac transplant outcome, Pediatr. Transplant. 16 (3) (2012) 265–268.

[118] D. Holmgren, H. Wahlander, B. Eriksson, A. Oldfors, E. Holme, M. Tulinius, Cardiomyopathy in children with mitochondrial disease clinical course and cardiological findings, Eur. Heart J. 24 (3) (February 2003) 280–288.

[119] F. Scaglia, J.A. Towbin, W.J. Craigen, J.W. Belmont, E.O. Smith, S.R. Neish, et al., Clinical spectrum, morbidity, and mortality in 113 pediatric patients with mitochondrial disease, Pediatrics 114 (4) (October 2004) 925–931.

[120] K.C. Chatfield, G.C. Sparagna, C.C. Sucharov, S.D. Miyamoto, J.E. Grudis, R.D. Sobus, et al., Dysregulation of cardiolipin biosynthesis in pediatric heart failure, J. Mol. Cell. Cardiol. 74 (2014) 251–259.

[121] S.L.N. Clarke, A. Bowron, I.L. Gonzalez, S.J. Groves, R. Newbury-Ecob, N. Clayton, et al., Barth syndrome, Orphanet J. Rare Dis. 8 (January 2013) 23.

[122] S.B. Wortmann, M. Duran, Y. Anikster, P.G. Barth, W. Sperl, J. Zschocke, et al., Inborn errors of metabolism with 3-methylglutaconic aciduria as discriminative feature: proper classification and nomenclature, J. Inherit. Metab. Dis. 36 (6) (November 2013) 923–928.

[123] T. Ojala, P. Polinati, T. Manninen, A. Hiippala, J. Rajantie, R. Karikoski, et al., New mutation of mitochondrial DNAJC19 causing dilated and noncompaction cardiomyopathy, anemia, ataxia, and male genital anomalies, Pediatr. Res. 72 (4) (2012) 432–437.

[124] U. Spiekerkoetter, Mitochondrial fatty acid oxidation disorders: clinical presentation of long-chain fatty acid oxidation defects before and after newborn screening, J. Inherit. Metab. Dis. 33 (5) (October 2010) 527–532.

[125] J. Baruteau, P. Sachs, P. Broué, M. Brivet, H. Abdoul, C. Vianey-Saban, et al., Clinical and biological features at diagnosis in mitochondrial fatty acid beta-oxidation defects: a French pediatric study of 187 patients, J. Inherit. Metab. Dis. 36 (5) (September 2013) 795–803.

[126] D. Bonnet, D. Martin, E. Villain, P. Jouvet, D. Rabier, M. Brivet, et al., Arrhythmias and conduction defects as presenting symptoms of fatty acid oxidation disorders in children, Circulation 100 (22) (November 30, 1999) 2248–2253.

[127] S. Dangwal, T. Thum, microRNA therapeutics in cardiovascular disease models, Annu. Rev. Pharmacol. Toxicol. 54 (January 6, 2014) 185–203.

[128] A. Carè, D. Catalucci, F. Felicetti, D. Bonci, A. Addario, P. Gallo, et al., MicroRNA-133 controls cardiac hypertrophy, Nat. Med. 13 (5) (May 29, 2007) 613–618 Nat. Publishing Group.

[129] T. Thum, P. Galuppo, C. Wolf, J. Fiedler, S. Kneitz, L.W. van Laake, et al., MicroRNAs in the human heart: a clue to fetal gene reprogramming in heart failure, Circulation 116 (3) (July 17, 2007) 258–267.

[130] A.S.M. Sayed, K. Xia, U. Salma, T. Yang, J. Peng, Diagnosis, prognosis and therapeutic role of circulating miRNAs in cardiovascular diseases, Heart Lung Circ. 23 (6) (June 2014) 503–510.

[131] S.D. Miyamoto, A. Karimpour-Fard, V. Peterson, S.R. Auerbach, K.R. Stenmark, B.L. Stauffer, et al., Circulating microRNA as a biomarker for recovery in pediatric dilated cardiomyopathy, J. Heart Lung Transplant. 34 (5) (2015) 724–733 Elsevier.

[132] E. Van Rooij, E.N. Olson, MicroRNA therapeutics for cardiovascular disease: opportunities and obstacles, Nat. Rev. Drug Discov. 11 (11) (November 2012) 860–872 Nature Publishing Group, a division of Macmillan Publishers Limited. All Rights Reserved.

[133] B.L. Stauffer, G. Russell, K. Nunley, S.D. Miyamoto, C.C. Sucharov, miRNA expression in pediatric failing human heart, J. Mol. Cell. Cardiol. 57 (2013) 43–46.

[134] W.G. Guntheroth, Improved outcomes of pediatric dilated cardiomyopathy and heart transplantation, J. Am. Coll. Cardiol. 45 (10) (May 17, 2005) 1733–1734 author reply 1734.

[135] A. Arola, J. Tuominen, O. Ruuskanen, E. Jokinen, Idiopathic dilated cardiomyopathy in children: prognostic indicators and outcome, Pediatrics 101 (3) (March 1, 1998) 369–376.

[136] J.H. Van Berlo, J.D. Molkentin, An emerging consensus on cardiac regeneration, Nat. Med. 20 (12) (2014) 1386–1393.

[137] R.S. Whelan, V. Kaplinskiy, R.N. Kitsis, Cell death in the pathogenesis of heart disease: mechanisms and significance, Annu. Rev. Physiol. 72 (January 11, 2010) 19–44.

[138] I. Bulatovic, A. Månsson-Broberg, C. Sylvén, K.-H. Grinnemo, Human fetal cardiac progenitors: the role of stem cells and progenitors in the fetal and adult heart, Best Pract. Res. Clin. Obstet. Gynaecol. (2015) 1–11.

[139] M.R. Rosen, R.J. Myerburg, D.P. Francis, G.D. Cole, E. Marbán, Translating stem cell research to cardiac disease therapies, J. Am. Coll. Cardiol. 64 (9) (2014) 922–937.

[140] E.R. Porrello, A.I. Mahmoud, E. Simpson, J.A. Hill, J.A. Richardson, E.N. Olson, et al., Transient regenerative potential of the neonatal mouse heart, Science 331 (6020) (February 25, 2011) 1078–1080.

[141] J.O. Oberpriller, J.C. Oberpriller, Response of the adult newt ventricle to injury, J. Exp. Zool. 187 (2) (February 1974) 249–253.

[142] R.O. Becker, S. Chapin, R. Sherry, Regeneration of the ventricular myocardium in amphibians, Nature 248 (5444) (March 8, 1974) 145–147.

[143] K.D. Poss, L.G. Wilson, M.T. Keating, Heart regeneration in zebrafish, Science 298 (5601) (December 13, 2002) 2188–2190.

[144] O. Bergmann, R.D. Bhardwaj, S. Bernard, S. Zdunek, F. Barnabé-Heider, S. Walsh, et al., Evidence for cardiomyocyte renewal in humans, Science 324 (5923) (April 3, 2009) 98–102.

[145] D. Orlic, J. Kajstura, S. Chimenti, I. Jakoniuk, S.M. Anderson, B. Li, et al., Bone marrow cells regenerate infarcted myocardium, Nature 410 (6829) (April 5, 2001) 701–705 Macmillian Magazines Ltd.

[146] L.B. Balsam, A.J. Wagers, J.L. Christensen, T. Kofidis, I.L. Weissman, R.C. Robbins, Haematopoietic stem cells adopt mature haematopoietic fates in ischaemic myocardium, Nature 428 (6983) (April 8, 2004) 668–673.

[147] C.E. Murry, M.H. Soonpaa, H. Reinecke, H. Nakajima, H.O. Nakajima, M. Rubart, et al., Haematopoietic stem cells do not transdifferentiate into cardiac myocytes in myocardial infarcts, Nature 428 (6983) (April 8, 2004) 664–668.

[148] G.M. Ellison, C. Vicinanza, A.J. Smith, I. Aquila, A. Leone, C.D. Waring, et al., Adult c-kit(pos) cardiac stem cells are necessary and sufficient for functional cardiac regeneration and repair, Cell 154 (4) (August 15, 2013) 827–842.

[149] K.S. Telukuntla, V.Y. Suncion, I.H. Schulman, J.M. Hare, The advancing field of cell-based therapy: insights and lessons from clinical trials, J. Am. Heart Assoc. 2 (5) (October 10, 2013) e000338.

[150] R.R. Makkar, R.R. Smith, K. Cheng, K. Malliaras, L.E.J. Thomson, D. Berman, et al., Intracoronary cardiosphere-derived cells for heart regeneration after myocardial infarction (CADUCEUS): a prospective, randomised phase 1 trial, Lancet (Lond. Engl.) 379 (9819) (March 10, 2012) 895–904.

[151] A.R. Chugh, G.M. Beache, J.H. Loughran, N. Mewton, J.B. Elmore, J. Kajstura, et al., Administration of cardiac stem cells in patients with ischemic cardiomyopathy: the SCIPIO trial: surgical aspects and interim analysis of myocardial function and viability by magnetic resonance, Circulation 126 (11 Suppl. 1) (September 11, 2012) S54–S64.

[152] B. Assmus, D.M. Leistner, V. Schächinger, S. Erbs, A. Elsässer, W. Haberbosch, et al., Long-term clinical outcome after intracoronary application of bone marrow-derived mononuclear cells for acute myocardial infarction: migratory capacity of administered cells determines event-free survival, Eur. Heart J. 35 (19) (May 14, 2014) 1275–1283.

[153] B. Assmus, J. Honold, V. Schächinger, M.B. Britten, U. Fischer-Rasokat, R. Lehmann, et al., Transcoronary transplantation of progenitor cells after myocardial infarction, N. Engl. J. Med. 355 (12) (September 21, 2006) 1222–1232.

[154] C. Ikebe, K. Suzuki, Mesenchymal stem cells for regenerative therapy: optimization of cell preparation protocols, Biomed. Res. Int. 2014 (1) (2014) 951512.

[155] B.A. Scruggs, J.A. Semon, X. Zhang, S. Zhang, A.C. Bowles, A.C. Pandey, et al., Age of the donor reduces the ability of human adipose-derived stem cells to alleviate symptoms in the experimental autoimmune encephalomyelitis mouse model, Stem Cells Transl. Med. 2 (10) (October 1, 2013) 797–807 AlphaMed Press.

[156] M.C. Capogrossi, Cardiac stem cells fail with aging: a new mechanism for the age-dependent decline in cardiac function, Circ. Res. 94 (4) (March 5, 2004) 411–413.

[157] D. Cesselli, A.P. Beltrami, F. D'Aurizio, P. Marcon, N. Bergamin, B. Toffoletto, et al., Effects of age and heart failure on human cardiac stem cell function, Am. J. Pathol. 179 (1) (July 2011) 349–366.

[158] D. Duscher, R.C. Rennert, M. Januszyk, E. Anghel, Z.N. Maan, A.J. Whittam, et al., Aging disrupts cell subpopulation dynamics and diminishes the function of mesenchymal stem cells, Sci. Rep. 4 (2014) 7144.

[159] R. Gao, J. Zhang, L. Cheng, X. Wu, W. Dong, X. Yang, et al., A Phase II, randomized, double-blind, multicenter, based on standard therapy, placebo-controlled study of the efficacy and safety of recombinant human neuregulin-1 in patients with chronic heart failure, J. Am. Coll. Cardiol. 55 (18) (May 4, 2010) 1907–1914.

[160] X. Lian, J. Zhang, S.M. Azarin, K. Zhu, L.B. Hazeltine, X. Bao, et al., Directed cardiomyocyte differentiation from human pluripotent stem cells by modulating Wnt/β-catenin signaling under fully defined conditions, Nat. Protoc. 8 (1) (January 2013) 162–175.

[161] C. Kim, J. Wong, J. Wen, S. Wang, C. Wang, S. Spiering, et al., Studying arrhythmogenic right ventricular dysplasia with patient-specific iPSCs, Nature 494 (7435) (February 7, 2013) 105–110 Nature Publishing Group, a division of Macmillan Publishers Limited. All Rights Reserved.

[162] S.I. Hashem, C.N. Perry, M. Bauer, S. Han, S.D. Clegg, K. Ouyang, et al., Brief report: oxidative stress mediates cardiomyocyte apoptosis in a human model of Danon disease and heart failure, Stem Cells 33 (7) (July 2015) 2343–2350.

[163] N. Sun, M. Yazawa, J. Liu, L. Han, V. Sanchez-Freire, O.J. Abilez, et al., Patient-specific induced pluripotent stem cells as a model for familial dilated cardiomyopathy, Sci. Transl. Med. 4 (130) (April 18, 2012) 130ra47.

[164] I. Itzhaki, L. Maizels, I. Huber, L. Zwi-Dantsis, O. Caspi, A. Winterstern, et al., Modelling the long QT syndrome with induced pluripotent stem cells, Nature 471 (7337) (March 10, 2011) 225–229 Nature Publishing Group.

[165] H.L. Li, N. Fujimoto, N. Sasakawa, S. Shirai, T. Ohkame, T. Sakuma, et al., Precise correction of the dystrophin gene in duchenne muscular dystrophy patient induced pluripotent stem cells by TALEN and CRISPR-Cas9, Stem Cell Rep. 4 (1) (January 13, 2015) 143–154 Elsevier.

[166] A.M. Martins, G. Vunjak-Novakovic, R.L. Reis, The current status of iPS cells in cardiac research and their potential for tissue engineering and regenerative medicine, Stem Cell Rev. 10 (2) (2014) 177–190.

[167] B.J. Maron, M.S. Maron, Hypertrophic cardiomyopathy, Lancet 381 (9862) (January 19, 2013) 242–255.

[168] M.J. Lohse, What is the role of beta-adrenergic signaling in heart failure? Circ. Res. 93 (10) (October 23, 2003) 896–906.

Chapter 2

Cardiovascular Receptors and Signaling in Heart Failure

Daniel Bernstein
Stanford University, Stanford, CA, United States

HISTORY OF ADRENERGIC SIGNALING AND THE HEART

The earliest description of the sympathetic nervous system can be traced back to the great anatomist Galen (AD 130–200), who described a set of "hollow nerves," originating in the brain, that carried the "animal spirits" from one organ to the other. This level of communication between organs was referred to as "sympathy" [1], a concept that lasted well into the 18th century, when Robert Whytt described "sympathies" traveling through the brain and spinal cord. John Newport Langley would be the first to use the term "autonomic nervous system" and to develop the central tenet of antagonism between the sympathetic and parasympathetic nervous systems. In 1884, George Oliver and Edward Albert Schäfer published the first description of physiologic changes (blood pressure increase, reflex bradycardia) after injection of adrenal gland extracts. Recognition of the chemical source of neurotransmission came with the work of Otto Loewi, who in 1921 described Vagusstoff (acetylcholine) and Accleransstoff (adrenaline). Within the next 10 years, Walter Bradford Cannon isolated an adrenalin-like substance, which he dubbed sympathin, and was the first to popularize the concept of sympathetic activation as the "fight or flight" response. In 1948, Raymond Ahlquist introduced the concept of α and β receptors, based on the potency of various drugs to stimulate physiologic responses [2]; and in 1958, Powell and Slater reported development of the first β-antagonist, dichloroisoproterenol [3]. The term β-blocker was introduced by Moran and Perkins that same year [4] and the first clinically utilized β-blocker, propranolol, was developed by Sir James Black in 1974 [5].

The role of the sympathetic nervous system as not just a regulator of physiologic responses but as a mechanism of disease was recognized in the early 1900s, when it was referred to as the body's "Mischief-Making Mechanism," but it was not until the early biomarker studies in the 1990s that plasma norepinephrine was identified as the best predictor of survival in patients with heart failure [6,7]. When cultured cardiomyocytes became available as a research tool, the mechanisms for catecholamine-induced injury could at last be investigated, and one of the best methods of inducing rapid cell death was exposure to norepinephrine [8].

TRANSLATION OF BASIC RESEARCH INTO CLINICAL PRACTICE

With advances in molecular cell signaling methodologies, our understanding of hormone–receptor interactions was greatly advanced, and adrenergic receptors became the most extensively studied model system [9–15]: the basic concept that β-receptors mediate their effects through coupling to a stimulatory guanylyl nucleotide-binding protein (G protein or G_s), stimulating adenylyl cyclase and leading to generation of the second messenger cyclic adenosine monophosphate (cAMP) (Fig. 2.1). The concepts of receptor desensitization and downregulation as an explanation for the clinically observed phenomenon of tachyphylaxis were elegantly described by Lefkowitz and coworkers [16]. β-adrenergic receptors were among the first G protein-coupled receptors to be cloned [17,18] and successfully knocked out in the mouse [19–23]. More recently, exacting studies by Kobilka and colleagues defined the crystal structure of the β2-receptor, leading to an understanding of how ligand–receptor interactions affect receptor structure and coupling to G proteins [24], and leading to the Nobel Prize shared by Brian Kobilka and Robert Lefkowitz in 2012.

Coincident with these advances in basic science was a revolution in clinical practice, beginning in the late 1970s, moving away from the use of β-agonists for chronic treatment of heart failure and the adoption of β-blockers. This paradigm switch was led by pioneering studies in 1975 by Waagstein et al. [25] and in 1980 by Swedberg et al. [26], although as with many new ideas, there was initially much skepticism and resistance. In the 1990s, several large adult clinical trials such as CIBIS-II (bisoprolol) [27], MERIT-HF (metoprolol-XL) [28], and Copernicus (carvedilol) [29] confirmed a dramatic 30%–35% reduction in mortality with

Heart Failure in the Child and Young Adult. http://dx.doi.org/10.1016/B978-0-12-802393-8.00002-8

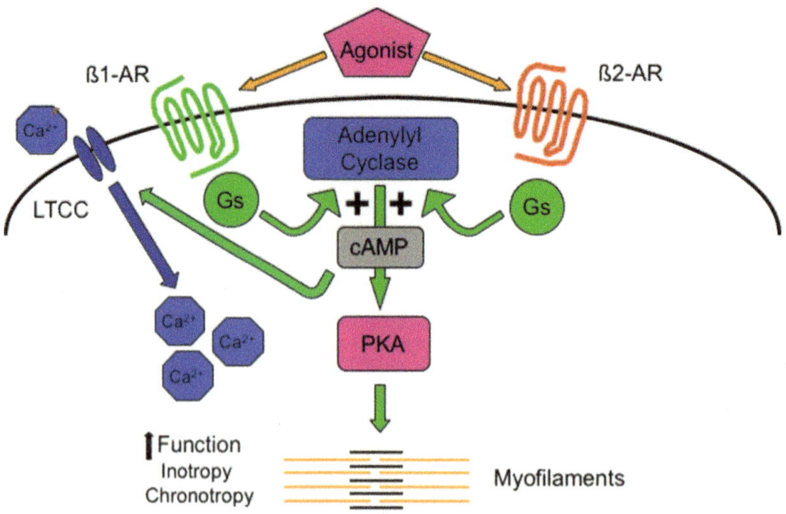

FIGURE 2.1 The classic (linear) model of β-adrenergic receptor signaling. *cAMP*, cyclic adenosine monophosphate; *Gs*, stimulatory guanylyl nucleotide-binding protein; *LTCC*, L-type calcium channel; *PKA*, protein kinase A; *β1-AR*, β1-adrenoceptor; *β2-AR*, β2-adrenoceptor. *(Adapted from Bernstein et al., The role of β-adrenergic receptors in heart failure: differential regulation of cardiotoxicity and cardioprotection, Prog. Pediatr. Card. 31 (2011) 35–38. Elsevier, Philadelphia, PA. PMID: 21765627, https://doi.org/10.1016/j.ppedcard.2010.11.007.)*

TABLE 2.1 Summary of Results From Large Multicenter-Controlled Trials of β-Blockers in Adults

Study	Year	Enrollment	β-Blocker	Reduction of All-Cause Mortality
MDC	1993	383	Metoprolol vs. placebo	34% [95]
CIBIS	1994	641	Bisoprolol vs. placebo	No difference [96]
USCHFS	1996	1094	Carvedilol vs. placebo	65% [97]
CIBIS-II	1999	2647	Bisoprolol vs. placebo	34% [27]
MERIT-HF	2000	3991	Metoprolol vs. placebo	34% [28]
BEST	2001	2708	Bucindolol vs. placebo	No difference [98]
Capricorn	2001	1959	Carvedilol vs. placebo	23% [99]
Copernicus	2002	2289	Carvedilol vs. placebo	35% [29]
COMET	2003	3029	Carvedilol vs. metoprolol	17% [100]
SENIORS	2005	2128	Nebivolol vs. placebo	14% [101]

Adapted from C. Kubon, N.B. Mistry, I. Grundvold, S. Halvorsen, S.E. Kjeldsen, A.S. Westheim, The role of beta-blockers in the treatment of chronic heart failure, Trends Pharmacol. Sci. 32 (4) (2011) 206–212.

β-blocker treatment (Table 2.1). In the world of adult heart failure, β-blocker therapy is now standard practice and widely used as a quality-of-care metric. Long-term but noncontrolled follow-up data on patients treated for at least 10 years show that carvedilol can produce a sustained improvement in left ventricular function and reduction in symptoms [30]. A recent metaanalysis of randomized, controlled, direct-comparison trials of adults found that carvedilol significantly reduced all-cause mortality when compared with atenolol, bisoprolol, metoprolol, or nebivolol [31].

ADVANCES IN OUR UNDERSTANDING OF β-ADRENERGIC SIGNALING: FROM LINEARITY TO CROSS TALK

Over the past two decades, our understanding of the mechanisms of β-AR signaling has changed radically and has maintained its role as a model system for understanding cell signaling in general. In the classic, linear model of hormone–receptor interaction (Fig. 2.1), β-ARs were understood to regulate changes in cardiac function (inotropy and chronotropy)

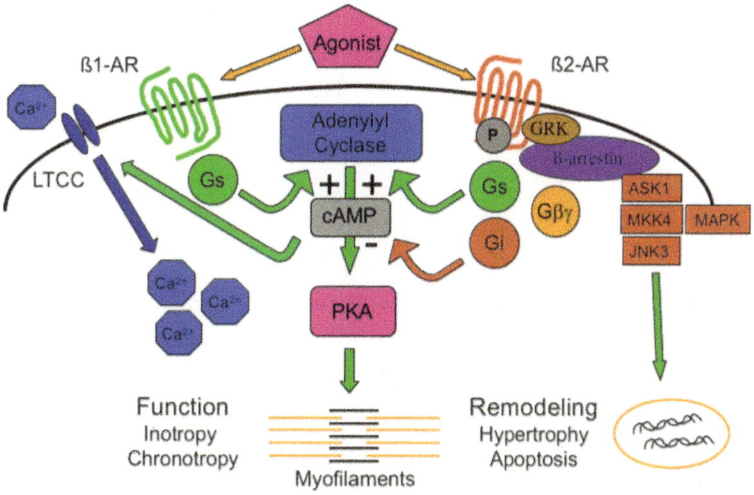

FIGURE 2.2 The model undergoes revision: β-adrenergic receptor signaling cross talk with remodeling signaling pathways. *ASK1*, apoptosis signal-regulating kinase 1; *cAMP*, cyclic adenosine monophosphate; *Gi*, inhibitory guanylyl nucleotide-binding protein; *GRK*, G protein receptor kinase (formerly βARK); *Gs*, stimulatory guanylyl nucleotide-binding protein; *Gβγ*, a subunit of Gs, which is dissociated from the α subunit after Gs is activated by the β-receptor; *JNK3*, c-Jun N-terminal kinase; *LTCC*, L-type calcium channel; *MAPK*, mitogen-activated protein kinase; *MKK4*, mitogen-activated protein kinase kinase 4; *PKA*, protein kinase A; *β1-AR*, β1-adrenoceptor; *β2-AR*, β2-adrenoceptor. *(Adapted from Bernstein et al., The role of β-adrenergic receptors in heart failure: differential regulation of cardiotoxicity and cardioprotection, Prog. Pediatr. Card. 31 (2011) 35–38. Elsevier, Philadelphia, PA. PMID: 21765627, https://doi.org/10.1016/j.ppedcard.2010.11.007.)*

through activation of the stimulatory guanylyl nucleotide-binding protein (Gs), adenylyl cyclase, and generation of the cAMP second messenger. cAMP then activates downstream signaling pathways including protein kinase A (PKA), which activates (through phosphorylation) phospholamban (PLB), and the sarcoplasmic/endoplasmic reticulum calcium ATPase (SERCA), enhancing SR calcium reuptake and L-type calcium channel activity. However, under this limited linear model, how β-receptors could stimulate heart function while also inducing cardiac injury was still incompletely understood.

A first breakthrough was made by Lefkowitz, who demonstrated the processes of β-receptor desensitization and downregulation after exposure to an agonist, where the density of receptors on the cell membrane decreased, thus explaining the clinical phenomenon of tachyphylaxis [16]. Translating this finding to the clinical realm, Bristow demonstrated that receptor downregulation occurs in the human heart, finding that β1-receptors were downregulated by 60% in failing human hearts explanted at the time of transplantation [32]. These studies ushered in an era of molecular signaling research in heart failure and also sparked a debate as to whether this downregulation of β-receptors played a role in the pathogenesis of heart failure or whether it was a homeostatic process by which the heart protected itself from the ravages of chronic sympathetic stimulation.

If β-AR downregulation was one of the causes of cardiac dysfunction, then it was logical to assume that restoring receptor density to normal levels would improve heart failure. Studies in transgenic mice overexpressing the β2-AR by 50- to 200-fold initially seemed to support this hypothesis, as contractility was dramatically enhanced in these animals when young [33]. However, as they aged, these mice developed myocardial fibrosis and eventually a severe dilated cardiomyopathy [34]. Overexpression of the β1-receptor resulted in an even more rapid deterioration in cardiac function [35,36], evidence that the β1-subtype was even more tightly linked to cardiotoxicity (see below). Additional support for the paradigm that β-receptor downregulation was not the direct cause of heart failure came from studies where both β1 and β2-ARs were knocked out in mice, in which cardiac development is normal, as is cardiac function and exercise capacity [21].

We now appreciate that β-AR signaling involves multiple pathways and multiple avenues of cross talk with other signaling pathways (Fig. 2.2). For example, β2-ARs can couple to both stimulatory (Gs) as well as inhibitory (Gi) pathways [37], via which they activate signaling pathways regulating the processes of cardiac remodeling (hypertrophy, cell death) [12,38]. As well, the process of receptor downregulation, thought initially to only be involved in desensitization, has now been linked to alternative cell signaling pathways mediating cardiac remodeling [12,39]. Downregulation occurs via phosphorylation of the β-receptor via two pathways, PKA and G protein receptor kinase (GRK), which recruits β-arrestin to the cell membrane, activating a cassette of signaling molecules, including mitogen-activated protein kinase (MAPK) family members, mediators of hypertrophy and apoptosis (see below for more details).

Despite this extensive knowledge base, the mechanisms by which β-blockers exert their beneficial effects in patients with heart failure are still not completely understood. At the time of the first clinical trials, it was assumed that β-blockade would mediate its protective effect by restoring and reversing the downregulation of β1-receptors in the heart. Although initial studies suggested this was the case [40], subsequent studies have failed to show a clear relationship between clinical response and changes in β-receptor expression in the heart [41]. Other mechanisms that have been proposed include a reversal of the induction of the "fetal" gene program, responsible for adverse remodeling and activation of pathways that inhibit programmed cell death (apoptosis) [41–43].

β1 VERSUS β2 SIGNALING: CLINICAL IMPLICATIONS

There are important differences between β1 and β2-receptor signaling, which may have clinical significance. One of the most intriguing is the intracellular compartment(s) in which each receptor mediates its effects. β-receptors tend to cluster in cellular microdomains adjacent to their downstream targets, e.g., PLB or calcium channels, mediated by scaffolding of A-kinase anchoring domains [44]. Thus, β1-receptor-induced cAMP activation occurs throughout the cell and activates both PKA and PLB. In contrast, β2-receptor-induced cAMP accumulation is highly compartmentalized, where it activates local pools of adenylyl cyclase and L-type calcium channels [45]. These cellular microdomains include many other signaling components, e.g., different isoforms of phosphodiesterase, which act to regulate local concentration of cAMP.

Recent studies have suggested that β1-receptors are largely responsible for the cardiotoxic effects of sympathetic stimulation (Fig. 2.3), mediated through PKA and calcium/calmodulin-dependent protein kinase (CaMK), increased intracellular calcium, inhibition of the antiapoptotic effects of Akt [42], and phosphorylation of the ryanodine receptor, increasing diastolic calcium leak and arrhythmogenesis [46,47]. The clinical therapeutic equivalence of selective β1-receptor blockade and nonselective β-blockade, at doses that equally block the β1-receptor, is additional evidence that the majority of cardiotoxic signaling is mediated by the β1-receptor [43].

In contrast, the β2-receptor can switch between cardiotoxic and cardioprotective signaling [48,49], the latter through activation of Gi, PI3K, and Akt [48,50]. Evidence for the cardioprotective effect initially came from in vitro studies, where β2-receptor agonists were shown to block apoptosis induced by catecholamines and other stressors [50,51]. As well, cardiomyocytes isolated from β2-receptor knockout mice show enhanced injury when treated with doxorubicin [52]. In vivo studies have confirmed some of these findings: β2-receptor agonists have been shown to reduce ischemic injury after coronary artery ligation [53,54]. Mice lacking the β2-receptor have increased susceptibility to isoproterenol [55] and doxorubicin [56] cardiotoxicity. β2-receptor signaling has also been shown to be a component of preconditioning [57].

These data have led some investigators to suggest that selective β1-blockade combined with selective β2-stimulation might be beneficial under certain circumstances [53,54,58]. In rats undergoing coronary artery ligation, Ahmet et al. have

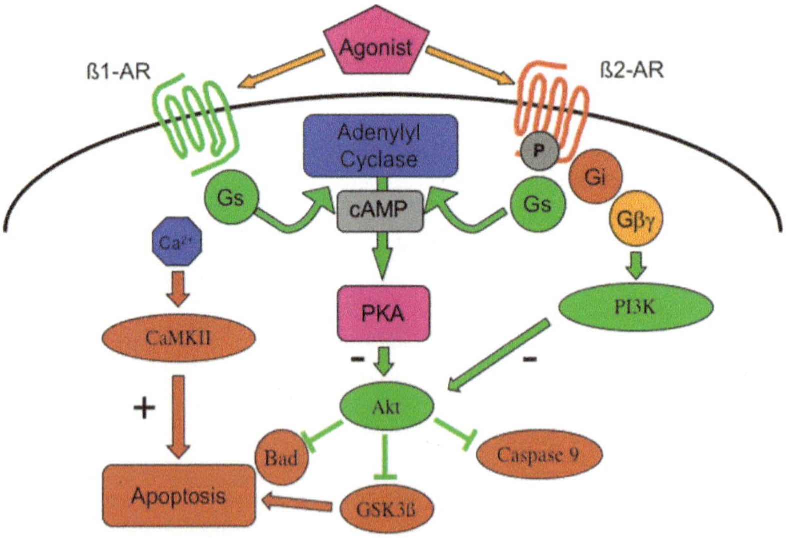

FIGURE 2.3 β-adrenergic receptors differentially regulate pro- and antiapoptotic signaling. *Akt*, protein kinase B; *Bad*, Bcl-2-associated death promoter; *CaMKII*, calcium/calmodulin-dependent protein kinase II; *cAMP*, cyclic adenosine monophosphate; *Gi*, inhibitory guanylyl nucleotide-binding protein; *Gs*, stimulatory guanylyl nucleotide-binding protein; *GSK3 β*, glycogen synthase kinase 3 β; *PI3K*, phosphoinositide 3-kinase; *PKA*, protein kinase A; *Gβγ*, a subunit of Gs; *β1-AR*, β1-adrenoceptor; *β2-AR*, β2-adrenoceptor. *(Adapted from Bernstein et al., The role of β-adrenergic receptors in heart failure: differential regulation of cardiotoxicity and cardioprotection, Prog. Pediatr. Card. 31 (2011) 35–38. Elsevier, Philadelphia, PA. PMID: 21765627, https://doi.org/10.1016/j.ppedcard.2010.11.007.)*

shown that a combination of the β1-blocker metoprolol with the β2-agonist fenoterol improves cardiac function compared to the use of metoprolol alone [53,59]. Although this specific combination has not been tested in clinical trials, celiprolol, a β1-antagonist and β2-partial agonist, was found not to be effective in treating heart failure [60]. Whether this discrepancy represents a difference in drugs or a difference in response between rodents and humans is not known. One potential beneficial effect of β2-blockade may be due to its sympatholytic effects, blocking prejunctional β2-receptors, which enhance norepinephrine release across the neuromuscular junction [61]. Currently utilized β-blockers induce varying degrees of sympatholysis, e.g., bucindolol to a greater degree than carvedilol; however, the additional clinical benefit from enhanced sympatholysis is still debated.

Not all data, however, show that β2-receptors are cardioprotective. Transgenic overexpression of the β2-receptor fails to rescue a genetic (muscle LIM protein (MLP)) cardiomyopathy [62] and over time, β2-overexpression induces cardiomyopathy in its own right [34]. Although mice with deletion of the β2-receptor have increased susceptibility to acute doxorubicin cardiotoxicity, when exposed to a low dose, chronic doxorubicin regimen, β2-receptor signaling switches from being cardioprotective to cardiotoxic: β2-knockout mice survived longer than controls in this chronic model. Using the genetic cardiomyopathy model (MLP knockout) that Rockman et al. had used and failed to rescue with β2-receptor overexpression, Fajardo et al. found that crossbreeding MLP mice with mice with a knockout of the β2-receptor rescued the MLP knockout mice from cardiomyopathy, suggesting that in this model the β2-receptor was acting in a cardiotoxic role [63]. Moreover, in contrast to its purported role as the "cardiotoxic receptor," when the β1-receptor knockout was crossed with the MLP knockout, it markedly enhanced cardiotoxicity, suggesting that in this model, the β1-receptor was acting in a cardioprotective fashion. Subtle ß-receptor-mediated changes in intracellular calcium transients and their effect on mitochondrial function were shown to play a critical role in this balance between beneficial/deleterious effect [63,64].

In conclusion, β1 versus β2-receptor subtypes regulate the balance between cardiotoxicity and cardioprotection through cross talk with signaling pathways, such as CaMK, PI3K, the MAPKs, PKC, and Akt, through alterations in intracellular calcium, and through regulation of mitochondrial cell death pathways. However, labeling one β-receptor subtype as the mediator of "cardiotoxic" effects and the other to "cardioprotective" effects is overly simplistic. The balance between cardiotoxicity and cardioprotection regulated by β-receptor subtypes is dependent both on the type of cardiac stressor (e.g., ischemia/reperfusion, pressure or volume overload, genetic mutation or cardiotoxins like doxorubicin) and also by the duration of the cardiac stress (acute vs. chronic).

BIASED SIGNALING VIA β-ARRESTIN: CLINICAL IMPLICATIONS

β-blockers not only inhibit β-receptor cardiotoxic signaling mediated by Gs activation but also act on non-Gs-dependent pathways. After β-receptors are activated by an agonist, they undergo phosphorylation by GRKs, which inhibit Gs binding (inducing desensitization). After receptor phosphorylation, the cytosolic protein β-arrestin is recruited to the plasma membrane. This process is not only responsible for receptor internalization (downregulation) but is also a signaling pathway in its own right. β-arrestin activates cardioprotective/antiapoptotic downstream signaling, in part through transactivation of the epidermal growth factor receptor, and activation of extracellular-signal receptor kinase (ERK), PI3K, and Akt [65]. This switch from Gs-mediated to β-arrestin-mediated cardioprotective signaling is highly time-dependent, with Gs signaling occurring early (within 2–5 min) and β-arrestin signaling occurring later after receptor activation.

Many of the β-blockers used in clinical practice inhibit both Gs- and β-arrestin-based signaling, therefore potentially blocking a cardioprotective pathway. This has led to the search for drugs that act as "biased agonists," activating the β-receptor preferentially through the "cardioprotective" β-arrestin pathway [66]. β-blockers in clinical use such as carvedilol, bucindolol, and labetolol activate Gs versus β-arrestin to various degrees, with carvedilol showing the greatest level of β-arrestin/ERK signaling [62,69,74]. β1-receptor polymorphisms (see below) have also been shown to affect this biased signaling [67]. Similar biased ligand activity has been observed for other clinically important cardiac receptor systems, such as angiotensin II type IA receptors [65].

PHARMACOGENOMICS OF β-RECEPTORS/β-BLOCKERS

There has been a recent explosion of interest in personalized medicine, and β-blocker pharmacogenomics (tailoring choice of drug treatment to a patient's genotype) has been an area of considerable research. Initial studies focused on whether β-receptor gene variants affected the risk for death or transplant in patients with dilated cardiomyopathy. Known as single nucleotide polymorphisms (SNPs), these variations in nucleotide sequence are generally defined as those that occur with an allele frequency of 1% or greater in a population. It has been estimated that there is one SNP every 300 bp or ~10 million

TABLE 2.2 Common Polymorphisms in β-Receptors and Associated Signaling Molecules

Gene	Nucleotide Change	Amino Acid Change	MAF (European Descent)	MAF (African–Americans)	Functional Effects of MA
β1-AR (ADRB1)	145 A/G	49 Ser/Gly	12%–16%	23%–28%	↑ downregulation with agonist [103,104]
	1165 C/G	389 Arg/Gly	24%–34%	39%–46%	↓ G protein coupling, ↓ β-blocker response [73,105]
β2-AR (ADRB2)	46 G/A	16 Gly/Arg	40%	50%	↑ downregulation [106]
	79 C/G	27 Gln/Glu	25%	19%	↓ downregulation [106]
α2C-AR (ADRA2C)	Del 964-975	Del 322-325	3.8%	40%	↓ inhibition of adenylyl cyclase [107]
GRK5	122 A/T	41 Gln/Leu	1.3%	23%	Endogenous β-blocking effect [78]

AR, adrenergic receptor; *Del*, deletion; *GRK5*, G protein receptor kinase; *MA*, minor (less common) allele; *MAF*, minor allele frequency.
Adapted from G.D. Femminella, V. Barrese, N. Ferrara, G. Rengo, Tailoring therapy for heart failure: the pharmacogenomics of adrenergic receptor signaling, Pharmacogenomics Personalized Med. 7 (2014) 267–273 and J.A. Johnson, S.B., Liggett, Cardiovascular pharmacogenomics of adrenergic receptor signaling: clinical implications and future directions, Clin. Pharmacol. Ther. 89 (3) (2011) 366–378.

total SNPs in the human genome. SNPs occurring in the noncoding region of a gene can affect gene splicing, transcription factor-binding sites, mRNA degradation, or microRNA sequences. SNPs occurring in the coding region can be nonsynonymous (affecting the translated protein) or synonymous (a base pair change that does not affect the translated protein) and which may have their effect through altering mRNA stability or a microRNA binding site.

Overall, there are 12 nonsynonymous SNPs in the β1-AR, of which Ser49Gly and Arg389Gly are the most common; and 5 nonsynonymous SNPs in the β2-AR, of which Arg16Gly, Gln27Glu, and Thr164Ile are the most common (Table 2.2). There are also SNPs in other components of the adrenergic signaling system that could potentially influence heart failure progression and response to therapy, including in the β3, α1A, α2A, α2B, and α2C adrenergic receptors, and in GRK4 and GRK5, which mediate desensitization and β-arrestin signaling. At present, there is no evidence that any of these SNPs actually predispose patients to the development of heart failure, the way that gene mutations in contractile proteins cause dilated or hypertrophic cardiomyopathy [68]. Initial studies by Liggett and colleagues on the Thr164Ile variant showed increased mortality in patients carrying the Ile164 variant, with a 2 year survival of 40% compared to 70% of those carrying the more common Thr164 [69]. Other studies have shown poorer outcomes for those carrying the β1-AR Arg389Arg, α2c-AR Del322-325, and GRK Gln41Gln genotypes [70]; however, the majority of larger studies have failed to show these effects [68], highlighting a principal caveat of all gene association studies: the need for replication in large populations. Thus, at present, there is no conclusive evidence that β-AR SNPs directly alter heart failure outcomes [68].

These initial studies sparked further interest in understanding the role of gene variants in response to β-blocker therapy. One catalyst for these studies was the disparity in results of patients treated with the β-blocker bucindolol. European clinical trials had shown a protective effect, whereas the BEST trial in the US did not, leading investigators to examine differences in racial/ethnic mix between the two trials. Reanalysis of data from the BEST trial showed a decreased beneficial response to bucindolol in African–American patients [71]. Subsequent research into the role of β1-AR SNPs in this response showed that the Arg-389 variant acts as a gain-of-function polymorphism, enhancing signaling through the β1-AR and leading to increased ventricular contractility [72]. The Arg variant, less common in African–Americans, has higher constitutive activity and is therefore more sensitive to β-blockers with inverse agonist activity. This hyperresponsiveness suggested that this SNP could affect response to treatment in patients with heart failure. This effect was most notable with bucindolol, which effectively antagonized the hyperfunctional β1-Arg-389 receptor, but not the β1-Gly-389 receptor. Translating these in vitro studies to patients, Liggett and colleagues went on to show that patients who were treated with bucindolol and were homozygous Arg/Arg had increased survival and decreased hospitalizations compared with placebo-treated patients. In contrast, Gly-389 carriers, more common in African–Americans, showed no benefit of bucindolol.

If this were a class effect, applicable to all β-blockers, it would have had a profound effect on medical therapy. For carvedilol, two small studies have shown better improvement in left ventricular ejection fraction (LVEF) in Arg389Arg carriers compared with Arg/Gly or Gly/Gly carriers [73,74]. However, subsequent larger studies have failed to show any association between β-receptor SNPs and clinical efficacy [75,76]. A recent study did show a gene–dose interaction for carvedilol, suggesting that patients who are Arg-389 homozygotes might require a higher dose of β-blocker to achieve a similar reduction in mortality as patients who are Gly-389 carriers [77].

In addition to SNPs within the β-AR themselves, there are also variants in several of the proteins that interact and regulate β-receptor signaling. One of these, GRK5 is part of the previously described pathway that desensitizes β-receptors, reducing the effect of sympathetic stimulation. African–American patients with a Leu-41 SNP in GRK5, a gain-of-function variant that produces a level of self-β-blockade, did show improved survival compared with those with the Gln-41 variant [78,79]. The prevalence of the Leu-41 SNP is 10-fold greater in the African–American population [68].

In conclusion, African–American patients have different minor allele frequencies for several key adrenergic receptor polymorphisms, which have been linked to a decreased response to β-blocker therapy. It is these genetic variants that appear to be responsible for the differential response of African–American patients to heart failure therapies such as β-blockers. Since these differences are in ratios and not absolute, and any individual patient may carry either the more common (major) or the variant (minor) allele, race alone cannot be used to guide drug therapy. Finally, the translation of these results to children is uncertain.

IMPLICATIONS FOR TREATING CHILDREN WITH HEART FAILURE

As we have discussed, multiple large, prospective, multicenter, randomized-controlled trials in adult patients with heart failure have convincingly demonstrated the benefit of β-blockers in reducing hospitalization and improving transplant-free survival. When β-blocker therapy initially began to be accepted in adults, several small mostly single center studies suggested that β-blockers were also efficacious in children with heart failure [80–85]. The pediatric carvedilol study, the largest multicenter, randomized-controlled trial of β-blockade in children, followed 161 patients with chronic symptomatic heart failure from 26 US centers for a period of 5 years. 60% of these patients had dilated cardiomyopathy, but in contrast to the adult studies, 40% had congenital heart disease. The primary end point, a composite measure of clinical heart failure, was not different between carvedilol- and placebo-treated patients [86]. Secondary end points, including death or transplantation, were also not different between treated and control patients. However, the mortality in this pediatric study was only 5%, compared to the much higher mortality rates (14%–30%) typical of adult studies. To achieve the same level of statistical power with this much lower mortality rate, a pediatric study would have had to enroll over 6000 patients, thus increasing the likelihood that these results represent a Type II error [87]. Other significant differences from adult studies include the small number of children with ischemic cardiomyopathy and the high number of pediatric patients whose systemic ventricle was not a morphologic left ventricle. Indeed, the response to β-blocker was greater (64%) in those with a systemic left ventricle than in those with a systemic right ventricle (35%), in whom there was a subset in which function may have actually worsened. Similarly, other commonly used "left ventricular" heart failure therapies (ACE inhibitors, angiotensin receptor blockers) have been shown to be ineffective or less effective when used in patients with a systemic right ventricle [88,89]. To explain these findings, there are data suggesting that the response of the β-AR system to heart failure may not be identical in adults and children. Miyamoto et al. have shown downregulation of both β1 and β2-ARs in children with heart failure, in contrast to adults where only the β1-AR is downregulated. Similarly, in children phosphatase expression and phospholamban phosphorylation do not change with heart failure, whereas phosphatase is upregulated and PLB phosphorylation decreased in adults with heart failure [90].

More recently, a smaller, prospective randomized clinical trial of carvedilol in 89 children with dilated cardiomyopathy demonstrated a beneficial effect on Ross heart failure score and left ventricular function [91]. Patients in this trial tended to have more severe heart failure than in the larger study by Shaddy et al. Two additional smaller trials of β-blockers in children with congenital heart disease also showed a benefit with β-blocker therapy [92,93]. A recent metaanalysis was performed of seven pediatric studies with 420 total participants. The analysis consisted of one large study (the previously cited study by Shaddy), two medium-sized studies with 80 children each, and four smaller studies with 20–30 children each. There was no significant difference in mortality or transplantation between the β-blocker and control groups, whereas LVEF showed a small improvement [94]. However, this analysis was influenced by the disproportionate contribution of patients from the one large negative study.

Thus, based on currently available data, Rossano and Shaddy have written that "it is difficult to conclude with any degree of certainty whether the medications that have been well established to be beneficial for adult heart failure patients are also beneficial for children." [87]. The likelihood of a sufficiently powered study, and one that accounts for all of the unique etiologies of pediatric heart failure, being performed in the future is unlikely. Thus, we are left to try to extrapolate data from adult studies to the pediatric population, with the understanding that differences in response may be due to differences in underlying disease etiology, developmental differences in response of the heart to similar stresses, or differences in pharmacodynamics between children and adults.

REFERENCES

[1] E.H. Ackerknecht, The history of the discovery of the vegetative (autonomic) nervous system, Med. Hist. 18 (1) (1974) 1–8.

[2] R.P. Ahlquist, A study of the adrenotropic receptors, Am. J. Physiol. 153 (3) (1948) 586–600.

[3] C.E. Powell, I.H. Slater, Blocking of inhibitory adrenergic receptors by a dichloro analog of isoproterenol, J. Pharmacol. Exp. Ther. 122 (4) (1958) 480–488.

[4] N.C. Moran, M.E. Perkins, Adrenergic blockade of the mammalian heart by a dichloro analogue of isoproterenol, J. Pharmacol. Exp. Ther. 124 (3) (1958) 223–237.

[5] J.W. Black, A.F. Crowther, R.G. Shanks, L.H. Smith, A.C. Dornhorst, A new adrenergic betareceptor antagonist, Lancet 1 (7342) (1964) 1080–1081.

[6] C. Benedict, B. Shelton, D. Johnstone, G. Francis, B. Greenberg, M. Konstam, et al., Prognostic significance of plasma norepinephrine in patients with asymptomatic left ventricular dysfunction. SOLVD Investigators, Circulation 94 (1996) 690–697.

[7] G. Francis, J. Cohn, G. Johnson, T. Rector, S. Goldman, A. Simon, Plasma norepinephrine, plasma renin activity, and congestive heart failure: relations to survival and the effects of therapy in V-HeFT II, Circulation 87 (Suppl VI) (1993) VI-40–48.

[8] D.L. Mann, R.L. Kent, B. Parsons, G. Cooper, Adrenergic effects on the biology of the adult mammalian cardiocyte, Circulation 85 (2) (1992) 790–804.

[9] R.J. Lefkowitz, W.P. Hausdorff, M.G. Caron, Role of phosphorylation in desensitization of the beta-adrenoceptor, Trends Pharmacol. Sci. 11 (5) (1990) 190–194.

[10] W.P. Hausdorff, M.G. Caron, R.J. Lefkowitz, Turning off the signal: desensitization of beta-adrenergic receptor function, FASEB J. 4 (11) (1990) 2881–2889.

[11] B.B. Hoffman, T. Michel, T.B. Brenneman, R.J. Lefkowitz, Interactions of agonists with platelet alpha 2-adrenergic receptors, Endocrinology 110 (3) (1982) 926–932.

[12] Y. Daaka, L.M. Luttrell, R.J. Lefkowitz, Switching of the coupling of the ß2-adrenergic receptor to different G proteins by protein kinase A, Nature 390 (6) (1997) 88–91.

[13] W. Koch, H. Rockman, P. Samama, R. Hamilton, R. Bond, C. Milano, et al., Cardiac function in mice overexpressing the ß-adrenergic receptor kinase or a ßARK inhibitor, Science 268 (1995) 1350–1353.

[14] W. Koch, B. Hawes, L. Allen, R. Lefkowitz, Direct evidence that Gi-coupled receptor stimulation of mitogen-activated protein kinase is mediated by Gbg activation of p21ras, Proc. Natl. Acad. Sci. U.S.A. 91 (1994) 12706–12710.

[15] J.R. Raymond, M. Hnatowich, R.J. Lefkowitz, M.G. Caron, Adrenergic receptors. Models for regulation of signal transduction processes, Hypertension 15 (2) (1990) 119–131.

[16] D.R. Sibley, R.J. Lefkowitz, Molecular mechanisms of receptor desensitization using the beta-adrenergic receptor-coupled adenylate cyclase system as a model, Nature 317 (6033) (1985) 124–129.

[17] T. Frielle, S. Collins, K. Daniel, M. Caron, R. Lefkowitz, B. Kobilka, Cloning of the cDNA for the human ß1-adrenergic receptor, Proc. Natl. Acad. Sci. U.S.A. 84 (1987) 7920–7924.

[18] R.A. Dixon, B.K. Kobilka, D.J. Strader, J.L. Benovic, H.G. Dohlman, T. Frielle, et al., Cloning of the gene and cDNA for mammalian beta-adrenergic receptor and homology with rhodopsin, Nature 321 (6065) (1986) 75–79.

[19] R.E. Link, K. Desai, L. Hein, M.E. Stevens, A. Chruscinski, D. Bernstein, et al., Cardiovascular regulation in mice lacking alpha2-adrenergic receptor subtypes b and c, Science 273 (5276) (1996) 803–805.

[20] D. Rohrer, K. Desai, J. Jasper, M. Stevens, D. Regula, G. Barsh, et al., Targeted disruption of the mouse ß1-adrenergic receptor gene: developmental and cardiovascular effects, Proc. Natl. Acad. Sci. U.S.A. 93 (1996) 7375–7380.

[21] D.K. Rohrer, D. Bernstein, A. Chruscinski, K.H. Desai, E. Schauble, B.K. Kobilka, The developmental and physiological consequences of disrupting genes encoding beta 1 and beta 2 adrenoceptors, Adv. Pharmacol. 42 (1998) 499–501.

[22] J.D. Altman, A.U. Trendelenburg, L. MacMillan, D. Bernstein, L. Limbird, K. Starke, et al., Abnormal regulation of the sympathetic nervous system in alpha2A-adrenergic receptor knockout mice, Mol. Pharmacol. 56 (1) (1999) 154–161.

[23] A.J. Chruscinski, D.K. Rohrer, E. Schauble, K.H. Desai, D. Bernstein, B.K. Kobilka, Targeted disruption of the beta2 adrenergic receptor gene, J. Biol. Chem. 274 (24) (1999) 16694–16700.

[24] S.G. Rasmussen, B.T. DeVree, Y. Zou, A.C. Kruse, K.Y. Chung, T.S. Kobilka, et al., Crystal structure of the beta2 adrenergic receptor-Gs protein complex, Nature 477 (7366) (2011) 549–555.

[25] F. Waagstein, A. Hjalmarson, E. Varnauskas, I. Wallentin, Effect of chronic beta-adrenergic receptor blockade in congestive cardiomyopathy, Br. Heart J. 37 (10) (1975) 1022–1036.

[26] K. Swedberg, A. Hjalmarson, F. Waagstein, I. Wallentin, Beneficial effects of long-term beta-blockade in congestive cardiomyopathy, Br. Heart J. 44 (2) (1980) 117–133.

[27] The cardiac insufficiency bisoprolol study II (CIBIS-II): a randomised trial, Lancet 353 (9146) (1999) 9–13.

[28] A. Hjalmarson, S. Goldstein, B. Fagerberg, H. Wedel, F. Waagstein, J. Kjekshus, et al., Effects of controlled-release metoprolol on total mortality, hospitalizations, and well-being in patients with heart failure: the Metoprolol CR/XL Randomized Intervention Trial in congestive heart failure (MERIT-HF). MERIT-HF Study Group, JAMA 283 (10) (2000) 1295–1302.

[29] M. Packer, M.B. Fowler, E.B. Roecker, A.J. Coats, H.A. Katus, H. Krum, et al., Effect of carvedilol on the morbidity of patients with severe chronic heart failure: results of the carvedilol prospective randomized cumulative survival (COPERNICUS) study, Circulation 106 (17) (2002) 2194–2199.

[30] J.F. MacGregor, S.B. Wachter, M. Munger, G. Stoddard, M.R. Bristow, E.M. Gilbert, Carvedilol produces sustained long-term benefits: follow-up at 12 years, Congest. Heart Fail. 15 (1) (2009) 5–8.

[31] J.J. DiNicolantonio, C.J. Lavie, H. Fares, A.R. Menezes, J.H. O'Keefe, Meta-analysis of carvedilol versus beta 1 selective beta-blockers (atenolol, bisoprolol, metoprolol, and nebivolol), Am. J. Cardiol. 111 (5) (2013) 765–769.
[32] M. Bristow, R. Ginsburg, V. Umans, M. Fowler, W. Minobe, R. Rasmussen, et al., ß1- and ß2-adrenergic-receptor subpopulations in nonfailing and failing human ventricular myocardium: coupling of both receptor subtypes to muscle contraction and selective down-regulation in heart failure, Circ. Res. 59 (1986) 297–309.
[33] C. Milano, L. Allen, H. Rockman, P. Dolber, T. McMinn, K. Chien, et al., Enhanced myocardial function in transgenic mice overexpressing the ß2-adrenergic receptor, Science 264 (1994) 582–586.
[34] S. Liggett, N. Tepe, J. Lorenz, A. Canning, T. Jantz, S. Mitarai, et al., Early and delayed consequences of ß2-adrenergic receptor overexpression in mouse hearts. Critical role for expression level, Circulation 101 (2000) 1707–1714.
[35] S. Engelhardt, L. Hein, F. Wisemann, M. Lohse, Progressive hypertrophy and heart failure in ß1-adrenergic receptor transgenic mice, Proc. Natl. Acad. Sci. U.S.A. 96 (1999) 7059–7064.
[36] J.D. Bisognano, H.D. Weinberger, T.J. Bohlmeyer, A. Pende, M.V. Raynolds, A. Sastravaha, et al., Myocardial-directed overexpression of the human ß1-adrenergic receptor in transgenic mice, J. Mol. Cell. Cardiol. 32 (2000) 817–830.
[37] R.-P. Xiao, X. Ji, E. Lakatta, Functional coupling of the ß2-adrenoceptor to a pertussis toxin-sensitive G protein in cardiac myocytes, Mol. Pharmacol. 47 (1995) 322–329.
[38] G. Post, J. Brown, G protein-coupled receptors and signalling pathways regulating growth responses, FASEB J. 10 (1996) 741–749.
[39] H. Zhu, M. Qi, S. McElwee-Witmer, L. Merkel-Jordan, M. Perrone, K. Clark, et al., The relationship between hypertrophy and apoptosis in cultured neonatal ventricular myocytes, Circulation 98 (1998) I-345.
[40] S.M. Heilbrunn, P. Shah, M.R. Bristow, H.A. Valantine, R. Ginsburg, M.B. Fowler, Increased beta-receptor density and improved hemodynamic response to catecholamine stimulation during long-term metoprolol therapy in heart failure from dilated cardiomyopathy, Circulation 79 (3) (1989) 483–490.
[41] B.D. Lowes, E.M. Gilbert, W.T. Abraham, W.A. Minobe, P. Larrabee, D. Ferguson, et al., Myocardial gene expression in dilated cardiomyopathy treated with beta- blocking agents, N. Engl. J. Med. 346 (18) (2002) 1357–1365.
[42] W.Z. Zhu, S.Q. Wang, K. Chakir, D. Yang, T. Zhang, J.H. Brown, et al., Linkage of beta1-adrenergic stimulation to apoptotic heart cell death through protein kinase A-independent activation of Ca2+/calmodulin kinase II, J. Clin. Investig. 111 (5) (2003) 617–625.
[43] M.R. Bristow, Treatment of chronic heart failure with beta-adrenergic receptor antagonists: a convergence of receptor pharmacology and clinical cardiology, Circ. Res. 109 (10) (2011) 1176–1194.
[44] K.L. Dodge-Kafka, L. Langeberg, J.D. Scott, Compartmentation of cyclic nucleotide signaling in the heart: the role of A-kinase anchoring proteins, Circ. Res. 98 (8) (2006) 993–1001.
[45] R.-P. Xiao, P. Avdonin, Y.-Y. Zhou, H. Cheng, S. Akhter, T. Eschenhagen, et al., Coupling of ß2-adrenoceptor to Gi proteins and its physiological relevance in murine cardiac myocytes, Circ. Res. 84 (1999) 43–52.
[46] M. Kohlhaas, T. Zhang, T. Seidler, D. Zibrova, N. Dybkova, A. Steen, et al., Increased sarcoplasmic reticulum calcium leak but unaltered contractility by acute CaMKII overexpression in isolated rabbit cardiac myocytes, Circ. Res. 98 (2) (2006) 235–244.
[47] J. Shan, M.J. Betzenhauser, A. Kushnir, S. Reiken, A.C. Meli, A. Wronska, et al., Role of chronic ryanodine receptor phosphorylation in heart failure and beta-adrenergic receptor blockade in mice, J. Clin. Investig. 120 (12) (2010) 4375–4387.
[48] W.Z. Zhu, M. Zheng, W.J. Koch, R.J. Lefkowitz, B.K. Kobilka, R.P. Xiao, Dual modulation of cell survival and cell death by beta(2)-adrenergic signaling in adult mouse cardiac myocytes, Proc. Natl. Acad. Sci. U.S.A. 98 (4) (2001) 1607–1612.
[49] M. Zheng, Q.D. Han, R.P. Xiao, Distinct beta-adrenergic receptor subtype signaling in the heart and their pathophysiological relevance, Acta Physiol. Sin. (Sheng li xue bao) 56 (1) (2004) 1–15.
[50] C. Communal, K. Singh, D.B. Sawyer, W.S. Colucci, Opposing effects of beta(1)- and beta(2)-adrenergic receptors on cardiac myocyte apoptosis: role of a pertussis toxin-sensitive G protein, Circulation 100 (22) (1999) 2210–2212.
[51] M. Zaugg, W. Xu, E. Lucchinetti, S.A. Shafiq, N.Z. Jamali, M.A. Siddiqui, Beta-adrenergic receptor subtypes differentially affect apoptosis in adult rat ventricular myocytes, Circulation 102 (3) (2000) 344–350.
[52] G. Fajardo, M. Zhao, J. Powers, D. Bernstein, Differential cardiotoxic/cardioprotective effects of beta-adrenergic receptor subtypes in myocytes and fibroblasts in doxorubicin cardiomyopathy, J. Mol. Cell. Cardiol. 40 (3) (2006) 375–383.
[53] I. Ahmet, M. Krawczyk, W. Zhu, A.Y.-H. Woo, C. Morrell, S. Poosala, et al., Cardioprotective and survival benefits of long-term combined therapy with beta2 adrenoreceptor (AR) agonist and beta1 AR blocker in dilated cardiomyopathy postmyocardial infarction, J. Pharmacol. Exp. Ther. 325 (2) (2008) 491–499.
[54] I. Ahmet, C. Morrell, E.G. Lakatta, M.I. Talan, Therapeutic efficacy of a combination of a beta1-adrenoreceptor (AR) blocker and beta2-AR agonist in a rat model of postmyocardial infarction dilated heart failure exceeds that of a beta1-AR blocker plus angiotensin-converting enzyme inhibitor, J. Pharmacol. Exp. Ther. 331 (1) (2009) 178–185.
[55] A.J. Patterson, W. Zhu, A. Chow, R. Agrawal, J. Kosek, R.P. Xiao, et al., Protecting the myocardium: a role for the beta2 adrenergic receptor in the heart, Crit. Care. Med. 32 (4) (2004) 1041–1048.
[56] D. Bernstein, G. Fajardo, M. Zhao, T. Urashima, J. Powers, G. Berry, et al., Differential cardioprotective/cardiotoxic effects mediated by beta-adrenergic receptor subtypes, Am. J. Physiol. Heart Circ. Physiol. 289 (6) (2005) H2441–H2449.
[57] H. Tong, D. Bernstein, E. Murphy, C. Steenbergen, Protective effect of ß-adrenergic receptor is through PKA-mediated switching of coupling of receptor, FASEB J. 19 (8) (June 2005) 983–985.
[58] W. Zhu, X. Zeng, M. Zheng, R.P. Xiao, The enigma of beta2-adrenergic receptor Gi signaling in the heart: the good, the bad, and the ugly, Circ. Res. 97 (6) (2005) 507–509.

[59] M.I. Talan, I. Ahmet, R.P. Xiao, E.G. Lakatta, beta(2) AR agonists in treatment of chronic heart failure: long path to translation, J. Mol. Cell. Cardiol. 51 (4) (2011) 529–533.

[60] S. Witchitz, A. Cohen-Solal, N. Dartois, N. Weisslinger, K. Juste, J.Y. Darmon, Treatment of heart failure with celiprolol, a cardioselective beta blocker with beta-2 agonist vasodilatory properties. The CELICARD Group, Am. J. Cardiol. 85 (12) (2000) 1467–1471.

[61] G.E. Newton, J.D. Parker, Acute effects of beta 1-selective and nonselective beta-adrenergic receptor blockade on cardiac sympathetic activity in congestive heart failure, Circulation 94 (3) (1996) 353–358.

[62] H.A. Rockman, K.R. Chien, D.J. Choi, G. Iaccarino, J.J. Hunter, J. Ross Jr., et al., Expression of a beta-adrenergic receptor kinase 1 inhibitor prevents the development of myocardial failure in gene-targeted mice, Proc. Natl. Acad. Sci. U.S.A. 95 (12) (1998) 7000–7005.

[63] G. Fajardo, M. Zhao, T. Urashima, S. Farahani, D.Q. Hu, S. Reddy, et al., Deletion of the beta2-adrenergic receptor prevents the development of cardiomyopathy in mice, J. Mol. Cell. Cardiol. 63 (2013) 155–164.

[64] G. Fajardo, M. Zhao, G. Berry, L.J. Wong, D. Mochly-Rosen, D. Bernstein, beta2-adrenergic receptors mediate cardioprotection through crosstalk with mitochondrial cell death pathways, J. Mol. Cell. Cardiol. 51 (5) (2011) 781–789.

[65] N. Noor, C.B. Patel, H.A. Rockman, Beta-arrestin: a signaling molecule and potential therapeutic target for heart failure, J. Mol. Cell. Cardiol. 51 (4) (2011) 534–541.

[66] S. Rajagopal, K. Rajagopal, R.J. Lefkowitz, Teaching old receptors new tricks: biasing seven-transmembrane receptors, Nat. Rev. Drug Disc. 9 (5) (2010) 373–386.

[67] F. Rochais, J.P. Vilardaga, V.O. Nikolaev, M. Bunemann, M.J. Lohse, S. Engelhardt, Real-time optical recording of beta1-adrenergic receptor activation reveals supersensitivity of the Arg389 variant to carvedilol, J. Clin. Investig. 117 (1) (2007) 229–235.

[68] M.R. Taylor, A.Y. Sun, G. Davis, M. Fiuzat, S.B. Liggett, M.R. Bristow, Race, common genetic variation, and therapeutic response disparities in heart failure, JACC Heart Fail. 2 (6) (2014) 561–572.

[69] S.B. Liggett, L.E. Wagoner, L.L. Craft, R.W. Hornung, B.D. Hoit, T.C. McIntosh, et al., The Ile164 beta2-adrenergic receptor polymorphism adversely affects the outcome of congestive heart failure, J. Clin. Investig. 102 (8) (1998) 1534–1539.

[70] J.A. Johnson, S.B. Liggett, Cardiovascular pharmacogenomics of adrenergic receptor signaling: clinical implications and future directions, Clin. Pharmacol. Ther. 89 (3) (2011) 366–378.

[71] D.E. Lanfear, T.N. Hrobowski, E.L. Peterson, K.E. Wells, T.V. Swadia, J.A. Spertus, et al., Association of beta-blocker exposure with outcomes in heart failure differs between African American and white patients, Circ. Heart Fail. 5 (2) (2012) 202–208.

[72] S.B. Liggett, J. Mialet-Perez, S. Thaneemit-Chen, S.A. Weber, S.M. Greene, D. Hodne, et al., A polymorphism within a conserved beta(1)-adrenergic receptor motif alters cardiac function and beta-blocker response in human heart failure, Proc. Natl. Acad. Sci. U.S.A. 103 (30) (2006) 11288–11293.

[73] J. Mialet Perez, D.A. Rathz, N.N. Petrashevskaya, H.S. Hahn, L.E. Wagoner, A. Schwartz, et al., Beta 1-adrenergic receptor polymorphisms confer differential function and predisposition to heart failure, Nat. Med. 9 (10) (2003) 1300–1305.

[74] L. Chen, D. Meyers, G. Javorsky, D. Burstow, P. Lolekha, M. Lucas, et al., Arg389Gly-beta1-adrenergic receptors determine improvement in left ventricular systolic function in nonischemic cardiomyopathy patients with heart failure after chronic treatment with carvedilol, Pharmacogenetics Genom. 17 (11) (2007) 941–949.

[75] A.J. Sehnert, S.E. Daniels, M. Elashoff, J.A. Wingrove, C.R. Burrow, B. Horne, et al., Lack of association between adrenergic receptor genotypes and survival in heart failure patients treated with carvedilol or metoprolol, J. Am. Coll. Cardiol. 52 (8) (2008) 644–651.

[76] P. de Groote, N. Helbecque, N. Lamblin, X. Hermant, E. Mc Fadden, C. Foucher-Hossein, et al., Association between beta-1 and beta-2 adrenergic receptor gene polymorphisms and the response to beta-blockade in patients with stable congestive heart failure, Pharmacogenetics Genom. 15 (3) (2005) 137–142.

[77] M. Fiuzat, M.L. Neely, A.Z. Starr, W.E. Kraus, G.M. Felker, M. Donahue, et al., Association between adrenergic receptor genotypes and beta-blocker dose in heart failure patients: analysis from the HF-ACTION DNA substudy, Eur. J. Heart Fail. 15 (3) (2013) 258–266.

[78] S.B. Liggett, S. Cresci, R.J. Kelly, F.M. Syed, S.J. Matkovich, H.S. Hahn, et al., A GRK5 polymorphism that inhibits beta-adrenergic receptor signaling is protective in heart failure, Nat. Med. 14 (5) (2008) 510–517.

[79] S. Cresci, R.J. Kelly, T.P. Cappola, A. Diwan, D. Dries, S.L. Kardia, et al., Clinical and genetic modifiers of long-term survival in heart failure, J. Am. Coll. Cardiol. 54 (5) (2009) 432–444.

[80] L.A. Bruns, M.K. Chrisant, J.M. Lamour, R.E. Shaddy, E. Pahl, E.D. Blume, et al., Carvedilol as therapy in pediatric heart failure: an initial multicenter experience, J. Pediatr. 138 (4) (2001) 505–511.

[81] R.V. Williams, L.Y. Tani, R.E. Shaddy, Intermediate effects of treatment with metoprolol or carvedilol in children with left ventricular systolic dysfunction, J. Heart Lung Transpl. 21 (8) (2002) 906–909.

[82] S. Laer, T.S. Mir, F. Behn, M. Eiselt, H. Scholz, A. Venzke, et al., Carvedilol therapy in pediatric patients with congestive heart failure: a study investigating clinical and pharmacokinetic parameters, Am. Heart J. 143 (5) (2002) 916–922.

[83] E. Azeka, J.A. Franchini Ramires, C. Valler, E. Alcides Bocchi, Delisting of infants and children from the heart transplantation waiting list after carvedilol treatment, J. Am. Coll. Cardiol. 40 (11) (2002) 2034–2038.

[84] P. Rusconi, O. Gomez-Marin, M. Rossique-Gonzalez, E. Redha, J.R. Marin, M. Lon-Young, et al., Carvedilol in children with cardiomyopathy: 3-year experience at a single institution, J. Heart Lung Transpl. 23 (7) (2004) 832–838.

[85] M. Nishiyama, I.S. Park, T. Yoshikawa, Y. Hatai, M. Ando, Y. Takahashi, et al., Efficacy and safety of carvedilol for heart failure in children and patients with congenital heart disease, Heart Ves. 24 (3) (2009) 187–192.

[86] R.E. Shaddy, M.M. Boucek, D.T. Hsu, R.J. Boucek, C.E. Canter, L. Mahony, et al., Carvedilol for children and adolescents with heart failure: a randomized controlled trial, JAMA 298 (10) (2007) 1171–1179.

[87] J.W. Rossano, R.E. Shaddy, Update on pharmacological heart failure therapies in children: do adult medications work in children and if not, why not? Circulation 129 (5) (2014) 607–612.
[88] A.A. Kouatli, J.A. Garcia, T.M. Zellers, E.M. Weinstein, L. Mahony, Enalapril does not enhance exercise capacity in patients after Fontan procedure, Circulation 96 (5) (1997) 1507–1512.
[89] T. van der Bom, M.M. Winter, B.J. Bouma, M. Groenink, H.W. Vliegen, P.G. Pieper, et al., Effect of valsartan on systemic right ventricular function: a double-blind, randomized, placebo-controlled pilot trial, Circulation 127 (3) (2013) 322–330.
[90] S.D. Miyamoto, B.L. Stauffer, S. Nakano, R. Sobus, K. Nunley, P. Nelson, et al., Beta-adrenergic adaptation in paediatric idiopathic dilated cardiomyopathy, Eur. Heart J. 35 (1) (2014) 33–41.
[91] M. Huang, X. Zhang, S. Chen, Y. Sun, Y. Xiao, J. Sun, et al., The effect of carvedilol treatment on chronic heart failure in pediatric patients with dilated cardiomyopathy: a prospective, randomized-controlled study, Pediatr. Cardiol. 34 (3) (2013) 680–685.
[92] R. Buchhorn, M. Hulpke-Wette, R. Hilgers, D. Bartmus, A. Wessel, J. Bursch, Propranolol treatment of congestive heart failure in infants with congenital heart disease: the CHF-PRO-INFANT Trial. Congestive heart failure in infants treated with propanol, Int. J. Cardiol. 79 (2–3) (2001) 167–173.
[93] N. Ishibashi, I.S. Park, T. Waragai, T. Yoshikawa, Y. Murakami, K. Mori, et al., Effect of carvedilol on heart failure in patients with a functionally univentricular heart, Circulation 75 (6) (2011) 1394–1399.
[94] S. Alabed, A. Sabouni, S. Al Dakhoul, Y. Bdaiwi, A.K. Frobel-Mercier, Beta-blockers for congestive heart failure in children, Cochrane Database Syst. Rev. (1) (2016) CD007037.
[95] F. Waagstein, M.R. Bristow, K. Swedberg, F. Camerini, M.B. Fowler, M.A. Silver, et al., Beneficial effects of metoprolol in idiopathic dilated cardiomyopathy. Metoprolol in Dilated Cardiomyopathy (MDC) Trial Study Group, Lancet 342 (8885) (1993) 1441–1446.
[96] A randomized trial of beta-blockade in heart failure. The Cardiac Insufficiency Bisoprolol Study (CIBIS). CIBIS Investigators and Committees, Circulation 90 (4) (1994) 1765–1773.
[97] M. Packer, M.R. Bristow, J.N. Cohn, W.S. Colucci, M.B. Fowler, E.M. Gilbert, et al., The effect of carvedilol on morbidity and mortality in patients with chronic heart failure. U.S. Carvedilol Heart Failure Study Group, N. Engl. J. Med. 334 (21) (1996) 1349–1355.
[98] Beta-Blocker Evaluation of Survival Trial I. A trial of the beta-blocker bucindolol in patients with advanced chronic heart failure, N. Engl. J. Med. 344 (22) (2001) 1659–1667.
[99] H.J. Dargie, Effect of carvedilol on outcome after myocardial infarction in patients with left-ventricular dysfunction: the CAPRICORN randomised trial, Lancet 357 (9266) (2001) 1385–1390.
[100] P.A. Poole-Wilson, K. Swedberg, J.G. Cleland, A. Di Lenarda, P. Hanrath, M. Komajda, et al., Comparison of carvedilol and metoprolol on clinical outcomes in patients with chronic heart failure in the Carvedilol or Metoprolol European Trial (COMET): randomised controlled trial, Lancet 362 (9377) (2003) 7–13.
[101] M.D. Flather, M.C. Shibata, A.J. Coats, D.J. Van Veldhuisen, A. Parkhomenko, J. Borbola, et al., Randomized trial to determine the effect of nebivolol on mortality and cardiovascular hospital admission in elderly patients with heart failure (SENIORS), Eur. Heart J. 26 (3) (2005) 215–225.
[102] C. Kubon, N.B. Mistry, I. Grundvold, S. Halvorsen, S.E. Kjeldsen, A.S. Westheim, The role of beta-blockers in the treatment of chronic heart failure, Trends Pharmacol. Sci. 32 (4) (2011) 206–212.
[103] D.A. Rathz, K.M. Brown, L.A. Kramer, S.B. Liggett, Amino acid 49 polymorphisms of the human beta1-adrenergic receptor affect agonist-promoted trafficking, J. Cardiovasc. Pharmacol. 39 (2) (2002) 155–160.
[104] M.C. Levin, S. Marullo, O. Muntaner, B. Andersson, Y. Magnusson, The myocardium-protective Gly-49 variant of the beta 1-adrenergic receptor exhibits constitutive activity and increased desensitization and down-regulation, J. Biol. Chem. 277 (34) (2002) 30429–30435.
[105] D.A. Mason, J.D. Moore, S.A. Green, S.B. Liggett, A gain-of-function polymorphism in a G-protein coupling domain of the human beta1-adrenergic receptor, J. Biol. Chem. 274 (18) (1999) 12670–12674.
[106] S.A. Green, J. Turki, M. Innis, S.B. Liggett, Amino-terminal polymorphisms of the human beta 2-adrenergic receptor impart distinct agonist-promoted regulatory properties, Biochemistry 33 (32) (1994) 9414–9419.
[107] K.M. Small, S.L. Forbes, F.F. Rahman, K.M. Bridges, S.B. Liggett, A four amino acid deletion polymorphism in the third intracellular loop of the human alpha 2C-adrenergic receptor confers impaired coupling to multiple effectors, J. Biol. Chem. 275 (30) (2000) 23059–23064.
[108] G.D. Femminella, V. Barrese, N. Ferrara, G. Rengo, Tailoring therapy for heart failure: the pharmacogenomics of adrenergic receptor signaling, Pharmacogenomics Personalized Med. 7 (2014) 267–273.

Chapter 3

Inflammatory Mediators in Heart Failure

Kory J. Lavine, Douglas L. Mann
Washington University School of Medicine, St. Louis, MO, United States

INTRODUCTION

In this chapter we will discuss the current state of knowledge regarding the importance of inflammation in heart failure. We will primarily focus on evidence that has provided insights into heart failure pathogenesis, prognosis, and therapy. We will initially concentrate on the relevance of inflammation in adult heart failure, as the majority of studies have been conducted in this population. We will then highlight important distinctions between the pediatric and adult immune system and discuss the ramifications of these differences as they relate to pediatric heart failure.

INFLAMMATION IN ADULT HEART FAILURE

It is well established that inflammation occurs in adult heart failure, is prognostically important, and represents a critical mechanism that contributes to disease progression. Local and systemic inflammation not only affects the heart but also plays important roles in peripheral tissues. For example, inflammatory mediators promote skeletal muscle atrophy and dysfunction, which are important components of the syndrome of heart failure. In this section, we will summarize evidence stemming from clinical studies that have implicated systemic inflammation in the pathogenesis of heart failure, cemented inflammatory mediators as biomarkers of heart failure, and discuss the mechanistic basis by which inflammation is generated and exerts its effects.

Prognosis and Biomarkers

Numerous clinical studies have revealed that adult patients with heart failure display signs of systemic inflammation [1–5]. Proinflammatory cytokines that are present in the serum of patients with heart failure include members of the tumor necrosis factor (TNF) superfamily (TNFSF), IL-6, and soluble ST2 (sST2) (an IL1 family member). In addition to cytokines, several other inflammatory mediators have been identified in the serum of patients with heart failure, most notably galectin-3 and pentraxin-3.

Tumor Necrosis Factor (TNFSF2) and IL-6

The link between heart failure and inflammation was first recognized in 1990 by Levine et al. who reported elevated levels of TNF in patients with heart failure with a reduced ejection fraction (HFrEF) [6]. Since this original report, there has been an increasing appreciation that cytokines and chemokines are upregulated in patients with acute and chronic systolic heart failure. Examination of biomarkers in the VEST trial, which was comprised of 1200 heart failure patients, demonstrated that serum levels of TNF and IL-6 are elevated in heart failure and are prognostically important. Patients with elevated levels of these cytokines display higher rates of mortality [2]. Further studies have shown that serum TNF and IL6 levels are predictive of the development of heart failure, increase with worsening heart failure class, and are reduced following initiation of aggressive medical therapy for heart failure [7,8]. Other cytokines and cytokine receptors that are increased in the serum of heart failure patients and associated with clinical outcomes include TWEAK/TNFSF12, FasL/TNFSF6, LIGHT/TNFSF-12, IL1β/IL-1F2, IL-2, IL-18/IL-1F8, and IL-33/IL-1F11 [9].

The exact sources of these cytokines is not well established, but likely includes both the myocardium and peripheral tissues including but not limited to the gastrointestinal tract, liver, and circulating monocytes [7,10,11]. While the failing heart releases TNF into the circulation [12,13] and previous reports have immunolocalized TNF to failing human cardiac myocytes, it remains unclear whether the primary source of TNF is cardiomyocytes, immune cells, endothelial cells, and/or

Heart Failure in the Child and Young Adult. http://dx.doi.org/10.1016/B978-0-12-802393-8.00003-X

fibroblasts. In addition, many cytokines are produced on the systemic level. One proposed mechanism is that reduced intestinal blood flow and increased venous congestion leads to increased gut permeability and systemic inflammation through either systemic lipopolysaccharides (LPS) exposure and/or dysregulated mucosal immune responses [14]. In the latter scenario, activation of innate immune cells results in elevated systemic levels of TNF, IL-6, IL-1β, and IL-2 with deleterious effects on the myocardium and peripheral tissues.

Soluble ST2

ST2/IL1RL1 is a member of the IL1 receptor family and serves as the receptor for IL-33. The ST2 protein has two isoforms including sST2 and the membrane-bound ST2 receptor, referred to as ST2L. Preclinical studies have demonstrated that binding of IL-33 to ST2L elicits a cardioprotective effect. Deletion of the ST2 gene in mice results in accelerated contractile dysfunction, cardiomyocyte hypertrophy, and myocardial fibrosis following pressure overload due to disruption of protective effects of ST2L receptor signaling [15]. sST2 is secreted by cardiomyocytes and that are subjected to mechanical strain or stretch and acts as a decoy receptor to inhibit IL-33 signaling by reducing ligand availability [16,17]. As such, soluble sST2 is an integrated marker of mechanical strain, inflammation, and adverse remodeling.

Patients with acute and chronic heart failure have increased serum concentrations of sST2. Importantly, sST2 serum levels are predictive of heart failure-associated mortality in acute heart failure, chronic heart failure, and following myocardial infarction [18–23]. As a result, sST2 was the first inflammatory biomarker to be approved by the Food and Drug Administration for the prognosis in heart failure.

Galectin-3 and Pentraxin-3

Galectin-3 is a member of the lectin family and contains a carbohydrate recognition–binding domain that binds specifically to β-galactosides. Galectin-3 has been shown to be involved in a diverse array of biological processes including cell–cell adhesion and cell–matrix interactions, chemoattraction, cell growth and differentiation, angiogenesis, immune cell activation, and apoptosis [24]. From a disease standpoint, Galectin-3 has been implicated in fibrosis, metastasis, and heart failure [25–27]. Galectin-3 is released by macrophages in response to tissue injury. Deletion of galectin-3 in mice attenuates contractile dysfunction, cardiomyocyte hypertrophy, and myocardial fibrosis in a model of hypertensive cardiomyopathy [28].

Galectin-3 is approved by the Food and Drug Administration as a biomarker for determining heart failure prognosis. Galectin-3 is elevated in the serum of heart failure patients and increases as a function of disease progression. Clinically, serum levels of galectin-3 are associated with myocardial fibrosis and predict higher risk of death in both acute and chronic heart failure patients [29–32].

Pentraxin-3 is a member of the pentraxin family of cytokines that also includes C-reactive protein (CRP), serum amyloid P component, and female protein. Collectively, pentraxins are acute phase reactants and may act as components of the humeral arm of the innate immune system. For example, CRP promotes agglutination, phagocytosis of bacteria, and activates the classical complement pathway by binding to phosphocholine [33]. Pentraxin-3 is an acute phase reactant that binds to apoptotic cells, triggers complement deposition, and restricts self-antigen cross presentation [34,35]. Pentraxin-3 is produced by monocytes, macrophages, dendritic cells, fibroblasts, and endothelial cells in response to toll-like receptor (TLR) engagement, TNF, and IL-1β signaling [36].

Pentraxin-3 has recently been examined as a biomarker for heart failure. Serum pentraxin-3 levels are increased following myocardial infarction and are associated with 3 month mortality. Examination of patients enrolled in the CORONA and GISSI-HF trials demonstrated that elevations in serum pentraxin-3 were associated with a higher risk of all-cause mortality, cardiovascular mortality, and hospitalization for worsening heart failure [37].

Mechanisms of Immune Activation

The systemic syndrome of heart failure results in multiple insults to the heart as well as peripheral tissues including skeletal muscle, liver, gastrointestinal tract, and nervous system [38]. Collectively, these perturbations contribute to progressive neurohormonal activation, systemic inflammation, and ultimately, result in progressive deterioration of cardiac function, cachexia, skeletal muscle wasting, and end organ dysfunction. Common to many forms of heart failure, intrinsic myocardial injury and systemic derangements in tissue perfusion stemming from increased venous congestion and inadequate cardiac output (either at rest or with exercise) contribute to the activation of the innate immune system. In the following section, we will discuss the mechanistic basis by which local and systemic inflammatory responses are generated in adult patients with heart failure.

Myocardial Inflammation

Within the myocardium, cardiomyocyte stretch, injury, and cell death represent common triggers of inflammation. For patients with ischemic cardiomyopathies, cardiomyocytes undergo necrosis and other forms of programmed cell death following episodes of coronary ischemia and/or ischemia reperfusion injury. Cardiomyocyte cell death has also been observed in various forms of nonischemic cardiomyopathies including dilated cardiomyopathy, muscular dystrophy, and cardiomyopathies associated with viral myocarditis, chemotherapeutic agents, and autoimmune diseases [39]. In addition, increased wall tension results in the release of immunomodulatory molecules such as sST2, which is secreted by cardiomyocytes in response to mechanical stretch [16,17].

In recent years, details have emerged clarifying the mechanisms by which cellular and tissue injury is recognized by the immune system and inflammatory responses are generated. It is now understood that cells that are injured or those that undergo cell death through necrosis, necroptosis, and aborted apoptosis release an array of intracellular signaling molecules with potent effects on tissue resident immune cells [9]. Dying cardiomyocytes release an array of signals collectively referred to as damage-associated molecular patterns (DAMPs) that encompass a variety of mediators including alarmins (HMGB1, S100A8/9/12, S100B, IL1α, HSPs), nucleotides (ATP, CpG, dsRNA), bioactive lipids, extracellular matrix fragments (glycans, heparin sulfate, hyaluronan), and lectins (Fig. 3.1) [40].

The majority of DAMPs are recognized by a set of germ line encoded pattern recognition receptors (PRRs) most prominently expressed on leukocytes, endothelial cells, and fibroblasts. However, these PRRs also are expressed by cardiac myocytes. PRRs are well known for their roles in recognizing pathogen-derived products referred to as pathogen-associated molecular patterns (PAMPs). Examples of PAMPs include gram-negative bacterial LPS, gram-positive bacterial teichoic acids, yeast zymosans, mycobacterial glycolipids, and viral dsRNAs [41]. Classically engagement of PRRs such as toll-like receptor 4 (TLR4) by pathogen-derived products (i.e., LPS) results in activation of mononuclear phagocytes and generation of profound inflammation responses aimed at eliminating both pathogens and infected cells [42–44].

A growing body of literature has provided substantial evidence indicating that recognition of DAMPs by PRRs is responsible for sterile injury-associated inflammation and, in some scenarios, tissue repair. PRRs implicated in sterile injury responses include TLRs (TLR2, 3, 4, and 9), NOD-like receptors (NOD, NLRs, NLRP3), RIG-I like receptors, C-type lectin receptors (CLRs), RAGE receptor, and formyl peptide receptors (FPRs) [45,46]. All of which are present in the heart. TLRs are found on either the plasma membrane (TLR2, 4) or endosomes (TLR3, 9) and recognize and array of DAMPs including HMGB1, S100A/B, HSPs, extracellular matrix fragments, and dsDNA including mitochondrial DNA and CpG fragments [46]. Engagement of TLR receptors by various DAMPS leads to the activation of a well-described cascade of signaling events culminating in the release of proinflammatory chemokines and cytokines [47]. Activation of the NOD-like receptors

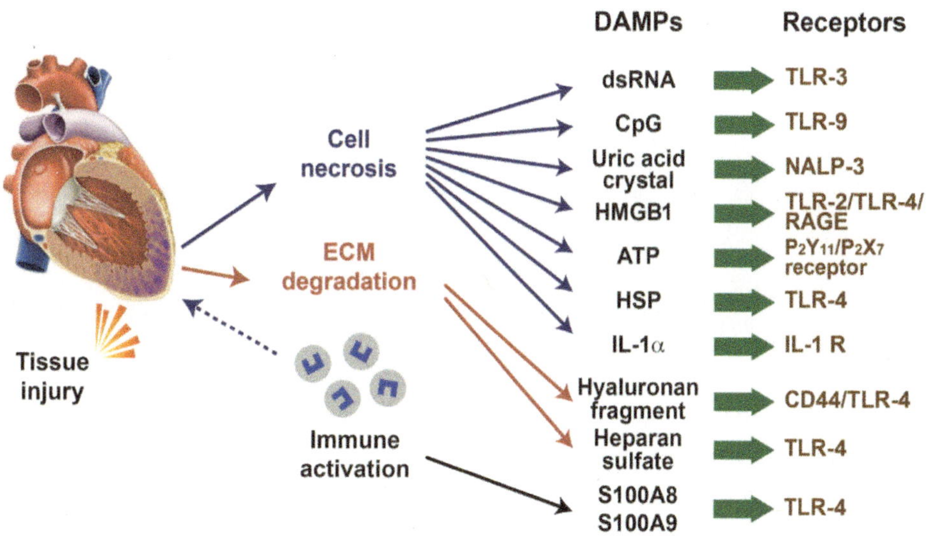

FIGURE 3.1 Damage-associated molecular patterns (DAMPs) are derived from dying cells that release their cytosolic content following myocardial injury, from degradation of the extracellular matrix, as well as by immune cells that become activated following tissue injury. *ATP*, adenosine triphosphate; *HMGB1*, high mobility box group 1 protein; *HSP*, heat shock protein; *IL-1R*, interleukin receptor; *IL-1α*, interleukin-1α; *NALP*, NACHT, LRR and PYD domains-containing protein 3 (cryopyrin); *RAGE*, receptor for advanced glycation end products; *TLR*, toll-like receptor. *(Reproduced with permission from D.L. Mann, Role of innate immunity in heart failure, in: D.L. Mann, G.M. Felker (Eds.), Heart Failure: A Companion to Braunwald's Heart Disease, third ed., Elsevier, Philadelphia, Pennsylvania, 2015, p. 109–126.)*

NOD1, NOD2, and NLRP3 by nucleotides and other metabolites including uric acid results in inflammasome activation and generation of robust inflammatory responses [48]. FPRs recognize products released from damaged mitochondrial and have been shown to trigger robust activation of neutrophils in the setting of sterile liver injury [49]. At this point in time considerably less is known regarding the roles of RIG-like receptors, CLRs, and RAGE receptors in sterile tissue injury.

With respect to the heart, multiple DAMPs have been implicated in heart failure pathogenesis. In general, DAMPs bind to and activate PRRs located on immune cells resident within and recruited to the heart following injury as well as endothelial cells and fibroblasts. Activation of these receptors represents a proximal step in the initiation of inflammation. TLR1-10 are expressed in the human heart [43,50], and TLR4 is upregulated in human heart failure [51,52]. Genetic deletion of TLR2 or TLR4 impairs adverse remodeling and impedes heart failure pathogenesis in mouse models of myocardial ischemia and infarction [42]. In addition, several NOD-like receptors including NOD1, NOD2, NLRP2, and NLRP3 are expressed in the human heart. NOD1 and NLRP3 activate the inflammasome and contribute to adverse remodeling following ischemia reperfusion injury or myocardial infarction [43,53].

Systemic Inflammation

Alterations in tissue perfusion also are sufficient to contribute to systemic inflammation. Reduced cardiac output (particularly during exercise) and increased venous pressure are central to all etiologies of heart failure and result in reduced end organ blood flow. Failure to augment blood flow during exercise due to reduced forward flow and impaired vasodilation leads to inadequate skeletal muscle, kidney, and liver perfusion and production of lactate, a hallmark of tissue ischemia [54]. Similarly, increased central venous pressure not only results in microvascular congestion and tissue edema but also reduced perfusion pressure across capillary beds [54,55]. As a consequence, peripheral tissues receive inadequate nutrient supply including oxygen and are either stressed, reversibly injured, or in more extreme conditions undergo apoptotic and/or necrotic cell death. Within ischemic tissue beds, injured and dying cells trigger the activation of immune cells (monocytes, macrophages, dendritic cells, and neutrophils) resulting in the elaboration of inflammatory chemokines and cytokines.

Extensive literature has established that patients with heart failure display evidence of neurohormonal activation, defined by activation of the systemic nervous system and the renin–angiotensin–aldosterone system [56]. In addition, to promoting cardiomyocyte cell death and myocardial adverse remodeling, neurohormonal activation has direct effects on peripheral tissues including skeletal myocytes leading to induction of oxidative injury, sarcomere loss, and cell death. Chronic epinephrine and norepinephrine exposure is sufficient to promote oxidative stress, capillary rarefaction, and skeletal muscle atrophy. These effects appear to occur through a combination of chronic β1-adrenergic stimulation and downregulation of β2-adrenergic signaling [57,58]. Moreover, norepinephrine may contribute to reduced tissue perfusion through exaggerated α-adrenergic-mediated vasoconstriction [59]. Lastly, increased local and systemic sympathetic nerve activity and reduce vagal tone have important effects on innate immune cell recruitment, proinflammatory signaling, and resolution of inflammatory responses. Sympathetic activation is an essential cue to mobilize monocytes from the bone marrow potentially through a β3-adrenergic mechanism, while parasympathetic signaling via nicotinic acetylcholine receptors is an important negative regulator of proinflammatory innate immune responses to sterile tissue injury [60–62].

Angiotensin II levels are also elevated in the setting of chronic heart failure and trigger the generation of damaging reactive oxygen species through direct stimulation of NADPH oxidase [63,64]. In addition, angiotensin II signaling directly contributes to immune activation through augmentation of inflammatory and inhibition of antiinflammatory signaling mechanisms. Angiotensin II signaling activates canonical NFκB–dependent proinflammatory gene expression in skeletal muscle myocytes and hepatocytes. Moreover, pathophysiologically relevant concentrations of angiotensin II are sufficient to provoke de novo TNF mRNA and protein synthesis in the adult heart through a NF-κB–dependent pathway [65]. Importantly, angiotensin II also suppresses insulin-like growth factor 1 (IGF1) signaling in skeletal myocytes, a central antiinflammatory signaling mechanism that governs skeletal muscle homeostasis and growth [64,66–69].

Contribution of Inflammation to the Syndrome of Heart Failure

Systemic inflammation has deleterious effects on the myocardium, peripheral vasculature, and end organ function that together contribute to the syndrome of heart failure. In the following section, we will discuss the mechanistic basis by which inflammatory mediators (cytokines, oxidative activity, matrix metalloproteases) drive adverse remodeling and heart failure pathogenesis.

Effects on the Myocardium

Inflammatory mediators have important biological effects on the heart and are key regulators of cardiomyocyte contractile dysfunction, cardiomyocyte cell death, adverse left ventricular (LV) remodeling, and myocardial fibrosis [70]. These effects have been demonstrated through genetic and pharmacological inhibition of DAMP receptors, inflammatory signaling pathways, and proinflammatory cytokines [42]. In addition, numerous cytokines have been observed to provoke cardiomyocyte contractile dysfunction in vitro and in vivo. TNF, IL-1β, IL-6, and IL-18 have profound negative inotropic effects on cardiomyocytes [70–72]. The effects of TNF and IL-1β are at least partially mediated through a nitric oxide-dependent pathway.

Chronic exposure to elevated cytokine signaling is sufficient to provoke a phenotype that closely mirrors heart failure. Transgenic overexpression of TNF is sufficient to mimic heart failure and results in a dose-dependent reduction in LV contractile function [73]. In addition, chronic administration of TNF to dogs led to the development of progressive LV remodeling and dilation through activation of matrix metalloproteases and collagen degradation [74,75]. Similarly, chronic exposure to IL-1β results in acute and progressive contractile dysfunction and LV remodeling [76]. Inhibition of IL-1β abrogates impairments in contractile dysfunction following myocardial infarction [77,78].

Effects on the Vasculature

Inflammatory cytokines have important and profound effects on the peripheral vasculature and are central mediators of endothelial cell dysfunction. Chronic inflammation results in reduced nitric oxide activity and impaired vasodilatory responses. These effects contribute to the increase in systemic vascular resistance present in patients with chronic heart failure [79]. TNF and other cytokines impair eNOS levels (essential enzyme for NO production) through reductions in eNOS mRNA expression and stability [80]. In addition, cytokine activity increases free radical levels and shortens NO half-life as a result of reduces superoxide dismutase expression [81].

Effects on Peripheral Tissues

Heart failure is a systemic syndrome with profound effects on multiple peripheral tissues; the best described being skeletal muscle [82]. Several clinical studies have convincingly demonstrated that impaired skeletal muscle physiology and function are largely responsible for exercise intolerance in patients with chronic systolic heart failure. Clinically, cachexia and skeletal muscle atrophy represent important comorbidities associated with poor prognosis [83]. Within the chronic heart failure population, skeletal muscle atrophy and intrinsic reductions in oxidative metabolism are tightly associated with reduced exercise capacity [84]. Patients with chronic heart failure not only have smaller peripheral muscle mass but also display reduced oxidative metabolism during exercise. Moreover, measurement of skeletal muscle lactate production during exercise demonstrated metabolic abnormalities in patients with chronic heart failure independent of tissue perfusion. Consistent with this, skeletal mitochondria density is reduced in patients with chronic heart failure; and the extent of mitochondrial loss correlates with peak exercise capacity [85,86].

Intriguingly, the pathology of heart failure-associated skeletal muscle myopathy closely resembles what has been observed in myopathies due to chronic inflammatory conditions, such as Crohn's disease. Examination of muscle biopsies obtained from patients with Crohn's disease revealed fiber atrophy, myocyte apoptosis, reduced type I fibers, increased type II fibers, and increased numbers of inflammatory cells. These findings were associated with elevated levels of the proinflammatory cytokines TNF, sphingosine, and LPS [1]. As numerous clinical studies have shown, patients with systolic heart failure also have elevated serum levels of proinflammatory cytokines including TNF, IL-1β, IL-6, and IL-2 [2–5]. These findings highlight a potentially shared pathogenesis of skeletal muscle atrophy in Crohn's disease and chronic systolic heart failure and implicate systemic and/or local inflammation as a potential causative mechanism in heart failure-associated skeletal muscle myopathy.

Indeed, cytokine signaling is sufficient to trigger skeletal myocyte injury, generation of reactive oxygen intermediates, and muscle atrophy [87,88]. IL-6 signaling via STAT3 has been reported to regulate myostatin, an important mediator of skeletal muscle catabolism [89]. In addition, muscle-specific TNF signaling through NF-kB results in a severe muscle wasting phenotype that is mediated by the ubiquitin ligase MuRF1 and suppression of IGF1 signaling [90,91]. The TNFSF member, TWEAK (TNF-like weak inducer of apoptosis), induces a similar phenotype by binding to the Fn14 receptor and activating NF-kB signaling [92].

Patients with heart failure also have reduced levels of circulating factors that are protective toward skeletal muscle, the most notable of which is IGF1 [93,94]. Serum IGF1 levels are inversely associated with LV systolic dysfunction, neurohormonal activation, cytokine production, and muscle atrophy [95–97]. IGF1 is expressed by multiple tissues in the body including liver, skeletal, and cardiac muscle. The exact mechanism by which systemic IGF1 is reduced in heart failure is not well defined. However, elevated angiotensin II activity may play an important role [69]. IGF1 signaling represents a well-established mechanism to stimulate muscle growth and regeneration [98]. IGF transgenic mice are resistant to angiotensin II and heart failure-induced muscle atrophy and local IGF1 treatment can reverse disuse atrophy [99–101]. These protective properties of IGF1 signaling are mediated through an AKT1, mTOR, and FoxO axis supporting cell survival, myofibril growth, and protein synthesis, while inhibiting protein degradation [94]. Importantly, IGF1 also possess significant immunomodulatory activity. Specifically, IGF1 is a robust inhibitor of proinflammatory responses through IL-10 dependent suppression of monocyte activation [102].

CLINICAL TRIALS OF IMMUNOMODULATION

In addition to providing information about patient prognosis, the measurement of inflammatory biomarkers in patients with heart failure may signify that inflammation could be a therapeutic target and identify subsets of patients most likely to benefit from this approach. In support of this concept, several small clinical trials have documented beneficial effects of nonselective and targeted antiinflammatory agents.

The first study to demonstrate that patients with dilated cardiomyopathy benefit from antiinflammatory therapies randomized 102 patients to placebo or 60mg/day of prednisone. Steroid therapy is thought to block cytokine synthesis at the transcriptional and translational level. Three months after therapy patients who received prednisone showed a modest improvement in LV systolic function. Interestingly, this effect was most evident in patients who displayed signs of ongoing myocardial inflammation as evidence by myocardial immune cell infiltration or immunoglobulin deposition on endomyocardial biopsy, positive gallium scan, or elevated erythrocyte sedimentation rate [103].

Other nonselective antiinflammatory agents investigated in heart failure include methotrexate and intravenous immunoglobulin (IVIg). Methotrexate was evaluated in a prospective clinical trial that randomized 71 patients to placebo or 7.5 mg of methotrexate administered on a weekly basis [104]. Patients receiving methotrexate had significant reductions in circulating levels of inflammatory mediators (TNF, IL-6, MCP1) and increased levels of antiinflammatory mediators (IL-10, soluble IL1 receptor antagonist). While methotrexate had no effect on LV function or remodeling at 12 weeks, patients receiving methotrexate reported improved heart failure symptoms documented by NYHA functional class, quality of life, and 6 min walk test. The clinical efficacy of methotrexate as a cardiovascular therapeutic is currently being tested in the Cardiovascular Inflammation Reduction Trial (CIRT; NCT1594333). IVIg is used in multiple autoimmune pathologies. In a small randomized trial of 20 ischemic and nonischemic heart failure patients, administration of IVIg resulted in a modest increase in LV ejection fraction and improved NYHA functional class compared to placebo. This was accompanied by a reduction in circulating TNF and increased levels of IL-10 and soluble IL-1 receptor antagonist (sIL-1Ra) [105]. Together these small studies formed the basis for further clinical investigation of antiinflammatory agents targeted against specific cytokines, most notably IL-1β and TNF signaling pathways.

IL-1 Signaling Inhibition

Anakinra (Kineret) is a recombinant version of sIL-1Ra that is approved for the treatment of rheumatoid arthritis. This agent functions by binding IL-1α and IL-1β and reducing ligand availability for the endogenous IL-1 receptor. The potential benefits of IL-1 receptor blockade in heart failure are supported by preclinical studies showing that administration of Anakinra reduces adverse remodeling in a mouse model of ischemic cardiomyopathy [43,77,78,106–108]. Currently, IL-1 receptor antagonists are under clinical investigation as novel therapeutics for adults with acute myocardial and chronic heart failure. Early results have indicated that although Anakinra did not prevent adverse remodeling in a small randomized clinical trial of patients with acute myocardial infarction [69], 2 small clinical trials demonstrated that Anakinra improves exercise capacity in patients with chronic heart failure [70,109]. Larger future studies will ultimately be required to determine of IL-1 receptor blockade represents a viable therapeutic target for adult heart failure.

Tumor Necrosis Factor Blockade

Two classes of therapeutics have been developed to block TNF signaling: decoy receptors and antibodies that neutralize circulating TNF. Etanercept (Enbrel) is a genetically engineered protein consisting of the human TNF receptor 2 fused in duplicate to the Fc portion of human IgG1. Etanercept functions by binding and sequestering TNF thereby competing with endogenous TNF receptors and reducing TNF signaling. Etanercept is approved for the treatment of ankylosing spondylitis, juvenile rheumatoid arthritis, psoriasis, psoriatic arthritis, and rheumatoid arthritis. The potential utility of TNF blockade in the treatment of heart failure was first documented by two early clinical trials revealing that etanercept improved quality of life, 6 min walking distance, and LV systolic performance following 3 months of treatment [70]. These results provided the basis for 2 multicenter trials (RENAISSANCE and RECOVER) examining the efficacy of etanercept in chronic heart failure Fig. 3.2. The primary endpoint of both trials was a clinical composite score that classified patients as improved,

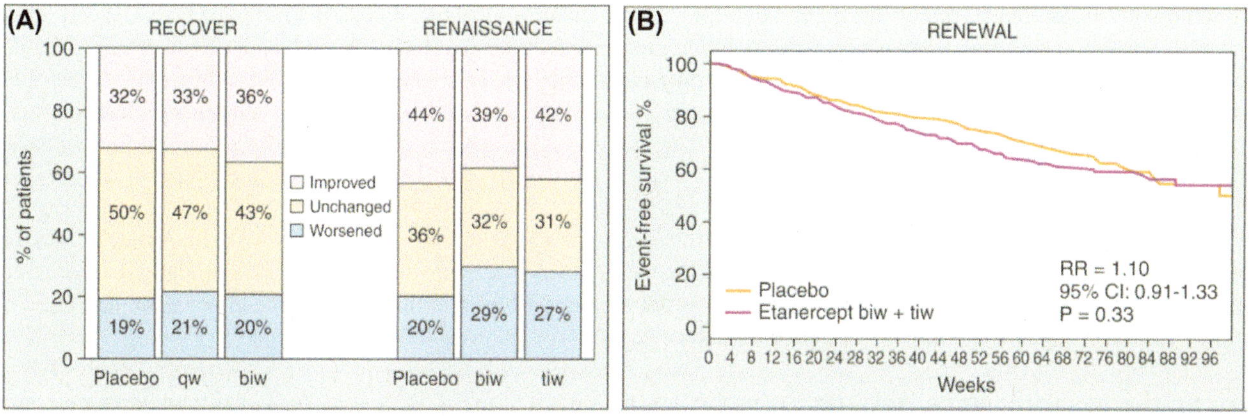

FIGURE 3.2 Results of the RENAISSANCE, RECOVER, and RENEWAL trials. (A) Analysis of the "clinical status" composite score for the RECOVER and RENAISSANCE trials in the placebo and etanercept groups. (B) Kaplan–Meier analysis of the time to death or heart failure hospitalizations in the placebo and etanercept group (biw and tiw) in the RENEWAL analysis. *(From D.L. Mann, J.J.V. McMurray, M. Packer, et al., Targeted anti-cytokine therapy in patients with chronic heart failure: results of the Randomized EtaNcercept Worldwide evALuation (RENEWAL), Circulation 109 (2004) 1594–1602; Reproduced with permission D.L. Mann, Activation of inflammatory mediators in heart failure. in: D.L. Mann (Ed.), Heart failure: A companion to Braunwald's heart disease, Second ed., Elsevier/Saunders, Philadelphia, 2011, p. 163–84.)*

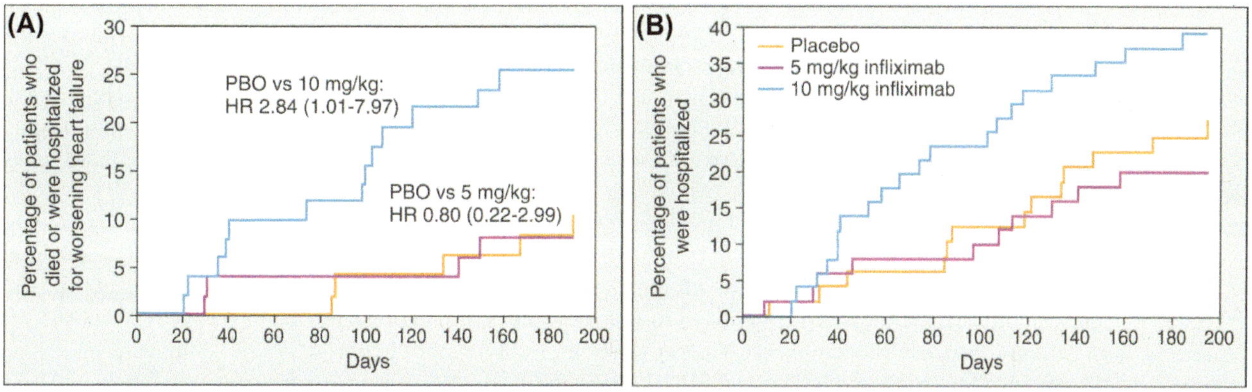

FIGURE 3.3 Results of the ATTACH trial. (A) Kaplan–Meier rates of death and hospitalization for heart failure. (B) Kaplan–Meier rates of hospitalization for any reason. *HR*, hazard ratio; *PBO*, placebo. *(From E.S. Chung, M. Packer, K.H. Lo, et al., Randomized, double-blind, placebo-controlled, pilot trial of infliximab, a chimeric monoclonal antibody to tumor necrosis factor-α, in patients with moderate-to-severe heart failure: results of the anti-TNF therapy against congestive heart failure (ATTACH) trial, Circulation 107 (2003) 3133–3140; Reproduced with permission D.L. Mann, Activation of inflammatory mediators in heart failure. in: D.L. Mann (Ed.), Heart failure: A companion to Braunwald's heart disease, Second ed., Elsevier/Saunders, Philadelphia, 2011, p. 163–84.)*

unchanged, or worsened after 24 weeks of treatment. RENAISSANCE and RECOVER each randomized 900 patients to either placebo or etanercept. Both studies were terminated prematurely due to lack of benefit of etanercept with respect to the primary endpoint. A third study (RENEWAL, n = 1500), used pool data from RENAISSANCE and RECOVER and determined that etanercept did not reduce the incidence of death or heart failure hospitalizations [110]. Importantly, post hoc analysis of the RENAISSANCE trial revealed that patients receiving etanercept were more likely to be categorized as having worsened heart failure compared to placebo and showed trends toward increased risk of death and heart failure hospitalizations. These findings were not evident in the RECOVER trial, which used a lower dose of etanercept. Infliximab (Remicade) is a chimeric monoclonal antibody consisting of a murine anti-TNF Fab fragment fused to the Fc portion of human IgG1 and is approved for the treatment of Crohn's disease, ulcerative colitis, psoriasis, psoriatic arthritis, ankylosing spondylitis, and rheumatoid arthritis. The efficacy of infliximab in chronic heart failure was evaluated in the phase II ATTACH trial, which randomized 150 patients with moderate to advanced heart failure to placebo or infliximab [13]. The primary endpoint consisted of the same clinical composite score used in RENAISSANCE and RECOVER. Patients receiving infliximab failed to demonstrate improved heart failure classification. Strikingly, patients receiving the highest doses of infliximab displayed increased rates of mortality and heart failure hospitalization (Fig. 3.3). As a result of these studies, the prescribing information for both etanercept and infliximab was updated to state that TNF blockade should be discontinued in individuals with symptoms of worsening heart failure and not used in patients previously diagnosed with heart failure.

While it is difficult to accurately decipher why TNF blockade may worsen outcomes for adult patients with heart failure, several plausible mechanisms have been proposed. With respect to etanercept, previous studies have suggested that TNF receptor antagonists may have intrinsic biological activity in that they stabilize TNF and increase its bioactivity, thus acting as stimulating antagonists [111]. Others have suggested that infliximab may bind to TNF located on the sarcolemma of failing cardiomyocytes and trigger complement-dependent cytolysis [112]. Consistent with ongoing myocardial injury and inflammation, patients receiving infliximab display increased serum CRP and IL-6 levels over the course of the ATTACH study. Alternatively, it is possible that TNF may have beneficially roles in the failing heart. In support of this scenario, TNF ligands have been shown to be important mediators of tissue repair across several model systems [113]. As such, it is likely that characterizing inflammation as a maladaptive response to tissue injury or disease is overly simplistic. Indeed, future studies are underway to delineate the mechanistic basis for why anti-TNF cytokine therapy proved not to be an efficacious strategy and to identify more refined therapeutic targets.

DIFFERENCES BETWEEN THE PEDIATRIC AND ADULT HEART AND IMMUNE SYSTEM

In the following sections, we will discuss differences between the pediatric and adult immune system and describe recently identified complexities within the innate immune system that account for why immune responses have both adverse and beneficial effects on the heart. Furthermore, we will expand on the concept that innate immunity is a critical and targetable mechanism to prevent disease progression and promote recovery of the failing heart, particularly in the pediatric population.

Important differences exist between the pediatric and adult immune system. In general, neonates and young children demonstrate increased susceptibility to bacterial and viral pathogens. The prevailing theory is that immaturity of the immune system in children renders them susceptible to infection. For example, HIV infection in young children results in rapid progression of disease compared to adults and is associated with impaired cellular and humeral immunity [114,115]. Studies in neonatal animal models (generally within the first week of life) have revealed impairments in adaptive immunity, specifically defective CD4 T cell responses. Neonatal animals also have fewer T-cells, delayed antibody production, and, in some cases, defective CD8+ cytotoxic lymphocyte responses [116]. The underlying mechanisms explaining these impairments are unknown.

Substantially less is known regarding the role of innate immunity in neonates and children. Monocytes and macrophages derived from neonatal mice and humans demonstrate blunted responses to TLR stimulation including impaired cytokine and type I interferon production [117,118]. Consistent with impaired innate immune responses in animal models, critically ill children infected with influenza A virus display blunted responses to TLR stimulation ex vivo [119]. The mechanistic basis explaining why pediatric and adult macrophages display differing inflammatory behavior is not completely understood. However, details are emerging supporting the possibility that pediatric and adult macrophages represent distinct cell types.

Macrophages

Within the heart, macrophages represent the most abundant resident innate immune cell and harbor an array of PRRs poised to recognize the release of an array of DAMPs. Macrophages are evolutionary conserved mononuclear phagocytes that were first discovered late in the 19th century by Ilya Metchnikoff [15,94]. In addition to engulfing pathogens, foreign bodies, and cell debris through phagocytosis, macrophages essentially function as gate keepers of the immune system. Macrophages are found in nearly all organs throughout the body and take on tissue-specific morphologies and functions. Examples include Kupffer cells (liver), alveolar macrophages (lung), microglia (brain), Langerhans cells (skin), osteoclasts (bone), and histiocytic (lymph nodes). Within these tissues, macrophages patrol for the presence of pathogens and sterile tissue injury through use of PRRs. On activation, macrophages trigger innate immune responses by secreting inflammatory cytokines and chemoattractants for monocytes and neutrophils (chemokines). Macrophages can also act as antigen-presenting cells and stimulate adaptive immune responses. Beyond stimulating innate and adaptive immune responses, macrophages can also have a reparative role where they function to limit inflammation and organize tissue repair and regeneration (discussed below) [120–123]. Other functions of macrophages include iron homeostasis, neural network maturation, and vascular remodeling [124–127].

Macrophage Diversity

In the 1960s, Van Furth proposed that tissue macrophages originated from circulating blood monocytes, which has been the prevailing view for the last 40 years. However, evolving evidence has challenged this dogma and has provided definitive evidence that numerous population of tissue macrophages exist independent of circulating monocytes [128–130]. A recent series of studies performed in model systems have drastically revised our understanding of macrophage origins.

Collectively, these publications demonstrated that many tissue resident macrophages are established during embryonic development and persist into adulthood independent of blood monocyte input [131–137]. This advancement in knowledge was dependent on the development and utilization of sophisticated genetic lineage tracing and monocyte-tracking strategies. Several detailed review articles have seen been published describing different aspects of macrophage ontogeny and related functions [138–140]. In the following section, we will describe the currently available knowledge regarding cardiac macrophage subsets, origins, and potential functions in the context of heart failure.

In the mouse, macrophages originating from embryonic and adult hematopoietic progenitors can be readily distinguished through genetic lineage tracing. Adult monocyte-derived macrophages are derived from definitive hematopoietic stem cells, which express FLT3 as they differentiate. Based on this finding, a Flt3-Cre mouse was developed to track the progeny of adult definitive hematopoietic stem cells [141]. Using this genetic lineage tracing tool, several studies have identified embryonic-derived (Flt3-Cre negative) and adult monocyte-derived (Flt3-Cre positive) macrophages in a variety of tissues including the brain, heart, lung, kidney, liver, and skin [142,143]. Macrophages of embryonic and adult hematopoietic origin may coexist within tissues. Intriguingly, in the context of aging, adult monocyte-derived macrophages increase in number and progressively replace embryonic-derived macrophages in some tissues including the heart [144]. Furthermore, detailed studies have better refined the composition of embryonic-derived macrophages suggesting that this population consists of a compellation of two lineages derived from progenitors located within the early yolk sac and those that migrate from the yolk sac to the fetal liver at later developmental stages [135].

Embryonic-derived macrophages are first observed during early gestation (embryonic day 6.5–8.5 in the mouse) in the extra-embryonic yolk sac where they arise from an early bipotent erythromyeloid progenitor. At this early stage of development, the yolk sac supports primitive hematopoiesis producing erythrocytes and yolk sac-derived macrophages [145]. In the mouse, primitive hematopoiesis can be distinguished from definitive hematopoiesis based on the requirement for the transcription factor MYB. $Myb^{-/-}$ embryos have a selective deficiency in definitive hematopoietic stems and are unable to support the development of definitive hematopoietic progeny (lymphocytes, granulocytes, monocytes, and megakaryocytes); however, their ability to produce early erythrocytes and yolk sac-derived macrophages is not perturbed [132]. Yolk sac-derived macrophages give rise to adult brain microglia, a subset of cardiac macrophages, and a transient population of skin Langerhans's cells [131–135,146].

Definitive hematopoietic stem cells emerge at later stages of embryonic development (embryonic day 8.5–10.5 in the mouse) from the aorta–gonads–mesonephros, hemogenic endothelium, and yolk sac giving rise to definitive fetal immune lineages. Hematopoietic stem cells migrate to the fetal liver, which then serves as the major hematopoietic organ during the remainder of embryonic development [131,147]. During this period, fetal monocytes emigrating from the liver take residence within multiple developing organs and likely constitute the primary origin of the majority of tissue resident embryonic-derived macrophages [142,143] located within the skin, liver, kidney, and lung [136,137,143]. Fetal liver monocytes contribute to a population of cardiac macrophages located within the endocardial trabeculae of the embryonic heart [135].

During the perinatal period, definitive hematopoietic stem cells take residence within the bone marrow where they establish the primary site of hematopoiesis for the remainder of life. Within this compartment, Flt3-Cre positive definitive hematopoietic stem cells produce the full complement of immune lineages including adult monocyte-derived macrophages [148]. Adult monocytes arise from definitive hematopoietic stem cells through a well-characterized cascade involving the progressive differentiation of committed progenitor cells including the monocyte–macrophage dendritic cell progenitor and $Ly6C^{+}$ monocyte-specific progenitor [149,150]. In the mouse and human there appear to be two principle monocyte subsets: classical $Ly6C^{high}$ monocytes and nonclassical $Ly6C^{low}$ monocytes [151]. $Ly6C^{high}$ monocytes are direct descendants of the Ly6C positive monocyte progenitor and give rise to adult monocyte-derived macrophages located within the heart and other tissues [137,142]. Nonclassical $Ly6C^{low}$ monocytes differentiate from $Ly6C^{high}$ monocytes through an Nr4a1-dependent transcriptional program [133,150,152]. Within the vasculature, nonclassical $Ly6C^{low}$ monocytes crawl over the endothelium in a LFA-1 integrin-dependent manner where they clear damaged endothelial cells and maintaining vascular integrity [153]. While some have considered these monocytes to be "vascular macrophages," they transcriptionally cluster with monocytes and do not express core macrophage transcripts, including Mer tyrosine kinase [137,154].

Functions of Embryonic and Adult Macrophages in the Heart and Periphery

Macrophage Heterogeneity in the Failing Heart

There are numerous examples of seemingly contradictory reports claiming that inflammation is both harmful following tissue injury and an essential mediator of tissue repair [155]. This paradox is well established in models of ischemic cardiac injury. Macrophages within the infarcted heart not only drive robust inflammatory responses and pathological remodeling but

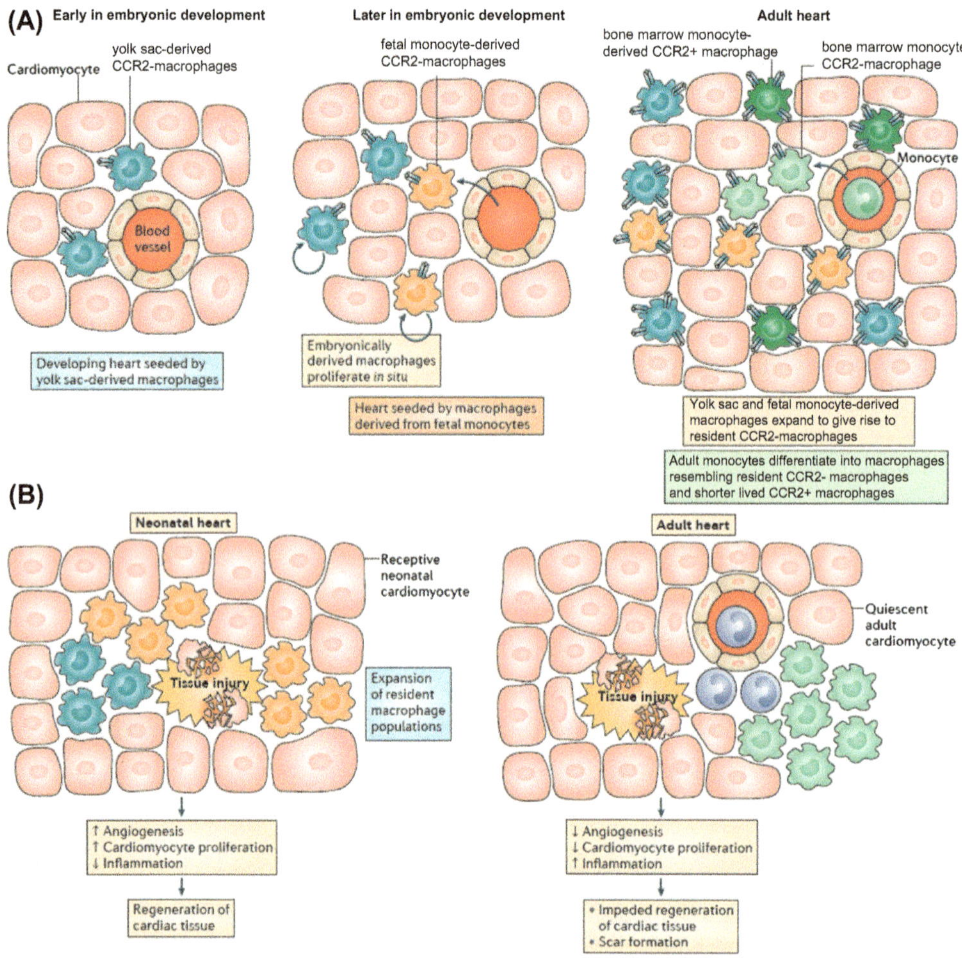

FIGURE 3.4 Macrophage diversity in the pediatric and adult heart. (A) During embryonic development, yolk sac-derived macrophages (shown in blue) initially seed the developing heart. These cells are CCR2⁻ and are derived from primitive hematopoiesis. Later during heart development, fetal monocyte-derived macrophages (shown in orange) originating from definitive hematopoiesis infiltrate the heart. These cells are also CCR2⁻ and together with yolk sac-derived macrophages expand through local proliferation. Yolk sac and fetal monocyte-derived macrophages give rise to resident CCR2⁻ macrophages present in the adult heart. In addition to these populations, the adult heart also contains macrophage populations that are derived from infiltrating monocytes derived from the bone marrow. Within this context, monocytes can differentiate into CCR2⁻ macrophages that resemble embryonic-derived subsets (light green) as well as a separate population of CCR2⁺ macrophages (dark green). Thus the adult heart contains an ontologically mixed population of macrophages. (B) The figure shows a comparison of the macrophage response to tissue injury in the neonatal and adult heart. In the neonate, embryonic-derived CCR2⁻ macrophages recognize injured cardiomyocytes, expand by local proliferation, and generate minimal inflammation and, instead, promote myocardial regeneration and tissue repair through coronary angiogenesis and myocardial proliferation. Following cardiac injury in the adult heart, there is a marked expansion of CCR2⁺ monocytes and macrophages. Importantly, CCR2⁺ macrophages possess a limited ability to stimulate tissue repair and, instead, generate robust inflammatory responses that ultimately lead to collateral tissue injury and impede tissue regeneration. Notably, the neonatal myocardium harbors a greater capacity for regeneration compared to the adult myocardium, as neonatal cardiomyocytes have greater potential for cardiomyocyte proliferation compared to adult cardiomyocytes. *(Adapted from S. Epelman, P. Liu, D.L. Mann, Nat. Rev. 15 (2015) 117–129.)*

also are required for the resolution of inflammation, tissue repair, and coronary angiogenesis [156]. One explanation for these findings is that distinct macrophage populations may mediate inflammatory (M1-like) and reparative (M2-like) macrophage behaviors [157]. Until recently, the exact identities of these proposed macrophage subsets have remained largely undefined.

Recently, we have demonstrated that distinct resident and recruited macrophages subsets derived from embryonic and definitive monocyte progenitors, respectively, govern tissue repair and inflammation in the context of acute heart failure [123] (Fig. 3.4). Under steady-state conditions, the heart contains several distinct resident macrophage populations that can be distinguished based on a combination of lineage tracing and cell surface expression of C-C chemokine receptor 2 (CCR2). By employing genetic lineage tracing using Flt3-Cre as a marker of the definitive hematopoietic lineage [141], we demonstrated that under steady-state conditions the mouse heart contains distinct populations of resident $CCR2^-$ and $CCR2^+$ macrophages. Resident $CCR2^-$ macrophages are derived from primitive yolk sac and definitive fetal monocyte progenitors that establish residency within the heart during embryonic and early postnatal development, respectively. These populations are maintained throughout adulthood independent of blood monocyte input [135]. Resident CCR2$^+$ macrophages are derived from definitive hematopoietic progenitors, enter the heart after the first week of life, and are maintained through a combination of local proliferation and gradual monocyte recruitment [135].

Resident CCR2$^-$ macrophages are critical regulators of coronary development, vascular expansion, and cardiac tissue repair [123,158]. In a model of acute pediatric heart failure, embryonic-derived CCR2$^-$ macrophages function to orchestrate tissue repair and functional recovery of the heart. Following pediatric cardiac injury, CCR2$^-$ macrophages expanded locally and home to sites of tissue injury. These cells produce minimal inflammation and, instead, promote myocardial regeneration through production of growth factors that stimulate angiogenesis, cardiomyocyte proliferation, and physiologic cardiac growth. In the absence of these cells, the pediatric mouse heart is unable to regenerate and, instead, undergoes adverse remodeling and ultimately progresses to end-staged heart failure.

In contrast to the pediatric heart, a dramatic shift in macrophage composition and ontogeny occurs in the setting of adult cardiac injury. In this context, monocytes infiltrate the myocardium, replace resident cardiac macrophage subsets, and differentiate into inflammatory monocyte-derived macrophages that lack the capacity to stimulate tissue repair. Instead, these cells generate robust quantities of inflammatory chemokines and cytokines, recruit neutrophils and additional monocytes, and ultimately contribute to the development and progression of cardiac dysfunction through resultant collateral tissue damage and adverse remodeling [123].

While the exact functions of CCR2$^+$ macrophages resident within the adult heart under steady-state conditions is incompletely defined, it is likely that activation of these cells represents a proximate mechanism driving inflammation in the failing adult heart. This concept is supported by the observation that resident CCR2$^+$ macrophages regulate neutrophil infiltration into the myocardium following ischemia reperfusion injury. Mechanistically, resident CCR2$^+$ macrophages are activated by mitochondrial DNA (presumably released from dying cardiomyocytes) through a TLR9-dependent signaling pathway that results in the release of the neutrophil chemokines, CXCL2 and CXCL5 [159]. Whether resident CCR2$^+$ macrophages similarly govern monocyte recruitment and macrophage ontogeny shifts through a similar molecular pathway is not yet clear, but represents an attractive hypothesis. Collectively, these findings have contributed to a new paradigm in macrophage biology and brought to light that distinct macrophage lineages/subsets have specific functions.

Macrophage Heterogeneity in Peripheral Tissues

Conceptually, it is unclear how these observations might apply to peripheral tissues in the context of chronic heart failure. For instance, do resident embryonic and recruited adult macrophages differentially contribute to end organ tissue repair and inflammatory responses, respectively? In support of this concept, monocyte-derived proinflammatory M1-like macrophages infiltrate injured skeletal muscle and secrete an array of inflammatory chemokines and cytokines including MCP1, IL1β, and TNF [160]. Each of these factors is sufficient to drive inflammation through recruitment of additional proinflammatory monocytes and collateral tissue injury. In addition, IL1β and TNF signaling to skeletal myocytes contribute to skeletal muscle atrophy and catabolism through reductions in oxidative metabolism and IGF1 signaling [64,91,161]. Furthermore, proinflammatory macrophages inhibit regeneration as persistence of these cells leads to ongoing damage and defective tissue healing [162–164]. Examination of a chronic model of skeletal muscle injury (i.e., muscular dystrophy) revealed the existence of proinflammatory M1-like and reparative alternatively activated "M2-like" macrophages [165–167], supporting the possibility that distinct macrophage subsets may also govern inflammation and regeneration in chronic skeletal muscle pathologies. M2-like skeletal muscle macrophages are required for skeletal muscle regeneration following cardiotoxin injury through augmentation of satellite cell proliferation and angiogenesis [160,168]. How these M2-like macrophages compare to embryonic-derived macrophages resident in cardiac muscle remains to be studied.

IMPLICATIONS FOR PEDIATRIC HEART FAILURE

Perhaps the most obvious distinction between pediatric and adult heart failure is the repeated observation that antiremodeling medications routinely used to treat adult heart failure patients do not significantly improve outcomes in children. The Pediatric Carvedilol Trial failed to demonstrate significant improvements in either clinical outcomes or echocardiographic parameters in children with dilated cardiomyopathy [169]. In addition, registry data revealed that children with dilated cardiomyopathy treated with ACE inhibitors or β-blockers had indistinguishable survival compared to those only receiving digoxin- and diuretic-based regimens [170,171]. One explanation for these findings is that remodeling is not a critical component of pediatric heart failure. This notion is consistent with prior studies showing that hallmarks of adverse remodeling including β-adrenergic receptor downregulation and fetal gene expression occur to a lesser extent in pediatric dilated cardiomyopathy [172]. These observations raise the question of what distinct disease mechanisms drive heart failure progression in children. In adult patients with ischemic and dilated cardiomyopathies, it is clear that inflammation contributes to heart failure initiation and progression [38,173]. Whether the failing pediatric heart follows a similar paradigm is unclear at this time. Future studies clarifying these mechanisms will be essential to guide effective therapeutic strategies for children with heart failure.

The capacity to recover cardiac function (i.e., cardiac recovery), represents an equally important difference between pediatric and adult heart failure. Approximately 20% of children diagnosed with pediatric dilated cardiomyopathy will spontaneously and completely recover LV systolic function over a 2 year follow-up period [174]. In contrast, cardiac recovery is a relatively infrequent outcome in the adult patients with chronic heart failure [175,176]. Indeed, in a recent study <15% of adult patients with dilated cardiomyopathy had complete recovery of function despite being placed on optimal medical management [177,178].

The observation that cardiac recovery occurs spontaneously in the pediatric population was further demonstrated in the Pediatric Carvedilol Study where children in both the placebo and carvedilol groups displayed improved LV systolic function through the course of the study [169]. These observations suggest that cardiac recovery represents an achievable outcome and a potential target for pediatric heart failure therapeutics. Consistent with this concept, previous reports have indicated that patients who experience cardiac recovery have improved quality of life and long-term survival [179].

The underlying mechanisms that dictate cardiac recovery and explain why children have a greater capacity for cardiac recovery compared to adults are poorly defined. Indeed, we and others have previously demonstrated that cardiac recovery can easily be reproduced in mouse models of acute pediatric heart failure. Within each of these models, embryonic-derived macrophages act as essential regulators of cardiac recovery, suppress inflammation and adverse remodeling, and orchestrate tissue repair through myocardial regeneration and expansion of the coronary vasculature [120,122]. In the absence of embryonic-derived macrophages, the failing pediatric heart acquires a phenotype reminiscent of the failing adult heart. Importantly, it has also been demonstrated that children have a greater capacity for cardiomyocyte proliferation compared to adults, suggestion that children possess an appropriate substrate for regeneration [180].

These findings have important implications for the treatment of pediatric heart failure. Few studies have investigated the relevance of inflammation in pediatric heart failure, and it is unclear if inflammation represents a prominent pathological mechanism driving the pathogenesis of pediatric heart failure. As such, it is equally unclear whether antiinflammatory therapeutics would be appropriate for children with heart failure. Furthermore, the observation that embryonic-derived macrophages govern tissue repair and recovery of the failing neonatal mouse heart suggests that innate immune cell activation is beneficial in the context of pediatric heart failure. Future studies investigating the molecular mechanisms by which these cells are activated and exert their effects will likely provide critical insights into whether therapeutics that modulate embryonic macrophage function could be used as a therapeutic approach to stimulate cardiac recovery in children with heart failure.

REFERENCES

[1] L. Cuoco, G. Vescovo, R. Castaman, B. Ravara, G. Cammarota, A. Angelini, et al., Skeletal muscle wastage in Crohn's disease: a pathway shared with heart failure? Int. J. Cardiol. 127 (2) (July 4, 2008) 219–227.

[2] A. Deswal, N.J. Petersen, A.M. Feldman, J.B. Young, B.G. White, D.L. Mann, Cytokines and cytokine receptors in advanced heart failure: an analysis of the cytokine database from the Vesnarinone trial (VEST), Circulation 103 (16) (April 24, 2001) 2055–2059.

[3] G. Torre-Amione, S. Kapadia, C. Benedict, H. Oral, J.B. Young, D.L. Mann, Proinflammatory cytokine levels in patients with depressed left ventricular ejection fraction: a report from the Studies of Left Ventricular Dysfunction (SOLVD), J. Am. Coll. Cardiol. 27 (5) (April 1996) 1201–1206.

[4] R. Ferrari, T. Bachetti, R. Confortini, C. Opasich, O. Febo, A. Corti, et al., Tumor necrosis factor soluble receptors in patients with various degrees of congestive heart failure, Circulation 92 (6) (September 15, 1995) 1479–1486.

[5] M. Rauchhaus, W. Doehner, D.P. Francis, C. Davos, M. Kemp, C. Liebenthal, et al., Plasma cytokine parameters and mortality in patients with chronic heart failure, Circulation 102 (25) (December 19, 2000) 3060–3067.

[6] B. Levine, J. Kalman, L. Mayer, H.M. Fillit, M. Packer, Elevated circulating levels of tumor necrosis factor in severe chronic heart failure, N. Engl. J. Med. 323 (4) (July 26, 1990) 236–241.

[7] R.S. Vasan, L.M. Sullivan, R. Roubenoff, C.A. Dinarello, T. Harris, E.J. Benjamin, et al., Inflammatory markers and risk of heart failure in elderly subjects without prior myocardial infarction: the Framingham Heart Study, Circulation 107 (11) (March 25, 2003) 1486–1491.

[8] T. Tsutamoto, T. Hisanaga, A. Wada, K. Maeda, M. Ohnishi, D. Fukai, et al., Interleukin-6 spillover in the peripheral circulation increases with the severity of heart failure, and the high plasma level of interleukin-6 is an important prognostic predictor in patients with congestive heart failure, J. Am. Coll. Cardiol. 31 (2) (February 1998) 391–398.

[9] D.L. Mann, Innate immunity and the failing heart: the cytokine hypothesis revisited, Circ. Res. 116 (7) (March 27, 2015) 1254–1268.

[10] S.R. Kapadia, K. Yakoob, S. Nader, J.D. Thomas, D.L. Mann, B.P. Griffin, Elevated circulating levels of serum tumor necrosis factor-alpha in patients with hemodynamically significant pressure and volume overload, J. Am. Coll. Cardiol. 36 (1) (July 2000) 208–212.

[11] S.R. Kapadia, H. Oral, J. Lee, M. Nakano, G.E. Taffet, D.L. Mann, Hemodynamic regulation of tumor necrosis factor-alpha gene and protein expression in adult feline myocardium, Circ. Res. 81 (2) (August 1997) 187–195.

[12] L. Gullestad, T. Ueland, J.G. Fjeld, E. Holt, T. Gundersen, K. Breivik, et al., Effect of thalidomide on cardiac remodeling in chronic heart failure: results of a double-blind, placebo-controlled study, Circulation 112 (22) (November 29, 2005) 3408–3414.

[13] E.S. Chung, M. Packer, K.H. Lo, A.A. Fasanmade, J.T. Willerson, Randomized, double-blind, placebo-controlled, pilot trial of infliximab, a chimeric monoclonal antibody to tumor necrosis factor-alpha, in patients with moderate-to-severe heart failure: results of the anti-TNF therapy against congestive heart failure (ATTACH) trial, Circulation 107 (25) (July 1, 2003) 3133–3140.

[14] J. Niebauer, H.D. Volk, M. Kemp, M. Dominguez, R.R. Schumann, M. Rauchhaus, et al., Endotoxin and immune activation in chronic heart failure: a prospective cohort study, Lancet 353 (9167) (May 29, 1999) 1838–1842.

[15] S. Sanada, D. Hakuno, L.J. Higgins, E.R. Schreiter, A.N. McKenzie, R.T. Lee, IL-33 and ST2 comprise a critical biomechanically induced and cardioprotective signaling system, J. Clin. Investig. 117 (6) (June 2007) 1538–1549.

[16] E.O. Weinberg, M. Shimpo, G.W. De Keulenaer, C. MacGillivray, S. Tominaga, S.D. Solomon, et al., Expression and regulation of ST2, an interleukin-1 receptor family member, in cardiomyocytes and myocardial infarction, Circulation 106 (23) (December 3, 2002) 2961–2966.

[17] J. Schmitz, A. Owyang, E. Oldham, Y. Song, E. Murphy, T.K. McClanahan, et al., IL-33, an interleukin-1-like cytokine that signals via the IL-1 receptor-related protein ST2 and induces T helper type 2-associated cytokines, Immunity 23 (5) (November 2005) 479–490.

[18] S.U. Rehman, T. Mueller, J.L. Januzzi Jr., Characteristics of the novel interleukin family biomarker ST2 in patients with acute heart failure, J. Am. Coll. Cardiol. 52 (18) (October 28, 2008) 1458–1465.

[19] E.O. Weinberg, M. Shimpo, S. Hurwitz, S. Tominaga, J.L. Rouleau, R.T. Lee, Identification of serum soluble ST2 receptor as a novel heart failure biomarker, Circulation 107 (5) (February 11, 2003) 721–726.

[20] B. Ky, B. French, K. McCloskey, J.E. Rame, E. McIntosh, P. Shahi, et al., High-sensitivity ST2 for prediction of adverse outcomes in chronic heart failure, Circ. Heart Fail. 4 (2) (March 2011) 180–187.

[21] R.A. Weir, A.M. Miller, G.E. Murphy, S. Clements, T. Steedman, J.M. Connell, et al., Serum soluble ST2: a potential novel mediator in left ventricular and infarct remodeling after acute myocardial infarction, J. Am. Coll. Cardiol. 55 (3) (January 19, 2010) 243–250.

[22] P. Kohli, M.P. Bonaca, R. Kakkar, A.Y. Kudinova, B.M. Scirica, M.S. Sabatine, et al., Role of ST2 in non-ST-elevation acute coronary syndrome in the MERLIN-TIMI 36 trial, Clin. Chem. 58 (1) (January 2012) 257–266.

[23] M.S. Sabatine, D.A. Morrow, L.J. Higgins, C. MacGillivray, W. Guo, C. Bode, et al., Complementary roles for biomarkers of biomechanical strain ST2 and N-terminal prohormone B-type natriuretic peptide in patients with ST-elevation myocardial infarction, Circulation 117 (15) (April 15, 2008) 1936–1944.

[24] J. Dumic, S. Dabelic, M. Flogel, Galectin-3: an open-ended story, Biochim. Biophys. Acta 1760 (4) (April 2006) 616–635.

[25] A.U. Newlaczyl, L.G. Yu, Galectin-3–a jack-of-all-trades in cancer, Cancer Lett. 313 (2) (December 27, 2011) 123–128.

[26] R.A. de Boer, A.A. Voors, P. Muntendam, W.H. van Gilst, D.J. van Veldhuisen, Galectin-3: a novel mediator of heart failure development and progression, Eur. J. Heart Fail. 11 (9) (September 2009) 811–817.

[27] N.C. Henderson, A.C. Mackinnon, S.L. Farnworth, F. Poirier, F.P. Russo, J.P. Iredale, et al., Galectin-3 regulates myofibroblast activation and hepatic fibrosis, Proc. Natl. Acad. Sci. U.S.A. 103 (13) (March 28, 2006) 5060–5065.

[28] L. Yu, W.P. Ruifrok, M. Meissner, E.M. Bos, G.H. van, B. Sanjabi, et al., Genetic and pharmacological inhibition of galectin-3 prevents cardiac remodeling by interfering with myocardial fibrogenesis, Circ. Heart Fail. 6 (1) (January 2013) 107–117.

[29] D.J. Lok, P. van der Meer, P.W. de la Porte, E. Lipsic, W.J. Van, H.L. Hillege, et al., Prognostic value of galectin-3, a novel marker of fibrosis, in patients with chronic heart failure: data from the DEAL-HF study, Clin. Res. Cardiol. 99 (5) (May 2010) 323–328.

[30] R.R. van Kimmenade, J.L. Januzzi Jr., P.T. Ellinor, U.C. Sharma, J.A. Bakker, A.F. Low, et al., Utility of amino-terminal pro-brain natriuretic peptide, galectin-3, and apelin for the evaluation of patients with acute heart failure, J. Am. Coll. Cardiol. 48 (6) (September 19, 2006) 1217–1224.

[31] R.V. Shah, A.A. Chen-Tournoux, M.H. Picard, R.R. van Kimmenade, J.L. Januzzi, Galectin-3, cardiac structure and function, and long-term mortality in patients with acutely decompensated heart failure, Eur. J. Heart Fail. 12 (8) (August 2010) 826–832.

[32] J.E. Ho, C. Liu, A. Lyass, P. Courchesne, M.J. Pencina, R.S. Vasan, et al., Galectin-3, a marker of cardiac fibrosis, predicts incident heart failure in the community, J. Am. Coll. Cardiol. 60 (14) (October 2, 2012) 1249–1256.

[33] I.R. Romero, C. Morris, M. Rodriguez, T.W. Du Clos, C. Mold, Inflammatory potential of C-reactive protein complexes compared to immune complexes, Clin. Immunol. Immunopathol. 87 (2) (May 1998) 155–162.

[34] P. Baruah, A. Propato, I.E. Dumitriu, P. Rovere-Querini, V. Russo, R. Fontana, et al., The pattern recognition receptor PTX3 is recruited at the synapse between dying and dendritic cells, and edits the cross-presentation of self, viral, and tumor antigens, Blood 107 (1) (January 1, 2006) 151–158.

[35] P. Rovere, G. Peri, F. Fazzini, B. Bottazzi, A. Doni, A. Bondanza, et al., The long pentraxin PTX3 binds to apoptotic cells and regulates their clearance by antigen-presenting dendritic cells, Blood 96 (13) (December 15, 2000) 4300–4306.

[36] C. Garlanda, B. Bottazzi, A. Bastone, A. Mantovani, Pentraxins at the crossroads between innate immunity, inflammation, matrix deposition, and female fertility, Annu. Rev. Immunol. 23 (2005) 337–366.

[37] R. Latini, L. Gullestad, S. Masson, S.H. Nymo, T. Ueland, I. Cuccovillo, et al., Pentraxin-3 in chronic heart failure: the CORONA and GISSI-HF trials, Eur. J. Heart Fail. 14 (9) (September 2012) 992–999.

[38] J. Hartupee, D.L. Mann, Neurohormonal activation in heart failure with reduced ejection fraction, Nat. Rev. Cardiol. 14 (1) (January 2017) 30–38.

[39] A. Briasoulis, E. Androulakis, T. Christophides, D. Tousoulis, The role of inflammation and cell death in the pathogenesis, progression and treatment of heart failure, Heart Fail. Rev. 21 (2) (March 2016) 169–176.

[40] J.K. Chan, J. Roth, J.J. Oppenheim, K.J. Tracey, T. Vogl, M. Feldmann, et al., Alarmins: awaiting a clinical response, J. Clin. Investig. 122 (8) (August 2012) 2711–2719.

[41] I.E. Muth, J. Zschuntzsch, K. Kleinschnitz, A. Wrede, E. Gerhardt, P. Balcarek, et al., HMGB1 and RAGE in skeletal muscle inflammation: implications for protein accumulation in inclusion body myositis, Exp. Neurol. 271 (September 2015) 189–197.
[42] D.L. Mann, V.K. Topkara, S. Evans, P.M. Barger, Innate immunity in the adult mammalian heart: for whom the cell tolls, Trans. Am. Clin. Climatol. Assoc. 121 (2010) 34–50.
[43] E. Mezzaroma, S. Toldo, D. Farkas, I.M. Seropian, B.W. Van Tassell, F.N. Salloum, et al., The inflammasome promotes adverse cardiac remodeling following acute myocardial infarction in the mouse, Proc. Natl. Acad. Sci. U.S.A. 108 (49) (December 6, 2011) 19725–19730.
[44] V.K. Topkara, S. Evans, W. Zhang, S. Epelman, L. Staloch, P.M. Barger, et al., Therapeutic targeting of innate immunity in the failing heart, J. Mol. Cell. Cardiol. 51 (4) (October 2011) 594–599.
[45] E. Venereau, C. Ceriotti, M.E. Bianchi, DAMPs from cell death to new life, Front. Immunol. 6 (2015) 422.
[46] O. Takeuchi, S. Akira, Pattern recognition receptors and inflammation, Cell 140 (6) (March 19, 2010) 805–820.
[47] A.M. Piccinini, K.S. Midwood, DAMPening inflammation by modulating TLR signalling, Mediators Inflamm. 2010 (2010).
[48] K. Geddes, J.G. Magalhaes, S.E. Girardin, Unleashing the therapeutic potential of NOD-like receptors, Nat. Rev. Drug Discov. 8 (6) (June 2009) 465–479.
[49] B. McDonald, K. Pittman, G.B. Menezes, S.A. Hirota, I. Slaba, C.C. Waterhouse, et al., Intravascular danger signals guide neutrophils to sites of sterile inflammation, Science 330 (6002) (October 15, 2010) 362–366.
[50] M. Nishimura, S. Naito, Tissue-specific mRNA expression profiles of human ATP-binding cassette and solute carrier transporter superfamilies, Drug Metab. Pharmacokinet. 20 (6) (December 2005) 452–477.
[51] E.J. Birks, L.E. Felkin, N.R. Banner, A. Khaghani, P.J. Barton, M.H. Yacoub, Increased toll-like receptor 4 in the myocardium of patients requiring left ventricular assist devices, J. Heart Lung Transplant. 23 (2) (February 2004) 228–235.
[52] S. Frantz, L. Kobzik, Y.D. Kim, R. Fukazawa, R. Medzhitov, R.T. Lee, et al., Toll4 (TLR4) expression in cardiac myocytes in normal and failing myocardium, J. Clin. Investig. 104 (3) (August 1999) 271–280.
[53] M. Kawaguchi, M. Takahashi, T. Hata, Y. Kashima, F. Usui, H. Morimoto, et al., Inflammasome activation of cardiac fibroblasts is essential for myocardial ischemia/reperfusion injury, Circulation 123 (6) (February 15, 2011) 594–604.
[54] M.J. Sullivan, J.D. Knight, M.B. Higginbotham, F.R. Cobb, Relation between central and peripheral hemodynamics during exercise in patients with chronic heart failure. Muscle blood flow is reduced with maintenance of arterial perfusion pressure, Circulation 80 (4) (October 1989) 769–781.
[55] I. Shiotani, H. Sato, H. Sato, H. Yokoyama, Y. Ohnishi, E. Hishida, et al., Muscle pump-dependent self-perfusion mechanism in legs in normal subjects and patients with heart failure, J. Appl. Physiol. 92 (4) (April 2002) 1647–1654 1985.
[56] R.J. Mentz, C.M. O'Connor, Pathophysiology and clinical evaluation of acute heart failure, Nat. Rev. Cardiol. 13 (1) (January 2016) 28–35.
[57] A.V. Bacurau, M.A. Jardim, J.C. Ferreira, L.R. Bechara, C.R. Bueno Jr., T.C. Alba-Loureiro, et al., Sympathetic hyperactivity differentially affects skeletal muscle mass in developing heart failure: role of exercise training, J. Appl. Physiol. 106 (5) (May 2009) 1631–1640 1985.
[58] V.A. Voltarelli, L.R. Bechara, A.V. Bacurau, K.C. Mattos, P.M. Dourado, C.R. Bueno Jr., et al., Lack of beta2-adrenoceptors aggravates heart failure-induced skeletal muscle myopathy in mice, J. Cell. Mol. Med. 18 (6) (June 2014) 1087–1097.
[59] M.J.N.N. Alves, M.R. dos Santos, T.S. Nobre, D.G. Martinez, A.C. Pereira Barretto, P.C. Brum, et al., Mechanisms of blunted muscle vasodilation during peripheral chemoreceptor stimulation in heart failure patients, Hypertension 60 (3) (September 2012) 669–676.
[60] G. Courties, F. Herisson, H.B. Sager, T. Heidt, Y. Ye, Y. Wei, et al., Ischemic stroke activates hematopoietic bone marrow stem cells, Circ. Res. 116 (3) (January 30, 2015) 407–417.
[61] P. Dutta, G. Courties, Y. Wei, F. Leuschner, R. Gorbatov, C.S. Robbins, et al., Myocardial infarction accelerates atherosclerosis, Nature 487 (7407) (July 19, 2012) 325–329.
[62] M.R. Pereira, P.E. Leite, The involvement of parasympathetic and sympathetic nerve in the inflammatory reflex, J. Cell. Physiol. **231** (9) (January 11, 2016) 1862–1869.
[63] I.L. Gomes-Santos, T. Fernandes, G.K. Couto, J.C. Ferreira-Filho, V.M. Salemi, F.B. Fernandes, et al., Effects of exercise training on circulating and skeletal muscle renin-angiotensin system in chronic heart failure rats, PLoS One 9 (5) (2014) e98012.
[64] N. Inoue, S. Kinugawa, T. Suga, T. Yokota, K. Hirabayashi, S. Kuroda, et al., Angiotensin II-induced reduction in exercise capacity is associated with increased oxidative stress in skeletal muscle, Am. J. Physiol. Heart Circ. Physiol. 302 (5) (March 1, 2012) H1202–H1210.
[65] D. Kalra, G. Baumgarten, Z. Dibbs, Y. Seta, N. Sivasubramanian, D.L. Mann, Nitric oxide provokes tumor necrosis factor-alpha expression in adult feline myocardium through a cGMP-dependent pathway, Circulation 102 (11) (September 12, 2000) 1302–1307.
[66] M. Brink, J. Wellen, P. Delafontaine, Angiotensin II causes weight loss and decreases circulating insulin-like growth factor I in rats through a pressor-independent mechanism, J. Clin. Investig. 97 (11) (June 1, 1996) 2509–2516.
[67] T. Yoshida, L. Semprun-Prieto, S. Sukhanov, P. Delafontaine, IGF-1 prevents ANG II-induced skeletal muscle atrophy via Akt- and Foxo-dependent inhibition of the ubiquitin ligase atrogin-1 expression, Am. J. Physiol. Heart Circ. Physiol. 298 (5) (May 2010) H1565–H1570.
[68] L.R. Bechara, J.B. Moreira, P.R. Jannig, V.A. Voltarelli, P.M. Dourado, A.R. Vasconcelos, et al., NADPH oxidase hyperactivity induces plantaris atrophy in heart failure rats, Int. J. Cardiol. 175 (3) (August 20, 2014) 499–507.
[69] S.T. Russell, S.M. Wyke, M.J. Tisdale, Mechanism of induction of muscle protein degradation by angiotensin II, Cell. Signal. 18 (7) (July 2006) 1087–1096.
[70] D.L. Mann, Inflammatory mediators and the failing heart: past, present, and the foreseeable future, Circ. Res. 91 (11) (November 29, 2002) 988–998.
[71] B.J. Pomerantz, L.L. Reznikov, A.H. Harken, C.A. Dinarello, Inhibition of caspase 1 reduces human myocardial ischemic dysfunction via inhibition of IL-18 and IL-1beta, Proc. Natl. Acad. Sci. U.S.A. 98 (5) (February 27, 2001) 2871–2876.
[72] S.D. Prabhu, Cytokine-induced modulation of cardiac function, Circ. Res. 95 (12) (December 10, 2004) 1140–1153.

[73] F. Franco, G.D. Thomas, B. Giroir, D. Bryant, M.C. Bullock, M.C. Chwialkowski, et al., Magnetic resonance imaging and invasive evaluation of development of heart failure in transgenic mice with myocardial expression of tumor necrosis factor-alpha, Circulation 99 (3) (January 26, 1999) 448–454.

[74] B. Bozkurt, S.B. Kribbs, F.J. Clubb Jr., L.H. Michael, V.V. Didenko, P.J. Hornsby, et al., Pathophysiologically relevant concentrations of tumor necrosis factor-alpha promote progressive left ventricular dysfunction and remodeling in rats, Circulation 97 (14) (April 14, 1998) 1382–1391.

[75] N. Sivasubramanian, M.L. Coker, K.M. Kurrelmeyer, W.R. MacLellan, F.J. DeMayo, F.G. Spinale, et al., Left ventricular remodeling in transgenic mice with cardiac restricted overexpression of tumor necrosis factor, Circulation 104 (7) (August 14, 2001) 826–831.

[76] B.W. Van Tassell, I.M. Seropian, S. Toldo, E. Mezzaroma, A. Abbate, Interleukin-1beta induces a reversible cardiomyopathy in the mouse, Inflamm. Res. 62 (7) (July 2013) 637–640.

[77] S. Toldo, E. Mezzaroma, B.W. Van Tassell, D. Farkas, C. Marchetti, N.F. Voelkel, et al., Interleukin-1beta blockade improves cardiac remodelling after myocardial infarction without interrupting the inflammasome in the mouse, Exp. Physiol. 98 (3) (March 2013) 734–745.

[78] S. Toldo, E. Mezzaroma, E. Bressi, C. Marchetti, S. Carbone, C. Sonnino, et al., Interleukin-1beta blockade improves left ventricular systolic/diastolic function and restores contractility reserve in severe ischemic cardiomyopathy in the mouse, J. Cardiovasc. Pharmacol. 64 (1) (July 2014) 1–6.

[79] R. Ferrari, T. Bachetti, L. Agnoletti, L. Comini, S. Curello, Endothelial function and dysfunction in heart failure, Eur. Heart J. 19 (Suppl. G) (July 1998) G41–G47.

[80] L. Agnoletti, S. Curello, T. Bachetti, F. Malacarne, G. Gaia, L. Comini, et al., Serum from patients with severe heart failure downregulates eNOS and is proapoptotic: role of tumor necrosis factor-alpha, Circulation 100 (19) (November 9, 1999) 1983–1991.

[81] J. McMurray, J. McLay, M. Chopra, A. Bridges, J.J. Belch, Evidence for enhanced free radical activity in chronic congestive heart failure secondary to coronary artery disease, Am. J. Cardiol. 65 (18) (May 15, 1990) 1261–1262.

[82] K.J. Lavine, O.L. Sierra, Skeletal muscle inflammation and atrophy in heart failure, Heart Fail. Rev. **22** (2) (January 14, 2017) 179–189.

[83] S.D. Anker, P. Ponikowski, S. Varney, T.P. Chua, A.L. Clark, K.M. Webb-Peploe, et al., Wasting as independent risk factor for mortality in chronic heart failure, Lancet 349 (9058) (April 12, 1997) 1050–1053.

[84] D.M. Mancini, G. Walter, N. Reichek, R. Lenkinski, K.K. McCully, J.L. Mullen, et al., Contribution of skeletal muscle atrophy to exercise intolerance and altered muscle metabolism in heart failure, Circulation 85 (4) (April 1992) 1364–1373.

[85] H. Drexler, U. Riede, T. Munzel, H. Konig, E. Funke, H. Just, Alterations of skeletal muscle in chronic heart failure, Circulation 85 (5) (May 1992) 1751–1759.

[86] J.R. Wilson, D.M. Mancini, W.B. Dunkman, Exertional fatigue due to skeletal muscle dysfunction in patients with heart failure, Circulation 87 (2) (February 1993) 470–475.

[87] L.L. Dalla, B. Ravara, V. Gobbo, B.D. Danieli, E. Germinario, A. Angelini, et al., Skeletal muscle myofibrillar protein oxidation in heart failure and the protective effect of Carvedilol, J. Mol. Cell. Cardiol. 38 (5) (May 2005) 803–807.

[88] K.A. Meadows, J.M. Holly, C.E. Stewart, Tumor necrosis factor-alpha-induced apoptosis is associated with suppression of insulin-like growth factor binding protein-5 secretion in differentiating murine skeletal myoblasts, J. Cell. Physiol. 183 (3) (June 2000) 330–337.

[89] L. Zhang, J. Pan, Y. Dong, D.J. Tweardy, Y. Dong, G. Garibotto, et al., Stat3 activation links a C/EBPdelta to myostatin pathway to stimulate loss of muscle mass, Cell Metab. 18 (3) (September 3, 2013) 368–379.

[90] D. Cai, J.D. Frantz, N.E. Tawa Jr., P.A. Melendez, B.C. Oh, H.G. Lidov, et al., IKKbeta/NF-kappaB activation causes severe muscle wasting in mice, Cell 119 (2) (October 15, 2004) 285–298.

[91] A.C. de, T. Teruel, R. Hernandez, M. Lorenzo, Tumor necrosis factor alpha produces insulin resistance in skeletal muscle by activation of inhibitor kappaB kinase in a p38 MAPK-dependent manner, J. Biol. Chem. 279 (17) (April 23, 2004) 17070–17078.

[92] C. Dogra, H. Changotra, N. Wedhas, X. Qin, J.E. Wergedal, A. Kumar, TNF-related weak inducer of apoptosis (TWEAK) is a potent skeletal muscle-wasting cytokine, FASEB J. 21 (8) (June 2007) 1857–1869.

[93] R.S. Vasan, L.M. Sullivan, R.B. D'Agostino, R. Roubenoff, T. Harris, D.B. Sawyer, et al., Serum insulin-like growth factor I and risk for heart failure in elderly individuals without a previous myocardial infarction: the Framingham Heart Study, Ann. Intern. Med. 139 (8) (October 21, 2003) 642–648.

[94] P. Bonaldo, M. Sandri, Cellular and molecular mechanisms of muscle atrophy, Dis. Model. Mech. 6 (1) (January 2013) 25–39.

[95] J. Ren, W.K. Samson, J.R. Sowers, Insulin-like growth factor I as a cardiac hormone: physiological and pathophysiological implications in heart disease, J. Mol. Cell. Cardiol. 31 (11) (November 1999) 2049–2061.

[96] S.D. Anker, M. Volterrani, C.D. Pflaum, C.J. Strasburger, K.J. Osterziel, W. Doehner, et al., Acquired growth hormone resistance in patients with chronic heart failure: implications for therapy with growth hormone, J. Am. Coll. Cardiol. 38 (2) (August 2001) 443–452.

[97] J. Niebauer, C.D. Pflaum, A.L. Clark, C.J. Strasburger, J. Hooper, P.A. Poole-Wilson, et al., Deficient insulin-like growth factor I in chronic heart failure predicts altered body composition, anabolic deficiency, cytokine and neurohormonal activation, J. Am. Coll. Cardiol. 32 (2) (August 1998) 393–397.

[98] A. Musaro, K. McCullagh, A. Paul, L. Houghton, G. Dobrowolny, M. Molinaro, et al., Localized Igf-1 transgene expression sustains hypertrophy and regeneration in senescent skeletal muscle, Nat. Genet. 27 (2) (February 2001) 195–200.

[99] P.C. Schulze, J. Fang, K.A. Kassik, J. Gannon, M. Cupesi, C. MacGillivray, et al., Transgenic overexpression of locally acting insulin-like growth factor-1 inhibits ubiquitin-mediated muscle atrophy in chronic left-ventricular dysfunction, Circ. Res. 97 (5) (September 2, 2005) 418–426.

[100] Y.H. Song, Y. Li, J. Du, W.E. Mitch, N. Rosenthal, P. Delafontaine, Muscle-specific expression of IGF-1 blocks angiotensin II-induced skeletal muscle wasting, J. Clin. Investig. 115 (2) (February 2005) 451–458.

[101] T.N. Stitt, D. Drujan, B.A. Clarke, F. Panaro, Y. Timofeyva, W.O. Kline, et al., The IGF-1/PI3K/Akt pathway prevents expression of muscle atrophy-induced ubiquitin ligases by inhibiting FOXO transcription factors, Mol. Cell 14 (3) (May 7, 2004) 395–403.

[102] R.T. Ge, L.H. Mo, R. Wu, J.Q. Liu, H.P. Zhang, Z. Liu, et al., Insulin-like growth factor-1 endues monocytes with immune suppressive ability to inhibit inflammation in the intestine, Sci. Rep. 5 (2015) 7735.
[103] J.E. Parrillo, R.E. Cunnion, S.E. Epstein, M.M. Parker, A.F. Suffredini, M. Brenner, et al., A prospective, randomized, controlled trial of prednisone for dilated cardiomyopathy, N. Engl. J. Med. 321 (16) (October 19, 1989) 1061–1068.
[104] K. Gong, Z. Zhang, X. Sun, X. Zhang, A. Li, J. Yan, et al., The nonspecific anti-inflammatory therapy with methotrexate for patients with chronic heart failure, Am. Heart J. 151 (1) (January 2006) 62–68.
[105] L. Gullestad, H. Aass, J.G. Fjeld, L. Wikeby, A.K. Andreassen, H. Ihlen, et al., Immunomodulating therapy with intravenous immunoglobulin in patients with chronic heart failure, Circulation 103 (2) (January 16, 2001) 220–225.
[106] A. Abbate, B.W. Van Tassell, I.M. Seropian, S. Toldo, R. Robati, A. Varma, et al., Interleukin-1beta modulation using a genetically engineered antibody prevents adverse cardiac remodelling following acute myocardial infarction in the mouse, Eur. J. Heart Fail. 12 (4) (April 2010) 319–322.
[107] A. Abbate, F.N. Salloum, B.W. Van Tassell, E. Vecile, S. Toldo, I. Seropian, et al., Alterations in the interleukin-1/interleukin-1 receptor antagonist balance modulate cardiac remodeling following myocardial infarction in the mouse, PLoS One 6 (11) (2011) e27923.
[108] B.W. Van Tassell, A. Varma, F.N. Salloum, A. Das, I.M. Seropian, S. Toldo, et al., Interleukin-1 trap attenuates cardiac remodeling after experimental acute myocardial infarction in mice, J. Cardiovasc. Pharmacol. 55 (2) (February 2010) 117–122.
[109] B.W. Van Tassell, R.A. Arena, S. Toldo, E. Mezzaroma, T. Azam, I.M. Seropian, et al., Enhanced interleukin-1 activity contributes to exercise intolerance in patients with systolic heart failure, PLoS One 7 (3) (2012) e33438.
[110] D.L. Mann, J.J. McMurray, M. Packer, K. Swedberg, J.S. Borer, W.S. Colucci, et al., Targeted anticytokine therapy in patients with chronic heart failure: results of the Randomized Etanercept Worldwide Evaluation (RENEWAL), Circulation 109 (13) (April 6, 2004) 1594–1602.
[111] B. Klein, H. Brailly, Cytokine-binding proteins: stimulating antagonists, Immunol. Today 16 (5) (May 1995) 216–220.
[112] J.W. Homeister, B.R. Lucchesi, Complement activation and inhibition in myocardial ischemia and reperfusion injury, Annu. Rev. Pharmacol. Toxicol. 34 (1994) 17–40.
[113] M. Karin, H. Clevers, Reparative inflammation takes charge of tissue regeneration, Nature 529 (7586) (January 21, 2016) 307–315.
[114] P.J. Goulder, P. Jeena, G. Tudor-Williams, S. Burchett, Paediatric HIV infection: correlates of protective immunity and global perspectives in prevention and management, Br. Med. Bull. 58 (2001) 89–108.
[115] K. Luzuriaga, J.L. Sullivan, Pediatric HIV-1 infection: advances and remaining challenges, AIDS Rev. 4 (1) (January 2002) 21–26.
[116] B. Adkins, C. Leclerc, S. Marshall-Clarke, Neonatal adaptive immunity comes of age, Nat. Rev. Immunol. 4 (7) (July 2004) 553–564.
[117] E. Aksoy, V. Albarani, M. Nguyen, J.F. Laes, J.L. Ruelle, W.D. De, et al., Interferon regulatory factor 3-dependent responses to lipopolysaccharide are selectively blunted in cord blood cells, Blood 109 (7) (April 1, 2007) 2887–2893.
[118] O. Levy, K.A. Zarember, R.M. Roy, C. Cywes, P.J. Godowski, M.R. Wessels, Selective impairment of TLR-mediated innate immunity in human newborns: neonatal blood plasma reduces monocyte TNF-alpha induction by bacterial lipopeptides, lipopolysaccharide, and imiquimod, but preserves the response to R-848, J. Immunol. 173 (7) (October 1, 2004) 4627–4634.
[119] M.W. Hall, S.M. Geyer, C.Y. Guo, A. Panoskaltsis-Mortari, P. Jouvet, J. Ferdinands, et al., Innate immune function and mortality in critically ill children with influenza: a multicenter study, Crit. Care Med. 41 (1) (January 2013) 224–236.
[120] J.W. Godwin, A.R. Pinto, N.A. Rosenthal, Macrophages are required for adult salamander limb regeneration, Proc. Natl. Acad. Sci. U.S.A. 110 (23) (June 4, 2013) 9415–9420.
[121] A.B. Aurora, E.R. Porrello, W. Tan, A.I. Mahmoud, J.A. Hill, R. Bassel-Duby, et al., Macrophages are required for neonatal heart regeneration, J. Clin. Investig. 124 (3) (February 24, 2014) 1382–1392.
[122] Y. Huang, M.R. Harrison, A. Osorio, J. Kim, A. Baugh, C. Duan, et al., Igf signaling is required for cardiomyocyte proliferation during zebrafish heart development and regeneration, PLoS One 8 (6) (2013) e67266.
[123] K.J. Lavine, S. Epelman, K. Uchida, K.J. Weber, C.G. Nichols, J.D. Schilling, et al., Distinct macrophage lineages contribute to disparate patterns of cardiac recovery and remodeling in the neonatal and adult heart, Proc. Natl. Acad. Sci. U.S.A. 111 (45) (November 11, 2014) 16029–16034.
[124] I.B. Lobov, S. Rao, T.J. Carroll, J.E. Vallance, M. Ito, J.K. Ondr, et al., WNT7b mediates macrophage-induced programmed cell death in patterning of the vasculature, Nature 437 (7057) (September 15, 2005) 417–421.
[125] W. Wang, D.D. Grier, J. Woo, M. Ward, G. Sui, S.V. Torti, et al., Ferritin H is a novel marker of early erythroid precursors and macrophages, Histopathology 62 (6) (May 2013) 931–940.
[126] M. Haldar, M. Kohyama, A.Y. So, W. Kc, X. Wu, C.G. Briseno, et al., Heme-mediated SPI-C induction promotes monocyte differentiation into iron-recycling macrophages, Cell 156 (6) (March 13, 2014) 1223–1234.
[127] M. Kohyama, W. Ise, B.T. Edelson, P.R. Wilker, K. Hildner, C. Mejia, et al., Role for Spi-C in the development of red pulp macrophages and splenic iron homeostasis, Nature 457 (7227) (January 15, 2009) 318–321.
[128] R. Van Furth, Z.A. Cohn, The origin and kinetics of mononuclear phagocytes, J. Exp. Med. 128 (3) (September 1, 1968) 415–435.
[129] A. Volkman, N.C. Chang, P.H. Strausbauch, P.S. Morahan, Differential effects of chronic monocyte depletion on macrophage populations, Lab. Investig. 49 (3) (September 1983) 291–298.
[130] R.T. Sawyer, P.H. Strausbauch, A. Volkman, Resident macrophage proliferation in mice depleted of blood monocytes by strontium-89, Lab. Investig. 46 (2) (February 1982) 165–170.
[131] F. Ginhoux, M. Greter, M. Leboeuf, S. Nandi, P. See, S. Gokhan, et al., Fate mapping analysis reveals that adult microglia derive from primitive macrophages, Science 330 (6005) (November 5, 2010) 841–845.
[132] C. Schulz, P.E. Gomez, L. Chorro, H. Szabo-Rogers, N. Cagnard, K. Kierdorf, et al., A lineage of myeloid cells independent of Myb and hematopoietic stem cells, Science 336 (6077) (April 6, 2012) 86–90.

[133] S. Yona, K.W. Kim, Y. Wolf, A. Mildner, D. Varol, M. Breker, et al., Fate mapping reveals origins and dynamics of monocytes and tissue macrophages under homeostasis, Immunity 38 (1) (January 24, 2013) 79–91.
[134] D. Hashimoto, A. Chow, C. Noizat, P. Teo, M.B. Beasley, M. Leboeuf, et al., Tissue-resident macrophages self-maintain locally throughout adult life with minimal contribution from circulating monocytes, Immunity 38 (4) (April 18, 2013) 792–804.
[135] S. Epelman, K.J. Lavine, A.E. Beaudin, D.K. Sojka, J.A. Carrero, B. Calderon, et al., Embryonic and adult-derived resident cardiac macrophages are maintained through distinct mechanisms at steady state and during inflammation, Immunity 40 (1) (January 16, 2014) 91–104.
[136] M. Guilliams, K.I. De, S. Henri, S. Post, L. Vanhoutte, P.S. De, et al., Alveolar macrophages develop from fetal monocytes that differentiate into long-lived cells in the first week of life via GM-CSF, J. Exp. Med. 210 (10) (September 16, 2013) 1977–1992.
[137] C. Jakubzick, E.L. Gautier, S.L. Gibbings, D.K. Sojka, A. Schlitzer, T.E. Johnson, et al., Minimal differentiation of classical monocytes as they survey steady-state tissues and transport antigen to lymph nodes, Immunity 39 (3) (September 19, 2013) 599–610.
[138] M.H. Sieweke, J.E. Allen, Beyond stem cells: self-renewal of differentiated macrophages, Science 342 (6161) (November 22, 2013) 1242974.
[139] L.C. Davies, S.J. Jenkins, J.E. Allen, P.R. Taylor, Tissue-resident macrophages, Nat. Immunol. 14 (10) (October 2013) 986–995.
[140] T.A. Wynn, A. Chawla, J.W. Pollard, Macrophage biology in development, homeostasis and disease, Nature 496 (7446) (April 25, 2013) 445–455.
[141] S.W. Boyer, A.V. Schroeder, S. Smith-Berdan, E.C. Forsberg, All hematopoietic cells develop from hematopoietic stem cells through Flk2/Flt3-positive progenitor cells, Cell Stem Cell 9 (1) (July 8, 2011) 64–73.
[142] S. Epelman, K.J. Lavine, G.J. Randolph, Origin and functions of tissue macrophages, Immunity 41 (1) (July 17, 2014) 21–35.
[143] G. Hoeffel, J. Chen, Y. Lavin, D. Low, F.F. Almeida, P. See, et al., C-Myb(+) erythro-myeloid progenitor-derived fetal monocytes give rise to adult tissue-resident macrophages, Immunity 42 (4) (April 21, 2015) 665–678.
[144] K. Molawi, Y. Wolf, P.K. Kandalla, J. Favret, N. Hagemeyer, K. Frenzel, et al., Progressive replacement of embryo-derived cardiac macrophages with age, J. Exp. Med. 211 (11) (October 20, 2014) 2151–2158.
[145] I.M. Samokhvalov, Deconvoluting the ontogeny of hematopoietic stem cells, Cell. Mol. Life Sci. 71 (6) (March 2014) 957–978.
[146] G. Hoeffel, Y. Wang, M. Greter, P. See, P. Teo, B. Malleret, et al., Adult Langerhans cells derive predominantly from embryonic fetal liver monocytes with a minor contribution of yolk sac-derived macrophages, J. Exp. Med. 209 (6) (June 4, 2012) 1167–1181.
[147] I.M. Samokhvalov, N.I. Samokhvalova, S. Nishikawa, Cell tracing shows the contribution of the yolk sac to adult haematopoiesis, Nature 446 (7139) (April 26, 2007) 1056–1061.
[148] S.H. Orkin, L.I. Zon, Hematopoiesis: an evolving paradigm for stem cell biology, Cell 132 (4) (February 22, 2008) 631–644.
[149] D.K. Fogg, C. Sibon, C. Miled, S. Jung, P. Aucouturier, D.R. Littman, et al., A clonogenic bone marrow progenitor specific for macrophages and dendritic cells, Science 311 (5757) (January 6, 2006) 83–87.
[150] J. Hettinger, D.M. Richards, J. Hansson, M.M. Barra, A.C. Joschko, J. Krijgsveld, et al., Origin of monocytes and macrophages in a committed progenitor, Nat. Immunol. 14 (8) (August 2013) 821–830.
[151] M.A. Ingersoll, R. Spanbroek, C. Lottaz, E.L. Gautier, M. Frankenberger, R. Hoffmann, et al., Comparison of gene expression profiles between human and mouse monocyte subsets, Blood 115 (3) (January 21, 2010) e10–e19.
[152] R.N. Hanna, L.M. Carlin, H.G. Hubbeling, D. Nackiewicz, A.M. Green, J.A. Punt, et al., The transcription factor NR4A1 (Nur77) controls bone marrow differentiation and the survival of Ly6C- monocytes, Nat. Immunol. 12 (8) (August 2011) 778–785.
[153] L.M. Carlin, E.G. Stamatiades, C. Auffray, R.N. Hanna, L. Glover, G. Vizcay-Barrena, et al., Nr4a1-dependent Ly6C(low) monocytes monitor endothelial cells and orchestrate their disposal, Cell 153 (2) (April 11, 2013) 362–375.
[154] E.L. Gautier, T. Shay, J. Miller, M. Greter, C. Jakubzick, S. Ivanov, et al., Gene-expression profiles and transcriptional regulatory pathways that underlie the identity and diversity of mouse tissue macrophages, Nat. Immunol. 13 (11) (November 2012) 1118–1128.
[155] T. Glaros, M. Larsen, L. Li, Macrophages and fibroblasts during inflammation, tissue damage and organ injury, Front. Biosci. (Landmark Ed.) 14 (2009) 3988–3993.
[156] S. Frantz, M. Nahrendorf, Cardiac macrophages and their role in ischaemic heart disease, Cardiovasc. Res. 102 (2) (February 24, 2014) 240–248.
[157] M. Nahrendorf, F.K. Swirski, E. Aikawa, L. Stangenberg, T. Wurdinger, J.L. Figueiredo, et al., The healing myocardium sequentially mobilizes two monocyte subsets with divergent and complementary functions, J. Exp. Med. 204 (12) (November 26, 2007) 3037–3047.
[158] J. Leid, J. Carrelha, H. Boukarabila, S. Epelman, S.E. Jacobsen, K.J. Lavine, Primitive embryonic macrophages are required for coronary development and maturation, Circ. Res. 118 (10) (May 13, 2016) 1498–1511.
[159] W. Li, H.M. Hsiao, R. Higashikubo, B.T. Saunders, A. Bharat, D.R. Goldstein, et al., Heart-resident $CCR2^+$ macrophages promote neutrophil extravasation through TLR9/MyD88/CXCL5 signaling, JCI Insight 1 (12) (August 4, 2016).
[160] L. Arnold, A. Henry, F. Poron, Y. Baba-Amer, R.N. van, A. Plonquet, et al., Inflammatory monocytes recruited after skeletal muscle injury switch into antiinflammatory macrophages to support myogenesis, J. Exp. Med. 204 (5) (May 14, 2007) 1057–1069.
[161] W. Li, J.S. Moylan, M.A. Chambers, J. Smith, M.B. Reid, Interleukin-1 stimulates catabolism in C2C12 myotubes, Am. J. Physiol. Cell Physiol. 297 (3) (September 2009) C706–C714.
[162] R. Mounier, M. Theret, L. Arnold, S. Cuvellier, L. Bultot, O. Goransson, et al., AMPKalpha1 regulates macrophage skewing at the time of resolution of inflammation during skeletal muscle regeneration, Cell Metab. 18 (2) (August 6, 2013) 251–264.
[163] D. Ruffell, F. Mourkioti, A. Gambardella, P. Kirstetter, R.G. Lopez, N. Rosenthal, et al., A CREB-C/EBPbeta cascade induces M2 macrophage-specific gene expression and promotes muscle injury repair, Proc. Natl. Acad. Sci. U.S.A. 106 (41) (October 13, 2009) 17475–17480.
[164] D. Sag, D. Carling, R.D. Stout, J. Suttles, Adenosine 5'-monophosphate-activated protein kinase promotes macrophage polarization to an anti-inflammatory functional phenotype, J. Immunol. 181 (12) (December 15, 2008) 8633–8641.
[165] S.A. Villalta, H.X. Nguyen, B. Deng, T. Gotoh, J.G. Tidball, Shifts in macrophage phenotypes and macrophage competition for arginine metabolism affect the severity of muscle pathology in muscular dystrophy, Hum. Mol. Genet. 18 (3) (February 1, 2009) 482–496.

[166] S.A. Villalta, B. Deng, C. Rinaldi, M. Wehling-Henricks, J.G. Tidball, IFN-gamma promotes muscle damage in the mdx mouse model of Duchenne muscular dystrophy by suppressing M2 macrophage activation and inhibiting muscle cell proliferation, J. Immunol. 187 (10) (November 15, 2011) 5419–5428.

[167] S.A. Villalta, C. Rinaldi, B. Deng, G. Liu, B. Fedor, J.G. Tidball, Interleukin-10 reduces the pathology of mdx muscular dystrophy by deactivating M1 macrophages and modulating macrophage phenotype, Hum. Mol. Genet. 20 (4) (February 15, 2011) 790–805.

[168] M. Summan, G.L. Warren, R.R. Mercer, R. Chapman, T. Hulderman, R.N. van, et al., Macrophages and skeletal muscle regeneration: a clodronate-containing liposome depletion study, Am. J. Physiol. Regul. Integr. Comp. Physiol. 290 (6) (June 2006) R1488–R1495.

[169] R.E. Shaddy, M.M. Boucek, D.T. Hsu, R.J. Boucek, C.E. Canter, L. Mahony, et al., Carvedilol for children and adolescents with heart failure: a randomized controlled trial, JAMA 298 (10) (September 12, 2007) 1171–1179.

[170] P.F. Kantor, J.R. Abraham, A.I. Dipchand, L.N. Benson, A.N. Redington, The impact of changing medical therapy on transplantation-free survival in pediatric dilated cardiomyopathy, J. Am. Coll. Cardiol. 55 (13) (March 30, 2010) 1377–1384.

[171] J.A. Towbin, A.M. Lowe, S.D. Colan, L.A. Sleeper, E.J. Orav, S. Clunie, et al., Incidence, causes, and outcomes of dilated cardiomyopathy in children, JAMA 296 (15) (October 18, 2006) 1867–1876.

[172] S.D. Miyamoto, B.L. Stauffer, S. Nakano, R. Sobus, K. Nunley, P. Nelson, et al., Beta-adrenergic adaptation in paediatric idiopathic dilated cardiomyopathy, Eur. Heart J. 35 (1) (July 26, 2012) 33–41.

[173] D.L. Mann, Basic mechanisms of left ventricular remodeling: the contribution of wall stress, J. Card. Fail. 10 (6 Suppl.) (December 2004) S202–S206.

[174] M.D. Everitt, L.A. Sleeper, M. Lu, C.E. Canter, E. Pahl, J.D. Wilkinson, et al., Recovery of echocardiographic function in children with idiopathic dilated cardiomyopathy: results from the pediatric cardiomyopathy registry, J. Am. Coll. Cardiol. 63 (14) (February 7, 2014) 1405–1413.

[175] D.L. Mann, P.M. Barger, D. Burkhoff, Myocardial recovery and the failing heart: myth, magic, or molecular target? J. Am. Coll. Cardiol. 60 (24) (December 18, 2012) 2465–2472.

[176] D.L. Mann, R. Bogaev, G.D. Buckberg, Cardiac remodelling and myocardial recovery: lost in translation? Eur. J. Heart Fail. 12 (8) (August 2010) 789–796.

[177] M. Merlo, D. Stolfo, M. Anzini, F. Negri, B. Pinamonti, G. Barbati, et al., Persistent recovery of normal left ventricular function and dimension in idiopathic dilated cardiomyopathy during long-term follow-up: does real healing exist? J. Am. Heart Assoc. 4 (1) (January 13, 2015) e001504.

[178] M. Merlo, S.A. Pyxaras, B. Pinamonti, G. Barbati, L.A. Di, G. Sinagra, Prevalence and prognostic significance of left ventricular reverse remodeling in dilated cardiomyopathy receiving tailored medical treatment, J. Am. Coll. Cardiol. 57 (13) (March 29, 2011) 1468–1476.

[179] D.M. McNamara, R.C. Starling, L.T. Cooper, J.P. Boehmer, P.J. Mather, K.M. Janosko, et al., Clinical and demographic predictors of outcomes in recent onset dilated cardiomyopathy: results of the IMAC (Intervention in Myocarditis and Acute Cardiomyopathy)-2 study, J. Am. Coll. Cardiol. 58 (11) (September 6, 2011) 1112–1118.

[180] M. Mollova, K. Bersell, S. Walsh, J. Savla, L.T. Das, S.Y. Park, et al., Cardiomyocyte proliferation contributes to heart growth in young humans, Proc. Natl. Acad. Sci. U.S.A. 110 (4) (January 22, 2013) 1446–1451.

Chapter 4

Mechanisms of Cardiac Hypertrophy

Matthew Zinn, Shawn West, Bernhard Kuhn
Children's Hospital of Pittsburgh of UPMC, Pittsburgh, PA, United States

INTRODUCTION

Definition and Significance of Myocardial Hypertrophy

Cardiac hypertrophy, the enlargement of heart muscle, is found in a diverse set of conditions and types of heart disease. Myocardial hypertrophy (MH) is the final common pathway of a diverse set of diseases and conditions and as a result has a high incidence in pediatric and congenital cardiology. MH is characterized by local and/or global enlargement of the myocardium. Local enlargement of the interventricular septum is typical of familial hypertrophic cardiomyopathy (HCM) due to mutations in genes encoding for sarcomere proteins, pathologic ventricular hypertrophy seen in infants of diabetic mothers (IDM), and after pulmonary artery banding (PAB). Global, or concentric left ventricular hypertrophy (LVH), is more commonly seen in the athlete's heart (AH) and other forms of HCM.

The gold standard for measuring cardiac hypertrophy is postmortem examination of the heart for weight and regional enlargement. Careful attention must be paid when obtaining the heart mass as the value is dependent on the specifics of resection and fluid removal. Clinically, myocardial mass is determined by imaging (echocardiography or MRI) and reported as left ventricular (LV) mass. In adults, the upper limit of normal for heart mass has been defined by postmortem examination as approximately 500 g, also known as the critical heart mass [1].

In the pediatric population, heart mass is indexed to body size and imaging-based normative data are used commonly [2,3]. The heart mass increases 20-fold between birth and adulthood [1,4], creating a unique challenge in the pediatric population. Increases in myocardial mass may be the result of simultaneous natural heart growth and pathologic hypertrophy. We currently lack advanced diagnostic tools to delineate between these mechanisms. In addition, MH is associated with arrhythmias, myocardial fibrosis, and heart failure. It is imperative to recognize hypertrophy early and understand the underlying mechanisms.

Cellular Mechanisms of Cardiac Hypertrophy

The basic cellular mechanisms of organ growth are enlargement and proliferation. Cardiomyocytes, the contractile cells of the heart, constitute approximately 20%–50% of all cardiac cells. However, because cardiomyocytes undergo developmental enlargement, they may contribute more than 90% of the heart mass. Historically, normal postnatal heart growth was thought to be solely based on the enlargement of cardiomyocytes. This view was based on indirect measurements of cardiomyocyte volume [5]. Direct measurements of cardiomyocyte volume have shown that, although it increases significantly after birth, this alone cannot fully account for the increase of heart muscle volume [6]. Bergmann and colleagues reported a 12- to 16-fold increase in cardiomyocyte volume between the first 6 months and 19 years of age [6]. We have found that the cardiomyocyte volume increases 8.6- to 11-fold after birth [7]. This contrasts with the more than 20-fold increase of heart mass seen after birth, making additional mechanisms, such as cellular proliferation, responsible for the remaining cardiac growth. Direct quantification of the number of cardiomyocytes has shown a 3.7-fold increase from approximately 1 billion at birth to 3.7 billion in adults [7]. These findings advance our understanding of growth mechanisms beyond hypertrophy [6,7].

This advanced cellular growth model is significant for pediatric cardiologists [7]. First, it suggests that infants and children may be able to regenerate myocardium on the basis of regulated cardiomyocyte proliferation. Second, abnormal cardiomyocyte hypertrophy and proliferation may be involved in myocardial diseases that affect this population. Third, it indicates the possibility that cardiomyocyte proliferation could be therapeutically stimulated for cardiac regeneration.

Heart Failure in the Child and Young Adult. http://dx.doi.org/10.1016/B978-0-12-802393-8.00004-1

Molecular Mechanisms of Cardiac Hypertrophy

A large body of research examined the molecular mechanisms of cardiac hypertrophy in adult animals and humans [8]. Comparatively little basic and translational research addresses the molecular mechanisms of cardiac growth and hypertrophy in the pediatric population or in relevant animal models. This knowledge gap has been recognized by a working group of the National Heart, Lung, and Blood Institute [9]. Several well-characterized molecular pathways control cardiac hypertrophy in pediatric conditions and diseases and will be discussed in this chapter. Others, such as the β-adrenergic and renin–angiotensin–aldosterone system will be discussed in subsequent chapters.

THE INFANT OF A DIABETIC MOTHER

Maternal hyperglycemia has long been recognized as a risk factor for congenital malformations. Multiple studies dating back 30years have linked maternal diabetes mellitus (DM), especially insulin-dependent diabetes mellitus, to congenital heart defects. The estimated incidence of congenital heart disease (CHD) in this population ranges from 3% to 6%, five times the risk of the general population [10–13]. The teratogenic effects of hyperglycemia on the fetal heart, specifically before the seventh week of gestation, are well-documented [14–18]. Hypoplastic left heart syndrome, tetralogy of Fallot, pulmonary atresia, tricuspid atresia, transposition of the great arteries, and septal defects have been reported in IDM [16,17,19,20].

Ventricular Hypertrophy

Beyond structural heart disease, IDM can develop ventricular hypertrophy. A 1944 autopsy study was one of the first to show increased heart weight in IDM [21]. Asymmetric septal hypertrophy was not reported in IDM until 32years later, when Gutgesell and colleagues showed transient "hypertrophic subaortic stenosis" in three IDM, all of which gradually improved or resolved [22]. Subsequent studies have confirmed the phenomenon and estimated the incidence of asymmetric ventricular hypertrophy (AVH) in IDM between 31% and 43% [10,13,23–26]. AVH in IDM has been further analyzed by diabetic type. Limited data show the highest incidence of AVH in type 1 DM, followed by type 2 DM, then gestational DM [10]. Microscopic evaluation of the septal myocardium has differentiated PVH from HCM, with the former lacking disorganized myocardial fibers and less than 5% cellular disarray [27,28]. The pattern of hypertrophy is not often useful in differentiating between the two disease processes. The interventricular septum is the primary and often solitary site of hypertrophy in AVH, while HCM may be present as either asymmetric septal hypertrophy or concentric LVH [29].

Mechanisms of Hypertrophy

Several potential mechanisms have been proposed for transient infantile AVH. Maternal hyperglycemia and the complex interplay between insulin, insulin-like growth factor 1 (IGF-1), and insulin-like growth factor-binding protein 1 (IGFBP-1) have been extensively studied. Elevated maternal blood glucose, primarily in the second and third trimester, is thought to induce fetal hyperinsulinemia, which increases fat and protein synthesis leading to MH and hyperplasia [30–33]. Several authors have suggested uncontrolled maternal blood glucose levels as the cause for CHD and AVH, noting elevated maternal hemoglobin A1c (HbA1c) levels in affected infants [10,13,25]. IDM with AVH are commonly born to mothers with HbA1c values ≥7% [10,13]. However, a clear link cannot be made as several studies have documented normal maternal HbA1c levels in the presence of PVH [10,26,34,35].

The question then arises as to a second mechanism responsible for AVH in IDM, separate from but potentially linked to maternal glycemic control. Insulin and its related growth factors are known mediators of fetal growth [36]. In fact, IGF-1 is the predominant fetal growth factor, impacting cell growth, division, and differentiation [36–40]. Maternal IGF-1 does not cross the placenta but instead exerts its effects on the fetus by regulating the levels of fetal IGFBP-1 [36,39]. Elevated maternal IGF-1 and fetal insulin downregulate fetal IGFBP-1, which in turn upregulates fetal IGF-1 [36,41]. MH, and macrosomia in general, are the end products of increased fetal IGF-1 and hyperinsulinemia [39,42]. Infants with congenital hyperinsulinism (HI), previously known as nesidioblastosis, show a similar course to IDM. Huang et al. reported on 68 infants with HI, 10 (15% incidence) of which developed severe symptomatic ventricular hypertrophy resembling HCM [43]. All 10 symptomatic infants were refractory to medical therapy and required a pancreatectomy, which was associated with resolution of ventricular hypertrophy.

Resolution of Hypertrophy

Resolution of the asymmetric septal hypertrophy is the hallmark of AVH in IDM. Affected infants are typically asymptomatic without significant LV outflow tract obstruction [22–24]. Complete resolution of AVH is commonly seen by

2–12 months of age [22,23,28], presumably due to normalized growth factor activity. While the majority of infants have a benign course, rare cases of fetal demise have been reported [27,44].

PULMONARY ARTERY BANDING

Banding of the main pulmonary artery (PA) was first described in dogs in 1924 [45]. Not until 27 years later did Muller and Dammann [46] report the procedure in humans. At a time when cardiopulmonary bypass was not widely available, PAB was initially used as a palliative treatment in left to right shunting cardiac lesions to decrease PA blood flow and increase systemic blood flow [46]. PAB has subsequently been adopted for palliation of complex congenital heart lesions, including transposition of the great arteries [47].

The target ventricular pressure is variable after banding. Success has been traditionally defined as a systolic ventricular pressure that is 30% of the systolic systemic blood pressure or a decrease in the PA size by two-thirds [47,48]. Banding increases afterload by reducing the effective outflow diameter of the PA, thereby increasing ventricular systolic pressure. Increased ventricular systolic pressure induces hypertrophy and collagen deposition, which may lead to myocardial fibrosis.

Human Studies

Early single site and multicenter studies in humans did not show ventricular hypertrophy after PAB [49,50]. Subsequent reports have described ventricular hypertrophy after PAB in both single and biventricular physiology [51–55]. A single center retrospective study by Hess et al. reviewed 36 patients with single ventricle physiology after PAB [54]. 12 of 26 patients (46%) developed subaortic obstruction with pressure gradients ranging from 5 to 75 mmHg. Only five patients demonstrated a left ventricle to aortic pressure gradient >20 mmHg. More recently, PA bands have been used to prepare the left ventricle for late presentation of d-transposition of the great arteries or in preparation of a double switch procedure for congenitally corrected transposition [55]. By postoperative day 7, the LV mass had increased by 95%.

Adult Animal Models

PAB has been thoroughly studied from a physiologic and cellular perspective in animal models, with multiple models showing right ventricular hypertrophy (RVH) following PAB. Increased right ventricular (RV) systolic pressure and RVH after PAB has been demonstrated in a rabbit model [56,57]. Histologic investigation of the study animals revealed increased cardiomyocyte diameter and collagen deposition in the RV as early as 5 weeks after banding. One report [57] included an additional study group that received losartan after PAB, which resulted in decreased RV hypertrophy, RV myocyte diameter, and collagen volume. Increased RV mass and myocyte cell length after PAB has also been seen in a dog model [58].

Juvenile Animal Models

Numerous studies on PAB have been conducted in young animals. RVH and histologic markers of increased cell death were seen 4 weeks after PAB in a 10-day-old rabbit model [59]. Similar findings have been reported in 4-week-old lambs [60]. In a study by Orito et al. [61], twenty-four 1-year-old beagles were found to have increased collagen fiber deposition 60 and 180 days after PA banding, but not at postoperative day 15. Collagen was found near both the epicardium and endocardium, and RV myocytes were slightly increased in diameter after banding. Goat and piglet models have also shown increased RV mass by echocardiogram and cardiac MRI after PAB [62–65].

Applicability of the above animal models to human use is limited as all studied animals possessed a structurally normal heart. PA banding in humans is intended as a step toward definitive surgery. Unfortunately, a reversible model has not been studied in animals. It is suspected, but not known, that hypertrophy would resolve in animals following removal of a PA band.

ATHLETE'S HEART

Not all causes of cardiac hypertrophy are pathologic. Sitting on the border between normal and abnormal, healthy and diseased, is the AH. Cardiac output may increase up to six times that of normal during peak exercise to meet the perfusion demands of skeletal muscle [66]. This amazing feat is initially achieved without lasting structural myocardial alterations. Simple observations dating back to the 1890s have noted baseline changes in the hearts of those who exercised regularly.

Physical exam findings suggestive of an "enlarged heart" were seen in Nordic skiers, American runners, and Chinese rickshaw pullers [67–69]. In animals, exercise studies show enlarged hearts in subjects compared to their sedentary siblings, even more so during growth spurts [70].

Mechanisms of Hypertrophy

The first detailed description of exercise-induced cardiac hypertrophy came in 1975 from Morganroth and colleagues [71]. They studied both endurance (swimmers and runners) and resistance (wrestlers, commonly referred to as strength athletes today) athletes and came to the conclusion that exercise type and pattern of hypertrophy are linked. Endurance (isotonic, dynamic, aerobic exercise) athletes developed increased stroke volume, LV mass, and end-diastolic volume while maintaining normal LV wall thickness. Strength (isometric, static, anaerobic exercise) athletes developed increased LV mass and LV wall thickness while maintaining normal end-diastolic volume [71,72]. The former became known as eccentric LVH secondary to volume overload, and the latter concentric LVH secondary to pressure overload [73]. Morganroth's theory has been validated by others [73], including a large metaanalysis on the type of cardiac adaptations seen in purely endurance versus purely strength athletes [74].

A significant degree of crossover is seen between the two types of exercise when the sport contains both endurance and strength components (cyclists and rowers) [74,75]. Pluim et al. concluded that AH "is not to be considered an absolute or dichotomous concept" [74]. In fact, some have questioned Morganroth's original theory by citing lack of randomized longitudinal designs and advanced imaging data in available studies [76]. Others have expanded this doubt by showing no concentric hypertrophy in strength-based training and an eccentric hypertrophy incidence of only 30% in endurance-based training [77–80].

LVH may occur in athletes due to mechanisms distinct from HCM. The hypertrophy of AH is most commonly symmetric, with a slightly greater involvement of the anterior ventricular septum. Thickness of the remaining LV wall segments typically varies by less than 2 mm [81–83]. The pattern of hypertrophy can help distinguish AH from HCM, where hypertrophy is commonly asymmetric and heterogeneous [82,83]. The upper limit of normal for left ventricular wall thickness (LVWT) is 12 mm [75], while the lower limit of abnormal is 16 mm [81]. A gap exists from 13 to 15 mm where the differentiation between AH and HCM is problematic [75,82–84]. This "gray zone" presents a diagnostic and management dilemma since the evaluation for both conditions includes restriction from all high-level athletics. Fortunately, a LVWT >12 mm is seen in only 2% of adult athletes [75] and 0.4% of adolescent athletes [85]. In fact, the LVWT of an athlete is only 10%–20% larger compared to nonathletes and often remains in the normal range for age and sex [82].

Additional features of AH include enlargement of the left atrium and LV end-diastolic dimension (LVEDD), both secondary to increased stroke volume. The left atrial transverse diameter is ≥40 mm in 20% of athletes while maintaining normal LV filling patterns on echocardiogram [83]. The LVEDD is commonly >55 mm but maintains its ellipsoid shape and normal mitral valve function [84,85]. These features, along with normal systolic and diastolic LV function on echocardiogram, lack of inverted T waves on EKG, and a negative family history help differentiate AH from HCM [82,83].

Factors Affecting Hypertrophy

Most data on AH originate from studies on white male athletes and control aged 18–40 [71,74,77,83]. Practical use of this information is limited in today's world where all genders, races, and ethnicities compete at the highest athletic levels. The same holds true for the field of pediatrics as an increasing number of adolescents are involved in elite level athletics. Sharma et al. [85] evaluated LVH in 720 elite junior athletes aged 14–18 years. All LVH was concentric with a LVWT >11 mm in only 4%, with only 0.4% between 13 and 14 mm. No female athlete (25% of those studied) or control patient demonstrated a LVWT over 11 mm. The threshold for concerning LVH should therefore be lower in adolescent athletes: >12 mm in males and >11 mm in females [85]. Dores et al. put forth several potential explanations including "less skeletal muscle mass, lower accumulated training, lack of testosterone before puberty and lower catecholamine responses to exercise" [66].

Elite adult female athletes also exhibit a different response to exercise than their male counterparts. Female athletes have a less pronounced increase in LV cavity dimensions and LVWT when compared to male athletes of the same age, ethnicity, and sport [75,86]. In fact, women rarely fall into the gray zone of AH versus HCM as nearly none exhibit a LVWT >11 mm in white athletes [86] and 3% in black athletes [87].

This distinction leads to the concept of racial variation in LV dimensions. In the United Kingdom, Basavarajaiah and colleagues [88] studied 300 elite collegiate black male athletes, 300 white athletes, and an equal number of black and white male sedentary controls. No control subject had a LVWT >12 mm or LVEDD >55 mm. An LVWT >12 mm was seen in 18% of black athletes and only 4% on white athletes ($P<.001$). Furthermore, 3% of black athletes, but no white athletes, had an

LVWT ≥15 mm but no other risk factors for HCM. As opposed to a lower limit in women, perhaps a higher upper limit of normal LVWT should exist in black male athletes who may possess greater predilection for LVH.

Genetic factors may also increase one's risk for AH. White male military recruits with an angiotensin-converting enzyme (ACE)-DD phenotype showed a 42.3% increase in LV mass after training, with only a 2% change in the ACE-II genotype [89]. In a Finnish study, AGT (angiotensinogen) M235T polymorphisms correlated with variable LV mass in elite endurance athletes [90]. Individuals with the AGT-TT genotype had greater LV mass compared to those with the AGT-MM genotype in both men and women. No difference in LV mass was seen between the ACE I/D polymorphisms, contrary to the previously mentioned study in military recruits.

Resolution of Hypertrophy

Similar to cardiac hypertrophy seen in IDM, the natural history of LVH associated with athletic training is one of complete resolution with detraining. In the short term, athletes with a LVWT of 13–15 mm at peak training can achieve a reduction in LVWT of 2–5 mm within 3 months of detraining [91]. In a longitudinal study of detraining in 40 elite male Italian athletes, 62% showed ≥2 mm decrease in LVWT, while 15% decreased by 0–1 mm [92]. All subjects had an anterior ventricular septal thickness of ≤12 mm at study completion. Interestingly, 85% continued to show a LVEDD ≥55 mm and 45% had elevated LV mass 6 years after cessation of training. A more recent MRI study showed a significant decrease in the LVWT of endurance athletes after detraining compared to preparticipation values [78]. No such change was seen in strength athletes as they did not exhibit a significant increase in LVWT with training. Persistent LV cavity dilatation was also seen in this report, prompting the suggestion that LV hypertrophy resolves before LV dilatation, if it resolves at all. There is also increasing evidence of arrhythmias, particularly atrial fibrillation, in older athletes compared to nonathlete age matched controls [93]. These data suggest that prolonged periods of high intensity athletic training in youth may not be without consequence in age.

CONCLUSION

Cardiac hypertrophy is a complex process that has challenged clinicians for decades. The heart is capable of responding to transient stressors with reversible hypertrophy. Genetic factors likely play a leading role in both the development and regression of hypertrophy, as aberrations in normal genetic pathways are increasingly demonstrated in all forms of cardiomyopathy. Chronic cardiac hypertrophy may lead to myocardial fibrosis, arrhythmia, and heart failure. These pathologic mechanisms of cardiac hypertrophy will be discussed in great detail in later chapters.

REFERENCES

[1] A.J. Linzbach, Heart failure from the point of view of quantitative anatomy, Am. J. Cardiol. 5 (1960) 370–382.

[2] T. Sluysmans, S.P. Sanders, M. van der Velde, A. Matitiau, I.A. Parness, P.J. Spevak, J.E. Mayer Jr., S.D. Colan, Natural history and patterns of recovery of contractile function in single left ventricle after Fontan operation, Circulation 86 (1992) 1753–1761.

[3] B.J. Foster, A.S. Mackie, M. Mitsnefes, H. Ali, S. Mamber, S.D. Colan, A novel method of expressing left ventricular mass relative to body size in children, Circulation 117 (2008) 2769–2775.

[4] R. Zak, Cell proliferation during cardiac growth, Am. J. Cardiol. 31 (1973) 211–219.

[5] A.J. Linzbach, The muscle fiber constant and the law of growth of the human ventricles, Virchows Arch. 318 (1950) 575–618.

[6] O. Bergmann, S. Zdunek, A. Felker, M. Salehpour, K. Alkass, S. Bernard, S.L. Sjostrom, M. Szewczykowska, T. Jackowska, C. Dos Remedios, T. Malm, M. Andra, R. Jashari, J.R. Nyengaard, G. Possnert, S. Jovinge, H. Druid, J. Frisen, Dynamics of cell generation and turnover in the human heart, Cell 161 (2015) 1566–1575.

[7] M. Mollova, K. Bersell, S. Walsh, J. Savla, L.T. Das, S.Y. Park, L.E. Silberstein, C.G. Dos Remedios, D. Graham, S. Colan, B. Kuhn, Cardiomyocyte proliferation contributes to heart growth in young humans, Proc. Natl. Acad. Sci. U.S.A. 110 (2013) 1446–1451.

[8] J. Heineke, J.D. Molkentin, Regulation of cardiac hypertrophy by intracellular signalling pathways, Nat. Rev. Mol. Cell Biol. 7 (2006) 589–600.

[9] K.M. Burns, B.J. Byrne, B.D. Gelb, B. Kuhn, L.A. Leinwand, S. Mital, G.D. Pearson, M. Rodefeld, J.W. Rossano, B.L. Stauffer, M.D. Taylor, J.A. Towbin, A.N. Redington, New mechanistic and therapeutic targets for pediatric heart failure: report from a National Heart, Lung, and Blood Institute Working Group, Circulation 130 (2014) 79–86.

[10] S. Ullmo, Y. Vial, S. Di Bernardo, M. Roth-Kleiner, Y. Mivelaz, N. Sekarski, J. Ruiz, E.J. Meijboom, Pathologic ventricular hypertrophy in the offspring of diabetic mothers: a retrospective study, Eur. Heart J. 28 (11) (June 2007) 1319–1325.

[11] J.L. Mills, R.H. Knopp, J.L. Simpson, L. Jovanovic-Peterson, B.E. Metzger, L.B. Holmes, J.H. Aarons, Z. Brown, G.F. Reed, F.R. Bieber, et al., Lack of relation of increased malformation rates in infants of diabetic mothers to glycemic control during organogenesis, N. Engl. J. Med. 318 (11) (March 17, 1988) 671–676.

[12] C. Ferencz, J.D. Rubin, R.J. McCarter, J.I. Brenner, C.A. Neill, L.W. Perry, S.I. Hepner, J.W. Downing, Congenital heart disease: prevalence at livebirth. The Baltimore-Washington Infant Study, Am. J. Epidemiol. 121 (1) (January 1985) 31–36.

[13] M.M. El-Ganzoury, S.A. El-Masry, R.A. El-Farrash, M. Anwar, R.Z. Abd Ellatife, Infants of diabetic mothers: echocardiographic measurements and cord blood IGF-I and IGFBP-1, Pediatr. Diabetes 13 (2) (March 2012) 189–196.
[14] J.A. Goldman, D. Dicker, D. Feldberg, A. Yeshaya, N. Samuel, M. Karp, Pregnancy outcome in patients with insulin-dependent diabetes mellitus with preconceptional diabetic control: a comparative study, Am. J. Obstet. Gynecol. 155 (2) (August 1986) 293–297.
[15] J.L. Mills, L. Baker, A.S. Goldman, Malformations in infants of diabetic mothers occur before the seventh gestational week. Implications for treatment, Diabetes 28 (4) (April 1979) 292–293.
[16] J.L. Kitzmiller, J.P. Cloherty, M.D. Younger, A. Tabatabaii, S.B. Rothchild, I. Sosenko, M.F. Epstein, S. Singh, R.K. Neff, Diabetic pregnancy and perinatal morbidity, Am. J. Obstet. Gynecol. 131 (5) (July 1, 1978) 560–580.
[17] L.E. Shields, E.A. Gan, H.F. Murphy, D.J. Sahn, T.R. Moore, The prognostic value of hemoglobin A1c in predicting fetal heart disease in diabetic pregnancies, Obstet. Gynecol. 81 (6) (June 1993) 954–957.
[18] N.G. Soler, S.M. Soler, J.M. Malins, Neonatal morbidity among infants of diabetic mothers, Diabetes Care 1 (6) (November–December 1978) 340–350.
[19] G. Gladman, B.W. McCrindle, C. Boutin, J.F. Smallhorn, Fetal echocardiographic screening of diabetic pregnancies for congenital heart disease, Am. J. Perinatol. 14 (2) (February 1997) 59–62.
[20] T.W. Rowland, J.P. Hubbell Jr., A.S. Nadas, Congenital heart disease in infants of diabetic mothers, J. Pediatr. 83 (5) (November 1973) 815–820.
[21] H.C. Miller, Cardiac hypertrophy in newborn infants, Yale J. Biol. Med. 16 (5) (May 1944) 509–518.1.
[22] H.P. Gutgesell, C.E. Mullins, P.C. Gillette, M. Speer, A.J. Rudolph, D.G. McNamara, Transient hypertrophic subaortic stenosis in infants of diabetic mothers, J. Pediatr. 89 (1) (July 1976) 120–125.
[23] G.L. Way, R.R. Wolfe, E. Eshaghpour, R.L. Bender, R.B. Jaffe, H.D. Ruttenberg, The natural history of hypertrophic cardiomyopathy in infants of diabetic mothers, J. Pediatr. 95 (6) (December 1979) 1020–1025.
[24] R.M. Abu-Sulaiman, B. Subaih, Congenital heart disease in infants of diabetic mothers: echocardiographic study, Pediatr. Cardiol. 25 (2) (March–April 2004) 137–140.
[25] M.J. Cooper, M.A. Enderlein, H. Tarnoff, C.L. Rogé, Asymmetric septal hypertrophy in infants of diabetic mothers. Fetal echocardiography and the impact of maternal diabetic control, Am. J. Dis. Child. 146 (2) (February 1992) 226–229.
[26] M. Vela-Huerta, A. Aguilera-López, S. Alarcón-Santos, N. Amador, C. Aldana-Valenzuela, A. Heredia, Cardiopulmonary adaptation in large for gestational age infants of diabetic and nondiabetic mothers, Acta Paediatr. 96 (9) (September 2007) 1303–1307.
[27] J.N. McMahon, P.J. Berry, H.S. Joffe, Fatal hypertrophic cardiomyopathy in an infant of a diabetic mother, Pediatr. Cardiol. 11 (4) (October 1990) 211–212.
[28] H.P. Gutgesell, M.E. Speer, H.S. Rosenberg, Characterization of the cardiomyopathy in infants of diabetic mothers, Circulation 61 (2) (February 1980) 441–450.
[29] J.P. Moak, J.P. Kaski, Hypertrophic cardiomyopathy in children, Heart 98 (14) (July 2012) 1044–1054.
[30] J.A. Breitweser, R.A. Meyer, M.A. Sperling, R.C. Tsang, S. Kaplan, Cardiac septal hypertrophy in hyperinsulinemic infants, J. Pediatr. 96 (3 Pt 2) (March 1980) 535–539.
[31] N.F. Butte, Carbohydrate and lipid metabolism in pregnancy: normal compared with gestational diabetes mellitus, Am. J. Clin. Nutr. 71 (5 Suppl.) (May 2000) 1256S–1261S.
[32] H. Narchi, N. Kulaylat, Heart disease in infants of diabetic mothers, Images Paediatr. Cardiol. 2 (2) (April 2000) 17–23.
[33] L.K. Hornberger, Maternal diabetes and the fetal heart, Heart 92 (8) (August 2006) 1019–1021.
[34] P.Q. Sheehan, T.W. Rowland, B.L. Shah, V.J. McGravey, E.O. Reiter, Maternal diabetic control and hypertrophic cardiomyopathy in infants of diabetic mothers, Clin. Pediatr. (Phila.) 25 (5) (May 1986) 266–271.
[35] G. Rizzo, D. Arduini, C. Romanini, Accelerated cardiac growth and abnormal cardiac flow in fetuses of type I diabetic mothers, Obstet. Gynecol. 80 (3 Pt 1) (September 1992) 369–376.
[36] R.S. Lindsay, J.A. Westgate, J. Beattie, N.S. Pattison, G. Gamble, L.F. Mildenhall, B.H. Breier, F.D. Johnstone, Inverse changes in fetal insulin-like growth factor (IGF)-1 and IGF binding protein-1 in association with higher birth weight in maternal diabetes, Clin. Endocrinol. (Oxf.) 66 (3) (March 2007) 322–328.
[37] R.G. Rosenfeld, Insulin-like growth factors and the basis of growth, N. Engl. J. Med. 349 (23) (December 4, 2003) 2184–2186.
[38] N.A. Martina, E. Kim, U. Chitkara, N.C. Wathen, T. Chard, L.C. Giudice, Gestational age-dependent expression of insulin-like growth factor-binding protein-1 (IGFBP-1) phosphoisoforms in human extraembryonic cavities, maternal serum, and decidua suggests decidua as the primary source of IGFBP-1 in these fluids during early pregnancy, J. Clin. Endocrinol. Metab. 82 (6) (June 1997) 1894–1898.
[39] A.R. Hayati, F.C. Cheah, A.E. Tan, G.C. Tan, Insulin-like growth factor-1 receptor expression in the placentae of diabetic and normal pregnancies, Early Hum. Dev. 83 (1) (January 2007) 41–46.
[40] S.W. Yang, J.S. Yu, Relationship of insulin-like growth factor-I, insulin-like growth factor binding protein-3, insulin, growth hormone in cord blood and maternal factors with birth height and birthweight, Pediatr. Int. 42 (1) (February 2000) 31–36.
[41] M. Loukovaara, P. Leinonen, K. Teramo, E. Nurminen, S. Andersson, E.M. Rutanen, Effect of maternal diabetes on phosphorylation of insulin-like growth factor binding protein-1 in cord serum, Diabet. Med. 22 (4) (April 2005) 434–439.
[42] F.L. Culler, R.F. Tung, R.A. Jansons, H.D. Mosier, Growth promoting peptides in diabetic and non-diabetic pregnancy: interactions with trophoblastic receptors and serum carrier proteins, J. Pediatr. Endocrinol. Metab. 9 (1) (January–February 1996) 21–29.
[43] T. Huang, A. Kelly, S.A. Becker, M.S. Cohen, C.A. Stanley, Hypertrophic cardiomyopathy in neonates with congenital hyperinsulinism, Arch. Dis. Child. Fetal Neonatal. Ed. 98 (4) (July 2013) F351–F354.

[44] M.G. Sardesai, A.A. Gray, M.M. McGrath, S.E. Ford, Fatal hypertrophic cardiomyopathy in the fetus of a woman with diabetes, Obstet. Gynecol. 98 (5 Pt 2) (November 2001) 925–927.

[45] M.R. Reid, Partial occlusion of the pulmonary aorta and inferior vena cava with the metallic band. Observations on changes in the vessel wall and in the in the heart, J. Exp. Med. 40 (1924) 289–292.

[46] W.H. Muller, J.F. Dammann, The treatment of certain congenital mal-formations of the heart by the creation of pulmonic stenosis to reduce pulmonary hypertension and excessive pulmonary blood flow, Surg. Gynecol. Obstet. 95 (2) (1952) 213–219.

[47] R. Sharma, Pulmonary artery banding: rationale and possible indications in the current era, Ann. Pediatr. Cardiol. 5 (1) (2012) 40–43.

[48] I.L. Kron, S.P. Nolan, T.L. Flanagan, H.P. Gutgesell, W.H. Muller, Pulmonary artery banding revisited, Ann. Surg. 209 (5) (1989) 642–647.

[49] A. Goldblatt, W.F. Bernhard, A.S. Nadas, R.E. Gross, Pulmonary artery banding: indications and results in infants and children, Circulation 32 (1965) 172–184.

[50] K.J. Dooley, L. Parisi-Buckley, D.C. Fyler, A.S. Nadas, Results of pulmonary arterial banding in infancy. Survey of 5 years' experience in the New England regional infant cardiac program, Am. J. Cardiol. 36 (4) (1975) 484–488.

[51] R.M. Freedom, H. Sondheimer, R. Dische, R.D. Rowe, Development of "subaortic stenosis" after pulmonary arterial banding for common ventricle, Am. J. Cardiol. 39 (1) (1977) 78–83.

[52] J. Somerville, L. Becu, D. Ross, Common ventricle with acquired subaortic obstruction, Am. J. Cardiol. 34 (1974) 206–214.

[53] R.M. Freedom, L.N. Benson, J.F. Smallhorn, W.G. Williams, G.A. Trusler, R.D. Rowe, Subaortic stenosis, the univentricular heart, and banding of the pulmonary artery: an analysis of the courses of 43 patients with univentricular heart palliated by pulmonary artery banding, Circulation 73 (4) (1986) 758–764.

[54] S.L. Hess, J.T. Bricker, A. Garson, D. Ott, G.J. Reul, D.A. Cooley, Pulmonary artery banding and subaortic stenosis in patients with single ventricle: surgical alternatives and clinical outcomes, Tex. Heart Inst. J. 19 (1992) 15–20.

[55] C. Boutin, R.A. Jonas, S.P. Sanders, G. Wernovsky, S.M. Mone, S.D. Colan, Rapid two-stage arterial switch operation. Acquisition of left ventricular mass after pulmonary artery banding in infants with transposition of the great arteries, Circulation 90 (1994) 1304–1309.

[56] C. Apitz, O. Honjo, T. Humpl, J. Li, R.S. Assad, M.Y. Cho, J. Hong, M.K. Friedberg, A.N. Redington, Biventricular structural and functional responses to aortic constriction in a rabbit model of chronic right ventricular pressure overload, J. Thorac. Cardiovasc. Surg. 144 (2012) 1494–1501.

[57] M.K. Friedberg, M.Y. Cho, J. Li, R.S. Assad, M. Sun, S. Rohailla, O. Honjo, C. Apitz, A.N. Redington, Adverse biventricular remodeling in isolated right ventricular hypertension is mediated by increased transforming growth factor–b1 signaling and is abrogated by angiotensin receptor blockade, Am. J. Respir. Cell Mol. Biol. 49 (6) (December 2013) 1019–1028.

[58] M.M. Laks, F. Morady, H.J.C. Swan, Canine right and left ventricular cell and sarcomere lengths after banding the pulmonary artery, Circ. Res. 24 (1969) 705–710.

[59] S. Minegishi, K. Kitahori, A. Murakami, M. Ono, Mechanism of pressure-overload right ventricular hypertrophy in infant rabbits, Int. Heart J. 52 (2011) 56–60.

[60] A. Azakie, J. Fineman, Y. He, Differential responses of the right ventricle to abnormal loading conditions in vivo: possible pathophysiologic mechanisms, J. Thorac. Cardiovasc. Surg. 145 (2013) 1335–1344.

[61] K. Orito, T. Yamane, T. Kanai, Y. Fujii, Y. Wakao, H. Matsuda, Time course sequences of angiotensin converting enzyme and chymase-like activities during development of right ventricular hypertrophy induced by pulmonary artery constriction in dogs, Life Sci. 75 (2004) 1135–1145.

[62] A.M. Sheikh, C. Barrett, N. Villamizar, O. Alzate, A.M. Valente, J.R. Herlong, D. Craig, A. Lodge, J. Lawson, C. Milano, J. Jaggers, Right Ventricular hypertrophy with early dysfunction: a proteomics study in a neonatal model, J. Thorac. Cardiovasc. Surg. 137 (2009) 1146–1153.

[63] E.P. Bauer, S. Kuki, M. Arras, R. Zimmerman, W. Schaper, Increased growth factor transcription after pulmonary artery banding, Eur. J. Cardiothorac. Surg. 11 (1997) 818–823.

[64] G.A. Favaro, R.S. Assad, M.C.D. Abduch, G.J.J. Silva, G.S. Gomes, J.L. Andrade, J.E. Krieger, L.F.P. Moreira, Reversible pulmonary trunk banding. VII: stress echocardiographic assessment of rapid ventricular hypertrophy in young goats, J. Thorac. Cardiovasc. Surg. 145 (2013) 1245–1251.

[65] R. Assad, F.A. Atik, F.S. Oliveira, M.H. Fonseca-Alaniz, M.C. Abduch, G.J.J. Silva, G.A. Favaro, J.E. Krieger, N.A.G. Stolf, Reversible pulmonary trunk banding. VI: glucose-6-phosphate dehydrogenase activity in rapid ventricular hypertrophy in young goats, J. Thorac. Cardiovasc. Surg. 142 (2011) 1108–1113.

[66] H. Dores, A. Freitas, A. Malhotra, M. Mendes, S. Sharma, The hearts of competitive athletes: an up-to-date overview of exercise-induced cardiac adaptations, Rev. Port. Cardiol. 34 (1) (January 2015) 51–64.

[67] S. Henschen, Skidlauf und skidwettlauf: eine medizinische sport-studie, Mitt Med. Klin. Upsala (1899) 2.

[68] E.A. Darling, The effects of training: a study of the Harvard University crews, Boston Med. Surg. J. 161 (1899) 229–233.

[69] C.L. Tung, C.K. Hsieh, C.W. Bien, F.R. Dieuaide, The heart in ricksha pullers. A study of the effect of chronic exertion on the cardiovascular system, Am. Heart J. 10 (1934) 79–100.

[70] P.D. White, Heart Disease, fourth ed., MacMillan Co., New York, 1951, p. 612.

[71] J. Morganroth, B.J. Maron, W.L. Henry, S.E. Epstein, Comparative left ventricular dimensions in trained athletes, Ann. Intern. Med. 82 (4) (April 1975) 521–524.

[72] J. Morganroth, B.J. Maron, The athlete's heart syndrome: a new perspective, Ann. N.Y. Acad. Sci. 301 (1977) 931–941.

[73] A. D'Andrea, G. Limongelli, P. Caso, B. Sarubbi, A. Della Pietra, P. Brancaccio, G. Cice, M. Scherillo, F. Limongelli, R. Calabrò, Association between left ventricular structure and cardiac performance during effort in two morphological forms of athlete's heart, Int. J. Cardiol. 86 (2–3) (December 2002) 177–184.

[74] B.M. Pluim, A.H. Zwinderman, A. van der Laarse, E.E. van der Wall, The athlete's heart. A meta-analysis of cardiac structure and function, Circulation 101 (3) (January 25, 2000) 336–344.

[75] P. Spirito, A. Pelliccia, M.A. Proschan, M. Granata, A. Spataro, P. Bellone, G. Caselli, A. Biffi, C. Vecchio, B.J. Maron, Morphology of the "athlete's heart" assessed by echocardiography in 947 elite athletes representing 27 sports, Am. J. Cardiol. 74 (8) (October 15, 1994) 802–806.

[76] L.H. Naylor, K. George, G. O'Driscoll, D.J. Green, The athlete's heart: a contemporary appraisal of the 'Morganroth hypothesis', Sports Med. 38 (1) (2008) 69–90.

[77] V. Utomi, D. Oxborough, E. Ashley, R. Lord, S. Fletcher, M. Stembridge, R. Shave, M.D. Hoffman, G. Whyte, J. Somauroo, S. Sharma, K. George, Predominance of normal left ventricular geometry in the male 'athlete's heart', Heart 100 (16) (August 2014) 1264–1271.

[78] A.L. Spence, L.H. Naylor, H.H. Carter, C.L. Buck, L. Dembo, C.P. Murray, P. Watson, D. Oxborough, K.P. George, D.J. Green, A prospective randomised longitudinal MRI study of left ventricular adaptation to endurance and resistance exercise training in humans, J. Physiol. 589 (Pt 22) (November 15, 2011) 5443–5452.

[79] M.J. Haykowsky, K.K. Teo, A.H. Quinney, D.P. Humen, D.A. Taylor, Effects of long term resistance training on left ventricular morphology, Can. J. Cardiol. 16 (1) (January 2000) 35–38.

[80] M.J. Haykowsky, H.A. Quinney, R. Gillis, C.R. Thompson, Left ventricular morphology in junior and master resistance trained athletes, Med. Sci. Sports Exerc. 32 (2) (February 2000) 349–352.

[81] A. Pelliccia, B.J. Maron, A. Spataro, M.A. Proschan, P. Spirito, The upper limit of physiologic cardiac hypertrophy in highly trained elite athletes, N. Engl. J. Med. 324 (5) (January 31, 1991) 295–301.

[82] A. Pelliccia, M.S. Maron, B.J. Maron, Assessment of left ventricular hypertrophy in a trained athlete: differential diagnosis of physiologic athlete's heart from pathologic hypertrophy, Prog. Cardiovasc. Dis. 54 (5) (March–April 2012) 387–396.

[83] S. Caselli, M.S. Maron, J.A. Urbano-Moral, N.G. Pandian, B.J. Maron, A. Pelliccia, Differentiating left ventricular hypertrophy in athletes from that in patients with hypertrophic cardiomyopathy, Am. J. Cardiol. 114 (9) (November 1, 2014) 1383–1389.

[84] B.J. Maron, Hypertrophic cardiomyopathy: a systematic review, JAMA 287 (10) (March 13, 2002) 1308–1320.

[85] S. Sharma, B.J. Maron, G. Whyte, S. Firoozi, P.M. Elliott, W.J. McKenna, Physiologic limits of left ventricular hypertrophy in elite junior athletes: relevance to differential diagnosis of athlete's heart and hypertrophic cardiomyopathy, J. Am. Coll. Cardiol. 40 (8) (October 16, 2002) 1431–1436.

[86] A. Pelliccia, B.J. Maron, F. Culasso, A. Spataro, G. Caselli, Athlete's heart in women. Echocardiographic characterization of highly trained elite female athletes, JAMA 276 (3) (July 17, 1996) 211–215.

[87] J. Rawlins, F. Carre, G. Kervio, M. Papadakis, N. Chandra, C. Edwards, G.P. Whyte, S. Sharma, Ethnic differences in physiological cardiac adaptation to intense physical exercise in highly trained female athletes, Circulation 121 (9) (March 9, 2010) 1078–1085.

[88] S. Basavarajaiah, A. Boraita, G. Whyte, M. Wilson, L. Carby, A. Shah, S. Sharma, Ethnic differences in left ventricular remodeling in highly-trained athletes relevance to differentiating physiologic left ventricular hypertrophy from hypertrophic cardiomyopathy, J. Am. Coll. Cardiol. 51 (23) (June 10, 2008) 2256–2262.

[89] H.E. Montgomery, P. Clarkson, C.M. Dollery, K. Prasad, M.A. Losi, H. Hemingway, D. Statters, M. Jubb, M. Girvain, A. Varnava, M. World, J. Deanfield, P. Talmud, J.R. McEwan, W.J. McKenna, S. Humphries, Association of angiotensin-converting enzyme gene I/D polymorphism with change in left ventricular mass in response to physical training, Circulation 96 (3) (August 5, 1997) 741–747.

[90] J. Karjalainen, U.M. Kujala, A. Stolt, M. Mäntysaari, M. Viitasalo, K. Kainulainen, K. Kontula, Angiotensinogen gene M235T polymorphism predicts left ventricular hypertrophy in endurance athletes, J. Am. Coll. Cardiol. 34 (2) (August 1999) 494–499.

[91] B.J. Maron, A. Pelliccia, A. Spataro, M. Granata, Reduction in left ventricular wall thickness after deconditioning in highly trained olympic athletes, Br. Heart J. 69 (2) (February 1993) 125–128.

[92] A. Pelliccia, B.J. Maron, R. De Luca, F.M. Di Paolo, A. Spataro, F. Culasso, Remodeling of left ventricular hypertrophy in elite athletes after long-term deconditioning, Circulation 105 (8) (February 26, 2002) 944–949.

[93] A. D'Andrea, A. La Gerche, E. Golia, R. Padalino, R. Calabrò, M.G. Russo, E. Bossone, Physiologic and pathophysiologic changes in the right heart in highly trained athletes, Herz 40 (3) (May 2015) 369–378.

FURTHER READING

[1] S.C. Gupta, K.D. Varian, N.C. Bal, J.L. Abraham, M. Periasamy, P.M.L. Janssen, Pulmonary artery banding alters the expression of Ca^{2+} transport proteins in the right atrium in rabbits, Am. J. Physiol. Heart Circ. Physiol. 296 (2009) H1933–H1939.

Chapter 5

Hemodynamic Adaptive Mechanisms in Heart Failure

Alexander Hussey[1], Lucas Eastaugh[1,2], Robert G. Weintraub[1,2,3]
[1]The Royal Children's Hospital, Melbourne, VIC, Australia; [2]Murdoch Children's Research Institute, Melbourne, VIC, Australia; [3]University of Melbourne, Melbourne, VIC, Australia

INTRODUCTION

To understand the pathophysiological processes that occur in heart failure we need to first understand the normal cardiovascular physiology. To facilitate the autoregulation of blood pressure, there is a complex interplay of circulatory, neurohormonal, and molecular changes to not only help maintain distal organ perfusion but also trigger cardiac muscle changes to compensate for any abnormality. In a healthy well-functioning heart these compensatory mechanisms are usually efficient and only transiently stimulated. However, in a failing heart these mechanisms are chronically overstimulated and change from being physiological and adaptive to pathophysiological and maladaptive.

CARDIAC FUNCTION

Stroke Volume

In a structurally and functionally normal heart, the right ventricle ejects a volume of blood into the pulmonary artery, and almost simultaneously the left ventricle (LV) ejects a volume into the aorta with each cardiac contraction. If these "stroke volumes" (SV) are averaged over time then the SV from each ventricle can be considered to be equal. In general terms, SV is defined as the volume of blood ejected by the LV into the aorta with each contraction. If the heart has an intracardiac shunt (e.g., atrioventricular (AV) septal defect, ventricular septal defect) or left AV valve regurgitation, then this definition becomes flawed, as some of the SV will not be ejected into the aorta. A more precise definition for SV is the difference between ventricular end-diastolic volume (EDV) and end-systolic volume (ESV).

$$SV = EDV - ESV$$

The three primary factors that regulate EDV and ESV, and therefore SV, are as follows:

- Preload
- Afterload
- Contractility (inotropy)

Preload

This is the force that stretches the cardiac myocytes prior to contraction and is dependent on sarcomere length.

Preload is increased by the following:

- Increased central venous pressure (CVP), e.g., from decreased venous compliance due to sympathetic activation; increased blood volume; respiratory augmentation; increased skeletal pump activity.
- Increased ventricular compliance.
- Increased atrial contraction.
- Reduced heart rate (increased ventricular filling time).
- Increased afterload (increased ESV, reduces SV, and leads to a secondary increase in preload).

Heart Failure in the Child and Young Adult. http://dx.doi.org/10.1016/B978-0-12-802393-8.00005-3

Preload is decreased by the following:

- Decreased CVP (e.g., hypovolemia).
- Impaired atrial contraction (e.g., due to atrial arrhythmias).
- Increased heart rate (decreased ventricular filling time).
- Decreased afterload (reduced ESV, increases SV, and leads to secondary decrease in preload).
- AV valve stenosis

The effect of preload on SV is described by the Frank–Starling mechanism (Fig. 5.1) eponymously attributed to the German-born doctor and physiologist, Otto Frank (1865–1944), and later work by the English physiologist, Ernest Starling (1866–1927). This is described as the "principal mechanism by which the heart adapts to changing inflow of blood. When the cardiac muscle becomes stretched an extra amount, as it does when extra amounts of blood enter the heart chambers, the stretched muscle contracts with a greatly increased force, thereby automatically pumping the extra blood into the arteries" [1].

In laboratory studies, when isolated cardiac muscle is stimulated to contract at a low resting length (low preload) with all other factors kept constant, the amount of active tension that develops is relatively small. If the cardiac muscle is stimulated to contract at a larger preload length, the active tension is greatly increased in a directly proportional way. There is an increased sensitivity of troponin C to calcium (Ca^{2+}) in the cardiac myocytes [2,3] and less spacing between the myofilaments, which allows a greater number of actin–myosin cross bridges to form. This results in a greater force of contraction and so increased SV [2,4,5].

When a normal cardiac muscle fiber is allowed to shorten against a fixed afterload (isotonic contraction), an increase in muscle length prior to contraction (increased preload) causes an increase in the amount of shortening but to the same minimal length, as well as an increase in the velocity of shortening. This response is intrinsic to the individual heart and can be modified by extrinsic neurohormonal mechanisms and by the afterload and inotropic state. Increasing afterload or decreasing inotropy shifts the curve downward and rightward, resulting in a lower SV at a given left ventricular end-diastolic pressure (LVEDP). Conversely, decreasing the afterload and increasing inotropy shifts the curve upward and leftward, resulting in a greater SV at a given LVEDP. The active tension that develops due to preload can increase but only to a maximal limit, which corresponds to the length of a sarcomere (1.6–2.2 μm) [6]. The greater stiffness of cardiac muscle normally prevents its sarcomeres from being stretched beyond their length, unlike sarcomeres in skeletal muscle, which can stretch beyond their length.

In the early stages of heart failure, the Frank–Starling mechanism has an important compensatory role to maintain SV. However, in established heart failure, the relevance of the Frank–Starling mechanism is controversial. Some studies have shown that the failing heart is unable to develop an appropriate increase in SV when subjected to increased preload (Fig. 5.2). This is shown by the Frank–Starling curve being so significantly flattened that the failing heart operates at the top or near the top of the curve already [7,8]. This is thought to be due to a failure in troponin C developing an increase in Ca^{2+} sensitivity [9].

Afterload

This is the "load" the heart must eject against following ventricular contraction and is affected by aortic pressure and systemic vascular resistance (SVR). SVR is the combined resistance to blood flow from all of the systemic vasculature (not the pulmonary vasculature). An isolated increase in afterload due to increased SVR should theoretically result in a decrease in SV due to

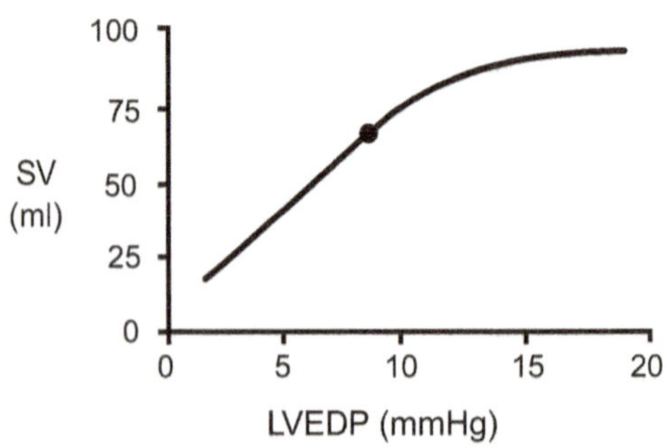

FIGURE 5.1 Frank–Starling mechanism—increasing preload increases LVEDP and SV. In an adult the mean operating point (dot on curve) occurs at LVEDP ~8 mmHg and SV ~70 ml. *LVEDP*, left ventricular end-diastolic pressure; *SV*, stroke volume.

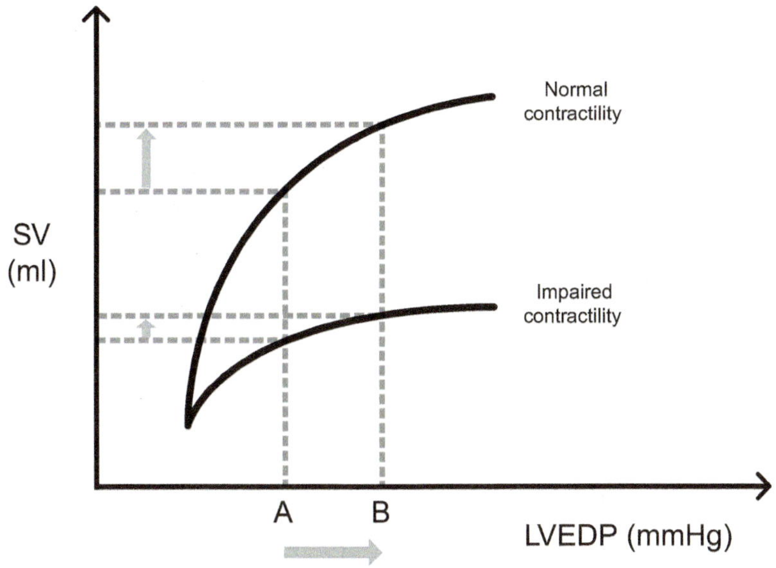

FIGURE 5.2 Effect of heart failure on the Frank–Starling curve. Increase in LVEDP (from A to B) can result either in a significant or in a negligible increase in SV depending on the steepness of the Frank–Starling curve. Thus preload responsiveness occurs in normal functioning hearts, and relative preload unresponsiveness occurs in impaired ventricular contractility. *LVEDP*, left ventricular end-diastolic pressure; *SV*, stroke volume. *(Adapted from Science Direct database: Guerin, Monnet, Teboul, Monitoring volume and fluid responsiveness: From static to dynamic indicators, Best Practice Res. Clin. Anaesthesiol. 27 (2) (2013) 177–185).*

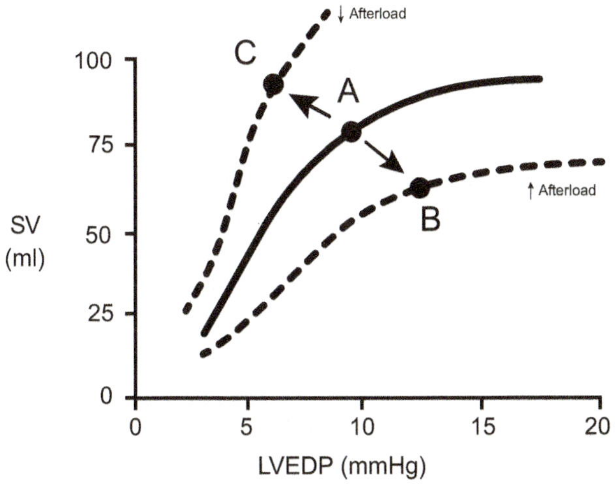

FIGURE 5.3 Effect of afterload on Frank–Starling curve. Increasing afterload shifts the curve down and to the right (from point A to B), which decreases SV and increases LVEDP. In contrast, a decrease in afterload shifts the Frank–Starling curve up and to the left (A to C), which increases SV and at the same time reduces LVEDP. *LVEDP*, left ventricular end-diastolic pressure; *SV*, stroke volume. *Adapted and used with permission by Dr Richard E. Klabunde, Cardiovascular Physiology Concepts (cvphysiology.com).*

diminished ventricular muscle fiber shortening (increased left ventricular end-systolic volume, LVESV). However, the process is a lot more complicated in a healthy heart due to the Anrep effect where homeostatic mechanisms try to maintain a relatively constant SV as the arterial blood pressure varies [10]. If there is a sudden increase in afterload, there is a compensatory rapid decrease in cardiac ejection and so increase in LVESV and LVEDV. The LV responds by initially increasing contractility (as per the Frank–Starling mechanism (Fig. 5.3)), which is largely due to increased troponin C sensitivity to Ca^{2+}. However, if this increased afterload is sustained for 10–15 min, contractility increases further and LVESV and LVEDV begin to decrease. This delayed compensatory response likely involves several mechanisms that promote increased calcium release by the sarcoplasmic reticulum mediated by various mediators (e.g., endothelin-1, angiotensin II) and increased calcium sensitivity with consequent rise in cross-bridge formation and myocardial force generation.

In heart failure, SV is very sensitive to changes in afterload due to the already impaired contractility and that the Anrep effect does not adequately compensate for the physiological changes. The ventricular wall is usually thin around a dilated cavity, and so at a given pressure, wall stress is increased and this leads to further maladaptive structural and molecular changes.

SVR is determined by vessel diameter, vessel length, and blood viscosity, which is represented by Poiseuille's equation:

$$F = \frac{\pi \Delta P \cdot r^4}{8\eta \cdot L}$$

F, flow; ΔP, pressure difference; r, radius of vessel; η, viscosity of fluid; L, length of vessel.

Jean Léonard Marie Poiseuille was a 19th century French physician who described that a decrease in vessel radius would increase the resistance to the power of four of the change in radius. This was assuming that the flow was laminar and constant velocity, and that the fluid was incompressible and Newtonian. So a reduction in the radius by 50% will increase resistance by a factor of 16 and thus decrease blood flow by a factor of 16 assuming the pressure gradient is constant, laminar flow conditions, and that the resistance of the segment studied is representative of the total resistance to flow.

Systemic vascular function curves (Fig. 5.4) compare the effects on right atrial pressure (RA_P) by changes in cardiac output (CO). If CO is stopped, then the aortic blood pressure falls and RA_P increases and peaks at the mean circulatory filling pressure (P_{mc}) if the baroreceptor response to the hypotension is blocked. In a healthy adult heart the P_{mc} is approximately 8 mmHg, which is due to the 10–20 times greater compliance of veins in comparison to arteries. So when the heart stops, the volume and pressure of blood in the arteries decreases and increases in the veins. If the CO is restarted, then RA_P decreases as CO increases (curve moves upward and leftward). When RA_P falls below 0 mmHg, the increase in CO plateaus because the venae cavae collapse, thus limiting venous return to the heart. The systemic vascular function curve is affected by blood volume, venous compliance, and SVR (graph A). If blood volume is increased, or venous compliance is decreased due to activation of the sympathetic division of the autonomic nervous system, there is a shift of the curve to the right. Then if the heart is stopped, the resultant P_{mc} value is increased. Conversely, if SVR is increased (graph B), the slope of the curve decreases with little or no change in the P_{mc} value due to the relatively less arterial compliance.

SVR is affected by local regulatory systems and by extrinsic mechanisms. Locally, organs are able to regulate their own blood flow through the vascular endothelium and by various vasoactive metabolites released by the tissue surrounding blood vessels. Important extrinsic mechanisms are the autonomic nervous system and circulating vasoactive hormones (e.g., angiotensin II, epinephrine, norepinephrine, vasopressin, atrial natriuretic peptide, and endothelin), which are all stimulated in heart failure.

SVR is also affected by blood viscosity. Viscosity is an intrinsic property of a fluid related to the internal friction (resistance) with adjacent fluid levels sliding past one another. Water is a homogenous fluid that is described as Newtonian, and therefore under nonturbulent conditions, its viscosity is independent of flow velocity. However, blood is a non-Newtonian fluid as it consists of plasma and cells, which means that its viscosity changes with flow velocity. Under normal conditions, red cells have the greatest effect on viscosity with an increase in hematocrit leading to a nonlinear increase in relative viscosity and an increase in blood flow resistance. This effect is enhanced in heart failure where the microcirculatory blood flow in the tissues is reduced because of reduced arterial pressures. Low flow states can lead to a large increase in viscosity and allow increased molecular interactions to occur between cells and plasma proteins. This may lead to rouleaux formation where red cells stick together to form chains within the microcirculation, which further increases blood viscosity and may lead to thrombus formation if the coagulation system is also stimulated [11].

Contractility

This is the intrinsic ability of a ventricle to contract at a defined preload and afterload. Skeletal muscle is able to modulate the contractile force generation through changes in motor nerve activity and motor unit recruitment. However, when cardiac muscle contracts then all the muscle fibers are activated and only changes in fiber length (preload) and changes in inotropy alter the amount of force generated. However in heart failure, contractility is often impaired, which will decrease SV. This will be exacerbated by the structural and molecular changes that occur to the myocytes due to the chronic overstimulation of the neurohormonal compensatory mechanisms as discussed later.

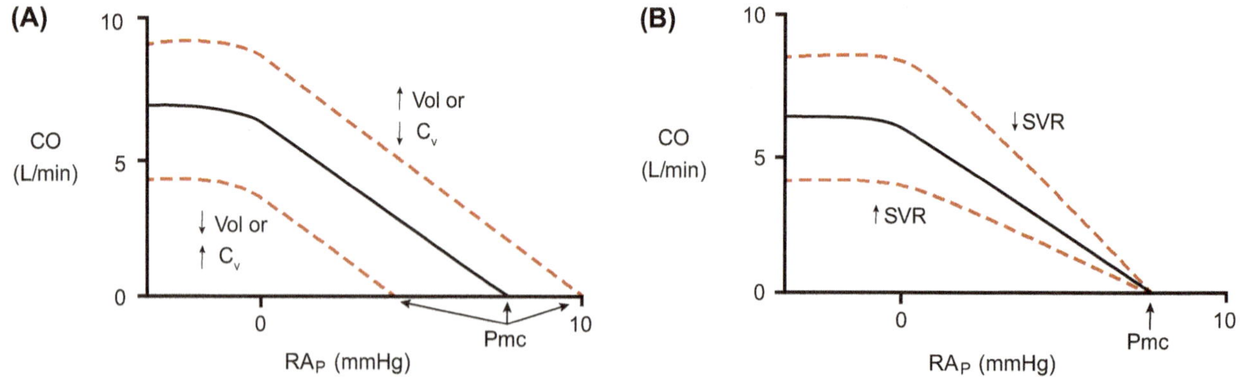

FIGURE 5.4 Systemic vascular function curves. *CO*, cardiac output; *C_V*, venous compliance; *Pmc*, mean circulating filling pressure; *RA_P*, right atrial pressure; *SVR*, systemic vascular resistance; *Vol*, blood volume. *(Adapted and used with permission by Dr Richard E. Klabunde, Cardiovascular Physiology Concepts (cvphysiology.com).)*

Cardiac Output/Cardiac Index

The CO is the cumulative SV over a minute and is measured in milliliters per minute (ml/min).

$$CO = SV \times HR = (EDV - ESV) \times HR.$$

CO, cardiac output; SV, stroke volume; HR, heart rate; EDV, end-diastolic volume; ESV, end-systolic volume.

Basal CO differs among individuals of different sizes and so cardiac index is a more useful measurement. This is the CO per body surface area and has unit, ml/min/m^2. The factors that affect heart rate and SV will affect CO. The maintenance and regulation of CO is normally proportional to the demand for oxygen and other nutrients by other tissues and organs. During exercise, the normal physiological response is to increase CO by increasing chronotropy and inotropy. If we consider heart failure where there is low CO due to poor contractility, various neurohormonal mechanisms are stimulated to compensate. The most rapid compensatory change is positive chronotropy, which is mainly achieved via various neurohormonal mechanisms but primarily stimulation of the sympathetic division of the autonomic nervous system. This is initially a helpful adaptive process to try to improve CO. However, as the heart rate increases it leads to reduced time for diastolic relaxation, reduced diastolic-dependent coronary perfusion and increased myocardial oxygen demand. If sustained this can lead to myocardial ischemia.

The American physiologist, Arthur Guyton, carried out animal studies in the 1950s and 1960s [11a,11b] assessing the relationship between cardiac function and SVR. These interactions were described in cardiac function curves Fig. 5.5, which are similar to Frank–Starling curves except have RA_P replacing LVEDP on the x-axis and CO replacing SV on the y-axis. The curves show that very small changes in RA_P, a matter of a few mmHg, can lead to large changes in CO. If cardiac function is enhanced (e.g., during exercise) by increased inotropy, increased chronotropy, or reduced afterload, then CO increases more with smaller changes in RA_P. When cardiac performance is depressed (e.g., in heart failure), then the changes are less marked.

When cardiac and vascular function curves are combined (Fig. 5.6), the intersect of the two curves (point A) represents the steady-state operating point for those particular physiological conditions. If cardiac function is depressed as in heart failure then the cardiac function curve shifts downward and rightward, and the intercept moves to point B. This describes the increase in RA_P and venous pressures along with a decrease in CO. If the depressed cardiac function is accompanied by an increase in blood volume, reduced venous compliance or increased SVR, which occurs in heart failure, the systemic function curve will shift rightward with a reduced slope gradient. The new operating point moves to point C where there is an improvement in CO in comparison to point B. This demonstrates how systemic vascular function changes help to partially restore CO despite depressed cardiac function. However, this comes at the expense of increased RA_P and venous pressures, which leads to worsening features of congestive cardiac failure.

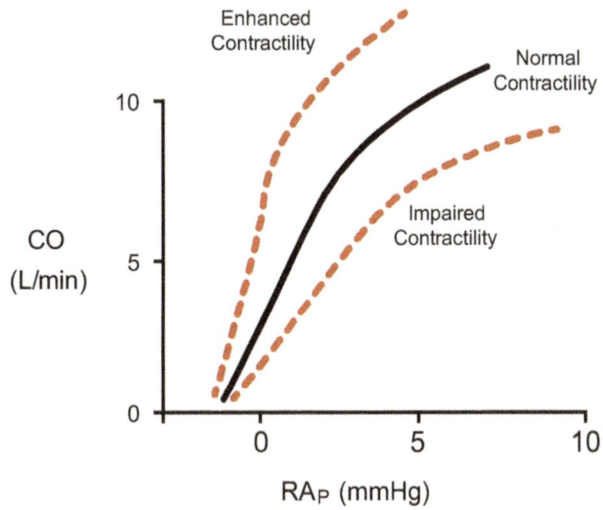

FIGURE 5.5 Cardiac function curves. *CO*, cardiac output; *RA_P*, right atrial pressure. *Adapted and used with permission by Dr Richard E. Klabunde, Cardiovascular Physiology Concepts (cvphysiology.com).*

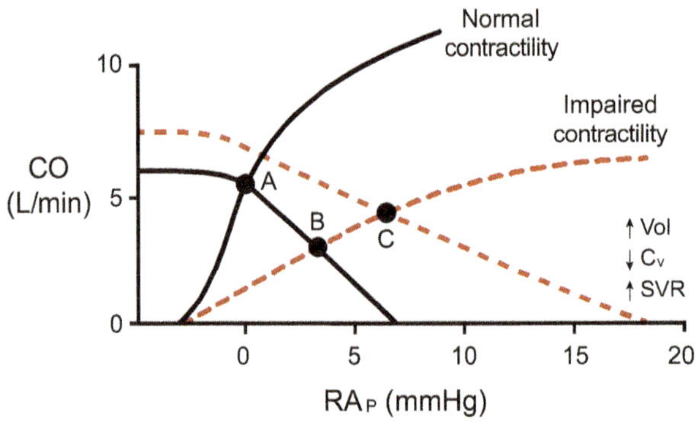

FIGURE 5.6 Combined cardiac and vascular function curves. *CO*, cardiac output; C_V, venous compliance; RA_P, right atrial pressure; *SVR*, systemic vascular resistance; *Vol*, volume. *(Adapted and used with permission by Dr Richard E. Klabunde, Cardiovascular Physiology Concepts (cvphysiology.com).)*

NEUROHORMONAL COMPENSATORY MECHANISMS

Neurohormonal mechanisms describe a complex interaction between the autonomic nervous system, catecholamines (epinephrine, norepinephrine), circulating hormones (renin-angiotensin-aldosterone system), and a variety of peptides, growth factors and cytokines. In response to the effects of reduced cardiac function from heart failure, these neurohormonal mechanisms are stimulated to help compensate. Neurohormonal is actually a historical misnomer originating from the early recognition that some of the early compensatory mechanisms were neuroendocrine and acted in an endocrine fashion. It is now recognized that some of these "neurohormones" are also produced by the myocardium and act in a paracrine and autocrine fashion and some are actually peptides, growth factors, or cytokines produced by a number of cell types.

Autonomic Nervous System and Circulating Catecholamines

The autonomic nervous system has many biological roles including an important rapid-acting autoregulatory effect on the cardiovascular system. It originates in the medulla oblongata in the brainstem and consists of two main divisions—sympathetic and parasympathetic nervous systems. These two divisions generally have antagonistic effects, but usually complement each other to modulate vital functions to achieve homeostasis. In simple terms, the sympathetic nervous system is a "quick response mobilizing system," while the parasympathetic nervous system is a "more slowly activated dampening system."

Sympathetic Nervous System

The preganglionic neurons of the sympathetic nervous system originate in the lateral gray column from the thoracic and lumbar spinal cord (T1 to L2-3) where they emerge and synapse with postganglionic neurons at ganglia before innervating various organs. The preganglionic neurons also synapse directly with the chromaffin cells of the adrenal medulla. The chromaffin cells are modified postganglionic sympathetic neurons that have lost their axon and dendrites and when stimulated secrete catecholamines into the bloodstream by exocytosis [12]. Sympathetic efferent nerves are present throughout the atria (especially the sinoatrial (SA) node) and ventricles, including the conduction system of the heart. They also innervate the vascular system by traveling along arteries and veins and are found in the adventitia (outer wall of a blood vessel). Small enlargements along the nerve fibers called varicosities, are the site of neurotransmitter (primarily norepinephrine) release stimulating vascular changes.

Circulating Catecholamines

When the sympathetic nervous system stimulates the chromaffin cells of the adrenal medulla, there is a release of catecholamines into the bloodstream. The two circulating catecholamines are epinephrine and norepinephrine, which are released in times of stress (e.g., exercise, heart failure, hemorrhage, and pain). About 80% of the total catecholamine released from the chromaffin cells is epinephrine and 20% is norepinephrine [13]. The primary source for norepinephrine is the sympathetic nerves innervating blood vessels, as described above [14].

The sympathetic nervous system is not just the only stimulant of the chromaffin cells, there are in fact a number of different receptors attached on the cell membrane, which when activated lead to catecholamine release. These include muscarinic cholinergic receptors [15], angiotensin II receptors [16], and histaminergic receptors [17].

When epinephrine binds to β1-adrenoceptors (β1-ARs) on myocytes, it rapidly causes an increase in the cytosolic Ca^{2+} concentration through Ca^{2+} influx, Ca^{2+} release from the sarcoplasmic reticulum, and also increases the rate up Ca^{2+} uptake by the sarcoplasmic reticulum through disinhibition of a protein called phospholamban. This results in increased heart rate (positive chronotropy), increased force of contraction (positive inotropy), increased speed of electrical conduction of AV node (positive dromotropy), and increased relaxation in diastole (positive lusitropy). In addition, at low-to-moderate concentrations of epinephrine, it preferentially binds to β2-ARs causing peripheral vasodilation (decreased SVR) and increased blood flow to the muscle and liver. However, at higher concentrations, there is an increased proportion of binding to α-ARs, which shifts the result to net vasoconstriction (increased SVR) and affecting blood flow to other organs and tissues.

When norepinephrine binds to β1-ARs on myocytes it transiently causes positive chronotropy, positive inotropy, positive dromotropy, and positive lusitropy but these actions are rapidly counteracted by the activation of baroreceptors and the parasympathetic branch of the autonomic nervous system. The predominant effect of norepinephrine is vasoconstriction of systemic blood vessels through stimulation of postjunctional α1-AR and α2-AR (increased SVR).

In the short term, activation of the sympathetic nervous system acts rapidly in providing beneficial homeostasis of many body systems [18]. However, when the sympathetic nervous system is chronically overstimulated, as is the case in heart failure, then it leads to negative pathophysiological consequences [19]. When overstimulated, there tends to be regional stimulation preferentially directed to the heart and kidneys rather than affecting all the normal target organs [20]. In normal conditions, most of the norepinephrine released by sympathetic nerves is reabsorbed and metabolized by the nerves and extra-neuronal tissues, and only a small amount spills over into the circulation. However, at times of high sympathetic nerve stimulation, this amount of spill-over dramatically increases [21], and there is good evidence that plasma concentration of norepinephrine is negatively associated with survival in heart failure patients [22].

The effects of the overstimulated sympathetic nervous system have been understood from patients suffering with pheochromocytoma. This is a rare neuroendocrine tumor usually of the chromaffin cells of the adrenal medulla. The effects include the following:

- Positive chronotropy and inotropy, which increases metabolic demand and reduced coronary perfusion [23].
- Increased risk of tachyarrhythmia
- Reduced diastolic function. This is related to the combined effects of less time for passive ventricular filling due to tachycardia and reduced myocardial compliance due to myocardial hypertrophy and fibrosis [24].
- Myocyte hypertrophy by direct action by binding to α–ARs and selective β-ARs on cardiac myocytes [25,26].
- Myocyte toxicity and associated cardiac structural changes through promotion of myocyte apoptosis and necrosis, free radical production monocytic inflammation, and calcium deposition [27,28].
- Fibroblast hyperplasia with increased collagen deposition and myocardial fibrosis [29].
- Stimulates release of proinflammatory cytokines [30].

The body responds to these deleterious effects by deactivating the β-ARs by a process called desensitization. This is achieved by reducing the number (downregulation) [31,32] and loss of function (receptor uncoupling) [32,33] of the β-ARs. In fact the β1-subtype undergoes more downregulation, while the β2-subtype undergoes more uncoupling [34,35]. Reduction in the receptor numbers occurs early on in heart failure [36] and correlates with disease severity [25]. Several mechanisms occur to cause receptor uncoupling. The most prominent mechanism involves firstly phosphorylation of the receptor by a specific G protein-coupled receptor kinase called β-AR kinase [37], which is then bound by the β-arrestin protein [38]. This final process inhibits the β-AR function by up to 70% [39,40]. This is also the first step in the internalization and downregulation of the receptor. This process of desensitization is considered to be cardioprotective to counteract the deleterious effects of chronic sympathetic nervous system overstimulation but at the detriment of reduced inotropy [41].

Parasympathetic Nervous System

The parasympathetic division of the autonomic nervous system has a craniosacral outflow with efferent nerves originating in the brainstem (cranial nerves III, VII, IX, X) and at the sacral spinal cord (S2-S4). The left and right vagus nerves (cranial nerve X) leave the medulla oblongata, pass through the jugular foramen, and enter into the carotid sheath between the internal carotid artery and the internal jugular vein down to the neck, thorax, and abdomen, where they innervate many organs including the heart, lungs, liver, and stomach. The right vagus nerve primarily innervates the SA node, whereas the left vagus nerve innervates the AV node; however, there can be significant overlap in the anatomical distribution. Atrial muscle is also innervated by vagal efferents, while the ventricular myocardium is only sparsely innervated.

In heart failure, activation of the parasympathetic nervous system is decreased by reduced vagal ganglionic transmission, reduced muscarinic receptor activity, altered receptor composition, and decreased acetylcholinesterase activity [42,43]. Therefore the sympathetic nervous system remains overstimulated without the dampening effect of the parasympathetic nervous system.

Renin–Angiotensin–Aldosterone System

The Renin–Angiotensin–Aldosterone System (RAAS) (Fig. 5.7) is an important hormonal compensatory mechanism, which helps regulate blood volume and SVR during periods of low arterial blood pressure. It has less immediate effects on the cardiovascular system in comparison to the other major compensatory mechanism, the sympathetic nervous system.

The main trigger for activation of RAAS is stimulation of baroreceptors within the wall of the glomerular afferent arterioles in the kidney. These respond to reduced perfusion pressure by stimulating the release of the proteolytic enzyme, renin, into the circulation by the juxtaglomerular cells of the kidneys [44]. Renin acts by cleaving amino acids from the circulating substrate, angiotensinogen, to form angiotensin I (AT I). AT I is then converted to angiotensin II (AT II) by angiotensin-converting enzyme (ACE). ACE is present in the vascular endothelium, particularly in the lungs. AT II is also synthesized locally by numerous body tissues, including the heart. This may lead to the chronic homeostasis of the cardiovascular system, which may be important in heart failure. AT II receptor-binding sites have been found on the myocardium and cardiac adrenergic nerves [45]. Studies on the denervated heart [46] and on hearts subject to β-adrenergic receptor blockade [47] have shown that AT II retains the positive inotropic effect, which suggests that the positive inotropic effect of AT II on the heart is likely to be direct. This effect is significant in heart failure as there is no decrease in ventricular AT II receptor levels with the condition [45].

AT II has a number of effects on the body:

- Potent vasoconstrictor causing an increase in SVR.
- Positive inotropy and chronotropy [48].
- Stimulates sodium reabsorption at several renal tubular sites, thereby increasing sodium and water retention [49].
- Stimulates the release of aldosterone from the adrenal cortex.
- Stimulates the release of vasopressin from the posterior pituitary.
- Stimulates thirst centers in the brain so increasing fluid intake.
- Stimulates norepinephrine release from the sympathetic nerve endings and inhibits norepinephrine reuptake by nerve endings, thereby enhancing sympathetic adrenergic function [45].
- Direct stimulation of prohypertrophic, proapoptotic, and profibrotic signaling pathways in cardiac myocytes [50,51].
- Stimulates the release of proinflammatory cytokines [52].

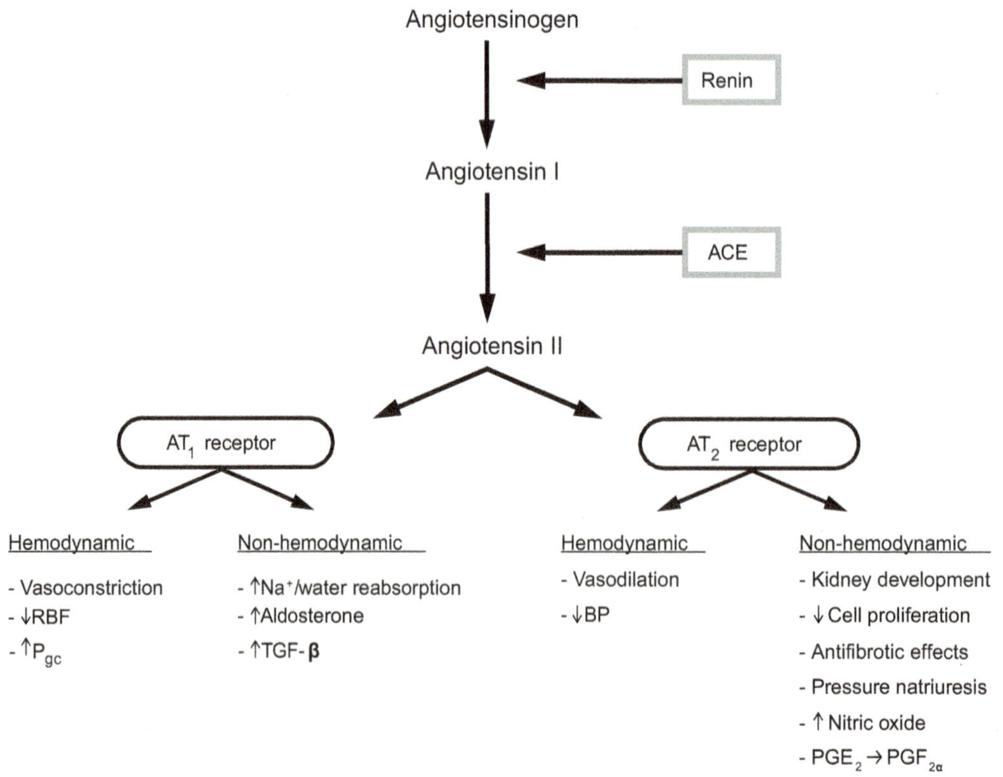

FIGURE 5.7 Renin–angiotensin–aldosterone system (RAAS). *ACE*, angiotensin-converting enzyme; *BP*, blood pressure; *PG*, prostaglandin; P_{gc}, glomerular capillary hydrostatic pressure; *RBF*, renal blood flow; *TGF-β*, transforming growth factor-β. *(Adapted from Science Direct database: M.W. Taal, B.M. Brenner, Renoprotective benefits of RAS inhibition: From ACEI to angiotensin II antagonists, Kidney Int. 57 (5) (2000) 1803–1817.)*

Aldosterone is a steroid hormone produced by the zona glomerulosa of the adrenal cortex of the adrenal gland. As we have mentioned, aldosterone synthesis is stimulated by plasma AT II; however, it is also stimulated by adrenocorticotropic hormone (ACTH) released from the anterior pituitary gland, acidemia, hyperkalemia, the sympathetic nervous system, and by stimulation of arterial and atrial baroreceptors. These baroreceptors are found in the vessel walls of all the large arteries of the thorax and neck, especially in the sinuses of the carotid arteries and the aortic arch. A low arterial blood pressure or low circulating volume is sensed by baroreceptors and atrial stretch receptors, stimulating the release of aldosterone to counteract the original abnormality.

Aldosterone acts by:

- Increasing sodium and water reabsorption (and potassium excretion) by upregulation and activation of the basolateral sodium/potassium ion pumps in the distal tubules and collecting ducts of the nephron.
- Increasing sodium and water reabsorption by upregulation of apical membrane epithelial sodium channels in the renal collecting ducts and the colon.
- Increasing sodium and water reabsorption by stimulating the sodium/potassium ion pump in the gut, salivary glands and sweat glands.
- Regulates acid–base balance by stimulating the secretion of hydrogen ions in exchange for potassium ions in the intercalated cells of the cortical collecting renal tubules.
- Important growth effects and is a key regulator of cardiac fibrosis by promoting collagen synthesis [53].

In heart failure, RAAS is chronically activated by reduced arterial blood pressure and renal blood flow. The effects of AT II and aldosterone are to promote sodium and water retention with vasoconstriction. The resultant increased preload and afterload is a compensatory process to improve the new steady-state operating point (see Fig. 5.6) and thus partially restore CO despite depressed cardiac function. However, this comes at the expense of increased RA_P and venous pressures, which leads to worsening features of congestive cardiac failure [54]. Unfortunately there are other effects of RAAS stimulation, which also become maladaptive in heart failure. These include direct and indirect stimulation of cardiac myocyte chronotropy and inotropy. This increases metabolic demand on the failing heart and can compromise coronary perfusion. Myocardial AT II is also involved in ventricular remodeling by augmenting apoptosis via increasing cytosolic calcium and by reactive oxygen species formation, and also stimulating cytokine synthesis (especially the proinflammatory cytokines, e.g., Transforming Growth Factor-β (TGF-β)). These play a key role in hypertrophic and fibrotic remodeling of the heart leading to cardiac myocyte growth, fibroblast activation, and extracellular matrix deposition [55–57].

Natriuretic Peptides

These are peptide hormones that are primarily produced by the brain and the heart. In simple terms they act as a counterregulatory system to RAAS and so help regulate blood volume and arterial blood pressure by promoting vasodilation, diuresis, and natriuresis [58]. There are three known natriuretic peptides: Atrial Natriuretic Peptide (ANP), Brain Natriuretic Peptide (BNP), and C-type Natriuretic Peptide (CNP).

ANP is a 28-amino acid peptide that is produced and stored by atrial myocytes as pre-pro-ANP. In response to atrial distension, AT II, ET-1, and sympathetic stimulation, pre-pro-ANP is cleaved to pro-ANP and finally the biologically active peptide, ANP.

BNP is a 32-amino acid peptide, which was first isolated in brain tissue but is predominantly made by the cardiac ventricles. Initially it is in the form pre-pro-BNP, which is then cleaved to pro-BNP in a similar response to physiological triggers as ANP. Pro-BNP is 108 amino acids long and is proteolysed by the enzyme corin to N-terminal piece of pro-BNP (NT-pro-BNP) and BNP. Both BNP and NT-pro-BNP are sensitive diagnostic markers for heart failure severity.

CNP is a 22-amino acid peptide that is widely expressed especially in the brain [59], chondrocytes, and endothelial cells. Initially it is in the form pre-pro-CNP, which is then cleaved to form pro-CNP, which in turn is cleaved by the enzyme furin to form CNP-53. This peptide has some biological activity but is normally further processed to CNP. CNP release is stimulated by proinflammatory cytokines (e.g., TNF, IL-1, TGF-β), bacterial lipopolysaccharide, and sheer stress. Unlike the other natriuretic peptides, CNP has predominantly local effects by acting as a paracrine and an autocrine regulator where it acts as a potent vasodilator but unlike ANP and BNP it does not have direct natriuretic activity [60].

The natriuretic peptides act on specific receptors of which three types have been identified, NPR-A, NPR-B, and NPR-C. ANP and BNP bind and activate NPR-A, while CNP binds and activates NPR-B. NPR-C functions as a clearance receptor by binding and sequestering the natriuretic peptides from the circulation. The natriuretic peptides are removed from the circulation by receptor-mediated endocytosis and lysosomal degradation via CNP, but also by enzymatic degradation by neural endopeptidase.

The effects of the natriuretic peptides are as follows:

- Venous vasodilation (increased venous compliance), which decreases preload and thus reduces SV [61].
- Arterial vasodilation, which decreases afterload and further reduces arterial blood pressure [62].
- Positive lusitropy. BNP only [63].
- Increasing glomerular filtration rate (GFR) and filtration fraction. This promotes natriuresis (increased sodium excretion) and diuresis (increased fluid excretion) [64]. ANP and BNP only.
- Inhibits renin release and so antagonizes RAAS, so decreasing circulating levels of AT II and aldosterone. This leads to further natriuresis and diuresis. ANP and BNP only.
- Inhibits vasopressin release.
- Blocks sympathetic nervous system activity [65,66].
- Inhibit myocardial fibrosis formation by inhibiting fibroblast proliferation and collagen synthesis [67–69].
- Inhibits cardiac myocyte hypertrophy [70,71].

In heart failure, the venous pressures are elevated due to increased preload from the effects of RAAS and other neurohormones Fig. 5.8. This causes chronically increased atrial and ventricular distension, which stimulates the increased myocardial secretion of the natriuretic peptides into the circulation [69,72]. The action of ANP and BNP acts not only as a counterregulatory mechanism to RAAS but also counteracts the other deleterious maladaptive changes that occur in heart failure albeit unsuccessfully. This includes attenuation of the hypertrophic signaling pathways in cardiac myocytes so can be considered as an endogenous "antiremodeling" hormone.

Vasopressin

Vasopressin, also known as antidiuretic hormone, is a peptide hormone that was first isolated in the 1950s [73]. The main actions of vasopressin are as follows:

- Increased water permeability and thus reabsorption by increased expression of aquaporin-2 water channels in the collecting ducts and distal convoluted tubules in the kidneys by stimulation of the cAMP-dependent V_2 receptors.
- Increase SVR by stimulation of V_{1a} receptors on the vascular smooth muscle [74].
- Increase ACTH release by binding to V_{1b} receptors on the anterior pituitary gland, which in turn stimulates aldosterone release [75].

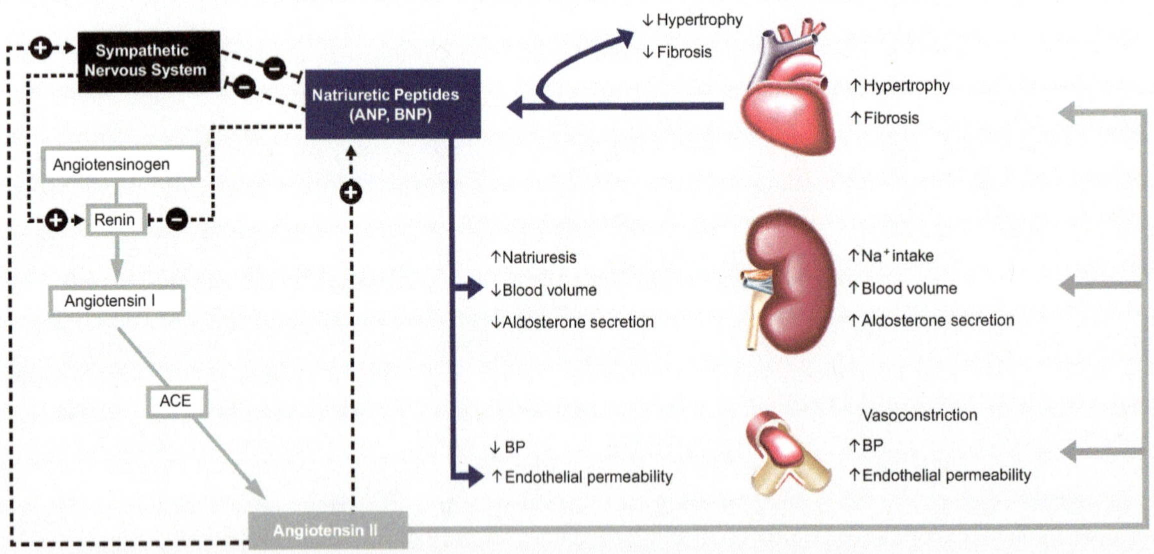

FIGURE 5.8 Interaction between the natriuretic peptides, renin-angiotensin-aldosterone system, and the sympathetic nervous system to maintain cardio–renal homeostasis. *ACE*, angiotensin-converting enzyme; *ANP*, atrial natriuretic peptide; *BNP*, brain natriuretic peptide; *BP*, blood pressure. *(Adapted from Science Direct database: M. Volpe, Natriuretic peptides and cardio-renal disease, Int. J. Cardiol. 176 (3) (2014) 630–639.)*

It is synthesized by the hypothalamus in the brain, transported by axons, and stored in vesicles in the posterior pituitary gland. Vasopressin release is stimulated by baroreceptors responding to low blood pressure and volume, osmoreceptors in the hypothalamus responding to hyperosmolality, sympathetic nervous system, and increased AT II levels. Vasopressin release is inhibited by ANP.

Paradoxically vasopressin secretion is stimulated in heart failure despite the normally inhibiting effect of increased blood volume and atrial pressures. It is thought that this occurs due to the more dominant effect of the sympathetic nervous system and RAAS activation on stimulating vasopressin release. In normal circumstances vasopressin has a compensatory homeostatic function, but in heart failure it has a negative pathophysiological effect by further increasing preload and afterload [76] (Fig. 5.9). At higher physiological circulating vasopressin concentrations, activation of the V_{1a} receptors mediate coronary vasoconstriction and thus reduced coronary blood flow [75]. Vasopressin induces myocyte hypertrophy indirectly by increasing afterload, but also directly by binding to V_{1a} receptors on the myocytes [77–80].

Endothelin

The endothelin family consists of three structurally and functionally similar 21 amino acid peptides. Endothelin-1 (ET-1) is the predominant isoform and was first identified in 1985 [81] from the culture media of bovine aortic endothelial cells and was found to be a potent vasoconstrictor. Four years later [82], two further isoforms were identified, endothelin-2 (ET-2) and endothelin-3 (ET-3). The latter of which we shall not cover in this chapter as it is considered to be the "brain" endothelin peptide.

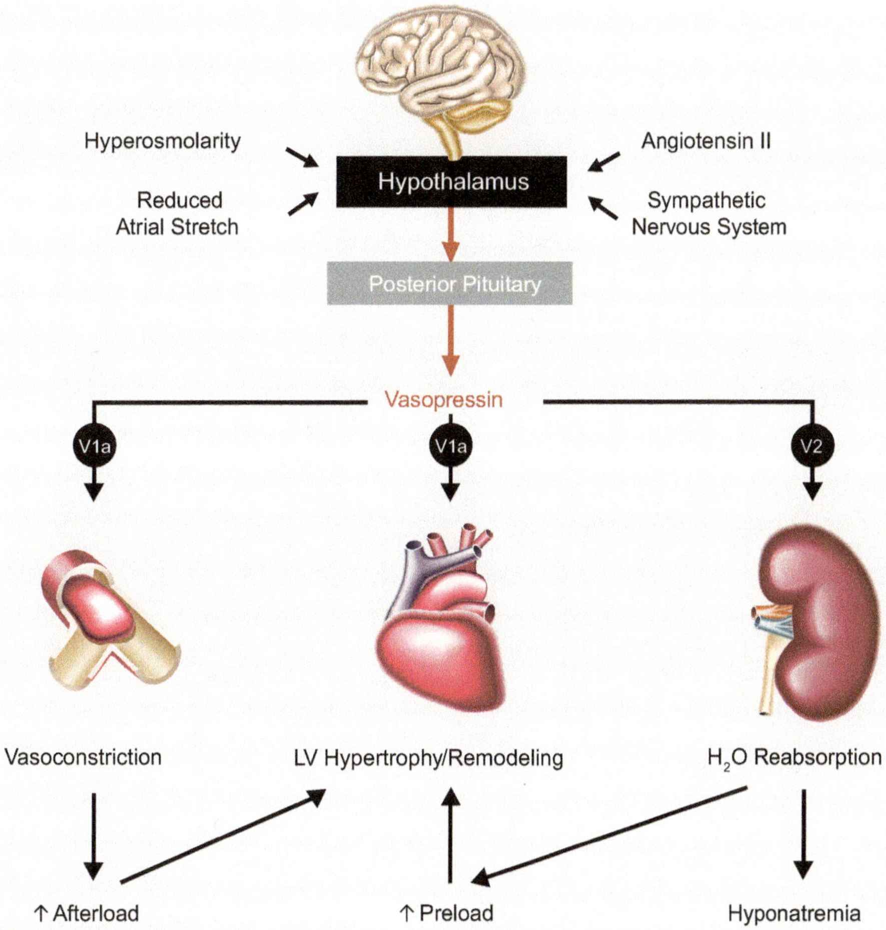

FIGURE 5.9 Schematic diagram of the triggers, synthesis, and function of vasopressin with the implications for chronic stimulation with heart failure. *LV*, left ventricular.

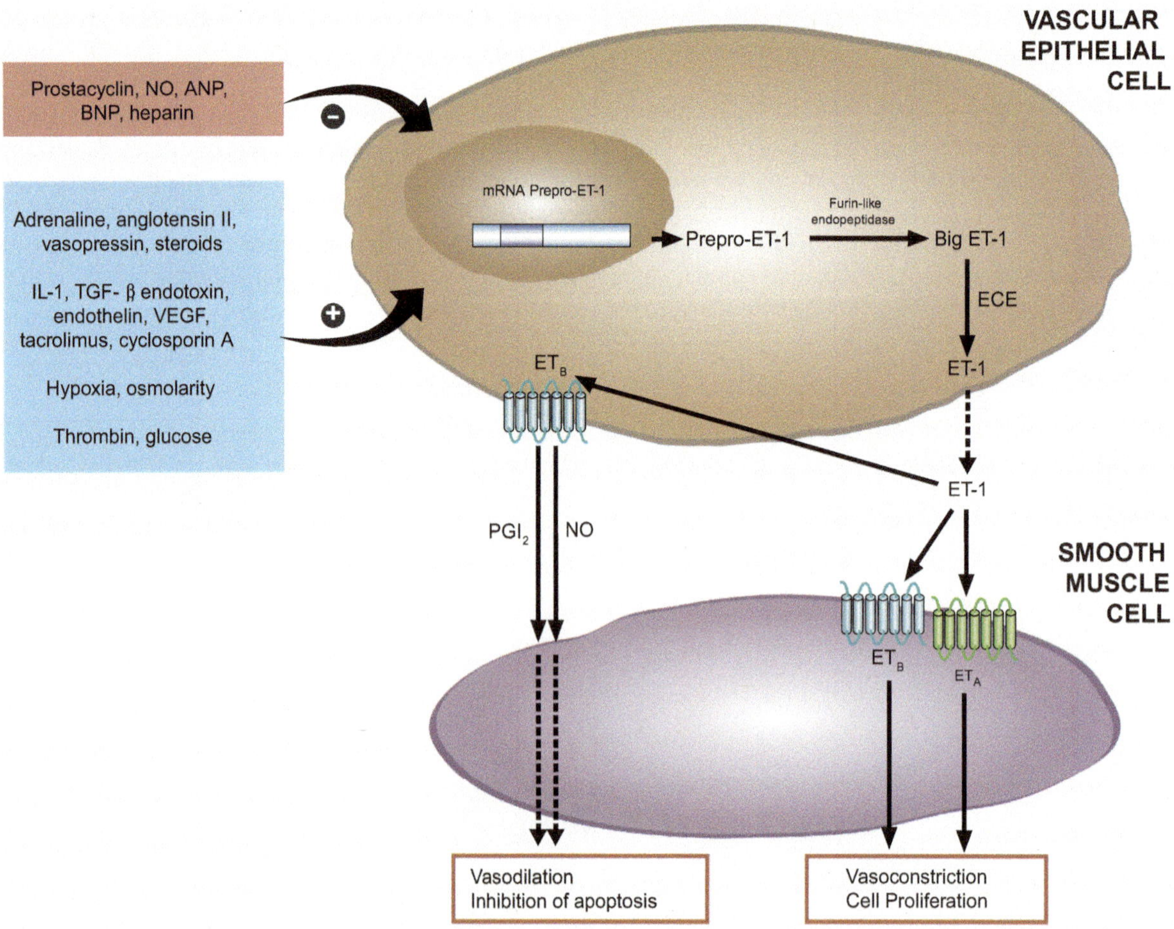

FIGURE 5.10 Schematic diagram of ET-1 synthesis and actions on smooth muscle cells. *ANP*, atrial natriuretic peptide; *BNP*, brain natriuretic peptide; *ECE*, endothelin converting enzyme; *ET*, endothelin; *IL-1*, interleukin-1; *NO*, nitric oxide; PGI_2, prostaglandin I_2 (prostacyclin); *TGF-β*, transforming growth factor-β; *VEGF*, vascular endothelial growth factor. *(Adapted from Science Direct database: Trow, Taichman, Endothelin receptor blockade in the management of pulmonary arterial hypertension: selective and dual antagonism, Respir. Med. 103 (7) 2009 951–962.)*

ET-1 is an extremely potent and long-acting vasoconstrictor that is likely to be involved in blood flow autoregulation throughout the body. It is primarily produced by the vascular endothelial cells but is also produced by various types of epithelial cells (e.g., in lungs, kidneys, and colon), inflammatory cells, and certain neurons and reactive glial cells in the central nervous system. ET-1 is synthesized and released continuously from endothelial cells. The endothelin pathway (Fig. 5.10) consists of an initial gene transcription to form preproendothelin, which is followed by proteolytic cleavage due to the enzyme furin. This forms the 39 amino acid peptide "Big endothelin." Big endothelin has three isoforms, 1–3, which are cleaved by endothelin converting enzyme to form the respective endothelin peptides. Levels of preproendothelin are predominantly affected not only at the level of transcription by various factors but also by certain physiological and pathophysiological conditions, e.g., AT II, vasopressin, thrombin, cytokines, hypoxia, and also by shearing forces acting on the vascular endothelium [83].

ET-2 is similar to ET-1 in the way it is synthesized, its location, and function. However, there is increasing evidence that ET-2 should be considered as having distinct physiologic and potentially pathophysiological role. In particular it has a distinct chemokine action, where at low concentrations it acts as a chemoattractant for neutrophils but an inhibitor at high concentrations [84].

The endothelin family binds to two types of G protein-coupled receptors, ET_A [85] and ET_B [86]. In studies on adult mouse tissues, endothelin receptor mRNA is detected in all tissues receiving a blood supply, reflecting the expression of ET_A on vascular smooth muscle (especially in heart and lungs) and ET_B on endothelial cells (especially in the brain and lung peripheries) [87]. In the human heart, ET_A comprises 90% of the endothelin receptor subtype in cardiac myocytes, while ET_B receptors are more abundant in the AV conducting system [88].

These two receptor subtypes have contrasting phenotypic actions on the cardiovascular system under normal physiologic conditions:

- Vasoconstriction via ET_A receptors in smooth muscle cells.
- Vasodilation via ET_B receptors in the endothelium by the release of nitric oxide [89].

When ET-1 binds to smooth muscle cell ET_A and ET_B receptors it triggers myosin light chain phosphorylation, which results in smooth muscle contraction. When ET-1 binds to ET_B on the endothelium then the formation of nitric oxide (NO) is stimulated. NO has a number of vascular effects including direct vasodilation, indirect vasodilation by vasoconstrictor inhibition (e.g., inhibits AT II), antithrombotic, antiinflammatory, and antiproliferative. In normal conditions, the predominant effect of ET receptor activation is vasoconstriction. However, in the absence of smooth muscle ET receptor stimulation, then NO formation predominates causing vasodilation.

ET-1 causes [90]:

- Smooth muscle contraction through stimulation of ET_A and ET_B receptors.
- Positive inotropy and chronotropy through stimulation of cardiac ET_A and ET_B receptors.
- Vasodilation through stimulation of vascular endothelial ET_B receptors in the absence of smooth muscle ET receptor stimulation.
- Stimulates aldosterone secretion.
- Decreases renal blood flow and GFR.
- Stimulates ANP release.

In heart failure, circulating ET-1 levels are increased [91] along with increased myocardial expression of ET-1, and both ET_A and ET_B receptors [92]. The elevated cardiac ET-1 levels have chronic deleterious effect on the already failing heart by inducing sustained vasoconstriction, severe cardiac inflammation, ventricular dysfunction, fibrosis, and cardiac hypertrophy [93–96].

CONCLUSION

The cardiovascular system undergoes a number of complex and interrelated changes in response to heart failure. The changes involve hemodynamic changes to improve the reduced SV (related to poor contractility) by increasing preload and afterload. The heart is also encouraged to work harder with increased chronotropy and inotropy. These hemodynamic changes are stimulated by a number of different, yet interrelated neurohormonal mechanisms. Unfortunately when these mechanisms are chronically stimulated their effects become pathophysiological and cause maladaptive changes. These changes often lead to cardiac structural alterations involving myocyte hypertrophy, cell death, and extracellular fibrosis. As a result, the patient usually becomes more symptomatic due to disease progression. Understanding the physiological mechanisms of cardiovascular homeostasis is the key to the pathophysiological mechanisms of heart failure and is the basis for drug development and pharmacotherapy to manage the condition.

REFERENCES

[1] J.P. Konhilas, T.C. Irving, P.P. de Tombe, Frank-Starling law of the heart and the cellular mechanisms of length-dependent activation, Pflugers Arch. 445 (3) (2002) 305–310.

[2] D.G. Allen, J.C. Kentish, The cellular basis of the length-tension relation in cardiac muscle, J. Mol. Cell Cardiol. 17 (9) (1985) 821–840.

[3] J. Gulati, Length-sensing function of troponin C and Starling's law of the heart, Circulation 85 (5) (1992) 1954–1955.

[4] T. Wannenburg, et al., Cross-bridge kinetics in rat myocardium: effect of sarcomere length and calcium activation, Am J Physiol Heart Circ Physiol 279 (2) (2000) H779–H790.

[5] N. Fukuda, et al., Length dependence of tension generation in rat skinned cardiac muscle: role of titin in the Frank-Starling mechanism of the heart, Circulation 104 (14) (2001) 1639–1645.

[6] G.H. Pollack, J.W. Krueger, Sarcomere dynamics in intact cardiac muscle, Eur. J. Cardiol. (4 Suppl.) (1976) 53–65.

[7] K. Komamura, et al., Exhaustion of Frank-Starling mechanism in conscious dogs with heart failure, Am. J. Physiol. 265 (4 Pt 2) (1993) H1119–H1131.

[8] R.H. Schwinger, et al., The failing human heart is unable to use the Frank-Starling mechanism, Circ. Res. 74 (5) (1994) 959–969.

[9] F. Fuchs, Y.P. Wang, Sarcomere length versus interfilament spacing as determinants of cardiac myofilament Ca2+ sensitivity and Ca2+ binding, J. Mol. Cell Cardiol. 28 (7) (1996) 1375–1383.

[10] R.G. Monroe, et al., Left ventricular pressure-volume relations and performance as affected by sudden increases in developed pressure, Circ. Res. 22 (3) (1968) 333–344.

[11] R. Skalak, et al., Mechanics of Rouleau formation, Biophys. J. 35 (3) (1981) 771–781.

[11a] A.C. Guyton, A.W. Lindsey, B.N. Kaufmann, Effect of mean circulatory filling pressure and other peripheral circulatory factors on cardiac output, Am. J. Physiol. 180 (1955) 463–468.
[11b] V.S. Bishop, H.L. Stone, A.C. Guyton, Cardiac function curves in conscious dogs, Am. J. Physiol. 207 (1964) 677–682.
[12] M. Haase, H.S. Willenberg, S.R. Bornstein, Update on the corticomedullary interaction in the adrenal gland, Endocr. Dev. 20 (2011) 28–37.
[13] A. Lymperopoulos, et al., Adrenal GRK2 upregulation mediates sympathetic overdrive in heart failure, Nat. Med. 13 (3) (2007) 315–323.
[14] A. Lymperopoulos, G. Rengo, W.J. Koch, Adrenal adrenoceptors in heart failure: fine-tuning cardiac stimulation, Trends Mol. Med. 13 (12) (2007) 503–511.
[15] O.L. Zaika, et al., Acetylcholine-induced calcium signalling in adrenaline- and noradrenaline-containing adrenal chromaffin cells, Arch. Biochem. Biophys. 424 (1) (2004) 23–32.
[16] I. Armando, et al., Angiotensin II AT1 and AT2 receptor types regulate basal and stress-induced adrenomedullary catecholamine production through transcriptional regulation of tyrosine hydroxylase, Ann. N. Y. Acad. Sci. 1018 (2004) 302–309.
[17] D.J. Wallace, C. Chen, P.D. Marley, Histamine promotes excitability in bovine adrenal chromaffin cells by inhibiting an M-current, J. Physiol. 540 (Pt 3) (2002) 921–939.
[18] O.E. Brodde, Pathophysiology of the beta-adrenoceptor system in chronic heart failure: consequences for treatment with agonists, partial agonists or antagonists? Eur. Heart J. (12 Suppl F) (1991) 54–62.
[19] D.M. Kaye, et al., Adverse consequences of high sympathetic nervous activity in the failing human heart, J. Am. Coll. Cardiol. 26 (5) (1995) 1257–1263.
[20] G.J. Hasking, et al., Norepinephrine spillover to plasma in patients with congestive heart failure: evidence of increased overall and cardiorenal sympathetic nervous activity, Circulation 73 (4) (1986) 615–621.
[21] I.T. Meredith, et al., Cardiac sympathetic nervous activity in congestive heart failure. Evidence for increased neuronal norepinephrine release and preserved neuronal uptake, Circulation 88 (1) (1993) 136–145.
[22] J.N. Cohn, et al., Plasma norepinephrine as a guide to prognosis in patients with chronic congestive heart failure, N. Engl. J. Med. 311 (13) (1984) 819–823.
[23] M.W. Dunser, W.R. Hasibeder, Sympathetic overstimulation during critical illness: adverse effects of adrenergic stress, J. Intensive Care Med. 24 (5) (2009) 293–316.
[24] K.T. Weber, Y. Sun, S.E. Campbell, Structural remodelling of the heart by fibrous tissue: role of circulating hormones and locally produced peptides, Eur. Heart J. (16 Suppl N) (1995) 12–18.
[25] S. Engelhardt, et al., Progressive hypertrophy and heart failure in beta1-adrenergic receptor transgenic mice, Proc. Natl. Acad. Sci. U.S.A. 96 (12) (1999) 7059–7064.
[26] P. Simpson, Norepinephrine-stimulated hypertrophy of cultured rat myocardial cells is an alpha 1 adrenergic response, J. Clin. Invest 72 (2) (1983) 732–738.
[27] G. Rona, Catecholamine cardiotoxicity, J. Mol. Cell Cardiol. 17 (4) (1985) 291–306.
[28] W.E. Radtke, et al., Cardiovascular complications of pheochromocytoma crisis, Am. J. Cardiol. 35 (5) (1975) 701–705.
[29] A. Roghi, et al., Adrenergic myocarditis in pheochromocytoma, J. Cardiovasc. Magn. Reson. 13 (2011) 4.
[30] D.R. Murray, S.D. Prabhu, B. Chandrasekar, Chronic beta-adrenergic stimulation induces myocardial proinflammatory cytokine expression, Circulation 101 (20) (2000) 2338–2341.
[31] M.R. Bristow, et al., Decreased catecholamine sensitivity and beta-adrenergic-receptor density in failing human hearts, N. Engl. J. Med. 307 (4) (1982) 205–211.
[32] M. Ungerer, et al., Altered expression of beta-adrenergic receptor kinase and beta 1-adrenergic receptors in the failing human heart, Circulation 87 (2) (1993) 454–463.
[33] M. Bohm, et al., Reduction of beta-adrenoceptor density and evaluation of positive inotropic responses in isolated, diseased human myocardium, Eur. Heart J. 9 (8) (1988) 844–852.
[34] O.E. Brodde, Beta 1- and beta 2-adrenoceptors in the human heart: properties, function, and alterations in chronic heart failure, Pharmacol. Rev. 43 (2) (1991) 203–242.
[35] M. Steinfath, et al., Distinct down-regulation of cardiac beta 1- and beta 2-adrenoceptors in different human heart diseases, Naunyn Schmiedebergs Arch. Pharmacol. 343 (2) (1991) 217–220.
[36] K. Kiuchi, et al., Myocardial beta-adrenergic receptor function during the development of pacing-induced heart failure, J. Clin. Invest 91 (3) (1993) 907–914.
[37] J.L. Benovic, et al., Purification and characterization of the beta-adrenergic receptor kinase, J. Biol. Chem. 262 (19) (1987) 9026–9032.
[38] M.J. Lohse, et al., beta-Arrestin: a protein that regulates beta-adrenergic receptor function, Science 248 (4962) (1990) 1547–1550.
[39] M.J. Lohse, et al., Multiple pathways of rapid beta 2-adrenergic receptor desensitization. Delineation with specific inhibitors, J. Biol. Chem. 265 (6) (1990) 3202–3211.
[40] M.J. Lohse, et al., Receptor-specific desensitization with purified proteins. Kinase dependence and receptor specificity of beta-arrestin and arrestin in the beta 2-adrenergic receptor and rhodopsin systems, J. Biol. Chem. 267 (12) (1992) 8558–8564.
[41] T. Noma, et al., Beta-arrestin-mediated beta1-adrenergic receptor transactivation of the EGFR confers cardioprotection, J. Clin. Invest 117 (9) (2007) 2445–2458.
[42] T. Kinugawa, M.E. Dibner-Dunlap, Altered vagal and sympathetic control of heart rate in left ventricular dysfunction and heart failure, Am. J. Physiol. 268 (2 Pt 2) (1995) R310–R316.
[43] E.R. Azevedo, J.D. Parker, Parasympathetic control of cardiac sympathetic activity: normal ventricular function versus congestive heart failure, Circulation 100 (3) (1999) 274–279.

[44] H.A. Bock, et al., Pressure dependent modulation of renin release in isolated perfused glomeruli, Kidney Int. 41 (2) (1992) 275–280.
[45] H. Urata, et al., Angiotensin II-forming pathways in normal and failing human hearts, Circ. Res. 66 (4) (1990) 883–890.
[46] P.J. Dempsey, et al., Direct myocardial effects of angiotensin II, Am. J. Physiol. 220 (2) (1971) 477–481.
[47] M. Kobayashi, Y. Furukawa, S. Chiba, Positive chronotropic and inotropic effects of angiotensin II in the dog heart, Eur. J. Pharmacol. 50 (1) (1978) 17–25.
[48] M.J. Peach, Renin-angiotensin system: biochemistry and mechanisms of action, Physiol. Rev. 57 (2) (1977) 313–370.
[49] A.M. DelliPizzi, S.D. Hilchey, C.P. Bell-Quilley, Natriuretic action of angiotensin(1-7), Br. J. Pharmacol. 111 (1) (1994) 1–3.
[50] C.P. Baines, J.D. Molkentin, STRESS signaling pathways that modulate cardiac myocyte apoptosis, J. Mol. Cell Cardiol. 38 (1) (2005) 47–62.
[51] P.J. Lijnen, V.V. Petrov, R.H. Fagard, Induction of cardiac fibrosis by angiotensin II, Methods Find Exp. Clin. Pharmacol. 22 (10) (2000) 709–723.
[52] M. Ruiz-Ortega, et al., Angiotensin II regulates the synthesis of proinflammatory cytokines and chemokines in the kidney, Kidney Int. Suppl. (82) (2002) S12–S22.
[53] P. Lijnen, V. Petrov, Induction of cardiac fibrosis by aldosterone, J. Mol. Cell Cardiol. 32 (6) (2000) 865–879.
[54] J. George, A.D. Struthers, C.C. Lang, Modulation of the renin-angiotensin-aldosterone system in heart failure, Curr. Atheroscler. Rep. 16 (4) (2014) 403.
[55] S.E. Campbell, L.C. Katwa, Angiotensin II stimulated expression of transforming growth factor-beta1 in cardiac fibroblasts and myofibroblasts, J. Mol. Cell Cardiol. 29 (7) (1997) 1947–1958.
[56] A. Desmouliere, et al., Transforming growth factor-beta 1 induces alpha-smooth muscle actin expression in granulation tissue myofibroblasts and in quiescent and growing cultured fibroblasts, J. Cell Biol. 122 (1) (1993) 103–111.
[57] M.O. Gray, et al., Angiotensin II stimulates cardiac myocyte hypertrophy via paracrine release of TGF-beta 1 and endothelin-1 from fibroblasts, Cardiovasc. Res. 40 (2) (1998) 352–363.
[58] G. Thibault, F. Amiri, R. Garcia, Regulation of natriuretic peptide secretion by the heart, Annu. Rev. Physiol. 61 (1999) 193–217.
[59] K. Totsune, et al., C-type natriuretic peptide in the human central nervous system: distribution and molecular form, Peptides 15 (1) (1994) 37–40.
[60] A.L. Clavell, et al., C-type natriuretic peptide: a selective cardiovascular peptide, Am. J. Physiol. 264 (2 Pt 2) (1993) R290–R295.
[61] A.M. Richards, et al., Atrial natriuretic hormone has biological effects in man at physiological plasma concentrations, J. Clin. Endocrinol. Metab. 67 (6) (1988) 1134–1139.
[62] G. Tonolo, et al., Low-dose infusion of atrial natriuretic factor in mild essential hypertension, Circulation 80 (4) (1989) 893–902.
[63] P.B. Clarkson, et al., Brain natriuretic peptide: effect on left ventricular filling patterns in healthy subjects, Clin. Sci. (Lond) 88 (2) (1995) 159–164.
[64] P.J. Harris, D. Thomas, T.O. Morgan, Atrial natriuretic peptide inhibits angiotensin-stimulated proximal tubular sodium and water reabsorption, Nature 326 (6114) (1987) 697–698.
[65] J.S. Floras, Sympathoinhibitory effects of atrial natriuretic factor in normal humans, Circulation 81 (6) (1990) 1860–1873.
[66] H.P. Brunner-La Rocca, et al., Effects of intravenous brain natriuretic peptide on regional sympathetic activity in patients with chronic heart failure as compared with healthy control subjects, J. Am. Coll. Cardiol. 37 (5) (2001) 1221–1227.
[67] L. Cao, D.G. Gardner, Natriuretic peptides inhibit DNA synthesis in cardiac fibroblasts, Hypertension 25 (2) (1995) 227–234.
[68] A.M. Kapoun, et al., B-type natriuretic peptide exerts broad functional opposition to transforming growth factor-beta in primary human cardiac fibroblasts: fibrosis, myofibroblast conversion, proliferation, and inflammation, Circ. Res. 94 (4) (2004) 453–461.
[69] C.J. Watson, et al., Mechanical stretch up-regulates the B-type natriuretic peptide system in human cardiac fibroblasts: a possible defense against transforming growth factor-beta mediated fibrosis, Fibrogenesis Tissue Repair 5 (1) (2012) 9.
[70] J.W. Knowles, et al., Pressure-independent enhancement of cardiac hypertrophy in natriuretic peptide receptor A-deficient mice, J. Clin. Invest 107 (8) (2001) 975–984.
[71] I. Kishimoto, K. Rossi, D.L. Garbers, A genetic model provides evidence that the receptor for atrial natriuretic peptide (guanylyl cyclase-A) inhibits cardiac ventricular myocyte hypertrophy, Proc. Natl. Acad. Sci. U.S.A. 98 (5) (2001) 2703–2706.
[72] M. Volpe, M. Carnovali, V. Mastromarino, The natriuretic peptides system in the pathophysiology of heart failure: from molecular basis to treatment, Clin. Sci. (Lond) 130 (2) (2016) 57–77.
[73] R.A. Turner, J.G. Pierce, V.V. du, The purification and the amino acid content of vasopressin preparations, J. Biol. Chem. 191 (1) (1951) 21–28.
[74] T. Aoyagi, T.A. Koshimizu, A. Tanoue, Vasopressin regulation of blood pressure and volume: findings from V1a receptor-deficient mice, Kidney Int. 76 (10) (2009) 1035–1039.
[75] K. Chatterjee, Neurohormonal activation in congestive heart failure and the role of vasopressin, Am. J. Cardiol. 95 (9A) (2005) 8B-13B.
[76] D.L. Xu, et al., Upregulation of aquaporin-2 water channel expression in chronic heart failure rat, J. Clin. Invest 99 (7) (1997) 1500–1505.
[77] M. Hiroyama, et al., Vasopressin promotes cardiomyocyte hypertrophy via the vasopressin V1A receptor in neonatal mice, Eur. J. Pharmacol. 559 (2–3) (2007) 89–97.
[78] X.D. Yang, et al., Effects of arginine vasopressin on growth of rat cardiac fibroblasts: role of V1 receptor, J. Cardiovasc. Pharmacol. 42 (1) (2003) 132–135.
[79] M.A. Brostrom, et al., Vasopressin-induced hypertrophy in H9c2 heart-derived myocytes, Int. J. Biochem. Cell Biol. 32 (9) (2000) 993–1006.
[80] Y. Nakamura, et al., Hypertrophic growth of cultured neonatal rat heart cells mediated by vasopressin V(1A) receptor, Eur. J. Pharmacol. 391 (1–2) (2000) 39–48.
[81] K.A. Hickey, et al., Characterization of a coronary vasoconstrictor produced by cultured endothelial cells, Am. J. Physiol. 248 (5 Pt 1) (1985) C550–C556.
[82] N. Inoue, et al., Angiotensin II-induced reduction in exercise capacity is associated with increased oxidative stress in skeletal muscle, Am. J. Physiol. Heart Circ. Physiol. 302 (5) (2012) H1202–H1210.
[83] L.R. Stow, et al., Endothelin-1 gene regulation, FASEB J. 25 (1) (2011) 16–28.
[84] J.G. Elferink, B.M. de Koster, The effect of endothelin-2 (ET-2) on migration and changes in cytosolic free calcium of neutrophils, Naunyn Schmiedebergs Arch. Pharmacol. 353 (2) (1996) 130–135.

[85] H. Arai, et al., Cloning and expression of a cDNA encoding an endothelin receptor, Nature 348 (6303) (1990) 730–732.

[86] T. Sakurai, et al., Cloning of a cDNA encoding a non-isopeptide-selective subtype of the endothelin receptor, Nature 348 (6303) (1990) 732–735.

[87] J.B. Regard, I.T. Sato, S.R. Coughlin, Anatomical profiling of G protein-coupled receptor expression, Cell 135 (3) (2008) 561–571.

[88] P. Molenaar, et al., Characterization and localization of endothelin receptor subtypes in the human atrioventricular conducting system and myocardium, Circ. Res. 72 (3) (1993) 526–538.

[89] M.C. Verhaar, et al., Endothelin-A receptor antagonist-mediated vasodilatation is attenuated by inhibition of nitric oxide synthesis and by endothelin-B receptor blockade, Circulation 97 (8) (1998) 752–756.

[90] A.P. Davenport, et al., Endothelin, Pharmacol. Rev. 68 (2) (2016) 357–418.

[91] D.J. Stewart, et al., Elevated endothelin-1 in heart failure and loss of normal response to postural change, Circulation 85 (2) (1992) 510–517.

[92] B. Pieske, et al., Functional effects of endothelin and regulation of endothelin receptors in isolated human nonfailing and failing myocardium, Circulation 99 (14) (1999) 1802–1809.

[93] L.L. Yang, et al., Conditional cardiac overexpression of endothelin-1 induces inflammation and dilated cardiomyopathy in mice, Circulation 109 (2) (2004) 255–261.

[94] R.V. Shohet, et al., Mice with cardiomyocyte-specific disruption of the endothelin-1 gene are resistant to hyperthyroid cardiac hypertrophy, Proc. Natl. Acad. Sci. U.S.A. 101 (7) (2004) 2088–2093.

[95] X.S. Zhao, et al., Endogenous endothelin-1 is required for cardiomyocyte survival in vivo, Circulation 114 (8) (2006) 830–837.

[96] J.L. Vachiery, A. Davenport, The endothelin system in pulmonary and renal vasculopathy: les liaisons dangereuses, Eur. Respir. Rev. 18 (114) (2009) 260–271.

Chapter 6

Neurohormonal Axis and Natriuretic Peptides in Heart Failure

Stephanie J. Nakano, Melanie D. Everitt
University of Colorado, Aurora, CO, United States

PROGRESSIVE MODEL OF HEART FAILURE

Following an initial decline in the pumping capacity of the heart, the progression of heart failure occurs as a result of excessive activation of compensatory mechanisms that, when chronically stimulated, exert detrimental effects on the heart and circulation [1,2]. In an attempt to preserve cardiac output, there is early activation of both the sympathetic/adrenergic nervous system and the renin–angiotensin–aldosterone system (RAAS). Vasoconstriction ensues which, in turn, stimulates vasodilatory molecules including natriuretic peptides. The transition to symptomatic heart failure is accompanied by further activation of the neurohormonal and cytokine pathways, as well as a series of adaptive changes within the myocardium (left ventricular remodeling) [2]. In adult heart failure, the magnitude of sympathetic and neurohormonal activation in congestive heart failure appears to predict survival [3,4].

NEUROHORMONAL RESPONSES SPECIFIC TO PEDIATRIC HEART FAILURE

In adults with heart failure, the same neurohormonal mechanisms are activated regardless of the cause of the initial decline in heart function. However, there is more diversity in pediatric heart failure with regard to disease etiology, rate of progression, and additional end organ dysfunction. While the neurohormonal mechanisms in adult heart failure appear to be consistently activated across etiologies, it is not clear that neurohormonal responses to heart failure in children is similar to what is seen in adults. Given the comparatively small number of pediatric heart failure patients as well as the heterogeneous nature of their disease, there is a paucity of pediatric-specific data with regard to the interplay between pump failure and neurohormonal responses, particularly at the molecular and mechanistic levels. Nevertheless, applying the adult heart failure knowledge base regarding neurohormonal responses to pediatric patients may provide a useful framework for further pediatric-specific investigation.

Sympathetic Nervous System

The sympathetic/adrenergic nervous system modulates cardiovascular function through regulation of heart rate, blood pressure, force of contraction, and cardiac myocyte hypertrophy [5]. The primary function of adrenergic stimulation of the heart is to promote a rapid increase in physical performance for immediate, short-term gain. However, prolonged adrenergic hyperactivity, as seen in chronic adult heart failure, leads to loss of adrenergic receptors from the cardiac cell surface (receptor down-regulation) [1], decreased adrenergic reserve, and cardiotoxicity. The net effect of a sustained increase in cardiac adrenergic activity in the failing heart is to promote myocardial disease progression and accelerate the natural history of heart failure [2].

Components and Activation

The autonomic nervous system, comprised of the sympathetic/adrenergic and parasympathetic/cholinergic limbs, supplies efferent regulation of the heart and circulation. Sympathetic fibers originating from the right stellate ganglion innervate the sinus and atrioventricular nodes, while sympathetic fibers originating from the left stellate ganglion innervate the left ventricle [6]. The ventricles receive almost exclusively sympathetic fiber innervations, with minimal connection to the parasympathetic system [7,8]; thus cardiac contraction and relaxation are controlled almost exclusively by the sympathetic nervous system. This is illustrated in (Fig. 6.1). Sympathetic stimulation also contributes to vascular tone via vasoconstrictor and vasodilator fibers.

Heart Failure in the Child and Young Adult. http://dx.doi.org/10.1016/B978-0-12-802393-8.00006-5

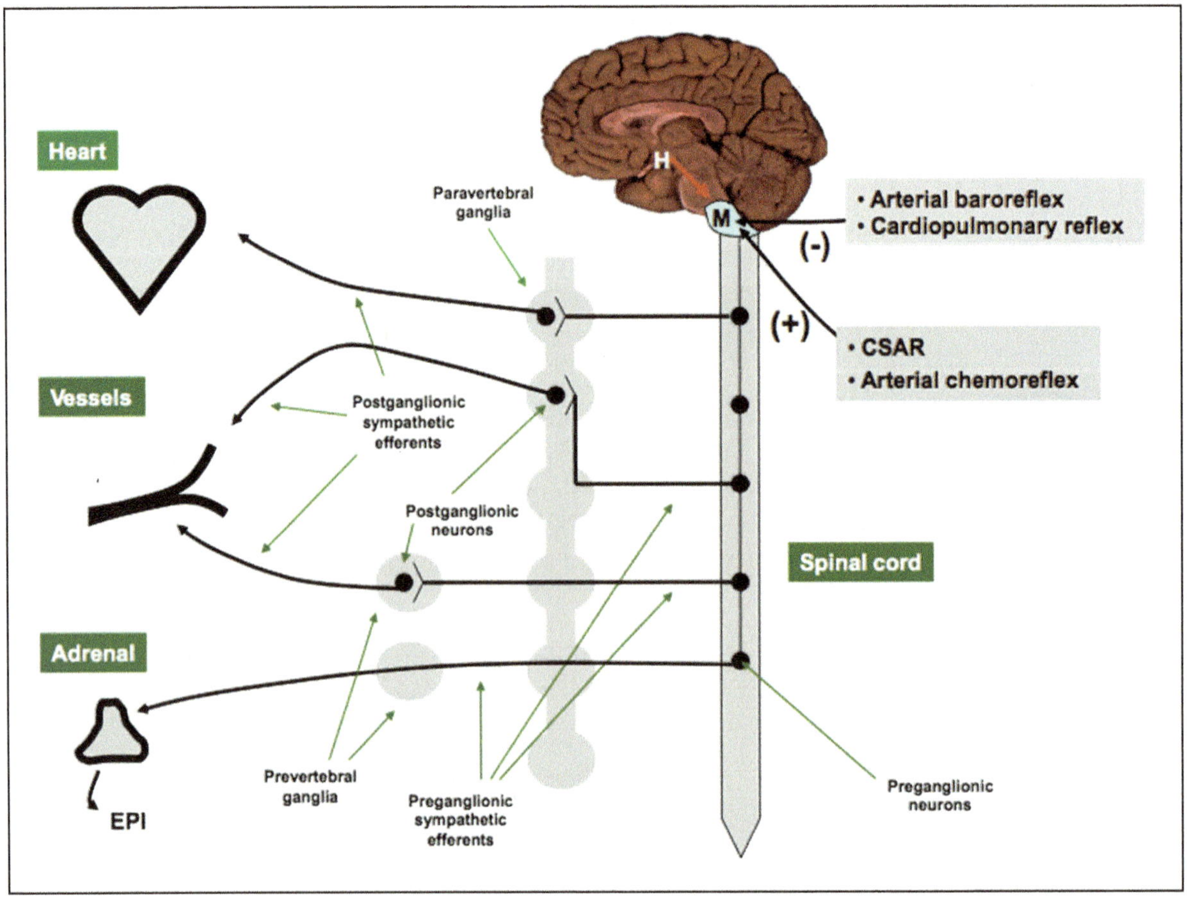

FIGURE 6.1 **The Sympathetic Nervous System.** The most important level of integration of sympathetic nervous system efferent activities to the cardiovascular system resides in the *dorsolateral reticular formation of the medulla.* The hypothalamus modifies the activity of the medullary centers and is important in stimulating cardiovascular responses to emotion and stress. The motor outflow of the sympathetic nervous system is formed by two serially connected sets of neurons. The first set (*preganglionic neurons*) originates in the brain stem or the spinal cord, and the second set (*postganglionic neurons*) lies outside the central nervous system in collections of nerve cells called *sympathetic ganglia.* The sympathetic preganglionic neurons originate in the lateral horns of the 12 thoracic and the first 2 or 3 lumbar segments of the spinal cord (*thoracolumbar outflow*). The axons of these neurons (short, myelinated) exit the spinal cord in the ventral roots and then synapse on either sympathetic ganglion cells or chromaffin cells in the adrenal gland that releases epinephrine (EPI). The sympathetic ganglia can be divided into two major groups: (1) the *paravertebral* (3 in the cervical region including the right and left stellate ganglia, 10–11 in the thoracic region, 4 in the lumbar region, 4 in the sacral region, and a single, unpaired ganglion lying in front of the coccyx), which lie on each side of the vertebrae and are connected to form the sympathetic chain or trunk; and (2) the *prevertebral (preaortic)*, which provide axons that are distributed with the three major gastrointestinal arteries arising from the aorta. The predominant neurotransmitter of the sympathetic preganglionic neurons is *acetylcholine*, whereas the predominant neurotransmitter of most sympathetic postganglionic neurons is *norepinephrine.* Sympathetic activity is attenuated (–) by the arterial baroreflex and the cardiopulmonary reflex and increased (+) by the cardiac sympathetic afferent reflex (CSAR) and the arterial chemoreceptor reflex. *H*, hypothalamus; *M*, medulla. *With permission from F. Triposkiadis, G. Karayannis, G. Giamouzis, J. Skoularigis, G. Louridas, J. Butler. The sympathetic nervous system in heart failure physiology, pathophysiology, and clinical implications. Journal of the American College of Cardiology. 54 (2009) 1747–1762.*

Sympathetic activation exerts its effects on the cardiovascular system via two catecholamines, norepinephrine and epinephrine. The predominant neurotransmitter of most sympathetic postganglionic neurons is norepinephrine. By contrast, epinephrine is released into the circulation by chromaffin cells in the adrenal medulla. Under normal conditions, epinephrine comprises 80% of the total adrenal catecholamine secretion, while norepinephrine accounts for the other 20% [9]. Interestingly, both norepinephrine and epinephrine can also be released locally by blood vessels and cardiac myocytes themselves, thus acting in an autocrine/paracrine manner [10,11]. The total amount of catecholamine seen by the cardiac adrenergic receptors at any given time is a combination of circulating norepinephrine and epinephrine plus norepinephrine released locally from sympathetic nerve terminals and myocytes within the heart [10].

Norepinephrine and epinephrine mediate their effects via cell surface adrenergic receptors, which belong to the superfamily of G protein-coupled receptors (discussed in greater detail in Chapter 2). Briefly, stimulation of β-adrenergic receptors in the heart increases cardiac contractility, frequency, and rate of relaxation, as well as accelerates impulse conduction through the atrioventricular node and pacemaker activity from the sinoatrial node [12]. Conversely, α-adrenergic receptor stimulation may actually reduce cardiac output by increasing peripheral resistance. Signaling from endogenous catecholamines is rapidly terminated through uptake and degradation in intraneuronal and extraneuronal sites. The norepinephrine transporter type 1 recycles approximately 80% of norepinephrine released by the sympathetic nerve terminals, with the remainder spilling over into the circulation [13]. Central α_2-adrenergic receptors also inhibit additional sympathetic nervous system outflow via an autocrine negative feedback mechanism [14].

Alterations in Chronic Heart Failure

In adult heart failure, increased activation of the adrenergic nervous system (measured by plasma norepinephrine levels) is inversely correlated with left ventricular function and is accompanied by progressive clinical deterioration [4,15]. Adrenergic nervous system hyperactivity is evidenced by increased plasma norepinephrine and epinephrine levels, elevated central sympathetic outflow, and heightened norepinephrine spillover into the circulation [16]. With chronic adrenergic stimulation, sympathetic neuronal density and function are reduced, neuronal norepinephrine stores are depleted, and presynaptic reuptake of norepinephrine is decreased secondary to norepinephrine transporter downregulation [17,18]. Additionally, cardiac myocyte β-adrenergic receptor signaling and function are significantly deranged and the adrenergic reserve of the heart is diminished [19–21]. Furthermore, the expected inhibitory effect of α_2-adrenergic stimulation on presynaptic norepinephrine release is markedly blunted with chronic heart failure [22]. Overall, the heart becomes progressively unresponsive to the stimulatory effects of catecholamines despite chronically elevated norepinephrine spillover, promoting myocardial disease progression and accelerating the natural history of heart failure [2].

Elevated plasma norepinephrine, however, is not simply a biomarker of chronic heart failure but is a direct contributor to disease progression. Both intravenous infusions of isoproterenol (a nonselective β-adrenergic receptor agonist) and norepinephrine result in detrimental cardiac myocyte effects, including acute contraction band lesions attributed to relative hypoxia, increased sarcolemmal permeability, calcium overload, elevation of cyclic adenosine monophosphate, activation of adrenergic receptors, and formation of oxidative catecholamine metabolites [23,24]. Chronic catecholamine administration in rats causes interstitial fibrosis, reduces β-adrenergic receptor-mediated inotropic responses (adrenergic inotropic reserve), promotes cardiac apoptosis, and induces contractile dysfunction primarily through left ventricular dilation [25,26]. Specifically, norepinephrine has been shown to induce cardiac apoptosis via β_1-adrenergic receptor-mediated and reactive oxygen species/tumor necrosis factor/caspase-mediated signaling pathways [27,28]. Furthermore, as part of the process of left ventricular remodeling, failing human cardiac myocytes undergo a number of changes including desensitization of β-adrenergic signaling [20] that may directly contribute to progressive loss of myocyte contractile function.

Pediatric-Specific Data

Based on the molecular and mechanistic findings generated from in vivo studies as well as the decidedly beneficial effect of β-blocker therapy in adults with heart failure, β-adrenergic receptor antagonism has been applied to pediatric heart failure patients. However, a randomized-control trial of β-blocker therapy in pediatric patients with symptomatic heart failure did not demonstrate any significant improvement in clinical heart failure outcomes with the nonselective β-blocker carvedilol [29]. As a contrast, carvedilol therapy in adults with chronic heart failure significantly reduced the risk of death as well as the risk of cardiovascular-related hospitalization [30]. Given this disparate response to β-blocker treatment, it is likely that the adrenergic response to heart failure in pediatric patients is unique: there is differential adaptation of β-adrenergic receptors and adrenergic signaling pathways in children with heart failure compared with adults [31]. Specifically, in a murine model of pediatric heart failure, selective β_1-adrenergic receptor blockade may be of particular benefit [32]. Furthermore, the adaptation of the β-adrenergic receptor system in the right ventricular myocardium of children with hypoplastic left heart syndrome is dissimilar from both adults and children with heart failure due to dilated cardiomyopathy, demonstrating a downregulation of the β_1-adrenergic receptor [33]. Thus, while pediatric data regarding the adrenergic response to heart failure are limited, there are likely both resemblances and divergences from the adrenergic adaptations seen in adult heart failure.

Renin–Angiotensin–Aldosterone System

The RAAS regulates the cardiovascular system through modulation of systemic blood pressure, water and electrolyte balance, and hormones; its activity significantly increases in the setting of left ventricular hypertrophy and heart failure [34]. Initially in a homeostatic mechanism, the increase in RAAS activity is an adaptive process to increase blood pressure and intravascular volume in the setting of low cardiac output. However, prolonged RAAS activation becomes maladaptive, leading to excessive vasoconstriction, fibrosis, and cardiac remodeling. Thus, activation of the RAAS is associated with increased morbidity and mortality among adult patients with hypertension and heart failure, and the degree of RAAS activation correlates with prognosis.

Renin–Angiotensin–Aldosterone System Components

Circulating effectors of the RAAS include angiotensin II (AT II), bradykinin, and aldosterone, which act in concert to modulate vascular tone on a minute-to-minute basis. From a physiological perspective, decreases in intravascular volume detected by baroreceptors (mediated by β-adrenergic receptor activation) and by reduced sodium concentration at the macula densa cause an increase in synthesis and release of the protease renin by juxtaglomerular cells in the afferent arteriole of the kidney. Renin catalyzes the hydrolysis of circulating angiotensinogen to angiotensin I. Angiotensin I is converted to AT II by angiotensin-converting enzyme (ACE), present predominantly in the lungs and vascular tissue [35]. AT II is the primary effector molecule of the RAAS, acting on cardiac myocytes, endothelial cells, vascular smooth muscle cells, and extracellular matrix molecules [34,36]. The majority of the physiologic effects of AT II are mediated by angiotensin type 1 receptors (AT1Rs), which are widely distributed in all organs, including the heart, brain, kidney, and vasculature. Acutely (within seconds to minutes), binding of AT II to local AT1Rs activates signaling pathways leading to vascular smooth muscle cell contraction and maintenance of vascular tone. Secondarily, ACE activity also promotes vasoconstriction through degradation of the vasodilatory peptide bradykinin. Additionally, AT II acts through AT1Rs remotely, in multiple organ systems, to help maintain blood pressure and perfusion. Specifically, AT II augments the inward calcium current through L-type calcium channels in cardiac myocytes [37], thus increasing both inotropy and chronotropy. AT II stimulates the synthesis and release of aldosterone from the adrenal glands, and increases renal sodium absorption. Furthermore, AT II acts on the central nervous system to maintain sympathetic outflow to the vasculature. With chronic elevation of AT II, pathologic effects eventually emerge.

Angiotensin II and Activation of Angiotensin Type 1 Receptors

Formation of Angiotensin II

In animal models [38–40] and adult heart failure patients [41], plasma renin activity is markedly elevated during severe, decompensated left ventricular failure, before the development of extracellular fluid volume expansion and restoration of systemic blood pressure. This increase in renin activity results in heightened conversion of angiotensinogen into angiotensin I (AT II precursor). AT II synthesis is primarily controlled by ACE activity, which becomes upregulated in the setting of both pressure-induced hypertrophy and volume overload models of heart failure [42–44]. Increased ACE activation results in augmented AT II synthesis and bradykinin degradation, disrupting the normal endothelial balance of vasoconstriction and vasodilation. While ACE in the lungs and vasculature is responsible for the majority of AT II synthesis, a small amount of angiotensin I is converted into AT II in the heart by chymase [45]. Thus, AT II acts in both endocrine and paracrine manners, activating AT1Rs in a variety of cell types and tissues that can contribute to disease progression.

Regulation and Activation of Angiotensin Type 1 Receptors

Modulation of AT1R density on the cell membrane regulates the ultimate effects of AT II on its target tissue. Acutely, increased levels of AT II lead to an increased level of AT1R activation; however, chronic exposure to AT II downregulates AT1Rs [46–48]. Thus, similar to the adrenergic system, target tissues are desensitized to further agonism following initial AT II stimulation via internalization of the AT1R [46,49]. Binding of AT II to AT1Rs activates a series of signaling cascades via classic G protein-mediated pathways (responsible for acute vasoconstriction) as well as several tyrosine kinases and activation of NADPH oxidases (with subsequent generation of reactive oxygen species) [50]. AT1R activation also activates downstream serine/threonine kinases such as protein kinase C and mitogen-activated protein kinases implicated in cell growth and hypertrophy [36]. Intracellular signaling responses to AT II are time dependent and are also influenced by differences in receptor/ligand affinity, alterations in trafficking patterns, AT1R structural modifications, and the local tissue environment.

Angiotensin II in Cardiovascular Pathology

Since AT II affects numerous cell types, including endothelial cells, smooth muscle cells, fibroblasts, monocytes/macrophages, and cardiac myocytes, it is not surprising that AT II is critical to disease progression. In adult subjects, and animal and cell culture models, AT II has been implicated in vascular smooth muscle cell proliferation, hypertrophy, differentiation, and apoptosis [51]. However, AT II also has multiple unfavorable effects on endothelial cells, including production of reactive oxygen species, activating apoptotic signaling pathways, and promoting thrombosis, all contributing to endothelial dysfunction [36]. Overall, these changes promote inflammation, atherosclerosis, fibrosis, and thrombosis. The effects of excessive AT II, through AT1R activation, also have direct, detrimental effects on cardiac cells, including myocyte hypertrophy, myofibroblast remodeling, and conduction system disturbances [36]. Interestingly, elevated AT II has independently been associated with the development of cardiac myocyte necrosis, which is preventable with ACE inhibitor treatment [52]. In addition, there is significant interplay between the RAAS and adrenergic systems: AT II enhances the release and inhibits the reuptake of norepinephrine at adrenergic presynaptic nerve terminals [53,54].

Aldosterone

The renin–angiotensin system also regulates the biosynthesis of aldosterone, which is intimately involved in blood pressure homeostasis through fluid and electrolyte balance. However, aldosterone also has marked effects on nonepithelial tissues including the myocardium. In the setting of excess RAAS activation, elevated aldosterone directly promotes adverse cardiac remodeling and heart failure progression, as well as mediates several of the cardiotoxic effects (fibrosis, increased oxidative stress, and inflammation) of AT II in the cardiovascular system [55–57].

Formation of Aldosterone and Mechanism of Action

The principal regulators of aldosterone synthesis and secretion are AT II, the concentration of extracellular potassium and adrenocorticotropic hormone. Nevertheless, a number of other factors have been shown to stimulate or inhibit aldosterone production, including epinephrine, vasoactive intestinal polypeptide, serotonin, atrial natriuretic peptide (ANP), and dopamine. Aldosterone is synthesized from cholesterol in the zona glomerulosa of the adrenal cortex by a series of enzymatic reactions. Aldosterone then binds to specific mineralocorticoid receptors located in the cytosol of target epithelial cells; this steroid-receptor complex then translocates to the cell nucleus where it modulates gene expression and translation of specific "aldosterone-induced" proteins that regulate electrolyte and fluid balance. Additionally, in the cardiovascular system, aldosterone can mediate rapid effects independent of gene transcription and translation [55].

Aldosterone in Cardiovascular Pathology

Plasma aldosterone levels may be elevated as high as 20-fold in adult heart failure patients, primarily due to increased production by the adrenal glands following stimulation by high plasma AT II concentrations [55–57]. Decreased metabolic clearance by the liver further contributes to increased plasma concentrations of aldosterone in patients with congestive heart failure [57,58]. In addition to its classic mineralocorticoid properties, aldosterone has other adverse effects that can contribute to the pathophysiology of heart failure, including coronary and renovascular remodeling, endothelial and baroreceptor dysfunction, and inhibition of myocardial norepinephrine reuptake [59–61]. Specifically, excess aldosterone increases responsiveness to catecholamines, impairs the vasodilatory response, and upregulates AT1Rs [62–64]. Aldosterone also promotes fibrosis through collagen deposition in the blood vessels and increased collagen I synthesis in cardiac fibroblasts [65]. Furthermore, aldosterone contributes to elevation of AT II levels by augmenting expression of vascular ACE [66].

Pediatric-Specific Data

Similar to our understanding regarding the adrenergic system, the vast majority of knowledge regarding the RAAS originates from adult heart failure patients, animal and cell culture models, and in vitro studies. Evaluations of the RAAS in pediatric heart failure have largely consisted of relatively small clinical trials of ACE inhibitors [67–71] or aldosterone antagonists [72] in pediatric patients with congenital heart disease. Genetic variations in the RAAS cascade have been associated with cardiovascular disease, and relevant to pediatric patients with single ventricle heart disease, there has been an association between RAAS genotype and cardiac and renal response to volume-unloading surgery [73].

Natriuretic Peptides

Natriuretic peptides directly protect against excess salt and water retention. However, particularly in the setting of heart failure, natriuretic peptides exert other beneficial effects including inhibition of vasoconstrictor peptides and sympathetic activation, assisting with vascular relaxation, and mitigating adverse cardiovascular remodeling. Additionally, circulating levels of natriuretic peptides are increasingly utilized as biomarkers to gauge severity of heart failure in adults [74], and modulation of natriuretic peptides represents potential therapeutic targets.

Biochemistry and Molecular Biology

The natriuretic peptide family consists of three peptides, each with unique tissue expression and regulation: ANP, brain natriuretic peptide (BNP), and C-type natriuretic peptide (CNP). The natriuretic peptides are synthesized as preprohormones, and cleaved to form prohormones; the prohormones are then cleaved into the C-terminal and N-terminal peptides. The C-terminal peptide is the biologically active molecule, while the N-terminal peptide circulates in the plasma, largely without a known, distinct biological function [75].

The stimulus for natriuretic peptide release is myocyte stretch [75–78]. ANP is secreted primarily from the cardiac atria in response to increased atrial wall tension, reflecting volume and pressure loads. Additionally, multiple hormones and neurotransmitters, such as endothelin, arginine vasopressin, and catecholamines, directly stimulate the secretion of ANP [77]. BNP is secreted primarily from the cardiac ventricles in response to increased left and/or right ventricular volume and pressure loads. The majority of CNP is found in the central nervous system, anterior pituitary, kidney, and vascular endothelial cells; the plasma concentration of CNP is very low [77].

The natriuretic peptides bind to specific receptors (natriuretic peptide receptors A, B, and C) on the surface of target cells. Natriuretic peptide receptors A and B are linked to a cyclic guanosine monophosphate-mediated signaling cascade. Natriuretic peptide receptor A is the most abundant natriuretic receptor type in large blood vessels and binds both ANP and BNP but has higher affinity for ANP. Natriuretic peptide receptor B is the predominant receptor in the brain and binds CNP. Binding of the natriuretic peptides to natriuretic peptide receptors A or B activates cyclic guanosine monophosphate formation by guanylyl cyclase [77]. Natriuretic peptide receptor C, however, is involved in peptide clearance [79]; binding of the natriuretic peptide to natriuretic peptide receptor C results in internalization and enzymatic degradation of the peptide, after which the receptor returns to the cell surface. Binding of ANP to its receptors and the effects of binding are shown in (Fig. 6.2). All three natriuretic peptides bind to natriuretic peptide C with equal affinity. Breakdown of circulating natriuretic peptides is also accomplished by neutral endopeptidases that are present within renal tubular and vascular cells [77].

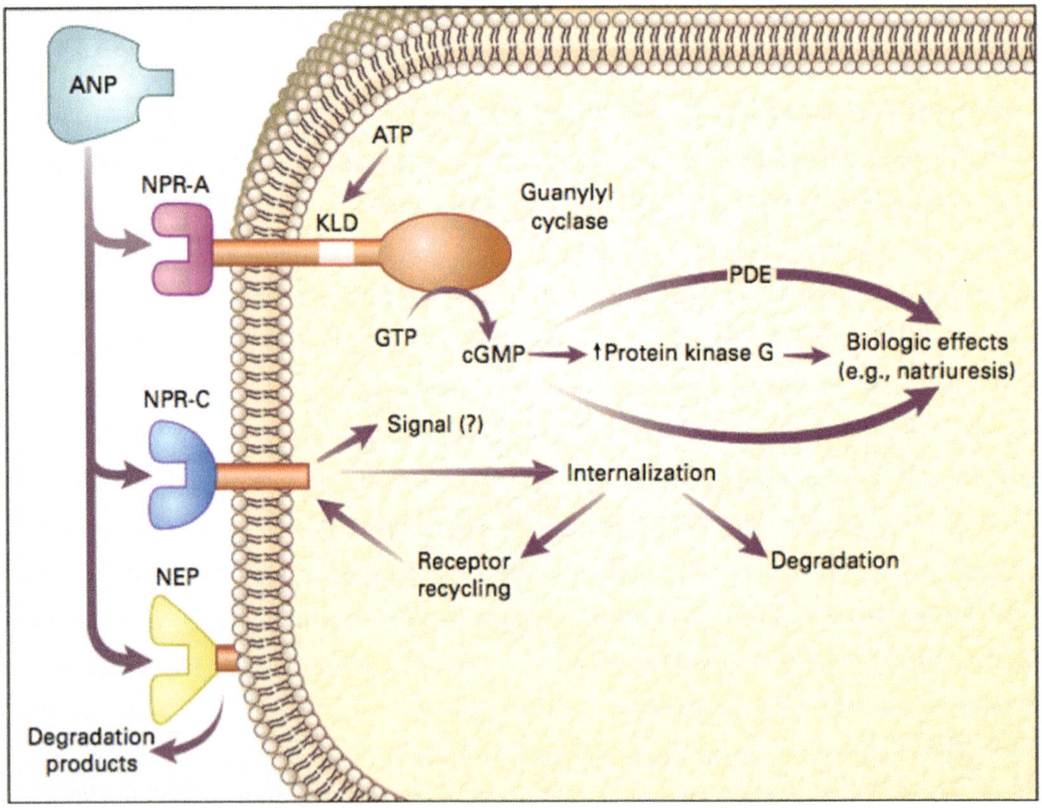

FIGURE 6.2 **Action of Atrial Natriuretic Peptide at Target Cells.** Atrial natriuretic peptide (ANP) binds to natriuretic peptide receptor A (NPR-A) and, in an ATP-dependent fashion, stimulates the intrinsic guanylyl cyclase activity of the receptor. Cyclic guanosine monophosphate (cGMP) exerts its biologic effects indirectly through cGMP-dependent protein kinase G or one or more phosphodiesterases (PDEs), or by direct action on effectors such as amiloride-sensitive sodium channels in the kidney. ATP dependence requires the kinase-like domain (KLD) of the receptor. ANP also binds to natriuretic peptide receptor C (NPR-C), after which it is internalized and degraded. The C receptor may also have independent signaling functions. Finally, ANP may be degraded by the extracellular neutral endopeptidases (NEPs) in the kidney and vasculature. GTP denotes guanosine triphosphate. *With permission from E.R. Levin, D.G. Gardner, W.K. Samson. Natriuretic peptides. The New England journal of medicine. 339 (1998) 321–8.*

Cardiovascular Actions

With an increase in venous return to the heart, the physiologic role of the natriuretic peptides is to provide a compensatory reduction in intravascular volume and blood pressure through a coordinated effect on the brain, adrenal gland, kidney, and vasculature. This decrease in preload is achieved through a number of mechanisms: (1) shifting of intravascular fluid into the extravascular compartment through increasing permeability of the vascular endothelium and increasing hydraulic pressure in the capillary bed [80], (2) increasing venous capacitance, and (3) decreasing extracellular fluid volume through effects on the kidney and from suppression of the RAAS [81]. Furthermore, the natriuretic peptides reduce sympathetic tone in the peripheral vasculature by suppressing catecholamine release from presynaptic nerve endings [82,83]. ANP and BNP have similar cardiovascular effects, while CNP is a more potent venous dilator than the other two peptides [77].

Renal and Central Nervous System Effects

ANP stimulates dilation of the afferent renal arterioles and constriction of efferent arterioles, leading to increased glomerular filtration [84]. However, ANP also has direct tubular actions, inhibiting AT II-stimulated sodium and water transport in the proximal convoluted tubules [85], inhibiting tubular water transport by antagonizing vasopressin in the cortical collecting ducts [86], and blocking sodium absorption in the inner medullary collecting duct by stimulating cyclic guanosine monophosphate production [87–90]. Importantly, infusions of ANP or BNP reduce plasma renin and aldosterone concentrations and inhibit AT II-stimulated aldosterone secretion [80].

Although plasma ANP and BNP do not cross the blood–brain barrier, the natriuretic peptides are also produced in the brain and thus have central nervous system actions. The natriuretic peptides act centrally to inhibit salt appetite and water drinking [91,92] and inhibit the secretion of vasopressin through effects on the brain and pituitary [77]. This interplay between the central nervous system and periphery are shown in (Fig. 6.3). Finally, natriuretic peptides also act in the brain stem to decrease sympathetic tone [82,83,93].

Natriuretic Peptides in Heart Failure

Patients with heart failure have elevated plasma concentrations of both ANP and BNP, rising to levels as much as 30 times normal in adult patients with New York Heart Association class IV symptoms [94]. In adults with heart failure, plasma BNP is an important predictor of both morbidity and mortality [95] and is routinely used to as a heart failure biomarker [96,97]. However, unlike norepinephrine and At II, the natriuretic peptides do not appear to have a direct effect on the cardiac myocyte in vivo that contributes to disease progression. Natriuretic peptide release is stimulated by myocyte stretch in the failing atria and ventricles, as well as by increased RAAS activation. Furthermore, cardiac remodeling and subsequent ventricular hypertrophy leads to augmented production of both ANP and BNP [77]. Increased natriuretic peptide synthesis and release attempts to counteract the effects of neurohormonal activation (increased catecholamines, AT II, aldosterone, and endothelin-1) through reducing systemic vascular resistance and decreasing intracardiac filling pressure to improve myocardial performance. Blocking the effects of ANP, for example, results in accelerated progression to overt heart failure [98]. However, renal responsiveness to natriuretic peptides decreases as heart failure worsens, likely secondary to changes in renal hemodynamics, receptor downregulation, and increased cyclic guanosine monophosphate hydrolysis by phosphodiesterases [99], which in turn exacerbates a deterioration in cardiac function [100].

Pediatric-Specific Data

Interestingly, plasma levels of BNP are elevated in healthy infants immediately after birth and gradually decrease to adult levels by 3 months of age [101]. Evaluation of natriuretic peptides in the pediatric heart failure population has consisted of several clinical studies demonstrating elevated natriuretic peptide levels in a variety of patient populations: dilated cardiomyopathy [102], left-to-right shunts (such as patent ductus arteriosus, atrial and ventricular septal defects) [103–106], right ventricular pressure or volume overload [104], and heart failure from heterogenous etiologies [107,108]. Several small pediatric studies demonstrate a correlation between higher BNP and lower left ventricular ejection fraction and more ventricular dilation. However, there is conflicting pediatric data related to BNP and exercise capacity or outcomes in single ventricle congenital heart disease. For children and young adults with heart failure, the establishment of age-specific and disease-specific diagnostic or prognostic cutoffs will likely be more informative.

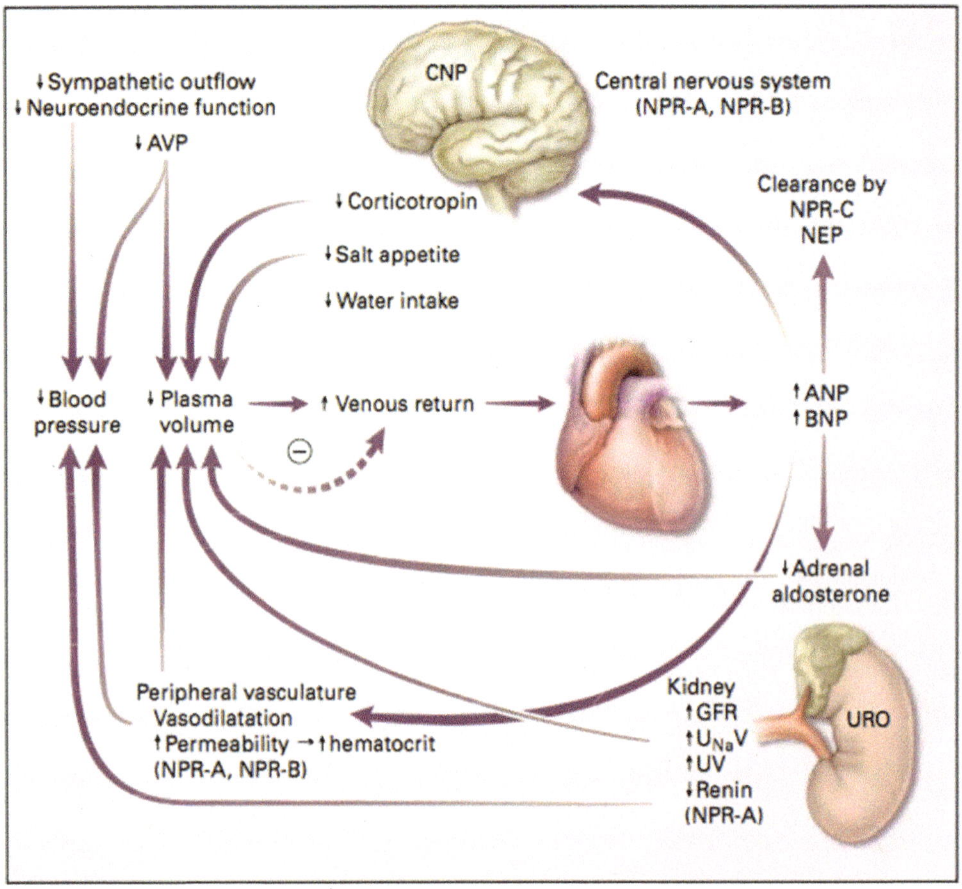

FIGURE 6.3 **Physiologic Effects of Natriuretic Peptides Released from the Heart When Venous Return Is Increased.** Increased secretion of the natriuretic peptides reduces blood pressure and plasma volume through coordinated actions in the brain, adrenal gland, kidney, and vasculature. The minus sign indicates that a decrease in plasma volume leads to a decrease in venous return, which in turn decreases the secretion of the natriuretic peptides. *BP*, blood pressure; *ANP* and *BNP*, atrial and brain natriuretic peptides, respectively; *AVP*, arginine vasopressin; *CNF*, C-type natriuretic peptide; *GFR*, glomerular filtration rate; *NEP*, neutral endopeptidase; *NPR-A*, *NPR-B*, and *NPR-C*, natriuretic peptide receptors A, B, and C, respectively; $U_{Na}V$, urinary sodium excretion; *URO*, urodilatin; and *UV*, urinary volume. The receptors that mediate the functions of the natriuretic peptides are indicated in parentheses. *With permission from E.R. Levin, D.G. Gardner, W.K. Samson. Natriuretic peptides. The New England journal of medicine. 339 (1998) 321–328.*

CONCLUSION

The sympathetic/adrenergic system and the RAAS work to preserve cardiac output and maintain perfusion to vital organs early in heart failure, but the chronic effects result in adverse remodeling and can even block the beneficial effects of other peptides. Understanding these adaptive and maladaptive processes has led to therapeutics that have improved outcomes in adult heart failure. While some of this understanding can be applied to pediatric heart failure, there appear to be important distinctions that require further elucidation with respect to age and maturation, organ-specific changes, and disease etiology.

REFERENCES

[1] M.R. Bristow, The adrenergic nervous system in heart failure, N. Engl. J. Med. 311 (13) (September 27, 1984) 850–851 PubMed PMID: 6472388.

[2] D.L. Mann, M.R. Bristow, Mechanisms and models in heart failure: the biomechanical model and beyond, Circulation 111 (21) (May 31, 2005) 2837–2849 PubMed PMID: 15927992.

[3] K. Swedberg, P. Eneroth, J. Kjekshus, L. Wilhelmsen, Hormones regulating cardiovascular function in patients with severe congestive heart failure and their relation to mortality. CONSENSUS Trial Study Group, Circulation 82 (5) (November 1990) 1730–1736 PubMed PMID: 2225374.

[4] J.N. Cohn, T.B. Levine, M.T. Olivari, V. Garberg, D. Lura, G.S. Francis, et al., Plasma norepinephrine as a guide to prognosis in patients with chronic congestive heart failure, N. Engl. J. Med. 311 (13) (September 27, 1984) 819–823 PubMed PMID: 6382011.

[5] E.J. Eichhorn, M.R. Bristow, Medical therapy can improve the biological properties of the chronically failing heart. A new era in the treatment of heart failure, Circulation 94 (9) (November 1, 1996) 2285–2296 PubMed PMID: 8901684.

[6] A. Lymperopoulos, G. Rengo, W.J. Koch, Adrenergic nervous system in heart failure: pathophysiology and therapy, Circ. Res. 113 (6) (August 30, 2013) 739–753 PubMed PMID: 23989716. Pubmed Central PMCID: 3843360.

[7] D.P. Zipes, Heart-brain interactions in cardiac arrhythmias: role of the autonomic nervous system, Clevel. Clin. J. Med. 75 (Suppl. 2) (March 2008) S94–S96 PubMed PMID: 18540155.
[8] F. Triposkiadis, G. Karayannis, G. Giamouzis, J. Skoularigis, G. Louridas, J. Butler, The sympathetic nervous system in heart failure physiology, pathophysiology, and clinical implications, J. Am. Coll. Cardiol. 54 (19) (November 3, 2009) 1747–1762 PubMed PMID: 19874988.
[9] M.J. Eaton, H. Duplan, Useful cell lines derived from the adrenal medulla, Mol. Cell. Endocrinol. 228 (1–2) (December 30, 2004) 39–52 PubMed PMID: 15541571.
[10] A. Lymperopoulos, G. Rengo, W.J. Koch, Adrenal adrenoceptors in heart failure: fine-tuning cardiac stimulation, Trends Mol. Med. 13 (12) (December 2007) 503–511 PubMed PMID: 17981507.
[11] A. Lymperopoulos, Ischemic emergency?: endothelial cells have their own "adrenaline shot" at hand, Hypertension 60 (1) (July 2012) 12–14 PubMed PMID: 22665125.
[12] W.S. Colucci, R.F. Wright, E. Braunwald, New positive inotropic agents in the treatment of congestive heart failure. Mechanisms of action and recent clinical developments. 1, N. Engl. J. Med. 314 (5) (January 30, 1986) 290–299 PubMed PMID: 2867470.
[13] K. Leineweber, T. Wangemann, C. Giessler, H. Bruck, S. Dhein, M. Kostelka, et al., Age-dependent changes of cardiac neuronal noradrenaline reuptake transporter (uptake1) in the human heart, J. Am. Coll. Cardiol. 40 (8) (October 16, 2002) 1459 PubMed PMID: 12392837.
[14] M. Philipp, M. Brede, L. Hein, Physiological significance of alpha(2)-adrenergic receptor subtype diversity: one receptor is not enough, Am. J. Physiol. Regul. Integr. Comp. Physiol. 283 (2) (August 2002) R287–R295 PubMed PMID: 12121839.
[15] J.A. Thomas, B.H. Marks, Plasma norepinephrine in congestive heart failure, Am. J. Cardiol. 41 (2) (February 1978) 233–243 PubMed PMID: 203177.
[16] G.S. Pepper, R.W. Lee, Sympathetic activation in heart failure and its treatment with beta-blockade, Arch. Intern. Med. 159 (3) (February 8, 1999) 225–234 PubMed PMID: 9989534.
[17] V. Regitz, B. Leuchs, C. Bossaller, J. Sehested, M. Rappolder, E. Fleck, Myocardial catecholamine concentrations in dilated cardiomyopathy and heart failure of different origins, Eur. Heart J. 12 (Suppl. D) (August 1991) 171–174 PubMed PMID: 1915450.
[18] J. Backs, A. Haunstetter, S.H. Gerber, J. Metz, M.M. Borst, R.H. Strasser, et al., The neuronal norepinephrine transporter in experimental heart failure: evidence for a posttranscriptional downregulation, J. Mol. Cell. Cardiol. 33 (3) (March 2001) 461–472 PubMed PMID: 11181015.
[19] M.R. Bristow, R. Ginsburg, V. Umans, M. Fowler, W. Minobe, R. Rasmussen, et al., Beta 1- and beta 2-adrenergic-receptor subpopulations in nonfailing and failing human ventricular myocardium: coupling of both receptor subtypes to muscle contraction and selective beta 1-receptor down-regulation in heart failure, Circ. Res. 59 (3) (September 1986) 297–309 PubMed PMID: 2876788.
[20] M.R. Bristow, R. Ginsburg, W. Minobe, R.S. Cubicciotti, W.S. Sageman, K. Lurie, et al., Decreased catecholamine sensitivity and beta-adrenergic-receptor density in failing human hearts, N. Engl. J. Med. 307 (4) (July 22, 1982) 205–211 PubMed PMID: 6283349.
[21] J.D. Port, M.R. Bristow, Altered beta-adrenergic receptor gene regulation and signaling in chronic heart failure, J. Mol. Cell. Cardiol. 33 (5) (May 2001) 887–905 PubMed PMID: 11343413.
[22] A. Aggarwal, M.D. Esler, F. Socratous, D.M. Kaye, Evidence for functional presynaptic alpha-2 adrenoceptors and their down-regulation in human heart failure, J. Am. Coll. Cardiol. 37 (5) (April 2001) 1246–1251 PubMed PMID: 11300430.
[23] G.L. Todd, G. Baroldi, G.M. Pieper, F.C. Clayton, R.S. Eliot, Experimental catecholamine-induced myocardial necrosis. II. Temporal development of isoproterenol-induced contraction band lesions correlated with ECG, hemodynamic and biochemical changes, J. Mol. Cell. Cardiol. 17 (7) (July 1985) 647–656 PubMed PMID: 4020881.
[24] D.L. Mann, R.L. Kent, B. Parsons, G. Cooper, Adrenergic effects on the biology of the adult mammalian cardiocyte, Circulation 85 (2) (February 1992) 790–804 PubMed PMID: 1370925.
[25] F. Brouri, N. Hanoun, O. Mediani, F. Saurini, M. Hamon, P.M. Vanhoutte, et al., Blockade of beta 1- and desensitization of beta 2-adrenoceptors reduce isoprenaline-induced cardiac fibrosis, Eur. J. Pharmacol. 485 (1–3) (February 6, 2004) 227–234 PubMed PMID: 14757145.
[26] O.E. Osadchii, G.R. Norton, R. McKechnie, D. Deftereos, A.J. Woodiwiss, Cardiac dilatation and pump dysfunction without intrinsic myocardial systolic failure following chronic beta-adrenoreceptor activation, Am. J. Physiol. Heart Circ. Physiol. 292 (4) (April 2007) H1898–H1905 PubMed PMID: 17158652.
[27] C. Communal, K. Singh, D.R. Pimentel, W.S. Colucci, Norepinephrine stimulates apoptosis in adult rat ventricular myocytes by activation of the beta-adrenergic pathway, Circulation 98 (13) (September 29, 1998) 1329–1334 PubMed PMID: 9751683.
[28] Y.C. Fu, C.S. Chi, S.C. Yin, B. Hwang, Y.T. Chiu, S.L. Hsu, Norepinephrine induces apoptosis in neonatal rat cardiomyocytes through a reactive oxygen species-TNF alpha-caspase signaling pathway, Cardiovasc. Res. 62 (3) (June 1, 2004) 558–567 PubMed PMID: 15158148.
[29] R.E. Shaddy, M.M. Boucek, D.T. Hsu, R.J. Boucek, C.E. Canter, L. Mahony, et al., Carvedilol for children and adolescents with heart failure: a randomized controlled trial, JAMA 298 (10) (September 12, 2007) 1171–1179 PubMed PMID: 17848651.
[30] M. Packer, M.R. Bristow, J.N. Cohn, W.S. Colucci, M.B. Fowler, E.M. Gilbert, et al., The effect of carvedilol on morbidity and mortality in patients with chronic heart failure. U.S. Carvedilol Heart Failure Study Group, N. Engl. J. Med. 334 (21) (May 23, 1996) 1349–1355 PubMed PMID: 8614419.
[31] S.D. Miyamoto, B.L. Stauffer, S. Nakano, R. Sobus, K. Nunley, P. Nelson, et al., Beta-adrenergic adaptation in paediatric idiopathic dilated cardiomyopathy, Eur. Heart J. 35 (1) (January 2014) 33–41 PubMed PMID: 22843448. Pubmed Central PMCID: 3877432.
[32] C.C. Sucharov, J.G. Hijmans, R.D. Sobus, W.F. Melhado, S.D. Miyamoto, B.L. Stauffer, beta-Adrenergic receptor antagonism in mice: a model for pediatric heart disease, J. Appl. Physiol. 115 (7) (October 1, 2013) 979–987 PubMed PMID: 23887897. Pubmed Central PMCID: 3798823.
[33] S.D. Miyamoto, B.L. Stauffer, J. Polk, A. Medway, M. Friedrich, K. Haubold, et al., Gene expression and beta-adrenergic signaling are altered in hypoplastic left heart syndrome, J. Heart Lung Transplant. 33 (8) (August 2014) 785–793 PubMed PMID: 24793904. Pubmed Central PMCID: 4111994.

[34] J.W. Wright, S. Mizutani, J.W. Harding, Pathways involved in the transition from hypertension to hypertrophy to heart failure. Treatment strategies, Heart Fail. Rev. 13 (3) (September 2008) 367–375 PubMed PMID: 17987382.

[35] H. Yamada, B. Fabris, A.M. Allen, B. Jackson, C.I. Johnston, A.O. Mendelsohn, Localization of angiotensin converting enzyme in rat heart, Circ. Res. 68 (1) (January 1991) 141–149 PubMed PMID: 1845851.

[36] P.K. Mehta, K.K. Griendling, Angiotensin II cell signaling: physiological and pathological effects in the cardiovascular system, Am. J. Physiol. Cell Physiol. 292 (1) (January 2007) C82–C97 PubMed PMID: 16870827.

[37] K.M. Baker, G.W. Booz, D.E. Dostal, Cardiac actions of angiotensin II: role of an intracardiac renin-angiotensin system, Annu. Rev. Physiol. 54 (1992) 227–241 PubMed PMID: 1562174.

[38] L. Watkins Jr., J.A. Burton, E. Haber, J.R. Cant, F.W. Smith, A.C. Barger, The renin-angiotensin-aldosterone system in congestive failure in conscious dogs, J. Clin. Investig. 57 (6) (June 1976) 1606–1617 PubMed PMID: 180056. Pubmed Central PMCID: 436820.

[39] R.H. Freeman, J.O. Davis, G.M. Williams, J.M. DeForrest, A.A. Seymour, B.P. Rowe, Effects of the oral converting enzyme inhibitor, SQ 14225, in a model of low cardiac output in dogs, Circ. Res. 45 (4) (October 1979) 540–545 PubMed PMID: 225056.

[40] B.J. Morris, J.O. Davis, M.L. Zatzman, G.M. Williams, The renin-angiotensin-aldosterone system in rabbits with congestive heart failure produced by aortic constriction, Circ. Res. 40 (3) (March 1977) 275–282 PubMed PMID: 837474.

[41] V.J. Dzau, W.S. Colucci, N.K. Hollenberg, G.H. Williams, Relation of the renin-angiotensin-aldosterone system to clinical state in congestive heart failure, Circulation 63 (3) (March 1981) 645–651 PubMed PMID: 7006851.

[42] A. Leri, P.P. Claudio, Q. Li, X. Wang, K. Reiss, S. Wang, et al., Stretch-mediated release of angiotensin II induces myocyte apoptosis by activating p53 that enhances the local renin-angiotensin system and decreases the Bcl-2-to-Bax protein ratio in the cell, J. Clin. Investig. 101 (7) (April 1, 1998) 1326–1342 PubMed PMID: 9525975. Pubmed Central PMCID: 508710.

[43] M. Ruzicka, V. Skarda, F.H. Leenen, Effects of ACE inhibitors on circulating versus cardiac angiotensin II in volume overload-induced cardiac hypertrophy in rats, Circulation 92 (12) (December 15, 1995) 3568–3573 PubMed PMID: 8521580.

[44] H. Schunkert, J.R. Ingelfinger, A.T. Hirsch, S.S. Tang, S.E. Litwin, C.E. Talsness, et al., Evidence for tissue-specific activation of renal angiotensinogen mRNA expression in chronic stable experimental heart failure, J. Clin. Investig. 90 (4) (October 1992) 1523–1529 PubMed PMID: 1401084. Pubmed Central PMCID: 443199.

[45] A. Wolny, J.P. Clozel, J. Rein, P. Mory, P. Vogt, M. Turino, et al., Functional and biochemical analysis of angiotensin II-forming pathways in the human heart, Circ. Res. 80 (2) (February 1997) 219–227 PubMed PMID: 9012744.

[46] K.K. Griendling, P. Delafontaine, S.E. Rittenhouse, M.A. Gimbrone Jr., R.W. Alexander, Correlation of receptor sequestration with sustained diacylglycerol accumulation in angiotensin II-stimulated cultured vascular smooth muscle cells, J. Biol. Chem. 262 (30) (October 25, 1987) 14555–14562 PubMed PMID: 2822694.

[47] B. Lassegue, R.W. Alexander, G. Nickenig, M. Clark, T.J. Murphy, K.K. Griendling, Angiotensin II down-regulates the vascular smooth muscle AT1 receptor by transcriptional and post-transcriptional mechanisms: evidence for homologous and heterologous regulation, Mol. Pharmacol. 48 (4) (October 1995) 601–609 PubMed PMID: 7476884.

[48] R.M. Touyz, G. He, L.Y. Deng, E.L. Schiffrin, Role of extracellular signal-regulated kinases in angiotensin II-stimulated contraction of smooth muscle cells from human resistance arteries, Circulation 99 (3) (January 26, 1999) 392–399 PubMed PMID: 9918526.

[49] S. Gunther, M.A. Gimbrone Jr., R.W. Alexander, Regulation by angiotensin II of its receptors in resistance blood vessels, Nature 287 (5779) (September 18, 1980) 230–232 PubMed PMID: 6253796.

[50] K.K. Griendling, D. Sorescu, M. Ushio-Fukai, NAD(P)H oxidase: role in cardiovascular biology and disease, Circ. Res. 86 (5) (March 17, 2000) 494–501 PubMed PMID: 10720409.

[51] V.J. Dzau, Theodore Cooper lecture: tissue angiotensin and pathobiology of vascular disease: a unifying hypothesis, Hypertension 37 (4) (April 2001) 1047–1052 PubMed PMID: 11304501.

[52] L.B. Tan, J.E. Jalil, R. Pick, J.S. Janicki, K.T. Weber, Cardiac myocyte necrosis induced by angiotensin II, Circ. Res. 69 (5) (November 1991) 1185–1195 PubMed PMID: 1834362.

[53] C. Sumners, M.K. Raizada, Angiotensin II stimulates norepinephrine uptake in hypothalamus-brain stem neuronal cultures, Am. J. Physiol. 250 (2 Pt 1) (February 1986) C236–C244 PubMed PMID: 3513605.

[54] M.A. Weber, R.E. Purdy, Catecholamine-mediated constrictor effects of aldosterone on vascular smooth muscle, Life Sci. 30 (23) (June 7, 1982) 2009–2017 PubMed PMID: 7109834.

[55] J.M. Connell, E. Davies, The new biology of aldosterone, J. Endocrinol. 186 (1) (July 2005) 1–20 PubMed PMID: 16002531.

[56] A.M. Marney, N.J. Brown, Aldosterone and end-organ damage, Clin. Sci. 113 (6) (September 2007) 267–278 PubMed PMID: 17683282.

[57] K.T. Weber, Aldosterone in congestive heart failure, N. Engl. J. Med. 345 (23) (December 6, 2001) 1689–1697 PubMed PMID: 11759649.

[58] J.F. Tait, B. Little, S.A. Tait, C. Flood, J. Bougas, Splanchnic extraction and clearance of aldosterone in subjects with minimal and marked cardiac dysfunction, J. Clin. Endocrinol. Metab. 25 (February 1965) 219–228 PubMed PMID: 14268489.

[59] C.S. Barr, C.C. Lang, J. Hanson, M. Arnott, N. Kennedy, A.D. Struthers, Effects of adding spironolactone to an angiotensin-converting enzyme inhibitor in chronic congestive heart failure secondary to coronary artery disease, Am. J. Cardiol. 76 (17) (December 15, 1995) 1259–1265 PubMed PMID: 7503007.

[60] C.A. Farquharson, A.D. Struthers, Spironolactone increases nitric oxide bioactivity, improves endothelial vasodilator dysfunction, and suppresses vascular angiotensin I/angiotensin II conversion in patients with chronic heart failure, Circulation 101 (6) (February 15, 2000) 594–597 PubMed PMID: 10673249.

[61] I.H. Zucker, W. Wang, M. Brandle, H.D. Schultz, K.P. Patel, Neural regulation of sympathetic nerve activity in heart failure, Prog. Cardiovasc. Dis. 37 (6) (May–June 1995) 397–414 PubMed PMID: 7777669.

[62] E.L. Schiffrin, D.J. Franks, J. Gutkowska, Effect of aldosterone on vascular angiotensin II receptors in the rat, Can. J. Physiol. Pharmacol. 63 (12) (December 1985) 1522–1527 PubMed PMID: 3006895.

[63] A. Jazayeri, W.J. Meyer 3rd, Mineralocorticoid-induced increase in beta-adrenergic receptors of cultured rat arterial smooth muscle cells, J. Steroid Biochem. 33 (5) (November 1989) 987–991 PubMed PMID: 2557490.

[64] W. Wang, J.M. McClain, I.H. Zucker, Aldosterone reduces baroreceptor discharge in the dog, Hypertension 19 (3) (March 1992) 270–277 PubMed PMID: 1532165.

[65] V. Robert, N. Van Thiem, S.L. Cheav, C. Mouas, B. Swynghedauw, C. Delcayre, Increased cardiac types I and III collagen mRNAs in aldosterone-salt hypertension, Hypertension 24 (1) (July 1994) 30–36 PubMed PMID: 8021005.

[66] J.E. Macdonald, N. Kennedy, A.D. Struthers, Effects of spironolactone on endothelial function, vascular angiotensin converting enzyme activity, and other prognostic markers in patients with mild heart failure already taking optimal treatment, Heart 90 (7) (July 2004) 765–770 PubMed PMID: 15201246. Pubmed Central PMCID: 1768327.

[67] D.T. Hsu, V. Zak, L. Mahony, L.A. Sleeper, A.M. Atz, J.C. Levine, et al., Enalapril in infants with single ventricle: results of a multicenter randomized trial, Circulation 122 (4) (July 27, 2010) 333–340 PubMed PMID: 20625111. Pubmed Central PMCID: 3692364.

[68] M. Frenneaux, R.A. Stewart, C.M. Newman, K.A. Hallidie-Smith, Enalapril for severe heart failure in infancy, Arch. Dis. Child. 64 (2) (February 1989) 219–223 PubMed PMID: 2539059. Pubmed Central PMCID: 1791876.

[69] Y. Mori, M. Nakazawa, H. Tomimatsu, K. Momma, Long-term effect of angiotensin-converting enzyme inhibitor in volume overloaded heart during growth: a controlled pilot study, J. Am. Coll. Cardiol. 36 (1) (July 2000) 270–275 PubMed PMID: 10898445.

[70] N.J. Shaw, N. Wilson, D.F. Dickinson, Captopril in heart failure secondary to a left to right shunt, Arch. Dis. Child. 63 (4) (April 1988) 360–363 PubMed PMID: 3284479. Pubmed Central PMCID: 1778804.

[71] K. Momma, ACE inhibitors in pediatric patients with heart failure, Paediatr. Drugs 8 (1) (2006) 55–69 PubMed PMID: 16494512.

[72] W.T. Mahle, A. Wang, A.A. Quyyumi, M.E. McConnell, W.M. Book, Impact of spironolactone on endothelial function in patients with single ventricle heart, Congenit. Heart Dis. 4 (1) (January–February 2009) 12–16 PubMed PMID: 19207397. Pubmed Central PMCID: 3907773.

[73] S. Mital, W.K. Chung, S.D. Colan, L.A. Sleeper, C. Manlhiot, C.B. Arrington, et al., Renin-angiotensin-aldosterone genotype influences ventricular remodeling in infants with single ventricle, Circulation 123 (21) (May 31, 2011) 2353–2362 PubMed PMID: 21576655. Pubmed Central PMCID: 3137902.

[74] A.S. Maisel, P. Krishnaswamy, R.M. Nowak, J. McCord, J.E. Hollander, P. Duc, et al., Rapid measurement of B-type natriuretic peptide in the emergency diagnosis of heart failure, N. Engl. J. Med. 347 (3) (July 18, 2002) 161–167 PubMed PMID: 12124404.

[75] N. Nasser, B. Bar-Oz, A. Nir, Natriuretic peptides and heart disease in infants and children, J. Pediatr. 147 (2) (August 2005) 248–253 PubMed PMID: 16126059.

[76] M.R. Cowie, G.F. Mendez, BNP and congestive heart failure, Prog. Cardiovasc. Dis. 44 (4) (January–February 2002) 293–321 PubMed PMID: 12007084.

[77] E.R. Levin, D.G. Gardner, W.K. Samson, Natriuretic peptides, N. Engl. J. Med. 339 (5) (July 30, 1998) 321–328 PubMed PMID: 9682046.

[78] J. Mair, A. Hammerer-Lercher, B. Puschendorf, The impact of cardiac natriuretic peptide determination on the diagnosis and management of heart failure, Clin. Chem. Lab. Med. 39 (7) (July 2001) 571–588 PubMed PMID: 11522102.

[79] T. Maack, M. Suzuki, F.A. Almeida, D. Nussenzveig, R.M. Scarborough, G.A. McEnroe, et al., Physiological role of silent receptors of atrial natriuretic factor, Science 238 (4827) (October 30, 1987) 675–678 PubMed PMID: 2823385.

[80] C.N. Wijeyaratne, P.J. Moult, The effect of alpha human atrial natriuretic peptide on plasma volume and vascular permeability in normotensive subjects, J. Clin. Endocrinol. Metab. 76 (2) (February 1993) 343–346 PubMed PMID: 8432776.

[81] P.J. Hunt, E.A. Espiner, M.G. Nicholls, A.M. Richards, T.G. Yandle, Differing biological effects of equimolar atrial and brain natriuretic peptide infusions in normal man, J. Clin. Endocrinol. Metab. 81 (11) (November 1996) 3871–3876 PubMed PMID: 8923831.

[82] H.D. Schultz, D.G. Gardner, C.F. Deschepper, H.M. Coleridge, J.C. Coleridge, Vagal C-fiber blockade abolishes sympathetic inhibition by atrial natriuretic factor, Am. J. Physiol. 255 (1 Pt 2) (July 1988) R6–R13 PubMed PMID: 2969196.

[83] R.H. Yang, H.K. Jin, J.M. Wyss, Y.F. Chen, S. Oparil, Pressor effect of blocking atrial natriuretic peptide in nucleus tractus solitarii, Hypertension 19 (2) (February 1992) 198–205 PubMed PMID: 1531332.

[84] M. Marin-Grez, J.T. Fleming, M. Steinhausen, Atrial natriuretic peptide causes pre-glomerular vasodilatation and post-glomerular vasoconstriction in rat kidney, Nature 324 (6096) (December 4–10, 1986) 473–476 PubMed PMID: 2946962.

[85] P.J. Harris, D. Thomas, T.O. Morgan, Atrial natriuretic peptide inhibits angiotensin-stimulated proximal tubular sodium and water reabsorption, Nature 326 (6114) (April 16–22, 1987) 697–698 PubMed PMID: 2951600.

[86] M.A. Dillingham, R.J. Anderson, Inhibition of vasopressin action by atrial natriuretic factor, Science 231 (4745) (March 28, 1986) 1572–1573 PubMed PMID: 3006248.

[87] H. Sonnenberg, U. Honrath, C.K. Chong, D.R. Wilson, Atrial natriuretic factor inhibits sodium transport in medullary collecting duct, Am. J. Physiol. 250 (6 Pt 2) (June 1986) F963–F966 PubMed PMID: 2940876.

[88] M.L. Zeidel, D. Kikeri, P. Silva, M. Burrowes, B.M. Brenner, Atrial natriuretic peptides inhibit conductive sodium uptake by rabbit inner medullary collecting duct cells, J. Clin. Investig. 82 (3) (September 1988) 1067–1074 PubMed PMID: 2458385. Pubmed Central PMCID: 303621.

[89] D.B. Light, E.M. Schwiebert, K.H. Karlson, B.A. Stanton, Atrial natriuretic peptide inhibits a cation channel in renal inner medullary collecting duct cells, Science 243 (4889) (January 20, 1989) 383–385 PubMed PMID: 2463673.

[90] M.L. Zeidel, Regulation of collecting duct Na+ reabsorption by ANP 31-67, Clin. Exp. Pharmacol. Physiol. 22 (2) (February 1995) 121–124 PubMed PMID: 7621604.

[91] R.E. Blackburn, W.K. Samson, R.J. Fulton, E.M. Stricker, J.G. Verbalis, Central oxytocin and ANP receptors mediate osmotic inhibition of salt appetite in rats, Am. J. Physiol. 269 (2 Pt 2) (August 1995) R245–R251 PubMed PMID: 7653644.

[92] L.M. Burrell, H.J. Lambert, P.H. Baylis, Effect of atrial natriuretic peptide on thirst and arginine vasopressin release in humans, Am. J. Physiol. 260 (3 Pt 2) (March 1991) R475–R479 PubMed PMID: 1825748.

[93] M.K. Steele, D.G. Gardner, P.L. Xie, H.D. Schultz, Interactions between ANP and ANG II in regulating blood pressure and sympathetic outflow, Am. J. Physiol. 260 (6 Pt 2) (June 1991) R1145–R1151 PubMed PMID: 1829337.

[94] J.C. Burnett Jr., P.C. Kao, D.C. Hu, D.W. Heser, D. Heublein, J.P. Granger, et al., Atrial natriuretic peptide elevation in congestive heart failure in the human, Science 231 (4742) (March 7, 1986) 1145–1147 PubMed PMID: 2935937.

[95] I.S. Anand, L.D. Fisher, Y.T. Chiang, R. Latini, S. Masson, A.P. Maggioni, et al., Changes in brain natriuretic peptide and norepinephrine over time and mortality and morbidity in the valsartan heart failure trial (Val-HeFT), Circulation 107 (9) (March 11, 2003) 1278–1283 PubMed PMID: 12628948.

[96] A. Harrison, L.K. Morrison, P. Krishnaswamy, R. Kazanegra, P. Clopton, Q. Dao, et al., B-type natriuretic peptide predicts future cardiac events in patients presenting to the emergency department with dyspnea, Ann. Emerg. Med. 39 (2) (February 2002) 131–138 PubMed PMID: 11823766.

[97] W.H. Tang, G.S. Francis, D.A. Morrow, L.K. Newby, C.P. Cannon, R.L. Jesse, et al., National academy of clinical biochemistry laboratory medicine practice guidelines: clinical utilization of cardiac biomarker testing in heart failure, Circulation 116 (5) (July 31, 2007) e99–109 PubMed PMID: 17630410.

[98] T.L. Stevens, J.C. Burnett Jr., M. Kinoshita, Y. Matsuda, M.M. Redfield, A functional role for endogenous atrial natriuretic peptide in a canine model of early left ventricular dysfunction, J. Clin. Investig. 95 (3) (March 1995) 1101–1108 PubMed PMID: 7883958. Pubmed Central PMCID: 441446.

[99] S.N. Rahman, G.E. Kim, A.S. Mathew, C.A. Goldberg, R. Allgren, R.W. Schrier, et al., Effects of atrial natriuretic peptide in clinical acute renal failure, Kidney Int. 45 (6) (June 1994) 1731–1738 PubMed PMID: 7933821.

[100] J.B. Smith, T.M. Lincoln, Angiotensin decreases cyclic GMP accumulation produced by atrial natriuretic factor, Am. J. Physiol. 253 (1 Pt 1) (July 1987) C147–C150 PubMed PMID: 2440311.

[101] M. Yoshibayashi, T. Kamiya, Y. Saito, K. Nakao, K. Nishioka, S. Temma, et al., Plasma brain natriuretic peptide concentrations in healthy children from birth to adolescence: marked and rapid increase after birth, Eur. J. Endocrinol. 133 (2) (August 1995) 207–209 PubMed PMID: 7655645.

[102] J.F. Price, A.K. Thomas, M. Grenier, B.W. Eidem, E. O'Brian Smith, S.W. Denfield, et al., B-type natriuretic peptide predicts adverse cardiovascular events in pediatric outpatients with chronic left ventricular systolic dysfunction, Circulation 114 (10) (September 5, 2006) 1063–1069 PubMed PMID: 16940194.

[103] Y. Kunii, M. Kamada, S. Ohtsuki, T. Araki, K. Kataoka, M. Kageyama, et al., Plasma brain natriuretic peptide and the evaluation of volume overload in infants and children with congenital heart disease, Acta Med. Okayama 57 (4) (August 2003) 191–197 PubMed PMID: 14627071.

[104] A. Nir, B. Bar-Oz, Z. Perles, R. Brooks, A. Korach, A.J. Rein, N-terminal pro-B-type natriuretic peptide: reference plasma levels from birth to adolescence. Elevated levels at birth and in infants and children with heart diseases, Acta Paediatr. 93 (5) (May 2004) 603–607 PubMed PMID: 15174780.

[105] K. Suda, M. Matsumura, M. Matsumoto, Clinical implication of plasma natriuretic peptides in children with ventricular septal defect, Pediatr. Int. 45 (3) (June 2003) 249–254 PubMed PMID: 12828576.

[106] J.L. Yeh, J.H. Hsu, Z.K. Dai, S.F. Liou, I.J. Chen, J.R. Wu, Increased circulating big endothelin-1, endothelin-1 and atrial natriuretic peptide in infants and children with heart failure secondary to congenital heart disease, Int. J. Cardiol. 104 (1) (September 15, 2005) 15–20 PubMed PMID: 16055212.

[107] T.S. Mir, S. Marohn, S. Laer, M. Eiselt, O. Grollmus, J. Weil, Plasma concentrations of N-terminal pro-brain natriuretic peptide in control children from the neonatal to adolescent period and in children with congestive heart failure, Pediatrics 110 (6) (December 2002) e76 PubMed PMID: 12456943.

[108] S.R. Auerbach, M.E. Richmond, J.M. Lamour, E.D. Blume, L.J. Addonizio, R.E. Shaddy, et al., BNP levels predict outcome in pediatric heart failure patients: post hoc analysis of the pediatric carvedilol trial, Circ. Heart Fail. 3 (5) (September 2010) 606–611 PubMed PMID: 20573993.

Chapter 7

Ventricular Pressure–Volume Relationships in Heart Failure

Daniel J. Penny
Texas Children's Hospital, Houston, TX, United States

INTRODUCTION AND HISTORY

The examination of the relationships between chamber pressure and volume has been used to describe the function of a pump for centuries. Indeed this framework was used by James Watt in the late 18th century to quantify the work of the steam engine, using his so-called "indicator diagram," which was published in The Quarterly Journal of Science in 1822 [1]. In 1899 Otto Frank published a theoretical paper entitled "Die Grundform des arteriellen Pulses" [2], an English translation of which was published by Sagawa in 1990 [3], which characterized the function of the frog ventricle in a pressure–volume domain. The work of Suga and coworkers [4], beginning in the late 1960s greatly extended previous work, using the pressure–volume loop to provide insights into cardiac contractility and myocardial energetics. The clinical application of the pressure–volume framework was greatly accelerated by the description by Baan of the "impedance" catheter, (subsequently referred to as the "conductance" catheter) to provide instantaneous measurement of ventricular volume [5]. Potentially, the next impetus will occur from the development of high-fidelity noninvasive or less-invasive methods [6].

Despite these advances it must be acknowledged that there are few studies, which examine the ventricular pressure–volume relationship in any type of cardiovascular disease in children and almost none in the setting of pediatric cardiac failure. As a result, while recognizing that children are not just small adults, many of the data and principles used in this chapter will be from the study of cardiac failure in adults.

THE LEFT VENTRICULAR PRESSURE–VOLUME RELATIONSHIP

Changes in Left Ventricular Pressure and Volume During the Cardiac Cycle

The traditional examination (for example, in the cardiac catheterization laboratory) of the hemodynamic events, which occur in the left ventricle during the cardiac cycle, can be represented by a plot of instantaneous ventricular pressure or volume on the y-axis and time on the x-axis. To examine the left ventricular pressure–volume relationship, a display is derived in which ventricular pressure is plotted on the y-axis and volume on the x-axis. Where conditions are maintained in steady state, a pressure–volume "loop" will be displayed, which repeats with every cardiac cycle [4]. End-diastole is represented by the pressure–volume point at the lower right corner of the loop, and with the pressure–volume points moving counterclockwise, end-systole by that at the upper left. Within the left ventricle, the four main phases of the cardiac cycle (isovolumic contraction, ventricular ejection, isovolumic relaxation, and filling) can usually be easily discerned (Fig. 7.1).

Left Ventricular External Work

Frank's classic paper produced a theoretical model of cardiac contraction in the pressure–volume plane, which provided a number of insights [2]. One of the most important of these was that the external work (EW) produced by the ventricle (the stroke work) could be easily represented by the area enclosed within the pressure–volume loop (Fig. 7.1).

Left Ventricular Contractility

The use of the pressure–volume relationship to gain insights into the function of the heart was slow to develop support, until interest in the area was revitalized through the work of Suga and coworkers on anesthetized dogs. These studies were initially

Heart Failure in the Child and Young Adult. http://dx.doi.org/10.1016/B978-0-12-802393-8.00007-7

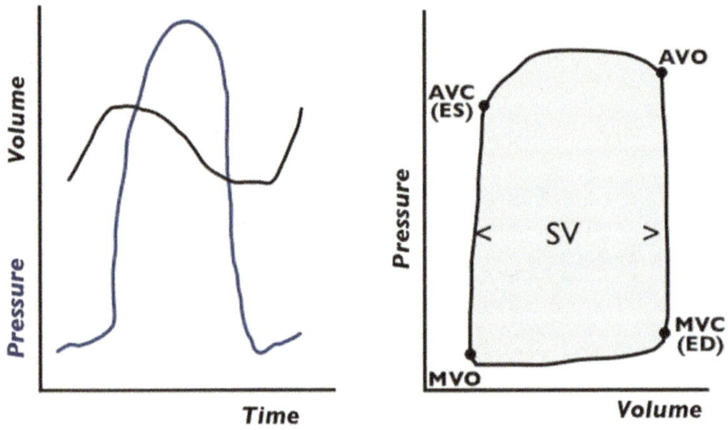

FIGURE 7.1 A plot of instantaneous ventricular pressure and volume on the y-axis and time on the x-axis (left-hand panel). To examine the left ventricular pressure–volume relationship, a display is derived in which ventricular pressure is plotted on the y-axis and volume on the x-axis (right-hand panel). Where conditions are maintained in steady state, a pressure–volume "loop" will be displayed, which repeats with every cardiac cycle. *AVC*, aortic valve closure; *AVO*, aortic valve opening; *ED*, end-diastole; *ES*, end-systole; *MVC*, mitral valve closure; *MVO*, mitral valve opening.

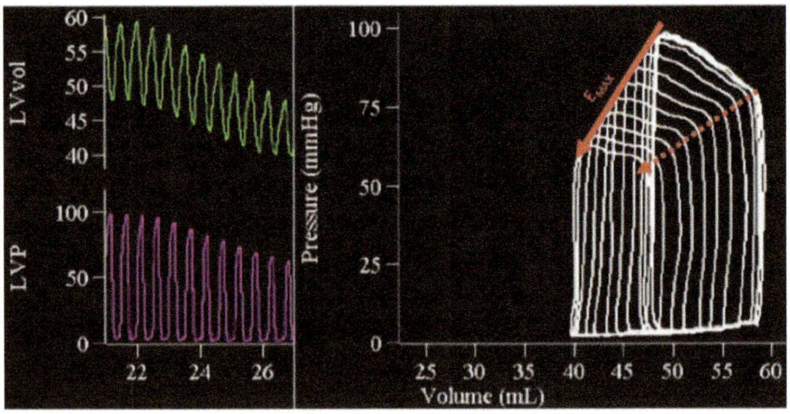

FIGURE 7.2 Changes in left ventricular pressure (LVP) and volume (LVvol) during preload reduction (left-hand panel). As ventricular volume is altered, at all times during the cardiac cycle, the ventricular pressure–volume points appeared to adopt a linear relationship (right-hand panel), so that ventricular contraction can be considered to be a "time-varying elastance." This elastance is maximal (E_{MAX}) around the time of end-systole.

published in the Japanese literature in the late 1960s and for the first time in English in 1971 [7]. They demonstrated that at a constant level of inotropy, at all times during the cardiac cycle, the ventricular pressure–volume points appeared to adopt a linear relationship as ventricular volume is altered, so that ventricular contraction could be considered to be a "time-varying elastance." This elastance appears to be maximal (E_{MAX}) around the time of end-systole (E_{es}) (The top left-hand corner of the pressure–volume display) (Fig. 7.2). Inotropic agents were seen to increase the slope of the end-systolic pressure–volume relationship (ESPVR), while by contrast, negative inotropes reduced it. The intercept of the ESPVR line with the volume axis (V_0) appeared to be constant and independent of the level of inotropy. As a result, E_{MAX} was considered to represent one of the "gold-standard" measures of cardiac contractility. Some of these principles appeared to be undermined, when it was demonstrated that under less well-controlled conditions in vivo, V_0 did sometimes appear to vary with changes in inotropic level and that the relationship between end-systolic pressure and volume may not always be truly linear, under extreme changes in load [8]. Nonetheless, for most clinical applications in humans in which changes in volume load are relatively modest, a linear relationship is usually observed. Furthermore, it must be acknowledged that nonlinearity does not in and of itself change the fact that the relationship does underline the limits of ventricular systolic performance, and, to some extent, linearity is merely a mathematical convenience, which allows a description of cardiac function in simple terms.

Diastolic Function

By contrast to the ESPVR, the relationship between pressure and volume at end-diastole is intrinsically nonlinear [9]. At low ventricular volumes, only a small increase in pressure occurs for a given increment in volume, while at higher volumes, pressure rises more steeply, reflecting the elastic characteristics of the ventricular chamber. A variety of curve fits have been applied to these observations to characterize the diastolic stiffness of the left ventricle. The simplest of these assumes an exponential relationship between pressure and volume, which may be applicable in carefully controlled circumstances (Fig. 7.3). In practice, however, several factors may influence this relationship, above and beyond the elastic characteristics of the ventricle, including the impacts of intrathoracic pressure, pericardial constraint, and the influence of cross talk between the ventricles during filling [9].

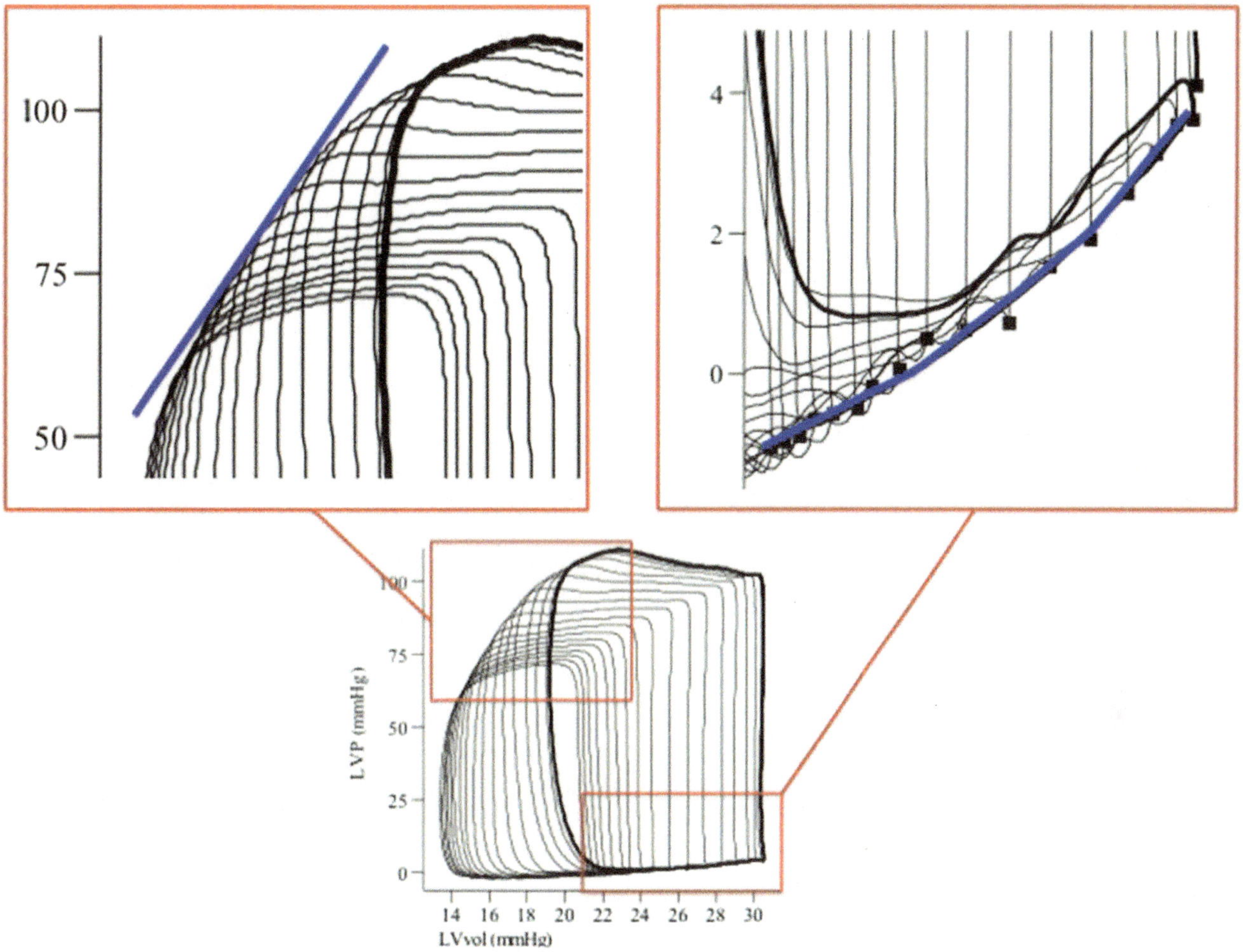

FIGURE 7.3 The relationship between left ventricular pressure (LVP) and volume (LVvol) during preload reduction. While the end-systolic pressure–volume relationship appears to adopt a linear relationship (top left-hand panel), the relationship at end-diastole is curvilinear and is usually modeled by an exponential equation (top right-hand panel).

Energy Consumption

Further examination of the elastance model by Suga, in the late 1970s, produced new insights into the energetic consequences of ventricular contraction [10]. He demonstrated that the model could not only provide a measure of the EW performed by the ventricle but also the elastic potential energy generated within the ventricle during cardiac contraction. Combined, these two are represented by the Pressure–Volume Area (PVA), which was subsequently confirmed to correlate with the O_2 consumption (VO_2) of the ventricle under various pre- and afterload conditions at constant levels of E_{MAX} (Fig. 7.4). The slope of the linear relationship between the VO_2 and PVA represents the oxygen cost of increases in PVA, and the intercept on the y-axis of the linear relationship represents the VO_2 required for basal metabolism and the requirements for excitation–contraction coupling (PVA-independent VO_2). At elevated levels of inotropy, the oxygen cost of increased PVA remains relatively constant, although the oxygen cost of excitation–contraction coupling increased with increased levels of E_{MAX} (Fig. 7.4).

Ventriculovascular Coupling

Once the ventricle contracts, it is necessary to convert pressure–work generated by the ventricle into flow in the aorta. The efficiency with which this conversion occurs cannot be taken for granted, and it is now recognized that this coupling between the ventricle and the vasculature is central to the regulation of cardiovascular performance in many disease states and is an important determinant of the response to therapeutic maneuvers.

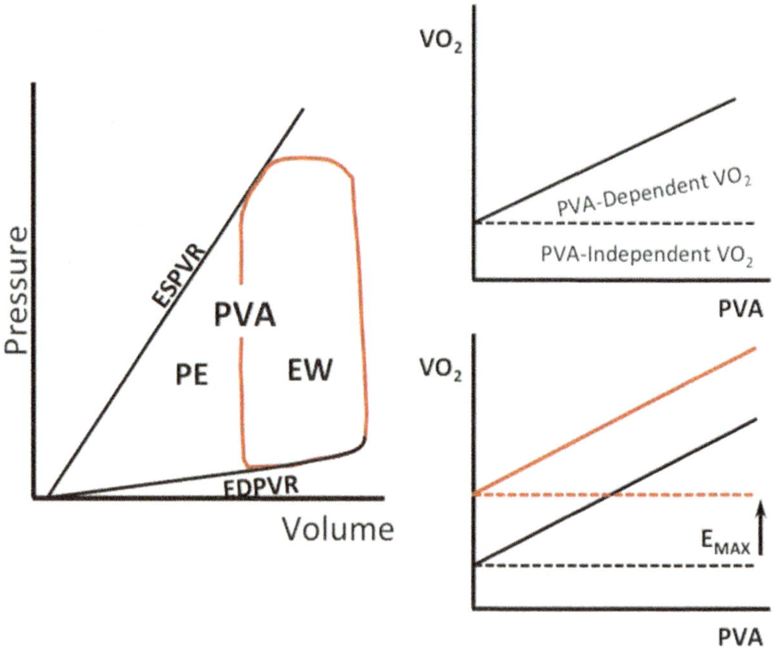

FIGURE 7.4 The relationship between left ventricular pressure and volume demonstrating the end-systolic pressure–volume relationship (ESPVR), the external work performed by the ventricle during a cardiac cycle (EW), and the elastic potential energy stored in the left ventricle (PE). The pressure–volume area (PVA) is the sum of the EW and PE (left-hand panel). There is a linear relationship between left ventricular O_2 consumption (VO_2) and the PVA, with the intercept on the y-axis representing the O_2 cost of basal metabolism and excitation–contraction coupling (top right-hand panel). The slope of the relationship is unchanged by alterations in E_{MAX}, but rather at elevated levels of inotropy, the cost of myocardial metabolism and excitation–contraction coupling is elevated (bottom right-hand panel).

The challenge in defining the nature of the coupling between the ventricle and the vasculature is to design a model, which can not only describe the independent properties of both the ventricle and the vasculature but also predict the changes in their interaction under changing physiological, pathological, and therapeutic conditions. While it is generally recognized that the properties of the vasculature are most accurately examined in the frequency domain, most measures of ventricular function have been derived in the time- or pressure–volume domain, making it complicated to compare the interactions between the two. One approach, based on the pressure–volume relationships, was derived by Sunagawa and coworkers [11]. In this framework vascular properties are condensed into the single measure of "effective arterial elastance" (E_a), which predicts that the ratio of end-systolic pressure (P_{es}) to stroke volume is constant under a given steady-state impedance load. It is then simple to use this model to not only examine the relationship between arterial (E_a) and ventricular elastance (E_{MAX}) but also the integration of ventricular and vascular properties and the changes in the level of this integration during physiological, pathological, and therapeutic changes (Fig. 7.5).

COMPARISON OF THE LEFT AND RIGHT PRESSURE–VOLUME RELATIONSHIPS

Although the output from the right ventricle is essentially almost equal to that of the left, the right ventricle differs from the left in a number of key aspects. Of major significance is that normally, the load placed on the right ventricle is significantly different to that on the left. Consequently, its work output will differ significantly, as will the timing of ejection. These differences, in turn, will have implications for the pressure–volume relationship.

Compared to the load on the left ventricle, the arterial load imposed on the right ventricle differs in that pulmonary vascular resistance and hydraulic impedance are lower and compliance typically higher. These will have important implications for the pattern of ventricular ejection and for its termination. As a result, while in the left ventricle, ejection is seen to terminate at the time of crossover between left ventricular (LV) and aortic pressures (the onset of isovolumic relaxation), by contrast, in right ventricle, ejection often continues long beyond this crossover point, during what has been termed the "hangout period," so that the pulmonary valve remains open well into "diastole" [12]. These differences between the right and left ventricles with respect to their interactions with their respective arterial loads can be seen from the pressure–volume relationship. Although as described, the LV acts essentially as a square-wave pump, the RV pressure–volume loop adopts a trapezoidal shape, with a less clear delineation of where the relaxing ventricle is truly isovolumic (Fig. 7.6). Given that the trapezoidal shape of the RV pressure–volume loop reflects its low hydraulic impedance, rather than an intrinsic difference in the physiology of the RV myocyte, as might be expected, when the RV is faced with increased arterial load, for example, when it is supporting the systemic circulation or in the setting of pulmonary arterial hypertension, its pressure–volume relationship assumes a square-wave pattern.

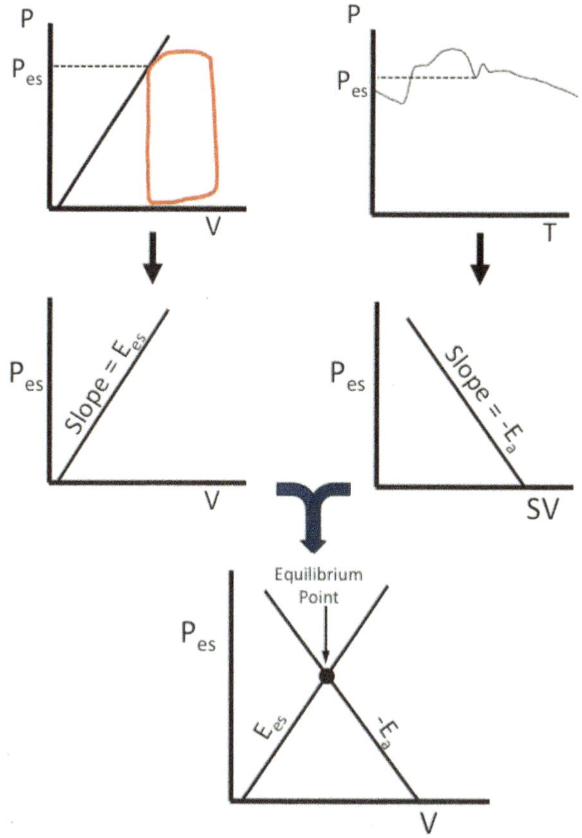

FIGURE 7.5 There is a linear relationship between left ventricular pressure and volume at end-systole. The slope of the relationship represents end-systolic ventricular elastance (E_{es}) (left-hand panels). There is also a linear relationship between aortic pressure and stroke volume at end-systole. The slope of this relationship represents the negative integer of the systemic arterial elastance (E_a). The intersection between these two lines represents the stroke volume resulting from the coupling between the ventricular and arterial systems (bottom panel).

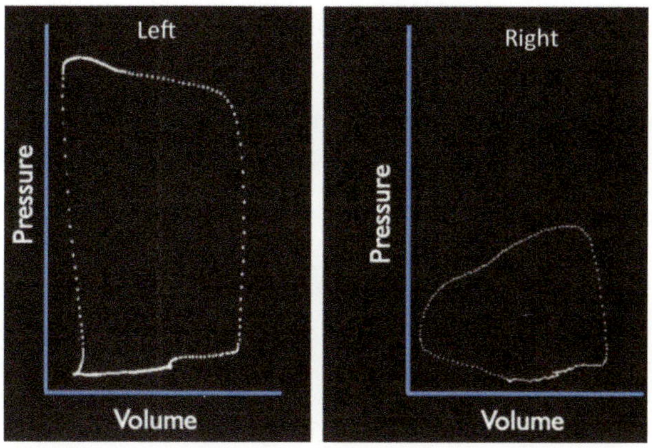

FIGURE 7.6 Comparison of the left- and right-ventricular pressure–volume relationships. The left ventricular pressure–volume relationship assumes a square-wave, with well-defined isovolumic periods (left-hand panel). By contrast, because of differences in load, the right ventricular pressure–volume relationship assumes a more triangular appearance, with a poorly delineated isovolumic relaxation period, such that there are ongoing reductions in volume during the period of pressure decay (right-hand panel). P_{es}, end-systolic pressure.

LEFT VENTRICULAR PRESSURE–VOLUME RELATIONSHIPS IN HEART FAILURE

Changes in the Left Ventricular Pressure–Volume Relationship in Heart Failure

There are few data in the literature, which examine the progressive changes in the pressure–volume relationships within patients as the severity of cardiac failure evolves. One "metaanalysis" digitized pressure–volume images provided in published papers representing more than 200 patients in different stages of heart failure [13]. Staging was performed according to the American Heart Association/American College of Cardiology Heart Failure Classification, ranging from Stage O, which represented the normal state, Stage A, a patient at risk of cardiac failure without structural heart disease, Stage B, an asymptomatic patient with structural changes, Stage C, a symptomatic patient with structural changes, to Stage D, a patient with refractory cardiac failure requiring high-level specialist intervention. Although there was a wide distribution of the PV loops within each stage, the study did demonstrate that as cardiac failure progressed, stroke volume and ejection fraction decreased, while LV volume and afterload increased. There was a progressive reduction in E_{MAX} at all stages, such that even asymptomatic patients (Stage B) demonstrated a reduction in E_{MAX} by 60% compared to Stage O. The onset of symptoms was heralded by a 50% further reduction in E_{MAX} [13].

It appears that alterations in ventricular afterload (E_a) occur early in patients with heart failure, occurring significantly earlier than the onset of symptoms. These alterations in afterload will not only impact on the efficiency of ventriculoarterial coupling but also on myocardial energetics. Thus, it appears that in normal subjects with an ejection fraction of 60% or more, E_{MAX} is typically nearly twice E_a. This relationship affords an optimal coupling between LV work and myocardial O_2 consumption. As cardiac failure develops such that ejection fraction has fallen to between 40% and 50%, as in the case of moderate cardiac failure, E_{MAX} and E_a approach equity. This maintains an optimal stroke work at a given end-diastolic volume (but at a lesser efficiency of O_2 utilization). As failure progresses and ejection fraction declines further, E_{MAX} is typically less than E_a, a situation, which provides suboptimal coupling between ventricular work and both oxygen consumption and stroke volume. It therefore appears that under normal circumstances, the coupling between the ventricle and vasculature is such that metabolic efficiency (relationship between work and O_2 consumption) is optimized; as cardiac function declines, this relationship is subordinated by an attempt to maintain stroke work in the face of declining ventricular function. As ventricular function declines further and compensation mechanisms are overwhelmed, the ventricle and vasculature become uncoupled to the detriment of both stroke work and metabolic efficiency [14].

The condition of cardiac failure, in the presence of a normal ejection fraction, is widely recognized in the adult clinical literature. It is commonly assumed that this reflects an abnormality of ventricular diastolic stiffness, with a leftward/upward shift of the end-diastolic pressure–volume relationship (diastolic dysfunction). Although this type of pathophysiology can be observed, it is by no means ubiquitous in patients with this syndrome [15]. Kass and coworkers have presented a novel formulation on the relationship between arterial stiffening (E_a) and ventricular stiffening (E_{MAX}) in patients with preserved "systolic function." In this phenomenon, which has been termed "ventricular–vascular stiffening," an elevation in E_a is associated with a concomitant increase in E_{MAX}. While this increase in E_{MAX} may serve to maintain ejection fraction, at least in the short term, the high level of E_{MAX} will potentially limit contractile reserve, increase the energetic cost of cardiac output, and worsen diastolic filling [16].

Effect of Therapies

Beta-adrenergic antagonists, for example, carvedilol, have been shown to reduce morbidity and delay mortality in adults (but not in children) [17] with chronic systolic heart failure. Chronic treatment with carvedilol has been demonstrated to result in an increase in LV ejection fraction. The mechanisms, which underscore this increase, appear to be a reduction in heart rate [18] as well as an increase in LV myocardial contractility [19] secondary to reverse remodeling. It also appears that chronic carvedilol treatment improves ventricular–vascular coupling by reducing arterial elastance, through a reduction in heart rate [20].

There is increasing use of cardiac resynchronization therapy (CRT) in patients with heart failure and increasing interest in determining the factors, which will determine the therapeutic response. In a small group of patients with heart failure and left bundle branch block, CRT acutely increased LV contractility both when the LV was stimulated using a coronary sinus electrode and an electrode placed on the LV endocardium [21]. In patients with similar levels of dyssynchrony, patients with preserved contractility assessed using the pressure–volume relationship demonstrated improved clinical outcomes at 12 months after CRT placement [22].

VENTRICULAR PRESSURE–VOLUME RELATIONSHIPS IN PEDIATRIC CARDIAC FAILURE

There is a paucity of examples in the literature in which ventricular pressure–volume relationships have been examined in the setting of cardiac failure in children. The numerous etiologies responsible for cardiac failure in children make extrapolations between disease conditions difficult, and the importance of right ventricular (RV) failure in many forms of pediatric cardiac failure demand increased attention to the function of the right ventricle in these patients. Furthermore, the requirement for general anesthesia in children has driven the search for less-invasive methods, and the large size of the standard conductance catheters has led the drive toward miniaturization of technologies [23].

Clearly the right ventricle is of considerable importance in the etiology of cardiac failure in many pediatric conditions. In many patients with complex disease the right ventricle is used to support the systemic circulation (as in certain patients after Fontan operation) or the right ventricle may sometimes support the systemic circulation in a biventricular circulation. Redington et al. examined the functions of the systemic right and subpulmonary left ventricles in patients after an atrial redirection procedure for transposition of the great arteries, demonstrating that effectively the pressure–volume loop of the systemic right ventricle in these patients assumed a square-wave pattern, similar to the normal systemic left ventricle and conversely, the loop from the subpulmonary left ventricle assumed that of a normal right ventricle, reiterating the conclusion that it is the loading conditions, rather than the intrinsic properties of the ventricular myocardium, which underpin the differences between right and left ventricular pressure–volume relationships [24]. In similar patients, Derrick and coworkers demonstrated a blunted increase in cardiac index and stroke volume in response to exercise and to dobutamine infusions [25]. This blunting was observed despite significantly improved indices of myocardial systolic function (E_{MAX}), enhanced ventriculoarterial coupling, and improved isovolumic relaxation. Rather, the key feature that appeared to underpin the blunted cardiac output response was an inability to augment ventricular filling during tachycardia, presumably related to a limitation of transit through the atrial baffle. In an attempt to consider whether less-invasive methods may be appropriate to examine RV function in these patients, Vogel and coworkers demonstrated that the changes in the ESPVRs of the systemic right ventricle during dobutamine infusion in this patient group could be relatively accurately represented by changes in the echocardiographic index of isovolumic acceleration [26].

Abnormalities of RV function superimposed with the effects of severe pulmonary regurgitation are important in the pathogenesis of cardiac failure in patients after repair of tetralogy of Fallot. RV pressure–volume relationships have been extensively used to quantify the severity of pulmonary regurgitation in this patient group, by examining the increases in RV volume during the decline in RV pressure [27]. Impaired right-sided ventricular–vascular coupling (as manifest by an altered relationship between E_a and E_{es}) has been demonstrated in patients after repair of tetralogy of Fallot, with abnormalities being more severe in patients with a transannular patch, compared to those after a valve-sparing transatrial–transpulmonary repair [28]. Most patients after tetralogy repair appear to display an increase in RV contractility during inotropic stimulation, as manifest by an increase in the RV E_{es}, although a subgroup does appear to have a blunted response. This impairment in myocardial reserve does not appear to be associated with elevations in plasma B-type natriuretic peptide levels [29].

Staged palliation of the patient with a functionally single ventricle imposes rapid and profound changes in ventricular loading and geometry. The effects of these changes on integrated cardiovascular performance have been assessed using the ventricular pressure–volume relationship. In an acute animal model of the Fontan operation, impaired ventricular performance and ventriculovascular coupling have been demonstrated as manifest by a reduction in E_{es}, an increase in E_a, and, as a result, a reduction in the E_{es}/E_a ratio. Furthermore, there was a reduction in LV mechanical efficiency [30]. Although there are clear limitations of the model, these observations do demonstrate the ability of the pressure–volume relationship to "tease out" complex changes in cardiovascular integration during alterations in hemodynamic state. In patients undergoing palliation with a Fontan operation, Tanoue et al. demonstrated more favorable matching of afterload (E_a) to contractility (E_{es}) in patients who had undergone a previous bidirectional cavopulmonary shunt, supporting the hypothesis that early correction of afterload with the cavopulmonary shunt may be important in optimizing the functional outcomes in the longer term after definitive palliation [31]. There have been a number of attempts to examine whether other less-invasive measures might replace invasive techniques. In a study of patients with one-functional ventricle, the fractional area change of the systemic ventricle on cross-sectional echocardiography correlated best with the ESPVR [32], while invasive measures of end-diastolic compliance correlated reasonably with the standard Doppler measures of atrioventricular flow (E/A ratio) and with tissue Doppler measures of E/E′ [33].

CONCLUSION

This chapter provides an introduction to the technique of pressure–volume analysis of left and RV performance. It is clear that this analysis provides useful insights into cardiovascular integration, above and beyond cardiac contractility. Although there is a growing literature on the use of ventricular pressure–volume relationships in the adult with heart failure, there remains a paucity of data in the pediatric patient.

REFERENCES

[1] Anonymous, Account of a steam-engine indicator, Quart. J. Sci. 13 (1822) 95.

[2] O. Frank, Die Grundform des arteriellen pulses, Z. Biol. 37 (1899) 483–526.

[3] K. Sagawa, R.K. Lie, J. Schaefer, Translation of Otto Frank's paper "Die Grundform des Arteriellen Pulses" Zeitschrift für Biologie 37: 483–526 (1899), J. Mol. Cell Cardiol. (22) (1990) 253–254.

[4] H. Suga, Cardiac energetics: from E(max) to pressure-volume area, Clin. Exp. Pharmacol. Physiol. 30 (2003) 580–585.

[5] J. Baan, T.T. Jong, P.L. Kerkhof, R.J. Moene, A.D. van Dijk, E.T. van der Velde, J. Koops, Continuous stroke volume and cardiac output from intraventricular dimensions obtained with impedance catheter, Cardiovasc. Res. 15 (1981) 328–334.

[6] W.R. Witschey, F. Contijoch, J.R. McGarvey, V.A. Ferrari, M.S. Hansen, M.E. Lee, S. Takebayashi, C. Aoki, J.A. Chirinos, P.A. Yushkevich, J.H. Gorman 3rd, R.C. Pilla JJ,Gorman, Real-time magnetic resonance imaging technique for determining left ventricle pressure-volume loops, Ann. Thorac. Surg. 97 (2014) 1597–1603.

[7] H. Suga, Theoretical analysis of a left-ventricular pumping model based on the systolic time-varying pressure-volume ratio, IEEE Trans. Biomed. Eng. 18 (1971) 47–55.
[8] D. Burkhoff, S. Sugiura, D.T. Yue, K. Sagawa, Contractility-dependent curvilinearity of end-systolic pressure-volume relations, Am. J. Physiol. 252 (1987) H1218–H1227.
[9] A. Pasipoularides, Right and left ventricular diastolic pressure-volume relations: a comprehensive review, J. Cardiovasc. Transl. Res. 6 (2013) 239–252.
[10] H. Suga, Total mechanical energy of a ventricle model and cardiac oxygen consumption, Am. J. Physiol. 236 (1979) H498–H505.
[11] K. Sunagawa, W.L. Maughan, K. Sagawa, Optimal arterial resistance for the maximal stroke work studied in isolated canine left ventricle, Circ. Res. 56 (1985) 586–595.
[12] J.A. Shaver, Clinical implications of the hangout interval, Int. J. Cardiol. 5 (1984) 391–398.
[13] D.R. Warriner, A.G. Brown, S. Varma, P.J. Sheridan, P. Lawford, D.R. Hose, A. Al-Mohammad, Y. Shi, Closing the loop: modelling of heart failure progression from health to end-stage using a meta-analysis of left ventricular pressure-volume loops, PLoS One 9 (2014) e114153.
[14] H. Asanoi, S. Sasayama, T. Kameyama, Ventriculoarterial coupling in normal and failing heart in humans, Circ. Res. 65 (1989) 483–493.
[15] T. Bench, D. Burkhoff, J.B. O'Connell, M.R. Costanzo, W.T. Abraham, M. St John Sutton, M.S. Maurer, Heart failure with normal ejection fraction: consideration of mechanisms other than diastolic dysfunction, Curr. Heart Fail. Rep. 6 (2009) 57–64.
[16] D.A. Kass, Ventricular arterial stiffening: integrating the pathophysiology, Hypertension 46 (2005) 185–193.
[17] R.E. Shaddy, M.M. Boucek, D.T. Hsu, R.J. Boucek, C.E. Canter, L. Mahony, R.D. Ross, E. Pahl, E.D. Blume, D.A. Dodd, D.N. Rosenthal, J. Burr, B. LaSalle, R. Holubkov, M.A. Lukas, L.Y. Tani, Pediatric Carvedilol Study Group, Carvedilol for children and adolescents with heart failure: a randomized controlled trial, JAMA 298 (2007) 1171–1179.
[18] M.S. Maurer, J.D. Sackner-Bernstein, L. El-Khoury Rumbarger, M. Yushak, D.L. King, D. Burkhoff, Mechanisms underlying improvements in ejection fraction with carvedilol in heart failure, Circ. Heart Fail. 2 (2009) 189–196.
[19] B. Bozkurt, M. Bolos, A. Deswal, S. Ather, W. Chan, D.L. Mann, B. Carabello, New insights into mechanisms of action of carvedilol treatment in chronic heart failure patients–a matter of time for contractility, J. Card. Fail. 18 (2012) 183–193.
[20] R. Razzolini, G. Tarantini, G.M. Boffa, S. Orlando, S. Iliceto, Effects of carvedilol on ventriculo-arterial coupling in patients with heart failure, Ital. Heart J. 5 (2004) 517–522.
[21] L. Padeletti, P. Pieragnoli, G. Ricciardi, L. Perrotta, G. Grifoni, M.C. Porciani, V. Lionetti, S. Valsecchi, Acute hemodynamic effect of left ventricular endocardial pacing in cardiac resynchronization therapy: assessment by pressure-volume loops, Circ. Arrhythm. Electrophysiol. 5 (2012) 460–467.
[22] Q. Ciampi, L. Pratali, R. Citro, B. Villari, E. Picano, R. Sicari, Clinical and prognostic role of pressure-volume relationship in the identification of responders to cardiac resynchronization therapy, Am. Heart J. 160 (2010) 906–914.
[23] U. Herberg, E. Gatzweiler, T. Breuer, J. Breuer, Ventricular pressure-volume loops obtained by 3D real-time echocardiography and mini pressure wire-a feasibility study, Clin. Res. Cardiol. 102 (2013) 427–438.
[24] A.N. Redington, M.L. Rigby, E.A. Shinebourne, P.J. Oldershaw, Changes in the pressure-volume relation of the right ventricle when its loading conditions are modified, Br. Heart J. 63 (1990) 45–49.
[25] G.P. Derrick, I. Narang, P.A. White, A. Kelleher, A. Bush, D.J. Penny, A.N. Redington, Failure of stroke volume augmentation during exercise and dobutamine stress is unrelated to load-independent indexes of right ventricular performance after the Mustard operation, Circulation 102 (19 Suppl. 3) (2000) III154–I159.
[26] M. Vogel, G. Derrick, P.A. White, S. Cullen, H. Aichner, J. Deanfield, A.N. Redington, Systemic ventricular function in patients with transposition of the great arteries after atrial repair: a tissue Doppler and conductance catheter study, J. Am. Coll. Cardiol. 43 (2004) 100–106.
[27] A.N. Redington, P.J. Oldershaw, E.A. Shinebourne, M.L. Rigby, A new technique for the assessment of pulmonary regurgitation and its application to the assessment of right ventricular function before and after repair of tetralogy of Fallot, Br. Heart J. 60 (1988) 57–65.
[28] H. Latus, W. Binder, G. Kerst, M. Hofbeck, L. Sieverding, C. Apitz, Right ventricular-pulmonary arterial coupling in patients after repair of tetralogy of Fallot, J. Thorac. Cardiovasc. Surg. 146 (2013) 1366–1372.
[29] C. Apitz, L. Sieverding, H. Latus, A. Uebing, S. Schoof, M. Hofbeck, Right ventricular dysfunction and B-type natriuretic peptide in asymptomatic patients after repair for tetralogy of Fallot, Pediatr. Cardiol. 30 (2009) 898–904.
[30] G. Szabó, V. Buhmann, A. Graf, S. Melnitschuk, S. Bährle, C.F. Vahl, S. Hagl, Ventricular energetics after the Fontan operation: contractility-afterload mismatch, J. Thorac. Cardiovasc. Surg. 125 (2003) 1061–1069.
[31] Y. Tanoue, A. Sese, Y. Ueno, K. Joh, T. Hijii, Bidirectional Glenn procedure improves the mechanical efficiency of a total cavopulmonary connection in high-risk fontan candidates, Circulation 103 (2001) 2176–2180.
[32] R.J. Butts, S.M. Chowdhury, J. Buckley, A.M. Hlavacek, T.Y. Hsia, S. Khambadkone, G.H. Baker, MOCHA investigators, Comparison of echocardiographic and pressure-volume loop indices of systolic function in patients with single ventricle physiology: a preliminary report, Congenit. Heart Dis. 10 (2015) E17–E24.
[33] S.M. Chowdhury, R.J. Butts, J. Buckley, A.M. Hlavacek, T.Y. Hsia, S. Khambadkone, G.H. Baker, MOCHA Investigators, Comparison of pressure-volume loop and echocardiographic measures of diastolic function in patients with a single-ventricle physiology, Pediatr. Cardiol. 35 (2014) 998–1006.

Chapter 8

Systolic and Diastolic Function

Aamir Jeewa[1], Antonio G. Cabrera[2]

[1]*The Hospital for Sick Children and the University of Toronto, Toronto, ON, Canada;* [2]*Baylor College of Medicine/Texas Children's Hospital, Houston, TX, United States*

INTRODUCTION

The concept of ventricular function, or what can also be termed ventricular performance, divides into two main components: systolic and diastolic function. However, both systolic and diastolic functions have determinants that arise from genetic, molecular, cellular, and histologic levels. In addition, assessment of ventricular performance can be done on multiple levels such (i.e., catheter-based hemodynamics) and noninvasive techniques (i.e., clinical exam, echocardiography, cardiac magnetic resonance imaging (CMR), or other imaging modalities). It is the use of a combination of techniques, which are required to make a complete assessment to differentiate between normal and abnormal ventricular performance.

In recent years, much has been learned now about the different functions of the myocardial fibers (orientation and force synchrony), the pumping function of the right and left ventricles (including suction and twist), and recoil or diastolic untwist [1]. Significant understanding of the myocardial mechanics has been attained by measuring myocardial deformation or strain [2]. The concept of myocardial strain heavily relates to the myocardial architecture. It has been proposed that the LV myocardial architecture is continuum of two helical fiber geometries [3,4]. These helical fibers are a continuum of transmural and opposing forces, one with a right handed orientation (subendocardial) and the other with a left-handed orientation (subepicardial) [5].

The objective of this chapter is to first lay the foundation for the normal components of systolic and diastolic function so that when derangement occurs the potential underlying root cause can also be determined.

SYSTOLIC FUNCTION

Systole is best described as the period that starts when the heart is maximally filled with blood and then subsequently ejected from the ventricle to the aorta whereupon the aortic valve closes. The volume of blood ejected from the heart is the stroke volume (SV). The SV when multiplied by the heart rate (HR) will give the cardiac output delivered. Oxygen delivery needs depend on energy consumption (i.e., the more the body utilizes energy the more oxygen delivery is required) and thus the ventricular performance may change when at rest compared to when exercising or under stress.

Just prior to a cardiac muscle contraction, an electrical signal causes the influx of Ca into the cell. Calcium then binds to troponin and releasing the complex from actin and making it available to interact with myosin. The myosin heads in the thick filaments bind with actin in the thin filaments and, after utilizing energy it the form of ATP, pulls the thin filaments to the center and thus pulling the ends of the sarcomere closer together, thereby shortening the length of the muscle fiber [6]. The concerted sarcomeric shortening results in ventricular contraction that generates pressure within the ventricle and eventually exceeds the pressure in the atria. At this time, the atrioventricular valves are closed, and this is referred to isovolumic contraction. Once the building pressure exceeds the aortic pressure, the aortic valve opens and blood ejected. Pressure measurement at that time will result in a rapid rise, peak, and then steady decline. Once the ventricular pressure falls below the aortic pressure, the aortic valve closes. Initial description of the basic relationships between, pressure, volume and flow events were reported by Carl John Wiggers almost a 100 years ago. Although there are different versions of these diagrams, the main tenet is to show the changes in pressure and flow in the left atrium, left ventricle, and aorta during both systole and diastole (see Fig. 8.1) [7,16].

Normal left ventricular performance is affected by: preload, afterload, and contractility. Preload is the distending force that cardiac muscle is in relaxed state. The effects of preload as seen in relation to the force–velocity relationship help explain that with an increase in muscle fiber length there is an increase in the velocity of fiber shortening or force of the contraction at a given afterload (Fig. 8.2 of force–velocity curves) [8]. This comprises the inherent aspect of Starling's Law that with an increase in preload there is further stretch of the myocardial fibers and thus resulting in a greater SV and force of contraction. Afterload is the pressure exerted on the heart to which the ventricle must overcome to eject blood.

Heart Failure in the Child and Young Adult. http://dx.doi.org/10.1016/B978-0-12-802393-8.00008-9

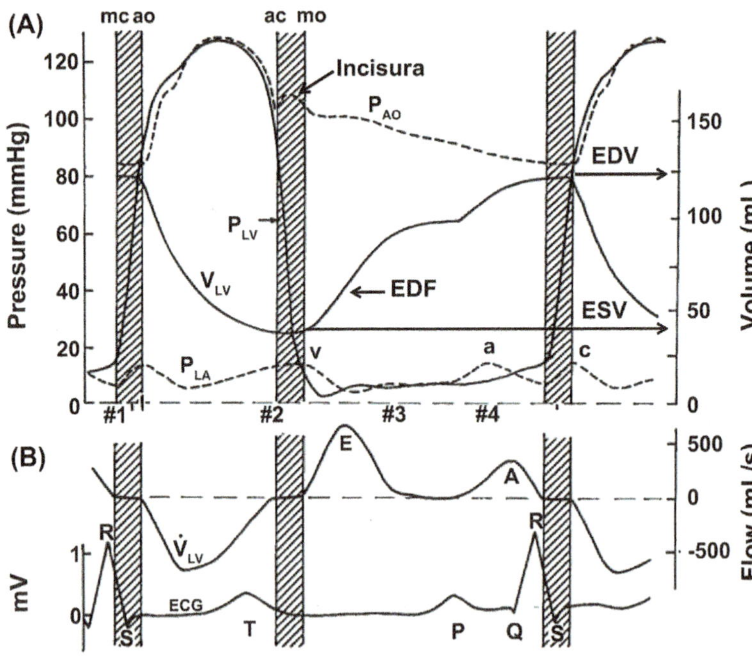

FIGURE 8.1 Wiggers diagram. (A) Temporal relationships between left ventricular (LV) pressure (P_{LV}), LV volume (V_{LV}), left atrial (LA) pressure (P_{LA}), and aortic pressure (P_{AO}). Shown in (A) are mitral valve opening and closing (mo and mc, respectively), aortic valve opening and closing (ao and ac, respectively), P_{AO} incisura, early diastolic filling (EDF), end-diastolic volume (EDV), end-systolic volume (ESV), and the a, c, and v waves of P_{LA}. Auditory events are shown in (A) for *sounds* 1 and 2 (mitral valve closure and aortic valve closure, respectively) and heart *sounds* 3 and 4. (B) Blood flow out of the LV during the ejection phase of systole ($\dot{V}_{LV}$), early diastolic blood flow into the LV (E wave), blood flow into the LV during LA contraction (A wave), and a standard lead II ECG showing LA depolarization, LV depolarization, and LV repolarization (P wave, QRS complex, and T wave, respectively). *(Unpublished figure provided courtesy of Dr. John V. Tyberg and Dr. Henk E. D. J. ter Keurs. Mitchell JR Adv. Physiol. Educ. 38, 170–175, 2014.)*

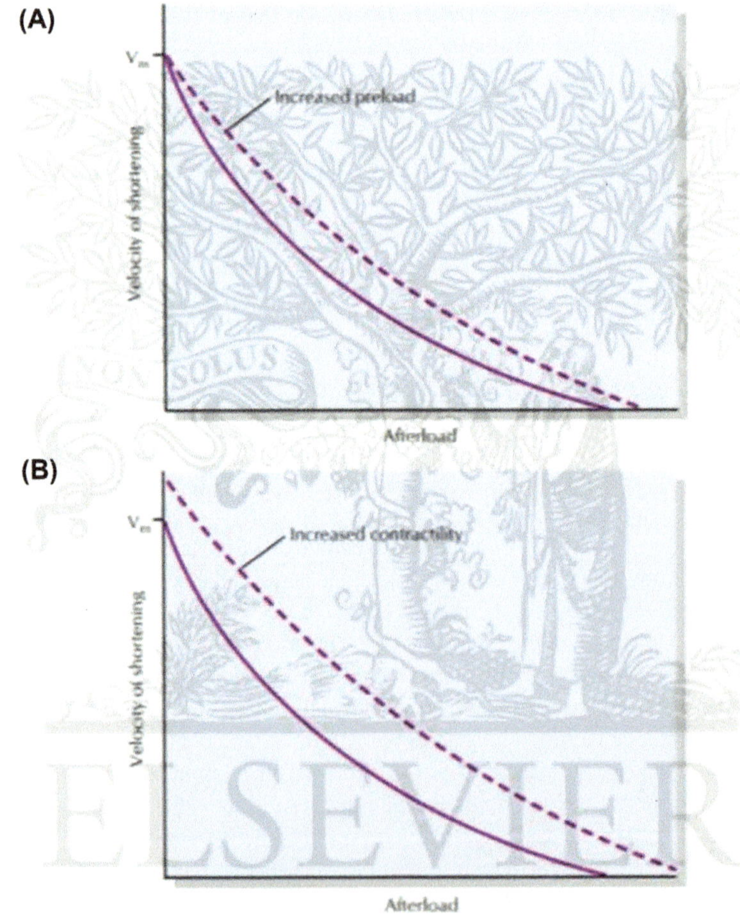

FIGURE 8.2 Force Velocity Relationship Curve. *Susan E. Mulroney, Adam K. The Cardiac Pump, 119.*

The higher the afterload (i.e., systolic pressure) the less of an ability to reduce the ventricular volume to a smaller state and thus results in a lower SV. The converse being the case for lower afterload states. Ventricular wall stress is also integral to the concept of afterload as this estimates the force that resists shortening or thickening of the myocardial fibers ("Law of Laplace") or even more simply the wall tension divided by the wall thickness [9]. Contractility is the inherent force of the myocardium to contract that is independent of both preload and afterload. The concept of contractility has also become synonymous with inotropy. The modulation of contractility begins at the cellular level with the influx of calcium before each contraction. The increase in available calcium to bind with troponin or the more sensitive troponin is to calcium will make more available myosin-binding sites to interact with actin. The force–velocity relationship again shows the effect of increasing contractility (i.e., inotropes, catecholamines, sympathetic stimulation, etc.) with an increase in the velocity of myofiber shortening [9] (Fig. 8.2).

The assessment of ventricular systolic function can be done both by invasive and noninvasive methods. Invasive monitoring with impedance catheters in a cardiac catheterization lab will yield direct pressure–volume curves [9].

The heart primary function is the ejection of blood through the circulation. The pressure–volume loop analysis offers a framework to better understand the variables that affect cardiac function. Although the continued measurement of pressure volume loops has been applied to the clinical setting, their implementation as a tool for bedside decision-making has been less frequent.

The pressure–volume loop has four characteristic phases (Fig. 8.3). Beginning at the bottom right corner of the loop, an initial upstroke 1–2 represents the rapid increase in ventricular pressure, with little volume change—isovolumic contraction. During this phase, ventricular pressure increases rapidly with ventricular pressure depending, almost exclusively by the myocardial contractile elements (sarcomeres) as they shorten. There is a rapid decrease in ventricular volume as ventricular ejection proceeds to the end-systolic point 2–3. Then, there is a rapid fall in ventricular pressure, with little volume change, as the ventricle enters into the isovolumic relaxation phase 3–4. After this phase, ventricular volume increases to its end-diastolic level, reflecting ventricular passive and active filling.

It has been proposed that cardiac contraction can me modeled as a time-varying elastance represented by the upper left-hand corner of the pressure volume loop during the end-systolic pressure–volume relationship (ESPVR) (Fig. 8.3). Although other measures have been proposed, ESPVR is considered the "gold standard" measure of ventricular contractility.

PRESSURE–VOLUME RELATIONSHIP AND CONGENITAL HEART DISEASE

The pressure volume relationship can provide important insights for the understanding of CHD. In these patients changes in cardiac load, cardiac function after cardiopulmonary bypass and response to inotropes are of utmost importance when determining cardiovascular performance. Left-to-right shunts and intracardiac valve insufficiency lead to a progressive increase in end-diastolic volume and a shift of the pressure volume to the right on the end-diastolic pressure–volume relationship. Pathophysiologic changes affect more than one parameter at once in the pressure volume relationship. The pressure volume loops in Fig. 8.4 highlight the differences in the loops in the setting of systolic and diastolic disease in comparison to normal hemodynamics [25].

When assessing systole, pressure–volume loop analysis assumes that the myocardium elastic properties when pressure and volume are increasing. Chamber compliance decreases as the ventricle fills. Placement of impedance catheters is invasive, costly, and not easily done in the routine functional assessment. Noninvasive measures to assess systolic function have become reasonable surrogates. Echocardiography parameters of systolic function can be done by the visual inspection ("eye-ball") method, which is essentially the qualitative and subjective assessment of two-dimensional function. There is reasonable correlation with this qualitative function assessment when the ventricular function is normal or near normal but loses accuracy once even subtle ventricular dysfunction has developed [10]. Other echocardiography parameters include "M-mode" assessment of shortening fraction (%SF) and ventricular dimensions in both systole and diastole. M-mode is the single plane, one-dimensional view of the heart with time on the x-axis [11]. The end-diastolic and systolic dimensions are often used to trend the chronic effects of the cavity size in the failing heart. Simpson's biplane and the Bullet method are examples of commonly used two-dimensional echocardiography techniques used to assess the ventricular dimension and ejection fraction, or EF. The determinants of EF include the LV end-diastolic dimension—LV end-systolic dimension/LV end-diastolic dimension. However, both techniques are based on assumptions of the ability to visualize the endocardium well and the overall "normalcy" of the ventricular geometry [11]. Thus, these methods are often challenging in instances of congenital heart disease. Newer techniques to assess ventricular systolic function include three-dimensional (3D) echocardiography, or 3D imaging, which allows capturing the ventricular shape in all three planes and in addition deriving a 3D volumetric assessment and EF [12]. Strain analysis by speckle tracking echocardiography allows for a more detailed assessment of myocardial deformation and regional wall motion measures. The multidimensional deformation, or "strain," which

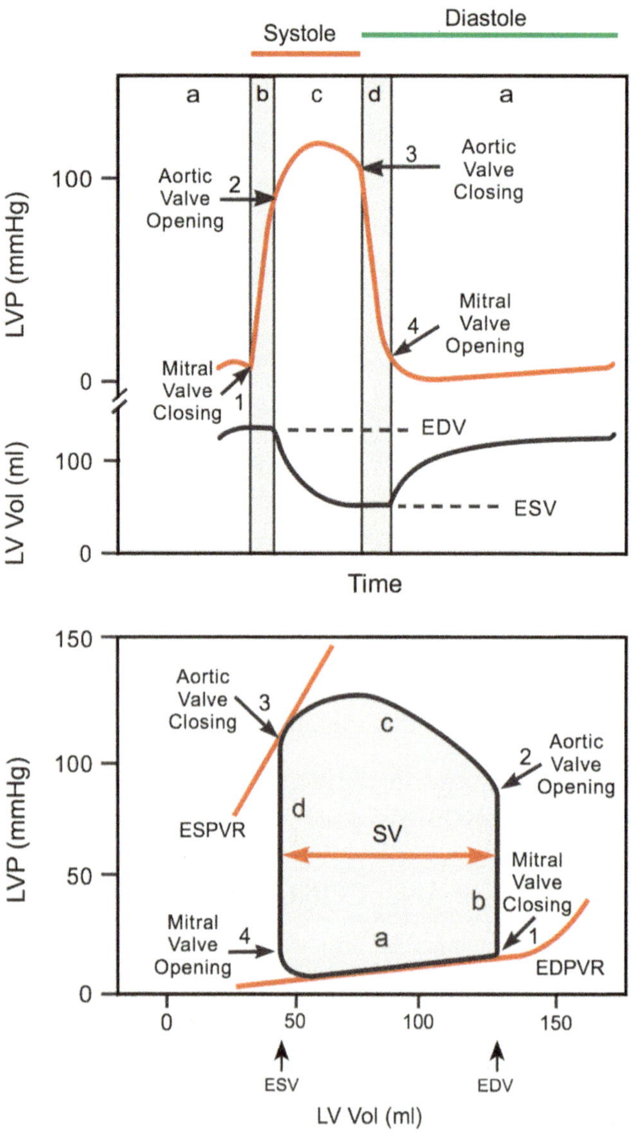

FIGURE 8.3 The pressure–volume loop. *(Cardiovascular Physiology Concepts, 2nd edition, a textbook published by Lippincott Williams & Wilkins (2012).)*

is exhibited by the heart can be quantified in longitudinal, circumferential, and radial changes of the respective cardiac fibers and thereby provide further detailed interpretation of ventricular function [13,14]. In patients with cancer-therapeutics cardiac dysfunction, the expert consensus in multimodality imaging from the American Society of echocardiography, has proposed that a decrease by >10% points on EF, from EF<53%, should be consider as dysfunction. Additionally, the document proposes to repeat the study 2–3 weeks after for further verification.

DIASTOLIC FUNCTION

Diastole is the period of the cardiac cycle that encompasses ventricular relaxation, passive and active filling of blood into the heart, and the period just prior to ejection. At the cellular level, the interplay of calcium within the cardiac myocytes is crucial to ventricular relaxation. The cessation of the troponin C/Calcium ion interaction results in the uptake of the calcium ions by the sarcoplasmic reticulum via the sarcoplasmic reticulum calcium ATPase ion pump. Calcium exits out of the myocyte via sodium/calcium exchange and an energy utilizing pathway (i.e., in the form of an ATP sarcolemmal transfer) across a concentration gradient and under the influence of activated phospholamban, which results in myocardial relaxation [15].

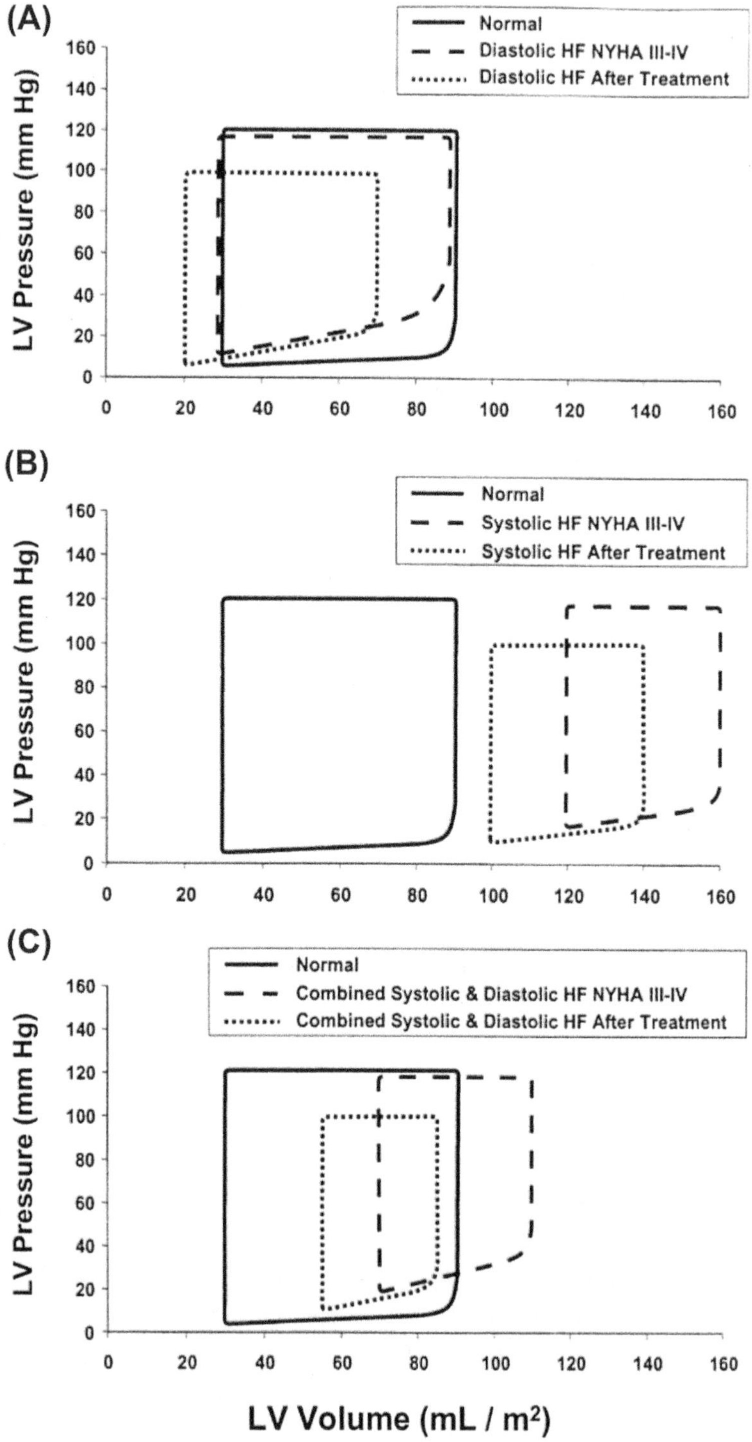

FIGURE 8.4 Pressure-volume loops contrasting isolated diastolic heart failure (A) with systolic heart failure (B) and combined systolic and diastolic heart failure (C). *Zile and Brutsaert [25].*

Understanding the role of the ion exchanges gives an insight for the problems that can occur when dysfunction develops; be it acquired such as after a myocardial infarction or congenital in the instance of familial cardiomyopathies. The four components of diastole include (1) isovolumic relaxation period (2) rapid filling (3) slow filling (4) atrial systole. However, factor that influence normal diastolic function also include myocardial relaxation or compliance, elastic recoil, passive ventricular filling, atrial function, and HR [16].

One can start the description of diastole with isovolumic relaxation, which is the period when left ventricular pressure is dropping (change in dP/dT) after the preceding systole and just prior to the opening of the mitral valve with the start of passive left ventricular filling. This relaxation period is inherent to the intrinsic nature of the myocardium and is affected by the cellular calcium regulation, contractile function, loading, and electromechanical conditions. The next phase is the rapid filling of the left ventricle, which is driven by the rapid untwisting, or torsion of the myocardium and dependent on its elastic recoil properties. This rapid filling phase is manifest by active suction of blood into the ventricle and is responsible for the majority of the filling during diastole [17]. Slow filling occurs from the passive filling of the heart from the pulmonary veins. The final phase of filling is regulated by atrial contraction, which occurs at the end of diastole. This "atrial kick" represents a last push of blood into the LV as end-diastolic pressure starts to rise and the oncoming systole is imminent. In addition the atrial surface area in relation to the ventricle generates a hydraulic force, which adds further insight to the role of the atria when there is diastolic dysfunction [18].

From a clinical standpoint, diastolic function may be best assessed by the direct measurement of left heart filling pressures such as during cardiac catheterization. However, this method is invasive and in young children may require mechanical ventilation and general anesthesia, which can increase the risk of the procedure especially if there is underlying clinical instability. Echocardiographic assessment of diastolic function can be done via multiple methods. From a two-dimensional standpoint, the left atrial volume is an excellent "marker" for the development of diastolic dysfunction as this a resultant feature of long-standing elevated filling pressures [19,20]. In children, left atrial dimension can be obtained by either routine two-dimensional echocardiography or CMR imaging. Enlargement of the left atrium can be a marker of chronically elevated filling pressures. Menon et al. studied 88 individuals under the age of 20 with hypertrophic cardiomyopathy and found on univariable analysis that an enlarged left atrium correlated with diastolic dysfunction grade, LV outflow tract gradient, mitral E/E', degree of mitral regurgitation. Multivariable analysis showed that left atrial volume was related to diastolic dysfunction grade and mean mitral regurgitation grade [21]. Doppler assessment of the mitral valve is another routinely used method of for evaluating diastolic function. This is done by measuring the Doppler velocity of blood flow across the mitral valve during filling phase and highlights the rapid filling and the atrial systole components of diastole, measured as the E and A waves, respectively (Fig. 8.5) [22].

In addition, Doppler velocities and waveforms can also be sampled at the level of the pulmonary veins (see Fig. 8.6).

Tissue Doppler imaging, or TDI, is a Doppler technique that samples the velocity of the myocardium as opposed to that of blood. The annular motion of the myocardium also behaves in a similar relationship to that of transmitral blood flow and the concomitant filling phases are labeled as E' and A' (see Fig. 8.7).

When annular velocities as measured by TDI are reduced, this suggests diastolic impairment. Nagueh et al. performed invasive hemodynamic assessment of 125 adults and found a significant correlation with an elevated E/E' ratio and elevated pulmonary capillary wedge pressures [23]. These findings have been corroborated in other adult studies are done routinely in most echocardiography labs [24,25].

However, similar studies have been attempted in pediatric patients with little success in reproducing adult findings. Ezon et al. in study of 38 children with cardiomyopathy found little correlation with TDI and their left ventricular filling

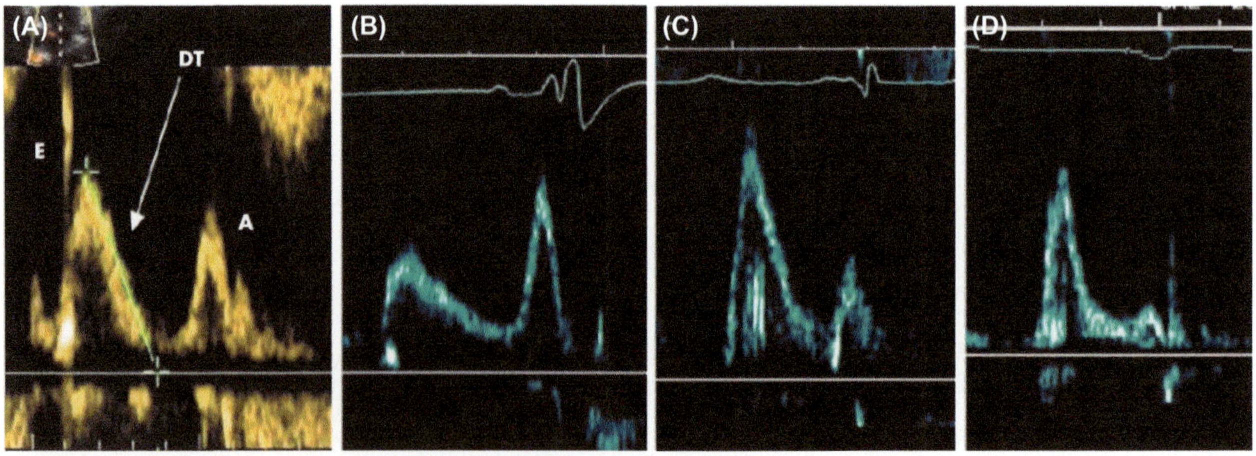

FIGURE 8.5 Pathophysiological characterization of left ventricular (LV) filling patterns. (A) Normal transmitral flow in a patient in sinus rhythm. (B) Impaired relaxation with normal filling pressures. (C) Pseudonormal filling. (D) Restrictive filling. *Mottram and Marwick [22].*

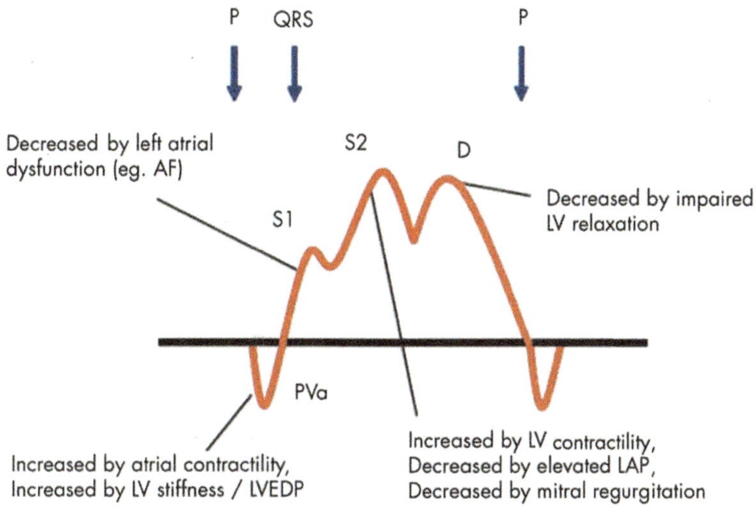

FIGURE 8.6 Pulmonary vein inflow pattern in relation to various hemodynamic conditions. *Mottram and Marwick [22] #466.*

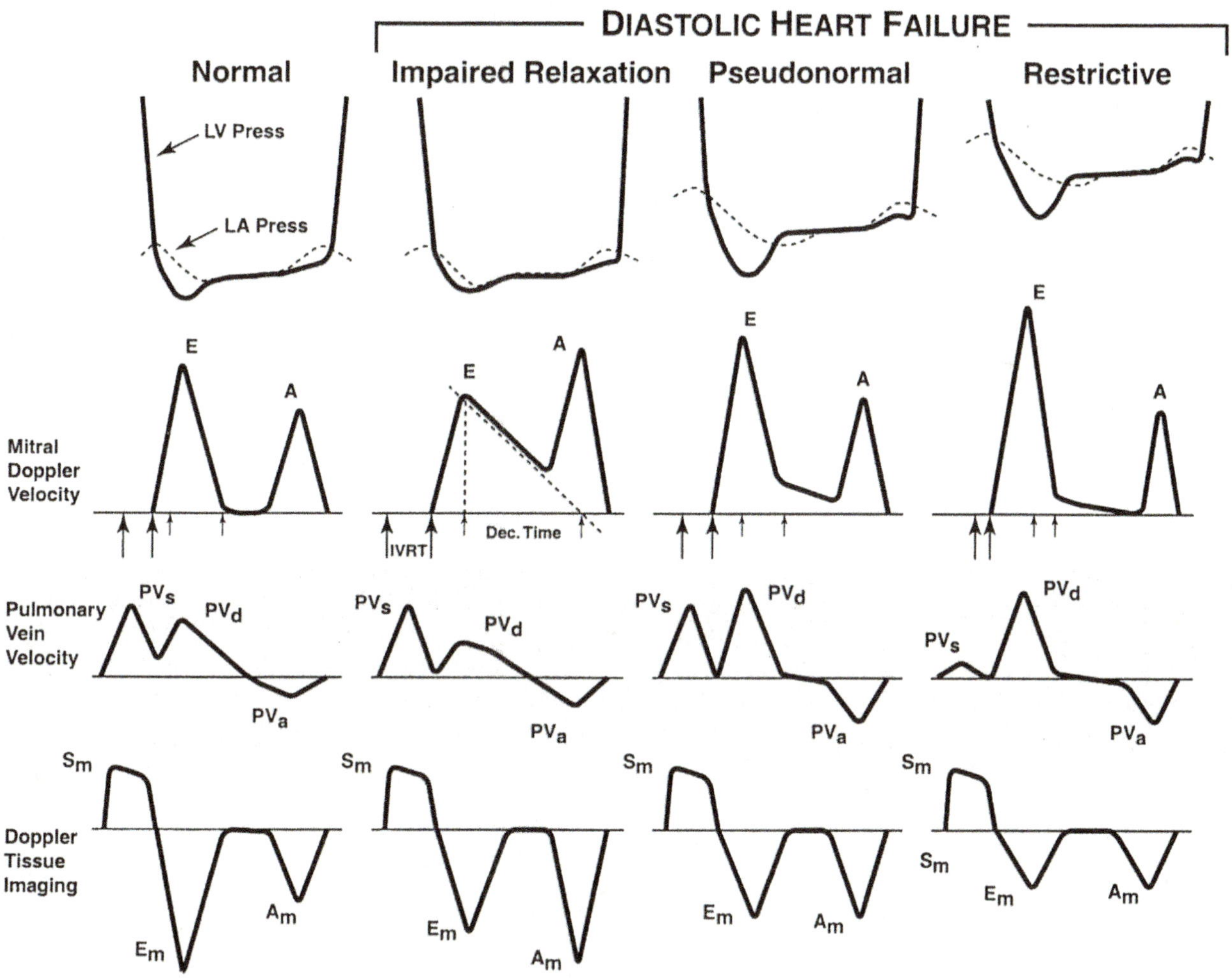

FIGURE 8.7 LV and left atrial (LA) pressures during diastole, transmitral Doppler LV inflow velocity, pulmonary vein Doppler velocity, and Doppler tissue velocity. *Zile and Brutsaert [25] #470.*

Diastology when ejection fraction is (near) normal (>45–50%)
1. Normal diastolic function.
2. Mild diastolic dysfunction with normal resting filling pressures (impaired relaxation)
3. Moderate diastolic dysfunction with elevated filling pressures (pseudonormal filling)
4. Severe diastolic dysfunction with notably elevated filling pressures (restrictive filling—reversible or non-reversible)
5. Indeterminate diastolic function (paced rhythm, atrial fibrillation, mitral valve disease)

Diastology when ejection fraction is reduced (<45%)
1. Diastolic dysfunction with normal filling pressures (impaired relaxation pattern)
2. Diastolic dysfunction with elevated filling pressures (pseudonormal filling pattern)
3. Diastolic dysfunction with severely elevated filling pressures (restrictive filling—reversible or non-reversible)
4. Diastolic dysfunction with indeterminate filling pressures

FIGURE 8.8 Practical classification of diastolic function. *Mottram and Marwick [22].*

pressures obtained at cardiac catheterization [26]. Dragulescu et al. retrospectively studied 175 children with lesions known to have diastolic dysfunction (i.e., dilated, hypertrophic, and restrictive cardiomyopathies) and compared them to normal controls. This study found diagnostic criteria for diastolic dysfunction discrepant in most patients with abnormal relaxation found in 14% of those with hypertrophic cardiomyopathy and never in the other cardiomyopathy types; even though half of the patients had coexisting evidence of elevated filling pressures. In addition, only approximately a third of patients were found to have agreement of diastolic parameters among investigators [27]. These studies highlight the challenges of incorporating adult diastolic norms to pediatric patients.

It must also be recognized that dysfunction in systole and diastole does not always occur in isolation and that they most likely represent a continuum of heart disease. In the presence of systolic heart failure and increased diastolic pressures, this is better classified as combined systolic and diastolic heart failure [25]. A reasonable approach to determining the type of diastolic dysfunction would be determine if it is in the setting of normal (or near normal) systolic function or in depressed systolic function. The Figure below provides a useful classification system (see Fig. 8.8).

The clinical entity described as heart failure with preserved ejection fraction or "HFpEF" is less commonly seen in children in comparison to adults but poses a challenge with regard to diagnosis and management. In adults with HFpEF, it is often sequelae of myocardial ischemia, obesity, or long-standing hypertension [28]. In children, this maybe a more unrecognized problem that may be seen in those with restrictive cardiomyopathy or who have had interventions for left-sided obstructive lesions with the possible development of endocardial fibroelastosis. As this represents a clinical challenge to adults, so it remains in the pediatric population and oft-times with the end result being consideration for cardiac transplantation.

REFERENCES

[1] P.P. Sengupta, A.J. Tajik, K. Chandrasekaran, B.K. Khandheria, Twist mechanics of the left ventricle: principles and application, JACC Cardiovasc. Imaging 1 (2008) 366–376.

[2] Y. Notomi, P. Lysyansky, R.M. Setser, et al., Measurement of ventricular torsion by two-dimensional ultrasound speckle tracking imaging, J. Am. Coll. Cardiol. 45 (2005) 2034–2041.

[3] L.P. Badano, M.H. Miglioranza, T. Edvardsen, et al., European Association of Cardiovascular Imaging/Cardiovascular Imaging Department of the Brazilian Society of Cardiology recommendations for the use of cardiac imaging to assess and follow patients after heart transplantation, Eur. Heart J. Cardiovasc. Imaging 16 (2015) 919–948.

[4] M. Sengelov, P.G. Jorgensen, J.S. Jensen, et al., Global longitudinal strain is a superior predictor of all-cause mortality in heart failure with reduced ejection fraction, JACC Cardiovasc. Imaging 8 (2015) 1351–1359.
[5] A.M. Omar, S. Vallabhajosyula, P.P. Sengupta, Left ventricular twist and torsion: research observations and clinical applications, Circ. Cardiovasc. Imaging 8 (2015).
[6] J.P. Morgan, Abnormal intracellular modulation of calcium as a major cause of cardiac contractile dysfunction, New Engl. J. Med. 325 (1991) 625–632.
[7] M.A. Fogel, Ventricular Function and Blood Flow in Congenital Heart Disease, John Wiley & Sons, 2008.
[8] W. Grossman, D.S. Baim, Grossman's Cardiac Catheterization, Angiography, and Intervention, Lippincott Williams & Wilkins, 2006.
[9] R. Klabunde, Cardiovascular Physiology Concepts, Wolters Kluwer Health, 2011.
[10] R. Melamed, M.D. Sprenkle, V.K. Ulstad, C.A. Herzog, J.W. Leatherman, Assessment of left ventricular function by intensivists using hand-held echocardiography, Chest 135 (2009) 1416–1420.
[11] J.F. Keane, J.E. Lock, D.C. Fyler, Nadas' Pediatric Cardiology, Saunders, 2006.
[12] M.J. Monaghan, Role of real time 3D echocardiography in evaluating the left ventricle, Heart 92 (2006) 131–136.
[13] M. Bansal, R.R. Kasliwal, How do I do it? Speckle-tracking echocardiography, Indian Heart J. 65 (2013) 117–123.
[14] H. Blessberger, T. Binder, Two dimensional speckle tracking echocardiography: basic principles, Heart 96 (2010) 716–722.
[15] T. Bombardini, Myocardial contractility in the echo lab: molecular, cellular and pathophysiological basis, Cardiovasc. Ultrasound 3 (2005) 27.
[16] J.R. Mitchell, J. Wang Jr., Expanding application of the Wiggers diagram to teach cardiovascular physiology, Adv. Physiol. Educ. 38 (2014) 170–175.
[17] M. Courtois, S.J. Kovacs Jr., P.A. Ludbrook, Transmitral pressure-flow velocity relation. Importance of regional pressure gradients in the left ventricle during diastole, Circulation 78 (1988) 661–671.
[18] E. Maksuti, M. Carlsson, H. Arheden, S.J. Kovacs, M. Broome, M. Ugander, Hydraulic forces contribute to left ventricular diastolic filling, Sci. Rep. 7 (2017) 43505.
[19] O. Issa, J.G. Peguero, C. Podesta, et al., Left atrial size and heart failure hospitalization in patients with diastolic dysfunction and preserved ejection fraction, J. Cardiovasc. Echography 27 (2017) 1–6.
[20] C.P. Appleton, J.M. Galloway, M.S. Gonzalez, M. Gaballa, M.A. Basnight, Estimation of left ventricular filling pressures using two-dimensional and Doppler echocardiography in adult patients with cardiac disease. Additional value of analyzing left atrial size, left atrial ejection fraction and the difference in duration of pulmonary venous and mitral flow velocity at atrial contraction, J. Am. Coll. Cardiol. 22 (1993) 1972–1982.
[21] S.C. Menon, M.J. Ackerman, F. Cetta, P.W. O'Leary, B.W. Eidem, Significance of left atrial volume in patients <20 years of age with hypertrophic cardiomyopathy, Am. J. Cardiol. 102 (2008) 1390–1393.
[22] P.M. Mottram, T.H. Marwick, Assessment of diastolic function: what the general cardiologist needs to know, Heart 91 (2005) 681–695.
[23] S.F. Nagueh, K.J. Middleton, H.A. Kopelen, W.A. Zoghbi, M.A. Quinones, Doppler tissue imaging: a noninvasive technique for evaluation of left ventricular relaxation and estimation of filling pressures, J. Am. Coll. Cardiol. 30 (1997) 1527–1533.
[24] S.R. Ommen, R.A. Nishimura, C.P. Appleton, et al., Clinical utility of Doppler echocardiography and tissue Doppler imaging in the estimation of left ventricular filling pressures: a comparative simultaneous Doppler-catheterization study, Circulation 102 (2000) 1788–1794.
[25] M.R. Zile, D.L. Brutsaert, New concepts in diastolic dysfunction and diastolic heart failure: Part I, Diagn. Progn. Meas. Diastolic Funct. 105 (2002) 1387–1393.
[26] D.S. Ezon, S.A. Maskatia, K. Sexson-Tejtel, W.J. Dreyer, A. Jeewa, S.W. Denfield, Tissue Doppler imaging measures correlate poorly with left ventricular filling pressures in pediatric cardiomyopathy, Congenit. Heart Dis. 10 (2015) E203–E209.
[27] A. Dragulescu, L. Mertens, M.K. Friedberg, Interpretation of left ventricular diastolic dysfunction in children with cardiomyopathy by echocardiography: problems and limitations, Circ. Cardiovasc. Imaging 6 (2013) 254–261.
[28] S.M. Dunlay, V.L. Roger, M.M. Redfield, Epidemiology of heart failure with preserved ejection fraction, Nat. Rev. Cardiol. (2017) 14, 591–602.

Chapter 9

Echocardiographic Quantitation of Ventricular Function

Mark K. Friedberg

The Hospital for Sick Children and the University of Toronto, Toronto, ON, Canada

INTRODUCTION

Echocardiographic assessment of ventricular function is one of the most important aspects in the initial assessment and follow-up of children with heart failure. Echocardiography can provide a noninvasive, accessible, real-time assessment of the underlying etiology, the degree and mechanism of ventricular dysfunction, and serial changes in ventricular dimensions and function over time. Multiple echocardiographic parameters have been found to provide prognostic information that can be used to guide patient management and counseling of families. On the initial assessment, echocardiography will provide an indication on whether the patient's cardiomyopathy phenotype is dilated, hypertrophic, restrictive, or noncompacted (Fig. 9.1) [1]. Within a specific diagnosis, such as left ventricular (LV) noncompaction, a dilated or hypertrophic phenotype has prognostic significance [2]. The bright echogenic appearance of endocardial fibroelastosis in a child with dilated cardiomyopathy (DCM) can be a poor prognostic sign [3]. The degree of posterior wall thickening has prognostic significance in hypertrophic cardiomyopathy (HCM) [4]. This type of information provides guidance for the differential diagnosis, patient management, prognostication, and context for the interpretation of ventricular function. Echocardiography is also crucial to evaluate for specific underlying etiologies, especially those amenable to intervention, such as the presence of anomalous coronary artery from the pulmonary artery.

Rather than detail an exhaustive list of all possible tools and methodologies, this chapter provides a broad practical overview and opinion on assessment of ventricular function by echocardiography with the heart failure specialist in mind. For a more in-depth view on the specific ultrasound methods, the reader is referred to pediatric echocardiography texts [5].

BACKGROUND TO ECHOCARDIOGRAPHIC ASSESSMENT OF VENTRICULAR FUNCTION

A text on echo assessment of ventricular function would not be complete without defining ventricular function. Various definitions target different aspects of function. At the organism level, cardiovascular function may be defined as the adequate delivery of blood and oxygen to the tissues to meet their metabolic needs. Note that this definition, while appropriate to heart failure, disregards the performance of the cardiac chambers themselves. At the organ level, cardiac function may be defined by the pump activity that yields sufficient cardiac output at low filling pressures, and the ability to augment cardiac output during increased metabolic need, such as during exercise [6]. Yet even this definition is incomplete, as patients may have impaired ventricular function yet adequately maintain cardiac output due to extracardiac compensatory mechanisms. At the myocardial level, myocardial function may be defined as the phasic shortening and force generation followed by lengthening and force decay. This definition is directly pertinent to echo imaging of myocardial deformation (strain) discussed later in this chapter.

Consequently, when assessing ventricular function by echocardiography, one should define the anatomical level of interrogation: (1) the myofiber (2) the myocardial wall (myocardial function), or (3) the ventricular cavity (pump function). In addition, regional (segmental) wall performance should be defined versus global (overall) pump function.

Whatever the anatomical level of assessment, cardiac function includes cardiac generation of force, stress, or pressure that leads to a change in shape or dimension. At the level of the myofiber, fiber stress is generated and the myofiber shortens in systole and lengthens in diastole. At the myocardial level, wall stress is generated and the myocardium shortens and thickens in systole and lengthens and thins in diastole. At the ventricular level, pressure is generated in systole with

Heart Failure in the Child and Young Adult. http://dx.doi.org/10.1016/B978-0-12-802393-8.00009-0

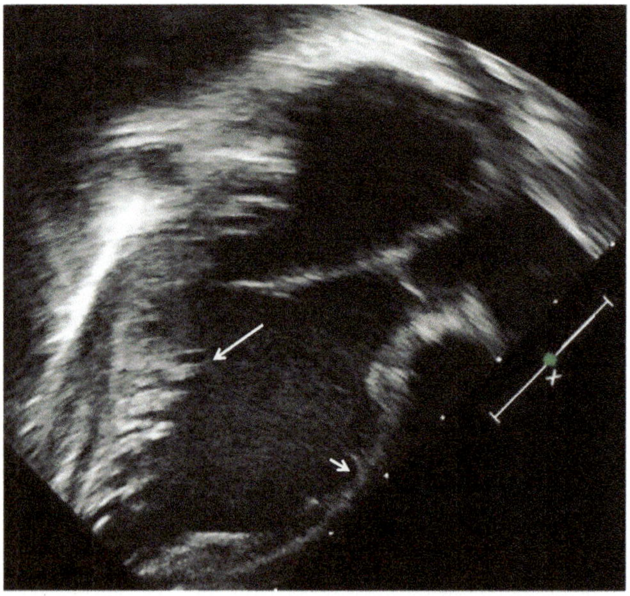

FIGURE 9.1 Apical three-chamber view in a child with a dilated cardiomyopathy phenotype. The left ventricle (LV) is dilated and globular. Note the heavy trabeculations along the posterior LV wall (*long arrow*) consistent with noncompaction cardiomyopathy. The interventricular septum is thin (*short arrow*).

cavity volumes/dimensions decreasing in systole during ejection; and enlarging in diastole during ventricular filling. This is directly relevant to the interpretation of various echo indices.

Current clinical imaging techniques, echocardiography included, do not directly assess function at the myofiber level. Rather, myofiber function is indirectly inferred from other parameters of regional or global function. In addition, at each of the anatomical levels detailed above, echocardiography assesses the change in shape or dimension; while wall stress or force generation has to be indirectly calculated or inferred. Nonetheless, wall stress, is a key determinant of myocardial shortening, hypertrophy, oxygen consumption, and myocardial injury [7,8]; and in DCM, high wall stress, predicts survival [9,10]. Thus, force/wall stress/pressure generation and dimension changes are intimately linked: on the one hand myocardial shortening determines pressure/stress generation and on the other hand end-systolic wall stress, determined by cavity pressure, dimensions, and wall thickness, influences the degree of myocardial shortening [11].

Other key factors need to be accounted for in the interpretation of cardiac function. These include, among others, ventricular preload, afterload, geometry, the presence of atrioventricular and semilunar valve insufficiency, heart rate, ventricular–vascular relations, myocardial segmental–segmental interactions, regional wall motion abnormalities, electromechanical dyssynchrony, and ventricular–ventricular interactions. Tissue elasticity directly affects ventricular function but is difficult to assess directly.

The following examples demonstrate some considerations when interpreting ventricular function by echocardiography. Changes in blood pressure (LV cavity pressure), and hence afterload is an obvious example. Likewise, if a child has a LV ejection fraction (EF) of 55% in the presence of severe mitral regurgitation, LV function may be depressed despite a normal EF numerical value, as the ventricle pumps blood into the low-impedance atrium. On the other hand, the presence of mitral regurgitation increases ventricular preload, which itself not only can increase contraction if contractility is preserved but also increase sphericity and wall stress, which reduce shortening. In children and adults with DCM, the presence of mitral regurgitation is an independent risk factor for transplant-free survival [12] (Fig. 9.2).

A faster heart rate can increase contractility through the force–frequency relationship [13]. Thus, function that appears similar in the same patient, at different heart rates, may indicate worse cardiac performance. It is also apparent from these examples that the various factors detailed above are intimately linked, and it is difficult, if not impossible, to separate them. Although assessment of cardiac contractility is perhaps the "holy grail" of functional assessment, in clinical practice cardiac performance is most commonly assessed in relation to the existing loading conditions [14]. Within this framework, it is important to consider whether changes in conditions and function are acute or chronic as chronicity profoundly impacts cardiac adaptation.

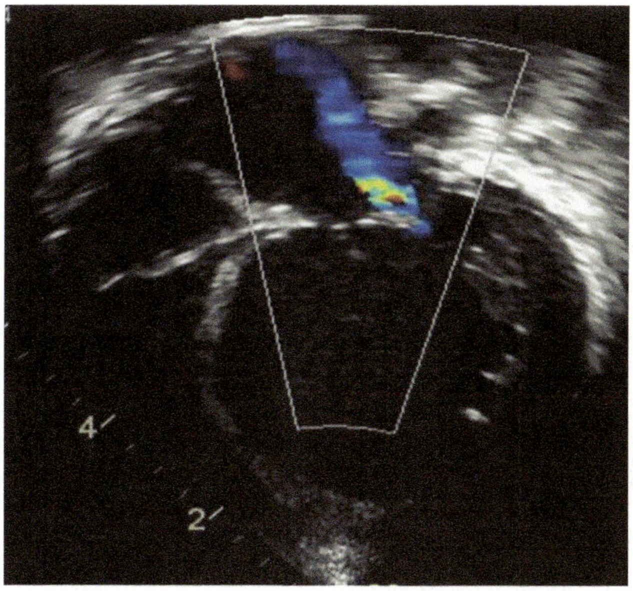

FIGURE 9.2 Dilated and globular left ventricle that underlie mitral regurgitation (blue jet) in a child with dilated cardiomyopathy. While the presence of mitral regurgitation may increase the ejection fraction value above the true underlying myocardial function, its presence is an independent risk factor for death or need for transplant.

SUBJECTIVE ASSESSMENT OF FUNCTION

Subjective assessment of ventricular function is obviously impacted by the experience and individual capabilities of the individual appraiser and consequently suffers from high interobserver variability and suboptimal reproducibility. Nonetheless, subjective assessment remains central to the assessment of ventricular function and is used widely in clinical practice [15]. Subjective assessment is an important parameter to use while understanding and acknowledging its pitfalls. Indeed, I believe that "objective" numerical parameters should be interpreted during subjective assessment of function. Currently, there is no computer algorithm that can adequately synthesize the various factors, especially in the context of the clinical information. It is the human operator's assessment and interpretation of the different "objective" parameters, in the context of the clinical scenario that renders the specialist's echocardiographic assessment of ventricular function. When subjectively interpreting function, the reader should account for the multiple factors detailed above including heart rate, ventricular geometry and dimensions, wall thickness and thickening, atrial versus ventricular size, ventricular cavity shortening, regional differences in appearance and motion, the presence of valvar/outflow stenosis and/or regurgitation, and the visual presence of intracavitary masses, aneurysms, trabeculations, and pericardial effusion.

QUANTITATIVE ASSESSMENT OF VENTRICULAR FUNCTION

Despite the continuing importance of subjective assessment, major advances have been made in quantitation of ventricular function, in particular the quantitative assessment of regional myocardial performance. The challenge often lies in deciding which parameter from a wide armamentarium is relevant, reliable, and reproducible; how to integrate these into a cohesive and useful summary of ventricular function for the clinician; and how to integrate relatively new and emerging techniques into the busy daily routine. Several technologies such as three-dimensional (3D) echocardiography and myocardial strain are now widely available on commercial ultrasound platforms. However, in many instances, the resources allocated to adequate training, integration, processing, and interpretation of these technologies remains inadequate.

From a scientific and practical standpoint so-called "conventional" parameters of ventricular function remain key components of quantitative assessment of ventricular function and central tools in assessment of disease progression, treatment effects, and prognosis.

EJECTION PHASE INDICES

As defined above, the heart ejects blood to meet the body's metabolic needs. Consequently, many echo functional parameters assess cardiac ejection. It is convenient to divide these into geometrical indices and blood flow indices.

Geometrical Indices

Ventricular Dimensions

Intrinsic to ventricular failure is the occurrence of ventricular remodeling [16]. As contractility diminishes, the heart dilates and becomes more spherical to maintain stroke volume and cardiac output (Fig. 9.3A and B). Ventricular dimensions at end-diastole reflect ventricular remodeling, correlate with clinical outcomes, and should be a routine part of functional assessment [17–19]. From a larger end-diastolic dimension and in the presence of reduced contractility, shortening is diminished and end-systolic dimensions enlarge. Thus both larger end-diastolic and end-systolic volumes/dimensions are used to reflect ventricular remodeling and predict outcomes [18,20]. Conversely, in children with DCM, a lower LV end-diastolic dimension (less remodeling) at presentation is associated with greater chance for recovery [21]. In our laboratory, M-mode echo from the parasternal short-axis view at the level of the mitral valve leaflet tips is used to derive LV dimensions (Fig. 9.4), although the American Society of Echocardiography pediatric guidelines promote two-dimensional (2D) over M-mode echocardiography [22]. To account for differences in body size across the pediatric age range, ventricular dimensions can be expressed as z-scores, i.e., the number of standard deviations from the mean of a normal population [23]. Nonetheless, standardization across studies varies [24]. When interpreting ventricular dimensions, it is important to account for the presence and severity of atrioventricular or semilunar valvar regurgitation as possible etiologies for ventricular remodeling [25]. With progressive LV dilatation there is usually relative thinning of the ventricular walls (reduced mass to volume ratio), for example, in DCM [26]. Thus, even if absolute myocardial mass is increased, the decreased mass to volume ratio leads results in increased wall stress, which further contributes to ventricular dysfunction. Wall stress can be derived from echocardiography [27] through measurement of ventricular cavity diameter, wall thickness, and systolic blood pressure (as a surrogate of chamber pressure). The velocity of fiber circumferential shortening (VCFC) relative to the wall stress is an indicator of contractility [27,28], although in our laboratory we do not routinely use wall stress or its relation to VCFC due to pitfalls and difficulty in obtaining accurate measurements. The failing ventricle assumes a more spherical shape.

(A) (B)

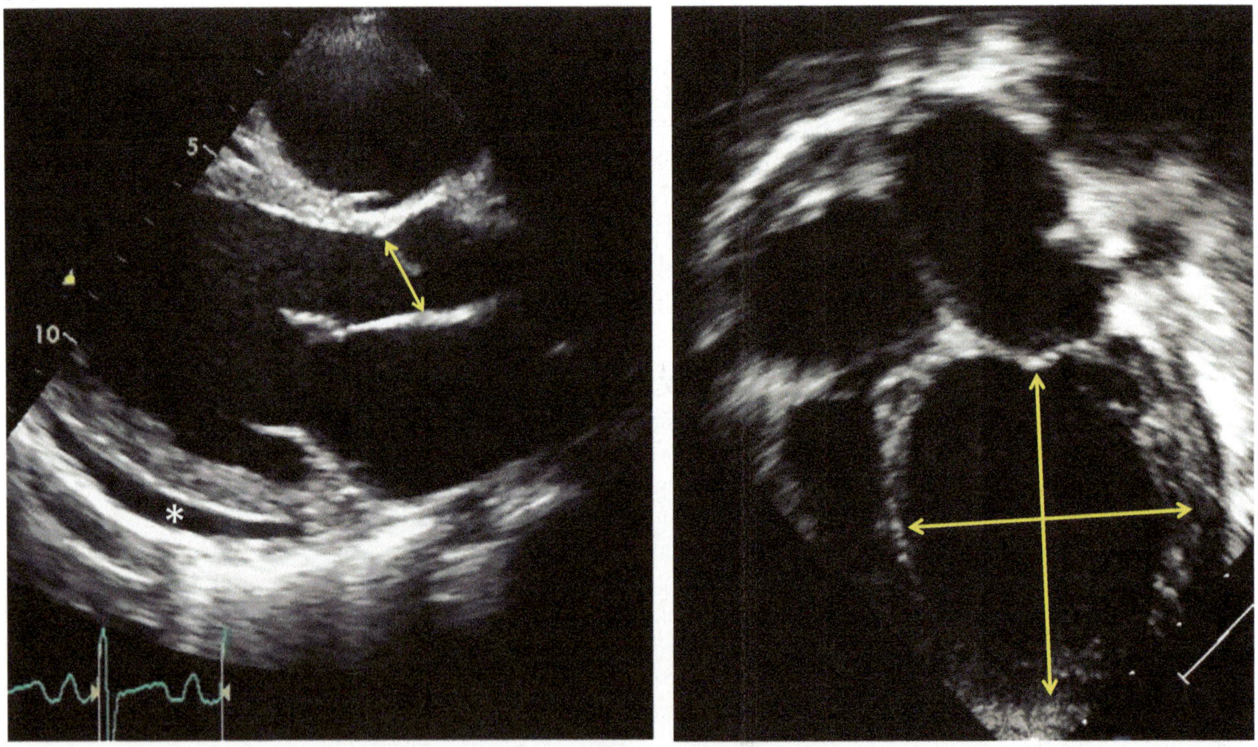

FIGURE 9.3 Panel (A): Parasternal long-axis view in a child with dilated cardiomyopathy. The left ventricle is dilated and spherical. Although not routinely performed, the aortic valve diameter (*yellow double arrow*) can be used together with the time velocity integral of the aortic outflow spectral Doppler jet to measure cardiac output. A small posterior pericardial effusion is present (*asterisks*). Panel (B): Apical four-chamber view in a different child with dilated cardiomyopathy. The left ventricle (LV) is dilated and globular. This remodeling, which ultimately lowers LV pump efficiency, can be simply expressed as the sphericity index the ratio of the LV short-to-long axis dimension ratio at end diastole. A decrease in the sphericity index is associated with improved LV function and reduction in mitral regurgitation.

A simple, but often overlooked parameter is the end-diastolic LV sphericity [29] index (LV minor/major axis dimension) (Fig. 9.3B). A decrease in LV sphericity may be associated with improved EF [29].

Left Ventricular Shortening and Ejection Fraction

The change in LV dimensions or volumes from diastole to systole reflect ejection and are among the most widely used and powerful parameters to quantitate LV function. When LV short-axis M-mode or 2D end-diastolic and end-systolic dimensions are used, these are expressed as the LV shortening fraction (SF% = (LVEDD − LVESD)/LVEDD × 100). A low SF at presentation and lack of improvement over time are risk factors for poor outcome in childhood DCM [30]. When volumes are extrapolated from these dimensions or more directly measured using the 5/6 area length method, the Simpson's method of discs or by 3D echocardiography, the EF is derived as the change in end-diastolic and end-systolic volumes expressed as a percentage (EF% = (LVEDV − LVESV)/LVEDV × 100) (Fig. 9.5). In essence, the EF% represents the stroke volume

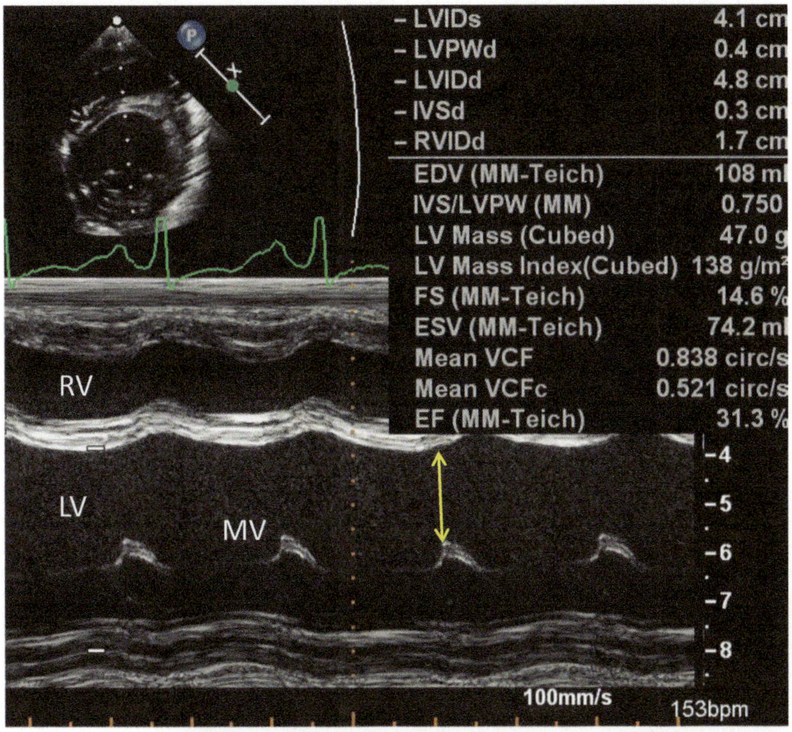

FIGURE 9.4 M-mode echocardiography in a parasternal short-axis view in a child with dilated cardiomyopathy. Left ventricular (LV) end-diastolic and end-systolic dimensions will yield fractional shortening, and through an extrapolation to volumes, ejection fraction. Septal and LV posterior wall thickness can be measured. LV dilatation and remodeling is also reflected in the increased distance between the maximal point of mitral valve (MV) excursion and septum (*double arrow*). End-diastolic right ventricular (RV dimension) can be measured and its z-score is used in our lab to reflect RV size. Also note in this example the thin septum with poor thickening.

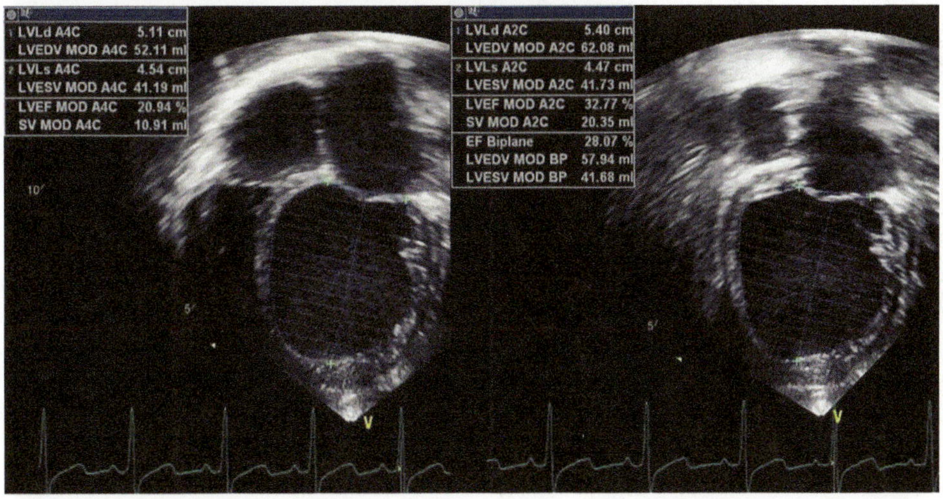

FIGURE 9.5 Left ventricular ejection fraction as calculated by the Simpson's method of discs from an apical four-chamber (left) and two-chamber (right) view in a child with dilated cardiomyopathy.

corrected for end-diastolic volume. This measure incorporates ventricular remodeling and contractility and is influenced by loading conditions. Mathematically, the EF is a reduced expression of formulas reflecting ventricular–vascular coupling (as expressed by the Ea/Ees ratio derived from pressure–volume loops) and as such incorporates ventricular function and its response to vascular impedance [31]. Thus, the EF, a measure of ventricular performance, correlates with mortality and other clinical outcomes in heart failure, including childhood DCM [4,32–34], and is used across diverse age range and clinical conditions as a determining parameter on which clinical management decisions are made. However, as mentioned previously, it is influenced by loading conditions and ventricular characteristics such as hypertrophy and mitral regurgitation, and these should be accounted for when interpreting the EF value.

There are important limitations to the use of each of the measures of shortening or ejection. EF by M-mode uses a local measurement through the basal posterior wall and interventricular septum at the level of the mitral valve leaflet tips and will not adequately reflect global LV function when regional wall or septal motion abnormalities are present. In addition, M-mode EF quantifies radial function and not longitudinal shortening. In many conditions that induce increased wall stress, longitudinal function is diminished relative to radial function [35]. This will not necessarily be detected by M-mode EF. Under these circumstances the Simpson's biplane or 5/6 AL method EF may be preferable (Fig. 9.5). Recent studies in children with DCM have found that the EF by 5/6 AL method is more reproducible than EF measured by the Simpson's method [36,37]. However, the 5/6 AL method also relies on regional measurements, which may not accurately reflect global LV EF. Moreover, M-mode, the 5/6 AL method and numerous other EF methods rely on mathematical formula that assume the LV holds a specific geometrical shape. These assumptions are almost always incorrect in the failing ventricle as the ventricular geometry changes during remodeling [38]. Minor variations in imputed measurements can lead to large differences in the calculated EF. The Simpson's method overcomes some of these pitfalls but can be technically challenging in trying to get a true (nonforeshortened) apical view, as well as a reliable two-chamber (2CH) view (Fig. 9.5). In addition, the Simpson's method can be inaccurate when the LV is hypertrabeculated, as occurs in LV noncompaction, as the endocardial border is poorly defined (Fig. 9.1). LV EF by 3D-echocardiography can overcome several of these problems, is reliable for LV volumes in children [39–43], and is now recommended as a standard method in adult guidelines [44] (Fig. 9.6). However, accurate 3D echo requires a true apical view, depends on adequate endocardial delineation, and the orthogonal 2CH plane may be difficult to obtain (Fig. 9.6). Thus, EF from 3D-echo, while beneficial, is prone to some of the same limitations of other techniques. In addition, 3D-echo has lower frame (volume) rates than M-mode or 2D echo, which may

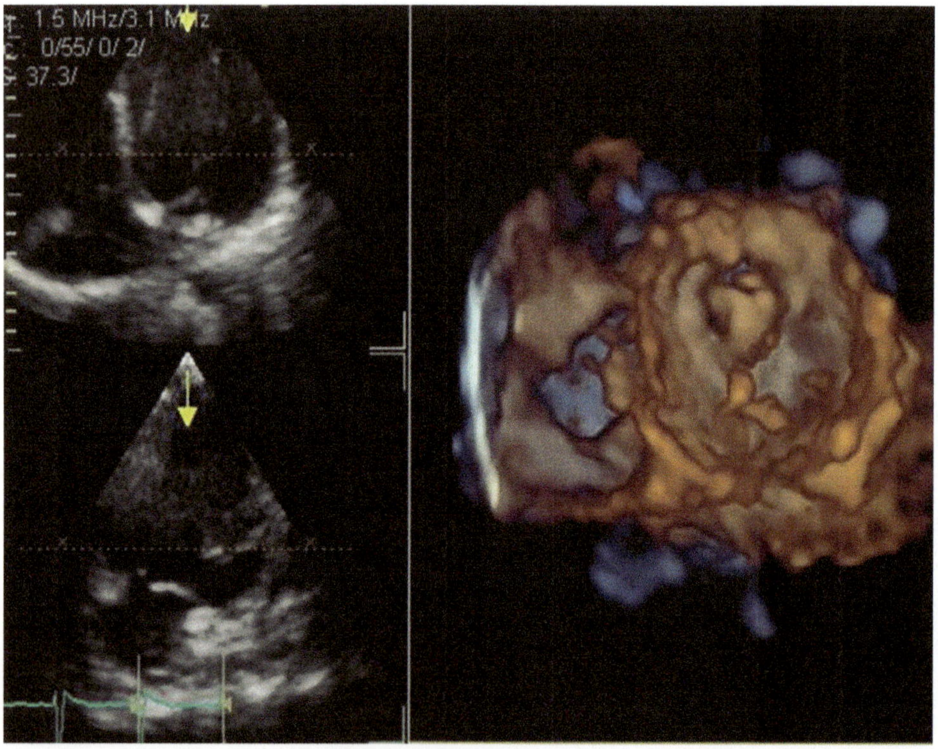

FIGURE 9.6 Left ventricular ejection fraction as calculated from a three-dimensional full-volume acquisition. The software automatically segments the ventricle and displays the two-dimensional four- and two-chamber (2CH) views as depicted in Fig. 9.5. Note that it may be difficult to visualize the endocardial borders in the orthogonal (2CH view equivalent) rendition.

lead to underestimation of the true end-diastolic and end-systolic ventricular volumes, especially in young children with heart failure in whom heart rates can be high.

In all techniques, the calculated EF value can be misleading in the presence of marked hypertrophy, such as occurs in HCM [45] (Fig. 9.7A and B). When the LV cavity is small, as occurs in HCM, any change in cavity dimension will lead to a large percentage change in EF that does not necessarily reflect good ventricular function [46]. Thus, the notion of "hyperdynamic" function in HCM based on a high LV EF is a misconception. This is demonstrated by strain imaging, which as discussed below, demonstrates severely reduced myocardial strain in hypertrophic regions [47,48] (Fig. 9.8). Thus, while EF is a key measure of function; loading conditions, ventricular geometry, and technical details need to be carefully accounted for.

Doppler Ejection and Timing Indices

Echo can quantify hemodynamics, including stroke volume and cardiac output from the measures of ventricular volumes detailed above or from Doppler flow. When derived from Doppler, the stroke volume is calculated as the product of the velocity time integral (VTI) of the LV outflow Doppler, easily obtained by tracing the spectral Doppler envelope, and the cross-sectional area of the aortic valve [49] (Fig. 9.3A). Measurement inaccuracies, predominantly in calculating the cross-sectional area of the valve, have limited use of echo-derived stroke volume in clinical practice; except in specific conditions such as in fetal echocardiography where serial measurement of combined cardiac output may be useful, and in pulmonary hypertension where some clinicians use serial assessment of the pulmonary VTI as a surrogate measure of RV stroke volume and cardiac output.

Cardiac Timing Intervals and Related Measures Assessed From Doppler Flow

Cardiac time intervals have been recognized for decades as being useful measures of ventricular systolic and diastolic function [50–53]. The time required for the ventricle to mount sufficient pressure to open the aortic valve and eject blood lengthens if contractility is reduced and/or afterload increased both common scenarios in heart failure. Consequently, the isovolumic contraction time (ICT), measured from the electrocardiogram (ECG) Q-wave onset to onset of LV/aortic Doppler flow prolongs. Normally, the ICT should be up to approximately one-third of the LV/aortic ejection time (measured as the duration of LV/aortic ejection from the spectral Doppler). In diastole, normal recoil and relaxation ensure a rapid isovolumic relaxation time (IVRT) when ventricular pressure falls below atrial pressure and the atrioventricular valve opens. IVRT is measured from termination of LV/aortic outflow to onset on mitral inflow from a spectral Doppler tracing, acquired in the apical, anteriorly angulated view, which simultaneously samples the LV inflow and outflow (Fig. 9.9). Both ICT and IVRT are heart rate dependent [54]. Also, the IVRT shortens with increased filling pressures on the one hand but prolongs with delayed relaxation on the other. Thus, a "normal" IVRT value may be the product of coexisting delayed

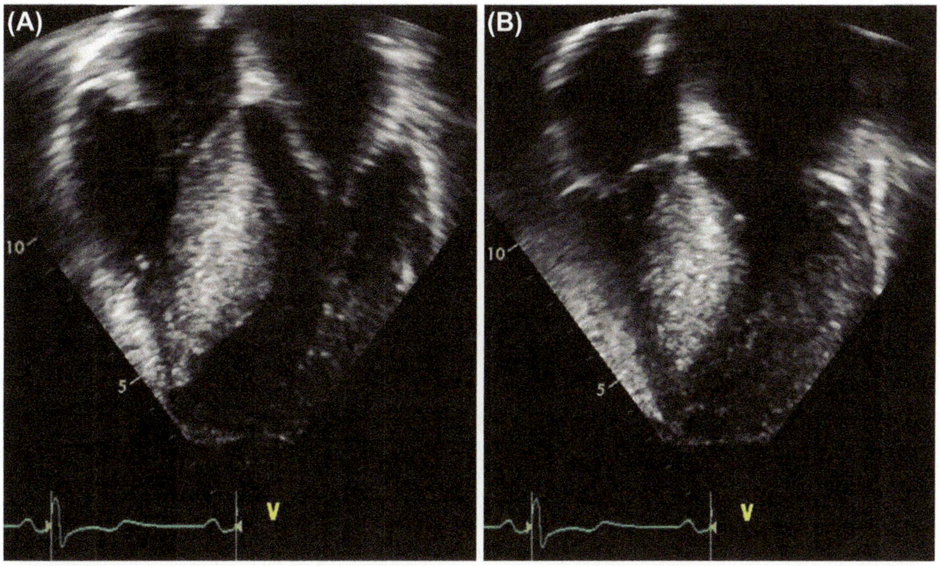

FIGURE 9.7 Apical four-chamber view at end diastole (panel A) and end systole (panel B) in an adolescent with severe hypertrophic cardiomyopathy. The marked septal hypertrophy causes a small LV cavity, which produces a high ejection fraction as the cavity dimension changes from diastole to systole. This does not necessarily accurately reflect underlying myocardial performance as shown in Fig. 9.8.

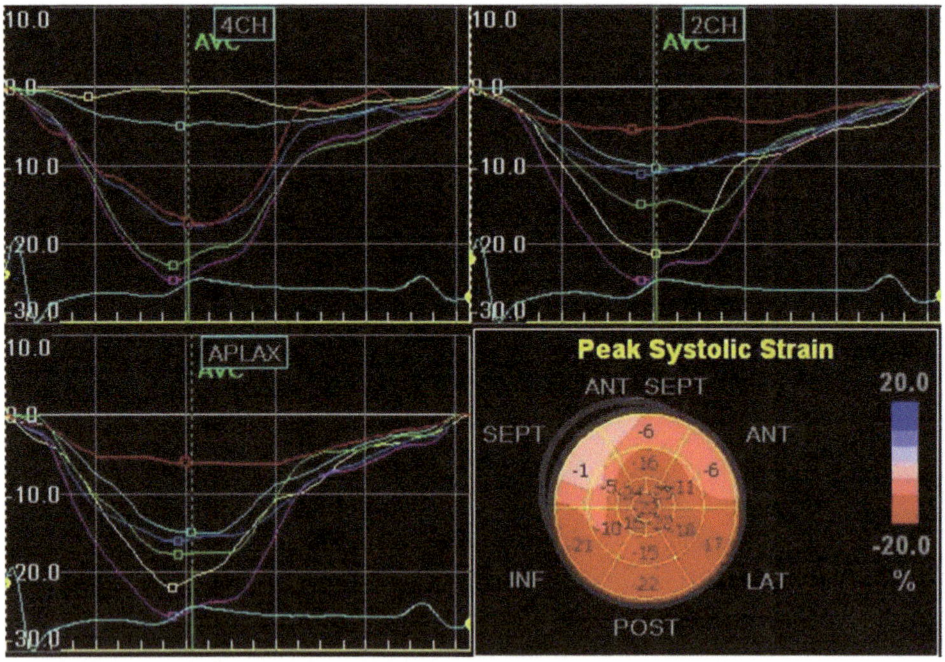

FIGURE 9.8 Speckle-tracking longitudinal strain echocardiography in an adolescent with hypertrophic cardiomyopathy. Regional strain from apical four-chamber (4CH), two-chamber (2CH) and long-axis (APLAX) views are displayed. LV peak systolic strain results are shown in a bull's-eye plot format in the right lower panel. The innermost circle depicts the apex, the middle circle depicts the midsegments, and the outer circle the basal LV segments. In the longitudinal direction, the percent of myocardial shortening is reflected by a negative value. The more negative the value, the more the segment has shortened in relation to its end-diastolic length. Note the low shortening in the hypertrophic basal, and to lesser extent mid-anteroseptal segments (yellow and cyan regional curves in the 4CH view and red curve in the long-axis views). Myocardial shortening is normal in the basal inferior and posterior segments. The green line marked as "AVC" depicts the software's estimation of the timing of aortic valve closure. *ANT*, anterior; *ANT SEPT*, anterior septal; *INF*, inferior; *LAT*, lateral; *POST*, posterior; *SEPT*, septal.

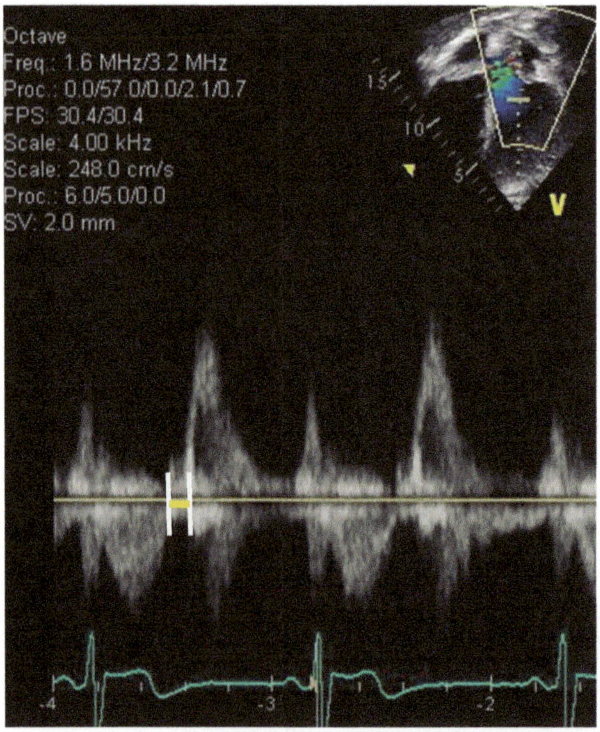

FIGURE 9.9 Spectral Doppler trace taken from an apical view where the sample volume straddles the mitral inflow and aortic outflow. The interval between cessation of LV outflow and beginning of mitral inflow (*horizontal yellow line* between the *vertical white lines*) is measured in milliseconds as the isovolumic relaxation time.

relaxation and increased filling pressures, which we found to be a common scenario in pediatric cardiomyopathies [55]. Nonetheless, a prolonged or short IVRT, in combination with other measures can be informative. It is popular in current practice to integrate the ICT and IVRT and express their sum as a ratio of ejection time, as a "global" measure of systolic and diastolic performance termed the myocardial performance index (MPI) [56]. While the MPI correlates with clinical outcomes in many conditions, a "global" measure does not differentiate between systolic and diastolic performance (and indeed the two are linked) [57]. Moreover, this measure reflects myocardial performance only in as much as the ICT and/or IVRT reflect myocardial performance, and we prefer to assess each component individually. Together with Dr. Norman Silverman, I have proposed the duration of systole over the duration of diastole (systolic: diastolic duration ratio) as an index of ventricular performance that is simple to acquire and measure (Fig. 9.10). In various heart failure conditions, including dilated and restrictive cardiomyopathy and pulmonary hypertension, we have observed that systole, as measured by the duration of mitral or tricuspid regurgitation (akin to the pan–systolic murmur heard on physical examination) prolongs at the expense of a shortened diastolic duration [58,59]. As diastolic duration is exponentially dependent on heart rate, the S:D duration ratio worsens with increasing heart rates, reducing the time available for ventricular filling and perhaps explaining why tachycardia may lead to adverse consequences in heart failure patients [60]. We recently found that in children with DCM, the S:D duration ratio as measured from tissue Doppler correlated with need for transplant and mortality and is thus a potentially useful index for prognostication [61]. Nonetheless, my preference is to assess the S:D duration ratio from the atrioventricular valve regurgitation Doppler (when present) rather than by tissue Doppler, as an index of ventricular pump, rather than regional myocardial, performance. In pulmonary hypertension, a prolonged RV S:D duration ratio reflects not only RV performance but also adverse ventricular–ventricular interactions [62]. As systole prolongs in the failing hypertensive RV, the septum is shifted leftward for a prolonged duration, well into LV diastole, thereby impeding LV filling and performance [63]. A high RV S:D duration ratio (>1.4) is associated with increased risk for death or lung transplant in pulmonary hypertension [64].

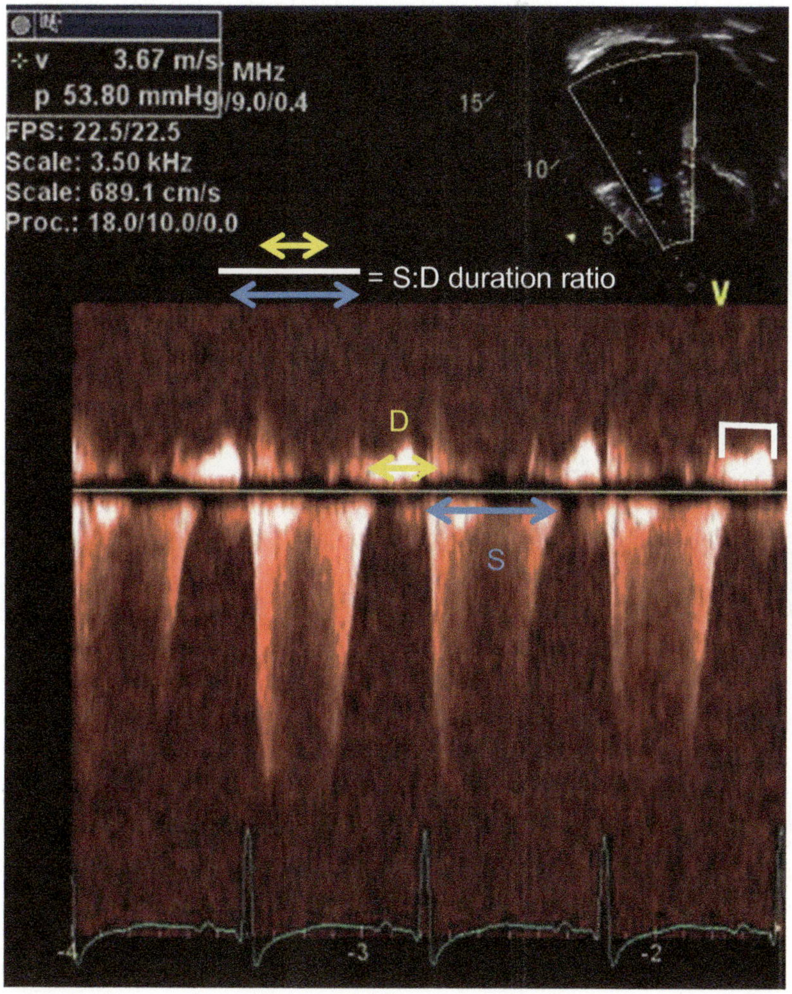

FIGURE 9.10 Spectral Doppler trace of tricuspid regurgitation taken from an apical view in a patient with pulmonary arterial hypertension. The figure depicts measurement of the systolic (S, *blue double arrow*) to diastolic (D, *yellow double arrow*) (S:D) duration ratio. Even though, the tricuspid spectral Doppler envelope is incomplete, the S:D duration ratio can be readily measured. In ventricular dysfunction systole prolongs at the expense of diastole also apparent in the short RV filling time delineated by the white bracket.

Tissue Doppler Imaging

Over the past years, echocardiographic techniques that more directly quantify myocardial performance have become available. Tissue Doppler, whether by pulsed or by color Doppler techniques, measures tissue velocities, and hence a component of myocardial performance at the region sampled. I will not detail the differences in pulsed versus color Doppler methodologies, but pulsed velocities are more commonly used in clinical practice and are more readily interpreted in the context of available normal pediatric values [65,66] (Fig. 9.11A and B). As an index of myocardial systolic and diastolic performance, myocardial systolic and diastolic velocities are influenced not only by myocardial contractility and recoil/relaxation, respectively, but also directly reflect changes in overall ventricular volumes [35]. Tissue velocities are easy to obtain, robust, and correlate with clinical outcomes in pediatric heart failure [17,18]. While tissue velocities can be measured anywhere in the myocardium, they are most commonly measured at the basal LV and RV lateral walls (or mitral and tricuspid annuli) and at the basal interventricular septum (Fig. 9.11A and B). These locations, when sampled from the apex, reflect the longitudinal motion, and hence performance, of these segments. Longitudinal motion is often compromised early in the disease process, as longitudinal fibers, due to their higher radius of circumference, are more sensitive to increased loading conditions and wall stress than circumferential fibers [35]. Thus tissue velocities are sensitive markers of dysfunction or response to increased pressure load. Most commonly, the peak systolic, early and late diastolic peak values are reported. However, it is also useful to qualitatively evaluate the tissue Doppler tracings beyond the absolute values. In failing hearts, tissue velocities are typically low, poorly defined, and poorly organized with indistinct peaks (Fig. 9.11A).

While tissue Doppler velocities are useful and have several advantages, they also have several inherent limitations that are important to remember. Firstly, tissue velocities only measure tissue motion; and motion is often equated with contraction. This is partly true, in that the myocardium obviously moves as it contracts and relaxes. However, myocardial motion is also influenced by noncontractile motion such as translational motion of the heart in the chest, the rocking motion that is commonly observed in the dilated failing ventricle and passive motion of tethered segments [67]. Only the component of the tissue velocity, which reflects contraction and relaxation, may be expected to correlate with intrinsic function and hence clinical outcomes. Even then, cardiac function is only one component of a more complex system of the heart failure syndrome that determines the clinical course. This should be remembered when assigning prognostic significance of a momentous event, such as death, to a single systolic or diastolic velocity measured at a single region in the ventricle at a single

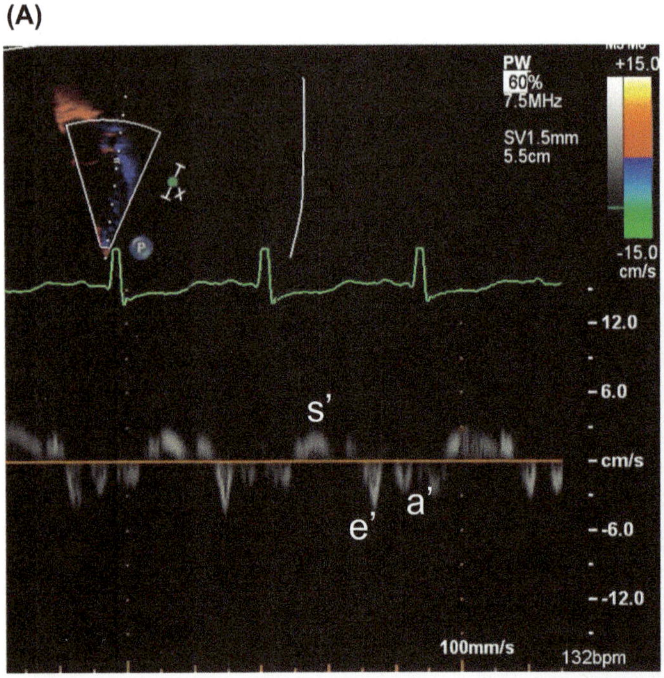

FIGURE 9.11 Pulsed tissue Doppler imaging sampled at the lateral mitral (panel A) and basal septal (panel B) annulus in two children with dilated cardiomyopathy. The systolic (s′), early diastolic (e′), and late diastolic (a′) signals are apparent. These reflect systolic and diastolic tissue motion (velocities) and function, respectively. Note the relatively poorly formed signals, low velocities, and reversed e′/a′ velocities in panel (B), reflecting systolic and diastolic dysfunction. The *arrow* in panel (B) marks the spike of isovolumic acceleration (IVA). The slope of the IVA signal, from baseline to peak, is reported to reflect myocardial contractility, but has poor interobserver measurement reproducibility.

point in time. In DCM, the spherical configuration of the ventricle causes a rounded basal segment. It is difficult to measure the longitudinal motion of this rounded basal segment from the apex due to the angle of the Doppler beam relative to the longitudinal axis of the ventricular wall at the rounded base. Moreover, while tissue velocities at the mitral or septal annulus are used to measure "global" ventricular performance; they are in essence a local velocity that reflects local dynamics. These local dynamics may not reliably reflect global performance if there are regional differences or other confounding factors. Nonetheless, TDI velocities have prognostic value for outcomes or disease progression in pediatric cardiomyopathies, including noncompaction, dilated, and HCMs [17,18,68,69], as well as graft failure in pediatric heart transplant recipients [70] (Fig. 9.12). It is notable that not only the systolic but also especially diastolic velocities have prognostic importance, notably the tricuspid early diastolic velocity [17]. In general, the impact of RV dysfunction on outcomes in LV failure in DCM is important to keep in mind and should be assessed during evaluation of "LV" cardiomyopathy by echo [71,72].

Myocardial Strain

Strain imaging allows for bedside quantification of the percent change in myocardial length or thickness, as a measure of its performance. Strain rate is the rate at which the myocardium changes its length or thickness. Two techniques are currently available in the clinical arena to measure myocardial strain and strain rate: (1) Strain derived from color tissue Doppler and (2) strain derived from speckle tracking, which is currently the most commonly used modality.

Both strain and strain rate are influenced by loading conditions, but as peak strain rate occurs early in systole, it is less influenced by afterload than strain, which normally peaks with aortic valve closure and is by definition an ejection phase index. Thus "global" strain, i.e., the average of regional strains across the ventricle, correlates with the change in ventricular volume (in essence with EF), while strain rate correlates more with contractility or the rapid buildup of force in early systole. As detailed at the beginning of the chapter, ventricular function is characterized by production of force, pressure, or wall stress that is followed by a change in dimension or length. For the myocardium, generation of wall stress is followed by shortening in the longitudinal and circumferential directions, and a resultant myocardial thickening in the radial (transverse) direction. Consequently, using speckle-tracking echocardiography, myocardial strain can be measured in the longitudinal direction from the apical views, in the circumferential direction from the parasternal short-axis views and in the radial direction from the parasternal and apical views (often termed transverse strain) [73]. It should be noted from this description that strain imaging only measures the change in myocardial dimension (from the original or end-diastolic myocardial length) and not the underlying wall stress (stress–strain relations). Nonetheless, myocardial performance is implied from the strain, but the loading conditions and ventricular dimensions need to be accounted for when interpreting the strain values and curves, as discussed above. Currently, global longitudinal strain, measured from apical 2CH, three-, and four-chamber (4CH) views is the most widely used strain index in clinical practice and one which we routinely utilize when assessing ventricular function in our daily practice (Fig. 9.8).

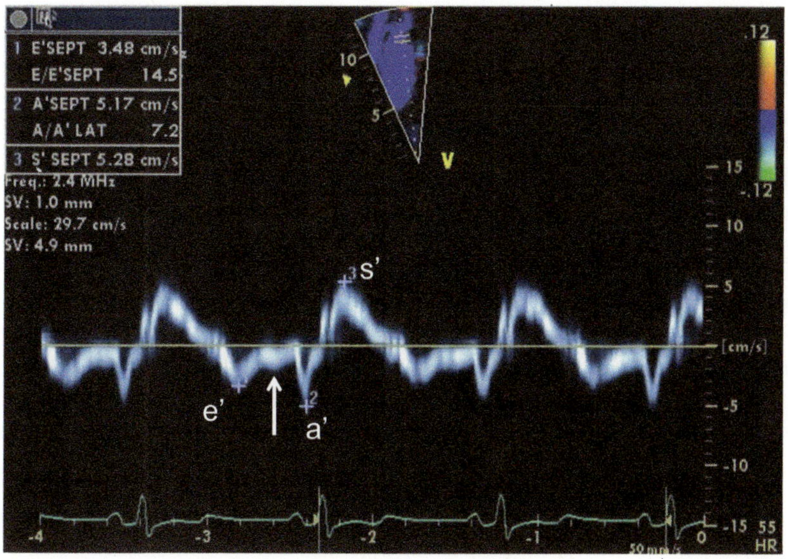

FIGURE 9.12 Pulsed tissue Doppler imaging at the basal septum in an adolescent with hypertrophic cardiomyopathy (same patient shown in Fig. 9.7). The early diastolic (e′) velocity is very low and the e′–a′ pattern is reversed with a higher a′ velocity. This is consistent with impaired relaxation in the sampled segment. There is an abnormal velocity during diastasis—an L′ wave (*arrow*), consistent with impaired relaxation and possibly increased filling pressures.

Assessment of Regional Wall Motion Abnormalities

Assessment of regional wall motion abnormalities is important and although seemingly simple, it is notoriously difficult. The presence of regional abnormalities is important to assess as they may indicate ischemia, scar or aneurysm. The adult classification of regional wall motion abnormalities classifies motion as (1) normal or hyperkinetic, (2) hypokinetic (reduced thickening), (3) akinetic (absent or negligible thickening, e.g., scar), and (4) dyskinetic (systolic thinning or stretching, e.g., aneurysm) [44]. These, and functional heterogeneity in general, should be noted. Indeed it is our experience that regional heterogeneity in myocardial function, in essence a form of regional wall motion abnormality, is very common in DCM [74–76] and in HCM when hypertrophy is not evenly distributed. In congenital heart disease (CHD), especially in single ventricles, regional heterogeneity in myocardial function is common [77–79]. Whether in the functionally biventricular or univentricular heart, regional abnormalities, and heterogeneity affect global function and may contribute to pump inefficiency [74,79]. Moreover, "global" assessment using M-mode EF or annular tissue Doppler velocities may be grossly inaccurate in the presence of regional differences in ventricular function as discussed above.

Ventricular Dyssynchrony

Dyssynchrony refers to timing differences (incoordination) between the contraction (and/or relaxation) of different ventricular segments. Electromechanical dyssynchrony refers to mechanical incoordination resulting from electrical conduction delay [80,81]. The prototype abnormality is left bundle branch block (LBBB), which commonly drives heart failure in adults with LBBB and LV dysfunction. Dyssynchrony can occur between atrial contraction and ventricular filling (A–V dyssynchrony), between different ventricular segments (most commonly septum and posterior/lateral wall; intraventricular dyssynchrony) and between the LV and RV (interventricular dyssynchrony) [82]. Echocardiography can assess all of these levels, but the best method is not yet established; and in pediatrics the prognostic significance of dyssynchrony and whether echo can predict response to cardiac resynchronization therapy (CRT) are not established [83].

A–V dyssynchrony is assessed by optimal ventricular filling using the Doppler signal of mitral or tricuspid inflow. Interventricular dyssynchrony is most commonly assessed by the mechanical interventricular delay, which is the delay between onset of pulmonary versus aortic ejection as measured by Doppler flow [84]. The main focus, however, is placed on assessment of intraventricular dyssynchrony [84]. Although published adult literature and previous guidelines were based on time to peak motion or contraction, these inform on mechanical dispersion (itself a risk factor for arrhythmia and sudden death in adult DCM) [85,86] but not electromechanical dyssynchrony that is expected to respond to CRT [87]. In our lab we assess for a wide ECG QRS duration associated with echo signs of early septal activation (septal flash) late termination and concomitant early stretch followed by late contraction of the opposing lateral or posterior wall [88] (Fig. 9.13). This can be assessed using visual assessment of the 2D echo clip, M-mode, tissue Doppler, and strain imaging [88].

Echo Assessment of Diastolic Function

Echo assessment of diastolic function in children is important as it has high prognostic value [68] but is difficult due to the wide range of normal values in children, changing values with age and heart rate, inapplicability of adult guidelines to children, absence of guidelines on how to classify diastolic dysfunction in children, presence of often apparently conflicting echo criteria, lack of correlation of echo criteria with invasively measure reference parameters, and the infrequent presence of isolated delayed relaxation in children [54,55]. Nonetheless, the same echo parameters that are used in adult patients to classify impaired relaxation and/or elevated filling pressures (restrictive physiology) are used in children [55,89]. In general, reduced E-wave velocity (and reversed E/A ratio), long deceleration time of the mitral valve E-wave, prolonged isovolumetric relaxation time, low E' (early diastolic) tissue Doppler annular velocity, presence of middiastolic filling (L-wave) and reduced color M-mode flow propagation of ventricular inflow are consistent with impaired ventricular recoil and/or relaxation (Fig. 9.14). Atrial enlargement, increased velocity and duration of pulmonary vein flow reversal during atrial contraction, increased RV systolic pressures (RVSps) (assessed from the tricuspid regurgitation jet), short IVRT, and short mitral E-wave deceleration time are indicators of decreased ventricular compliance and increased filling pressures [90] (Fig. 9.15). However, values can be affected in opposite directions by impaired relaxation and increased filling pressures. For example, mitral E-wave deceleration time lengthens with impaired relaxation but shortens with increased filling pressures. The concomitant presence of both may render values in the normal range and difficult to interpret. Therefore, as stated above, often only some of these are present, and it is the interpretation of multiple factors taken together, and taking into account other factors such as ventricular hypertrophy, which determines interpretation of diastolic function.

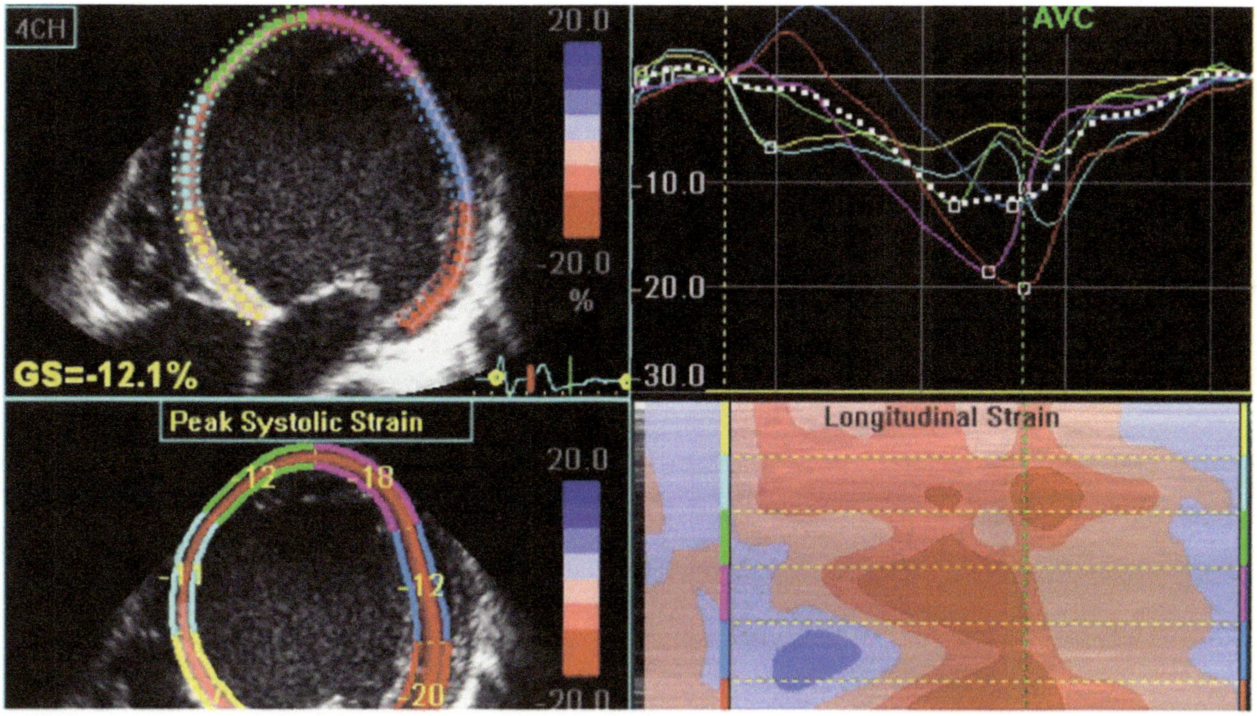

FIGURE 9.13 Child after surgical repair of double outlet right ventricle with subaortic ventricular septal defect and left bundle branch block. The child experienced progressive heart failure symptoms with low left ventricular (LV) ejection fraction. Note the dilated LV in the reference image. Speckle-tracking strain echocardiography shows electromechanical dyssynchrony with early septal activation (*yellow and cyan curves*) with concomitant left lateral wall stretch (*red and blue curves*). The lateral segments then contract late with termination of septal shortening. Note that total deformation is relatively good in the prestretched lateral wall.

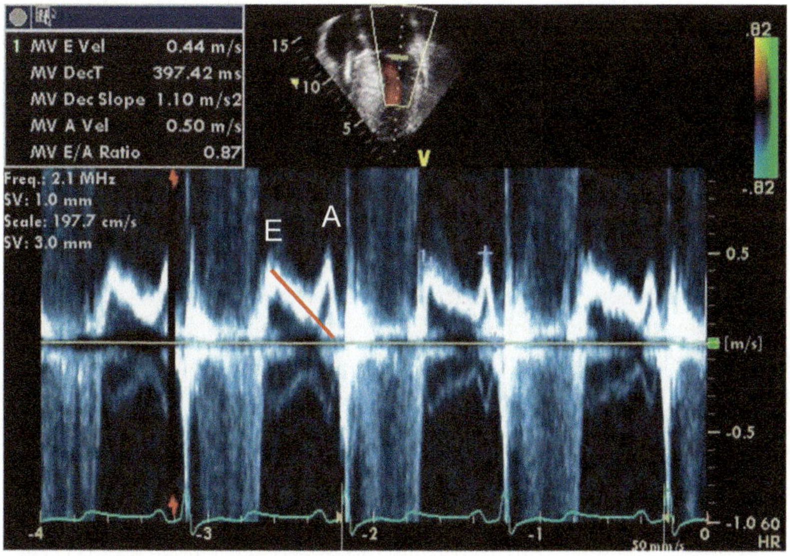

FIGURE 9.14 Pulsed Doppler of the mitral inflow in an adolescent with hypertrophic cardiomyopathy (same patient shown in Figs. 9.7 and 19.2). The early diastolic velocity (E) is low and the early to late (A) diastolic velocity (E/A) pattern is reversed with a higher A velocity. The mitral valve deceleration time (*red line*) is markedly prolonged. These findings are consistent with diastolic dysfunction due to impaired relaxation; a pattern that we observed (in isolation) almost exclusively in adolescents with hypertrophic cardiomyopathy.

Echo Assessment of Right Ventricular Function

Functional assessment of the RV is important as concomitant RV dysfunction in left-sided failure is associated with increased risk for mortality [91,92]. RV dysfunction may arise from increased LV filling pressures leading to increased pulmonary vascular resistance, primary involvement by the disease process or adverse ventricular–ventricular interactions. Assessment of RV function poses a unique challenge due to the RVs anterior location behind the sternum (complicating its visualization by echo), its complex geometry, its thin and heterogeneous walls, and its trabeculated nature. Assessment of RV function should account for pulmonary artery pressures using the configuration of the interventricular septum (rightward

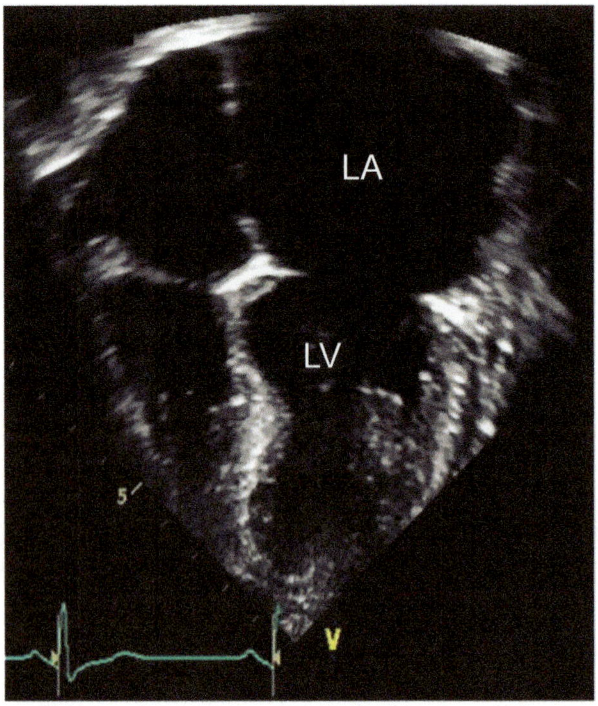

FIGURE 9.15 Apical four-chamber view in a patient with hypertrophic cardiomyopathy and a restrictive phenotype. Note the markedly enlarged left atrium (LA), which in the absence of mitral regurgitation indicates chronically increased left ventricular (LV) filling pressures.

position is consistent with less than half systemic RVSp, flat-half systemic, and leftward-systemic or suprasystemic RVSp), and the velocity of the spectral Doppler envelope of the TR jet. As for evaluation of diastolic function, there is no single echo parameter that can adequately encapsulate RV function. Subjective (eyeball) assessment of RV dilatation, shortening, myocardial thickening, and motion and RA enlargement should be combined with quantitative measures of function, which predominantly evaluate longitudinal function of the lateral wall and lateral tricuspid annulus from the apical 4CH view. These include tricuspid annular planar systolic excursion, a measure of annular displacement, usually measured by M-mode, and tissue Doppler systolic and diastolic velocities at the tricuspid lateral annulus by pulsed tissue Doppler (Fig. 9.16) [22,93]. As annular motion alone may be misleading and inadequate a singular parameter of RV function (there is often substantial translational motion and in addition the annulus may move relatively well even when other RV segments, particularly apical segments are hypokinetic), we add assessment of fractional area of change (FAC, RV end-diastolic area end-systolic area/end-diastolic area, expressed as a percent) from the apical 4CH view (Fig. 9.16). FAC is a surrogate of RV EF, but one should be cognizant of its low interobserver reliability that arises from the difficulty in defining the RV endocardial border (Fig. 9.16). One may add Doppler-derived parameters to this assessment. As for the LV, the MPI sums the isovolumic contraction and relaxation periods over the ejection duration as a measure of combined ventricular systolic and diastolic function and correlates with morbidity and mortality in various heart failure conditions (Fig. 9.16). While in the LV, the MPI can be assessed in a single cardiac cycle by a Doppler sample straddling the mitral inflow and LV outflow, in the RV, the inflow and outflow tracts are anatomically distant, and measurement of the MPI requires two separate views and hence two separate cardiac cycles. Tissue Doppler–derived MPI is an alternative to obtain the MPI in a single cardiac cycle, but adequate validation is lacking is not equal to Doppler flow–derived MPI. As described above for the LV, I also measure the S:D duration ratio from the tricuspid regurgitation jet (Fig. 9.10) Measuring the maximal slope of the TR Doppler jet is proposed as a measure of the change in RV pressure over time (dP/dt) and hence contractility. While theoretically sound, measurement of a slope is highly variable, the dP/dT is affected by loading conditions and heart rate and normal values published for the RV span a wide range in different studies and are uncertain. Therefore, we do not report this parameter routinely in our clinical practice.

In certain patient groups such as tetralogy of Fallot and pulmonary hypertension we now incorporate 2D speckle longitudinal strain to assess RV myocardial performance (Fig. 9.17). It would also be beneficial to assess RV volumes and EF using 3D echocardiography (Fig. 9.18). A body of validation studies in children, predominantly in patients with CHD, suggests that echo approximates magnetic resonance imaging evaluation for RV functional assessment, but its incorporation into clinical practice still lags far behind that for 3D assessment of LV function in most labs due to availability of equipment, lack of proficiency and practical difficulties incorporating these modalities into the existing routine [42].

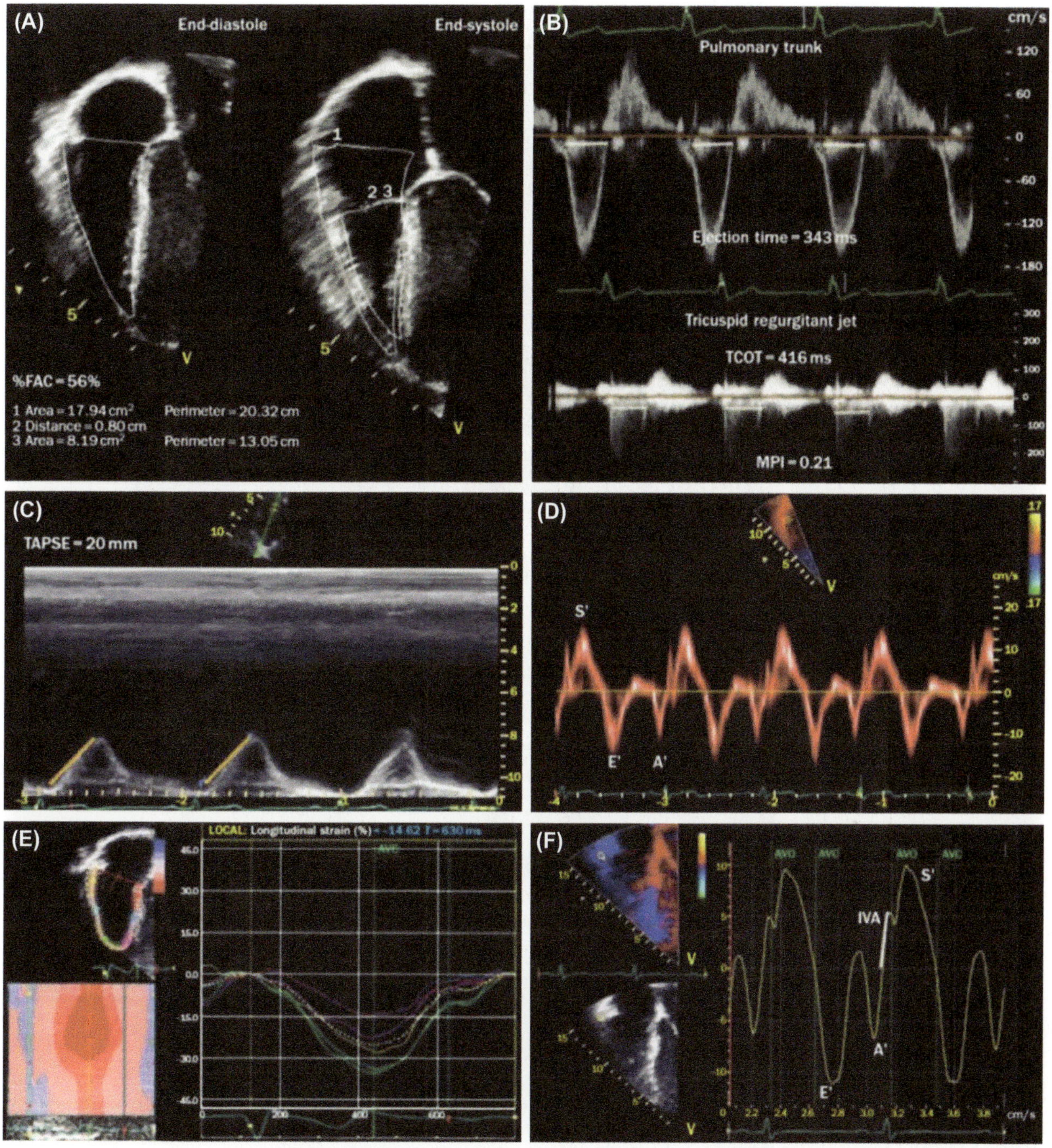

FIGURE 9.16 Assessment of right ventricular (RV) function by echocardiography. (A) %FAC, calculated from the apical four-chamber view measures the change in RV area between end diastole and end systole. The importance of longitudinal shortening can be appreciated in this image. (B) MPI calculated by measuring the ejection time on the pulmonary artery tracing and the time between closure and opening of the tricuspid valve on the tricuspid inflow tracing. MPI=(TCOT−ET)/ET. In this patient, the MPI was normal after tetralogy of Fallot repair. (C) TAPSE. An M-mode echocardiogram through the tricuspid annulus is obtained and the excursion of the tricuspid annulus is measured as illustrated. This index is a measure of longitudinal RV function. (D) Tissue Doppler velocities of the tricuspid annulus as a parameter of systolic and diastolic longitudinal RV function. (E) Longitudinal RV strain measurements by speckle-tracking echocardiography. By convention, systolic longitudinal shortening is represented as a negative value and is measured here in six lateral wall and septal segments. The mean values of these segments represent the mean longitudinal strain curve (*white dotted line*). (F) Color tissue Doppler at the lateral tricuspid valve annulus and measurement of IVA. Aortic valve opening and closure are depicted by green lines for event timing. The timing of these events may be taken as that of pulmonary valve opening and closure. The slope of IVA is shown (*white line*). Note that IVA occurs within the QRS complex and peaks before pulmonary valve opening in the isovolumic period. *A'*, late diastolic tissue velocity; *AVC*, aortic valve closure; *AVO*, aortic valve opening; *E'*, early diastolic tissue velocity; *ET*, ejection time; *IVA*, isovolumic acceleration; *MPI*, myocardial performance index; *S'*, systolic tissue velocity; *TAPSE*, tricuspid annular systolic plane excursion; *TCOT*, tricuspid valve closure–opening time; *%FAC*, percentage fractional area change. *Reproduced from L.L. Mertens, M.K. Friedberg, Imaging the right ventricle–current state of the art, Nat. Rev. Cardiol. 7(10) (October 2010) 551–563. PubMed PMID: 20697412. Epub 2010/08/11. eng.*

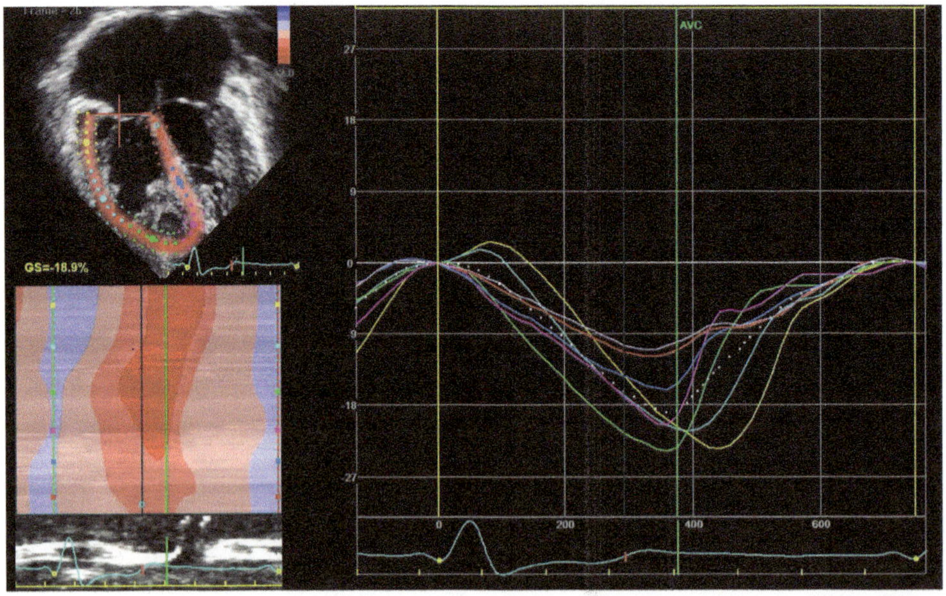

FIGURE 9.17 Right ventricular (RV) longitudinal strain by speckle-tracking echocardiography in a patient after surgical repair of tetralogy of Fallot. Note the relatively low peak strain values and marked mechanical dispersion, partly arising from RV right bundle branch block electromechanical dyssynchrony. Note the early activation of septal apical segments (*purple and green curves*) with concomitant right lateral wall stretch (*yellow and cyan curves*).

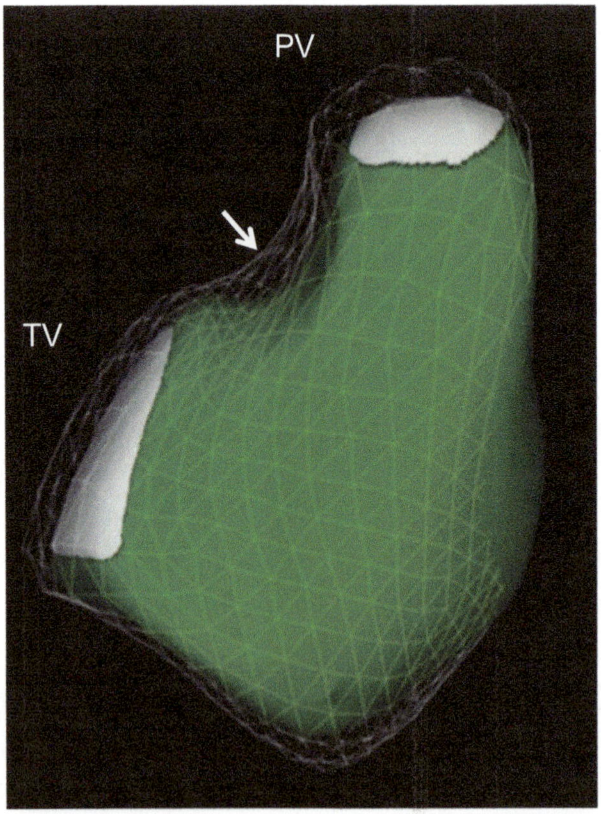

FIGURE 9.18 Three-dimensional echocardiography full-volume acquisition of the right ventricle (RV). The tricuspid (TV) and pulmonary (PV) valves are annotated. The mesh (*arrow*) reflects the end-diastolic RV volume. From such acquisitions, the software can calculate RV ejection fraction with good comparison to cardiac magnetic resonance imaging-derived measurements.

CONCLUSION

In summary, echocardiographic assessment of cardiac function is an integral part of heart failure assessment in children providing information on the etiology, prognosis, and serial changes in ventricular function and remodeling. These impact heart failure management. Subjective assessment, together with use of quantitative measures, should be combined to assess LV and RV systolic function, diastolic function, regional wall motion abnormalities, and the presence and impact of pericardial effusion.

REFERENCES

[1] R.H. Pignatelli, C.J. McMahon, W.J. Dreyer, S.W. Denfield, J. Price, J.W. Belmont, et al., Clinical characterization of left ventricular noncompaction in children: a relatively common form of cardiomyopathy, Circulation 108 (21) (November 25, 2003) 2672–2678 PubMed PMID: 14623814.

[2] J.L. Jefferies, J.D. Wilkinson, L.A. Sleeper, S.D. Colan, M. Lu, E. Pahl, et al., Cardiomyopathy phenotypes and outcomes for children with left ventricular myocardial noncompaction: results from the pediatric cardiomyopathy registry, J. Cardiac Fail. 21 (11) (November 2015) 877–884 PubMed PMID: 26164213. Pubmed Central PMCID: 4630116.

[3] A. Arola, J. Tuominen, O. Ruuskanen, E. Jokinen, Idiopathic dilated cardiomyopathy in children: prognostic indicators and outcome, Pediatrics 101 (3 Pt 1) (March 1998) 369–376 PubMed PMID: 9480999. Epub 1998/03/14. eng.

[4] T. Bharucha, K.J. Lee, P.E. Daubeney, A.W. Nugent, C. Turner, G.F. Sholler, et al., Sudden death in childhood cardiomyopathy: results from a long-term national population-based study, J. Am. Coll. Cardiol. 65 (21) (June 2, 2015) 2302–2310 PubMed PMID: 26022819.

[5] W.W. Lai, L.L. Mertens, M.S. Cohen, T. Geva, J. D'hooge, S. Drant, et al., Echocardiography in Pediatric and Congenital Heart Disease: From Fetus to Adult, second ed., Wiley Blackwell, New Delhi, India, 2016. 914 p.

[6] J.D. Thomas, Z.B. Popovic, Assessment of left ventricular function by cardiac ultrasound, J. Am. Coll. Cardiol. 48 (10) (November 21, 2006) 2012–2025 PubMed PMID: 17112991.

[7] W.K. Laskey, N. Reichek, M. St John Sutton, W.J. Untereker, J.W. Hirshfeld Jr., Matching of myocardial oxygen consumption to mechanical load in human left ventricular hypertrophy and dysfunction, J. Am. Coll. Cardiol. 3 (2 Pt 1) (February 1984) 291–300 PubMed PMID: 6229568.

[8] H. Suga, Y. Goto, T. Nozawa, Y. Yasumura, S. Futaki, N. Tanaka, Force-time integral decreases with ejection despite constant oxygen consumption and pressure-volume area in dog left ventricle, Circ. Res. 60 (6) (June 1987) 797–803 PubMed PMID: 3594752.

[9] Y. Hara, M. Hamada, K. Hiwada, Left ventricular end-systolic wall stress is a potent prognostic variable in patients with dilated cardiomyopathy, Jpn. Circ. J. 63 (3) (March 1999) 196–200 PubMed PMID: 10201621.

[10] W.K. Laskey, M.S. Sutton, G. Zeevi, J.W. Hirshfeld Jr., N. Reichek, Left ventricular mechanics in dilated cardiomyopathy, Am. J. Cardiol. 54 (6) (September 1, 1984) 620–625 PubMed PMID: 6433689.

[11] H. Suga, A. Kitabatake, K. Sagawa, End-systolic pressure determines stroke volume from fixed end-diastolic volume in the isolated canine left ventricle under a constant contractile state, Circ. Res. 44 (2) (February 1979) 238–249 PubMed PMID: 761306.

[12] F.P. Fernandes, C. Manlhiot, B.W. McCrindle, L. Mertens, P.F. Kantor, M.K. Friedberg, Usefulness of mitral regurgitation as a marker of increased risk for death or cardiac transplantation in idiopathic dilated cardiomyopathy in children, Am. J. Cardiol. 107 (10) (May 15, 2011) 1517–1521 PubMed PMID: 21377646. Epub 2011/03/08. eng.

[13] N.R. Alpert, B.J. Leavitt, F.P. Ittleman, G. Hasenfuss, B. Pieske, L.A. Mulieri, A mechanistic analysis of the force-frequency relation in non-failing and progressively failing human myocardium, Basic Res. Cardiol. 93 (Suppl. 1) (1998) 23–32 PubMed PMID: 9833127.

[14] G.G. Sandor, Echocardiographic tests of left ventricular function in pediatric cardiology: are we searching for the holy grail? Can. J. Cardiol. 32 (10) (October 2016) 1186–1192 PubMed PMID: 26922289.

[15] H.R. Bellsham-Revell, J.M. Simpson, O.I. Miller, A.J. Bell, Subjective evaluation of right ventricular systolic function in hypoplastic left heart syndrome: how accurate is it? J. Am. Soc. Echocardiogr. 26 (1) (January 2013) 52–56 PubMed PMID: 23098782. Pubmed Central PMCID: 3548410.

[16] J.N. Cohn, R. Ferrari, N. Sharpe, Cardiac remodeling–concepts and clinical implications: a consensus paper from an international forum on cardiac remodeling. Behalf of an International Forum on Cardiac Remodeling, J. Am. Coll. Cardiol. 35 (3) (March 1, 2000) 569–582 PubMed PMID: 10716457.

[17] C.J. McMahon, S.F. Nagueh, R.S. Eapen, W.J. Dreyer, I. Finkelshtyn, X. Cao, et al., Echocardiographic predictors of adverse clinical events in children with dilated cardiomyopathy: a prospective clinical study, Heart (Br. Card. Soc.) 90 (8) (August 2004) 908–915 PubMed PMID: 15253966. eng.

[18] K.M. Molina, P. Shrader, S.D. Colan, S. Mital, R. Margossian, L.A. Sleeper, et al., Predictors of disease progression in pediatric dilated cardiomyopathy, Circ. Heart Fail. 6 (6) (November 2013) 1214–1222 PubMed PMID: 24132734. Epub 2013/10/18. eng.

[19] T.P. Singh, L.A. Sleeper, S. Lipshultz, A. Cinar, C. Canter, S.A. Webber, et al., Association of left ventricular dilation at listing for heart transplant with postlisting and early posttransplant mortality in children with dilated cardiomyopathy, Circ. Heart Fail. 2 (6) (November 2009) 591–598 PubMed PMID: 19919984. Epub 2009/11/19. eng.

[20] J.A. Alvarez, E.J. Orav, J.D. Wilkinson, L.E. Fleming, D.J. Lee, L.A. Sleeper, et al., Competing risks for death and cardiac transplantation in children with dilated cardiomyopathy: results from the pediatric cardiomyopathy registry, Circulation 124 (7) (August 16, 2011) 814–823 PubMed PMID: 21788591. Epub 2011/07/27. eng.

[21] M.D. Everitt, L.A. Sleeper, M. Lu, C.E. Canter, E. Pahl, J.D. Wilkinson, et al., Recovery of echocardiographic function in children with idiopathic dilated cardiomyopathy: results from the pediatric cardiomyopathy registry, J. Am. Coll. Cardiol. 63 (14) (April 15, 2014) 1405–1413 PubMed PMID: 24561146. Pubmed Central PMCID: 4030008.

[22] L. Lopez, S.D. Colan, P.C. Frommelt, G.J. Ensing, K. Kendall, A.K. Younoszai, et al., Recommendations for quantification methods during the performance of a pediatric echocardiogram: a report from the pediatric measurements writing group of the American society of echocardiography pediatric and congenital heart disease council, J. Am. Soc. Echocardiogr. 23 (5) (May 2010) 465–495 PubMed PMID: 20451803. Epub 2010/05/11. eng.

[23] T. Sluysmans, S.D. Colan, Theoretical and empirical derivation of cardiovascular allometric relationships in children, J. Appl. Physiol. 99 (2) (August 2005) 445–457 PubMed PMID: 15557009.

[24] M. Cantinotti, M. Scalese, S. Molinaro, B. Murzi, C. Passino, Limitations of current echocardiographic nomograms for left ventricular, valvular, and arterial dimensions in children: a critical review, J. Am. Soc. Echocardiogr. 25 (2) (February 2012) 142–152 PubMed PMID: 22101087.

[25] W.A. Zoghbi, M. Enriquez-Sarano, E. Foster, P.A. Grayburn, C.D. Kraft, R.A. Levine, et al., Recommendations for evaluation of the severity of native valvular regurgitation with two-dimensional and Doppler echocardiography, J. Am. Soc. Echocardiogr. 16 (7) (July 2003) 777–802 PubMed PMID: 12835667. Epub 2003/07/02. eng.

[26] S. Yuda, V. Khoury, T.H. Marwick, Influence of wall stress and left ventricular geometry on the accuracy of dobutamine stress echocardiography, J. Am. Coll. Cardiol. 40 (7) (October 2, 2002) 1311–1319 PubMed PMID: 12383580.

[27] S.D. Colan, K.M. Borow, A. Neumann, Left ventricular end-systolic wall stress-velocity of fiber shortening relation: a load-independent index of myocardial contractility, J. Am. Coll. Cardiol. 4 (4) (October 1984) 715–724 PubMed PMID: 6207218.

[28] G.G. Sandor, R. Popov, E. De Souza, S. Morris, B. Johnston, Rate-corrected mean velocity of fiber shortening-stress at peak systole as a load-independent measure of contractility, Am. J. Cardiol. 69 (4) (February 1, 1992) 403–407 PubMed PMID: 1734656.

[29] L.Y. Tani, L.L. Minich, R.V. Williams, R.E. Shaddy, Ventricular remodeling in children with left ventricular dysfunction secondary to various cardiomyopathies, Am. J. Cardiol. 96 (8) (October 15, 2005) 1157–1161 PubMed PMID: 16214456.

[30] P.E. Daubeney, A.W. Nugent, P. Chondros, J.B. Carlin, S.D. Colan, M. Cheung, et al., Clinical features and outcomes of childhood dilated cardiomyopathy: results from a national population-based study, Circulation 114 (24) (December 12, 2006) 2671–2678 PubMed PMID: 17116768. eng.

[31] P.S. Saba, M.J. Roman, A. Ganau, R. Pini, E.C. Jones, T.G. Pickering, et al., Relationship of effective arterial elastance to demographic and arterial characteristics in normotensive and hypertensive adults, J. Hypertens. 13 (9) (September 1995) 971–977 PubMed PMID: 8586832.

[32] S.A. Hollander, D. Bernstein, J. Yeh, D. Dao, H.Y. Sun, D. Rosenthal, Outcomes of children following a first hospitalization for dilated cardiomyopathy, Circ. Heart Fail. 5 (4) (July 1, 2012) 437–443 PubMed PMID: 22570362.

[33] D.B. McElhinney, S.D. Colan, A.M. Moran, D. Wypij, M. Lin, J.A. Majzoub, et al., Recombinant human growth hormone treatment for dilated cardiomyopathy in children, Pediatrics 114 (4) (October 2004) e452–e458 PubMed PMID: 15466071.

[34] M.S. Patel, A.M. Berg, R.N. Vincent, W.T. Mahle, Serum parameters and echocardiographic predictors of death or need for transplant in newborns, children, and young adults with heart failure, Am. J. Cardiol. 105 (12) (June 15, 2010) 1798–1801 PubMed PMID: 20538133.

[35] B.H. Bijnens, M. Cikes, P. Claus, G.R. Sutherland, Velocity and deformation imaging for the assessment of myocardial dysfunction, Eur. J. Echocardiogr. 10 (2) (March 2009) 216–226 PubMed PMID: 19098303. Epub 2008/12/23. eng.

[36] S.D. Colan, G. Shirali, R. Margossian, D. Gallagher, K. Altmann, C. Canter, et al., The ventricular volume variability study of the pediatric heart network: study design and impact of beat averaging and variable type on the reproducibility of echocardiographic measurements in children with chronic dilated cardiomyopathy, J. Am. Soc. Echocardiogr. 25 (8) (August 2012) 842–854 e6. PubMed PMID: 22677278. Epub 2012/06/09. eng.

[37] R. Margossian, S. Chen, L.A. Sleeper, L.Y. Tani, G. Shirali, F. Golding, et al., The reproducibility and absolute values of echocardiographic measurements of left ventricular size and function in children are algorithm dependent, J. Am. Soc. Echocardiogr. 28 (5) (May 2015) 549–558 e1. PubMed PMID: 25728351. Pubmed Central PMCID: 4426088.

[38] M.H. Picard, R.L. Popp, A.E. Weyman, Assessment of left ventricular function by echocardiography: a technique in evolution, J. Am. Soc. Echocardiogr. 21 (1) (January 2008) 14–21 PubMed PMID: 18165124.

[39] L. Bu, S. Munns, H. Zhang, M. Disterhoft, M. Dixon, A. Stolpen, et al., Rapid full volume data acquisition by real-time 3-dimensional echocardiography for assessment of left ventricular indexes in children: a validation study compared with magnetic resonance imaging, J. Am. Soc. Echocardiogr. 18 (4) (April 2005) 299–305 PubMed PMID: 15846155.

[40] X. Lu, M. Xie, D. Tomberlin, B. Klas, V. Nadvoretskiy, N. Ayres, et al., How accurately, reproducibly, and efficiently can we measure left ventricular indices using M-mode, 2-dimensional, and 3-dimensional echocardiography in children? Am. Heart J. 155 (5) (May 2008) 946–953 PubMed PMID: 18440346. eng.

[41] T.J. Riehle, W.T. Mahle, W.J. Parks, D. Sallee 3rd, D.A. Fyfe, Real-time three-dimensional echocardiographic acquisition and quantification of left ventricular indices in children and young adults with congenital heart disease: comparison with magnetic resonance imaging, J. Am. Soc. Echocardiogr. 21 (1) (January 2008) 78–83 PubMed PMID: 17628400. eng.

[42] J. Simpson, L. Lopez, P. Acar, M. Friedberg, N. Khoo, H. Ko, et al., Three-dimensional echocardiography in congenital heart disease: an expert consensus document from the European association of cardiovascular imaging and the American society of echocardiography, Eur. Heart J. Cardiovasc. Imaging 17 (10) (October 2016) 1071–1097 PubMed PMID: 27655864.

[43] K. Ylanen, A. Eerola, K. Vettenranta, T. Poutanen, Three-dimensional echocardiography and cardiac magnetic resonance imaging in the screening of long-term survivors of childhood cancer after cardiotoxic therapy, Am. J. Cardiol. 113 (11) (June 1, 2014) 1886–1892 PubMed PMID: 24837269.

[44] R.M. Lang, L.P. Badano, V. Mor-Avi, J. Afilalo, A. Armstrong, L. Ernande, et al., Recommendations for cardiac chamber quantification by echocardiography in adults: an update from the American society of echocardiography and the European association of cardiovascular imaging, J. Am. Soc. Echocardiogr. 28 (1) (January 2015) 1–39 e14. PubMed PMID: 25559473.

[45] K.A. Connelly, D.L. Prior, D.J. Kelly, M.P. Feneley, H. Krum, R.E. Gilbert, Load-sensitive measures may overestimate global systolic function in the presence of left ventricular hypertrophy: a comparison with load-insensitive measures, Am. J. Physiol. Heart Circ. Physiol. 290 (4) (April 2006) H1699–H1705 PubMed PMID: 16272203.

[46] G.P. Aurigemma, K.H. Silver, M.A. Priest, W.H. Gaasch, Geometric changes allow normal ejection fraction despite depressed myocardial shortening in hypertensive left ventricular hypertrophy, J. Am. Coll. Cardiol. 26 (1) (July 1995) 195–202 PubMed PMID: 7797752.

[47] M. Cikes, G.R. Sutherland, L.J. Anderson, B.H. Bijnens, The role of echocardiographic deformation imaging in hypertrophic myopathies, Nat. Rev. Cardiol. 7 (7) (July 2010) 384–396 PubMed PMID: 20458340. Epub 2010/05/12. eng.

[48] J. Ganame, L. Mertens, B.W. Eidem, P. Claus, J. D'Hooge, L.M. Havemann, et al., Regional myocardial deformation in children with hypertrophic cardiomyopathy: morphological and clinical correlations, Eur. Heart J. 28 (23) (December 2007) 2886–2894 PubMed PMID: 17971400. eng.

[49] J.F. Lewis, L.C. Kuo, J.G. Nelson, M.C. Limacher, M.A. Quinones, Pulsed Doppler echocardiographic determination of stroke volume and cardiac output: clinical validation of two new methods using the apical window, Circulation 70 (3) (September 1984) 425–431 PubMed PMID: 6744546.

[50] A.S. Ghafour, H.P. Gutgesell, Echocardiographic evaluation of left ventricular function in children with congestive cardiomyopathy, Am. J. Cardiol. 44 (7) (December 1979) 1332–1338 PubMed PMID: 506936.

[51] D. Golde, L. Burstin, Systolic phases of the cardiac cycle in children, Circulation 42 (6) (December 1970) 1029–1036 PubMed PMID: 5492536. Epub 1970/12/01. eng.

[52] B.S. Lewis, N. Lewis, D. Sapoznikov, M.S. Gotsman, Isovolumic relaxation period in man, Am. Heart J. 100 (4) (October 1980) 490–499 PubMed PMID: 7415937.

[53] S.E. Meiler, H. Boudoulas, D.V. Unverferth, C.V. Leier, Diastolic time in congestive heart failure, Am. Heart J. 114 (5) (November 1987) 1192–1198 PubMed PMID: 3673886.

[54] P.W. O'Leary, K. Durongpisitkul, T.M. Cordes, K.R. Bailey, D.J. Hagler, J. Tajik, et al., Diastolic ventricular function in children: a Doppler echocardiographic study establishing normal values and predictors of increased ventricular end-diastolic pressure, Mayo Clin. Proc. 73 (7) (July 1998) 616–628 PubMed PMID: 9663189.

[55] A. Dragulescu, L. Mertens, M.K. Friedberg, Interpretation of left ventricular diastolic dysfunction in children with cardiomyopathy by echocardiography: problems and limitations, Circ. Cardiovasc. Imaging 6 (2) (March 1, 2013) 254–261 PubMed PMID: 23343514. Epub 2013/01/25. eng.

[56] C. Tei, New non-invasive index for combined systolic and diastolic ventricular function, J. Cardiol. 26 (2) (August 1995) 135–136 PubMed PMID: 7674144. Epub 1995/08/01. eng.

[57] M.K. Friedberg, R. Margossian, M. Lu, L. Mercer-Rosa, H.T. Henderson, A. Nutting, et al., Systolic-diastolic functional coupling in healthy children and in those with dilated cardiomyopathy, J. Appl. Physiol. 120 (11) (June 1, 2016) 1301–1318 PubMed PMID: 26940654. Pubmed Central PMCID: 4891930.

[58] M.K. Friedberg, N.H. Silverman, The systolic to diastolic duration ratio in children with heart failure secondary to restrictive cardiomyopathy, J. Am. Soc. Echocardiogr. 19 (11) (November 2006) 1326–1331 PubMed PMID: 17098134. eng.

[59] M.K. Friedberg, N.H. Silverman, Cardiac ventricular diastolic and systolic duration in children with heart failure secondary to idiopathic dilated cardiomyopathy, Am. J. Cardiol. 97 (1) (January 1, 2006) 101–105 PubMed PMID: 16377292. eng.

[60] C.S. Chung, M. Karamanoglu, S.J. Kovacs, Duration of diastole and its phases as a function of heart rate during supine bicycle exercise, Am. J. Physiol. Heart Circ. Physiol. 287 (5) (November 2004) H2003–H2008 PubMed PMID: 15217800. eng.

[61] T. Mondal, C. Slorach, C. Manlhiot, W. Hui, P.F. Kantor, B.W. McCrindle, et al., Prognostic implications of the systolic to diastolic duration ratio in children with idiopathic or familial dilated cardiomyopathy, Circ. Cardiovasc. Imaging 7 (5) (September 2014) 773–780 PubMed PMID: 25140066.

[62] M.K. Friedberg, A.N. Redington, Right versus left ventricular failure: differences, similarities, and interactions, Circulation 129 (9) (March 4, 2014) 1033–1044 PubMed PMID: 24589696. Epub 2014/03/05. eng.

[63] D.A. Burkett, C. Slorach, S.S. Patel, A.N. Redington, D.D. Ivy, L. Mertens, et al., Impact of pulmonary hemodynamics and ventricular interdependence on left ventricular diastolic function in children with pulmonary hypertension, Circ. Cardiovasc. Imaging 9 (9) (September 2016) PubMed PMID: 27581953. Pubmed Central PMCID: 5012318.

[64] J. Alkon, T. Humpl, C. Manlhiot, B.W. McCrindle, J.T. Reyes, M.K. Friedberg, Usefulness of the right ventricular systolic to diastolic duration ratio to predict functional capacity and survival in children with pulmonary arterial hypertension, Am. J. Cardiol. 106 (3) (August 1, 2010) 430–436 PubMed PMID: 20643259. Epub 2010/07/21. eng.

[65] B.W. Eidem, C.J. McMahon, R.R. Cohen, J. Wu, I. Finkelshteyn, J.P. Kovalchin, et al., Impact of cardiac growth on Doppler tissue imaging velocities: a study in healthy children, J. Am. Soc. Echocardiogr. 17 (3) (March 2004) 212–221 PubMed PMID: 14981417. eng.

[66] D.A. Roberson, W. Cui, Z. Chen, L.F. Madronero, B.F. Cuneo, Annular and septal Doppler tissue imaging in children: normal z-score tables and effects of age, heart rate, and body surface area, J. Am. Soc. Echocardiogr. 20 (11) (November 2007) 1276–1284 PubMed PMID: 17596911. eng.

[67] M.K. Friedberg, L. Mertens, Tissue velocities, strain, and strain rate for echocardiographic assessment of ventricular function in congenital heart disease, Eur. J. Echocardiogr. 10 (5) (July 2009) 585–593 PubMed PMID: 19401299. Epub 2009/04/30. eng.

[68] C.J. McMahon, S.F. Nagueh, R.H. Pignatelli, S.W. Denfield, W.J. Dreyer, J.F. Price, et al., Characterization of left ventricular diastolic function by tissue Doppler imaging and clinical status in children with hypertrophic cardiomyopathy, Circulation 109 (14) (April 13, 2004) 1756–1762 PubMed PMID: 15023880. eng.

[69] C.J. McMahon, R.H. Pignatelli, S.F. Nagueh, V.V. Lee, W. Vaughn, S.O. Valdes, et al., Left ventricular non-compaction cardiomyopathy in children: characterisation of clinical status using tissue Doppler-derived indices of left ventricular diastolic relaxation, Heart (Br. Card. Soc.) 93 (6) (June 2007) 676–681 PubMed PMID: 17135224. Epub 2006/12/01. eng.

[70] D.A. Fyfe, D. Ketchum, R. Lewis, J. Sabatier, K. Kanter, W. Mahle, et al., Tissue Doppler imaging detects severely abnormal myocardial velocities that identify children with pre-terminal cardiac graft failure after heart transplantation, J. Heart Lung Transplant. 25 (5) (May 2006) 510–517 PubMed PMID: 16678028. Epub 2006/05/09. eng.

[71] A. Gulati, T.F. Ismail, A. Jabbour, F. Alpendurada, K. Guha, N.A. Ismail, et al., The prevalence and prognostic significance of right ventricular systolic dysfunction in nonischemic dilated cardiomyopathy, Circulation 128 (15) (October 8, 2013) 1623–1633 PubMed PMID: 23965488.

[72] C. Venner, C. Selton-Suty, O. Huttin, M.L. Erpelding, E. Aliot, Y. Juilliere, Right ventricular dysfunction in patients with idiopathic dilated cardiomyopathy: prognostic value and predictive factors, Arch. Cardiovasc. Dis. 109 (4) (April 2016) 231–241 PubMed PMID: 26782624.
[73] J. Forsey, M.K. Friedberg, L. Mertens, Speckle tracking echocardiography in pediatric and congenital heart disease, Echocardiography (Mt. Kisco N.Y.) 30 (4) (April 2013) 447–459 PubMed PMID: 23551605. Epub 2013/04/05. eng.
[74] D. Forsha, C. Slorach, C.K. Chen, A. Sherman, L. Mertens, P. Barker, et al., Patterns of mechanical inefficiency in pediatric dilated cardiomyopathy and their relation to left ventricular function and clinical outcomes, J. Am. Soc. Echocardiogr. 29 (3) (March 2016) 226–236 PubMed PMID: 26711366.
[75] M. Friedberg, S.L. Roche, A.F. Mohammed, M. Balasingam, E.G. Atenafu, P.F. Kantor, Left ventricular diastolic mechanical dyssynchrony and associated clinical outcomes in children with dilated cardiomyopathy, Circ. Cardiovasc. Imaging 1 (2008) 50–57.
[76] M.K. Friedberg, S.L. Roche, M. Balasingam, E. Stephenson, C. Slorach, C. Fackoury, et al., Evaluation of mechanical dyssynchrony in children with idiopathic dilated cardiomyopathy and associated clinical outcomes, Am. J. Cardiol. 101 (8) (April 15, 2008) 1191–1195 PubMed PMID: 18394457. eng.
[77] T. Bharucha, R. Khan, L. Mertens, M.K. Friedberg, Right ventricular mechanical dyssynchrony and asymmetric contraction in hypoplastic heart syndrome are associated with tricuspid regurgitation, J. Am. Soc. Echocardiogr. 26 (10) (October 2013) 1214–1220 PubMed PMID: 23876994.
[78] M.K. Friedberg, N.H. Silverman, A.M. Dubin, D.N. Rosenthal, Right ventricular mechanical dyssynchrony in children with hypoplastic left heart syndrome, J. Am. Soc. Echocardiogr. 20 (9) (June 11, 2007) 1073–1079 PubMed PMID: 17566698. eng.
[79] N.S. Khoo, J.F. Smallhorn, S. Kaneko, K. Myers, S. Kutty, E.B. Tham, Novel insights into RV adaptation and function in hypoplastic left heart syndrome between the first 2 stages of surgical palliation, JACC Cardiovasc. Imaging 4 (2) (February 2011) 128–137 PubMed PMID: 21329896. Epub 2011/02/19. eng.
[80] N.H. Kuijpers, E. Hermeling, J. Lumens, H.M. ten Eikelder, T. Delhaas, F.W. Prinzen, Mechano-electrical coupling as framework for understanding functional remodeling during LBBB and CRT, Am. J. Physiol. Heart Circ. Physiol. 306 (12) (June 15, 2014) H1644–H1659 PubMed PMID: 24748591.
[81] J. Lumens, B. Tayal, J. Walmsley, A. Delgado-Montero, P.R. Huntjens, D. Schwartzman, et al., Differentiating electromechanical from non-electrical substrates of mechanical discoordination to identify responders to cardiac resynchronization therapy, Circ. Cardiovasc. Imaging 8 (9) (September 2015) e003744 PubMed PMID: 26338877.
[82] C. Parsai, B. Bijnens, G.R. Sutherland, A. Baltabaeva, P. Claus, M. Marciniak, et al., Toward understanding response to cardiac resynchronization therapy: left ventricular dyssynchrony is only one of multiple mechanisms, Eur. Heart J. 30 (8) (November 11, 2009) 940–949 PubMed PMID: 19004844. eng.
[83] M.K. Friedberg, Echocardiography for assessment of mechanical dyssynchrony in children: the search must go on, J. Am. Soc. Echocardiogr. 26 (2) (February 2013) 160–164 PubMed PMID: 23352085.
[84] J. Gorcsan 3rd, T. Abraham, D.A. Agler, J.J. Bax, G. Derumeaux, R.A. Grimm, et al., Echocardiography for cardiac resynchronization therapy: recommendations for performance and reporting–a report from the American society of echocardiography dyssynchrony writing group endorsed by the heart rhythm society, J. Am. Soc. Echocardiogr. 21 (3) (March 2008) 191–213 PubMed PMID: 18314047. eng.
[85] K.H. Haugaa, B.L. Grenne, C.H. Eek, M. Ersboll, N. Valeur, J.H. Svendsen, et al., Strain echocardiography improves risk prediction of ventricular arrhythmias after myocardial infarction, JACC Cardiovasc. Imaging 6 (8) (August 2013) 841–850 PubMed PMID: 23850251.
[86] S.I. Sarvari, K.H. Haugaa, O.G. Anfinsen, T.P. Leren, O.A. Smiseth, E. Kongsgaard, et al., Right ventricular mechanical dispersion is related to malignant arrhythmias: a study of patients with arrhythmogenic right ventricular cardiomyopathy and subclinical right ventricular dysfunction, Eur. Heart J. 32 (9) (May 2011) 1089–1096 PubMed PMID: 21406439.
[87] E.S. Chung, A.R. Leon, L. Tavazzi, J.P. Sun, P. Nihoyannopoulos, J. Merlino, et al., Results of the predictors of response to CRT (PROSPECT) trial, Circulation 117 (20) (May 20, 2008) 2608–2616 PubMed PMID: 18458170. eng.
[88] D. Forsha, C. Slorach, C.K. Chen, E.A. Stephenson, N. Risum, C. Hornik, et al., Classic-pattern dyssynchrony and electrical activation delays in pediatric dilated cardiomyopathy, J. Am. Soc. Echocardiogr. 27 (9) (September 2014) 956–964 PubMed PMID: 25063467.
[89] S.F. Nagueh, O.A. Smiseth, C.P. Appleton, B.F. Byrd 3rd, H. Dokainish, T. Edvardsen, et al., Recommendations for the evaluation of left ventricular diastolic function by echocardiography: an update from the American society of echocardiography and the European association of cardiovascular imaging, J. Am. Soc. Echocardiogr. 29 (4) (April 2016) 277–314 PubMed PMID: 27037982.
[90] P.C. Frommelt, Echocardiographic measures of diastolic function in pediatric heart disease, Curr. Opin. Cardiol. 21 (3) (May 2006) 194–199 PubMed PMID: 16601456.
[91] A. Groner, J. Yau, I.D. Lytrivi, H.H. Ko, J.C. Nielsen, I.A. Parness, et al., The role of right ventricular function in paediatric idiopathic dilated cardiomyopathy, Cardiol. Young 23 (3) (June 2013) 409–415 PubMed PMID: 22914442.
[92] L. Grosse-Wortmann, S.L. Roche, S.J. Yoo, M. Seed, P. Kantor, Early changes in right ventricular function and their clinical consequences in childhood and adolescent dilated cardiomyopathy, Cardiol. Young 20 (4) (August 2010) 418–425 PubMed PMID: 20420745.
[93] L.L. Mertens, M.K. Friedberg, Imaging the right ventricle–current state of the art, Nat. Rev. Cardiol. 7 (10) (October 2010) 551–563 PubMed PMID: 20697412. Epub 2010/08/11. eng.

Chapter 10

MRI Assessment of Heart Failure

Michael Taylor
Cincinnati Children's Medical Center, Cincinnati, OH, United States

CARDIAC MAGNETIC RESONANCE

Over the past two decades, cardiovascular magnetic resonance (CMR) has become a standard for anatomical and functional evaluation for pediatric cardiomyopathy. CMR is not used as the initial imaging modality. Echocardiography is the primary modality used for initial evaluation. As an addition to echocardiography, CMR provides excellent quantitative volumetry and functional assessment and unique myocardial characterization information. Advances in CMR provide the potential to identify potentially treatable conditions, risk stratifying patients, and monitoring therapy in a single setting and complementing other noninvasive tests. In a single study, CMR provides cardiac anatomy, function, tissue characterization, and coronary and microvascular perfusion data without ionizing radiation. There is little substantive difference in the cardiac MR protocols used for adult and pediatric cardiomyopathy evaluation. However, there are certain age-dependent technical considerations for pediatric evaluations. These include the need for sedation or nonbreath-hold studies, better spatial resolution to account for the relatively smaller myocardium, and sequence modifications to account for relative increases in heart rate.

Pediatric Examinations

As with other medical procedures, the parents should be provided with a description of the CMR study. They should be encouraged to discuss it with their child in an age-appropriate manner. Before bringing the patient into the MRI room, the patient's history and safety screening form is reviewed for implanted devices known to be hazardous in the CMR environment. All patients who have undergone procedures and have elements of the medical history that are not well documented should have a chest radiograph prior to undergoing CMR. After screening the physiological monitoring devices and hearing protection are placed. Care should be taken to account for the relatively increased heat dissipation of smaller children. A high-fidelity electrocardiogram (ECG) signal is essential for data acquisition in cardiac-gated sequences required by CMR. The ECG should be evaluated before placing the patient in the magnet bore and again after moving the patient into the bore. The imaging receiver coil is chosen to maximize the signal-to-noise (SNR) ratio over the heart. In small pediatric patients, specialized coils may be preferable. As is standard, appropriate coil coverage should be confirmed after obtaining the initial localizer images.

Sedation

Patients undergoing CMR are required to not move and follow directions for up to 60 min to minimize motion artifact. Young children (typically less than 7 years old) and cognitively impaired older patients typically require some form of sedation. There are multiple factors to consider when deciding whether a patient requires sedation. These include the anticipated examination length, developmental state, the patient's experience with prior procedures, the sedation risks, and the possible benefits of the CMR information.

Strategies for sedation and anesthesia during CMR vary and often depend on institutional preference and availability of resources such as pediatric anesthesiologists with experience in CHD. Exams of very young infants can be attempted with tight bundling while sleeping immediately after a feeding [**1,2]. This technique does not allow for breath holding and is susceptible to motion artifacts. Deep sedation can be used as an alternative. The patients are allowed to spontaneously breath. This is done under the supervision of a sedation team including anesthesiology or ICU physicians. Although most of these studies are performed without an artificial airway, a laryngeal mask airway may be used if the aspiration risk is though to be high. Again, these patients will not suspend respiration during image acquisition. The images have slightly increased respiratory motion artifacts but are typically of diagnostic quality. Also, since the respiratory motion is very regular, compensating for the motion by triggering acquisition to the diaphragm or the chest wall is straightforward and

Heart Failure in the Child and Young Adult. http://dx.doi.org/10.1016/B978-0-12-802393-8.00010-7

available on all CMR platforms. For either safety or image quality requirements, some patients require general anesthesia with endotracheal intubation and mechanical ventilation. If the patients are administered neuromuscular paralytics, the respiratory motion can be eliminated by acquisition during suspended ventilation. Deep sedation and general anesthesia are both safe in young patients (Fig. 10.3) [**3–8].

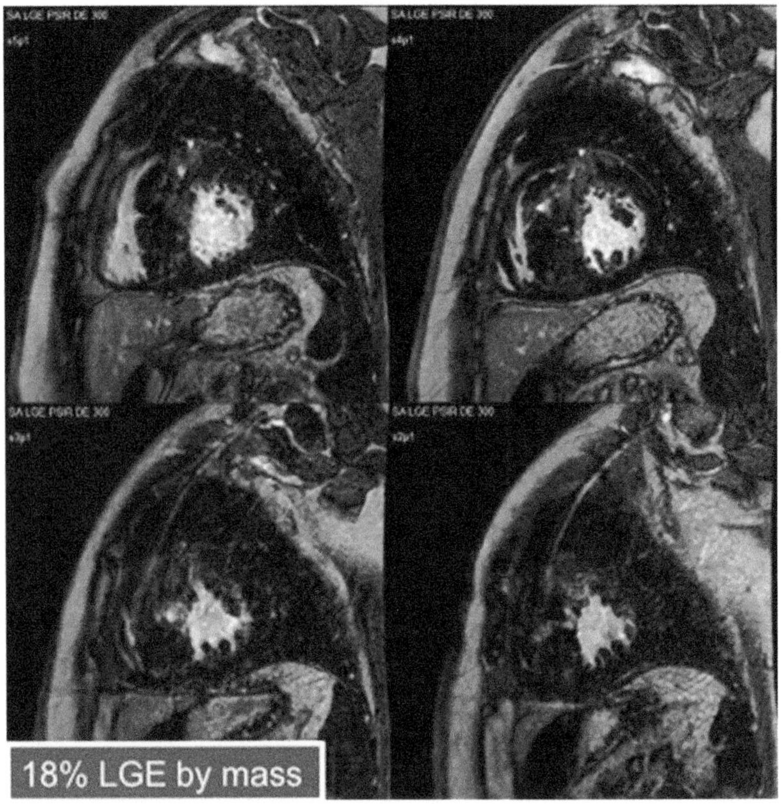

FIGURE 10.1 Late gadolinium enhancement of hypertrophic cardiomyopathy.

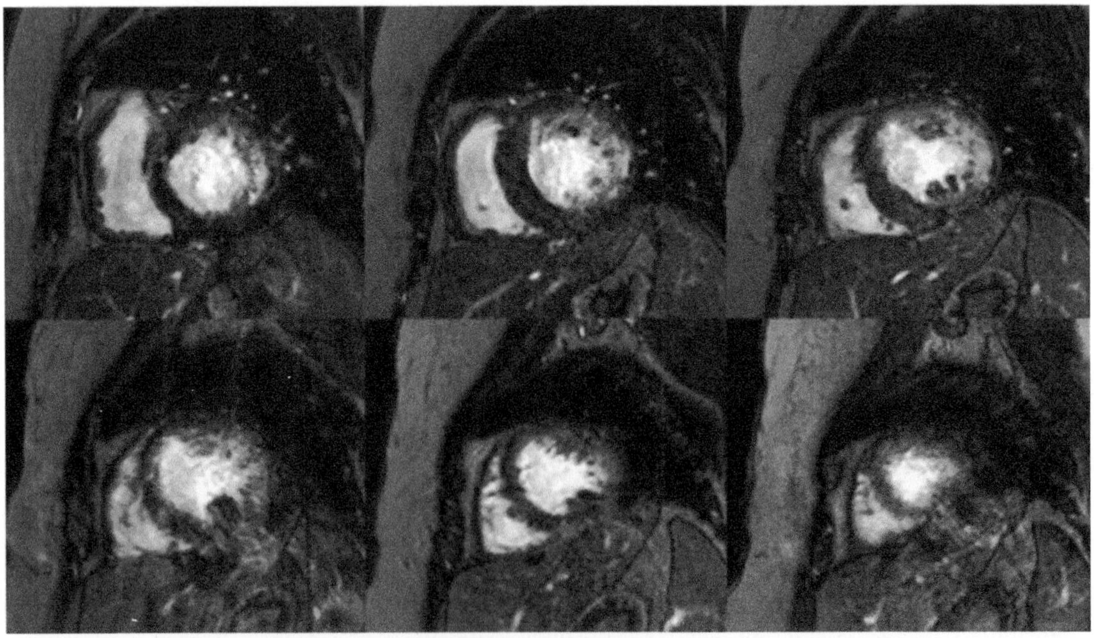

FIGURE 10.2 Short-axis late gadolinium enhancement image of Anderson-Fabry disease.

Scanner Field Strength

Clinical MRI systems are most often either 1.5 or 3 T in strength. Pediatric CMR can be accomplished in either system. The 3T systems provide higher SNR ratio, allowing for better spatial resolution. The imaging that benefits the most from this increased SNR includes coronary angiography, myocardial tagging, myocardial perfusion, and late gadolinium enhancement (LGE) imaging. However, the MR imaging at 3 T has significantly more artifacts. Also, at 3 T implanted metal devices encountered in CHD patients referred for CMR cause increased artifacts [**9]. The device-related signal loss artifact from T2* effects is more pronounced at higher field strengths. Also, CMR compatibility information for devices is more commonly available at the 1.5 T than the 3 T field strength.

CARDIOVASCULAR MAGNETIC RESONANCE TECHNIQUES

Imaging of pediatric heart failure utilizes range of sequences acquired according to dedicated protocols tuned to the particular clinical scenario [10–13]. The sequences are detailed below. The following section describes specific clinical scenarios and how these sequences might be used in a particular situation.

Anatomic Imaging

An overview of the thoracic anatomy can be done with either black blood or bright-blood sequences. The black-blood images are acquired with spin-echo pulse sequences in which flowing blood appears dark and stationary tissues appear as varying shades of gray or white. The variants of this technique are termed fast or turbo-spin echo and single-shot fast turbo-spin echo. Both versions use ECG triggering to compensate for cardiac motion. Respiratory motion can be addressed by breath holding, acquiring multiple signal averages, triggering from respiratory bellows, or respiratory-navigator gating. The fast spin-echo technique collects data for one image over multiple heartbeats and thus takes longer than the single-shot technique, but it produces higher resolution images. Black-blood images can be acquired in the transaxial, coronal, and sagittal planes for complete delineation of the anatomy.

Alternatively, bright blood images using a gradient echo sequence, typically steady-state free precession (SSFP) can be acquired in the three planes. These images are acquired using the ECG triggering during short (<12 s) breath-holds.

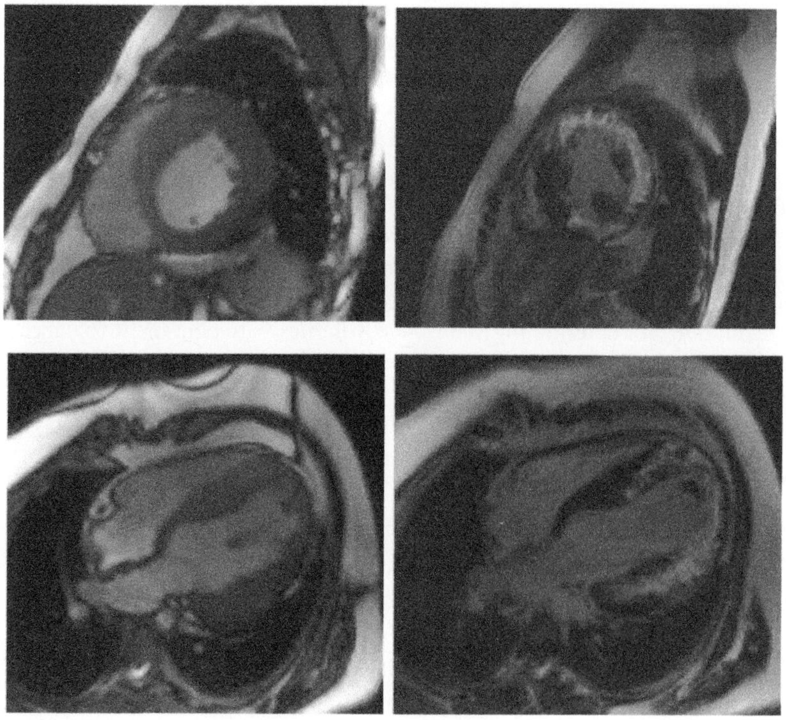

FIGURE 10.3 Cardiovascular magnetic resonance of patient with Danon disease.

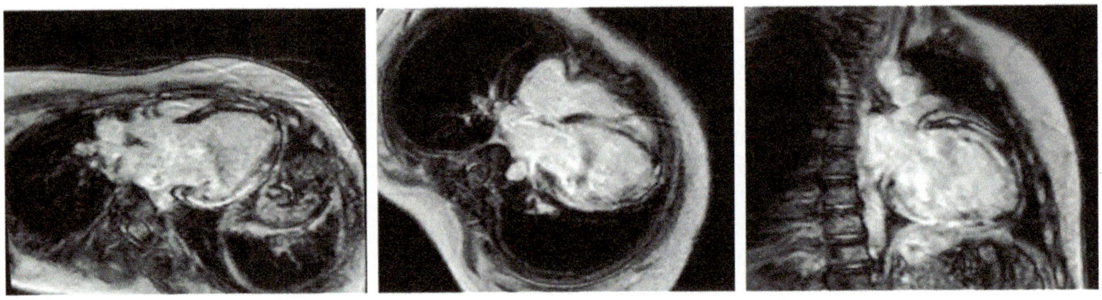

FIGURE 10.4 Three long-axis Late gadolinium enhancement images of DMD patient with extensive fi.

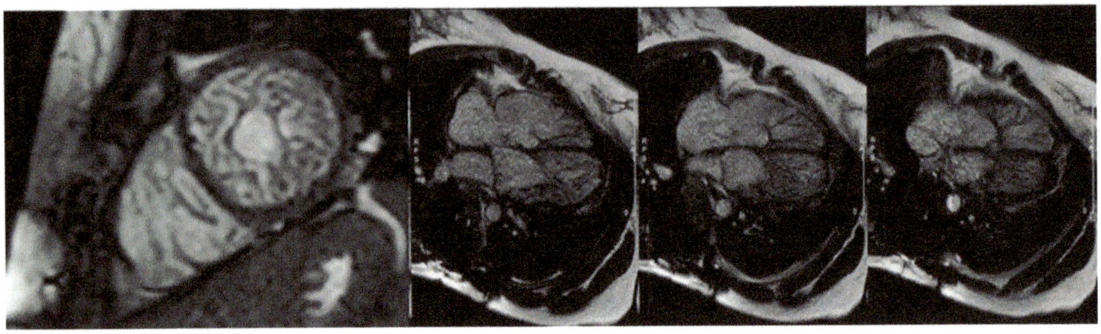

FIGURE 10.5 Steady-state free precession images of left ventricle noncompaction.

Functional Cine Imaging

The workhorse sequences for functional imaging are breath-hold SSFP sequences. These fast gradient echo sequences generate images in which flowing blood appears bright. With the use of ECG-gating, it produces multiple images across the cardiac cycle with excellent spatial and temporal spatial resolution. Respiratory motion is compensated by breath holding (preferred when possible) or by acquiring multiple signal averages during quiet respiration. SSFP images are acquired in specific orientations relative to the heart anatomy of interest to yield a stack of contiguous cross-sectional slices that can be displayed in a multilocation, multiphase format. Gradient echo cine imaging can be performed using a standard spoiled gradient echo pulse sequence or the faster SSFP sequence. SSFP imaging is faster and yields better contrast between endocardium and blood pool. The SSFP sequence is relatively less sensitive to flow disturbances by stenotic or regurgitant jets. Conversely, it is also more prone to artifacts caused by motion or implanted devices. Thus, the standard gradient echo technique may be preferred for visualization of flow jets or imaging near implanted devices such as stents and mechanical valves. The spatial resolution requirements of pediatric imaging require a careful balance of signal, voxel size, contrast, and temporal resolution. A detailed discussion of the parameter trade-offs is beyond the scope of this chapter.

Cine SSFP imaging is the gold standard for accurate and reproducible quantification of left and right ventricular volumes, ejection fractions, and ventricular mass. These values are obtained through manual or semiautomated planimetry using widely available software [**14]. The availability of reference values for wide age ranges normalized to body surface area allows for objective evaluation [**15]. The techniques for determining ventricular volumes with cine CMR (balanced SSFP or gradient echo sequences) have been standardized for both adults and children [***10–12], and reasonable sets of normal values for children are available in the literature [***1,13–15].

Noncontrast Myocardial Characterization

Special sequences allow myocardial tissue characterization without the need for contrast agents. These include both sequences that generate images with gray values representing different tissue states and so-called parametric images with pixel values representing different modes of proton relaxation.

T2- and T1-Weighted Images

The T2-weighted sequence called short-tau inversion recovery (STIR) is a sequence that suppresses signal from flowing blood and from fat that is sensitive to edema in the myocardium. The relatively long T2 relaxation times of water-bound

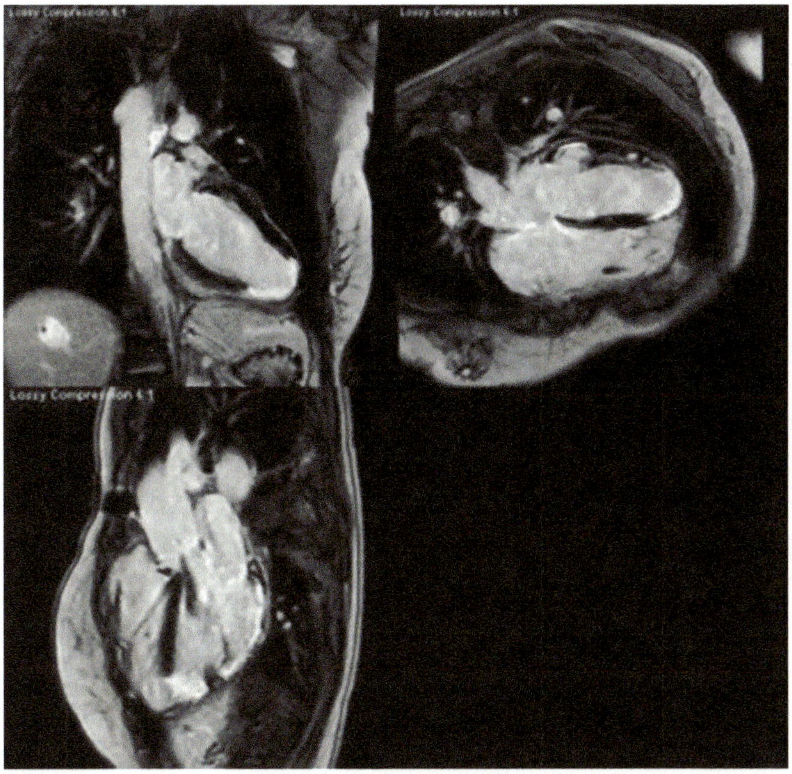

FIGURE 10.6 Apical ischemia in tetralogy of Fallot patient repaired as.

protons are used to generate a water-specific contrast resulting in high signal intensity of tissue with increased water content. Consequently, STIR imaging can detect both acute myocyte swelling and interstitial fluid accumulation. The sequence was initially used in the evaluation of acute ischemia but has found extensive use in nonischemic cardiomyopathy, myocarditis, and transplant rejection [16,17]. The sequence is plagued by low SNR ratio, surface coil intensity variation, interfering bright signal from slow flowing blood, motion artifacts, and nonquantitative interpretation. A similar sequence, but without the extra fat-suppression pulse using T1-weighted and turbo-spin echo is useful to assess the pericardium and to look for fat infiltration (Fig. 10.6).

T1 Parametric Imaging—Noncontrast

It is now possible to obtain images that represent the longitudinal or spin-lattice relaxation of the myocardium. The T1 map can be obtained in a single breath hold with the modified look-locker inversion recovery sequence or its variants. It has been shown that T1 mapping without contrast agent can provide information on diffuse fibrosis [17]. Native T1 values can discriminate between normal and diffuse fibrosis in nonischemic dilated and hypertrophic cardiomyopathy (HCM) [18]. T1 imaging without contrast is termed native T1. Avoiding contrast has benefit in pediatrics with the new concerns about amygdala deposits after repeated administration of gadolinium-based MR contrast agents (GBCAs). The primary limitation is that changes in T1 in affected myocardium can be very small.

T2 Parametric Imaging

The T2 time constant is a measure of spin–spin relaxation. It is lengthened in areas of edema. T2 mapping has been shown to correlate with the region of acute ischemic injury. Also in patients the T2 relaxation time provides an effective parameter to detect myocardial edema in the case of acute myocardial infarction [19]. It has also been shown to be abnormal in acute myocarditis [16,18].

T2 Parametric Images*

The T2* time constant characterizes the rapid relaxation of the proton transverse magnetization as a result of static magnetic field inhomogeneities [13]. Therefore, T2* mapping enables the measurement of macro- and mesoscopic magnetic field inhomogeneities. The macroscopic inhomogeneities are caused by inhomogeneity of the primary magnetic field.

The mesoscopic field inhomogeneities, however, are induced by local biological structure and ferromagnetic ion concentrations. The primary use of T2* mapping cardiac MR is for assessment of myocardial iron deposition. T2* mapping can provide accurate measurement of myocardial iron concentration in iron overload syndromes including thalassemia and hemochromatosis [16]. It is an effective and quantitative method for evaluating chelation therapy.

T1 Rho Parametric Images

T1 ρ is a less well-known magnetic relaxation parameter. It is commonly applied to study the musculoskeletal system. T1 ρ describes relaxation in the transverse plane. In standard T1 ρ relaxation, energy is exchanged from spins to the surrounding environment near the resonant frequency. However, in T1 relaxation, the interaction between water and other molecules are at a different frequency. Fortuitously, macromolecules are in the order of the correct frequency, so T1 ρ relaxation is sensitive to water—macromolecule interactions and indirectly to fibrosis burden in of the myocardium [18].

Gadolinium Contrast Agents

GBCA are commonly administered in patients for angiography, coronary evaluation, assessment of myocardial perfusion and viability. In pediatrics, the agents are often used "off-label" as several of them are not approved by the US Food and Drug Administration or the European Medicines Agency, for pediatric-age patients. The incidence of GBCA-related adverse events in both adults and children is very low. The severe, life-threatening anaphylactoid or nonallergic anaphylactic reactions are rare (0.001%–0.01%). There is no evidence indicating acute nephrotoxicity at approved dosages. However, GBCA administration to patients with acute renal failure or severe chronic kidney disease is associated with the development of nephrogenic systemic fibrosis (NSF), a rare and serious condition that involves fibrosis of primarily the skin and subcutaneous tissue Patients with a glomerular filtration rate $<30\,mL/min/1.73\,m^2$ are considered at highest risk. Thus, all patients who are candidates for GBCA administration should be screened for renal dysfunction. There are only a small number of reported cases of NSF in children, the youngest of which was 8 years of age and all had significant renal dysfunction [17]. No NSF cases have been reported in preterm or term neonates despite their immature kidney function.

Late Gadolinium Enhancement

Myocardial LGE detects focal regions increased volume of distribution in myocardial regions with fibrosis and increased extracellular volume (ECV). These appear brighter than normal myocardium on LGE images. Areas of LGE are correlated with the distribution of histological myocardial fibrosis in both animal models and in humans. It has utility in both acute and chronic ischemic heart disease, nonischemic cardiomyopathies, myocarditis, and tumors.

LGE imaging is performed 6–20 min following injection of 0.1–0.2 mmol/kg of a GBCA. For LGE imaging, an ECG-gated 2D segmented inversion recovery gradient echo pulse sequence is used with data acquisition timed to coincide with diastasis. Breath-hold imaging is preferred respiratory-navigator gating or single-shot imaging can be used. Imaging planes

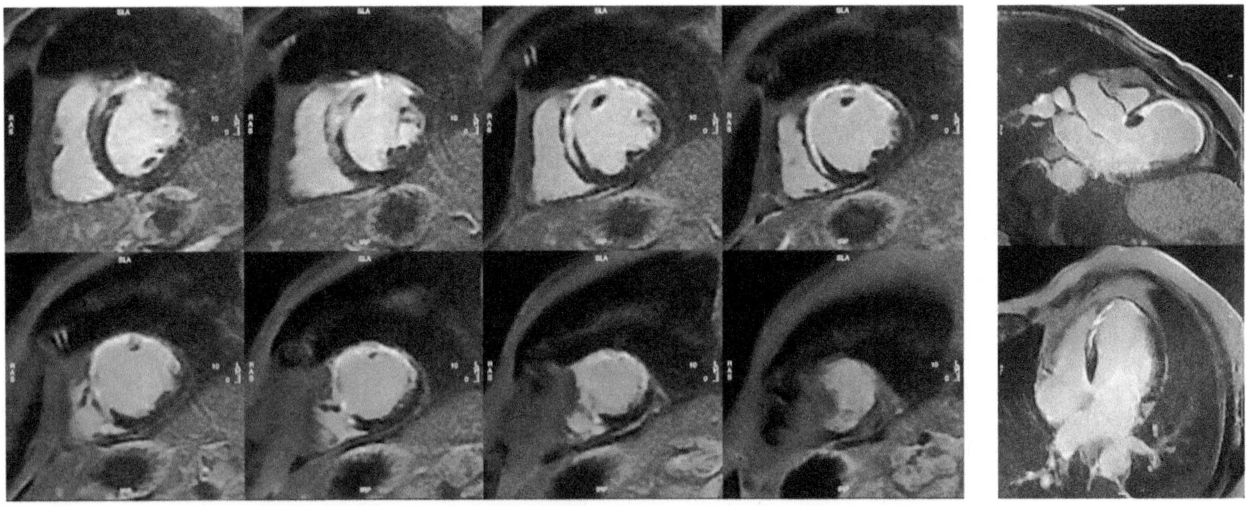

FIGURE 10.7 Coronary occlusion in an SLE patient with diffuse systemic.

are matched with the cine imaging planes for comparison. A typical examination would include LGE imaging in short-axis and multiple long-axis imaging planes. The imaging sequence is based on using an inversion pulse to enhance contrast between myocardium and the blood pool. The time between the inversion pulse and image acquisition, known as the inversion time (TI), should be set to make normal myocardium black. Performing LGE in pediatrics requires modifications for the smaller myocardium and faster heart rates. The voxel size should be 1.0–1.5 mm in-plane with a thickness of <5 mm. At higher heart rates (>100 bpm), the interval between data acquisition should be increased from every second cardiac cycle to every third or fourth cycle. In addition, the data acquisition (shot) duration should be decreased to minimize blurring from faster cardiac motion. Selection of the TI is important for producing high quality LGE images, maximizing the differences between normal and abnormal myocardium. If the TI is too short, the image intensity of normal myocardium will be increased and that of abnormal myocardium decreased. If the TI is set too long, the relative contrast between normal and abnormal myocardium will be reduced and sensitivity diminished. Selection of the appropriate TI is crucial for producing valid LGE images and maximizing the image intensity difference between normal and infarcted/fibrotic myocardium. If the TI is too short, the image intensity of normal myocardium will be increased and that of abnormal myocardium decreased (or even nulled) leading to gross misinterpretation. If the TI is set too long, the relative contrast between normal and abnormal myocardium will be reduced and sensitivity diminished (Figs. 10.4 and 10.8).

T1 Parametric Mapping and Extracellular Volume Fraction Imaging—Postcontrast

Similar to the LGE technique, a T1 parametric relaxation image acquired after gadolinium shows differences in focal Gd volume of distribution. However, the parametric map is proportional to the T1 relaxation time per voxel. By directly estimating pixel by pixel T1 time constants, it is possible to detect diffuse myocardial fibrosis. Combing the pre- and postcontrast T1 of myocardium and blood and adjusting for the hematocrit, the ECV can be calculated according to the formula

$$ECV = (1 - HCT) \times \frac{R_{myo}^{post} - R_{myo}^{pre}}{R_{bld}^{post} - R_{bld}^{pre}} \tag{1}$$

Using contrast-enhanced T1 mapping allows noninvasive quantification of diffuse myocardial fibrosis by the calculation of an ECV map [10]. Although the application of contrast-enhanced myocardial T1 mapping and ECV mapping is a valuable tool to study fibrosis, it needs to be validated in further clinical studies. There are significant limitations to its widespread application. Calculation of an ECV map requires the acquisition of two different parametric T1 maps, one before and one 15–20 min after contrast injection and motion correction between the two acquisitions can be challenging. The technique also requires measurement of the hematocrit.

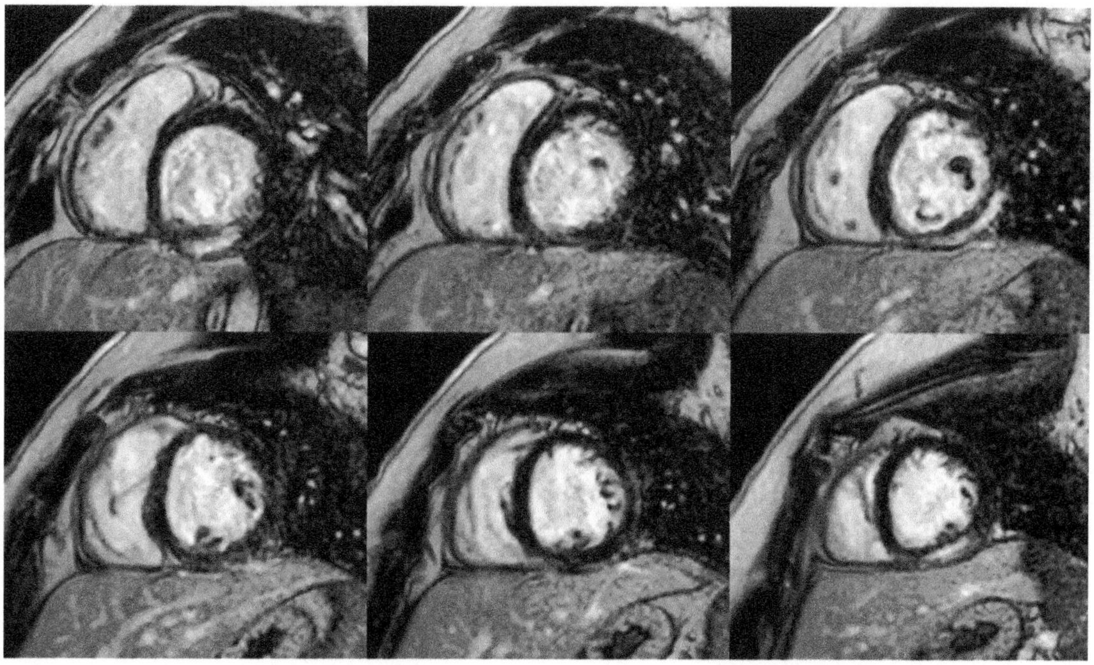

FIGURE 10.8 Teenager with myocaridits. Late gadolinium enhancement images show inferolateral an.

SPECIFIC DISEASE ENTITIES

Myocarditis

Cardiac magnetic resonance is now the standard noninvasive modality for initial diagnosis and longitudinal follow-up of both adult and pediatric myocarditis [19]. Cardiac MR is able to differentiate myocarditis from dilated cardiomyopathy (DCM) with good specificity. CMR can image three different features of myocarditis in pediatrics. First, using black-blood T2-weighted images, the extent of edema can be delineated. Using standard T2 sequences, the myocardial images can be normalized to the skeletal muscle as a measure of the myocardial specific edema. Using T2 parametric images may provide a more accurate measure of edema using a cut-off value of 59?? ms [14]. Second, the hyperemia that results from localized tissue inflammation can be measured by administering the partially extractable Gd contrast agent. Again, the relative myocardial uptake compared with skeletal muscle gives a quantitative measure of myocardial hyperemia. Finally, LGE imaging shows area of myocardial necrosis, extracellular space expansion that can be present in severe myocarditis [17]. The pattern of LGE is typically epicardial or midmyocardial partial thickness in the inferolateral or anterolateral segments of the left ventricular (LV); however, any segments can be affected. CMR with LGE can also be used to monitor recovery from myocarditis. It has been noted that persistence of LGE, likely representing replacement fibrosis, is a poor prognostic sign [4]. Putting the three parameters together according to the Lake Louise criteria gives sensitivity and specificity values that can be used clinically [18]. Moving from these criteria to quantitative myocardial characterization may be particularly useful. Using T1 mapping provides incremental benefit in myocarditis. This includes both precontrast and postcontrast imaging as well as calculation of the ECV parameter.

The most challenging situation is differentiation of myocarditis from idiopathic DCM. Myocardial edema as seen on T2-weighted images may be suggestive of myocarditis. The diagnosis of myocarditis is also suggested by typical subepicardial LGE versus the thin areas of midmyocardial enhancement seen on idiopathic DCM. However, there is significant overlap between the two phenotypes as seen by CMR.

Each CMR technique might require specific modifications to adjust for small body size and high heart rate in young children or even infants. While cine imaging usually yields good image quality with free breathing (using two or three averages), black-blood techniques, such as STIR, are very sensitive to breathing artifacts and might better be replaced by T2-prepared gradient echo techniques.

Neuromuscular Disease

The first report of cardiac MR in neuromuscular disease associated cardiomyopathy was in 2007 [5]. They reported on 10 patients with a mix of Duchenne and Becker muscular dystrophy. 7 of the 10 patients were positive for LGE, all in a nonischemic pattern. Cardiac MR is now the preferred modality for longitudinal monitoring of neuromuscular patients [1,2,7,11,12]. First, cardiac MR allows accurate ventricular function assessment in neuromuscular patients throughout their disease course. As these patients age, they become increasingly difficult to image by echocardiography secondary to skeletal muscle degeneration. Second, cardiac MR yields myocardial characterization information not available by echocardiography. It was shown by Tandon et al. that the appearance of new LGE in these patients portends the development of decreased cardiac function [20]. Third, MR allows assessment of skeletal muscle involvement in a single setting. Imaging biomarker endpoints are now endorsed as valid endpoints for neuromuscular clinical trials.

Hypertrophic Cardiomyopathy

HCM is characterized by asymmetric increased LV hypertrophy with a normal or small ventricular chamber without systemic cause of hypertrophy. The pathophysiology of HCM may include LV outflow tract obstruction, diastolic dysfunction, mitral regurgitation, myocardial ischemia, and arrhythmias. CMR is increasingly used in the diagnosis and prognosis stratification of HCM. The primary objective of the CMR exam for a patient with suspected HCM is to characterize the right and LV myocardium. CMR can define with great detail the pattern of LV hypertrophy, assess the LVOT and mitral valve apparatus, and define extent of LGE. CMR has been used to suggest which patients may have a higher likelihood of malignant ventricular dysrhythmias. There is excellent evidence the LGE by CMR confers excessive risk of arrhythmia in these patients (Fig. 10.1) [21].

Dilated Cardiomyopathy

CMRI is used extensively in DCM. CMR can differentiate between ischemic and nonischemic etiologies; determine ventricular size, function, and mass; detect intracardiac thrombus; and assess for LGE as a marker of fibrosis and for prognostic stratification. Children with nonischemic DCM may have a noncoronary pattern of LGE with patchy or longitudinal midwall enhancement, subepicardial, or diffuse subendocardial distribution. CMR studies on pediatric DCM have focused on the early detection of myocardial involvement in children at high risk for developing ventricular dysfunction, such as pediatric cancer survivors exposed to anthracyclines and radiation. Reduced global circumferential strain can be seen in pediatric cancer survivors. In addition, T1 Mapping and ECV were found to possibly represent diffuse fibrosis in pediatric cancer survivors with normal LV ejection fraction. As mentioned earlier, the primary benefit of CMR in DCM may be in its ability to distinguish inflammatory causes of DCM, i.e., myocarditis, from other chronic conditions. The diagnosis of midwall LGE is technically challenging, because of the thin myocardial walls in children. In addition, midwall fibrosis is generally considered a nonspecific finding, and its clinical impact in the care of pediatric DCM requires further investigation.

Arrhythmogenic Right Ventricular Cardiomyopathy

The goal of the CMR exam for the suspected arrhythmogenic right ventricular cardiomyopathy (ARVC) is to assess RV size, systolic function, RV and LV regional function, and tissue characterization. Assessment should include a description of RV dilation, RV regional wall motion abnormalities, RV wall thinning, RV outflow tract dyskinesis, and fatty infiltration. Qualitative assessment of myocardial fat infiltration, while challenging, was the most sensitive (84%), yet the least specific feature (79%). Due in part to resolution issues present from motion artifact and from the thinness of the RV wall, it may be difficult to delineate myocardial from pericardial fat. Furthermore, fatty infiltration is not currently an ARVC Task Force criterion.

Axial cine images are optimal for RV-free wall evaluation, short-axis views for evaluation of the inferior wall and angle of the RV, and RVOT views for the inferior wall. Regional wall motion abnormalities should be confirmed in multiple planes. Subtle aneurysms of the RV wall that becomes more prominent during systole can be seen in patients who later go on to develop more phenotypic evidence for ARVC. Wall motion abnormalities are described as (1) hypokinesis when an area has reduced thickening of less than 40%, (2) akinesis when wall thickening is less than 10%, and (3) dyskinesis when there is abnormal outward movement of a region during systole. Regional RV wall motion abnormalities alone—in the absence of RV dilation or reduced RV systolic function—though, should not be taken as criteria for establishing the diagnosis of ARVC. Establishing that a patient meets ARVC Task Force criteria requires comparison with age- and gender-appropriate data.

Myocardial LGE is not part of the revised ARVC Task Force criteria because detection of this for the thin RV wall can be challenging. Nonetheless, some have advocated assessment for areas of LGE, which have been shown to correlate with histological findings of myocardial fibrosis and inducible ventricular arrhythmias by electrical stimulation. Because this is often a biventricular disease, the LV should be analyzed carefully for fibro-fatty myocardial infiltration, regional wall motion abnormalities, LV dilation, and global dysfunction.

Ischemic Cardiomyopathy

Cardiac MR is used in pediatric ischemic cardiomyopathies for diagnosis, prognosis, and risk assessment. Although cardiac MR is used for the initial diagnosis in these lesions, the primary focus here is the use once ischemic cardiomyopathy has developed. The ischemic cardiomyopathy entities for which cardiac MR has utility include Kawasaki disease [20], anomalous coronary arteries [19], coronary fistula, coronary artery dissection [10], myocardial bridge, iatrogenic coronary artery injury. In general cardiac MR can show the coronary anatomy itself, although distal coronary artery assessment can be challenging particularly in young patients. The global and regional myocardial perfusion can also be measured with cardiac MR. Perfusion is performed both at rest and during pharmacologic stress to evaluate areas of both fixed and reversible perfusion defects. After determining the extent of perfusion defect, the myocardial LGE pattern is determined. The location and extent of LGE are useful in determining the long-term viability of myocardium injured by ischemic events. The LGE images combined with T2-weighted edema images show areas of myocardium at risk (Fig. 10.7).

Anderson-Fabry

Cardiac MR findings in Anderson-Fabry include concentric LV hypertrophy, decreased LV ejection fraction. Cardiac MR in these patients can be challenging in the face of persistent atrial arrhythmias. Cardiac MR has significant utility for Fabry in differentiating it from symmetric HCM. Since Fabry can be treated with enzyme replacement therapy, the differentiation is critical. The hypertrophy pattern does not provide discrimination between the two entities. The LGE pattern may differentiate them. Fabry patients will have midmyocardial enhancement in the basal inferolateral segment whereas HCM patients typically have LGE restricted to the interventricular septum [7,10]. Cardiac MR with LGE has been associated with poor prognosis in these patients [1]. LGE and quantitative function by MR is also useful in monitoring their response to enzyme replacement therapy (Fig. 10.2).

Left Ventricular Noncompaction Cardiomyopathy

Left ventricular noncompaction cardiomyopathy (LVNC) is characterized by a thin compacted epicardial layer with a thick spongiform endocardium. CMR adds value to echocardiography as it significantly easier to visualize all ventricular segments. The goal of CMR is to image the LV from four-chamber and short-axis imaging planes. There are two CMR methods for assessing the NC:C myocardial ratio. The first method uses SSFP cine imaging of three LV long-axis diastolic images to identify the myocardial segment with the most pronounced trabeculations. Measuring the trabeculation depth allows calculation of the NC:C ratio can be determined for any LV segment. A ratio of greater than 2.3:1 is used as the cut-off. The second method uses planimetry of short-axis SSFP cine diastolic images. The compacted myocardium is traced as usual. These are compared with tracings around all the trabeculations and the trabeculated mass calculated as the difference between the two masses. When the trabeculated LV myocardial mass is above 20% of the total LV mass, this is suggestive of LVNC. Novel CMR methods being employed for suspected LVNC patients include fractal analysis (a method of quantifying complex geometric patterns in biological structures) of end-diastolic short-axis images to quantify LV trabeculae. The fractal dimension of the endocardial border provides a quantitative parameter that can be used to distinguish normal from abnormal trabecular patterns. The presence of LGE in LVNC is variable but difficult to quantify secondary to the thinned compacted myocardium (Fig. 10.5).

REFERENCES

[1] J. Krämer, M. Niemann, S. Störk, S. Frantz, M. Beer, G. Ertl, et al., Relation of burden of myocardial fibrosis to malignant ventricular arrhythmias and outcomes in Fabry disease, Am. J. Cardiol. 114 (2014) 895–900.

[2] C. Krieghoff, M.J. Barten, L. Hildebrand, M. Grothoff, L. Lehmkuhl, C. Lücke, et al., Assessment of sub-clinical acute cellular rejection after heart transplantation: comparison of cardiac magnetic resonance imaging and endomyocardial biopsy, Eur. Radiol. 24 (2014) 2360–2371.

[3] S. Liu, J. Han, M.S. Nacif, J. Jones, N. Kawel, P. Kellman, et al., Diffuse myocardial fibrosis evaluation using cardiac magnetic resonance T1 mapping: sample size considerations for clinical trials, J. Cardiovasc. Magn. Reson. 14 (2012) 90.

[4] Ł.A. Małek, K. Werys, M. Kłopotowski, M. Śpiewak, B. Miłosz-Wieczorek, Ł. Mazurkiewicz, et al., Native T1-mapping for non-contrast assessment of myocardial fibrosis in patients with hypertrophic cardiomyopathy – comparison with late enhancement quantification, Magn. Reson. Imaging 33 (2015) 718–724.

[5] W. Mazur, K.N. Hor, J.T. Germann, R.J. Fleck, H.R. Al-Khalidi, J.P. Wansapura, et al., Patterns of left ventricular remodeling in patients with duchenne muscular dystrophy: a cardiac MRI study of ventricular geometry, global function, and strain, Int. J. Cardiovasc. Imaging (2011) NaN–NaN.

[6] E.M. McNally, J.R. Kaltman, D.W. Benson, C.E. Canter, L.H. Cripe, D. Duan, et al., Contemporary cardiac issues in duchenne muscular dystrophy. Working Group of the National Heart, Lung, and Blood Institute in collaboration with parent project muscular dystrophy, Circulation 131 (2015) 1590–1598.

[7] D.R. Messroghli, A. Radjenovic, S. Kozerke, D.M. Higgins, M.U. Sivananthan, J.P. Ridgway, Modified look-locker inversion recovery (MOLLI) for high-resolution T1 mapping of the heart, Magn. Reson. Med. 52 (2004) 141–146.

[8] J.C. Moon, M. Sheppard, E. Reed, P. Lee, P.M. Elliott, D.J. Pennell, The histological basis of late gadolinium enhancement cardiovascular magnetic resonance in a patient with Anderson-Fabry disease, J. Cardiovasc. Magn. Reson. 8 (2006) 479–482.

[9] Z. Weng, J. Yao, R.H. Chan, J. He, X. Yang, Y. Zhou, et al., Prognostic value of LGE-CMR in HCM: a meta-analysis, JACC Cardiovasc. Imaging 9 (2016) 1392–1402.

[10] F. De Cobelli, A. Esposito, E. Belloni, M. Pieroni, G. Perseghin, C. Chimenti, et al., Delayed-enhanced cardiac MRI for differentiation of Fabry's disease from symmetric hypertrophic cardiomyopathy, Am. J. Roentgenol. 192 (2009).

[11] M. Etesami, R.C. Gilkeson, P. Rajiah, Utility of late gadolinium enhancement in pediatric cardiac MRI, Pediatr. Radiol. 46 (2016) 1096–1113.

[12] M.G. Friedrich, U. Sechtem, J. Schulz-Menger, G. Holmvang, P. Alakija, L.T. Cooper, et al., Cardiovascular magnetic resonance in myocarditis: a JACC white paper, J. Am. Coll. Cardiol. 53 (2009) 1475–1487.

[13] S. Giri, Y.-C. Chung, A. Merchant, G. Mihai, S. Rajagopalan, S.V. Raman, et al., T2 quantification for improved detection of myocardial edema, J. Cardiovasc. Magn. Reson. 11 (2009) 56.

[14] S.C. Hagenbuch, W.M. Gottliebson, J. Wansapura, W. Mazur, R. Fleck, D.W. Benson, et al., Detection of progressive cardiac dysfunction by serial evaluation of circumferential strain in patients with duchenne muscular dystrophy, Am. J. Cardiol. 105 (2010) 1451–1455.

[15] K.N. Hor, J. Wansapura, L.W. Markham, W. Mazur, L.H. Cripe, R. Fleck, et al., Circumferential strain analysis identifies strata of cardiomyopathy in Duchenne muscular dystrophy: a cardiac magnetic resonance tagging study, J. Am. Coll. Cardiol. 53 (2009) 1204–1210.

[16] L.J. Anderson, S. Holden, B. Davis, E. Prescott, C.C. Charrier, N.H. Bunce, et al., Cardiovascular T2-star (T2*) magnetic resonance for the early diagnosis of myocardial iron overload, Eur. Heart J. 22 (2001) 2171–2179.

[17] G. Barone-Rochette, C. Augier, M. Rodière, J-L. Quesada, A. Foote, H. Bouvaist, et al., Potentially simple score of late gadolinium enhancement cardiac MR in acute myocarditis outcome, (2013).
[18] A.Y.-Y. Chen, M.J. Zirwas, M.P. Heffernan, Nephrogenic systemic fibrosis: a review, J. Drugs Dermatol. 9 (2010) 829–834.
[19] L.P. Browne, D. Kearney, M.D. Taylor, T. Chung, T.C. Slesnick, A.C. Nutting, et al., ALCAPA: the role of myocardial viability studies in determining prognosis, Pediatr. Radiol. 40 (2010) 163–167.
[20] J. Potet, A. Rahmouni, J. Mayer, A. Vignaud, P. Lim, A. Luciani, et al., Detection of myocardial edema with low-b-value diffusion-weighted echo-planar imaging sequence in patients with acute myocarditis, Radiology 269 (2013) 362–369.
[21] M.D. Puchalski, R.V. Williams, B. Askovich, C.T. Sower, K.H. Hor, J.T. Su, et al., Late gadolinium enhancement: precursor to cardiomyopathy in duchenne muscular dystrophy? Int. J. Cardiovasc. Imaging 25 (2009) 57–63.

FURTHER READING

[1] C.H. Park, E.-Y. Choi, A. Greiser, M.Y. Paek, S.H. Hwang, T.H. Kim, Diagnosis of acute global myocarditis using cardiac MRI with quantitative t1 and t2 mapping: case report and literature review, Korean J. Radiol. 14 (2013) 727–732.
[2] A.R. Payne, M. Casey, J. McClure, R. McGeoch, A. Murphy, R. Woodward, et al., Bright-blood T2-weighted MRI has higher diagnostic accuracy than dark-blood short tau inversion recovery MRI for detection of acute myocardial infarction and for assessment of the ischemic area at risk and myocardial salvage, Circ. Cardiovasc. Imaging 4 (2011) 210–219.
[3] V.O. Puntmann, T. Voigt, Z. Chen, M. Mayr, R. Karim, K. Rhode, et al., Native T1 mapping in differentiation of normal myocardium from diffuse disease in hypertrophic and dilated cardiomyopathy, JACC Cardiovasc. Imaging 6 (2013) 475–484.
[4] S. Sachdeva, X. Song, N. Dham, D.M. Heath, R.L. DeBiasi, Analysis of clinical parameters and cardiac magnetic resonance imaging as predictors of outcome in pediatric myocarditis, Am. J. Cardiol. 115 (2015) 499–504.
[5] M.C. Silva, Z.M.A. Meira, J. Gurgel Giannetti, M.M. da Silva, A.F.O. Campos, M. Mde Barbosa, et al., Myocardial delayed enhancement by magnetic resonance imaging in patients with muscular dystrophy, J. Am. Coll. Cardiol. 49 (2007) 1874–1879.
[6] C.E. Tacke, S. Romeih, I.M. Kuipers, A.M. Spijkerboer, M. Groenink, T.W. Kuijpers, Evaluation of cardiac function by magnetic resonance imaging during the follow-up of patients with kawasaki disease, Circ. Cardiovasc. Imaging 6 (2013) 67–73.
[7] A. Tandon, C.R. Villa, K.N. Hor, J.L. Jefferies, Z. Gao, J.A. Towbin, et al., Myocardial fibrosis burden predicts left ventricular ejection fraction and is associated with age and steroid treatment duration in duchenne muscular dystrophy, J. Am. Heart Assoc. 4 (2015) e001338.
[8] M. Westwood, L.J. Anderson, D.N. Firmin, P.D. Gatehouse, C.C. Charrier, B. Wonke, et al., A single breath-hold multiecho T2* cardiovascular magnetic resonance technique for diagnosis of myocardial iron overload, 18 (2003) 33–39.

Chapter 11

Assessment of Heart Failure by Invasive Methods

Michael L. O'Byrne, Jonathan J. Rome
Division of Cardiology, The Children's Hospital of Philadelphia and Perelman School of Medicine University of Pennsylvania, Philadelphia, PA, United States

Hemodynamic evaluation (measurement of cardiac output, pressures, and resistances) by right and left heart catheterization has been the gold standard for assessment of patients with heart failure. However, as noninvasive assessment techniques have evolved, the role for invasive assessment has changed. Echocardiographic and cardiac magnetic resonance imaging have generated a host of noninvasive metrics, some of which produce information parallel to that measured in a catheterization (e.g., cardiac output by MRI), while others assess other aspects of myocardial function without clear analogues in the catheterization laboratory (e.g., strain or tissue Doppler). To date, there have been little data to suggest that titrating therapy to specific pressure measurements improves outcome with heart failure therapy. Complicating matters, there are no evidence-based guidelines for the use of invasive assessment in children and young adults. However, heart catheterization remains useful to resolve diagnostic uncertainty in patients without a clear diagnosis (with special utility in patients with congenital heart disease) and also for identification of pulmonary arterial hypertension. Invasive assessment also may provide a means to assess for suitability of novel therapies and to guide these therapies.

HISTORY

Famously, Werner Forssmann performed the first right heart catheterization in a human being on himself in 1929 at August Victoria Home in Eberswalde, Germany. Andrew Cournand and Dickinson Richards of Columbia University's College of Physicians and Surgeons and the Bellevue Hospital in New York City refined these techniques, for which they were awarded the Nobel Prize for Medicine in 1956. The development of the balloon-tipped, flow-directed catheter by John Abbott, Melvin Scheinman, and Elliott Rapaport at the University of California at San Francisco in 1969 simplified the technique of right heart catheterization, as these catheters could be advanced to the pulmonary artery (PA) without the use of the use of X-ray guidance [1]. H.J.C. Swan, William Ganz, and colleagues at the University of California of Los Angeles reported in 1970 the use of balloon-tipped catheters for bedside evaluation of hemodynamics. This is widely credited as the impetus for widespread use of right heart catheterization in clinical applications for evaluation of critically ill patients [2]. In 1976, Forrester and colleagues proposed a classification system of hemodynamic profiles in patients postmyocardial infarction based on bedside PA catheters [3,4]. By the 1980s, 20%–40% of adult patients in intensive care units in the United States were monitored using bedside PA catheters [5].

However, more recently direct measurement of hemodynamics in adult patients with heart failure has become less common. Several studies starting with the SUPPORT trial found no improvement in outcomes in patients monitored with PA catheters compared to those without PA catheters [5–9]. In the wake of these results, there has been a dramatic reduction in the use of PA catheter monitoring in this population. A review of National Inpatient Database demonstrated a 65% reduction in PA catheter monitoring from 1993 to 2004 [10]. More recently, an analysis of data from The Acute Decompensated Heart Failure National Registry, a large US heart failure registry, demonstrated that less than 10% of patients hospitalized with heart failure symptoms were assessed with right heart catheterization and PA catheters [11].

CURRENT INDICATIONS

The trend away from routine hemodynamic evaluation and monitoring is reflected in current American Heart Association guidelines from 2013 for older adult patients with heart failure (Table 11.1), which recommend monitoring with a PA

Heart Failure in the Child and Young Adult. http://dx.doi.org/10.1016/B978-0-12-802393-8.00011-9

TABLE 11.1 Recommendations for Heart Catheterization in Adults With Heart Failure

Recommendation	COR	LOE
Monitoring with a pulmonary artery catheter should be performed in patients with respiratory distress or impaired systemic perfusion when clinical assessment is inadequate	I	C
Invasive hemodynamic monitoring can be useful for carefully selected patients with acute heart failure with persistent symptoms and/or when hemodynamics are uncertain	IIa	C
When ischemia may be contributing to heart failure, coronary angiography is reasonable	IIa	C
Endomyocardial biopsy can be useful in patients with heart failure when a specific diagnosis is suspected that would influence therapy	IIa	C
Routine use of invasive hemodynamic monitoring is not recommended in normotensive patients with acute heart failure	III: No benefit	B
Endomyocardial biopsy should not be performed in the routine evaluation of heart failure	III: Harm	C

COR, class of recommendation; *LOE*, level of evidence.
Adapted from C.W. Yancy, et al., ACCF/AHA guideline for the management of heart failure, Circulation 128 (2013) e240–e327.

catheter only in those patients "with respiratory distress or impaired systemic perfusion in whom the adequacy or excess of intracardiac filling pressures cannot be determined from clinical assessment" to delineate central venous pressures (COR: I, LOE: C) or in select patients with acute heart failure in whom there is diagnostic uncertainty (COR: IIa, LOE: C) [12]. PA catheter monitoring is actually contraindicated in normotensive patients (COR: III, LOE B).

The recommendations for hemodynamic evaluation in the catheterization laboratory are even more limited. Right heart catheterization is not indicated for assessment of heart failure, with guideline authors stating that the benefits of heart failure medications in terms of survival and symptom reduction are not dependent on achieving any specific pressure. Left heart catheterization is recommended only for adults in whom there is suspicion for coronary artery disease contributing to symptoms (COR: IIA, LOE: C). Endomyocardial biopsy (EMB) is contraindicated in routine evaluation (COR: III, LOE: C) and only indicated when a specific diagnosis made using it would influence therapy (COR: IIa, and LOE: C). Thus, in adults with heart failure, though direct measurement of pressure is the gold standard, it is no longer a part of routine evaluation. To date, there is no evidence that titrating therapies to hemodynamic parameters improve outcomes. At this time, efficacy of heart failure treatment is judged at the patient level by symptom reduction and at the population level by risk of hospitalization and mortality. Thus, for patients with "straightforward" heart failure, the authors write, heart catheterization provides no benefit and represents a source of small but real risk of an adverse outcome. It is reserved (1) to clarify diagnostic uncertainty in patients with a cryptic presentation, (2) to determine suitability and guide efficacy of novel therapies, and (3) to identify and classify pulmonary hypertension.

The recommendations from the American Heart Association are intended for older adult patients, and it is important to interpret these guidelines with caution in children and young adults, for whom the epidemiology of heart failure is dramatically different. Heart failure in older adults is overwhelmingly the result of adaptive and maladaptive changes to chronic hypertension and ischemic insult. In children and young adults, the prevalence of ischemic cardiomyopathy is extremely low, with most heart failure attributable to congenital heart disease and cardiomyopathies. Children receiving heart transplantation are a surrogate population for those with severe heart failure. In this group, cardiomyopathy and congenital heart disease account for 97% of the population with the relative proportions varying by age group [13]. This reinforces that adult guidelines are not applicable to the pediatric population. In 2004, the International Society for Heart and Lung Transplantation published practice guidelines focused on heart failure in children [14], but these do not address how children with suspected heart failure should be evaluated. Specifically, they do not address the indications or contraindications for right heart catheterization, left heart catheterization, or EMB. The decision to pursue heart catheterization is therefore at the discretion of the team caring for the patient. Cardiac catheterization is an invasive test and as such is not without risk. These risks should be balanced against the possible benefit derived from the information gathered via catheterization. Relative to catheterizations in which an intervention is performed, diagnostic catheterization are associated with lower risk of major adverse event [15]. However, analyses of data from C3PO registry [16,17], the IMPACT database [18], and Pediatric Health Information Systems database [19,20] have demonstrated that patient-level characteristics are also independent markers of adverse outcomes, including death. Specifically, preprocedural hemodynamic embarrassment, receipt of vasoactive medications, and young patient age/small patient size are all associated with increased risk of periprocedural adverse events. The degree to which these factors are modifiable is an area of active research, but multicenter series have demonstrated that larger center procedural volume are associated with reduced risk of adverse outcomes [18–20]. There may be modifiable aspects of care performed at more experienced centers that are responsible for improved outcomes, but at this time these practices have not been well defined. All of this reinforces that the risk of diagnostic catheterization must be considered when deciding whether to pursue this strategy.

Therefore, clear objectives need to be defined before pursuing a cardiac catheterization. Generally, clarifying the etiology of heart failure in patients with cryptic presentation (especially if there is potential to identify a modifiable cause of heart failure) is the main reason for heart catheterization. Special attention should be paid to patients with congenital heart disease with or without previous surgery, in whom a careful hemodynamic evaluation can identify anatomic lesions that may contribute to heart failure symptoms and which are potentially amenable to intervention. Pulmonary hypertension also remains an important issue in children with heart failure. At this time there are no indications for heart catheterization as a guide for novel therapies, though these may be introduced as the range of advanced heart failure therapies continues to grow.

HEMODYNAMIC EVALUATION

A complete hemodynamic evaluation includes measurement of cardiac output, pressures throughout the cardiovascular system, and determination of systemic and pulmonary vascular resistance. The technique and procedures for obtaining a precise and accurate evaluation of individual hemodynamics have been reviewed in detail elsewhere [21–23], but there is utility in reviewing some key aspects of this evaluation. The conduct of catheterization includes several aspects that influence the data collected. Hemodynamic measurements are generally made with the patient at rest in a supine position, often with the patients either sedated or anesthetized. This does not directly reflect the patients's physiology for most of their life, when they are awake, stimulated, ambulatory, and exerting themselves. At the same time, almost all published data and the accompanying clinical experience of the field are derived from studies performed under these conditions, with recommendations based on extrapolation from resting studies under sedation or anesthesia. Upright or exercise/stress studies (as well as pharmacologic stress with inotropic or chronotropic medications) can be obtained and may have value. They are not often performed routinely in most catheterization laboratories (and their interpretation is hampered by a dearth of reference data).

The equipment used to measure pressures also can introduce error. To measure pressure, fluid-filled catheters are typically coupled to a remote transducer and recording system. Pressure is transmitted through the fluid column in the catheter to the transducer. Error can be introduced by factors such as transducer and patient positions. The transducer should be centered at the level of the right atrium (usually assumed to be the midpoint between the sternum and the spine). Dampening (false reduction in the peak pressures of the tracing) and poor frequency response are related to catheter diameter, length, stiffness, the presence of air bubbles in the catheter, and the number of stopcocks. Partial obstruction of the catheter lumen can also result in the propagation of standing waves and "fling" with a falsely elevated peak pressure. Complex pressure waveforms such as ventricular tracings are particularly subject to these factors.

Regardless of whether the patient is breathing freely or receiving positive pressure breaths from a ventilator, ventilation induces changes in the intrathoracic pressure that are reflected in the pressure measurements. The range of these fluctuations is usually between −1 and 5 mmHg, but the magnitude of these fluctuations can be much greater with obstructive pulmonary disease (e.g., asthma or obstructive sleep apnea). Care should be taken in patients with a natural airway to optimize patient position to minimize airway obstruction. Finally, digital systems frequently average measurements over a set number of seconds or cardiac cycles or can pick an individual pressure measurement, but this can introduce error. By convention, pressures are measured at end-expiration (where the effect of negative pressure ventilation on intrathoracic pressure is minimized) to be used.

All techniques for measuring cardiac output rely on techniques that measure the velocity and dilution of an indicator substance. In the current era, the two major techniques for measurement of cardiac output are (1) direct application of the Fick Principle and (2) thermodilution. In the past, other indicator dilution methods (e.g., Indocyanine Green and other dye dilution techniques) were used, but are primarily of historical interest. The Fick principle applies conservation of mass to the process of oxygen transport in the blood. Cardiac output can be calculated by dividing the patient's oxygen consumption (mL/min/m^2) by the difference in oxygen content of the systemic artery and systemic venous return (a mixed venous sample).

$$\text{CO} = \text{oxygen consumption}/(\text{systemic artery oxygen content} - \text{systemic vein oxygen content}).$$

The definition of the mixed venous sample is the most distal chamber on the right side of the heart proximal to a hemodynamically significant step-up. Because of streaming of different sources of venous blood, there are small variations in the saturation of blood in the cavae, right atrium, right ventricle, and pulmonary arteries. Early studies of subjects without shunt

TABLE 11.2 Detection of a Shunt by Oximetry

Chambers Sampled	Minimum Saturation Difference (%)	Multiple Samples (%)[a]
SVC-RA	8.7	7
RA-RV	5.2	4
RV-PA	5.6	4

PA, pulmonary artery; *RA*, right atrial; *RV*, right ventricular; *SVC*, superior vena cava.
[a]*Studies by Dexter et al. demonstrated that multiple measurements within 1 min narrow the difference detected that is needed to identify a hemodynamically significant shunt with confidence [25].*
Adapted from Diagnostic and interventional catheterization in congenital heart disease, in: J.E. Lock, J.F. Keane, S.B. Perry (Eds.), Hemodynamic Evaluation of Congenital Heart Disease, second ed., Kluwer Publications, 2000, pp. 37–72.

lesions defined the normal saturation in these chambers, including normal range of variation (Table 11.2) [24,25]. In patients with shunting between systemic and pulmonary circulations, saturations should be measured in chambers that provide saturations for mixed venous, pulmonary venous, systemic artery, and PA saturations. This is not especially important in patients with structurally normal hearts but is especially important in patients with congenital heart disease (See section below). Oxygen consumption can be measured using mask in spontaneously breathing patients or through the endotracheal tube where available. Often, oxygen consumption is estimated based on nomograms or formulae [26], which may introduce substantial error. There are also situations in which no true mixed saturation can be obtained (e.g., heterogeneous lung disease with variable desaturation in the pulmonary veins). A range of possible approaches exist to dealing with this, but the most stringent is calculating a range of outputs using the available data and recognizing that the degree of uncertainty represented by this range.

Thermodilution measurement of cardiac index uses a bolus cold saline as the indicator material through a specially designed catheter. A thermodilution catheter has three lumens (a balloon lumen, a distal port at the tip of the catheter, a proximal port, a variable length back from the tip). It also has an imbedded thermistor in the tip of the catheter. With the tip of the catheter in the PA and the proximal port in the right atrium, a bolus of saline of known temperature is injected. The temperature at the tip is measured and the temperature decay curve analyzed to determine cardiac output. Three or more consistent measurements are usually performed and averaged. Relative to dye dilution techniques, the cold saline bolus clears after passing through 1–2 capillary beds, so there is no recirculation phase as is seen in indocyanine green or other dye dilution techniques. This technique is most effective in patients with normal cardiac anatomy. In patients with poor mixing of venous blood (e.g., Fontan circulation), measurements are not accurate. Significant pulmonary regurgitation or tricuspid regurgitation can also make measurement unreliable. Intracardiac shunt confounds the interpretation of thermodilution, and care should be used in utilizing this technique in patients with anatomic shunts. Several other common problems, including (1) prolonged handling of the injectate, (2) proximal or distal port is in a position where there is not free-flowing blood, and (3) and an insufficiently brisk injection, result in relative warming of the injected saline and overestimation of cardiac output. Similarly in low cardiac output states, transit through the heart is delayed (allowing for relative warming), again leading to overestimation of cardiac output.

A complete right heart catheterization includes measurement of pressures in the right atrium, right ventricle, PA, and wedged in the PA as close in time as possible to one another. The right atrial pressure (RA, normal mean pressure: 3 mmHg) is composed of "a" and "v" waves coinciding with atrial and ventricular systole, respectively. A third wave, the "c" wave, occurs during early ventricular systole and does not have significant clinical utility. The RA pressure reflects the filling pressure in the right ventricle and fluid status. In addition, an accentuated v wave is consistent with tricuspid valve regurgitation, while the a-wave can be elevated in isolation due to diastolic dysfunction of the right ventricle. The RA trace is subject to respiratory variation, which is exaggerated in obstructive pulmonary disease. The important features of right ventricular pressure are the peak in systole and the end-diastolic pressure. Normal values include a systolic pressure of 24 mmHg and end-diastolic pressure of 5 mmHg. PA tracings reflect the systolic pressure in the right ventricle and usually have a low diastolic pressure. Since left atrial pressure is often not directly measured, the pulmonary capillary wedge pressure (normal mean pressure is 8 mmHg) is usually used as an estimate of left atrial pressure. Wedge tracings can, however, be misleading and must be carefully performed and interpreted. A number of conditions render the wedge pressures poor surrogates for left atrial pressure including pulmonary vein disease, severe pulmonary arterial hypertension, or lung disease. There is a delay in the wedge waveform of between 50 and 100 ms. In addition, the amplitude of a- and v-peaks can be attenuated. The pulmonary capillary wedge pressure provides insight into fluid status and left ventricular diastolic function, analogous to the RA. Along with the mean PA tracing the mean pulmonary capillary wedge tracing provides the means of calculating pulmonary vascular resistance (see subsequent section on pulmonary hypertension).

TABLE 11.3 Differentiating Constrictive Pericarditis From Restrictive Cardiomyopathy

	Constrictive Pericarditis	Restrictive Cardiomyopathy
Atrial pressures	Right and left atrial pressure equalization (within 5 mmHg)	Atrial pressures tend to be higher
Kussmaul's sign Loss of normal right atrial pressure decline with inspiration	Present	a
M or W-sign Right atrial a and v waves are equal in pressure	Present	a
Square root sign Prominent ventricular diastolic dip and rise	Present	a
LV and RV end-diastolic pressure	Equal	LV tends to be greater than RV
RV pressures	RVEDP > 1/3 RV systolic pressure	Secondary pulmonary hypertension and markedly elevated RV/PA pressures are more common
PA pressures	Moderately elevated	
Ventricular interdependence with spontaneous breathing	Present: with inspiration RV systolic pressure rises and LV systolic pressure drops	Absent: RV and LV systolic pressures increase and decreased over the respiratory cycle in parallel

LV, left ventricular; *PA*, pulmonary artery; *RV*, right ventricular; *RVEDP*, right ventricular end-diastolic pressure.
[a] *Though not characteristic, these signs can be present in patients with restrictive cardiomyopathy.*

Provocative testing to determine the effect of increased cardiac output can be performed either with controlled exercise (with reports of catheterization performed using recumbent bike ergometers) or with pharmacologic or fluid challenges. However, virtually all contemporaneous series and epidemiologic data in the field rely on catheterizations performed under the conditions described above. Therefore, provocative testing should be reserved for special circumstances (i.e., evaluation of possible restrictive physiology (see section below)).

RESTRICTIVE PHYSIOLOGY VERSUS CONSTRICTIVE PERICARDITIS

Differentiating restrictive myopathy, constrictive pericarditis, and effusions has long been an issue that is resolved through hemodynamic evaluation. Evaluation of effusions and tamponade is the domain of echocardiography in the current era [27]. Though there are MRI and echocardiographic measures that have been proposed, catheterization remains necessary in some cases to assess these etiologies of diastolic dysfunction [27–30]. Constrictive pericarditis is rare in children, especially those with congenital heart disease, but in patients with other systemic disease (e.g., oncologic diagnoses) and in adults with congenital heart disease, it remains an important etiology of diastolic dysfunction. Loss of pericardial compliance occurs reducing atrial compliance, and elevated filling pressures are necessary to maintain filling and cardiac output. Characteristic hemodynamic findings are summarized in Table 11.3 [27–30]. These rules of thumb are reportedly sensitive, but are non-specific, with several occurring in both constrictive pericarditis and restrictive cardiomyopathy. Identification of these findings (especially the square root sign) can be challenging because of shortened diastolic filling. The prolonged diastole after an iatrogenic premature ventricular contraction can make this easier to appreciate. In addition, relative hypovolemia (e.g., from prolonged "nothing-by-mouth" duration) can mask pressure findings. Rapid bolus infusion of intravenous fluid can make these findings more marked. Characteristic respiratory variation can be used to assess constrictive pericarditis in patients breathing spontaneously. Ventricular interdependence (inspiration accompanied by an increase in systolic right ventricular pressure with decrease in left ventricular systolic pressure) is a contrast to the normal response in which the left and right ventricular pressures rise and fall together. This reportedly is a more specific finding in patients who can be evaluated while breathing spontaneously.

The challenge is that restrictive myocardial disease (restrictive physiology) has significant overlap with pericardial disease. Findings that are typical of constrictive pericarditis (Kussmaul, M, and square root signs) are all potentially present in patients with restrictive cardiomyopathy. Absence of ventricular interdependence more specifically identifies restrictive cardiomyopathy. Also, left and right atrial pressures tend to be higher. Finally, secondary pulmonary vascular disease is also more common, so pulmonary arterial and right ventricular pressures are commonly markedly elevated (Table 11.3).

PULMONARY ARTERIAL HYPERTENSION

In the adult population the evaluation of pulmonary hypertension is indicated with heart failure, largely to differentiate between that caused by pulmonary vascular disease and that caused by elevated left atrial pressure [31,32]. This is particularly relevant in this population in whom elevated left ventricular end-diastolic pressure and concomitant left atrial hypertension is prevalent. In several forms of cardiomyopathy and congenital heart disease, pulmonary arterial hypertension and pulmonary vascular disease are especially important concerns. In these patients, identification and classification of pulmonary hypertension has ramifications for (1) pharmacotherapy, (2) prognosis, and (3) suitability for heart transplantation.

Therefore, when pulmonary arterial hypertension is suspected (based on the patient's diagnosis and clinical history and/or noninvasive imaging), a right heart catheterization with pulmonary vasodilator testing is indicated. In patients with structurally normal hearts, right heart catheterization (with access in either the femoral vein or internal jugular/subclavian vein) is performed with measurement of cardiac index and pressure measurements of one or both pulmonary arteries and pulmonary capillary wedge pressure, right ventricle and right atrium in a rest condition (without additional pulmonary vasodilator therapy). In patients with congenital heart disease, additionally detailed hemodynamic evaluation may be necessary. In this case, measuring PA and pulmonary capillary pressures in both lungs is necessary. In patients whose transpulmonary gradient is different in each lung, these data must be considered along with the distribution of pulmonary blood flow from cardiac MRI or nuclear medicine lung perfusion scan to measure total indexed pulmonary vascular resistance (PVRI).

Vasoreactivity testing is then performed by administering pulmonary vasodilators (commonly increasing the fraction of inspired oxygen and adding inhaled nitric oxide to the gas inspired by the patient). After a wash-in period to achieve a steady state (3–10 min) repeat measurements are performed. Hemodynamic measurements (cardiac index, pulmonary capillary wedge pressure, PA pressure, and pulmonary vascular resistance) are repeated under the second condition and compared. The presence of pulmonary hypertension with responsive pulmonary vascular resistance indicates (1) that pulmonary vasodilator therapy has the potential to improve symptoms and even longevity [31,32] and (2) ramifications for possible orthotopic heart transplantation. Current recommendations are to perform pulmonary vasodilator testing on patients who might undergo heart transplant and who have an indexed pulmonary vascular resistance greater than >3 Woods units per square meter [33,34]. Previously, there was a reticence to perform a heart transplant on patients with pulmonary vascular resistance greater than 6 Woods units per square meter. Though this threshold has been questioned [35,36], multiple studies have demonstrated that elevated pulmonary vascular resistance is a risk factor for right heart failure and early post-transplant mortality, and that this risk is reduced in subjects who with responsive pulmonary vasculature during catheterization [36–40].

An important situation is the assessment of a patient with elevated pulmonary capillary wedge pressure and pulmonary arterial hypertension. Pulmonary vasodilator testing is useful in these patients, in theory, to determine the degree to which their pulmonary vasculature disease is reversible. However, pulmonary vasodilator testing can exacerbate left atrial hypertension and cause flash pulmonary edema. To our knowledge there are no data guiding how/when to avoid performing pulmonary vasodilator testing. Care should be taken to perform pulmonary vasodilator testing in this subgroup of patients with caution and with appropriate precautions taken (e.g., endotracheal intubation with positive pressure ventilation allows for control over FiO_2 and the ability to increase positive end-expiratory and mean airway pressure to react rapidly to the development of pulmonary edema).

The additional risk of performing a catheterization in a child with pulmonary hypertension is a relevant concern. Studies using registry data suggest that catheterization in children and adults with pulmonary hypertension is relatively low risk [41–46]. However, studies using administrative data (which potentially identifies trends in broader practice than in registries) found that the risk of a catastrophic adverse event is markedly higher than in children without pulmonary hypertension [20]. This risk should be considered when considering whether hemodynamic evaluation is warranted.

HEMODYNAMIC EVALUATION IN PATIENTS WITH CONGENITAL HEART DISEASE

The evaluation of hemodynamics in a patient with congenital heart disease deserves special attention, relative to the evaluation in a patient with structurally normal heart. Residual shunts, anatomic obstruction, or valvar regurgitation impose pressure and volume loads on either ventricle. The interplay between these anatomic lesions and myocardial disease are complex, but they certainly can result in signs and symptoms of heart failure. Diagnosis of these lesions requires a detailed approach over and above that used in patients with a structurally normal heart. Diagnosis of these lesions is important because anatomic lesions can be responsive to transcatheter or operative intervention.

This detailed evaluation begins as described above, subsequently augmenting initial data with maneuvers to more completely understand specific lesions. A careful saturation run (with repeated saturations if necessary) needs to be performed to assess for intracardiac shunts that may result in a volume load. In cases where there is cyanosis, pulmonary venous desaturation needs to be differentiated from right-to-left shunt by measuring pulmonary vein saturations. If no mixed pulmonary vein saturation can be measured, then samples of each vein may be necessary to determine the range of possible saturations (and magnitude of pulmonary blood flow). Calculation of systemic and pulmonary blood flow, effective pulmonary blood flow, and magnitude of left-to-right and right-to-left shunting is vital to understanding the patient's physiology.

The measurement of pressures is similar to that described above. However, one cannot make assumptions that are more reasonable in structurally normal hearts. PA pressures should be measured in both lungs, and in patients with complicated stenosis it may be relevant to measure it in multiple lobar or even segmental branches. In patients with elevated pulmonary arterial pressures, one can no longer assume that the wedge pressure is equivalent to the left atrial pressure. The presence of a pulmonary capillary wedge pressure to left ventricular end-diastolic pressure gradient is a helpful adjunct, but even in this case it is important to determine whether that gradient, when present, is the result of stenosis of the pulmonary veins or mitral stenosis. PA wedge angiography can help identify pulmonary vein stenosis, but left atrial and pulmonary vein pressure measurements are superior (and may require transseptal puncture or other maneuvers in patients with an intact atrial septum). In patients with obstruction, detailed pullbacks with an end-hole catheter or multiport catheters may be necessary to isolate pressure gradients. Angiography should be used to confirm and augment data from hemodynamic measurements, specifically to confirm the location of anatomic stenoses and to grade valvar regurgitation. Hemodynamic evaluation of a patient with congenital heart disease requires gathering all of the information described and synthesizing the data in a cogent "story" of the patient's hemodynamics.

Pulmonary vascular disease and resultant pulmonary hypertension is an important concern in patients with congenital heart disease. In patients with elevated right ventricular or pulmonary arterial pressure it is important to differentiate between diastolic dysfunction with elevated left ventricular end-diastolic pressure, mitral stenosis, pulmonary vein stenosis, and pulmonary vascular disease with resultant increased PVRI. In patients with prolonged or persistent intracardiac left-to-right shunts, pulmonary vascular disease can occur. In patients with acquired or congenital stenosis of the branch pulmonary arteries, severe maldistribution of pulmonary blood flow can result in pulmonary vascular disease in the lung vasculature, which fed is by arteries without stenoses. Evaluation of this can require detailed pressure measurements in multiple lobar or segmental branches of each PA, wedge pressures in each lobe (or direct measurement of left atrial and pulmonary vein pressures). Again directed angiography can help isolate stenosis. As noted above additional data from nuclear medicine perfusion or MRI studies are required to determine pulmonary arteriolar resistance.

The circulation in patients who have undergone staged palliation resulting in a Fontan circulation deserves special attention. As has been reviewed elsewhere [47,48], heart failure in a Fontan patient differs from heart failure in biventricular circulation because of the absence of a subpulmonary ventricle. The cavopulmonary connections (and absence of subpulmonary ventricle) limit the ability of the heart to augment flow in response to stimuli. This results in variable degrees of venous congestion and decreased cardiac output. In addition, any impediment to the systemic ventricular function only exacerbates this. In addition, passive flow through the Fontan circuit can easily be impeded by poor function of any component of the circuit. Ventricular diastolic dysfunction (elevated end-diastolic pressure), atrioventricular valve stenosis or regurgitation, pulmonary vein stenosis, restrictive atrial communication in association with left atrioventricular valve atresia, pulmonary vascular disease with increased pulmonary vascular resistance, or PA stenosis all impair the ability of the circuit to function appropriately and can result in increased venous pressure and low cardiac output. Hemodynamic evaluation of Fontan patients must include careful evaluation of each of these variables through direct measurement followed by focused angiography. Identification of issues in any of these areas and appropriate intervention (either through medical therapy, transcatheter, or operative intervention) have the potential of reducing symptoms and may improve transplant-free survival. A Fontan fenestration sacrifices decreased arterial oxygen saturation for increased cardiac output but often results in increased tissue oxygen delivery. In some patients with high Fontan pressures and symptoms of heart failure, creation of a fenestration can result in improved oxygen delivery (reflected in increased mixed venous saturation, despite decreased systemic arterial saturation). However, in some patients the right-to-left shunt can result in debilitating desaturation. Typically, to determine if the patient will tolerate fenestration closure, test occlusion of the fenestration and remeasurement of arterial saturation and Fontan circuit pressure and saturation should be performed. With effective test occlusion, systemic arterial saturation will rise and in almost all patients Fontan pressure will rise. If the resultant Fontan pressure is acceptable and mixed venous saturation increases, tissue delivery of oxygen has increased and the patient may well benefit from device closure of his or her fenestration. However, these measurements are all performed in patients under conditions of minimal oxygen expenditure. There have clearly been cases where patients developed Fontan failure syndrome (such as protein losing enteropathy) immediately after fenestration closure. In general when heart failure occurs in a Fontan patient with a fenestration, fenestration closure is ill-advised. Whether patients with heart failure benefit from fenestration creation depends on a number of factors including the underlying cause and clinical manifestations of heart failure, and patient age.

ENDOMYOCARDIAL BIOPSY

EMB is sometimes requested as part of a catheterization procedure in children and young adults with heart failure. EMB samples can provide histologic data with high specificity for a subset of myocardial disorders that (to date) are not diagnosed by other modalities. The prognoses and treatments for these conditions differ enough that EMB may have utility. Typically the right internal jugular vein is used as a site for right ventricular EMB, though the femoral vein can be used [49]. Fluoroscopic guidance is commonly used, but several series have described performing the procedure guided by transthoracic echocardiography [50–53] with recent reports using three-dimensional transthoracic echocardiography [54]. Most data on safety of the procedure are derived from series of EMBs performed after heart transplantation. The risk of complications in adults is between 1% and 3% (higher in studies of dilated cardiomyopathy (DCM) and lower in series of subjects who have undergone transplant) [55–57]. The largest series in pediatric patients, which included data from multiple centers, was restricted to heart transplant recipients; it demonstrated an overall adverse event rate of 3.3% with severe adverse events in 1.1% [58]. The applicability of these observed risks to a pediatric patient presenting with acute heart failure (potentially due to myocarditis or cardiomyopathy) is limited. Small series from individual centers report a small but significant risk of mortality (0.6%–1.5%) and cardiac perforation (4%–5%) [59–61]. These series highlight the risk in infants with acute heart failure (14%), which is dramatically higher [62] than in older children. The risk of cardiac perforation in infants was very high in the small number of patients reported: 33%–50% [60,61]. It should be noted that these high rates may not be applicable to current practice. As of this time, registry data (such as the IMPACT registry) has not been used to evaluate this risk.

Myocardial disease can have a heterogeneous distribution, so sampling error is an issue of concern [63]. The marginal risk of each additional biopsy should be balanced against the potential incremental improvement in the sensitivity of the study. Joint American Heart Association/American College of Cardiology recommendations call for four to five samples per patient [49], but no references are cited as the basis for this recommendation.

Joint recommendations from the American Heart Association, American College of Cardiology, and European Society of Cardiology for the role of EMB in children and adults are summarized in Table 11.4 [49]. The rationale behind these is to differentiate between DCM and myocarditis for both prognostic reasons and to identify the subset of myocarditis patients

TABLE 11.4 Recommendations for Endomyocardial Biopsy in Children and Adults

Recommendation	COR	LOE
New onset heart failure (HF) <2 weeks with normal-sized LV and hemodynamic compromise	I	B
New onset HF of 2 weeks–3 months with dilated LV and new arrhythmia, second or complete heart block, or failure to respond within 1–2 weeks	I	B
HF >3 months with dilated LV and new arrhythmia, second or complete heart block, or failure to respond within 1–2 weeks	IIA	C
Suspicion of any of the following • DCM with suspected allergic reaction or eosinophilia • Anthracycline toxicity • Unexplained restrictive cardiomyopathy • Suspected cardiac tumor	IIA	C
New onset HF 2 weeks–3 months with dilated LV without arrhythmia, heart block, and which fails to respond within 1–2 weeks	IIB	B
HF >3 months with dilated LV without new arrhythmia, without second- or third-degree heart block that does not respond within 1–2 weeks	IIB	C
HF with unexplained HCM	IIB	C
Suspected ARVD/C	IIB	C
Unexplained ventricular arrhythmia	IIB	C
Unexplained atrial fibrillation	III[a]	C

ARVD/C, arrhythmogenic right ventricular dysplasia/cardiomyopathy; *COR*, class of recommendation; *DCM*, dilated cardiomyopathy; *HCM*, hypertrophic cardiomyopathy; *LOE*, level of evidence; *LV*, left ventricular
[a]*The authors do not state whether biopsy in this context is associated with Harm or No Benefit.*
Adapted from L.T. Cooper, et al., AHA/ACCF/ESC role of endomyocardial biopsy in the management of cardiovascular disease, Circulation 116 (2007) 2216–2233.

who may respond to immunomodulatory therapy. In adults, nonfulminant lymphocytic myocarditis has a reasonable prognosis, and there has not been sufficient evidence that intravenous immunoglobulin or other immunosuppressive medications provide significant improvement in outcome [64]. However, fulminant myocarditis, giant cell myocarditis, and necrotizing eosinophilic myocarditis have significantly worse outcomes and some evidence supports immunomodulatory therapy. The authors of the guidelines write that in cases where the pretest risk of either is higher than EMB, then EMB may be of benefit. This includes patients with (1) rapid and new symptoms, (2) an allergic reaction or eosinophilia, and (3) patients with arrhythmia or heart block (markers in adults of giant cell myocarditis).

In children, data regarding prevalence of these conditions and the efficacy of therapy are limited. As noted earlier, the risk of complication is 5–10 times greater than in adult patients (though this risk is skewed toward the infant population). In addition, the pretest probability of identifying myocarditis should be considered. In one series, 20% of infants and children with acute heart failure who were referred for EMB had myocarditis [59]. The pretest probability in children with arrhythmia was only 9%. For each patient, physicians have to balance the risk of adverse event with the potential prognostic benefit of the procedure, particularly in critically ill patients.

CORONARY ANGIOGRAPHY

In guidelines for adults with heart failure, coronary angiography is one of the indications for catheterization specifically for adults with heart failure in whom coronary pathology may contribute to heart failure symptoms (COR: IIa, LOE: C). The incidence of atherosclerosis in children is infinitesimally small. However, there is a subsegment of patients in whom heart failure symptoms are potentially attributable to coronary pathology either because of ostial stenosis/atresia or anomalous origin of the coronary artery from a PA (ALCAPA sometimes referred to as Bland–Garland–White syndrome). Use of coronary angiography in children is not addressed in the pediatric heart failure guidelines.

Several series report signs of subendomyocardial ischemia on electrocardiogram and echocardiogram (mitral regurgitation, echo-bright papillary muscle, characteristic electrocardiographic pattern) suggestive of ALCAPA [65–67] as well as the use of Doppler echocardiography to differentiate between ALCAPA and other etiologies of DCM. However, in all of these, cases were confirmed by coronary angiography, which remains the gold standard for diagnosis. To our knowledge no study has validated the predictive value of noninvasive imaging in the identification of ALCAPA. The low incidence of anomalous coronary origin from the PA or congenital atresia or severe ostial stenosis must be weighed against the possibility of identifying a surgically correctable lesion (and the cost of not identifying it expeditiously). The risks of transport, anesthesia, catheterization, and coronary angiography should be weighed against the patient specific pretest probability of a coronary anomaly (depending on age, presentation, and evidence on electrocardiograms and echocardiograms) and the benefit of identifying a reversible anatomic lesion as the etiology of heart failure symptoms.

CONCLUSION

Invasive hemodynamic evaluation in heart failure lies at a crossroads, especially in children. Right and left heart catheterization along with EMB have a role in the evaluation of some children with heart failure, but the decision regarding which children depends on weighing the balance of the potential benefit of the information derived and the risk of the procedure. At this time, data guiding this decision are limited, introducing uncertainty. To date no modality has replaced invasive hemodynamic assessment, which remains the gold standard. It is incumbent on practitioners to be judicious in choosing patients to send for invasive evaluation.

At the same time, current therapies are not titrated to specific hemodynamic parameters. It may be possible that in the development and testing of advanced heart failure therapy (whether in the form of mechanical support devices, resynchronization therapy, cellular or locally targeted therapies, or more traditional pharmacotherapies) invasive assessment will be necessary to guide development as well as longitudinal follow-up of these patients.

REFERENCES

[1] M.M. Scheinman, J.A. Abbott, E. Rapaport, Clinical uses of a flow-directed right heart catheter, Arch. Intern. Med. 124 (1969) 19–24.

[2] H.J.C. Swan, W. Ganz, J. Forrester, H. Marcus, G. Diamond, D. Chonette, Catheterization of the heart in man with use of a flow-directed balloon-tipped catheter, N. Engl. J. Med. 283 (1970) 447–451.

[3] J.S. Forrester, G. Diamond, K. Chatterjee, H.J. Swan, Medical therapy of acute myocardial infarction by application of hemodynamic subsets (first of two parts), N. Engl. J. Med. 295 (1976) 1356–1362.

[4] J.S. Forrester, G. Diamond, K. Chatterjee, H.J. Swan, Medical therapy of acute myocardial infarction by application of hemodynamic subsets (second of two parts), N. Engl. J. Med. 295 (1976) 1404–1413.

[5] A.F. Connors, T. Speroff, N.V. Dawson, C. Thomas, The effectiveness of right heart catheterization in the initial care of critically Ill patients, JAMA 276 (1996) 889–897.

[6] National Heart, Lung, and Blood Institute Acute Respiratory Distress Syndrome (ARDS) Clinical Trials Network, A.P. Wheeler, G.R. Bernard, B.T. Thompson, D. Schoenfeld, H.P. Wiedemann, B. deBoisblanc, A.F. Connors, R.D. Hite, A.L. Harabin, Pulmonary-artery versus central venous catheter to guide treatment of acute lung injury, N. Engl. J. Med. 354 (2006) 2213–2224.

[7] C. Binanay, R.M. Califf, V. Hasselblad, C.M. O'Connor, M.R. Shah, G. Sopko, L.W. Stevenson, G.S. Francis, C.V. Leier, L.W. Miller, ESCAPE Investigators and ESCAPE Study Coordinators, Evaluation study of congestive heart failure and pulmonary artery catheterization effectiveness: the ESCAPE trial, JAMA 294 (2005) 1625–1633.

[8] J.D. Sandham, R.D. Hull, R.F. Brant, L. Knox, G.F. Pineo, C.J. Doig, D.P. Laporta, S. Viner, L. Passerini, H. Devitt, A. Kirby, M. Jacka, Canadian Critical Care Clinical Trials Group, A randomized, controlled trial of the use of pulmonary-artery catheters in high-risk surgical patients, N. Engl. J. Med. 348 (2003) 5–14.

[9] M.R. Shah, V. Hasselblad, L.W. Stevenson, C. Binanay, C.M. O'Connor, G. Sopko, R.M. Califf, Impact of the pulmonary artery catheter in critically ill patients: meta-analysis of randomized clinical trials, JAMA 294 (2005) 1664–1670.

[10] R.S. Wiener, H.G. Welch, Trends in the use of the pulmonary artery catheter in the United States, 1993–2004, JAMA 298 (2007) 423–429.

[11] K.F. Adams Jr., G.C. Fonarow, C.L. Emerman, T.H. LeJemtel, M.R. Costanzo, W.T. Abraham, R.L. Berkowitz, M. Galvao, D.P. Horton, Characteristics and outcomes of patients hospitalized for heart failure in the United States: rationale, design, and preliminary observations from the first 100,000 cases in the Acute Decompensated Heart Failure National Registry (ADHERE), Am. Heart J. 149 (2005) 209–216.

[12] W.H. Stevenson, E.J. Tsai, B.L. Wilkoff, 2013 ACCF/AHA guideline for the management of heart failure: a report of the American College of Cardiology Foundation/American Heart Association Task Force on Practice Guidelines, Circulation 128 (2013) e240–e327.

[13] R. Kirk, A.I. Dipchand, L.B. Edwards, A.Y. Kucheryavaya, C. Benden, J.D. Christie, F. Dobbles, A.O. Rahmel, J. Stehlik, M.I. Hertz, International Society for Heart and Lung Transplantation, The Registry of the International Society for Heart and Lung Transplantation: fifteenth pediatric heart transplantation report–2012, J. Heart Lung Transplant. 31 (2012) 1065–1072.

[14] D. Rosenthal, M.R.K. Chrisant, E. Edens, L. Mahony, C. Canter, S. Colan, A. Dubin, J. Lamour, R. Ross, R. Shaddy, L. Addonizio, L. Beerman, S. Berger, D. Bernstein, E. Blume, M. Boucek, P. Checchia, A. Dipchand, J. Drummond-Webb, J. Fricker, R. Friedman, S. Hallowell, R. Jaquiss, S. Mital, E. Pahl, B. Pearce, L. Rhodes, K. Rotondo, P. Rusconi, J. Scheel, T. Pal Singh, J. Towbin, International Society for Heart and Lung Transplantation: practice guidelines for management of heart failure in children, J. Heart Lung Transplant. 23 (2004) 1313–1333.

[15] L. Bergersen, K. Gauvreau, A. Marshall, J. Kreutzer, R. Beekman, R. Hirsch, S. Foerster, D. Balzer, J. Vincent, W. Hellenbrand, R. Holzer, J. Cheatham, J. Moore, J. Lock, K. Jenkins, Procedure-type risk categories for pediatric and congenital cardiac catheterization, Circ. Cardiovasc. Interv. 4 (2011) 188–194.

[16] L. Bergersen, K. Gauvreau, J.E. Lock, K.J. Jenkins, A risk adjusted method for comparing adverse outcomes among practitioners in pediatric and congenital cardiac catheterization, Congenit. Heart Dis. 3 (2008) 230–240.

[17] L. Bergersen, K. Gauvreau, S.R. Foerster, A.C. Marshall, D.B. McElhinney, R.H. Beekman, R. Hirsch, J. Kreutzer, D. Balzer, J. Vincent, W.E. Hellenbrand, R. Holzer, J.P. Cheatham, J.W. Moore, G. Burch, L. Armsby, J.E. Lock, K.J. Jenkins, Catheterization for congenital heart disease adjustment for risk method (CHARM), JACC Cardiovasc. Interv. 4 (2011) 1037–1046.

[18] A.C. Glatz, N.M. Jayaram, M.L. O'Byrne, Y. Li, P.S. Chan, P.K. Sharma, L. Bergersen, J.A. Spertus, Abstract 19074: relationship between hospital procedure volume and complications following congenital cardiac catheterization: a report from the IMPACT® registry, Circulation 130 (2014) A19074. (Internet) Available from: http://circ.ahajournals.org/content/130/Suppl_2/A19074.abstract.

[19] M.L. O'Byrne, A.C. Glatz, R.T. Shinohara, N. Jayaram, M.J. Gillespie, Y. Dori, J.J. Rome, S. Kawut, Effect of center catheterization volume on risk of catastrophic adverse event after cardiac catheterization in children, Am. Heart J. 169 (2015) 823–832.e5.

[20] M.L. O'Byrne, A.C. Glatz, B.D. Hanna, R.T. Shinohara, M.J. Gillespie, Y. Dori, J.J. Rome, S.M. Kawut, Predictors of catastrophic adverse outcomes in children with pulmonary hypertension undergoing cardiac catheterization: a multi-institutional analysis from the pediatric Health information systems database, J. Am. Coll. Cardiol. 66 (2015) 1261–1269.

[21] J.F. Keane, J.E. Lock, Hemodynamic evaluation of congenital heart disease, in: J.E. Lock (Ed.), Diagnostic and Interventional Catheterization in Congenital Heart Disease, Springer, Norwell, 2000, pp. 37–72.

[22] C.E. Mullins, Hemodynamics, data acquisition, and interpretation and presentation of data, in: Cardiac Catheterization in Congenital Heart Disease, Wiley-Blackwell, Malden, 2006, pp. 272–324.

[23] C.J. Davidson, R.O. Bonow, Cardiac catheterization, in: D.L. Mann, D.P. Zipes, P. Libby, R.O. Bonow (Eds.), Braunwalds Heart Disease, Elsevier, Philadelphia, 2015, pp. 364–385.

[24] M.D. Freed, O.S. Miettinen, A.S. Nadas, Oximetric detection of intracardiac left-to-right shunts, Br. Heart J. 42 (1979) 690–694.

[25] L. Dexter, F.W. Haynes, C.S. Burwell, E.C. Eppinger, R.P. Sagerson, J.M. Evans, Studies of congenital heart disease. II. The pressure and oxygen content of blood in the right auricle, right ventricle, and pulmonary artery in control patietns, with observations on the oxygen saturation and source of pulmonary "capillary" blood, J. Clin. Investig. 26 (1947) 554–560.

[26] C.G. LaFarge, O.S. Miettinen, The estimation of oxygen consumption, Cardiovasc. Res. 4 (1970) 23–30.

[27] J.A. Goldstein, Cardiac tamponade, constrictive pericarditis, and restrictive cardiomyopathy, Curr. Probl. Cardiol. 29 (2004) 503–567.

[28] F.F. Syed, H.V. Schaff, J.K. Oh, Constrictive pericarditis–a curable diastolic heart failure, Nat. Rev. Cardiol. 11 (2014) 530–544.

[29] R. Shabetai, N.O. Fowler, W.G. Guntheroth, The hemodynamics of cardiac tamponade and constrictive pericarditis, Am. J. Cardiol. 26 (1970) 480–489.

[30] R.A. Nishimura, B.A. Carabello, Hemodynamics in the cardiac catheterization laboratory of the 21st century, Circulation 125 (2012) 2138–2150.

[31] N. Galiè, A. Torbicki, R. Barst, P. Dartevelle, S. Haworth, T. Higenbottam, H. Olschewski, A. Peacock, G. Pietra, L.J. Rubin, G. Simonneau, S.G. Priori, M.A.A. Garcia, J.-J. Blanc, A. Budaj, M. Cowie, V. Dean, J. Deckers, E.F. Burgos, J. Lekakis, B. Lindahl, G. Mazzotta, K. McGregor, J. Morais, A. Oto, O.A. Smiseth, J.A. Barbera, S. Gibbs, M. Hoeper, M. Humbert, R. Naeije, J. Pepke-Zaba, Task Force, Guidelines on diagnosis and treatment of pulmonary arterial hypertension. The task force on diagnosis and treatment of pulmonary arterial hypertension of the European Society of cardiology, Eur. Heart J. 25 (2004) 2243–2278.

[32] G. Simonneau, N. Galiè, L.J. Rubin, D. Langleben, W. Seeger, G. Domenighetti, S. Gibbs, D. Lebrec, R. Speich, M. Beghetti, R. Stuart, A. Fishman, Clinical classification of pulmonary hypertension, J. Am. Coll. Cardiol. 43 (2004) S5–S12.

[33] M.R. Costanzo, M.R. Costanzo, A. Dipchand, R. Starling, A. Anderson, M. Chan, S. Desai, S. Fedson, P. Fisher, G. Gonzales-Stawinski, L. Martinelli, D. McGiffin, F. Parisi, J. Smith, D. Taylor, B. Meiser, S. Webber, D. Baran, M. Carboni, T. Dengler, D. Feldman, M. Frigerio, A. Kfoury, D. Kim, J. Kobashigawa, M. Shullo, J. Stehlik, J. Teuteberg, P. Uber, A. Zuckermann, S. Hunt, M. Burch, G. Bhat, C. Canter, R. Chinnock, M. Crespo-Leiro, R. Delgado, F. Dobbels, K. Grady, W. Kao, J. Lamour, G. Parry, J. Patel, D. Pini, S. Pinney, J. Towbin, G. Wolfel, D. Delgado, H. Eisen, L. Goldberg, J. Hosenpud, M. Johnson, A. Keogh, C. Lewis, J. O'Connell, J. Rogers, H. Ross, S. Russell, J. Vanhaecke, The International Society of Heart and Lung Transplantation Guidelines for the care of heart transplant recipients, J. Heart Lung Transplant. 29 (2010) 914–956.

[34] C.E. Canter, R.E. Shaddy, D. Bernstein, D.T. Hsu, M.R.K. Chrisant, J.K. Kirklin, K.R. Kanter, R.S.D. Higgins, E.D. Blume, D.N. Rosenthal, M.M. Boucek, K.C. Uzark, A.H. Friedman, A.H. Friedman, J.K. Young, American Heart Association Council on Cardiovascular Disease in the Young, American Heart Association Council on Clinical Cardiology, American Heart Association Council on Cardiovascular Nursing, American Heart Association Council on Cardiovascular Surgery and Anesthesia, Quality of Care and Outcomes Research Interdisciplinary Working Group, Indications for heart transplantation in pediatric heart disease: a scientific statement from the American Heart Association Council on Cardiovascular Disease in the Young; the Councils on Clinical Cardiology, Cardiovascular Nursing, and Cardiovascular Surgery and Anesthesia; and the Quality of Care and Outcomes Research Interdisciplinary Working Group, Circulation 115 (2007) 658–676.

[35] P. Chiu, J.M. Schaffer, A.Y. Sheikh, R. Ha, O. Reinhartz, R. Mainwaring, B.A. Reitz, Elevated pretransplant pulmonary vascular resistance index does not predict mortality after isolated orthotopic heart transplantation in children: a retrospective analysis of the UNOS database, Pediatr. Transplant. 19 (2015) 623–633.

[36] P. Chiu, M.J. Russo, R.R. Davies, L.J. Addonizio, M.E. Richmond, J.M. Chen, What is high risk? Redefining elevated pulmonary vascular resistance index in pediatric heart transplantation, J. Heart Lung Transplant. 31 (2012) 61–66.

[37] G. Ofori-Amanfo, D. Hsu, J.M. Lamour, S. Mital, M.L. O'Byrne, A.J. Smerling, J.M. Chen, R. Mosca, L.J. Addonizio, Heart transplantation in children with markedly elevated pulmonary vascular resistance: impact of right ventricular failure on outcome, J. Heart Lung Transplant. 30 (2011) 659–666.

[38] A. Hoskote, C. Carter, P. Rees, M. Elliott, M. Burch, K. Brown, Acute right ventricular failure after pediatric cardiac transplant: predictors and long-term outcome in current era of transplantation medicine, J. Thorac. Cardiovasc. Surg. 139 (2010) 146–153.

[39] S.R. Auerbach, M.E. Richmond, J.M. Chen, R.S. Mosca, J.M. Quaegebeur, L.J. Addonizio, D.T. Hsu, J.M. Lamour, Multiple risk factors before pediatric cardiac transplantation are associated with increased graft loss, Pediatr. Cardiol. 33 (2011) 49–54.

[40] R.R. Davies, M.J. Russo, S. Mital, T.M. Martens, R.S. Sorabella, K.N. Hong, A.C. Gelijns, A.J. Moskowitz, J.M. Quaegebeur, R.S. Mosca, J.M. Chen, Predicting survival among high-risk pediatric cardiac transplant recipients: an analysis of the United Network for organ sharing database, J. Thorac. Cardiovasc. Surg. 135 (2008) 147–155.e2.

[41] C.J. Taylor, G. Derrick, A. McEwan, S.G. Haworth, M.R.J. Sury, Risk of cardiac catheterization under anaesthesia in children with pulmonary hypertension, Br. J. Anaesth. 98 (2007) 657–661.

[42] M.M. Hoeper, S.H. Lee, R. Voswinckel, M. Palazzini, X. Jais, A. Marinelli, R.J. Barst, H.A. Ghofrani, Z.-C. Jing, C. Opitz, H.-J. Seyfarth, M. Halank, V. McLaughlin, R.J. Oudiz, R. Ewert, H. Wilkens, S. Kluge, H.-C. Bremer, E. Baroke, L.J. Rubin, Complications of right heart catheterization procedures in patients with pulmonary hypertension in experienced centers, J. Am. Coll. Cardiol. 48 (2006) 2546–2552.

[43] K.D. Hill, D.S. Lim, A.D. Everett, D.D. Ivy, J.D. Moore, Assessment of pulmonary hypertension in the pediatric catheterization laboratory: current insights from the magic registry, Catheter. Cardiovasc. Interv. 76 (2010) 865–873.

[44] R.J. Barst, M. Beghetti, R. Berger, D. Kronmal, J. Berger, R. Geiger, G. Mallory, I. Schulze-Neick, T. Humpl, Complications related to heart catheterization (HC) in children with pulmonary hypertension (PH): factors identified from the TOPP registry (tracking outcomes and practice in pediatric PH), Am. J. Respir. Crit. Care Med. 187 (2015) A2090.

[45] M. Beghetti, R.M.F. Berger, I. Schulze-Neick, R.W. Day, T. Pulido, J. Feinstein, R.J. Barst, T. Humpl, On Behalf of the TOPP Registry Investigators, Diagnostic evaluation of paediatric pulmonary hypertension in current clinical practice, Eur. Respir. J. 42 (2013) 689–700.

[46] M.J. Carmosino, R.H. Friesen, A. Doran, D.D. Ivy, Perioperative complications in children with pulmonary hypertension undergoing noncardiac surgery or cardiac catheterization, Anesth. Analg. 104 (2007) 521–527.

[47] M. Gewillig, D.J. Goldberg, Failure of the fontan circulation, Heart Fail. Clin. 10 (2014) 105–116.

[48] M. Gewillig, S.C. Brown, B. Eyskens, R. Heying, J. Ganame, W. Budts, A. La Gerche, M. Gorenflo, The Fontan circulation: who controls cardiac output? Interact. Cardiovasc. Thorac. Surg. 10 (2010) 428–433.

[49] L.T. Cooper, K.L. Baughman, A.M. Feldman, A. Frustaci, M. Jessup, U. Kuhl, G.N. Levine, J. Narula, R.C. Starling, J. Towbin, R. Virmani, Endorsed by the Heart Failure Society of America and the Heart Failure Association of the European Society of Cardiology, The role of endomyocardial biopsy in the management of cardiovascular disease: a scientific statement from the American Heart Association, the American College of Cardiology, and the European Society of Cardiology, Circulation 116 (2007) 2216–2233.

[50] H. Bedanova, J. Necas, E. Petrikovits, P. Pokorny, S. Kovalova, P. Malik, J. Ondrasek, J. Cerny, Echo-guided endomyocardial biopsy in heart transplant recipients, Transpl. Int. 17 (2004) 622–625.

[51] A.M. Grande, G. Minzioni, L. Martinelli, C. Campana, M. Rinaldi, A.M. D'Armini, T. Ragni, C. Pederzolli, E. Ardemagni, N. Pederzolli, G. De Pieri, N. Castiglione, M. Viganò, Echo-controlled endomyocardial biopsy in orthotopic heart transplantation with bicaval anastomosis, G. Ital. Cardiol. 27 (1997) 877–880.

[52] R.S. Appleton, L.W. Miller, S. Nouri, G. Pennington, T.E. Bunchman, Endomyocardial biopsies in pediatric patients with no irradiation. Use of internal jugular venous approach and echocardiographic guidance, Transplantation 51 (1991) 309–311.

[53] S.Y. Jang, Y. Cho, J.H. Song, S.S. Cheon, S.H. Park, M.H. Bae, J.H. Lee, D.H. Yang, H.S. Park, S.C. Chae, Complication rate of transfemoral endomyocardial biopsy with fluoroscopic and two-dimensional echocardiographic guidance: a 10-year experience of 228 consecutive procedures, J. Korean Med. Sci. 28 (2013) 1323–1326.

[54] M. Scheurer, V. Bandisode, P. Ruff, A. Atz, G. Shirali, Early experience with real-time three-dimensional echocardiographic guidance of right ventricular biopsy in children, Echocardiography 0 (2015) 1–5.

[55] A.I. Fiorelli, L. Benvenuti, V. Aielo, A.Q. Coelho, J.F. Palazzo, R. Rossener, A.C.P. Barreto, C. Mady, F. Bacal, E. Bocchi, N.A.G. Stolf, Comparative analysis of the complications of 5347 endomyocardial biopsies applied to patients after heart transplantation and with cardiomyopathies: a Single-center Study, Transplant. Proc. 44 (2012) 2473–2478.

[56] M. Holzmann, A. Nicko, U. Kuhl, M. Noutsias, W. Poller, W. Hoffmann, A. Morguet, B. Witzenbichler, C. Tschope, H.P. Schultheiss, M. Pauschinger, Complication rate of right ventricular endomyocardial biopsy via the femoral approach: a retrospective and prospective study analyzing 3048 diagnostic procedures over an 11-year period, 118 (2008) 1722–1728. Available from: http://circ.ahajournals.org/cgi/doi/10.1161/CIRCULATIONAHA.107.743427.

[57] F. Saraiva, V. Matos, L. Gonçalves, M. Antunes, L.A. Providência, Complications of endomyocardial biopsy in heart transplant patients: a retrospective study of 2117 consecutive procedures, Transplant. Proc. 43 (2011) 1908–1912.

[58] K.P. Daly, A.C. Marshall, J.A. Vincent, W.A. Zuckerman, T.M. Hoffman, C.E. Canter, E.D. Blume, L. Bergersen, Endomyocardial biopsy and selective coronary angiography are low-risk procedures in pediatric heart transplant recipients: results of a multicenter experience, J. Heart Lung Transplant. 31 (2012) 398–409.

[59] S.A. Webber, G.J. Boyle, R. Jaffe, R.M. Pickering, L.B. Beerman, F.J. Fricker, Role of right ventricular endomyocardial biopsy in infants and children with suspected or possible myocarditis, Br. Heart J. 72 (1994) 360–363.

[60] T. Yoshizato, W.D. Edwards, Safety and utility of endomyocardial biopsy in infants, children and adolescents: a review of 66 procedures in 53 patients, J. Am. Coll. Cardiol. 15 (1990) 436–442.

[61] S.G. Pophal, G. Sigfusson, K.L. Booth, S.A. Bacanu, S.A. Webber, J.A. Ettedgui, W.H. Neches, S.C. Park, Complications of endomyocardial biopsy in children, J. Am. Coll. Cardiol. 34 (1999) 2105–2110. (Internet) Available from: http://eutils.ncbi.nlm.nih.gov/entrez/eutils/elink.fcgi?dbfrom=pubmed&id=10588231&retmode=ref&cmd=prlinks.

[62] D. Zhorne, C.J. Petit, F.F. Ing, H. Justino, J.L. Jefferies, W.J. Dreyer, D. Kearney, M.A. Crystal, A 25-year experience of endomyocardial biopsy safety in infants, Catheter. Cardiovasc. Interv. 82 (2013) 797–801.

[63] L.H. Chow, S.J. Radio, T.D. Sears, B.M. McManus, Insensitivity of right ventricular endomyocardial biopsy in the diagnosis of myocarditis, J. Am. Coll. Cardiol. 14 (1989) 915–920.

[64] J. Robinson, L. Hartling, B. Vandermeer, T.P. Klassen, Intravenous immunoglobulin for presumed viral myocarditis in children and adults (review), Cochrane Libr. (2015) 1–30.

[65] V.M. Blanco, S.E. Blalock, C. Ramaciotti, M. Lemler, L. Heistein, J. Moore, C. Ikemba, Oxygen supplementation is helpful for the echocardiographic detection of anomalous left coronary artery from the pulmonary artery, J. Am. Soc. Echocardiogr. 23 (2010) 1099–1102.

[66] R.K.R. Chang, V. Allada, Electrocardiographic and echocardiographic features that distinguish anomalous origin of the left coronary artery from pulmonary artery from idiopathic dilated cardiomyopathy, Pediatr. Cardiol. 22 (2001) 3–10.

[67] Y.-L. Yang, N.C. Nanda, X.-F. Wang, M.-X. Xie, Q. Lu, L. He, X.-F. Lu, Echocardiographic diagnosis of anomalous origin of the left coronary artery from the pulmonary artery, Echocardiography 24 (2007) 405–411.

Section II

Clinical Diagnosis and Management of Pediatric Heart Failure

Chapter 12

Epidemiology and Economics of Pediatric Heart Failure

Deipanjan Nandi[1], Christopher S. Almond[2], Joseph W. Rossano[1]
[1]*Perelman School of Medicine at the University of Pennsylvania, Philadelphia, PA, United States;* [2]*Stanford University, Palo Alto, CA, United States*

INTRODUCTION: CURRENT US HEALTH-CARE EXPENDITURES AND COST OF HEART DISEASE

United States (US) national health-care expenditures have been growing at approximately 5% per year over the last 5 decades, with costs in 2015 of $3 trillion yearly, and are expected to increase to more than $5 trillion by 2024 [1]. This figure represents approximately 18% of the US gross domestic product (GDP), one of the highest total expenditures in the world, compared to a global average of 9.9%. Despite the increased spending, average life span in the US remains at 78.8 years, with global life span of 70.9 years. In comparison, the Japanese life span is presently at 83 years, with 10.3% of GDP spent on health-care expenses [2]. In the industrialized world, including the US, the leading cause of death remains cardiovascular disease (CVD), and not surprisingly, almost 20% of the national health expenditure is focused on the prevention, treatment, and sequelae of CVD [3–5]. These expenditures, in addition to changes in population-level risk factors, such as decreased smoking, efforts at treating hypertension and improving lipid profiles, have reduced overall CVD prevalence and mortality significantly [6–9].

Heart failure, defined as a clinical syndrome with impaired ventricular filling or ejection of blood with inadequate end organ perfusion, is a significant subset of all CVD, representing on the order of 10% of all CVD costs. Pediatric heart failure, in lives, mortality and economic costs, has hitherto remained largely unstudied but is certainly not an insignificant part of the national CVD burden. This chapter seeks to describe the epidemiology, outcomes, and costs of pediatric heart failure within the context of the adult heart failure and the overall costs to society.

ADULT HEART FAILURE: COSTS AND EPIDEMIOLOGY

Among US patients, the prevalence of heart failure is expected to increase to 8 million adults by 2030, at a cost of $70 billion annually, accounting for approximately 10% of the costs of all CVD (Fig. 12.1) [4,10]. Heart failure admissions make up 1%–2% of all hospitalizations in the US and are responsible for significant mortality [11]. In the US and other western countries, the majority of heart failure in adults can be traced to ischemic heart disease and hypertension, driven by the rise in obesity, insulin resistance, and associated heightened inflammatory states [12]. Cardiomyopathies play an important role as well, with recent data supporting as high an incidence of hypertrophic cardiomyopathy (HCM) as 1 in 200 in the US, a significant proportion of which is found in adulthood [13]. The prevalence of other genetic or infectious cardiomyopathies is less well studied.

PEDIATRIC HEART FAILURE: EPIDEMIOLOGY AND OUTCOMES

Heart failure in the pediatric setting stems from a heterogeneous set of diagnoses, including congenital heart disease (CHD), cardiomyopathies, rhythm disorders, and acquired heart diseases secondary to infection, chemotherapeutic exposure, or coronary inflammation (Kawasaki disease) [14,15]. Each of these diagnoses carries variable outcomes and prognoses, but some statements can be made about the pediatric heart failure population as a whole. These children face substantial mortality and morbidity, with significant rates of hospitalization, readmission, and disability. Patients often have long, complicated hospital stays, during which they can develop life-threatening comorbidities, including respiratory failure, renal failure, and sepsis, which substantially increase their risk of in-hospital mortality, compared to patients without heart failure (Fig. 12.2). Mortality for patients hospitalized with heart failure in 2009 was 6.7%, compared to other hospitalized pediatric patients

Heart Failure in the Child and Young Adult. http://dx.doi.org/10.1016/B978-0-12-802393-8.00012-0

FIGURE 12.1 The projected increase in direct and indirect costs attributable to heart failure from 2012 to 2030 is displayed. Direct costs (cost of medical care) are expected to increase at a faster rate than indirect costs because of lost productivity and early mortality. *(Reproduced from P.A. Heidenreich, N.M. Albert, L.A. Allen, et al, Forecasting the impact of heart failure in the United States: a policy statement from the American Heart Association. Circ. Heart Fail. 6 (2013) 606–619. Circ. Heart Fail. published by Wolters Kluwer Health/ Lippincott Williams Wilkins – STM Association member and signatory, listed as "notification required," website: http://www.journals.lww.com.)*

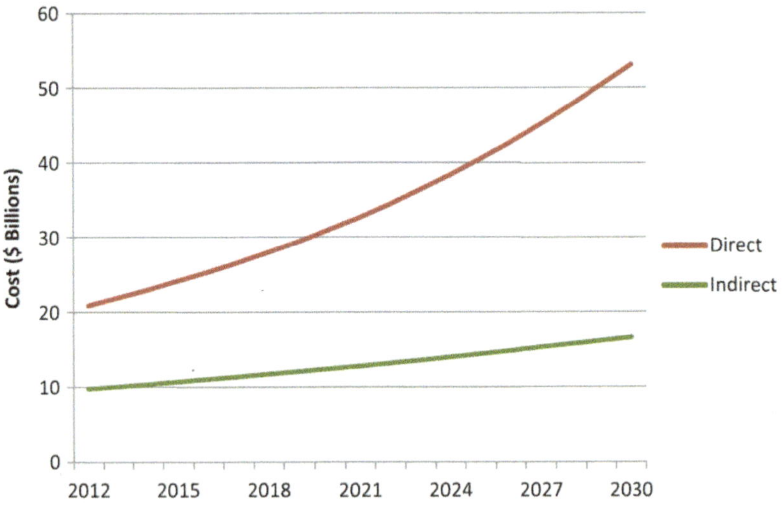

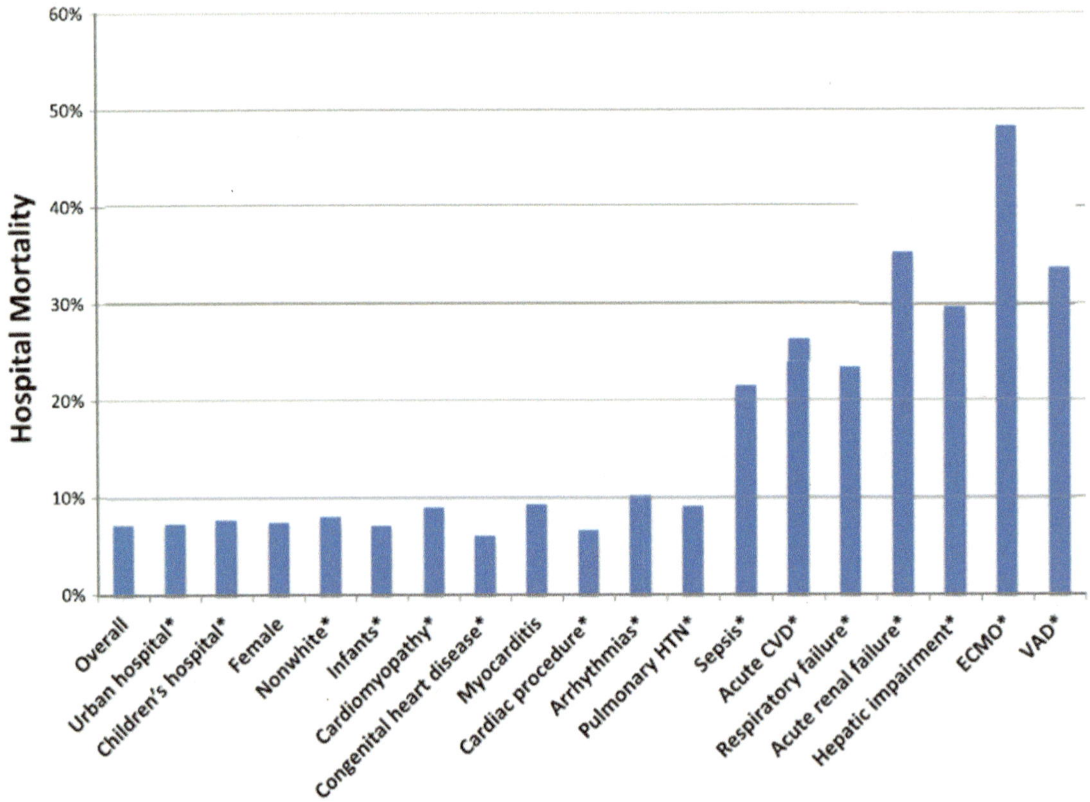

FIGURE 12.2 Hospital mortality for children with heart failure-related hospitalizations. *Factor associated with increased hospital mortality (*P* less than 0.05). *CVD*, cardiovascular disease; *ECMO*, extracorporeal membrane oxygenation; *HTN*, hypertension; *VAD*, ventricular assist device. *(Reproduced from J.W. Rossano, et al, Prevalence, morbidity, and mortality of heart failure–related hospitalizations in children in the United States: A Population-Based Study. J. Card. Fail. 18 (2012) 459–470. J. Card. Fail. published by Elsevier, STM Association member and signatory, listed as Notification not required, "automatic process." Also, Rossano is author.)*

with a 0.4% mortality rate [16]. The mortality rate for infants hospitalized with heart failure is even higher, at approximately 11% [17]. However, there has been a decrease in overall inpatient mortality over time, at least among patients with cardiomyopathy [17]. This may be due to advances in supportive therapies, and with somewhat improved survival, there has also been a rise in the prevalence of comorbidities, including respiratory and renal failure, contributing to increased morbidity in these patients [18].

Congenital Heart Disease

Approximately 50%–65% of all heart failure hospitalizations for Belgian and American children are associated with CHD, lending credence to the idea that CHD is the most common etiology of pediatric heart failure [16,19]. CHD leading to failure can vary widely, from so-called "simple" lesions such as ventricular septal defects to the "complex" conditions such as univentricular physiologies. Some "simple" lesions can lend themselves to curative correction, such as a surgical intervention to close a septal defect, while "complex" lesions may be treatable with only palliative interventions, with progressive and chronic heart failure being resultant. It is estimated that 10%–14% of univentricular physiology admissions are complicated by heart failure, with frequent need for mechanical circulatory support and/or heart transplantation [20]. Of note, most types of CHD are diagnosed during infancy, thus accounting for the higher percentage of heart failure admissions among children less than 1 year of age, approximately 55%–60% [16].

As would be expected for such a heterogeneous group of patients, outcomes vary as widely as the individual lesions. Univentricular patients have a higher rate of mortality at 12% compared to their biventricular CHD counterparts at 7.9% as well as higher rates of comorbidity [20]. Furthermore, although most pediatric heart transplants overall occur in cases of dilated cardiomyopathy (DCM), the majority of transplants performed among children in the first year of life occur in those with underlying CHD [21].

Cardiomyopathies

The myriad etiologies leading to a cardiomyopathy can be categorized as primary or acquired, and several etiologies will be discussed in detail below. However, the overall incidence of primary cardiomyopathies in children is an estimated 1.13–1.24 cases per 100,000. The highest incidence is in infancy, with cardiomyopathy being observed between 7.84 and 8.34 cases per 100,000 infants less than 1 year of age [22,23]. A study from the United Kingdom demonstrated an incidence of new-onset heart failure of 0.87 per 100,000 in patients younger than 16-years old diagnosed with cardiomyopathy, inclusive of DCM, HCM, and secondary causes such as myocarditis, anthracycline-induced cardiomyopathy, and arrhythmia [24]. It should be noted that cardiomyopathy is not necessarily synonymous with the clinical entity of heart failure, but rather that a cardiomyopathy certainly increases the risk of progression toward heart failure. Furthermore, such rate of progression is again dependent on the underlying condition. For example, only 13% of those with HCM present with heart failure, as compared to 71% of children with DCM [25]. Several major forms of cardiomyopathy are reviewed below.

Cardiomyopathy: Dilated

DCM is the most common cardiomyopathy diagnosed in childhood and the leading indication for pediatric heart transplantation [26]. The incidence of DCM has been reported as 0.57–0.76 per 100,000 [22–24]. However, this is likely an underestimate of the true burden of disease due to DCM given that many patients may go unrecognized until later in the disease course. The etiology of DCM is itself somewhat diverse. In one study from the Pediatric Cardiomyopathy Registry when a cause of DCM was found, myocarditis (46%) was the most common etiology, followed by neuromuscular disease (26%); however, the majority of cases were without an identifiable diagnosis and deemed idiopathic (66%) [25]. Inborn errors of metabolism and inherited familial cardiomyopathies comprised only 3% and 4% of all cases, respectively.

These patients have substantial morbidity and mortality, especially in the period just after DCM is diagnosed. In the United Kingdom experience, by 1 year after diagnosis, approximately 34% of patients experienced cardiac transplantation or death [24]. This is similar to the Australian and American experience, which found similar rates of mortality and transplantation at, respectively, 29% and 31% [27].After this initial period of more significant risk, the yearly event rate for transplant or death drops significantly to 1% [28]. However, as most of these events are transplantation, the natural history without transplantation is difficult to assess. Some proportion of these events are due to sudden death, with a 5-year incidence of sudden death in pediatric patients with DCM of approximately 3% based on data from the Pediatric Cardiomyopathy Registry [29] and 5% at 15-year follow-up in the Australian registry [30]. Despite these relatively high rates of mortality and morbidity, it is important to note that many pediatric patients with DCM who present with significant ventricular dysfunction will have significant improvement over time with a substantial minority of patients experiencing normalization of function [31,32]. Except for myocarditis, which can resolve within 1–2 weeks, the recovery time period for DCM can vary from as little as 6 months to as long as 2 years after initial presentation with heart failure (Fig. 12.3) [28,33,34].

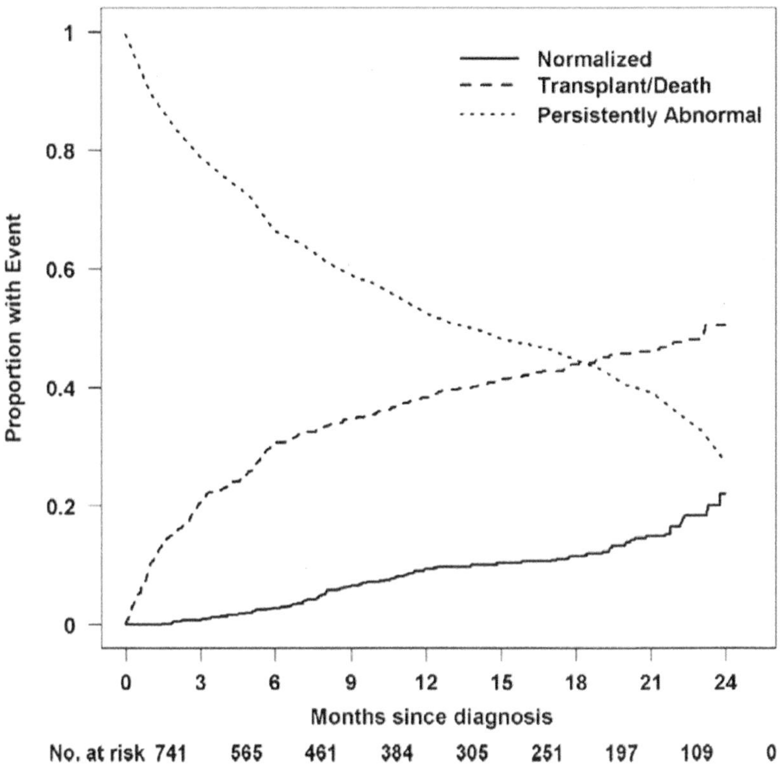

FIGURE 12.3 Cumulative incidence of echocardiographic normalization in children with idiopathic dilated cardiomyopathy (N=741), in the presence of the competing risk for death or transplantation. At any given time point, the estimated cumulative incidence rates associated with the 3 states totals to 1.0. At 2 years, 22% of children had normal echocardiographic values, 51% had died or undergone transplantation, and 27% remained abnormal with respect to left ventricular size and function. *(Reproduced from M.D. Everitt, L.A. Sleeper, M. Lu, et al, Recovery of echocardiographic function in children with idiopathic dilated cardiomyopathy. J. Am. Coll. Cardiol. 63 (14) (2014) 1405–1413, http://dx.doi.org/10.1016/j.jacc.2013.11.059. JACC published by Elsevier, STM Association member and signatory, listed as Notification not required, "automatic process." Also, Rossano is author.)*

Cardiomyopathy: Hypertrophic

HCM is one of the most common of all heart defects, with a prevalence ranging from 1 in 200 to 1 in 500 in the US, although many patients may remain unaware of their diagnoses for some time [13,35]. HCM can have diverse etiologies as well, although a cause was only found in roughly a quarter of patients in one study, with roughly equal distribution among malformation syndromes, inborn errors of metabolism, and neuromuscular disorders [36].

As noted previously, a cardiomyopathy diagnosis does not mean necessarily heart failure, and it is estimated that only 13% of patients with HCM present with heart failure [36]. This is particularly important, in that outcomes for HCM patients seem to vary directly with heart failure status and age at presentation, as well as the underlying cause. Presentation with heart failure at time of diagnosis, regardless of age or cause, is itself associated with a higher rate of death or transplantation [37]. Infants with idiopathic hypertrophy diagnosed prior to 1 year of age have a 15% 1-year mortality, compared to a 1% 1-year mortality for those diagnosed after 1 year of age [37]. For all those with idiopathic HCM surviving 1 year from diagnosis, the mortality rate is relatively stable at 1% annually. Those HCM patients with an underlying neuromuscular disorder have relatively good short-term outcomes, with an initial 98% 5-year survival rate. Yet, mortality increases substantially into the second decade of life [36]. Those with HCM secondary to malformation syndromes or inborn errors of metabolism have poor initial outcomes in comparison with 5-year survival rates as low as 74% and 41%, respectively. Of course, there is also a continued mortality risk attributable to sudden death. The risk of sudden death for all patients with HCM was 6% over a mean follow-up period of 8 years in an American cohort [38] and 6% at 15-years follow-up in an Australian cohort [30].

Cardiomyopathy: Other Types

Restrictive cardiomyopathy (RCM) accounts for less than 5% of all cardiomyopathies in the Pediatric Cardiomyopathy Registry [39]. The overall incidence of RCM by the Australian registry was 0.03 cases per 100,000 children [23]. RCM can present as a pure form in approximately two-thirds of all cases, or with hypertrophic features, commonly called mixed restrictive-HCM, accounting for the remaining one-third.

Reported 1-year and 5-year survival rates for the pure RCM and mixed RCM/HCM phenotypes are, respectively, 20% and 32%. Patients with a mixed phenotype are less likely to go on to require heart transplantation, compared to those with pure RCM [39]. Many centers consider listing for transplantation at the time of diagnosis the poor outcomes and inability to accurately risk stratify patients. There is limited understanding of the efficacy of conventional medical therapy or for the utility of ventricular assist devices (VADs), although some centers have reported some success with continuous flow VADs with restrictive patients [40].

Secondary cardiomyopathies and heart failure can occur from a variety of causes, including exposure to chemotherapy. Anthracyclines in particular are associated with acute and chronic heart failure. Acute decrement in ventricular function occurs in less than 1% of patients and is often reversible. Beyond the acute phase, heart failure has been found to occur within the first year of exposure at a rate of 1.6%–2.1% of patients within the first year of therapy but may also develop beyond a year after exposure, in as many as 2%–5% of patients [41]. Outcomes for these patients are not well delineated. There are limited other data regarding incidence or prevalence of other forms of acquired cardiomyopathy or heart failure, such as secondary to thyroid disease, Kawasaki disease, and acquired or anatomic coronary disease.

PEDIATRIC HEART FAILURE: COSTS

As noted above, the expected annual cost of heart failure in adults is forecast to increase to $70 billion by 2030 or 10% of all adult health-care costs. It is clear that the prevalence, poor outcomes, and complex therapies afforded the pediatric population and will similarly yield a high overall burden of cost. However, the heterogeneity of etiology, severity, and outcomes, noted above, makes a concrete study of the economics of this population and diagnosis particularly difficult to approximate. While the total cost is unknown, current cost data and the state of this field of study are described below.

Costs of Inpatient Admissions

US pediatric heart failure hospitalizations in 2009 averaged just over $70,000 in charges. With over 14,000 pediatric heart failure admissions yearly, this yields $1 billion in yearly charges for inpatient charges alone [16,17].

Length of stay is a major driver of increasing hospital charges. Stays longer than 18 days in pediatric heart failure hospitalizations have in the past been associated with 20-fold higher charges compared to lengths of stay of less than or equal to 4 days [17]. Inpatient admissions stays have increased over the last decade by almost 2 days from an average of 15 days in 2000 to 17 days in 2009. Infants, who comprise the greatest proportion of pediatric heart failure patients, have particularly long lengths of stay, average 26 days per admission in 2009 [17,18]. Indirect costs of these admissions are not accounted for fully; indeed, these admissions represent more than 240,000 inpatient hospital days for children, with substantial missed school days and parental work days, posing a significant burden to society. Of course, the other driver of cost is the increasing complexity of the care of these patients. Comorbidities have increased over time, likely reflecting our ability to treat patients successfully through the acute phase of their disease to reach a chronic and/or relapsing phase of disease where they can accrue multiple comorbidities. The presence of renal failure, respiratory failure, and stroke are each independently associated with two- to threefold increase in mean charges per hospitalization.

Costs of Outpatient Care

Inpatient costs likely reflect only a fraction of the total costs of heart failure. Necessarily, inpatient costs do not reflect the costs associated prior to diagnosis, namely that of screening. The Heart Failure Society of America has clear guidelines in place for the screening of first-degree family members of patients with cardiomyopathies with a suspected genetic basis, which include genetic testing, echocardiograms, electrocardiograms, and exercise testing, although the costs of this screening are largely unknown [42]. Genetic testing may have significant downstream cost and other effect on not only affected patients and family members but also on unaffected patients.

Once diagnosed, patients undergo routine examinations by cardiologists, frequent laboratory testing, and echocardiograms and may require cardiac MRI or catheterization. As noted above, heart failure patients have had increasing rates of comorbidities, which require further visits to specialty clinics (Nephrology, Pulmonology, Neurology to name a few) or therapeutic centers (i.e., hemodialysis). Patients also have significant use of emergency care, and pediatric heart failure visits have approximately twofold higher emergency care charges than those without heart failure [43]. At the present time, the scope of these additional costs has not been fully explored.

Specific Heart Failure Therapies

In the rapidly changing landscape of care for pediatric patients with heart failure, specific therapies warrant special mention. Heart transplantation for instance continues to advance, with more than 500 pediatric heart transplants performed internationally in each of the last 3 years [21]. The mean hospital charge for heart transplantation was $450,000 in 2009 [44]. This would yield nearly $250 million in transplant hospitalization charges annually. The cost (as opposed to charge) of the lifelong care of these complex patients has estimated at roughly $465,000 for primary transplant and $380,000 for retransplant [45]. Outcomes for heart transplantation have grown more favorable over time as well [46,47].

Mechanical circulatory support for pediatric patients with heart failure has grown substantially over time, first with the use of extracorporeal membrane oxygenation (ECMO) support and, increasingly, with the use of VADs. Charges associated with ECMO and VAD use are high, as much as $450,000 for hospitalizations, which require them, independent of transplant costs [18]. Newer generation VADs have had increasingly favorable risk–benefit profiles, especially in comparison to ECMO as bridge to transplantation [48,49]. As VADs continue to improve, there has also been greater use of VADs as destination therapy, rather than as bridge to transplantation, although the costs and value of this indication have not yet been fully explored.

Exploring Value in Pediatric Heart Failure

There has been a shift in recent years to provide not only effective care for patients but also in maximizing this care while minimizing costs to patients, payors, and health-care systems. This first necessitated the definition of cost-effective care, using quality-adjusted life years (QALYs) as a measure of effectiveness. QALYs seek to describe the impact of disease not only in terms of years of life lost (mortality) but also years of life lived with suboptimal quality. For instance, patients with HCM suffer from sudden cardiac death, but frequently also suffer from heart failure, worry regarding sudden death, poor quality of life from sequelae of medicines, implantable cardioverter-defibrillators (ICDs), inappropriate shocks, etc. One study of ICDs in adult patients with HCM estimated that ICDs increased quality-adjusted survival by 4.7 QALYs over a lifetime [50]. Cost-per-QALY calculations are thus frequently used to compare and justify costs of therapies, although the use of QALYs in pediatric populations can be very difficult from a methodological perspective [51]. Recent efforts in pediatric heart failure have specifically found that pediatric heart transplantation and VADs cost between $50,000 and $100,000 per QALY, and justifiably spent health care dollars, similar in cost per QALY for renal replacement therapy and adult heart transplantation [45,52,53]. Adult ICDs in HCM are estimated to cost $30,000 per QALY, while ICDs in children with DCM have been estimated to cost $280,000 per QALY, suggesting that ICDs may not be as cost-effective in this population [50,54].

While cost-effectiveness studies allow for comparisons of therapies, they do not necessarily demonstrate the value of treatment. Value has been defined previously as the effect achieved per unit of cost and can be considered an inverse proposition of cost-effectiveness [55]. Thus, value optimization necessitates cost reduction, outcome improvement, or both. With inpatient mortality decreasing over time for pediatric heart failure patients, but with higher rates of morbidity (see Fig. 12.4), and increasing costs, it is unlikely that the field of pediatric heart failure is meeting the value proposition.

Barriers to Understanding Costs and Value

The vast degree of data for pediatric heart failure costs is derived from administrative database analyses of charges, necessarily a proxy of actual costs. Also, these databases are for hospital-associated care (inpatient and emergency department) and thus are incomplete estimates. Indirect costs to society from educational loss, missed parental work days, and opportunity costs have never been described in the literature. Without prospective study of heart failure outcomes across health-care settings and incorporation of quality-of-life indicators, our estimates of mortality and morbidity remain simply estimates.

However, even with perfect knowledge of the costs and outcomes associated with heart failure and its treatment, optimizing value for this population would be difficult given the high variability of the care afforded these patients. It is well established that great variability in treatment and complication rates exists in congenital heart surgery, with resultant variability in cost [56–58]. When variability exists in treatment, it becomes difficult to assess what parts of that care are associated with the costs, especially with the complex levels of care, such as exists in congenital heart surgery and pediatric heart failure treatments. Variability in pediatric heart failure treatment has begun to be assessed, with recent analysis demonstrating variability in the treatment of myocarditis, with some US centers never using intravenous immunoglobulin, while one center used in 96% of all cases [59]. Similarly, with variability among centers regarding the timing of VAD placement or listing for transplant in pediatric patients, it is difficult to assess the value of these disparate strategies [60].

Future Directions

We must as a field move toward greater understanding of the value of care obtained for pediatric heart failure patients. At a minimum, a greater understanding of outpatient costs of treatment and current screening strategies must be explored.

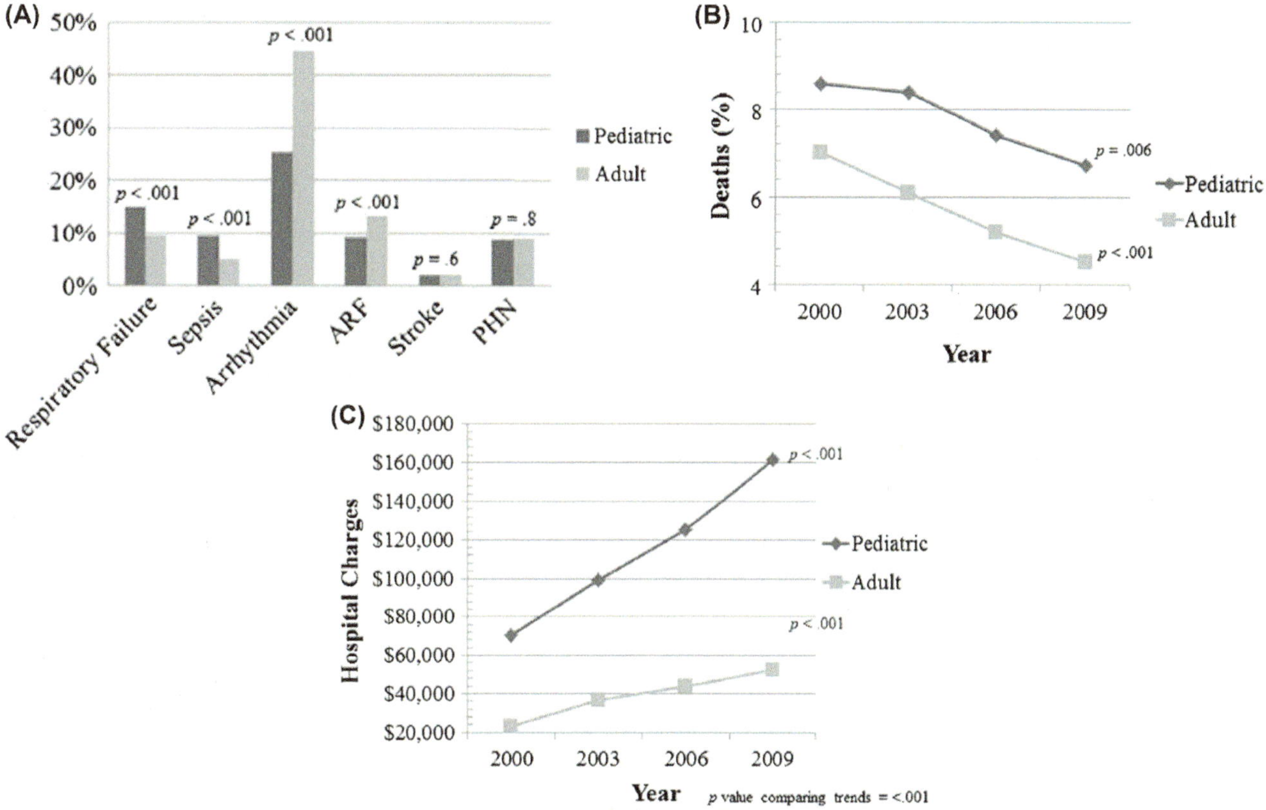

FIGURE 12.4 (A) Frequency of comorbidities occurring during pediatric and adult cardiomyopathy and heart failure hospitalizations; (B) Mortality (as a percentage of the cohort) over time for pediatric and adult cardiomyopathy and heart failure hospitalizations according to year; (C) Hospital charges over time for pediatric and adult cardiomyopathy and heart failure hospitalizations according to year. *ARF*, acute renal failure; *PHN*, pulmonary hypertension. *(Reproduced from C.A. Wittlieb-Weber, et al, Pediatric versus adult cardiomyopathy and heart failure–related hospitalizations: a value-based analysis. J. Card. Fail. 21 (2015) 76–82. J. Car. Fail. published by Elsevier, STM Association member and signator, listed as Notification not required, "automatic process." Also, Rossano is author.)*

Without understanding the quality of life we are incurring for our patients, we may be worsening the value our patients derive, despite our best intentions. Practice variability, within and among centers, is likely driving not only variability in costs but also hampering our ability to understand more subtly the drivers of cost and which parts of our care are adding value.

CONCLUSION

Pediatric heart failure is relatively rare, but with increasing use of national cardiomyopathy and heart failure registries, we have a greater understanding of the incidence and epidemiology of these varied diseases. Mortality rates are relatively low at 6%–7% overall, and with the advent of medical and advanced mechanical therapies, mortality is decreasing. However, this is at significant cost of more than $70,000 per admission, and almost $450,000 for admissions requiring mechanical support or heart transplant, with more than $1 billion in-hospital charges alone, without current meaningful estimates of the cost of outpatient therapies. With decreasing mortality, there is also increasing morbidity, with greater rates of respiratory and renal and neurologic complications. It is difficult to assess the value that our patients receive from their care. The assessment of care and value is complicated by the high variability in the application of advanced therapies. We must endeavor to understand more fully the costs, outcomes, and variability of care in the treatment of these complex patients.

REFERENCES

[1] S.P. Keehan, G.A. Cuckler, A.M. Sisko, A.J. Madison, S.D. Smith, D.A. Stone, et al., National health expenditure projections, 2014–24: spending growth faster than recent trends, Health Aff. (Millwood) 34 (8) (2015) 1407–1417.

[2] (Internet), Health | Data, November 11, 2015. Available from: http://data.worldbank.org/topic/health.

[3] D.L. Hoyert, (US) NC for HS, et al., 75 Years of Mortality in the United States, 1935–2010(Internet) US Department of Health and Human Services, Centers for Disease Control and Prevention, National Center for Health Statistics, 2012. Available from: http://stacks.cdc.gov/view/cdc/11884/cdc_11884_DS1.pdf.

[4] P.A. Heidenreich, J.G. Trogdon, O.A. Khavjou, J. Butler, K. Dracup, M.D. Ezekowitz, et al., Forecasting the future of cardiovascular disease in the United States: a policy statement from the American Heart Association, Circulation 123 (8) (March 1, 2011) 933–944.

[5] J.G. Trogdon, E.A. Finkelstein, I.A. Nwaise, F.K. Tangka, D. Orenstein, The economic burden of chronic cardiovascular disease for major insurers, Health Promot. Pract. 8 (3) (July 1, 2007) 234–242.

[6] E.S. Ford, U.A. Ajani, J.B. Croft, J.A. Critchley, D.R. Labarthe, T.E. Kottke, et al., Explaining the decrease in U.S. deaths from coronary disease, 1980–2000, N. Engl. J. Med. 356 (23) (June 7, 2007) 2388–2398.

[7] D.C. Goff, G. Howard, G.B. Russell, D.R. Labarthe, Birth cohort evidence of population influences on blood pressure in the United States, 1887–1994, Ann. Epidemiol. 11 (4) (May 2001) 271–279.

[8] D.C. Goff, D.R. Labarthe, G. Howard, G.B. Russell, Primary prevention of high blood cholesterol concentrations in the United States, Arch. Intern. Med. 162 (8) (April 22, 2002) 913–919.

[9] Dietary fat and its relation to heart attacks and strokes. Report by the Central Committee for Medical and Community Program of the American Heart Association, JAMA 175 (February 4, 1961) 389–391.

[10] P.A. Heidenreich, N.M. Albert, L.A. Allen, D.A. Bluemke, J. Butler, G.C. Fonarow, et al., Forecasting the impact of heart failure in the United States: a policy statement from the American Heart Association, Circ. Heart Fail. 6 (3) (May 2013) 606–619.

[11] A.P. Ambrosy, G.C. Fonarow, J. Butler, O. Chioncel, S.J. Greene, M. Vaduganathan, et al., The global health and economic burden of hospitalizations for heart failure, J. Am. Coll. Cardiol. 63 (12) (April 2014) 1123–1133.

[12] D.S. Frankel, R.S. Vasan, R.B. D'Agostino, E.J. Benjamin, D. Levy, T.J. Wang, et al., Resistin, adiponectin, and risk of heart failure, J. Am. Coll. Cardiol. 53 (9) (March 2009) 754–762.

[13] C. Semsarian, J. Ingles, M.S. Maron, B.J. Maron, New perspectives on the prevalence of hypertrophic cardiomyopathy, J. Am. Coll. Cardiol. 65 (12) (March 2015) 1249–1254.

[14] A. Damasceno, B.M. Mayosi, M. Sani, O.S. Ogah, C. Mondo, D. Ojji, et al., The causes, treatment, and outcome of acute heart failure in 1006 Africans from 9 countries, Arch. Intern. Med. 172 (18) (October 8, 2012) 1386–1394.

[15] J.W. Rossano, R.E. Shaddy, Heart failure in children: etiology and treatment, J. Pediatr. 165 (2) (August 2014) 228–233.

[16] J.W. Rossano, J.J. Kim, J.A. Decker, J.F. Price, F. Zafar, D.E. Graves, et al., Prevalence, morbidity, and mortality of heart failure-related hospitalizations in children in the United States: a population-based study, J. Card. Fail. 18 (6) (June 2012) 459–470.

[17] C.A. Wittlieb-Weber, K.Y. Lin, T.E. Zaoutis, M.J. O'Connor, K. Gerald, S.M. Paridon, et al., Pediatric versus adult cardiomyopathy and heart failure–related hospitalizations: a value-based analysis, J. Card. Fail. 21 (1) (January 2015) 76–82.

[18] D. Nandi, K. Lin, M. O'Connor, O. Elci, J. Kim, J. Decker, et al., Hospital charges for pediatric heart failure related hospitalization admissions in the United States from 2000 to 2009, J. Am. Coll. Cardiol. 63 (12) (April 1, 2014). (Internet) Available from: http://dx.doi.org/10.1016/S0735-1097(14)60601-X.

[19] M.M. Massin, I. Astadicko, H. Dessy, Epidemiology of heart failure in a tertiary pediatric center, Clin. Cardiol. 31 (8) (August 2008) 388–391.

[20] J.W. Rossano, D.J. Goldberg, A.R. Mott, J.W. Gaynor, K.Y. Lin, C.B. Falkensammer, et al., The burden of heart failure related hospitalizations in children with single ventricle heart disease in the United States (abstract), Circulation 126 (21 Suppl.) (November 20, 2012) A11975.

[21] A.I. Dipchand, L.B. Edwards, A.Y. Kucheryavaya, C. Benden, F. Dobbels, B.J. Levvey, et al., The registry of the international society for heart and lung transplantation: seventeenth official pediatric heart transplantation report-2014; focus theme: retransplantation, J. Heart Lung Transpl. 33 (10) (October 2014) 985–995.

[22] S.E. Lipshultz, L.A. Sleeper, J.A. Towbin, A.M. Lowe, E.J. Orav, G.F. Cox, et al., The incidence of pediatric cardiomyopathy in two regions of the United States, N. Engl. J. Med. 348 (17) (April 24, 2003) 1647–1655.

[23] A.W. Nugent, P.E. Daubeney, P. Chondros, J.B. Carlin, M. Cheung, L.C. Wilkinson, et al., The epidemiology of childhood cardiomyopathy in Australia, N. Engl. J. Med. 348 (17) (2003) 1639–1646.

[24] R.E. Andrews, M.J. Fenton, D.A. Ridout, M. Burch, British Congenital Cardiac Association, New-onset heart failure due to heart muscle disease in childhood: a prospective study in the United Kingdom and Ireland, Circulation 117 (1) (January 1, 2008) 79–84.

[25] J.D. Wilkinson, D.C. Landy, S.D. Colan, J.A. Towbin, L.A. Sleeper, E.J. Orav, et al., The pediatric cardiomyopathy registry and heart failure: key results from the first 15 years, Heart Fail. Clin. 6 (4) (October 2010) 401–413.

[26] A.E. Tsirka, K. Trinkaus, S.C. Chen, S.E. Lipshultz, J.A. Towbin, S.D. Colan, et al., Improved outcomes of pediatric dilated cardiomyopathy with utilization of heart transplantation, J. Am. Coll. Cardiol. 44 (2) (July 21, 2004) 391–397.

[27] J.A. Towbin, A.M. Lowe, S.D. Colan, L.A. Sleeper, E.J. Orav, S. Clunie, et al., Incidence, causes, and outcomes of dilated cardiomyopathy in children, JAMA 296 (15) (October 18, 2006) 1867–1876.

[28] P.M.A. Alexander, P.E.F. Daubeney, A.W. Nugent, K.J. Lee, C. Turner, S.D. Colan, et al., Long-term outcomes of dilated cardiomyopathy diagnosed during childhood: results from a national population-based study of childhood cardiomyopathy, Circulation 128 (18) (October 29, 2013) 2039–2046.

[29] E. Pahl, L.A. Sleeper, C.E. Canter, D.T. Hsu, M. Lu, S.A. Webber, et al., Incidence of and risk factors for sudden cardiac death in children with dilated cardiomyopathy, J. Am. Coll. Cardiol. 59 (6) (February 2012) 607–615.

[30] T. Bharucha, K.J. Lee, P.E.F. Daubeney, A.W. Nugent, C. Turner, G.F. Sholler, et al., Sudden death in childhood cardiomyopathy, J. Am. Coll. Cardiol. 65 (21) (June 2015) 2302–2310.

[31] M.D. Everitt, L.A. Sleeper, M. Lu, C.E. Canter, E. Pahl, J.D. Wilkinson, et al., Recovery of echocardiographic function in children with idiopathic dilated cardiomyopathy, J. Am. Coll. Cardiol. 63 (14) (April 2014) 1405–1413.

[32] R.E. Shaddy, M.M. Boucek, D.T. Hsu, R.J. Boucek, C.E. Canter, L. Mahony, et al., Carvedilol for children and adolescents with heart failure: a randomized controlled trial, JAMA 298 (10) (September 12, 2007) 1171–1179.

[33] P.E. Daubeney, A.W. Nugent, P. Chondros, J.B. Carlin, S.D. Colan, M. Cheung, et al., Clinical features and outcomes of childhood dilated cardiomyopathy: results from a national population-based study, Circulation 114 (24) (December 12, 2006) 2671–2678.

[34] J.J. O'Sullivan, S.L. Roche, D.S. Crossland, M.P. Chaudhari, R.C. Kirk, H. Asif, Recovery of heart function in children with acute severe heart failure, Transplantation 85 (7) (April 15, 2008) 975–979.

[35] B.J. Maron, W.J. McKenna, G.K. Danielson, L.J. Kappenberger, H.J. Kuhn, C.E. Seidman, et al., American College of Cardiology/European Society of Cardiology clinical expert consensus document on hypertrophic cardiomyopathy, J. Am. Coll. Cardiol. 42 (9) (November 2003) 1687–1713.

[36] S.D. Colan, S.E. Lipshultz, A.M. Lowe, L.A. Sleeper, J. Messere, G.F. Cox, et al., Epidemiology and cause-specific outcome of hypertrophic cardiomyopathy in children: findings from the pediatric cardiomyopathy registry, Circulation 115 (6) (February 13, 2007) 773–781.

[37] S.E. Lipshultz, E.J. Orav, J.D. Wilkinson, J.A. Towbin, J.E. Messere, A.M. Lowe, et al., Risk stratification at diagnosis for children with hypertrophic cardiomyopathy: an analysis of data from the Pediatric Cardiomyopathy Registry, Lancet 382 (9908) (2013) 1889–1897.

[38] B.J. Maron, I. Olivotto, P. Spirito, S.A. Casey, P. Bellone, T.E. Gohman, et al., Epidemiology of hypertrophic cardiomyopathy-related death: revisited in a large non-referral-based patient population, Circulation 102 (8) (August 22, 2000) 858–864.

[39] S.A. Webber, S.E. Lipshultz, L.A. Sleeper, M. Lu, J.D. Wilkinson, L.J. Addonizio, et al., Outcomes of restrictive cardiomyopathy in childhood and the influence of phenotype: a report from the Pediatric Cardiomyopathy Registry, Circulation 126 (10) (September 4, 2012) 1237–1244.

[40] A. Grupper, S.J. Park, N.L. Pereira, S.D. Schettle, Y. Gerber, Y. Topilsky, et al., Role of ventricular assist therapy for patients with heart failure and restrictive physiology: improving outcomes for a lethal disease, J. Heart Lung Transplant. (March 26, 2015).

[41] K.A. Wouters, L.C.M. Kremer, T.L. Miller, E.H. Herman, S.E. Lipshultz, Protecting against anthracycline-induced myocardial damage: a review of the most promising strategies, Br. J. Haematol. 131 (5) (December 2005) 561–578.

[42] R.E. Hershberger, J. Lindenfeld, L. Mestroni, C.E. Seidman, M.R. Taylor, J.A. Towbin, et al., Genetic evaluation of cardiomyopathy–a Heart Failure Society of America practice guideline, J. Card. Fail. 15 (2) (March 2009) 83–97.

[43] E. Mejia, M.J. O'Connor, K.Y. Lin, C.E. Mascio, A.J. Donoghue, C. Ravishankar, et al., Characteristics and Outcomes of Pediatric Heart Failure Related Emergency Department Visits in the United States: A Population-Based Study (2015 AAP National Conference and Exhibition)(Internet) American Academy of Pediatrics National Conference and Exhbition, October 23, 2015. Available from: https://aap.confex.com/aap/2015/webprogrampress/Paper28465.html.

[44] S.P. Law, J.J. Kim, J.A. Decker, J.F. Price, A.G. Cabrera, D.E. Graves, et al., Hospital charges for pediatric heart transplant hospitalizations in the United States from 1997 to 2006, J. Heart Lung Transpl. 31 (5) (May 2012) 485–491.

[45] J.D. Dayton, K.R. Kanter, R.N. Vincent, W.T. Mahle, Cost-effectiveness of pediatric heart transplantation, J. Heart Lung Transpl. 25 (4) (April 2006) 409–415.

[46] C.S. Almond, K. Gauvreau, C.E. Canter, S.K. Rajagopal, G.E. Piercey, T.P. Singh, A risk-prediction model for in-hospital mortality after heart transplantation in US children: risk prediction in pediatric heart transplant, Am. J. Transplant. 12 (5) (May 2012) 1240–1248.

[47] K.R. Schumacher, C. Almond, T.P. Singh, R. Kirk, R. Spicer, T.M. Hoffman, et al., Predicting graft loss by 1 year in pediatric heart transplantation candidates: an analysis of the pediatric heart transplant study database, Circulation 131 (10) (March 10, 2015) 890–898.

[48] C.S. Almond, T.P. Singh, K. Gauvreau, G.E. Piercey, F. Fynn-Thompson, P.T. Rycus, et al., Extracorporeal membrane oxygenation for bridge to heart transplantation among children in the United States: analysis of data from the Organ Procurement and Transplant Network and Extracorporeal Life Support Organization Registry, Circulation 123 (25) (June 28, 2011) 2975–2984.

[49] D.L.S. Morales, C.S.D. Almond, R.D.B. Jaquiss, D.N. Rosenthal, D.C. Naftel, M.P. Massicotte, et al., Bridging children of all sizes to cardiac transplantation: the initial multicenter North American experience with the Berlin Heart EXCOR ventricular assist device, J. Heart Lung Transplant. 30 (1) (January 2011) 1–8.

[50] J.J. You, A. Woo, D.T. Ko, D.A. Cameron, A. Mihailovic, M. Krahn, Life expectancy gains and cost-effectiveness of implantable cardioverter/defibrillators for the primary prevention of sudden cardiac death in patients with hypertrophic cardiomyopathy, Am. Heart J. 154 (5) (November 2007) 899–907.

[51] I. Griebsch, Quality-adjusted life-years lack quality in pediatric care: a critical review of published cost-utility studies in child health, Pediatrics 115 (5) (May 1, 2005) e600–e614.

[52] W.T. Mahle, G. Ianucci, R.N. Vincent, K.R. Kanter, Costs associated with ventricular assist device use in children, Ann. Thorac. Surg. 86 (5) (November 2008) 1592–1597.

[53] W.T. Mahle, J.M. Forbess, P.M. Kirshbom, A.R. Cuadrado, J.M. Simsic, K.R. Kanter, Cost-utility analysis of salvage cardiac extracorporeal membrane oxygenation in children, J. Thorac. Cardiovasc. Surg. 129 (5) (May 2005) 1084–1090.

[54] B. Feingold, G. Arora, S.A. Webber, K.J. Smith, Cost-effectiveness of implantable cardioverter-defibrillators in children with dilated cardiomyopathy, J. Card. Fail. 16 (9) (September 2010) 734–741.

[55] M.E. Porter, What is value in health care? N. Engl. J. Med. 363 (26) (December 23, 2010) 2477–2481.

[56] J.P. Jacobs, S.M. O'Brien, S.K. Pasquali, M.L. Jacobs, F.G. Lacour-Gayet, C.I. Tchervenkov, et al., Variation in outcomes for benchmark operations: an analysis of the Society of Thoracic Surgeons Congenital Heart Surgery Database, Ann. Thorac. Surg. 92 (6) (December 2011) 2184–2191 discussion 2191–2192.

[57] S.K. Pasquali, J.P. Jacobs, E.L. Bove, J.W. Gaynor, X. He, M.G. Gaies, et al., Quality-cost relationship in congenital heart surgery, Ann. Thorac. Surg. (July 2015). (Internet) Available from: http://linkinghub.elsevier.com/retrieve/pii/S000349751500819X.

[58] S.K. Pasquali, M.L. Jacobs, X. He, S.S. Shah, E.D. Peterson, M. Hall, et al., Variation in congenital heart surgery costs across hospitals, Pediatrics 133 (3) (March 2014) e553–560.

[59] D. Nandi, P. Shamszad, M.J. O'Connor, K.Y. Lin, A.T. Costarino Jr., R.E. Shaddy, et al., Abstract: Variability of Utilization of Intravenous Immunoglobulin for Acute Myocarditis Amongst U.S. Children's Hospitals (2015 AAP National Conference and Exhibition)(Internet) American Academy of Pediatrics National Conference and Exhibition, Washington, DC, October 23, 2015. Available from: https://aap.confex.com/aap/2015/webprogrampress/Paper31577.html.

[60] M.J. O'Connor, J.W. Rossano, Ventricular assist devices in children, Curr. Opin. Cardiol. 29 (1) (January 2014) 113–121.

Chapter 13

Clinical Recognition of Congestive Heart Failure in Children

Jonathan N. Johnson, David J. Driscoll
Mayo Clinic, Rochester, MN, United States

INTRODUCTION

Heart failure (HF) in children can result from primary cardiomyopathies, infections, drug/toxin exposure, and congenital heart disease [1–4]. Descriptions of each cause are presented in later chapters of this textbook. We will focus here on the clinical presentation of children with HF.

HF is a condition that results from the reduced ability of the heart to fill with or to eject blood [1,4,5]. Clinically, the symptoms of HF are related directly to impairment of cardiac output or pulmonary or cardiac overcirculation. Impairment of cardiac output may result in fatigue, exercise intolerance, and/or end organ hypoperfusion. Left ventricular failure results in increased left ventricular end-diastolic pressure, elevated left atrial, and pulmonary venous pressure, causing shortness of breath, cough, and orthopnea. Right ventricular failure causes hepatomegaly, peripheral edema, and abdominal discomfort. In this chapter, we will detail the clinical presentation of pediatric HF patients across the spectrum of ages and diagnoses.

HISTORY

History—Age

The clinical history is a critical part of any evaluation. The specific findings on historical interrogation, however, largely depend on the age at presentation and the diagnosis.

Infants (Age <2)

One of the largest energy expenditures in infants is feeding, and infants with HF often present with symptoms related to feeding. Infants may take less formula or breast milk per feed [2] or may have symptoms apparent to their parents with feeding, including irritability, tachypnea, tachycardia, or diaphoresis [6]. In the original Ross study from 1992, the volume of each feed was the most sensitive historical variable associated with a clinical diagnosis of congestive heart failure (CHF) [2]. As the degree of HF worsens, poor growth may ensue. Further symptoms may occur at rest and depend on the cause of HF [1,7].

Children (Age 2–10)

HF presentation in children can be subtle, as children can compensate extremely well despite very abnormal myocardial contractility. Common symptoms may include shortness of breath, particularly with activity, or new-onset fatigue. Chronic cough may be present due to pulmonary congestion. Often, a mild intercurrent illness may prompt the presentation, as it may be enough to cause underlying hemodynamic abnormalities to become apparent [6]. Abdominal pain, nausea, or anorexia related to poor cardiac output and elevated systemic venous pressure may be the first presenting sign [8]. Chronic symptoms of fatigue, tachypnea at rest, or cardiac cachexia are rare in the newly diagnosed patient in First World countries.

Older Children/Adolescents (Ages 6–18)

Though older children and adolescents may present with similar symptoms as younger children, they also may present with symptoms more akin to adults, including shortness of breath, fatigue, and exercise intolerance [6]. Abdominal complaints may be the sole symptom present in up to a quarter of adolescents presenting with HF [8].

Heart Failure in the Child and Young Adult. http://dx.doi.org/10.1016/B978-0-12-802393-8.00013-2

History—Diagnosis

Primary Cardiomyopathy

Presenting symptoms for patients with primary cardiomyopathies will be dependent on the type of cardiomyopathy. The "classic" HF presentation is that of the patient with dilated cardiomyopathy, primarily affecting the left ventricle [7]. Poor feeding is common in infants, while exercise intolerance, shortness of breath, and abdominal complaints are common in children and adolescents. Patients with left ventricular noncompaction cardiomyopathy may present with similar symptoms; however, the clinician should inquire about palpitations due to an increased risk for arrhythmias and sudden death in this condition [9].

Idiopathic restrictive cardiomyopathy (IRCM) most commonly presents in children with indolent symptoms, including increasing dyspnea at rest and with exertion, generalized fatigue and weakness, or cough [10,11]. More severe cases may present with complaints of peripheral edema or abdominal distension/ascites, or syncope. Often, patients with IRCM are diagnosed secondarily due to an abnormal chest X-ray performed due to mild respiratory symptoms by noncardiologists [11].

The presentation of hypertrophic cardiomyopathy (HCM) also is dependent on the age at presentation. Infants with HCM may present with a murmur, failure to thrive, or as a result of screening because of a known genetic condition (family history of HCM or a personal or family history of Noonan Syndrome, Noonan Syndrome with Multiple Lentigines, Friedreich's ataxia, or other genetic syndrome) [12–14]. Older children may be asymptomatic, or have symptoms ranging from syncope to aborted sudden cardiac arrest [13].

Secondary "Cardiomyopathy" or Myocardial Dysfunction

The history is paramount for the diagnosis of secondary cardiomyopathies. A thorough history and review of symptoms should be performed to assess for historical details or symptoms consistent with the causes of myocardial dysfunction noted in Table 13.1 [1,15]. For instance, a history of chemotherapy, especially anthracycline medications, should prompt concern for anthracycline cardiotoxicity [16] (see Chapter 33). A history of frequent palpitations suggests tachycardia-induced cardiomyopathy. Notably, cardiac infiltrative disorders such as amyloidosis and sarcoidosis occur rarely, if ever, in children.

Myocarditis

Children with myocarditis can present with signs and symptoms ranging from no symptoms to cardiogenic shock, cardiac arrest, and sudden death [17] (see Chapter 17). Tachypnea and respiratory distress are classically the most common presenting symptoms [17–19]. Patients may complain of chest pain or palpitations, particularly teenagers [17,19]. Gastrointestinal complaints such as pain, vomiting, or poor appetite may be present [20]. Patients may have had symptoms of an upper

TABLE 13.1 Elements to be Addressed During a History and Review of Systems for the New Pediatric Patient With Heart Failure, to Rule Out Secondary Causes of Myocardial Dysfunction

Subtype	Diagnoses
Endocrine	Hypothyroidism, hyperthyroidism, pheochromocytoma, hypoglycemia
Hematologic	Thalassemia, sickle cell anemia
Rheumatological/vascular	Systemic lupus erythematosus, dermatomyositis, Kawasaki disease
Genetic/metabolic	Glycogen-storage diseases, fatty acid oxidation defects, mucopolysaccharidoses
Pharmacologic/toxic	History of anthracycline chemotherapy, iron overload, amphetamines, alcohol, medication hypersensitivity reactions
Nutritional	Pellagra, thiamine or selenium deficiency, carnitine deficiency
Fetal	High output states including twin–twin transfusion syndrome and arteriovenous malformations
Cardiac	Congenital heart disease (volume or pressure-overloading lesions), arrhythmias, coronary artery anomalies, postoperative coronary compromise, hypertension

respiratory tract infection in the prior 1–3 weeks. These patients often are misdiagnosed with a respiratory or gastrointestinal condition prior to the correct diagnosis of myocarditis [19,21].

Congenital Heart Disease

HF associated with congenital heart disease can be highly variable in terms of presenting history and symptoms, and largely depends on the specific anatomic lesion involved [1]. For instance, volume-overloading lesions such as a large ventricular septal defect will present in infancy after transition from fetal to neonatal circulation. These patients will present with tachypnea, poor feeding, and subsequently poor weight gain. Other volume-overloading lesions include: atrioventricular canal defect, patent ductus arteriosus, aortopulmonary window, Ebstein anomaly, and significant atrioventricular valve or semilunar valve regurgitation.

Pressure-overloading lesions such as severe aortic stenosis, severe HCM with obstruction, or coarctation of the aorta can present with HF. The mechanism of HF with these lesions often involves poor perfusion, acidosis, subendocardial ischemia, and subsequent systemic ventricular dilatation and dysfunction.

Please see Chapters 23–27 for a review of HF in structural heart disease.

History—Family History

The family history is critical to obtain for a patient in HF, as it suggests the diagnosis and allows for appropriate treatment before diagnostic testing has been completed. For all patients, a family history of any form of myocardial dysfunction should be acquired, as well as any history of congenital heart disease, genetic syndromes with associated cardiomyopathies, or early coronary artery disease. Finally, a family history of sudden unexplained death of any kind should be obtained, including any unexplained drowning, car accident, or sudden infant death syndrome. Genetics consultation should be considered for most patients with cardiomyopathy, particularly if there is a family history of cardiomyopathy or unexplained sudden death.

PHYSICAL EXAMINATION

A complete physical examination including four extremity blood pressures and measurement of systemic arterial blood oxygen saturation should be performed. One should assess the quality of the peripheral pulses, capillary refill, temperature, and any color changes such as mottling. Pulmonary evaluation may reveal rales. Right ventricular failure is suggested by hepatomegaly or jugular venous distension. Precordial evaluation may show prominence of the right ventricular impulse in the presence of right ventricular failure or pulmonary hypertension. With pulmonary hypertension, the second heart sound may be pronounced. A prominent left ventricular impulse suggests left ventricular dilatation or dysfunction. A gallop rhythm frequently will be present. However, an S3 heart sound is normal in children. An S4 heart sound or a summation gallop is not normal in children and indicates the need for further evaluation. Importantly, children with HF may not have a murmur; thus, the absence of a murmur should not be seen as proof of absence of HF [4].

Physical Examination—Age

Similar to the history, the specific findings on physical examination also depend on the age of the patient.

Infants (Age <2)

Common physical examination findings of infants in HF include tachycardia, tachypnea, and an abnormal respiratory pattern (grunting, retractions, etc.). Hepatomegaly is present commonly, with palpation of the liver at least 2 cm below the right costal margin. An S3 heart sound or diastolic filling sound may be present [22]. In the original Ross study from 1992, while the volume of each feed was the most sensitive historical variable associated with a clinical diagnosis of CHF, there were several examination measures that were similarly sensitive [2]. This included a respiratory rate greater than 50 breaths per minute, an abnormal respiratory pattern, a diastolic filling sound, and hepatomegaly.

Infants often present with symptoms related to feeding [2]. As such, in the absence of symptoms at rest, observation of the infant during a feeding can be helpful and may reveal irritability, tachypnea, tachycardia, or diaphoresis with feeds [6,22].

Children (Age 2–10)

In contrast to symptoms with feeding, toddlers and small children more often present with nausea, vomiting, and poor appetite. In these situations, the cardiac examination may be subtly abnormal, with a displaced apical impulse but no murmurs.

However, the liver will be enlarged, and there may be abdominal discomfort and/or distension apparent on examination. A chronic cough may be present. True cardiac cachexia is rare in First World countries but may be seen often in regions of the world with endemic rheumatic fever and other illnesses.

Older Children (Ages 6–18)

Older children and adolescents often have similar symptoms and examination findings as young adults, including pulmonary rales, a displaced apical impulse, and an S4 heart sound. Peripheral edema may be present but is rarely the presenting symptom or examination finding. Similar to younger children, patients may present with recurrent abdominal symptoms of nausea, vomiting, and pain. Fatigue, cachexia, and weakness are late findings.

Physical Examination—Diagnosis

Primary Cardiomyopathy

Patients with dilated or left ventricular noncompaction cardiomyopathy often have fairly typical findings on physical exam, including hepatomegaly, pulmonary rales, and a gallop rhythm. Patients with restrictive cardiomyopathy may have an S4 heart sound, a prominent second heart sound (due to elevated pulmonary artery pressures in the setting of increased left ventricular filling pressures), or a murmur of tricuspid regurgitation. Severe cases may present with peripheral edema, chronic cough, abdominal distension, or ascites.

Pediatric patients with HCM can have a myriad of presentations and examination findings. Some patients may have a normal physical examination, while others may have a murmur of left ventricular outflow tract obstruction, a prominent and displaced left ventricular impulse, or an S4 heart sound. All patients newly diagnosed with HCM should have their gait evaluated, looking for Friedreich's ataxia. A full genetics evaluation and examination may be warranted to look for signs of other associated genetic syndromes [13].

Secondary Cardiomyopathy

Patients with a presumed secondary cause of myocardial dysfunction must undergo a full and complete physical examination to ensure all possible etiologies are considered. For example, the patients' skin should be examined for evidence of rheumatologic diseases such as lupus or dermatomyositis or evidence of nutritional deficiencies. From a cardiac perspective, the examination findings are similar to those of the primary cardiomyopathies.

Myocarditis

The physical examination in a patient with myocarditis is similar to a patient with a primary dilated cardiomyopathy. A gallop may be present, and other signs of left ventricular dysfunction including pulmonary rales may be heard. In the acute setting, there may be mitral regurgitation, which can be heard as a systolic murmur on examination. Patients also may present with pallor, hypotension, and other signs of hemodynamic compromise due to the acute onset of their myocardial dysfunction. In a study of emergency department patients who were eventually diagnosed with myocarditis, however, the most frequent examination finding was an abnormal respiratory exam [19].

Congenital Heart Disease

The physical examination findings in a patient with congenital heart disease and HF are largely dependent on the anatomy and the operations that have been performed. For instance, a patient with aortic stenosis and HF will have a typical left ventricular outflow tract murmur radiating to the right upper sternal border, with a diastolic component if significant aortic regurgitation also is present. Notably, an outflow tract murmur may be decreased in intensity in the setting of low cardiac output and poor ventricular function.

The patient who has had a Fontan operation is of particular interest to the HF community and often has unique examination findings depending on their pathophysiologic state. Ascites, abdominal distension, pubertal delay, and short stature often are present in the patient with protein-losing enteropathy. The pulmonary examination findings are important for the patient with plastic bronchitis [23]. Hepatic evaluation by examination often is difficult in these patients, and liver imaging is crucial in the long-term follow-up of a Fontan patient [24]. Cyanosis may be present and may be indicative of systemic venous to pulmonary venous collateral formation.

SCORING SYSTEMS

Many scoring systems incorporating aspects of these presenting symptoms and signs have been developed and are validated for use in the pediatric population [2,22,25]. These classification systems will be discussed in more detail in Chapter 15 of this text.

CONCLUSION

The clinical evaluation of the children with HF begins with the history and physical examination. Clinical presentation and examination findings are dependent on both the age of the patient and the diagnosis.

ABBREVIATIONS

HCM Hypertrophic cardiomyopathy
HF Heart failure
IRCM Idiopathic restrictive cardiomyopathy

REFERENCES

[1] D.T. Hsu, G.D. Pearson, Heart failure in children: part I: history, etiology, and pathophysiology, Circ. Heart Fail. 2 (2009) 63–70.
[2] R.D. Ross, R.O. Bollinger, W.W. Pinsky, Grading the severity of congestive heart failure in infants, Pediatr. Cardiol. 13 (1992) 72–75.
[3] D. Rosenthal, M.R. Chrisant, E. Edens, L. Mahony, C. Canter, S. Colan, A. Dubin, J. Lamour, R. Ross, R. Shaddy, L. Addonizio, L. Beerman, S. Berger, D. Bernstein, E. Blume, M. Boucek, P. Checchia, A. Dipchand, J. Drummond-Webb, J. Fricker, R. Friedman, S. Hallowell, R. Jaquiss, S. Mital, E. Pahl, F.B. Pearce, L. Rhodes, K. Rotondo, P. Rusconi, J. Scheel, T. Pal Singh, J. Towbin, International Society for heart and lung transplantation: practice guidelines for management of heart failure in children, J. Heart Lung Transplant. 23 (2004) 1313–1333.
[4] J.W. Rossano, R.E. Shaddy, Heart failure in children: etiology and treatment, J. Pediatr. 165 (2014) 228–233.
[5] E. Madriago, M. Silberbach, Heart failure in infants and children, Pediatr. Rev. 31 (2010) 4–12.
[6] Clinical manifestations of heart failure, in: R. Kirk, A. Dipchand, D. Rosenthal (Eds.), ISHLT Guidelines for the Management of Pediatric Heart Failure, ISHLT, Birmingham, AL, 2014.
[7] B.D. Kaufman, R.E. Shaddy, G.S. Shirali, R. Tanel, J.A. Towbin, Assessment and management of the failing heart in children, Cardiol. Young 3 (18 Suppl.) (2008) 63–71.
[8] S.A. Hollander, L.J. Addonizio, C. Chin, J.M. Lamour, D.T. Hsu, D. Bernstein, D.N. Rosenthal, Abdominal complaints as a common first presentation of heart failure in adolescents with dilated cardiomyopathy, Am. J. Emerg. Med. 31 (2013) 684–686.
[9] S.T. Brescia, J.W. Rossano, R. Pignatelli, J.L. Jefferies, J.F. Price, J.A. Decker, S.W. Denfield, W.J. Dreyer, O. Smith, J.A. Towbin, J.J. Kim, Mortality and sudden death in pediatric left ventricular noncompaction in a tertiary referral center, Circulation 127 (2013) 2202–2208.
[10] S.A. Webber, S.E. Lipshultz, L.A. Sleeper, M. Lu, J.D. Wilkinson, L.J. Addonizio, C.E. Canter, S.D. Colan, M.D. Everitt, J.L. Jefferies, P.F. Kantor, J.M. Lamour, R. Margossian, E. Pahl, P.G. Rusconi, J.A. Towbin, Outcomes of restrictive cardiomyopathy in childhood and the influence of phenotype: a report from the Pediatric Cardiomyopathy Registry, Circulation 126 (2012) 1237–1244.
[11] F. Cetta, P.W. O'Leary, J.B. Seward, D.J. Driscoll, Idiopathic restrictive cardiomyopathy in childhood: diagnostic features and clinical course, Mayo Clin. Proc. 70 (1995) 634–640.
[12] S.D. Colan, Hypertrophic cardiomyopathy in childhood, Heart Fail. Clin. 6 (2010) 433–444 vii-iii.
[13] R.W. Loar, J.M. Bos, M.L. Will, S.R. Ommen, M.J. Ackerman, Genotype-phenotype correlations of hypertrophic cardiomyopathy when diagnosed in children, adolescents, and young adults, Congenit. Heart Dis. 10 (2015) 529–536.
[14] V.V. Michels, T.M. Olson, F.A. Miller, K.V. Ballman, A.G. Rosales, D.J. Driscoll, Frequency of development of idiopathic dilated cardiomyopathy among relatives of patients with idiopathic dilated cardiomyopathy, Am. J. Cardiol. 91 (2003) 1389–1392.
[15] D.T. Hsu, G.D. Pearson, Heart failure in children: part II: diagnosis, treatment, and future directions, Circ. Heart Fail. 2 (2009) 490–498.
[16] S.E. Lipshultz, T.R. Cochran, V.I. Franco, T.L. Miller, Treatment-related cardiotoxicity in survivors of childhood cancer, Nat. Rev. Clin. Oncol. 10 (2013) 697–710.
[17] C.E. Canter, K.E. Simpson, Diagnosis and treatment of myocarditis in children in the current era, Circulation 129 (2014) 115–128.
[18] S. Press, R.S. Lipkind, Acute myocarditis in infants. Initial presentation, Clin. Pediatr. 29 (1990) 73–76.
[19] S.B. Freedman, J.K. Haladyn, A. Floh, J.A. Kirsh, G. Taylor, J. Thull-Freedman, Pediatric myocarditis: emergency department clinical findings and diagnostic evaluation, Pediatrics 120 (2007) 1278–1285.
[20] Y.J. Chang, H.C. Chao, S.H. Hsia, D.C. Yan, Myocarditis presenting as gastritis in children, Pediatr. Emerg. Care 22 (2006) 439–440.
[21] Y. Durani, M. Egan, J. Baffa, S.M. Selbst, A.L. Nager, Pediatric myocarditis: presenting clinical characteristics, Am. J. Emerg. Med. 27 (2009) 942–947.
[22] R.D. Ross, The Ross classification for heart failure in children after 25 years: a review and an age-stratified revision, Pediatr. Cardiol. 33 (2012) 1295–1300.
[23] J.N. Johnson, D.J. Driscoll, P.W. O'Leary, Protein-losing enteropathy and the Fontan operation, Nutr. Clin. Pract. 27 (2012) 375–384.
[24] K. Pundi, K.N. Pundi, P.S. Kamath, F. Cetta, Z. Li, J.T. Poterucha, D.J. Driscoll, J.N. Johnson, Liver disease in patients after the Fontan operation, Am. J. Cardiol. 117 (2016) 456–460.
[25] D. Connolly, M. Rutkowski, M. Auslender, M. Artman, The New York University pediatric heart failure index: a new method of quantifying chronic heart failure severity in children, J. Pediatr. 138 (2001) 644–648.

Chapter 14

Classification of Heart Failure

Robert D. Ross
Children's Hospital of Michigan, Cardiology Division, Wayne State University School of Medicine, Detroit, MI, United States

The ability to accurately describe and classify the signs and symptoms of heart failure (HF) is critical to the study of and communication about the condition. This is particularly challenging in children in whom these variables change dramatically from infancy through adolescence. The ideal classification system would take into account these age-related changes as well as be reproducible and accurately reflect improvement with or without therapy or clinical worsening. It would be most useful if the system is correlated with risks and outcomes so that treatment could be tailored to the class and risk category.

Prior to 1987, research on HF in children relied on the New York Heart Association (NYHA) classification, which was ill-suited for children, especially infants and younger-aged patients with HF. A modification of the NYHA classification was utilized to study norepinephrine concentrations in children with HF, and this was subsequently named for the author as the "Ross Classification" for grading HF in children (Table 14.1) [1]. The system worked well in that progressive symptom class correlated with a step-wise increase in plasma norepinephrine levels and beta receptor down-regulation [1,2]. In addition, the Ross class correlated with the severity of mitral regurgitation in children with dilated cardiomyopathy, which predicted outcomes in terms of death or cardiac transplantation [3].

A study of infants under 6 months of age found 8 variables that were most sensitive and specific for HF in this age range. Based on these historical and physical examination findings, a numerical scoring system to grade HF in infants was proposed (Table 14.2) [4]. Several authors have modified this version of the Ross Classification to extend its utility to older children [5,6]. During the same time frame, a new system for grading HF in children was proposed called the New York University Pediatric Heart Failure Index (PHFI) [7]. This is a 30 point scale that incorporates signs and symptoms of HF and adds medications and single ventricle physiology to the mix (Table 14.3). The only comparison study was done in 20 children with HF from rheumatic heart disease between the NYHA, the modified Ross Classification, and the PHFI [8]. All three correlated with cardiothoracic index on chest X-ray, while the PHFI faired better when compared to left ventricular mass, end-systolic wall stress, left atrium to aortic size, and N-terminal pro brain natriuretic peptide (NT-proBNP).

In the 2004 "Practice Guidelines for Management of HF in Children" from the International Society for Heart and Lung Transplantation, a HF classification was proposed for staging infants and children, which distinguishes those at risk for HF from those with overt clinical symptoms (Table 14.4) [9]. While this is a valuable method for putting patients into broad categories of potential for HF versus those with symptoms, it does not provide enough gradations in symptoms to be useful for comparison with disease severity.

Multiple recent studies have shown NT-proBNP to be an indicator of HF of all ages [10,11]. It is the N-terminal fragment of BNP, which is released in response to ventricular volume and pressure overload. Normal values decrease with age, and newborns have high levels. Several reports have shown good correlation of NT-proBNP with progressive Ross Class of HF and cutoffs have been established for Ross Classes I through IV [12–14]. Others have noted that the trend in NT-proBNP correlates with HF symptoms and in predicting the need for mechanical circulatory support and/or transplantation [15–19].

Other parameters of HF in children that factor into disease severity or symptom class are exercise capacity and ventricular function [20–24]. The latter does not have a direct correlation with HF symptoms but does have predictive value

TABLE 14.1 Original Ross Classification [1]

I: No limitations or symptoms
II: Mild tachypnea or diaphoresis with feedings in infants; dyspnea on exertion in older children; no growth failure
III: Marked tachypnea or diaphoresis with feedings or exertion and prolonged feeding times with growth failure from CHF
IV: Symptomatic at rest with tachypnea, retractions, grunting, or diaphoresis

Heart Failure in the Child and Young Adult. http://dx.doi.org/10.1016/B978-0-12-802393-8.00014-4

TABLE 14.2 Ross Scoring System for Heart Failure in Infants [5]

	Score		
	0	1	2
Feeding History			
Volume consumed per feeding	>3.5 oz.	2.5–3.5 oz.	<2.5 oz.
Time taken per feeding	<40 min	>40 min	–
Physical Exam			
Respiratory rate	<50/min	50–60/min	>60/min
Heart rate	<160/min	160–170/min	>170/min
Respiratory pattern	Normal	Abnormal	–
Peripheral perfusion	Normal	Decreased	–
S_3 or diastolic rumble	Absent	Present	–
Liver edge from right costal margin	<2 cm	2–3 cm	>3 cm

Total score: *0–2*, no CHF; *3–6*, mild CHF; *7–9*, moderate CHF; *10–12*, severe CHF; *CHF*, congestive heart failure.

for outcomes. In older children who can perform an exercise test, those with a peak oxygen consumption ≤62% of predicted based on age and sex had a much worse prognosis than those above 62% of predicted values [22].

The most recent classification system proposed was age specific from infancy through adolescence and utilized the time-tested symptoms and signs of HF in children. In addition, parameters of exercise capacity, ventricular function, and the neurohumoral response to HF were incorporated. This "Age-based Ross Classification for HF in Children" is shown in Table 14.5 [25]. The five age groups were selected for ranges where the normal values for the variables are stable within each age group but vary between groups.

This system utilizes data from the history, physical exam, echocardiogram, the NT-proBNP levels, and in the older children exercise testing. Thus, it incorporates many of the complex contributing factors that make up HF. Each age grouping has 10 variables that are graded from 0 to 2 with a possible total score of 0–20. These scores can be used to study outcomes either as continuous variables or by Ross Classes: I = 0–5, II = 6–10, III = 11–15, and IV = 16–20.

Each age range has respiratory and heart rates adjusted to reported normal values at rest, and moderately–to-severely increased rates score 1 or 2 points, respectively. The normal levels for NT-proBNP are higher through age 3 years, thus the cutoffs have been adjusted down for those 4 years and older. The cutoffs in the older children coincide well with data obtained on adults with congenital heart disease where 646 patients aged 35 ± 12 years were followed for 6 ± 3 years. There was a 1% mortality rate in the 388 patients with a NT-proBNP less than 220 pg/mL, while there was 41% mortality in the 54 patients with a NT-proBNP greater than 1548 pg/mL, and the deaths were predominately from HF [26].

From newborns to 3 months of age, feeding is the main cause for increased metabolic demands, which may not be met when significant HF is present. Therefore, the volume of feeding and time for the feeding reflect these demands. For breast fed infants, the volume is subjectively rated as normal, decreased or gavage fed, and/or supplemented. From 4 to 12 months of age, diets vary but HF begins to affect weight gain. If there is enough HF to cause a fall off of 1 weight curve percentile on the growth curve, 1 point is awarded, whereas a fall off of ≥2 curve percentiles is given 2 points. If serial measurements are not available, a weight <5% for age from HF merits 2 points.

In the children 1–3 years of age and 4–8 years when growth rates normally decline, recent weight loss qualifies for a point, while cachexia earns 2 points. Over 4 years of age, gastrointestinal symptoms of HF predominate. Thus feeding history at these ages changes from intake amounts to symptoms of nausea and/or vomiting, graded none, intermittent, or frequent. By age 9, most children can do an exercise stress test so in the oldest group, stress testing has replaced growth failure as an objective measure of the response to increased metabolic demands. One point is given for a maximal oxygen consumption between 60% and 80% of predicted for age and sex, and 2 points for <60% predicted. If the HF is too far advanced to be able to perform this test, then 2 points are awarded.

Finally, if the HF has progressed to hospitalization with the requirement for intravenous support, mechanical circulatory support with extracorporeal membrane oxygenation, or a ventricular assist device, then they should be rated Ross Class IV.

TABLE 14.3 New York University Pediatric Heart Failure (HF) Index

Score	Signs and Symptoms
+2	Abnormal ventricular function by echocardiogram or gallop
+2	Dependent edema or pleural effusion or ascites
+2	Failure to thrive or cachexia
+1	Marked cardiomegaly by X-ray or by physical examination
+1	Reported physical activity intolerance or prolonged feeding time
+2	Poor perfusion by physical examination
+1	Pulmonary edema by X-ray or by auscultation
+2	Resting sinus tachycardia
+2	Retractions
	Hepatomegaly
+1	<4 cm below costal margin
+2	>4 cm below costal margin
	Observed tachypnea or dyspnea
+1	Mild to moderate
+2	Moderate to severe
Medications	
+1	Digoxin
	Diuretics
+1	Low–to-moderate dose
+2	High dose or more than one diuretic
+1	ACE inhibitors or non-ACE inhibitor vasodilators or angiotensin receptor blockers
+1	Beta-blockers
+2	Anticoagulants not related to prosthetic valve
+2	Antiarrhythmic agents or ICD
Physiology	
+2	Single ventricle

Scores can range from 0 (no HF) to 30 (severe HF).
ACE, Angiotensin-converting enzyme; *ICD*, implantable cardiac defibrillator.

TABLE 14.4 Heart Failure (HF) Staging for Infants and Children

Stage	Interpretation
A.	Patients with increased risk of developing HF, but who have normal cardiac function and no evidence of cardiac chamber volume overload. Examples: previous exposure to cardiotoxic agents, family history of heritable cardiomyopathy, univentricular heart, congenitally corrected transposition of the great arteries.
B.	Patients with abnormal cardiac morphology or cardiac function, with no symptoms of HF, past or present. Examples: aortic insufficiency with left ventricular (LV) enlargement, history of anthracycline exposure with decreased LV systolic function.
C.	Patients with underlying structural or functional heart disease and past or current symptoms of HF.
D.	Patients with end-stage HF requiring continuous infusion of inotropic agents, mechanical circulatory support, cardiac transplantation, or hospice care.

TABLE 14.5 Age-Based Ross Classification for Heart Failure in Children

	0–3 months				**4–12 months**		
	0	**1**	**2**		**0**	**1**	**2**
Oz/feed	>3.5	2.5–3.5	<2.5	**Feeding**	Nl	Decreased	Gavaged
Time/feed	<20 min	20–40	>40	**Wt%**	Nl	≥1 curve	≥2 curves
Breathing	Nl	Tachypnea	Retractions		Nl	Tachypnea	Retractions
RR/min	<50	50–60	>60		<40	40–50	>50
HR/min	<160	160–170	>170		<120	120–130	>130
Perfusion	Nl	Reduced	Shocky		Nl	Reduced	Shocky
Hepatomegaly	<2 cm	2–3 cm	>3 cm		<2 cm	2–3 cm	>3 cm
NT-proBNP (pg/mL)	<450 (>4d)	450–1700	>1700		<450	450–1700	>1700
EF%	>50	30–50	<30		>50	30–50	<30
AV insufficiency	None	Mild	Moderate/severe		None	Mild	Moderate/severe
		1–3 years				**4–8 years**	
	0	**1**	**2**		**0**	**1**	**2**
Feeding	Nl	Decreased	Gavaged	**N/V**	None	Intermittent	Frequent
Growth	Nl	Weight loss	Cachexia		Nl	Weight loss	Cachexia
Breathing	Nl	Tachypnea	Retractions		Nl	Tachypnea	Retractions
RR/min	<30	30–40	>40		<25	25–35	>35
HR/min	<110	110–120	>120		<100	90–100	>100
Perfusion	Nl	Reduced	Shocky		Nl	Reduced	Shocky
Hepatomegaly	<2 cm	2–3 cm	>3 cm		<2 cm	2–3 cm	>3 cm
NT-proBNP (pg/mL)	<450	450–1700	>1700		<300	300–1500	>1500
EF%	>50	30–50	<30		>50	30–50	<30
AV insufficiency	None	Mild	Moderate/severe		None	Mild	Moderate/severe
		9–18 years					
	0	**1**	**2**				
N/V	Nl	Intermittent	Frequent				
Breathing	Nl	Tachypnea	Retractions				
RR/min	<20	20–30	>30				
HR/min	<90	90–100	>100				
Perfusion	Nl	Reduced	Shocky				
Hepatomegaly	<2 cm	2–3 cm	>3 cm				
NT-proBNP (pg/mL)	<300	300–1500	>1500				
EF%	>50	30–50	<30				
Max% VO_2	>80%	60–80%	<60%				
AV insufficiency	None	Mild	Moderate/severe				

AV, systemic atrioventricular valve; *EF*, ejection fraction; *HR*, heart rate; *m*, meters; *Max% VO_2*, % of predicted maximal oxygen uptake for age and sex; *NT-proBNP*, N-terminal pro brain natriuretic peptide; *N/V*, nausea/vomiting; *Oz*, ounce; *RR*, respiratory rate; *Wt%*, fall off on weight growth curve %; */min*, per minute.

CONCLUSION

In summary, precise grading of the severity of HF is crucial to the study of the diseases that lead to HF and for accurate communication between clinicians and investigators. In children, signs and symptoms of HF vary with age, and therefore an age-stratified approach is required. Continued testing of these grading systems and comparing severity class with outcomes will help validate their utility and accuracy.

REFERENCES

[1] R.D. Ross, S.R. Daniels, D.C. Schwartz, D.W. Hannon, R. Shukla, S. Kaplan, Plasma levels of norepinphrine in infants and children with congestive heart failure, Am. J. Cardiol. 59 (1987) 911–914.

[2] J.R. Wu, H.R. Chang, T.Y. Huang, C.H. Chiang, S.S. Chen, Reduction in lymphocyte B-adrenergic receptor density in infants and children with heart failure secondary to congenital heart disease, Am. J. Cardiol. 77 (1996) 170–174.

[3] F.P. Fernandes, C. Manlhiot, B.W. McCrindle, L. Mertens, P.F. Kantor, M.K. Friedberg, Usefulness of mitral regurgitation as a marker of increased risk for death or cardiac transplantation in idiopathic dilated cardiomyopathy in children, Am. J. Cardiol. 107 (2011) 1517–1521.

[4] R.D. Ross, R.O. Bollinger, W.W. Pinsky, Grading the severity of congestive heart failure in infants, Pediatr. Cardiol. 13 (1992) 72–75.

[5] C. Reithmann, D. Reber, R. Kozlik-Feldmann, et al., A post-receptor defect of adenylyl cyclase in severely failing myocardium from children with congenital heart disease, Eur. J. Pharmcol. 330 (1997) 79–86.

[6] S. Laer, T.S. Mir, F. Behn, et al., Carvedilol therapy in pediatric patients with congestive heart failure: a study investigating clinical and pharmacokinetic parameters, Am. Heart J. 143 (2002) 916–922.

[7] D. Connelly, M. Rutkowski, M. Auslender, M. Artman, The New York University pediatric heart failure index: a new method of quantifying chronic heart failure severity in children, J. Pediatr. 138 (2001) 644–648.

[8] P. Tissieres, Y. Aggouon, E. Da Cruz, et al., Comparison of heart failure classifications in children undergoing valvular surgery, J. Pediatr. 149 (2006) 210–215.

[9] D. Rosenthal, M.R.K. Chrisant, E. Edens, L. Mahony, C. Canter, S. Colan, A. Dubin, J. Lamour, R. Ross, et al., International society for heart and lung transplantation: practice guidelines for management of heart failure in children, J. Heart Lung Transplant. 23 (2004) 1313–1333.

[10] M.S. Evim, B. Ucar, Z. Kilic, O. Colak, The value of serum N-terminal pro-brain natriuretic peptide levels in the differential diagnosis and follow-up of congestive cardiac failure and respiratory distress due to pulmonary aetiologies in infants and children, Cardiol. Young 20 (2010) 495–504.

[11] C. Ratnasamy, D.D. Kinnamon, S.E. Lipshultz, P. Rusconi, Associations between neurohormonal and inflammatory activation and heart failure in children, Am. Heart J. 155 (2008) 527–533.

[12] M. Sugimoto, H. Manabe, K. Nakau, et al., The role of N-terminal pro-B type natriuretic peptide in the diagnosis of congestive heart failure in children, Circ. J. 74 (2010) 998–1005.

[13] P.G. Rusconi, D.A. Ludwig, C. Ratnasamy, et al., Serial measurements of serum NT-proBNP as markers of left ventricular function and remodeling in children with heart failure, Am. Heart J. 160 (2010) 776–783.

[14] C.W. Lin, X.L. Zeng, J.F. Zhang, X.H. Meng, Determining the optimal cutoff values of plasma N-terminal pro-B-type natriuretic peptide levels for the diagnosis of heart failure in children of age up to 14 years, J. Cardiac Fail. 2 (2014) 168–173.

[15] D.T.H. Wong, K. George, J. Wilson, et al., Effectiveness of serial increases in Amino-terminal Pro-B-type natriuretic peptide levels to indicate the need for mechanical circulatory support in children with acute decompensated heart failure, Am. J. Cardiol. 107 (2011) 573–578.

[16] N. Narin, B. Hekimoglu, A. Baykan, A. Ozyurt, G. Zararsiz, S. Sezer, S.H. Onan, M. Argun, O. Pamukcu, K. Uzum, The role of N-terminal proBNP in the clinical scoring of heart failure due to dilated cardiomyopathy in children, Clin. Lab. 60 (2014) 563–570.

[17] S.R. Aurbach, M.E. Richmond, J.M. Lamour, et al., BNP levels predict outcome in pediatric heart failure patients: post hoc analysis of the pediatric cardvelilol trial, Circ. Heart Fail. 3 (2010) 606–611.

[18] A. Shah, A.M. Feraco, C. Harmon, T. Tacy, J.R. Fineman, H.S. Bernstein, Usefulness of various plasma biomarkers for diagnosis of heart failure in children with single ventricle physiology, Am. J. Cardiol. 104 (2009) 1280–1284.

[19] E. Lechner, R. Gitter, R. Mair, et al., Aminoterminal brain natriuretic peptide levels in children and adolescents after Fontan operation correlate with congestive heart failure, Pediatr. Cardiol. 29 (2008) 901–905.

[20] J. Butler, G. Khadim, K.M. Paul, et al., Selection of patients for heart transplantation in the current era of heart failure therapy, J. Am. Coll. Cardiol. 43 (2004) 787–793.

[21] B.B. Das, A.L. Taylor, M.M. Boucek, R.W. Wolfe, A.T. Yetman, Exercise capacity in pediatric heart transplant candidates: is there any role for the 14 ml/kg/min guideline? Pediatr. Cardiol. 27 (2006) 226–229.

[22] A. Giardini, M. Fenton, R.E. Andrews, G. Derrick, M. Burch, Peak oxygen uptake correlates with survival without clinical deterioration in ambulatory children with dilated cardiomyopathy, Circulation 124 (2011) 1713–1718.

[23] G.V. Guimaraes, V.M. d'Avila, P.R. Camargo, L.F.P. Moreira, J.R.L. Luces, E.A. Bocchi, Prognostic value of cardiopulmonary exercise testing in children with heart failure secondary to idiopathic dilated cardiomyopathy in a non-B-blocker setting, Eur. J. Heart Fail. 10 (2008) 560–565.

[24] M.S. Patel, A.M. Berg, R.N. Vincent, W.T. Mahle, Serum parameters and echocardiographic predictors of death of need for transplant in newborns, children, and young adults with heart failure, Am. J. Cardiol. 105 (2010) 1798–1801.

[25] R.D. Ross, The Ross classification for heart failure in children after 25 years: a review and an age-stratified revision, Pediatr. Cardiol. 33 (2012) 1295–1300.

[26] J. Rubackova, K. Kotaska, M. Tomkova, J. Tomek, Usefulness of N-terminal pro-brain natriuretic peptide to predict mortality in adults with congenital heart disease, Am. J. Cardiol. 116 (2015) 1425–1430.

Chapter 15

Right Ventricular Dysfunction

Andrew N. Redington
Cincinnati Children's Hospital Medical Center, Cincinnati, OH, United States

INTRODUCTION

Although once considered to be of secondary importance, few would now disagree that the right ventricle is fundamental to the pathogenesis and outcomes of almost all categories of heart disease. Clearly, heart failure is no exception. In this book, the relevance of the right ventricle in individual diseases will be discussed in detail. It has long been known to be the key driver of outcomes in various forms of congenital heart disease, and in patients with primary pulmonary hypertension, for example. While its role in the long-term outcomes of single ventricle physiology are perhaps sometimes overstated, emerging data in regard to the uniqueness of the right ventricle in this circulation are also appearing. Thus, instead of rehearsing the influence of right ventricular (RV) dysfunction in each of these circumstances, this brief chapter will serve to emphasize the fundamental physiology of the right ventricle and, perhaps most importantly, how it works with its counterpart on the left as essentially a single unit. The importance of these ventricular–ventricular interactions is already being appreciated in adult and pediatric heart failure, and their influence is likely to become even more relevant as more data become available.

THE UNSTRESSED RIGHT VENTRICLE AND ITS INFLUENCE ON THE LEFT SIDE OF THE HEART

The basic physiology of RV function is now well described [1] and need not be recapitulated in great detail here. Suffice it to say, that the right ventricle is uniquely adapted to the low hydraulic impedance of the pulmonary vasculature and generates its cardiac output at approximately one-fifth of the work cost and approximately one-sixth of the energy consumption of the left ventricle. More so than the left ventricle it is highly susceptible to its varying preload, for example, during normal respiration, although it's preload sensitively is fully intact. In this regard, while it's diastolic pressure–volume responses (Starling Mechanism) follow a slightly different trajectory to that of the left ventricle, the output of the right and left ventricles is closely matched within the usual physiologic boundaries. For example, extreme exercise can lead to a quadrupling, or more, of the cardiac output and both right and left ventricles achieve this, at relatively modest increment in ventricular end-diastolic pressure.

Conversely, the responses to afterload are quite different in the two ventricles [2]. Their afterload sensitivity is markedly disparate. An acute change in left ventricular (LV) afterload results in a relatively modest fall in stoke volume, over a wide physiologic range. Furthermore, its Anrep effect restores LV stoke volume within a few minutes (Fig. 15.1).

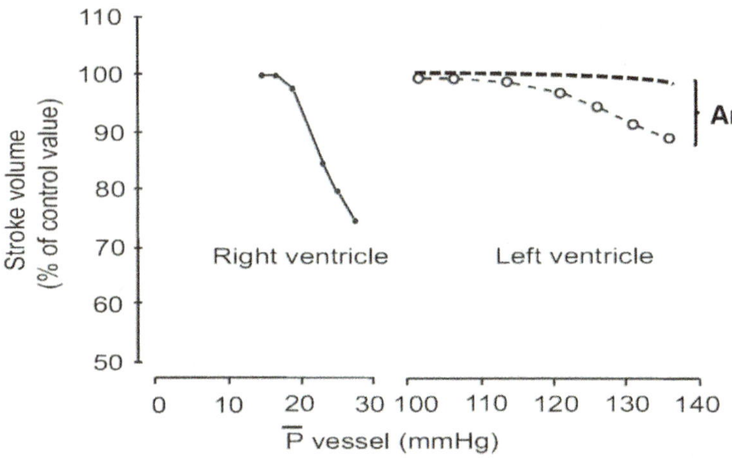

FIGURE 15.1 The acute responses to increased afterload in the right and left ventricle. The right ventricle is far more susceptible to changes in afterload, in terms of its stroke volume responses. Furthermore, stroke volume is restored in the left ventricle as a result of the Anrep effect (see text for details) that leads to an adaptive increase in contractility over approximately 5 min after a modest left ventricular afterload. The Anrep effect has not been demonstrated in the normal right ventricle. *(Adapted from E. Braunwald, Pathophysiology of heart failure, in: E. Braunwald (Ed.), Heart Disease. A Textbook of Cardiovascular Medicine, Saunders, Philadelphia, 1980, pp. 453–471.)*

Heart Failure in the Child and Young Adult. http://dx.doi.org/10.1016/B978-0-12-802393-8.00015-6

Consequently cardiac output is relatively independent of afterload over a wide range, in the normal circulation. The normal right ventricle, however, is much more sensitive to even modest changes in its afterload. It has been estimated that the afterload sensitivity of the right ventricle is 4 or 5 times that of the left ventricle, there being a sustained and precipitous falling cardiac output, as afterload is increased. With more dramatic change, for example, with acute massive pulmonary embolism, the limitation of the right ventricle are further exposed, there being a potentially fatal fall in cardiac output with only relatively modest increase in developed RV systolic pressure (the maximum pressure developed in acute pulmonary hypertension being just 40–50 mmHg). While an Anrep mechanism has only recently been described in the stressed right ventricle [3], no such demonstration has been made in the normal right ventricle. Its ability, at least in the relatively short term, to adapt to changes in afterload is relatively small therefore.

VENTRICULAR–VENTRICULAR INTERACTIONS IN THE NORMAL HEART

Given the lack of shunting in the normal circulation, changes in the left side of the heart necessarily must be matched by changes in the right side of the heart, at least in terms of cardiac output. These series effects are intuitive and adaptive over a wide range of physiologic cardiac output. Less obvious are the parallel interactions that are occurring on a beat-by-beat basis. Some of these interactions even call into question the utility of the right ventricle itself. For example, resection of the RV free wall, and replacement with a non-contractile patch, can be associated with relatively little perturbation in cardiac output in animal models [4]. It appears under these circumstances that shortening of the LV free wall during systole, "pulls" the noncontractile right ventricle free wall around the septum, provides for robust stroke volume from the right ventricle. Interestingly this positive ventricular–ventricular interaction is obviated by increasing size of the right ventricle (or at least the RV free wall patch). This emphasizes the geometric dependence of the right ventricle on the left ventricle in the physiologically normal heart and helps us understand why such mechanisms may be less effective in diseases that modify RV volume.

An even more elegant demonstration of this ventricular cross talk in the normal heart came from Damiano and coworkers [5]. Electrical isolation of the two sides of the heart, maintaining the contiguity of the shared myofibers between the right and left sides allowed them to examine the contributions of ventricular contraction on the contralateral ventricle. Electrical stimulation of RV free wall contraction under these circumstances led to very little change in LV pressure. However, the converse was quite different. Pacing of the left ventricle was associated, again, with a robust RV pressure development and stroke volume from the right ventricle, even in the absence of a contracting RV free wall. The authors estimated that over 50% of the stoke volume from the normal right ventricle is entirely dependent on LV contraction, again presumably by the mechanism of RV shortening generated by the LV free wall. These data serve to emphasize the biventricular nature of all ventricular function. Indeed, morphologic examination of the myocardium shows contiguous myofibers stretching from the RV outflow tract to the LV apex. Furthermore, the two ventricles share a common septum, and so it would be naïve to suggest that events on one side of the heart do not affect the other side by these parallel mechanisms. In pathophysiologic states one might imagine these interactions become even more crucial to overall cardiovascular physiology.

VENTRICULAR INTERDEPENDENCE IN DISEASE

Acute Right Ventricular Dysfunction

As discussed above, this is most likely to occur in response to acute changes in RV afterload, with additional burden being placed in the setting of recent cardiopulmonary bypass, ischemia, or systemic disease such as sepsis and inflammation. The management of such dysfunction primarily revolves around lowering RV afterload via pulmonary vasodilation and careful manipulation of preload so as not to over extend the right ventricle and push it toward the descending limb of its Starling curve. Indeed, the two most frequently used maneuvers to improve cardiac output in children with "low cardiac output syndrome," that of preload augmentation via fluid administration and the use of systemic afterload reduction via ino- and vasodilators, may be fundamentally adverse to RV function when there is isolated RV failure. This is particularly the case in settings such as postoperative cardiac transplantation where the right ventricle is particularly vulnerable (especially when the explant is from a donor after traumatic brain death where RV contractility is depressed [6]). Overexuberant fluid administration can lead to a vicious spiral of worsening RV function and dilatation. So profound can this effect be, that venesection can be a life-saving maneuver, by reducing preload the RV moves leftward and upward in terms of its Starling curve (Fig. 15.2), thereby restoring stroke volume and cardiac output. Another manifestation, which may also have important clinical consequences, of this phenomenon is seen in the convalescent phase after transplantation. In a study of the effects of inotropic reserve, using conductance catheter assessment of RV volume and contractility, administration of dopamine to

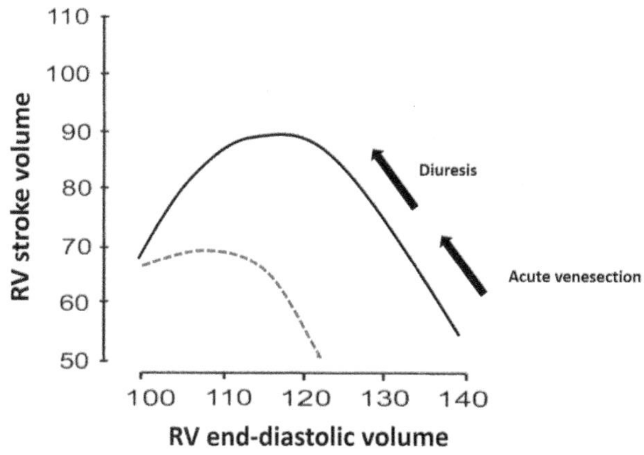

FIGURE 15.2 Schematic to show the RV Starling curve. With overdistension, RV stroke volume can fall precipitously. When profound and life-threatening, venesection may lead to a "paradoxical" prompt improvement in cardiac output. For less acute situations, cardiac output may increase with diuresis. Understanding biventricular interactions is crucial to the recognition and management of patients on the down-sloping part of the curve (see text for discussion). *RV*, right ventricular.

increase cardiac output led to a paradoxical increase in RV end-diastolic and end-systolic volumes [7], suggesting that the RV is working at the limits of its Starling curve and emphasizing the "contractility mismatch" between the right and left ventricles under these circumstances.

There may also be beneficial ventricular–ventricular interactions that can be harnessed under such circumstances. As we have already discussed, a significant portion of RV work is generated by the left ventricle. It may be possible to increase this LV contribution in the setting of acute RV failure. Experimentally, several studies [8,9] have shown that after-loading the left ventricle can generate benefit to the right ventricle by harnessing the LV Anrep effect. The Anrep effect is an autoregulatory response that leads to increased LV contractility in response to an increase in its afterload. While not demonstrable in the normal RV, the LV component can be harnessed to the benefit of the right ventricle, via ventricular–ventricular interactions. In animal experiments aortic banding has been shown to improve RV stroke volume in the setting of acute RV failure. Increasing the force of contraction in the LV, to overcome the aortic obstruction, appears to increase RV contractility via the shared fibers between the two ventricles. In one study, the right coronary flow was kept constant, obviating enhanced coronary perfusion as a mechanism for improved RV function [9]. This is clearly not a therapeutic option in children, but in a subsequent animal study [10], systemic vasoconstriction using norepinephrine similarly leads to increased RV stroke volume in experimental acute right heart failure. While it is often the case that systemic vasodilation is used in the failing circulation, this is one circumstance where a vasoconstrictive policy may be ultimately of benefit to the cardiac output, and the reverse might be expected with systemic vasodilation. Such a strategy is only viable if there is preserved LV function however.

VENTRICULAR–VENTRICULAR INTERACTIONS IN CHRONIC RIGHT VENTRICULAR DYSFUNCTION

Once again, it is beyond the scope of this chapter to discuss every disease state that is associated with chronic RV dysfunction. Instead, we will generally consider two situations, chronic RV volume overload and chronic RV pressure overload. The archetypes of these two states, at least in terms of their frequency and impact, are being postoperative tetralogy of Fallot and primary pulmonary hypertension, respectively.

We have learned a tremendous amount regarding the impact of chronic RV dilatation in response to pulmonary incompetence in the long-term follow-up of patients with tetralogy of Fallot repair. While remarkably well tolerated over years or even decades, ultimately the right ventricle will fail, and overt symptoms and signs appear. Consequently, worsening exercise tolerance, congestive cardiac failure, and ventricular arrhythmia are all sinister features in these patients. The aim of surveillance in these patients is to relieve the volume overload by surgical or transcatheter pulmonary valve replacement, before such symptoms arise. Again, it is beyond the scope of this chapter to discuss such matters in detail, but it is of interest to discuss the emerging understanding of the biventricular consequences of what has traditionally been considered to be a uniquely RV problem. In this regard, it is quite interesting to note that in studies of the long-term outcome in tetralogy of Fallot, when measured, LV indices of dysfunction are powerful predictors of poor outcome, sometimes more powerful than "traditional" RV indices.

It has long been known that there is a relatively linear correlation between RV ejection fraction and LV ejection fraction in these patients [11,12]. Conceptually, this is entirely to be expected given our earlier discussions regarding the shared myocardial fibers between the two ventricles. Furthermore, outcomes are worst in those with the most severely reduced LV ejection fraction [12]. There may also be important diastolic interactions. One of the strongest predictors for ventricular arrhythmia, late after repair of Tetralogy of Fallot, is the LV end-diastolic pressure [13]. There are several reasons why left ventricular end-diastolic pressure (LVEDP) may be increased in chronic RV volume overload. First, there is the simple geometric interaction that takes place whenever one of the heart cavities dilates. Depending on the degree of pericardial constraint, dilatation of one chamber will inevitably have a reciprocal effect on the others. The "squashed" left ventricle subsequently becomes relatively difficult to fill during early rapid filling, increasingly relies on atrial systole for its preloading, and ultimately its filling pressure will rise. That said, this must be a relatively rare cause of a raised end-diastolic pressure under basal conditions. Instead, in the setting of a failing RV one might consider it more usual for the LV pressure to fall (as its preload falls), and conversely for the end-diastolic volume and pressure to rise in response to improved cardiac output—following pulmonary valve replacement, for example. This is indeed the case, and several hemodynamic reports after transcatheter pulmonary valve replacement have demonstrated this phenomenon [14]. Furthermore, the relationship between RV end-diastolic volume and LVEDP is weak, almost idiosyncratic, in one study [15].

Consequently, there is likely to be an alternative explanation for a raised LVEDP, at least in some patients, and it may lay within the LV myocardium itself. Indeed, there appears to be a subset of patients that are predisposed to worsening LV compliance, and this may be related to progressive LV fibrosis. There is increasing experimental evidence to suggest that not only is there a ventricular–ventricular interaction at a hemodynamic and physiologic level but also at a biologic level. Conditions associated with fibrosis on one side of the heart can lead to fibrosis on the other side of the heart even if the contralateral ventricle is not subjected to significantly abnormal hemodynamic load. For example, in an animal preparation associated with chronic RV pressure load, we showed that not only did the right ventricle show increased fibrosis but there was increased LV fibrosis also [16]. Our enhanced ability to delineate fibrosis within the living human heart, using gadolinium enhancement during cardiac MRI, has greatly augmented our understanding of pathologic fibrosis in disease. Tetralogy of Fallot is no exception. In the first study of its kind, there was increased diffuse fibrosis within the left ventricle, measured by T1 mapping of late gadolinium enhancement [17], but not the right ventricle late after Tetralogy repair. While assessment of RV fibrosis is undoubtedly a challenge, in a recent study, there was increased fibrosis in both ventricles, the degree of which was correlated, and its extent was related to the incidence of arrhythmia on Holter monitoring [18]. It remains to be seen whether this diffuse fibrosis is correlated with hard clinical outcomes or is truly a manifestation of adverse ventricular–ventricular interactions. Nonetheless further studies will no doubt help us understand the mechanisms of its generation and its importance in risk stratification.

There are some similarities, but obvious differences, when it comes to the chronic pressure loaded right ventricle. Just as with chronic volume overload, there is a long preclinical period of adaptive remodeling before symptoms and signs appear. If the increase in afterload is slowly progressive, RV remodeling can be adaptive, with a commensurate increase in RV contractility [19]. Global RV function can be preserved, as can cardiac output, for many years or decades. This is somewhat akin to the situation when the right ventricle is in the systemic position. Ultimately, however, the remodeling becomes maladaptive. The ventricle dilates, the cardiac output falls, and symptoms of progressive exercise intolerance, congestive cardiac failure, and syncope with sudden death can occur. While superficially, these outcomes are similar to those seen with right heart volume overload, the pathogenesis and underlying physiology is different. Again, questions arise as to whether this is a uniquely RV problem or whether ventricular–ventricular interactions may, at least in part, be driving some of the adverse events. We can turn to functional magnetic resonance studies to help answer some of these questions. In a beautiful paper by Gan et al. [20] the relationship between RV remodeling and cardiac output was explored in patients with primary pulmonary hypertension. Interestingly there was only a rather loose inverse relationship between RV end-diastolic volume and stroke volume. Intriguingly, the relationship between LV end-diastolic volume and stroke volume was much closer, as LV end-diastolic volume fell so did stroke volume. Although ultimately a consequence of adverse RV remodeling, it appeared that the impact of that remodeling on the left ventricle is not predictable.

Nonetheless once the right ventricle begins to impose on the left ventricle volume, for whatever reason, cardiac output is more directly affected. Interestingly, there also appeared to be a relationship between RR interval (heart rate) and LV end-diastolic volume, the higher the heart rate, the lower the LV volume. This suggests factors over and above purely geometric considerations are at play. Indeed, there are reasons to believe that it is RV physiology, particularly as it pertains to its response to afterload, which drives some of these changes in the left ventricle. While it is true to say that RV ejection time is often abbreviated in chronic pulmonary hypertension, RV contraction time is often grossly prolonged. This is demonstrable by the difference in the duration of pulmonary artery flow, compared to the duration of the tricuspid regurgitant jet (Fig. 15.3). Prolongation of ventricular contraction time is a predictable and linear response to afterload increase in the RV. The greater the afterload, the longer the duration of ventricular contraction. The consequence of this is that ventricular septal tension is maintained for much longer in the RV than is required in the LV. Indeed, at the very time the left ventricle

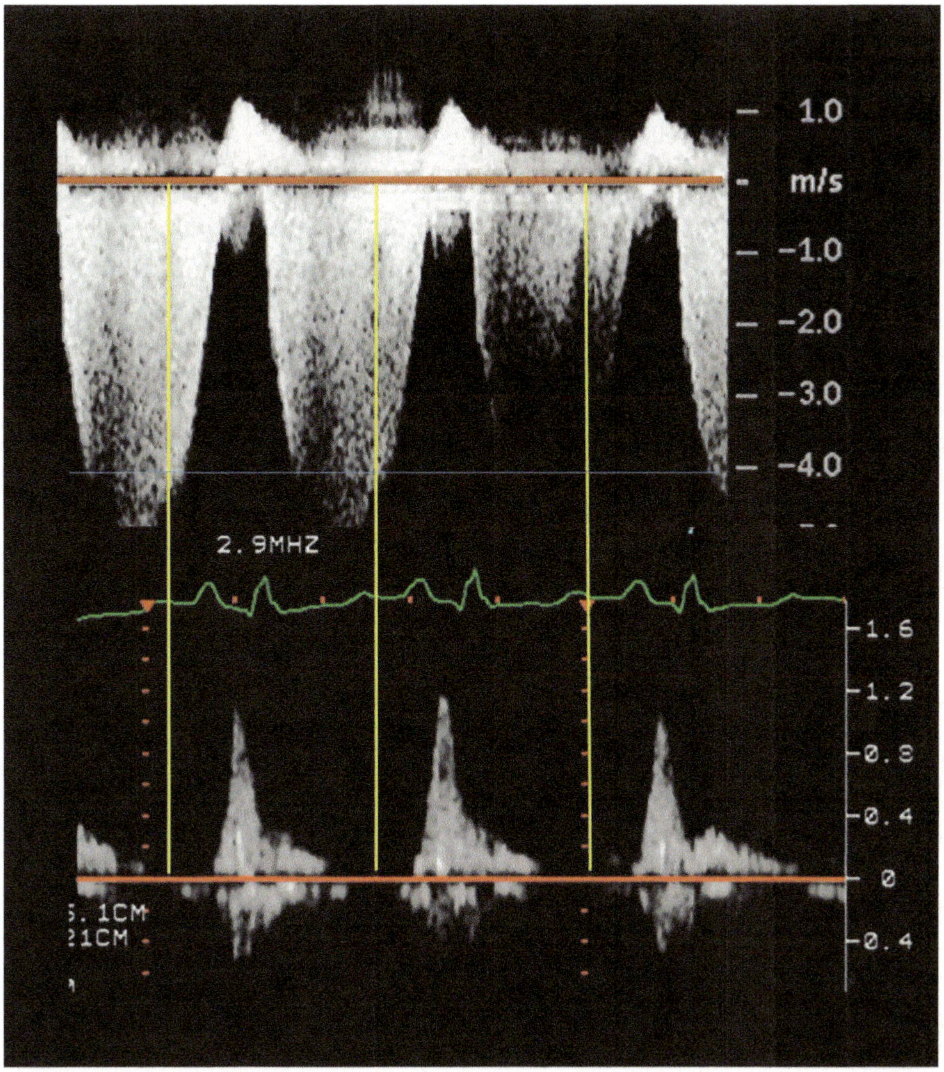

FIGURE 15.3 Spectral Doppler recordings of the tricuspid regurgitant jet velocity (top panel) and transmitral flow velocities (bottom panel) in a patient with severe pulmonary hypertension. The *yellow lines* demarcate the end of the T-wave on the electrocardiogram (onset of left ventricular (LV) relaxation). Note that at this time, the right ventricular (RV) pressure is estimated at approximately 70 mmHg (*blue line*). Consequently there is absence of the early rapid filling phase of transmitral flow because of loss of LV restoring forces. LV filling occurs exclusively with atrial systole.

should be filling during early rapid filling (a process driven by myocardial relaxation and restoring forces) the septum is still in systole with right ventricle. Consequently early rapid filling of the LV is reduced and there is a reciprocal increase in LV filling during atrial contraction. Reversal of transmitral E–A ratio by blood pool Doppler is a prominent feature of patients with pulmonary hypertension. This situation is clearly exacerbated by increase heart rate. The shortened RR interval, in the setting of a prolonged contraction time, has the ultimate consequence of a reduced diastolic filling time. LV end-diastolic volume falls, stroke volume falls, and the cardiac output falls linearly with increase heart rates above a certain level. This may explain some of the adverse effects of exercise in these patients, the exquisite sensitively to arrhythmia, and the tremendously adverse effects of traditional inotropic agents (which nearly always concomitantly increase heart rate) in these patients. While cause and effect can never be demonstrated, it is well known that the use of inotropes in patients with primary pulmonary hypertension requiring intensive care is associated with a massive increase in odds ratio for death (in excess of 130-fold) [21].

Interestingly, this physiology can be relatively easily measured by assessing the systolic to diastolic (S–D) time ratio from the tricuspid regurgitant jet [24]. When measured in children, the S–D ratio was predictive of not only poor functional outcome but also death, in a relatively small group of children with primary pulmonary hypertension. It may therefore not only be reflective of adverse physiology but also a useful tool for risk stratification.

RIGHT VENTRICLE IN DILATED LEFT VENTRICULAR CARDIOMYOPATHY

Just as some congenital diseases are thought of as uniquely RV in consequence, LV dilated cardiomyopathy is sometimes considered to be a uniquely LV disease. There is increasing evidence to suggest that biventricular consequences are equally important in this patient group also. Outcomes for dilated cardiomyopathy are worse when LV remodeling is associated with poor RV systolic function and are affected even more adversely when poor RV function is additionally associated with pulmonary hypertension [22]. In some ways, this is intuitive, and while helpful in terms of risk stratification and prognostication, its relevance is relatively limited in terms of its impact on day-to-day management. When it does become an issue, however, is when contemplating the use of a left ventricular assist device (LVAD). There is ongoing controversy as to how best to assess the ability of the right ventricle to perform when cardiac output is augmented using mechanical support. This remains a hot topic, and one that is largely impossible to address with the current level of mechanistic data. However, given that RV dysfunction may be intrinsic or secondary, the responses to LVAD may be significantly different depending on the underlying cause of the RV dysfunction. For many patients, RV dysfunction is secondary to increased RV afterload as a consequence of high downstream pressures. Under these circumstances a reduction in left atrial pressure might be expected to lead to a prompt improvement in RV function. However, if there is a fixed element to the RV afterload, as sometimes occurs with chronic left heart disease, a reduction in left atrial pressure may not necessarily reduce the hydraulic impedance on the right ventricle. Under these circumstances an improved LV output may add to the preload of an already failing ventricle as a consequence of its afterload [23]. RV failure may similarly be observed in the setting of RV dysfunction that is primarily related to RV myocardial disease. Again, an increase in LV output may be associated with a paradoxical increase in RV preload and worsening RV dysfunction, similar to the "contractility mismatch" phenomenon described earlier. As yet, there is no magic bullet that allows us to define, at least with any degree of accuracy, those patients that will or will not have important RV failure and require biventricular support. Nonetheless, within improved understanding of these physiologic responses, it is reasonable to anticipate that our ability to risk stratify will improve.

CONCLUSION

In summary, the right and left ventricles are inextricably linked in terms of their function, and consequently almost all causes of heart failure have a biventricular component to their pathogenesis. Although relatively understudied, these interactions have already been shown to have potentially profound influences on cardiovascular physiology and long-term outcomes of disease. A better understanding of the beneficial and adverse ventricular–ventricular interactions that occur under these circumstances may be the key to improved outcome in the future.

REFERENCES

[1] R. Naeije, S. Brimioulle, L. Dewachter, Biomechanics of the right ventricle in health and disease (2013 grover conference series), Pulm. Circ. 4 (3) (September 2014) 395–406.

[2] E. Braunwald, Pathophysiology of heart failure, in: E. Braunwald (Ed.), Heart Disease. A Textbook of Cardiovascular Medicine, Saunders, Philadelphia, 1980, pp. 453–471.

[3] R.C. Johnson, S.A. Datar, P.E. Oishi, S. Bennett, J. Maki, C. Sun, M. Johengen, Y. He, G.W. Raff, A.N. Redington, J.R. Fineman, Adaptive right ventricular performance in response to acutely increased afterload in a lamb model of congenital heart disease: evidence for enhanced Anrep effect, Am. J. Physiol. Heart Circ. Physiol. 306 (8) (April 15, 2014) H1222–H1230.

[4] D. Hoffman, D. Sisto, R.W. Frater, S.D. Nikolic, Left-to-right ventricular interaction with a noncontracting right ventricle, J. Thorac. Cardiovasc. Surg. 107 (6) (June 1994) 1496–1502.

[5] R.J. Damiano Jr., P. La Follette Jr., J.L. Cox, J.E. Lowe, W.P. Santamore, Significant left ventricular contribution to right ventricular systolic function, Am. J. Physiol. 261 (5 Pt 2) (November 1991) H1514–H1524.

[6] S.C. Stoica, D.K. Satchithananda, P.A. White, J. Parameshwar, A.N. Redington, S.R. Large, Noradrenaline use in the human donor and relationship with load-independent right ventricular contractility, Transplantation 78 (8) (October 27, 2004) 1193–1197.

[7] S.C. Stoica, D.K. Satchithananda, P.A. White, L. Sharples, J. Parameshwar, A.N. Redington, S.R. Large, Brain death leads to abnormal contractile properties of the human donor right ventricle, J. Thorac. Cardiovasc. Surg. 132 (1) (July 2006) 116–123.

[8] H. Yamashita, S. Onodera, T. Imamoto, A. Obara, S. Tanazawa, T. Takashio, H. Morimoto, H. Inoue, Functional and geometrical interference and interdependency between the right and left ventricle in cor pulmonale: an experimental study on simultaneous measurement of biventricular geometry of acute right ventricular pressure overload, Jpn. Circ. J. 53 (10) (October 1989) 1237–1244.

[9] I. Belenkie, S.G. Horne, R. Dani, E.R. Smith, J.V. Tyberg, Effects of aortic constriction during experimental acute right ventricular pressure loading. Further insights into diastolic and systolic ventricular interaction, Circulation 92 (3) (August 1, 1995) 546–554.

[10] C. Apitz, O. Honjo, M.K. Friedberg, R.S. Assad, G. Van Arsdell, T. Humpl, A.N. Redington, Beneficial effects of vasopressors on right ventricular function in experimental acute right ventricular failure in a rabbit model, Thorac. Cardiovasc. Surg. 60 (1) (February 2012) 17–23.

[11] P.A. Davlouros, P.J. Kilner, T.S. Hornung, W. Li, J.M. Francis, J.C. Moon, G.C. Smith, T. Tat, D.J. Pennell, M.A. Gatzoulis, Right ventricular function in adults with repaired tetralogy of Fallot assessed with cardiovascular magnetic resonance imaging: detrimental role of right ventricular outflow aneurysms or akinesia and adverse right-to-left ventricular interaction, J. Am. Coll. Cardiol. 40 (11) (December 4, 2002) 2044–2052.

[12] A. Ghai, C. Silversides, L. Harris, G.D. Webb, S.C. Siu, J. Therrien, Left ventricular dysfunction is a risk factor for sudden cardiac death in adults late after repair of tetralogy of Fallot, J. Am. Coll. Cardiol. 40 (9) (November 6, 2002) 1675–1680.

[13] P. Khairy, L. Harris, M.J. Landzberg, S. Viswanathan, A. Barlow, M.A. Gatzoulis, S.M. Fernandes, L. Beauchesne, J. Therrien, P. Chetaille, E. Gordon, I. Vonder Muhll, F. Cecchin, Implantable cardioverter-defibrillators in tetralogy of Fallot, Circulation 117 (3) (January 22, 2008) 363–370.

[14] P. Lurz, J. Nordmeyer, A. Giardini, S. Khambadkone, V. Muthurangu, S. Schievano, J.B. Thambo, F. Walker, S. Cullen, G. Derrick, A.M. Taylor, P. Bonhoeffer, Early versus late functional outcome after successful percutaneous pulmonary valve implantation: are the acute effects of altered right ventricular loading all we can expect? J. Am. Coll. Cardiol. 57 (6) (February 8, 2011) 724–731.

[15] M.C. Schwartz, J.J. Rome, M.J. Gillespie, K. Whitehead, M.A. Harris, M.A. Fogel, A.C. Glatz, Relation of left ventricular end diastolic pressure to right ventricular end diastolic volume after operative treatment of tetralogy of fallot, Am. J. Cardiol. 109 (3) (February 1, 2012) 417–422.

[16] M.K. Friedberg, M.Y. Cho, J. Li, R.S. Assad, M. Sun, S. Rohailla, O. Honjo, C. Apitz, A.N. Redington, Adverse biventricular remodeling in isolated right ventricular hypertension is mediated by increased transforming growth factor-β1 signaling and is abrogated by angiotensin receptor blockade, Am. J. Respir. Cell Mol. Biol. 49 (6) (December 2013) 1019–1028.

[17] M.F. Kozak, A. Redington, S.J. Yoo, M. Seed, A. Greiser, L. Grosse-Wortmann, Diffuse myocardial fibrosis following tetralogy of Fallot repair: a T1 mapping cardiac magnetic resonance study, Pediatr. Radiol. 44 (4) (April 2014) 403–409.

[18] C.A. Chen, S.M. Dusenbery, A.M. Valente, A.J. Powell, T. Geva, Myocardial ECV fraction assessed by CMR is associated with type of hemodynamic load and arrhythmia in repaired tetralogy of fallot, JACC Cardiovasc. Imaging 9 (1) (January 2016) 1–10.

[19] S.L. Gaynor, H.S. Maniar, J.B. Bloch, P. Steendijk, M.R. Moon, Right atrial and ventricular adaptation to chronic right ventricular pressure overload, Circulation 112 (9 Suppl.) (August 30, 2005) I212–I218.

[20] C. Gan, J.W. Lankhaar, J.T. Marcus, N. Westerhof, K.M. Marques, J.G. Bronzwaer, A. Boonstra, P.E. Postmus, A. Vonk-Noordegraaf, Impaired left ventricular filling due to right-to-left ventricular interaction in patients with pulmonary arterial hypertension, Am. J. Physiol. Heart Circ. Physiol. 290 (4) (April 2006) H1528–H1533.

[21] A. Campo, S.C. Mathai, J. Le Pavec, A.L. Zaiman, L.K. Hummers, D. Boyce, T. Housten, N. Lechtzin, H. Chami, R.E. Girgis, P.M. Hassoun, Outcomes of hospitalisation for right heart failure in pulmonary arterial hypertension, Eur. Respir. J. 38 (2) (August 2011) 359–367.

[22] S. Ghio, A. Gavazzi, C. Campana, C. Inserra, C. Klersy, R. Sebastiani, E. Arbustini, F. Recusani, L. Tavazzi, Independent and additive prognostic value of right ventricular systolic function and pulmonary artery pressure in patients with chronic heart failure, J. Am. Coll. Cardiol. 37 (1) (January 2001) 183–188.

[23] A. Pavie, P. Leger, Physiology of univentricular versus biventricular support, Ann. Thorac. Surg. 61 (1) (January 1996) 347–349.

[24] J. Alkon, T. Humpl, C. Manlhiot, B.W. McCrindle, J.T. Reyes, M.K. Friedberg, Usefulness of the right ventricular systolic to diastolic duration ratio to predict functional capacity and survival in children with pulmonary arterial hypertension, Am. J. Cardiol. 106 (3) (August 1, 2010) 430–436.

Chapter 16

Pediatric Myocarditis

Charles E. Canter, Kathleen E. Simpson
Washington University School of Medicine, St. Louis Children's Hospital, St Louis, MO, United States

INTRODUCTION

Despite advances over the past decades, myocarditis remains a challenging disease. Myocarditis has been defined as an inflammatory myocardial disease diagnosed by specific immunological, histological, and immunohistochemical criteria [1]. However, in practice, myocarditis is associated with a wide range of clinical presentations that lend to the difficulty of a timely diagnosis in both children and adults. Clinicians should be familiar with the varied phenotypes as well as appropriate diagnostic tools and therapeutic options in patients with myocarditis.

EPIDEMIOLOGY

Myocarditis has been recognized as a global disease with a substantial impact on the development of chronic heart failure and sudden death [2]. The incidence of myocarditis varies by continent, likely related to differences in the most prevalent causes among regions. Worldwide, myocarditis is estimated to account for 10%–50% of newly diagnosed dilated cardiomyopathy (DCM) in adults [2]. However, the actual incidence of myocarditis in children and adults is likely underestimated due to subclinical disease and the presentation of sudden death in some patients. Based on autopsy studies, the incidence of myocarditis is approximately 0.05%–0.1% in the general population [3,4] and 0.6%–1.8% in children and young adults [4,5]. Among patients with suspected sudden cardiac death (SCD), myocarditis accounted for 14.8% [6] of deaths in adults, while another study found evidence of myocarditis in 7.4% of autopsy subjects between 1 and 40 years of age [7]. In the review of cardiac deaths from the National Center for Review and Prevention of Child Deaths database, myocarditis was responsible for 4.6% of deaths, most commonly in the 3- to 10-year-old age group [8].

Several studies have noted age and gender differences in the incidence of myocarditis. In respect to age differences, there appears to be a bimodal distribution of myocarditis with peaks in very young children and young adults [9]. Autopsy studies have noted the majority of adults with evidence of myocarditis are in the late teens to early 30s, especially among men [4–7]. Myocarditis has been noted to be more common in males compared to females [7,10,11], with a peak incidence for males in early adulthood compared to a relatively even distribution among age groups in females [10]. The reason for the differences in incidence of myocarditis among different genders is unclear but may be related to differences in host immune response, cell signaling, and gene expression [11].

PATHOPHYSIOLOGY

Causes

Globally, myocarditis has been associated with various causes, from infectious agents to toxins, as noted in Table 16.1. Acute myocarditis is classically associated with viral infections in children and adults, often with common viruses known for causing relatively mild respiratory or gastrointestinal symptoms in the general population. In the past, enterovirus (especially Coxsackievirus) and adenovirus were the most commonly associated viral agents in pediatric myocarditis. Coxsackievirus B, in particular, has been associated with higher mortality and more severe disease in infants, thought to be due to more diffuse coxsackievirus and adenovirus receptor expression in immature myocardial tissue [12]. However, over the past decade, parvovirus B19 and human herpes virus-6 (HHV6) have been increasingly recognized as a major cause of myocarditis in children and adults. Interestingly, HHV6 may increase parvovirus B19 activity in the setting of coinfection, leading to higher viral loads than infection with parvovirus B19 alone [13]. The shift in viral etiology may be due to changes in virus characteristics or simply advances in viral detection by technology such as polymerase chain reaction (PCR) testing on cardiac tissue. Several other viruses have also been reportedly associated with myocarditis, such as Epstein–Barr virus,

Heart Failure in the Child and Young Adult. http://dx.doi.org/10.1016/B978-0-12-802393-8.00016-8

TABLE 16.1 Causative Agents Associated With Acute Myocarditis in Children and Adults

Infectious	
Viral	**Fungal**
Adenovirus	*Nocardia*
Enterovirus	*Histoplasma*
Coxsackievirus A and B	*Cryptococcus*
Echovirus	*Aspergillus*
Parvovirus B19	*Candida*
Influenza A and B viruses	*Actinomyces*
Respiratory syncytial virus	*Blastomyces*
Varicella virus	**Rickettsial**
Herpes viruses	*Rickettsia prowazekii*
Human herpes virus 6	*Rickettsia rickettsee*
Cytomegalovirus	*Coxiella burnetii*
Epstein–Barr virus	**Spirochetal**
Hepatitis B and C viruses	*Treponema pallidum*
Human immunodeficiency virus	*Borelia burgdorferi*
Bacterial	*Leptospira*
Listeria monocytogenes	**Protozoal**
Staphylococcus	*Entamoeba histolytica*
Streptococcus A	*Toxoplasmosis gondii*
Streptococcus pneumoniae	*Leishmania*
Chlamydia	*Trypanosoma cruzi*
Corynebacterium diphtheria	**Helminths**
Mycoplasma pneumonia	*Trichinella spiralis*
Mycobacterium tuberculosis	*Schistosoma*
Legionella	*Strongyloides stercoralis*

Autoimmune	
Systemic lupus erythemathosus	Celiac disease
Hypereosinophilic syndrome	Rheumatoid arthritis
Churg–Strauss syndrome	Kawasaki disease

Toxins and exposures	
Aminophylline	Lead
Cocaine	Arsenic
Ethanol	Radiotherapy
Copper	Thyrotoxicosis
Iron	Chloramphemicol
Anthracyclines	Zidovudine
Doxorubicin	Methysergide
Trastuzumab	Phenytoin

Hypersensitivity reactions	
Penicillin	Clozapine
Ampicillin	Benzodiazepines
Tetracyclines	Methyldopa
Sulfonamides	NSAIDS
Cephalosporins	Tricyclic antidepressants
Diuretics	Tetanus toxoid
Loop	Venom
Thiazides	Snake, wasp, scorpion, black widow spider, bee

cytomegalovirus (CMV), hepatitis C virus, human immunodeficiency virus, influenza A virus, and respiratory syncytial virus [14,15]. During the 2009 influenza A H1N1 outbreak, several cases of myocarditis were reported [16,17] and was a significant independent predictor of death [18].

Other infectious causes include bacterial, fungal, and parasitic infectious agents, although less common than viral causes in acute myocarditis [15]. Associated bacterial causes include *Listeria monocytogenes*, *Staphylococcus*, *Mycobacterium tuberculosis*, and *Streptococcus*. Parasites are a less common cause of myocarditis and are notably associated with an eosinophilic infiltrate on histology and often peripheral eosinophilia, such as with Chagas disease due to infection from *Trypanosoma cruzi* in endemic areas of Africa and South America [19,20]. Toxocariasis from helminthiasis, particularly in areas of Asia, has also been associated with development of eosinophilic myocarditis [21].

Beyond parasitic infections, eosinophilic myocarditis has also been associated with hypersensitivity reactions, toxin exposure, and autoimmune diseases [15]. Myocarditis due to a hypersensitivity reaction has been described with exposure to medications, such as clozapine or penicillin, as well as vaccines, including the smallpox vaccine. Toxins, such as copper and ethanol, and venom from various species have also been reported as causative agents. In addition, several autoimmune diseases have known cardiac involvement and can include myocarditis, such as systemic lupus erythematosus (SLE), Churg–Strauss syndrome, and hypereosinophilic syndrome (HES). Churg–Strauss syndrome (also referred to as eosinophilic granulomatosis with polyangiitis) leads to inflammation of blood vessels and, in some patients, myocarditis, which is associated with increased risk of death [22]. HES is a multiorgan disease associated with cardiac involvement including eosinophilic myocarditis, mural thrombi, coronary inflammation, and endocardial fibrosis [23]. Notably, with cases of eosinophilic myocarditis, peripheral eosinophilia may not be present in all patients, but most patients respond well to steroid therapy with good long-term outcomes [24].

Giant cell myocarditis (GCM) is a rare cause of myocarditis characterized by a lymphocytic infiltrate, multinucleated giant cells, and fibrosis on endomyocardial biopsy (EMB) [25]. Patients present with severe heart failure, ventricular tachyarrhythmias, and/or heart block. Survival is typically poor and dramatically worse compared to classic myocarditis patients, especially in children. A previous report from the GCM registry revealed an overall median survival of 5.5 months and rate of death or transplant of 89% [26]. However, a more recent small prospective adult study reported 73% 1-year transplant free survival using a standardized immunosuppression protocol [27]. Unfortunately, GCM recurrence has been also been reported in long-term survivors [28] and even after heart transplantation [26,29].

Mechanisms of Cellular Damage and Cardiac Dysfunction

Based on murine models, cardiac damage in myocarditis occurs through an intricate relationship between the inciting agent, usually a virus, and the host immune response [30] (Fig. 16.1). During the *acute phase*, viral titers increase due to viral replication in the blood and various tissues, including the myocardium. Cardiac myocytes are damaged through direct viral-mediated injury and inflammatory cytokines. In the *subacute phase*, natural killer cells and macrophages migrate to the area of injured tissue in response to virus, followed by further release of inflammatory cytokines and infiltration of B and T cells [30]. CD4+ Th17 cells play a role in enhancing the inflammatory response and stimulating B cell production of virus-specific antibodies [31]. Treg cells also affect the host inflammatory response but may have either proinflammatory effects or act to suppress cardiac fibrosis [31]. Overall, this response not only leads to viral clearance but also lysis of infected myocytes. After removal of virus, the chronic phase includes resolution of the inflammatory response and recovery of damage tissue [30]. However, in some patients, there may be ongoing viral persistence and/or immune activation leading to a chronic DCM phenotype. Maladaptive responses from immune cells, such as activated macrophages and cardiac fibroblasts, may lead to excessive collagen production and fibrosis of the myocardium, contributing to diastolic dysfunction and heart failure [31].

Autoimmunity

Part of the host immune response in myocarditis, as well as other inflammatory diseases, involves autoimmune activation and B cell production of autoantibodies [32–34]. With lysis of the cardiac myocytes during the acute and subacute phase of disease, cardiac proteins are released, which in some cases share similar epitopes with viral components, leading to the development of autoantibodies through the process of molecular mimicry [35,36]. Autoantibodies are thought to play a role in inflammation and cellular injury through the interaction with cell receptors and subsequent release of inflammatory cytokines. In murine models, antibodies to cardiac myosin were found to target cardiac myocytes, leading to apoptosis and development of a DCM phenotype [33,36]. Both myosin and beta-adrenergic receptor antibodies were found to activate beta-adrenergic receptors and cause increased activation of protein-kinase A, which has been associated with apoptosis in the setting of excessive stimulation [37,38]. Antimyosin antibodies have also been found in children [39] and adults [32] with myocarditis. Although not clearly associated with outcomes in children, a small study in adults found the presence of antimyosin antibodies at baseline, and follow-up was associated with worse parameters of systolic and diastolic function at follow-up compared to antibody negative patients [32].

Additional antibodies have been described, including antibodies to muscarinic-2 receptors. In rats, antimuscarinic-2 receptor antibodies were associated with lymphocyte infiltration and cell destruction leading to decreased systolic function

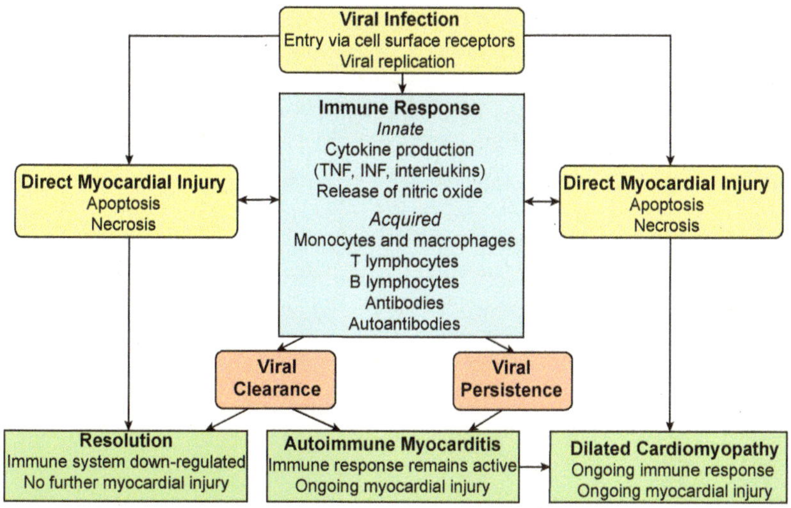

FIGURE 16.1 Mechanisms of injury, recovery, and chronic cardiomyopathy with myocarditis. INF, interferon; *TNF*, tumor necrosis factor *(Image from L.A. Blauwet, L.T. Cooper, Myocarditis, Prog. Cardiovasc. Dis. 42 (4) (January–February 2010) 274–288.)*

and changes in action potential duration [40]. Muscarinic-2 antibodies were associated with atrial fibrillation and sinus node dysfunction in adults with DCM, possibly through negative chronotropic effects and inducing supraventricular arrhythmias [41,42]. Antiadenine nucleotide translocator antibodies in murine models led to the development of cardiac dysfunction and have also been found in patients with myocarditis [43], but levels in humans did not correlate with left ventricular (LV) dysfunction or dilation [44]. The role of autoantibodies in myocarditis in the acute and chronic setting is evolving, but the use of assays remains experimental and not available for routine clinical evaluation.

CLINICAL PRESENTATIONS

Sudden Death

As mentioned above, much of the reported incidence of myocarditis comes from autopsy studies and reviews of sudden death in children and adults. Among adults with nonischemic heart disease and sudden death, myocarditis was found in 5.3% of patients in series from the United Kingdom [45]. Myocarditis was also found in 12% of patients less than 35-years old who presented with sudden death in an Australian review [46]. In a pediatric autopsy study, histological evidence consistent with myocarditis was found in 1.8% of patients, of which 57% presented with sudden death [47]. For deaths during sports or athletic events, myocarditis was found in 8% among all participants in a German registry, but in 24% of deaths among athletes less than 35-years old [48]. Other autopsy reviews of athletes and sudden death reported myocarditis in 3% of all deaths [49,50] and 8% of SCDs [49,51]. In children, myocarditis has also been recognized as a cause of death in infants with sudden infant death syndrome (SIDS), with a recent review finding 2% of SIDS patients met the histologic diagnosis of myocarditis [52].

Dilated Cardiomyopathy

The typical clinical phenotype for myocarditis in children is heart failure symptoms in the setting of DCM after a recent viral syndrome. Worldwide, myocarditis is known to be a common cause of cardiomyopathy in children. Among children in the United Kingdom, myocarditis is thought to account for 22% of new-onset LV dysfunction [53]. Pediatric cardiomyopathy registries in Australia and the United States have reported myocarditis as the cause of 27%–46% of DCM in children [54–56].

Fulminant Myocarditis

An important subset of children present with a more severe form of disease, known as fulminant myocarditis, with distinct clinical features and outcomes compared to classic acute lymphocytic myocarditis. Typically, patients will report a recent viral illness within approximately 2–4 weeks prior to presentation with sudden onset heart failure [57]. Symptoms are often severe, with cardiogenic shock, arrhythmias, and/or multiorgan failure frequency present requiring aggressive resuscitation and cardiac support, including short-term mechanical circulatory support (MCS) [58,59]. In fulminant myocarditis, characteristic echocardiographic findings include severely depressed ventricular systolic function, increased ventricular septal wall thickness, and normal LV dimensions [60]. Compared to classic myocarditis, long-term outcomes are superior after the initial period of illness, with reported 80%–90% transplant-free survival [58,59] in pediatric patients and 60%–70% in an adults [61,62], even after requiring MCS.

Acute Coronary Syndrome

A more recently recognized myocarditis phenotype in children and adults is signs and symptoms suggestive of acute coronary syndrome (ACS) in the absence of coronary artery disease. In children, ACS presentation of myocarditis appears to be more common in adolescents, particularly males, but typically both older children and adults complain of chest pain with or without dyspnea. Serum troponin levels are often elevated, and patients may have electrocardiographic changes suggestive of cardiac ischemia [63]. Cardiac function may be mildly depressed or even normal, with normal LV dimensions on echocardiogram at presentation. Angiographic evaluation is negative for significant coronary artery disease, although vasospasm has been demonstrated in up to 70% of patients [64]. For this population, cardiac magnetic resonance imaging (CMR) to evaluate for characteristic changes consistent with myocarditis is frequently helpful [65,66]. Interestingly, parvovirus B19 has been associated with the ACS phenotype [67], possibly due to specific targeting of myocardial endothelial cells by the virus [68].

DIAGNOSIS AND WORKUP

Differential Diagnosis

Many of the initial clinical symptoms and findings in children with myocarditis are nonspecific, and clinicians must have a high degree of suspicion for accurate diagnosis of myocarditis. Depending on the age, history, and associated extracardiac organ involvement, the differential diagnosis varies. Possible etiologies that may have a similar presentation to myocarditis in children include mitochondrial or metabolic diseases, familial cardiomyopathies, genetic syndromes, autoimmune disorders, ischemic cardiomyopathy, or toxin exposure.

History and Physical Exam

Classically, children with myocarditis present after a viral prodrome within several days to weeks before presenting with heart failure symptoms. Symptoms are often nonspecific, and patients may be initially misdiagnosed [69]. The majority of patients will have a history of recent gastrointestinal or upper respiratory tract infection prior to diagnosis [70,71]. Clinical history and physical exam typically suggests cardiac dysfunction, including tachypnea, tachycardia, poor appetite, emesis, abdominal pain, hepatomegaly, decreased perfusion, pallor, orthopnea, irritability, and/or lethargy [72,73]. Conversely, other patients may present in cardiogenic shock as the initial manifestation of myocarditis [71]. Initial laboratory testing may reveal elevated inflammatory markers, liver enzymes, and/or cell counts, but none are specific to the diagnosis of myocarditis in children [69,70,72,74,75].

Serum Biomarkers

Routine screening for cardiac disease, including myocarditis, with troponin levels in children with acute viral infection but no cardiac symptoms appears to be low yield, with elevated troponin levels noted in 0.05% of children tested that subsequently all had normal electrocardiograms (ECGs) and echocardiograms [76]. When used as a screening test in children and young adults presenting emergently with chest pain, 17% had elevated troponin levels, of which roughly half had cardiac disease in one case series [77]. In that study, cardiac disease was more likely if the ECG was abnormal, and significantly higher levels of troponin elevation were associated with a diagnosis of myocarditis. Similarly, troponin levels have been found to be elevated in children with a clinical presentation of myocarditis compared to controls [78], with significantly higher troponin levels in fulminant myocarditis patients compared to other myocarditis patients [79]. Troponin levels have also been correlated with extent of late gadolinium enhancement (LGE) on CMR [80]. However, the predictability of elevated troponin levels and patient outcomes is unclear, as studies have reported varied results in children and adults [78,79,81,82].

Similar to adults, B-type natriuretic peptide (BNP) has been reported to help differentiate cardiac and primary respiratory disease in children presenting with respiratory distress, with levels higher in those with primary ventricular dysfunction compared to volume overload [83]. N-terminal proBNP (NT-proBNP) levels may also be higher in children with myocarditis compared to children with idiopathic DCM [84]. Higher NT-proBNP (>4225 ng/mL) was associated with higher risk of death or heart transplant in adults [81], and very high BNP (>10,000 ng/L) was also associated with risk for death or heart transplant in children, with an odds ratio of 27.7 [82]. However, the relationship of either BNP or NT-proBNP levels and clinical prognosis in children with acute myocarditis is unclear.

Serum antibodies to cardiac proteins, such as myosin or beta-adrenergic receptors, can be measured in patients with myocarditis, but testing remains primarily confined to research. Antimyosin antibodies have been reported in adults with both clinical myocarditis and DCM [32,33,85] and children with myocarditis [39]. Persistence of antimyosin antibodies was associated with worse outcomes in adults with chronic myocarditis [32]. Currently, lack of wide availability and information regarding usefulness in diagnosis and outcomes limits the practical use of anticardiac antibodies.

Infection

As mentioned, the majority of myocarditis in children and adults is thought to be secondary to a viral infection. To that end, patients are often evaluated for possible infectious agents. Clinicians should also be sensitive to regional differences or immunocompromised states that require evaluation for specific pathogens based on known exposure or risk [57]. The gold standard for diagnosis of associated viral causes is analysis of endomyocardial tissue obtained by EMB. Previous techniques to identity viruses, such as cell culture, have been largely replaced by newer technology, such as PCR, at most institutions.

EMB PCR was positive for associated viruses in 68% of children in one study, but negative in all control tissue samples [86]. Similarly, 50% of children with biopsy-proven myocarditis also had positive viral PCR in another study; however, 35% of DCM patients without criteria for myocarditis also had positive viral results [87].

Reports have varied on the utility of peripheral samples in the absence of available endomyocardial tissue, such as from nasopharyngeal or serum samples, to accurately identify the causative infectious agent. One study reported identifying known cardiotropic viruses in up to 29% of children from either blood or cardiac tissue [82], while another reported positive viral studies in nearly 22% of patients from a wide range of sample types [71]. Another reported 43% of children with clinically suspected myocarditis tested had positive blood viral PCR, mainly in infants, compared to only 3.5% of controls [88]. An adult study in clinically suspected myocarditis reported 38% of patients were positive for virus from peripheral leukocytes, with 84% agreement of viral positivity and myocardial edema by CMR but not LGE [89]. However, comparison between viral serology and EMB PCR found poor correlation between viral testing results from serum and EMB samples [90]. It remains unclear if peripheral samples can be routinely used to accurately identify associated infectious agents in children with suspected myocarditis.

Radiography

Chest X-rays are frequently obtained in both children and adults with myocarditis due the frequent respiratory symptoms and chest pain noted during the initial presentation. The majority of children will not only have some abnormal findings on chest X-ray, most commonly cardiomegaly, but also may include pulmonary edema, pleural effusion, and/or cardiomegaly [69,70]. Notably, patients who present with the ACS clinical phenotype may have a normal chest X-ray at presentation [63].

Electrocardiogram

Nearly all patients will have some abnormality on ECG at presentation, making it a useful and sensitive, although not always specific, diagnostic tool in children with suspected myocarditis [69]. The classic finding on ECG is decreased QRS voltage, but other findings include atrial or ventricular tachyarrhythmias, various degrees of heart block, sinus tachycardia, ST- and T-wave abnormalities, abnormal Q waves, and QT prolongation [70,72,91] (Fig. 16.2). ECG in some cases may mimic acute myocardial infection in patients with the ACS phenotype [92,93]. Of those children and young adults who develop advanced atrioventricular block associated with myocarditis, normal conduction reportedly can return within a week, but permanent pacing may be required in those patients with prolonged heart block [94].

Echocardiogram

In children and adults with suspected myocarditis, an echocardiogram is typically obtained during the diagnostic evaluation. No one echocardiographic finding is specific to myocarditis, and findings may vary with clinical phenotype. Classically, patients with myocarditis present with a dilated left ventricle and a varying degree of decreased LV systolic function [60,72,73,95] (Fig. 16.3). Patients with fulminant myocarditis often have severely decreased systolic function but normal or only mildly dilated LV chamber size and thickened ventricular septal wall [60]. With the ACS phenotype, LV systolic function may be normal or only mildly depressed, with regional wall motion abnormalities in a noncoronary distribution and normal coronary angiography [67,75,93,96]. Even in those patients with normal systolic function, parameters of diastolic function may be abnormal during the initial evaluation [97]. Symptomatic diastolic dysfunction in the setting of normal systolic function has also been described in adults during follow-up several years after the diagnosis of myocarditis [98]. Speckle tracking can also be used to evaluate strain as well as regional wall abnormalities in myocarditis and is often abnormal in acute myocarditis [99,100]. Other findings include atrioventricular valve regurgitation, pericardial effusion, intramural thrombi, and/or evidence of pulmonary hypertension [72,101]. Ventricular aneurysms may also be found in patients with Chagas disease who develop associated heart disease [20].

Several studies have found that more severe ventricular dysfunction at presentation is associated with worse patient outcomes in children and adults. A shortening fraction <15% or ejection fraction (EF) <30% in children at admission was associated with persistent heart failure and poor outcomes [72,82]. Right ventricular dysfunction may accompany LV dysfunction and has been associated with increased risk for death or heart transplant [102].

Endomyocardial Biopsy

EMB is considered the gold standard diagnostic procedure for diagnosis of myocarditis in children and adults. Initially reported in 1987, the "Dallas criteria" describe the histologic criteria for diagnosis of myocarditis, including inflammatory

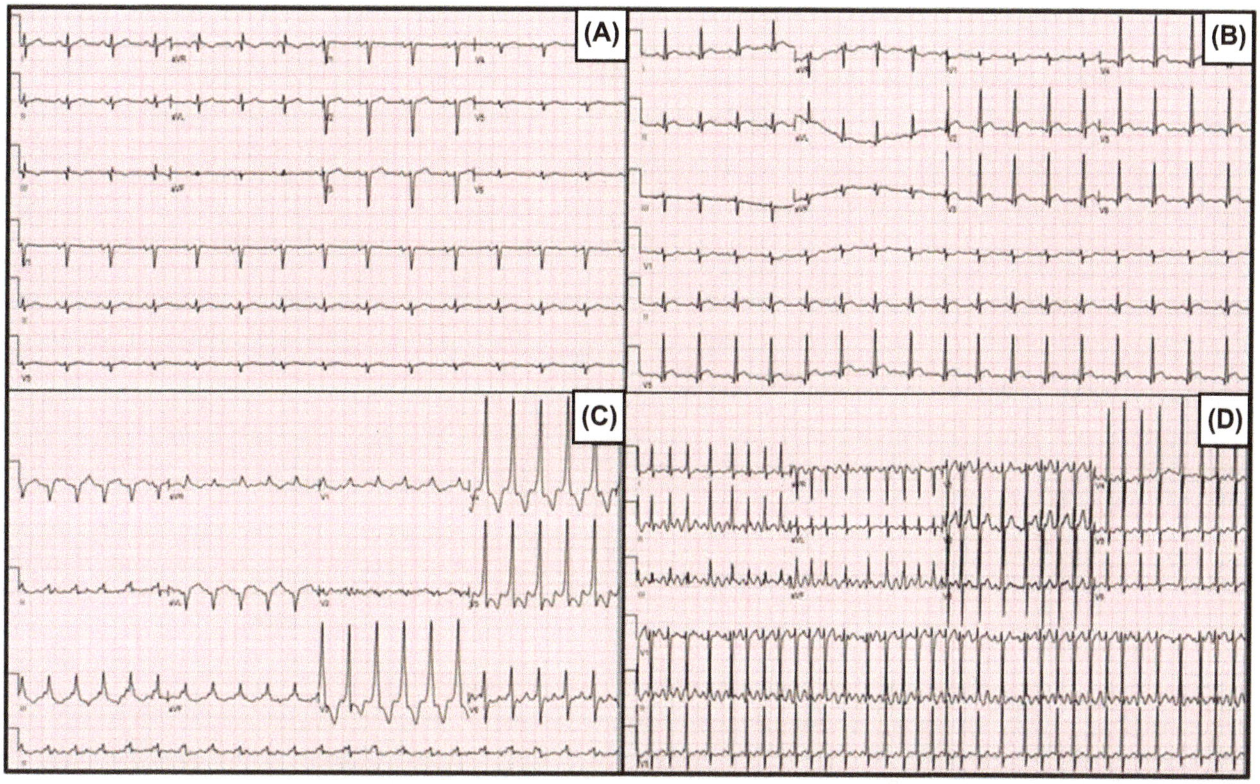

FIGURE 16.2 Examples of ECG findings in myocarditis. Panel (A): Low QRS voltage in a 16-year old; panel (B): sinus tachycardia and ST segment elevation in a 16-year old; panel (C): ventricular tachycardia in a 9-year old; and panel (D): atrial fibrillation with rapid ventricular response in a 7-month old.

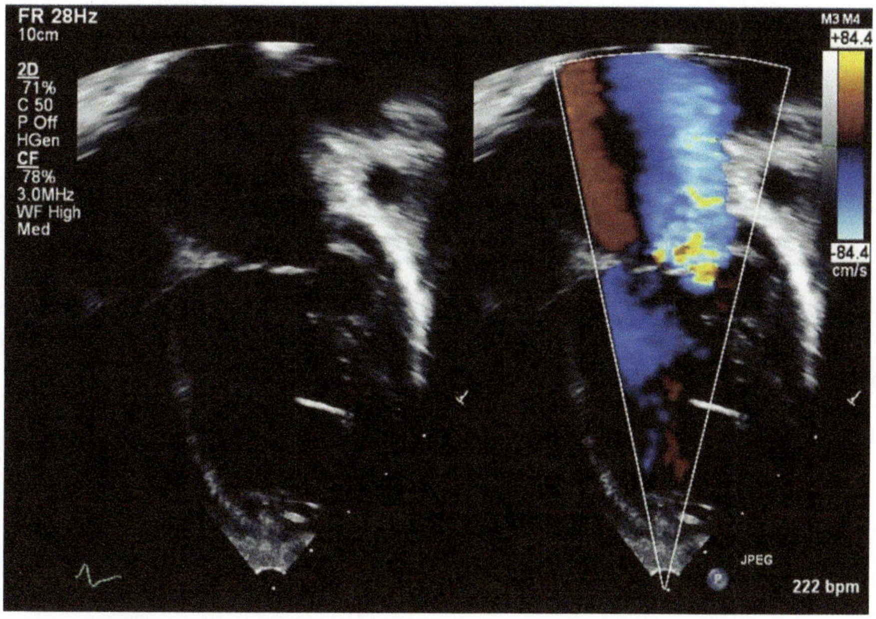

FIGURE 16.3 Apical view from an echocardiogram demonstrating a dilated left atrium, dilated left ventricle, and severe mitral valve regurgitation in a 7-month-old infant with human herpes virus-6 viral myocarditis.

infiltrate and cardiac myocyte necrosis and/or degeneration not typical of coronary artery disease or another cause [103] (Fig. 16.4). Histologic findings can be defined as (1) acute myocarditis with inflammation and myocyte necrosis, (2) borderline myocarditis with inflammation but lacking necrosis, or (3) persistent myocarditis with ongoing inflammation on serial biopsies without necrosis [30]. Evidence for the prognostic value of EMB varies, and the Dallas criteria alone may not predict response to therapy [104–106]. Evaluation of EMB samples from adults with acute myocarditis failed to find an association between immunohistochemical stains and long-term outcomes, although lymphocytic predominance and borderline myocarditis with fibrosis were associated with poorer outcomes [24].

Despite being considered the standard for diagnosis, practically the use of routine EMB in patients with suspected myocarditis has some important limitations. Myocarditis involvement in the myocardium is patchy and predominately affects the left ventricle as noted from autopsy studies and CMR. However, biopsy samples are usually obtained from the right ventricle, which may limit diagnostic yield in some cases [107]. There is some evidence to suggest LV biopsies or even biventricular biopsies may add higher diagnostic yield and not add any substantial procedural risk [108,109]. In addition, a large pediatric registry review found no significant difference in outcomes between biopsy confirmed and clinically diagnosed myocarditis, although both groups had better outcomes compared to idiopathic DCM [110]. Even with adequate sample in cases of suspected myocarditis, substantial interobserver variability and differences in interpretation of EMB samples among pathologists has been reported [111].

With the advent of improved CMR techniques and CMR-based criteria for diagnosis of myocarditis, there has been a noted shift to the decrease use of EMB and increase use of CMR in children and adults [9]. In 2007, the joint scientific statement from the American Heart Association, American College of Cardiology, and European Society of Cardiology did not recommend routinely obtaining EMB samples in adults but did give specific scenarios in which EMB would be particularly recommended: (1) new-onset heart failure of less than 2-weeks duration with either a normal or dilated left ventricle and hemodynamic compromise and (2) new-onset heart failure between 2-weeks and 3-months duration with a dilated left ventricle and new ventricular arrhythmias, heart block, or failure to respond to therapy in 1–2 weeks [112]. These guidelines also highlighted additional scenarios in which EMB may be useful in diagnosis and management, including clinical presentations suggestive of giant cell or eosinophilic myocarditis, for which prompt therapy is necessary. In the 2015 diagnostic recommendations from the European Society of Cardiology, the task force recommended testing EMB in adults for viruses and autoantibodies in addition to the Dallas criteria to evaluate for virus-negative inflammatory myocarditis, as there is some evidence this subset of patients may benefit from immunosuppressive therapy if unresponsive to standard therapy [57]. However, in children with suspected myocarditis, clear guidelines are lacking, and indications for EMB are more controversial, but a similar algorithm to evaluate for autoimmune myocarditis or viral persistence in the myocardium has been proposed [113].

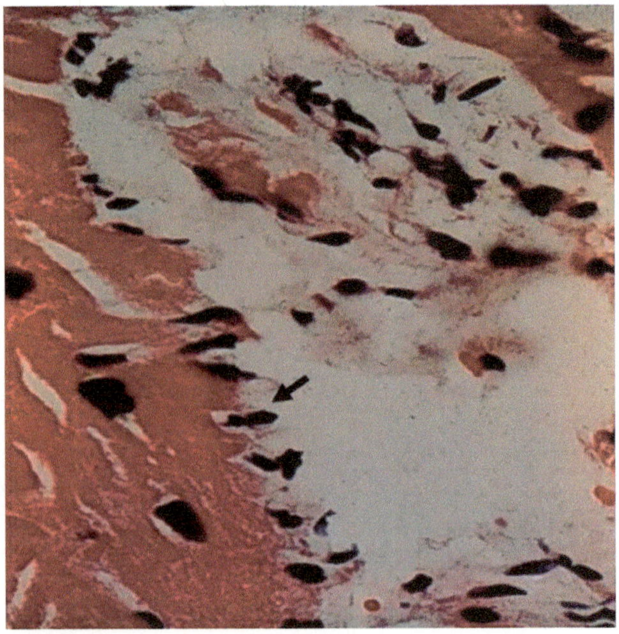

FIGURE 16.4 Representative histopathological findings compatible with myocarditis from an endomyocardial biopsy specimen. Inflammatory (mononuclear) elements are seen in close association with damaged cell membrane of myocardial fibers (*arrow*). In the interstitium, fragments of a myocardial fiber are seen in association with macrophages and fibroblasts (hematoxylin–eosin stain × 400). *(Image from P.R. Camargo, et al., Myocarditis in children and detection of viruses in myocardial tissue: implications for immunosuppressive therapy, Int. J. Cardiol. 148 (2) (April 14, 2011) 204–208.)*

Cardiac Magnetic Resonance Imaging

Over the past couple of decades, CMR has emerged as an important noninvasive imaging tool for the diagnosis of myocarditis in children and adults. CMR allows accurate evaluation of ventricular volumes and systolic function, including regional wall abnormalities [114]. Specialized sequences are also used to evaluate for the characteristic findings of myocarditis: myocardial edema, hyperemia, and fibrosis or scarring [115]. Edema is typically evaluated with T2-weighted imaging, which can also identify associated pericardial effusions [116,117] (Fig. 16.5). Hyperemia or myocardial inflammation is seen by ECG-triggered T1-weighted images obtained before and immediately after intravenous gadolinium-diethylenetriaminepentaacetate administration [116,118] (Fig. 16.6). T1-weighted segmented inversion–recovery gradient-echo sequences evaluate for LGE to detect areas of myocardial fibrosis, since areas of scar retain gadolinium contrast [119] (Fig. 16.7A and B). LGE can also be seen in other cardiac diseases leading to fibrosis, such as ischemic from coronary artery disease. However, the pattern of injury from coronary ischemia is subendocardial or transmural seen in a typical coronary perfusion distribution. The characteristic LGE pattern in myocarditis is typically patchy and subepicardial, and also may be transmural, but not in the pattern of a coronary distribution [67,116]. Areas of LGE identified by CMR in myocarditis can also be used to identify areas of myocardium for targeted EMB in attempt to increase diagnostic yield [107].

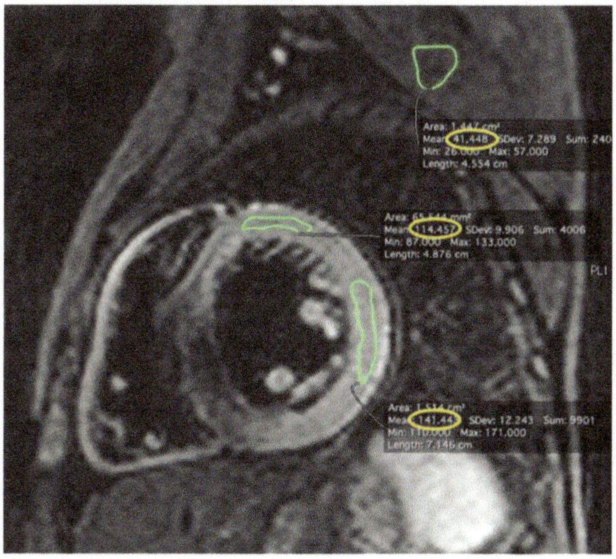

FIGURE 16.5 Cardiac MRI, midshort-axis view. T2-weighted sequence showing a >2x increase in signal intensity in the myocardium compared to skeletal muscle. This is consistent with myocardial edema in a patient with myocarditis.

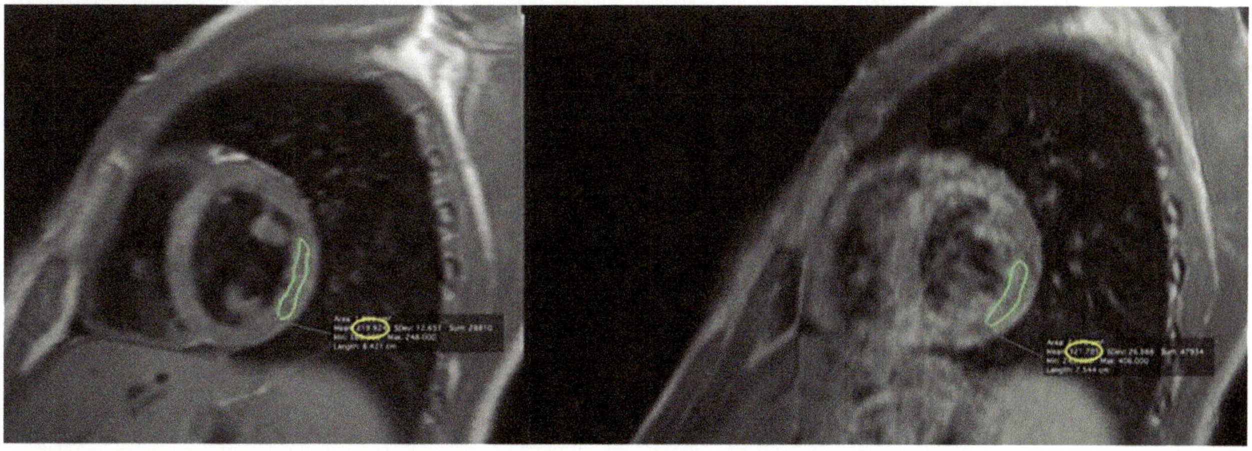

FIGURE 16.6 Cardiac MRI, midshort-axis view. Pre- (left panel) and postcontrast (right panel) T1-weighted sequence showing a >45% increase in signal intensity in the same region of the left ventricular posterior–lateral wall following administration of contrast. This is consistent with hyperemia or capillary leak in a patient with myocarditis.

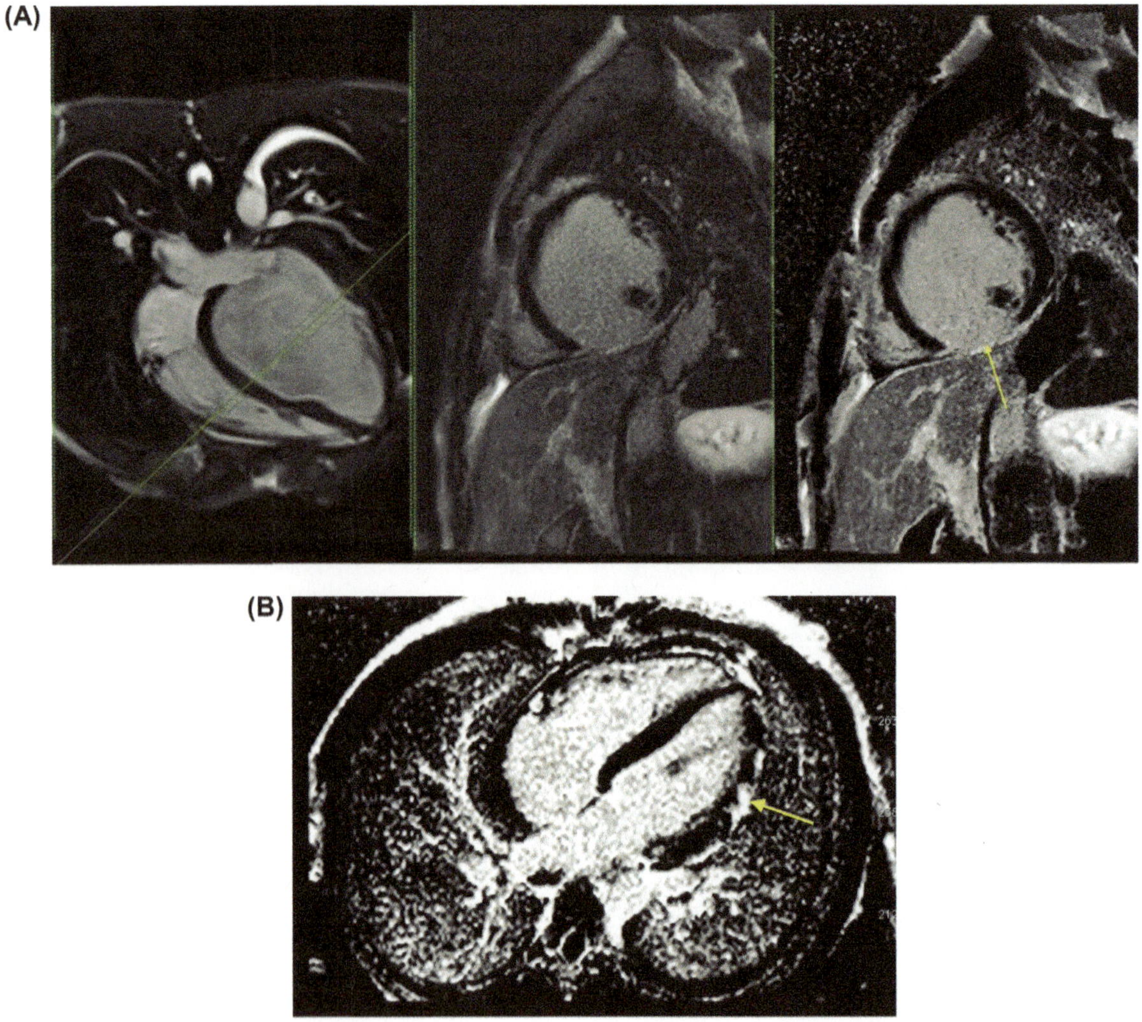

FIGURE 16.7 (A) Cardiac MRI case of dilated cardiomyopathy and active myocarditis. This image at the left ventricle midshort axis shows late gadolinium enhancement (*yellow arrow*) and wall thinning of the inferior wall. (B). Cardiac MRI, 4-chamber view. Phase Sensitive Inversion Recovery sequence showing patchy regions of late gadolinium enhancement in the left ventricular free wall (*yellow arrow*), indicating fibrosis or scarring in a patient with myocarditis.

The combined use of the imaging sequences above has the greatest diagnostic utility in myocarditis. To that end, the International Consensus Group on CMR diagnosis of myocarditis proposed the "Lake Louise" criteria in 2009, which includes T2-weighted images for evaluation of edema, pre- and postgadolinium T1-weighted images to evaluate hyperemia/capillary leak, and gadolinium-enhanced T1-weighted images for late enhancement for fibrosis [118] (Table 16.2). The combination of at least two or more findings in a patient with clinical suspicion for myocarditis is considered consistent with a diagnosis of myocarditis, giving a sensitivity of 67%, specificity of 91%, and diagnostic accuracy of 78%, compared to 68% accuracy for LGE alone. The authors also acknowledged that the timing of obtaining a CMR in suspected myocarditis may affect the sensitivity of the test, as findings may not all be evident very early on in the disease course [120]. There is some evidence that the optimal timing for CMR is between 2 and 4 weeks after onset of symptoms [121]. Repeated imaging in 1–2 weeks after initial CMR has been recommended in patients with a nondiagnostic test but high clinical suspicion [118]. However, sensitivity may also be affected by clinical presentation, with a sensitivity of 80% in the ACS phenotype compared to 57% in the DCM phenotype in a recent small series of CMR in 57 adults with biopsy-proven myocarditis [66].

Since publication of the Lake Louise criteria, additional CMR imaging techniques have been proposed to aid in diagnostic accuracy for patients with suspected myocarditis. In adults with myocarditis, the quantification of global myocardial extracellular volume in addition to LGE gave a reported 90% accuracy compared to 79% accuracy using the Lake Louise criteria [122]. T1 mapping to detect edema and relaxation by CMR has been proposed to also increase sensitivity and specificity in adults with acute myocarditis, with the possibility to detect more subtle changes in the myocardium and the added advantages of image quality being heart rate independent and not requiring contrast [123–125].

TABLE 16.2 Cardiac MRI (CMR) Diagnosis Criteria for Acute Myocarditis Based on the "Lake Louise Criteria"

1. In the case of clinically suspected myocarditis, CMR findings are consistent with a diagnosis of myocardial inflammation (myocarditis) if 2 or more of the following are present:
   a. Regional or global myocardial signal intensity is increased in T2-weighted images (indicating myocardial edema)
   b. Increased global myocardial early gadolinium enhancement ratio between myocardium and skeletal muscle in gadolinium-enhanced T1-weighted images (indicating hyperemia/capillary leak)
   c. At least 1 focal lesion of late gadolinium-enhanced enhancement is seen in a nonischemic distribution in inversion recovery-prepared gadolinium-enhanced T1-weighted images (indicating myocyte injury and/or fibrosis)
2. CMR study is consistent with myocyte injury and/or scar by myocardial inflammation if criterion A3 is present on CMR evaluation
3. CMR should be repeated between 1 and 2 weeks after initial CMR if:
   a. None of the above criteria are present at time of initial CMR, but onset of symptoms are very recent and there is strong clinical evidence for myocarditis
   b. Only one of the above criteria is present
4. The presence of left ventricular dysfunction or pericardial effusion on CMR provides additional, supportive evidence for a diagnosis of myocarditis.

Adapted from M.G. Friedrich, et al., Cardiovascular magnetic resonance in myocarditis: a JACC white paper, J. Am. Coll. Cardiol. 53 (17) (April 28, 2009) 1465–1487.

CMR findings in patients with myocarditis may also have prognostic value. In a study of 34 children with myocarditis who underwent CMR, LGE was found in 50% of patients and predictive of worse outcomes, including need for MCS, transplant, and/or death [82]. Similar findings have been reported in adult studies, with LGE and lower EF associated with poor outcomes and/or significant adverse cardiac events [80,126–128]. LGE may persist in some patients on serial CMR, consistent with irreversible tissue injury, but the extent of LGE reportedly decreases in many patients over time, which may be attributed to scar contraction [129,130]. Persistent T1-weighted myocardial enhancement at 28 days has also been associated with ventricular dysfunction and clinical symptoms at 2.5-year follow-up in adults [121]. However, more research on the use of serial CMR, including the prognostic value in children and adults, is needed.

Classification

The diagnosis of myocarditis remains challenging, even with the available diagnostic tools, and patients may exhibit any combination of clinical findings. To that end, Sagar et al. described a tiered clinical classification for the diagnosis of myocarditis based on the level of diagnostic certainty [75]. In *possible subclinical acute myocarditis*, patients are asymptomatic but have elevated biomarkers consistent with cardiac damage, ECG findings suggesting cardiac injury, and/or abnormal cardiac function by echocardiogram or CMR imaging. *Probable acute myocarditis* includes the findings of possible myocarditis with the addition of clinical symptoms of heart failure. Finally, *definite myocarditis* included the presence of histological and/or immunohistological evidence of myocarditis.

TREATMENT

The mainstay of treatment for children with myocarditis is supportive. As the clinical phenotypes vary, the extent of needed support for each patient also varies with the severity of their symptoms and presence of any hemodynamic compromise. Historically, as a whole, the majority of children will be admitted to the intensive care, 25%–50% will require mechanical ventilation, and around 45%–70% will be placed on inotropic support [9,72,73,131]. MCS may be required in more advanced cases of heart failure and cardiogenic shock, with use of extracorporeal membrane oxygenation (ECMO) reported in 7%–19% and ventricular assist devices (VAD) in 2%–4% [73,110,131].

Heart Failure and Rhythm Management

Patients with stable symptomatic heart failure should be treated with standard therapy per guidelines from the American College of Cardiology and American Heart Association [74,132]. Typical therapy includes diuretics, angiotensin-converting enzyme inhibitors (ACEI), angiotensin receptor blockers (ARB) if intolerant to ACEI, and beta-blockers. Over 90% of adults were on ACEI and beta-blocker therapy in one recent outcomes study [133]. However, limited studies have evaluated the use of heart failure medications specifically in myocarditis, and the majority of data are from animal models of myocarditis. Digoxin was associated with increased production of proinflammatory cytokines and mortality in mice [134] and is generally not recommended in patients with myocarditis [74]. ACEI and ARB medications in murine myocarditis models were associated with decreased inflammation, myocardial fibrosis, and autoantibody production [135–138]. Similarly, the aldosterone receptor antagonist eplerenone was associated with decreased fibrosis in mice, particularly when started at the beginning of the disease course [139]. Carvedilol, but not metoprolol, has been associated with antioxidant effects and improved function, fibrosis, and survival in murine models [140–142]. Use of metoprolol in murine models was associated with increased mortality, inflammation, and necrosis [143]. Calcium channel blockers also appear to have beneficial effects in mice with myocarditis, possibly through decrease in production of inflammatory cytokines and inhibition of nitric oxide production [144–146]. In humans, similar data on the effects of heart failure medications in patients with myocarditis are limited. A prospective observational adult study found lack of beta-blocker therapy was a risk factor for poorer outcomes, including death or heart transplant [106]. Similar studies in pediatric populations are not available [147].

As mentioned, rhythm disturbances are not uncommon in patients with myocarditis. Both tachyarrhythmias and various degrees of heart block may be observed, with a reported increased risk of mortality associated with tachyarrhythmias in children with myocarditis [148]. Evidence from murine models suggests amiodarone may not only have antiarrhythmic effects but also beneficial effects on development of myocardial necrosis and inflammation [147,149]. Some patients may require permanent pacemaker implantation for refractory clinically significant heart block. Batra et al. reported a series of 40 children with myocarditis and atrioventricular heart block, with return of conduction in 67%, all within a week, and need for pacemaker in 28% [94]. A small series of children with fulminant myocarditis reported resolution of arrhythmias and heart block in all the long-term survivors [91].

Antiinflammatory and Immunomodulatory Therapy

Myocarditis is marked by the activation of the patient immune response and presence of inflammatory changes in the myocardium with associated myocyte injury. The use of antiinflammatory medications and immunomodulatory therapy in patients with myocarditis, therefore, appears logical. However, data supporting various treatments are often limited by retrospective analysis, small sample size, inconsistent regimens, lack of control groups, variable results, and/or limited long-term follow-up. Although these treatments are widely used, therapeutic regimens often vary by institution and clinician experience.

In general, the routine use of NSAIDS is not recommended based on available animal models that found increased inflammation, myocardial necrosis, and mortality, regardless of the timing of administration during the disease course [150]. Some studies have suggested potential benefit of steroid therapy in murine models of myocarditis. Use of dexamethasone in mice before or right after inducing the myocarditis phenotype was associated with decreased mortality, relative LV dimensions, and fibrosis, but not in mice treated later [151]. Evidence in humans is inconsistent despite relatively common use. In a database review of pediatric myocarditis patients between 2006 and 2011, nearly a third of patients received steroids [110] and successful short-term use has been reported with minimal side effects in a case series of children [152]. A small randomized study of steroids versus standard therapy in children with clinical myocarditis of greater than 3-months duration found a greater percent of treated children had normal EF at follow-up compared to controls [153]. However, according to a recent Cochrane review, routine use of steroids in patients with myocarditis is not recommended [154]. The review found no reduction in mortality among treated patients. Although there was some possible improvement in EF, the supporting studies were poor in quality.

Other studies have evaluated the combination of steroids with immunosuppressants in acute myocarditis. Camargo et al. described improved hemodynamics and histologic findings on follow-up of children treated with prednisone plus cyclosporine or azathioprine (AZA) compared to conventional treatment or steroids alone, but the study was limited by a small sample size [155]. Camargo et al. later reported improved EF and cardiac index in 10 children treated with prednisone and AZA compared to a historical control group [87]. Kleinert et al. described improved echocardiographic parameters [156], and Gagliardi et al. reported superior event-free survival at follow-up [157] in children with myocarditis treated with prednisone and cyclosporine. However, these studies and their conclusions are limited by the use of noninflammatory DCM control groups, which have known inferior long-term outcomes [110].

Several adult studies of chronic myocarditis and DCM have reported findings of improved EF and decreased LV dimensions at follow-up with combination therapy, although there was no difference in survival or need for heart transplantation [158,159]. However, other studies with similar regimens failed to find differences in outcomes after treatment compared to controls [160]. Overall data are insufficient to recommend routine use due to lack of clear and consistent evidence [161], but further research may identify patient subgroups that could potentially benefit from immunosuppressant therapy. For instance, in adults, there are some data to support that patients with virus-negative inflammatory cardiomyopathy may benefit from immunosuppressive therapy [162].

Intravenous Immunoglobulin

Similar to steroids, intravenous immunoglobulin (IVIG) is commonly used in children and adults with myocarditis but with conflicting supporting data. Despite its widespread use in many inflammatory and autoimmune disorders, the exact mechanism of IVIG is not completely understood [163]. Typical dosing is 2 g/kg intravenously in children. A small case series of 13 children with clinical myocarditis admitted to the ICU and treated with IVIG found improved survival compared to conventional therapy [164]. Drucker et al. reported improved LV function and dimensions in 21 children given IVIG compared to historical controls, with a nonsignificant trend toward improved survival at 1 year [165]. In a review of the Pediatric Cardiomyopathy Registry (PCMR), IVIG was used in 70% of patients with myocarditis, although no difference in outcomes was noted based on IVIG therapy [110]. Other retrospective pediatric analyses also failed to find a significant difference in outcomes based on IVIG therapy, even in patients with more severe disease presentation [73,131]. Similarly, IVIG was not associated with survival to discharge in a series of 603 fulminant myocarditis adults supported with MCS [166]. In adults, a controlled trial of IVIG in myocarditis and recent onset DCM failed to find a difference in improvement of cardiac function based on IVIG treatment, although both treated and control groups had improvement in EF over time [167]. IVIG therapy in adults with chronic DCM had similar findings, despite some early improvements in inflammatory markers and function with IVIG [168]. To that end, the most recent 2015 Cochrane review found no evidence for routine use of IVIG in acute myocarditis based on current available data [169].

Immunoadsorption

As cardiac injury is related to production of autoantibodies and antibody-mediated cell signaling triggering host immune activation, immunoadsorption has been suggested as a potential adjunct therapy in myocarditis and DCM. However, immunoadsorption is not currently commonly used in children with acute myocarditis, and experience is mainly from trials in adults with DCM. Several studies in adults reported significantly increased EF and cardiac index at follow-up [170–172], although others have not found similar improvements in outcomes [173]. Type of immunoadsorption may affect outcomes after therapy. Staudt et al. reported targeted removal of immunoglobulin subclass IgG-3, which is associated with complement activation, was associated with significantly improved cardiac index and LV EF compared to patients with Ig removal that excluded IgG-3 [174]. The exact frequency and length of therapy is variable, but at least one study found no difference in 6-month outcomes between monthly and one time treatment in adults [175].

Antiviral Therapy

Although most cases of acute lymphocytic myocarditis in children and adults are thought to be secondary to viruses, specific antiviral therapy is not routinely used. Practical use of antiviral therapy is challenging due to difficulty in identifying the causative agent, even with EMB, and limited number of available targeted antiviral therapies. However, there is an increasing interest in the presence of detectable virus at diagnosis and the relationship of viral persistence on patient outcomes. In adults with DCM and detectable virus by EMB, persistence of positive virus on serial EMB was associated with decreased LV function compared to patients who demonstrated viral clearance at follow-up [176].

Published experience of antiviral therapy in myocarditis in humans consists mainly of case reports and small single center series. In a murine model of CMV myocarditis, treatment with cidofovir or ganciclovir led to decreased viral load and inflammation, but only if treatment was initiated in the acute phase of disease [177]. Successful treatment of CMV myocarditis with ganciclovir has been published in case reports of children and adults [178,179]. Pleconaril is an inhibitor of enteroviruses and rhinoviruses [180] with reported successful use in several children with enterovirus-related illness, including myocarditis [181,182]. Interferon (INF) has been shown to have antiviral activity in human myocardial fibroblasts [183] with demonstrated reduction of inflammatory cytokines [184]. INF-alpha was associated with improvement in cardiac function and viral clearance in several cases of adults with enterovirus myocarditis [185,186]. In addition, INF-beta was successfully used in adults with LV dysfunction and either adenovirus or enterovirus on EMB with noted elimination of viral genomes in all patients and improvement in LV function at 6-months follow-up [187].

Future Therapeutic Targets

Several possible future therapeutic targets in myocarditis are being investigated, mainly in animal models. In murine models of coxsackievirus myocarditis, use of a 3C protease inhibitor led to decreased mortality and myocardial damage [188]. Mice were also less likely to develop a chronic DCM phenotype after coxsackievirus infection with treatment [189]. Galectin-3 is thought to play an important role in cardiac inflammation and fibrosis as well as a biomarker for heart failure in adults [190]. Inhibition of galectin-3 function in knock-out mice infected with coxsackievirus demonstrated decreased cardiac inflammation despite no significant change in detected viral load [191]. Toll-like receptors (TLRs) are also thought to be involved in cardiac inflammation and myocyte injury during acute myocarditis, although effects are variable depending on the particular TLR activity [192]. Cardiac myosin, potentially released from damaged cardiac myocytes, was found to stimulate TLR-2 and TLR-8, leading to monocyte activation and inflammatory cytokine release [193]. TLR-4 has also been associated with proinflammatory effects in cardiac myocytes. TLR-4 knockout mice models of autoimmune myocarditis and inhibition of TLR-4 signaling were both associated with less severe myocarditis and myocyte apoptosis compared to wild-type mice [194,195]. Although these novel targets are promising, experience in humans is lacking and further development of therapies is needed.

Mechanical Circulatory Support

Patients with severe and refractory disease may require more advanced cardiac support with MCS. Options include short-term support with ECMO or temporary VAD. According to the Pediatric Health Information System database analysis from 2006 to 2011, nearly 19% of children with myocarditis required ECMO support, which was associated with 8 times increased risk of mortality [9]. An earlier review of the Extracorporeal Life Support Organization registry database (ELSO) from 1995 to 2006 reported myocarditis was the diagnosis in 1.3% of supported patients with a noted 61% survival to discharge [196]. Higher risk for death was associated with arrhythmias and dialysis-dependent renal failure. Unfortunately, prolonged support >2 weeks was associated with only 47% survival. A more recent pediatric ELSO analysis from 2012 found myocarditis accounted to 4% of diagnosis with notably worse survival in newborns, 49%, compared to 66%–74% in older children [197].

For patients presenting with the fulminant myocarditis phenotype and acute cardiovascular collapse, ECMO has been reported as a viable option as a bridge to recovery. In one series, 50% of patients with fulminant myocarditis required ECMO support [59]. As noted, children with fulminant myocarditis often have a more severe clinical presentation, but relatively good long-term cardiac recovery and survival [61,198,199]. Several studies have reported survival to discharge in 80% in children and 60%–70% in adults after ECMO support for fulminant myocarditis [61,198–201].

When children and young adults require more prolonged support as either a bridge to recovery or transplantation, durable VAD support should be considered. Implantable continuous flow devices, such as the Heartware HVAD or Heartmate II, have been used in children with similar outcomes to adults [202,203]. Options for younger and/or smaller children include the Berlin EXCOR VAD, which has been proven superior to ECMO support in children with 75% 1-year survival and 64% bridge to heart transplant [204]. Review of the multicenter Berlin EXCOR trial experience revealed a diagnosis of myocarditis in 13.9% and 14% overall mortality among children with myocarditis [204]. Explant of a VAD for recovery is relatively uncommon, accounting for only 6% of all Berlin VAD implants. Unfortunately, adverse events on Berlin VAD support were common, with major bleeding occurring in 44% and neurologic dysfunction in 29% of children.

RECOVERY, CARDIOMYOPATHY, AND HEART TRANSPLANTATION

Worldwide, reported rates of recovery, death, and heart transplant vary, but estimated rate of death or transplant in adults with myocarditis is 20%–22% with approximately 20%–50% of new diagnosis DCM attributable to myocarditis [2]. Kinderman et al. described 181 adults with clinical myocarditis, of which 22% had either died or undergone heart transplant at a mean follow-up of 5 years [106]. Worse outcomes were associated with higher New York Heart Association heart failure classification, inflammation on biopsy, and lack of beta-blocker therapy. Other studies have reported transplant-free 5-year survival in adults ranging from 45% to 56% [105,160,205].

Outcomes in children appear to be superior to adults with a greater chance of normalization of function over time [2]. Reports from the long-term National Australian Childhood Cardiomyopathy Study (NACCS) of children <10-years old found evidence of myocarditis in approximately 40% of children with DCM who underwent EMB [206]. An early NACCS report from 1987 to 1996 found 48% of myocarditis was diagnosed on autopsy, with half of the deaths occurring within a few days after presentation [55]. A later NACCS report found that although myocarditis may present with sudden death as the initial symptoms, there were no additional episodes of sudden death in biopsy-proven myocarditis patients during long-term follow-up [207]. One of the largest reports on outcomes of children with myocarditis in North America was from the PCMR in which outcomes were compared between children <18-years old with either biopsy-confirmed myocarditis, clinically suspected myocarditis, or idiopathic DCM [110]. Outcomes did not significantly differ between the myocarditis groups, with reported 6%–7% death, 17%–19% transplant, and 52%–54% normalization of cardiac function at 3 years compared to 17% death, 33% transplant, and 21% normalization in the idiopathic DCM group.

Overall survival in children ranges from approximately 75% to 90% [9,72,73,131], with majority of normalization of systolic function occurring over the course of 1–4 months after presentation in some studies [72,73]. However, the PCMR study revealed that normalization can continue to occur over the course of long-term follow-up, especially in the first 3 years after diagnosis [110]. Not surprisingly, worse outcomes have been associated with high severity of illness at presentation [131]. Analysis of the Pediatric Health Information System database from 2006 to 2011 found the risk of death or transplant was not only associated with use of vasoactive medication, ECMO or VAD support, but also noted higher mortality in children <12-years old [9]. For children with fulminant myocarditis, transplant-free survival has been reported between 50% and 80% and need for heart transplant in 1%–3% [59,71,196]. Of nontransplanted survivors, recovery of normal systolic function is expected in the majority of both children and adults with fulminant myocarditis, substantially better than patients with acute lymphocytic myocarditis [58,62,199,201,205,208].

For patients with heart failure secondary to myocarditis that is refractory to medical therapy, heart transplantation may be necessary. The reported rate of heart transplantation in children with myocarditis varies, but ranges from 4% to 19% [9,73,110]. In an analysis of merged data from the PCMR and Pediatric Heart Transplant Study, children with myocarditis had 97% waitlist survival prior to transplant [209]. However, posttransplant, children with prior myocarditis had worse 1- and 3-year survival compared to other children with DCM, with a surprising 2.7× increased risk of death. Death was secondary to rejection in 17% of myocarditis patients compared to 3% in the DCM patients. Although it is unclear why myocarditis patients had more death and fatal rejection episodes, the authors hypothesized that these outcomes may be related to ongoing infectious or immune mechanisms posttransplant. These results vary from a single center study of 759 adults that found no difference in survival or antibody-mediated rejection compared to other adults with either ischemic or idiopathic DCM [210]. Although early acute cellular rejection was also not different, rate of late cellular rejection was higher in myocarditis patients compared to ischemic cardiomyopathy.

ACTIVITY RESTRICTIONS

Patients are typically restricted from strenuous physical activity and competitive sports for a period after the diagnosis of myocarditis, mainly based on concern of sudden death from noted autopsy studies in athletes. No prospective studies regarding the risk of strenuous activity have been performed in humans, but mice with myocarditis were noted to have higher mortality with activity compared to wild-type mice [211]. According to the most recent sports participation guidelines from the American Heart Association and American College of Cardiology in 2015, athletes with a diagnosis of myocarditis may consider return to competitive sports within 3–6 months after diagnosis if (1) ventricular systolic function is normal, (2) serum markers of myocardial injury/inflammation and heart failure have normalized, and (3) there is no evidence of current clinically relevant arrhythmias [212]. These guidelines recommended that patients have a normal documented echocardiogram, 24-h Holter monitor, and exercise ECG prior to return to competitive sports. The authors did not include resolution of LGE by CMR as criteria for return to sports, acknowledging that the relationship of residual LGE and risk in athletes is unclear.

REFERENCES

[1] P. Richardson, W. McKenna, M. Bristow, B. Maisch, B. Mautner, J. O'Connell, et al., Report of the 1995 World Health Organization/International Society and Federation of cardiology task force on the definition and classification of cardiomyopathies, Circulation 93 (5) (1996) 841–842.

[2] L.T. Cooper Jr., A. Keren, K. Sliwa, A. Matsumori, G.A. Mensah, The global burden of myocarditis: part 1: a systematic literature review for the Global Burden of Diseases, Injuries, and Risk Factors 2010 study, Global Heart 9 (1) (2014) 121–129.

[3] S. Wakafuji, R. Okada, Twenty year autopsy statistics of myocarditis incidence in Japan, Jpn. Circ. J. 50 (12) (1986) 1288–1293.

[4] V. Kyto, A. Saraste, L.M. Voipio-Pulkki, P. Saukko, Incidence of fatal myocarditis: a population-based study in Finland, Am. J. Epidemiol. 165 (5) (2007) 570–574.

[5] R. Puranik, C.K. Chow, J.A. Duflou, M.J. Kilborn, M.A. McGuire, Sudden death in the young, Heart Rhythm 2 (12) (2005) 1277–1282.

[6] H. Wang, Q. Yao, S. Zhu, G. Zhang, Z. Wang, Z. Li, et al., The autopsy study of 553 cases of sudden cardiac death in Chinese adults, Heart Vessels 29 (4) (2014) 486–495.

[7] M. Vassalini, A. Verzeletti, M. Restori, F. De Ferrari, An autopsy study of sudden cardiac death in persons aged 1–40 years in Brescia (Italy), J. Cardiovasc. Med. 17 (6) (2016) 446–453.

[8] V.L. Vetter, T.M. Covington, N.P. Dugan, D.M. Haley, H. Dykstra, M. Overpeck, et al., Cardiovascular deaths in children: general overview from the National Center for the Review and Prevention of Child Deaths, Am. Heart J. 169 (3) (2015) 426–437 e23.

[9] S.J. Ghelani, M.C. Spaeder, W. Pastor, C.F. Spurney, D. Klugman, Demographics, trends, and outcomes in pediatric acute myocarditis in the United States, 2006 to 2011, Circ. Cardiovasc. Qual. Outcomes 5 (5) (2012) 622–627.

[10] V. Kyto, J. Sipila, P. Rautava, The effects of gender and age on occurrence of clinically suspected myocarditis in adulthood, Heart 99 (22) (2013) 1681–1684.

[11] D. Fairweather, L.T. Cooper Jr., L.A. Blauwet, Sex and gender differences in myocarditis and dilated cardiomyopathy, Curr. Probl. Cardiol. 38 (1) (2013) 7–46.
[12] T. Kashimura, M. Kodama, Y. Hotta, J. Hosoya, K. Yoshida, T. Ozawa, et al., Spatiotemporal changes of coxsackievirus and adenovirus receptor in rat hearts during postnatal development and in cultured cardiomyocytes of neonatal rat, Virchows Arch. 444 (3) (2004) 283–292.
[13] C.T. Bock, A. Duchting, F. Utta, E. Brunner, B.T. Sy, K. Klingel, et al., Molecular phenotypes of human parvovirus B19 in patients with myocarditis, World J. Cardiol. 6 (4) (2014) 183–195.
[14] L. Andreoletti, N. Leveque, C. Boulagnon, C. Brasselet, P. Fornes, Viral causes of human myocarditis, Arch. Cardiovasc. Dis. 102 (6–7) (2009) 559–568.
[15] L.J. May, D.J. Patton, D.S. Fruitman, The evolving approach to paediatric myocarditis: a review of the current literature, Cardiol. Young 21 (3) (2011) 241–251.
[16] M. Cabral, M.J. Brito, M. Conde, M. Oliveira, G.C. Ferreira, Fulminant myocarditis associated with pandemic H1N1 influenza A virus, (Revista portuguesa de cardiologia: orgao oficial da Sociedade Portuguesa de Cardiologia) Port. J. Cardiol. 31 (7–8) (2012) 517–520.
[17] A.E. Baruteau, N. Boimond, D. Ramful, Myocarditis associated with 2009 influenza A (H1N1) virus in children, Cardiol. Young 20 (3) (2010) 351–352.
[18] A.G. Randolph, F. Vaughn, R. Sullivan, L. Rubinson, B.T. Thompson, G. Yoon, et al., Critically ill children during the 2009–2010 influenza pandemic in the United States, Pediatrics 128 (6) (2011) e1450–e1458.
[19] J.A. Blum, M.J. Zellweger, C. Burri, C. Hatz, Cardiac involvement in African and American trypanosomiasis, Lancet Infect. Dis. 8 (10) (2008) 631–641.
[20] A. Rassi Jr., A. Rassi, J.A. Marin-Neto, Chagas heart disease: pathophysiologic mechanisms, prognostic factors and risk stratification, Mem. Inst. Oswaldo Cruz 104 (Suppl. 1) (2009) 152–158.
[21] K.H. Sohn, W.J. Song, B.K. Kim, M.K. Kang, S.Y. Lee, J.W. Suh, et al., Eosinophilic myocarditis: case series and literature review, Asia Pac. Allergy 5 (2) (2015) 123–127.
[22] L. Mouthon, B. Dunogue, L. Guillevin, Diagnosis and classification of eosinophilic granulomatosis with polyangiitis (formerly named Churg-Strauss syndrome), J. Autoimmun. 48-49 (2014) 99–103.
[23] P.U. Ogbogu, D.R. Rosing, M.K. Horne 3rd, Cardiovascular manifestations of hypereosinophilic syndromes, Immunol. Allergy Clin. N. Am. 27 (3) (2007) 457–475.
[24] J.C. Youn, H.S. Shim, J.S. Lee, A.Y. Ji, J. Oh, N. Hong, et al., Detailed pathologic evaluation on endomyocardial biopsy provides long-term prognostic information in patients with acute myocarditis, Cardiovasc. Pathol. 23 (3) (2014) 139–144.
[25] L.A. Blauwet, L.T. Cooper, Idiopathic giant cell myocarditis and cardiac sarcoidosis, Heart Fail. Rev. 18 (6) (2013) 733–746.
[26] L.T. Cooper Jr., G.J. Berry, R. Shabetai, Idiopathic giant-cell myocarditis–natural history and treatment. Multicenter Giant Cell Myocarditis Study Group Investigators, N. Engl. J. Med. 336 (26) (1997) 1860–1866.
[27] L.T. Cooper Jr., J.M. Hare, H.D. Tazelaar, W.D. Edwards, R.C. Starling, M.C. Deng, et al., Usefulness of immunosuppression for giant cell myocarditis, Am. J. Cardiol. 102 (11) (2008) 1535–1539.
[28] J.J. Maleszewski, V.M. Orellana, D.O. Hodge, U. Kuhl, H.P. Schultheiss, L.T. Cooper, Long-term risk of recurrence, morbidity and mortality in giant cell myocarditis, Am. J. Cardiol. 115 (12) (2015) 1733–1738.
[29] L.T. Cooper Jr., C. ElAmm, Giant cell myocarditis. Diagnosis and treatment, Herz 37 (6) (2012) 632–636.
[30] M. Esfandiarei, B.M. McManus, Molecular biology and pathogenesis of viral myocarditis, Annu. Rev. Pathol. 3 (2008) 127–155.
[31] B.P. Amoah, H. Yang, P. Zhang, Z. Su, H. Xu, Immunopathogenesis of myocarditis: the interplay between cardiac fibroblast cells, dendritic cells, macrophages and CD4+ T cells, Scand. J. Immunol. 82 (1) (2015) 1–9.
[32] B. Lauer, M. Schannwell, U. Kuhl, B.E. Strauer, H.P. Schultheiss, Antimyosin autoantibodies are associated with deterioration of systolic and diastolic left ventricular function in patients with chronic myocarditis, J. Am. Coll. Cardiol. 35 (1) (2000) 11–18.
[33] A. Mascaro-Blanco, K. Alvarez, X. Yu, J. Lindenfeld, L. Olansky, T. Lyons, et al., Consequences of unlocking the cardiac myosin molecule in human myocarditis and cardiomyopathies, Autoimmunity 41 (6) (2008) 442–453.
[34] M.W. Cunningham, H.C. Meissner, J.S. Heuser, B.A. Pietra, D.K. Kurahara, D.Y. Leung, Anti-human cardiac myosin autoantibodies in Kawasaki syndrome, J. Immunol. 163 (2) (1999) 1060–1065.
[35] A.L. Caforio, F. Tona, S. Bottaro, A. Vinci, G. Dequal, L. Daliento, et al., Clinical implications of anti-heart autoantibodies in myocarditis and dilated cardiomyopathy, Autoimmunity 41 (1) (2008) 35–45.
[36] Y. Li, J.S. Heuser, L.C. Cunningham, S.D. Kosanke, M.W. Cunningham, Mimicry and antibody-mediated cell signaling in autoimmune myocarditis, J. Immunol. 177 (11) (2006) 8234–8240.
[37] S. Saito, Y. Hiroi, Y. Zou, R. Aikawa, H. Toko, F. Shibasaki, et al., beta-Adrenergic pathway induces apoptosis through calcineurin activation in cardiac myocytes, J. Biol. Chem. 275 (44) (2000) 34528–34533.
[38] Y. Shizukuda, P.M. Buttrick, D.L. Geenen, A.C. Borczuk, R.N. Kitsis, E.H. Sonnenblick, beta-Adrenergic stimulation causes cardiocyte apoptosis: influence of tachycardia and hypertrophy, Am. J. Physiol. 275 (3 Pt 2) (1998) H961–H968.
[39] K.E. Simpson, C.K. Lee, M.W. Cunningham, C. Simon, J. Delaney, K. Ward, et al., The prevelance of autoimmunity and relationship to cardiac status in pediatric myocarditis and recent onset dilated cardiomyopathy, JACC 61 (10) (2013) E1265.
[40] A. Yoshizawa, S. Nagai, Y. Baba, T. Yamada, M. Matsui, H. Tanaka, et al., Autoimmunity against M(2) muscarinic acetylcholine receptor induces myocarditis and leads to a dilated cardiomyopathy-like phenotype, Eur. J. Immunol. 42 (5) (2012) 1152–1163.
[41] A. Baba, T. Yoshikawa, Y. Fukuda, T. Sugiyama, M. Shimada, M. Akaishi, et al., Autoantibodies against M2-muscarinic acetylcholine receptors: new upstream targets in atrial fibrillation in patients with dilated cardiomyopathy, Eur. Heart J. 25 (13) (2004) 1108–1115.

[42] P.A. Chiale, I. Ferrari, E. Mahler, M.A. Vallazza, M.V. Elizari, M.B. Rosenbaum, et al., Differential profile and biochemical effects of antiautonomic membrane receptor antibodies in ventricular arrhythmias and sinus node dysfunction, Circulation 103 (13) (2001) 1765–1771.

[43] H.P. Schultheiss, K. Schulze, A. Dorner, Significance of the adenine nucleotide translocator in the pathogenesis of viral heart disease, Mol. Cell. Biochem. 163–164 (1996) 319–327.

[44] M. Takemoto, S. Kusachi, N. Urabe, K. Inoue, T. Tsuji, Auto-antibody against adenine nucleotide translocator in dilated cardiomyopathy and myocarditis–incidence and relation to cardiac function and morphology, Jpn. Circ. J. 57 (12) (1993) 1150–1158.

[45] A. Fabre, M.N. Sheppard, Sudden adult death syndrome and other non-ischaemic causes of sudden cardiac death, Heart 92 (3) (2006) 316–320.

[46] A. Doolan, N. Langlois, C. Semsarian, Causes of sudden cardiac death in young Australians, Med. J. Aust. 180 (3) (2004) 110–112.

[47] M.A. Weber, M.T. Ashworth, R.A. Risdon, M. Malone, M. Burch, N.J. Sebire, Clinicopathological features of paediatric deaths due to myocarditis: an autopsy series, Arch. Dis. Child. 93 (7) (2008) 594–598.

[48] P. Bohm, J. Scharhag, T. Meyer, Data from a nationwide registry on sports-related sudden cardiac deaths in Germany, Eur. J. Prev. Cardiol. 23 (6) (2016) 649–656.

[49] B.J. Maron, J.J. Doerer, T.S. Haas, D.M. Tierney, F.O. Mueller, Sudden deaths in young competitive athletes: analysis of 1866 deaths in the United States, 1980–2006, Circulation 119 (8) (2009) 1085–1092.

[50] M.P. Suarez-Mier, B. Aguilera, R.M. Mosquera, M.S. Sanchez-de-Leon, Pathology of sudden death during recreational sports in Spain, Forensic Sci. Int. 226 (1–3) (2013) 188–196.

[51] K.G. Harmon, J.A. Drezner, J.J. Maleszewski, M. Lopez-Anderson, D. Owens, J.M. Prutkin, et al., Pathogeneses of sudden cardiac death in national collegiate athletic association athletes, Circ. Arrhythm. Electrophysiol. 7 (2) (2014) 198–204.

[52] S. Grasmeyer, B. Madea, Immunohistochemical diagnosis of myocarditis on (infantile) autopsy material: does it improve the diagnosis? Forensic Sci. Med. Pathol. 11 (2) (2015) 168–176.

[53] R.E. Andrews, M.J. Fenton, D.A. Ridout, M. Burch, British congenital cardiac A. New-onset heart failure due to heart muscle disease in childhood: a prospective study in the United Kingdom and Ireland, Circulation 117 (1) (2008) 79–84.

[54] S.E. Lipshultz, L.A. Sleeper, J.A. Towbin, A.M. Lowe, E.J. Orav, G.F. Cox, et al., The incidence of pediatric cardiomyopathy in two regions of the United States, N. Engl. J. Med. 348 (17) (2003) 1647–1655.

[55] P.E. Daubeney, A.W. Nugent, P. Chondros, J.B. Carlin, S.D. Colan, M. Cheung, et al., Clinical features and outcomes of childhood dilated cardiomyopathy: results from a national population-based study, Circulation 114 (24) (2006) 2671–2678.

[56] J.A. Towbin, A.M. Lowe, S.D. Colan, L.A. Sleeper, E.J. Orav, S. Clunie, et al., Incidence, causes, and outcomes of dilated cardiomyopathy in children, JAMA 296 (15) (2006) 1867–1876.

[57] A.L. Caforio, R. Marcolongo, C. Basso, S. Iliceto, Clinical presentation and diagnosis of myocarditis, Heart 101 (16) (2015) 1332–1344.

[58] N. Amabile, A. Fraisse, J. Bouvenot, P. Chetaille, C. Ovaert, Outcome of acute fulminant myocarditis in children, Heart 92 (9) (2006) 1269–1273.

[59] S.A. Teele, C.K. Allan, P.C. Laussen, J.W. Newburger, K. Gauvreau, R.R. Thiagarajan, Management and outcomes in pediatric patients presenting with acute fulminant myocarditis, J. Pediatr. 158 (4) (2011) 638–643 e1.

[60] G.M. Felker, J.P. Boehmer, R.H. Hruban, G.M. Hutchins, E.K. Kasper, K.L. Baughman, et al., Echocardiographic findings in fulminant and acute myocarditis, J. Am. Coll. Cardiol. 36 (1) (2000) 227–232.

[61] Y. Asaumi, S. Yasuda, I. Morii, H. Kakuchi, Y. Otsuka, A. Kawamura, et al., Favourable clinical outcome in patients with cardiogenic shock due to fulminant myocarditis supported by percutaneous extracorporeal membrane oxygenation, Eur. Heart J. 26 (20) (2005) 2185–2192.

[62] K. Ishida, H. Wada, K. Sakakura, N. Kubo, N. Ikeda, Y. Sugawara, et al., Long-term follow-up on cardiac function following fulminant myocarditis requiring percutaneous extracorporeal cardiopulmonary support, Heart Vessels 28 (1) (2013) 86–90.

[63] D.A. Kane, D.R. Fulton, S. Saleeb, J. Zhou, J.E. Lock, R.L. Geggel, Needles in hay: chest pain as the presenting symptom in children with serious underlying cardiac pathology, Congenit. Heart Dis. 5 (4) (2010) 366–373.

[64] A. Yilmaz, H. Mahrholdt, A. Athanasiadis, H. Vogelsberg, G. Meinhardt, M. Voehringer, et al., Coronary vasospasm as the underlying cause for chest pain in patients with PVB19 myocarditis, Heart 94 (11) (2008) 1456–1463.

[65] A. Florian, T. Schaufele, A. Ludwig, S. Rosch, I. Wenzelburger, H. Yildiz, et al., Diagnostic value of CMR in young patients with clinically suspected acute myocarditis is determined by cardiac enzymes, Clin. Res. Cardiol. 104 (2) (2015) 154–163.

[66] M. Francone, C. Chimenti, N. Galea, F. Scopelliti, R. Verardo, R. Galea, et al., CMR sensitivity varies with clinical presentation and extent of cell necrosis in biopsy-proven acute myocarditis, JACC Cardiovasc. Imaging 7 (3) (2014) 254–263.

[67] U. Kuhl, M. Pauschinger, T. Bock, K. Klingel, C.P. Schwimmbeck, B. Seeberg, et al., Parvovirus B19 infection mimicking acute myocardial infarction, Circulation 108 (8) (2003) 945–950.

[68] B.D. Bultmann, K. Klingel, K. Sotlar, C.T. Bock, H.A. Baba, M. Sauter, et al., Fatal parvovirus B19-associated myocarditis clinically mimicking ischemic heart disease: an endothelial cell-mediated disease, Human Pathol. 34 (1) (2003) 92–95.

[69] Y. Durani, M. Egan, J. Baffa, S.M. Selbst, A.L. Nager, Pediatric myocarditis: presenting clinical characteristics, Am. J. Emerg. Med. 27 (8) (2009) 942–947.

[70] S.B. Freedman, J.K. Haladyn, A. Floh, J.A. Kirsh, G. Taylor, J. Thull-Freedman, Pediatric myocarditis: emergency department clinical findings and diagnostic evaluation, Pediatrics 120 (6) (2007) 1278–1285.

[71] T. Saji, H. Matsuura, K. Hasegawa, T. Nishikawa, E. Yamamoto, H. Ohki, et al., Comparison of the clinical presentation, treatment, and outcome of fulminant and acute myocarditis in children, Circ. J. 76 (5) (2012) 1222–1228.

[72] H.J. Kim, G.H. Yoo, H.R. Kil, Clinical outcome of acute myocarditis in children according to treatment modalities, Korean J. Pediatr. 53 (7) (2010) 745–752.

[73] R.F. English, J.E. Janosky, J.A. Ettedgui, S.A. Webber, Outcomes for children with acute myocarditis, Cardiol. Young 14 (5) (2004) 488–493.

[74] I. Kindermann, C. Barth, F. Mahfoud, C. Ukena, M. Lenski, A. Yilmaz, et al., Update on myocarditis, J. Am. Coll. Cardiol. 59 (9) (2012) 779–792.
[75] S. Sagar, P.P. Liu, L.T. Cooper Jr., Myocarditis, Lancet 379 (9817) (2012) 738–747.
[76] M. Renko, M. Leskinen, T. Kontiokari, T. Tapiainen, P. Hedberg, M. Uhari, Cardiac troponin-I as a screening tool for myocarditis in children hospitalized for viral infection, Acta Paediatr. 99 (2) (2010) 283–285.
[77] J.L. Brown, D.A. Hirsh, W.T. Mahle, Use of troponin as a screen for chest pain in the pediatric emergency department, Pediatr. Cardiol. 33 (2) (2012) 337–342.
[78] J. Soongswang, K. Durongpisitkul, A. Nana, D. Laohaprasittiporn, C. Kangkagate, K. Punlee, et al., Cardiac troponin T: a marker in the diagnosis of acute myocarditis in children, Pediatr. Cardiol. 26 (1) (2005) 45–49.
[79] M. Al-Biltagi, M. Issa, H.A. Hagar, M. Abdel-Hafez, N.A. Aziz, Circulating cardiac troponins levels and cardiac dysfunction in children with acute and fulminant viral myocarditis, Acta Paediatr. 99 (10) (2010) 1510–1516.
[80] N. Mewton, A. Dernis, D. Bresson, O. Zouaghi, P. Croisille, E. Flocard, et al., Myocardial biomarkers and delayed enhanced cardiac magnetic resonance relationship in clinically suspected myocarditis and insight on clinical outcome, J. Cardiovasc. Med. 16 (10) (2015) 696.
[81] C. Ukena, M. Kindermann, F. Mahfoud, J. Geisel, P.M. Lepper, R. Kandolf, et al., Diagnostic and prognostic validity of different biomarkers in patients with suspected myocarditis, Clin. Res. Cardiol. 103 (9) (2014) 743–751.
[82] S. Sachdeva, X. Song, N. Dham, D.M. Heath, R.L. DeBiasi, Analysis of clinical parameters and cardiac magnetic resonance imaging as predictors of outcome in pediatric myocarditis, Am. J. Cardiol. 115 (4) (2015) 499–504.
[83] S. Koulouri, R.J. Acherman, P.C. Wong, L.S. Chan, A.B. Lewis, Utility of B-type natriuretic peptide in differentiating congestive heart failure from lung disease in pediatric patients with respiratory distress, Pediatr. Cardiol. 25 (4) (2004) 341–346.
[84] E. Mlczoch, F. Darbandi-Mesri, D. Luckner, U. Salzer-Muhar, NT-pro BNP in acute childhood myocarditis, J. Pediatr. 160 (1) (2012) 178–179.
[85] U. Nussinovitch, Y. Shoenfeld, The clinical and diagnostic significance of anti-myosin autoantibodies in cardiac disease, Clin. Rev. Allergy Immunol. 44 (1) (2013) 98–108.
[86] A.B. Martin, S. Webber, F.J. Fricker, R. Jaffe, G. Demmler, D. Kearney, et al., Acute myocarditis. Rapid diagnosis by PCR in children, Circulation 90 (1) (1994) 330–339.
[87] P.R. Camargo, T.S. Okay, L. Yamamoto, G.M. Del Negro, A.A. Lopes, Myocarditis in children and detection of viruses in myocardial tissue: implications for immunosuppressive therapy, Int. J. Cardiol. 148 (2) (2011) 204–208.
[88] K.E. Simpson, G.A. Storch, C.K. Lee, M.W. Cunningham, K. Ward, A. Tong, et al., Blood viral PCR frequently identifies cardiotropic viruses in pediatric patients with clinical myocarditis or recent onset dilated cardiomyopathy at time of presentation, Am. J. Cardiol. 1988 (62) (2013) 285–291.
[89] M. Jeserich, E. Brunner, R. Kandolf, M. Olschewski, S. Kimmel, M.G. Friedrich, et al., Diagnosis of viral myocarditis by cardiac magnetic resonance and viral genome detection in peripheral blood, Int. J. Cardiovasc. Imaging 29 (1) (2013) 121–129.
[90] F. Mahfoud, B. Gartner, M. Kindermann, C. Ukena, K. Gadomski, K. Klingel, et al., Virus serology in patients with suspected myocarditis: utility or futility? Eur. Heart J. 32 (7) (2011) 897–903.
[91] R. Ichikawa, N. Sumitomo, A. Komori, Y. Abe, T. Nakamura, J. Fukuhara, et al., The follow-up evaluation of electrocardiogram and arrhythmias in children with fulminant myocarditis, Circ. J. 75 (4) (2011) 932–938.
[92] J. Kern, R. Modi, M.K. Atalay, L.K. Kochilas, Clinical myocarditis masquerading as acute coronary syndrome, J. Pediatr. 154 (4) (2009) 612–615.
[93] L. Sarda, P. Colin, F. Boccara, D. Daou, R. Lebtahi, M. Faraggi, et al., Myocarditis in patients with clinical presentation of myocardial infarction and normal coronary angiograms, J. Am. Coll. Cardiol. 37 (3) (2001) 786–792.
[94] A.S. Batra, D. Epstein, M.J. Silka, The clinical course of acquired complete heart block in children with acute myocarditis, Pediatr. Cardiol. 24 (5) (2003) 495–497.
[95] H.N. Skouri, G.W. Dec, M.G. Friedrich, L.T. Cooper, Noninvasive imaging in myocarditis, J. Am. Coll. Cardiol. 48 (10) (2006) 2085–2093.
[96] G.W. Dec Jr., H. Waldman, J. Southern, J.T. Fallon, A.M. Hutter Jr., I. Palacios, Viral myocarditis mimicking acute myocardial infarction, J. Am. Coll. Cardiol. 20 (1) (1992) 85–89.
[97] N.S. Khoo, J.F. Smallhorn, J. Atallah, S. Kaneko, A.S. Mackie, I. Paterson, Altered left ventricular tissue velocities, deformation and twist in children and young adults with acute myocarditis and normal ejection fraction, J. Am. Soc. Echocardiogr. 25 (3) (2012) 294–303.
[98] F. Escher, D. Westermann, R. Gaub, J. Pronk, T. Bock, N. Al-Saadi, et al., Development of diastolic heart failure in a 6-year follow-up study in patients after acute myocarditis, Heart 97 (9) (2011) 709–714.
[99] F. Escher, M. Kasner, U. Kuhl, J. Heymer, U. Wilkenshoff, C. Tschope, et al., New echocardiographic findings correlate with intramyocardial inflammation in endomyocardial biopsies of patients with acute myocarditis and inflammatory cardiomyopathy, Mediat. Inflamm. 2013 (2013) 875420.
[100] S.C. Uppu, A. Shah, J. Weigand, J.C. Nielsen, H.H. Ko, I.A. Parness, et al., Two-dimensional speckle-tracking-derived segmental peak systolic longitudinal strain identifies regional myocardial involvement in patients with myocarditis and normal global left ventricular systolic function, Pediatr. Cardiol. 36 (5) (2015) 950–959.
[101] L.A. Blauwet, L.T. Cooper, Myocarditis, Prog. Cardiovasc. Dis. 52 (4) (2010) 274–288.
[102] L.A. Mendes, G.W. Dec, M.H. Picard, I.F. Palacios, J. Newell, R. Davidoff, Right ventricular dysfunction: an independent predictor of adverse outcome in patients with myocarditis, Am. Heart J. 128 (2) (1994) 301–307.
[103] H.T. Aretz, M.E. Billingham, W.D. Edwards, S.M. Factor, J.T. Fallon, J.J. Fenoglio Jr., et al., Myocarditis. A histopathologic definition and classification, Am. J. Cardiovasc. Pathol. 1 (1) (1987) 3–14.
[104] K.L. Baughman, Diagnosis of myocarditis: death of Dallas criteria, Circulation 113 (4) (2006) 593–595.

[105] J.W. Magnani, H.J. Danik, G.W. Dec Jr., T.G. DiSalvo, Survival in biopsy-proven myocarditis: a long-term retrospective analysis of the histopathologic, clinical, and hemodynamic predictors, Am. Heart J. 151 (2) (2006) 463–470.
[106] I. Kindermann, M. Kindermann, R. Kandolf, K. Klingel, B. Bultmann, T. Muller, et al., Predictors of outcome in patients with suspected myocarditis, Circulation 118 (6) (2008) 639–648.
[107] H. Mahrholdt, C. Goedecke, A. Wagner, G. Meinhardt, A. Athanasiadis, H. Vogelsberg, et al., Cardiovascular magnetic resonance assessment of human myocarditis: a comparison to histology and molecular pathology, Circulation 109 (10) (2004) 1250–1258.
[108] F. Escher, D. Lassner, U. Kuhl, U. Gross, D. Westermann, W. Poller, et al., Analysis of endomyocardial biopsies in suspected myocarditis–diagnostic value of left versus right ventricular biopsy, Int. J. Cardiol. 177 (1) (2014) 76–78.
[109] A. Yilmaz, I. Kindermann, M. Kindermann, F. Mahfoud, C. Ukena, A. Athanasiadis, et al., Comparative evaluation of left and right ventricular endomyocardial biopsy: differences in complication rate and diagnostic performance, Circulation 122 (9) (2010) 900–909.
[110] S.R. Foerster, C.E. Canter, A. Cinar, L.A. Sleeper, S.A. Webber, E. Pahl, et al., Ventricular remodeling and survival are more favorable for myocarditis than for idiopathic dilated cardiomyopathy in childhood: an outcomes study from the Pediatric Cardiomyopathy Registry, Circ. Heart Fail. 3 (6) (2010) 689–697.
[111] J.G. Shanes, J. Ghali, M.E. Billingham, V.J. Ferrans, J.J. Fenoglio, W.D. Edwards, et al., Interobserver variability in the pathologic interpretation of endomyocardial biopsy results, Circulation 75 (2) (1987) 401–405.
[112] L.T. Cooper, K.L. Baughman, A.M. Feldman, A. Frustaci, M. Jessup, U. Kuhl, et al., The role of endomyocardial biopsy in the management of cardiovascular disease: a scientific statement from the American Heart Association, the American College of Cardiology, and the European Society of Cardiology, Circulation 116 (19) (2007) 2216–2233.
[113] B.B. Das, Role of endomyocardial biopsy for children presenting with acute systolic heart failure, Pediatr. Cardiol. 35 (2) (2014) 191–196.
[114] P.M. Pattynama, A. De Roos, E.E. Van der Wall, A.E. Van Voorthuisen, Evaluation of cardiac function with magnetic resonance imaging, Am. Heart J. 128 (3) (1994) 595–607.
[115] M.G. Friedrich, F. Marcotte, Cardiac magnetic resonance assessment of myocarditis, Circ. Cardiovasc. Imaging 6 (5) (2013) 833–839.
[116] H. Abdel-Aty, P. Boye, A. Zagrosek, R. Wassmuth, A. Kumar, D. Messroghli, et al., Diagnostic performance of cardiovascular magnetic resonance in patients with suspected acute myocarditis: comparison of different approaches, J. Am. Coll. Cardiol. 45 (11) (2005) 1815–1822.
[117] A.H. Aletras, P. Kellman, J.A. Derbyshire, A.E. Arai, ACUT2E TSE-SSFP: a hybrid method for T2-weighted imaging of edema in the heart, Magn. Reson. Med. 59 (2) (2008) 229–235.
[118] M.G. Friedrich, U. Sechtem, J. Schulz-Menger, G. Holmvang, P. Alakija, L.T. Cooper, et al., Cardiovascular magnetic resonance in myocarditis: A JACC white paper, J. Am. Coll. Cardiol. 53 (17) (2009) 1475–1487.
[119] O.P. Simonetti, R.J. Kim, D.S. Fieno, H.B. Hillenbrand, E. Wu, J.M. Bundy, et al., An improved MR imaging technique for the visualization of myocardial infarction, Radiology 218 (1) (2001) 215–223.
[120] M.G. Friedrich, O. Strohm, J. Schulz-Menger, H. Marciniak, F.C. Luft, R. Dietz, Contrast media-enhanced magnetic resonance imaging visualizes myocardial changes in the course of viral myocarditis, Circulation 97 (18) (1998) 1802–1809.
[121] A. Wagner, J. Schulz-Menger, R. Dietz, M.G. Friedrich, Long-term follow-up of patients paragraph sign with acute myocarditis by magnetic paragraph sign resonance imaging, Magma 16 (1) (2003) 17–20.
[122] U.K. Radunski, G.K. Lund, C. Stehning, B. Schnackenburg, S. Bohnen, G. Adam, et al., CMR in patients with severe myocarditis: diagnostic value of quantitative tissue markers including extracellular volume imaging, JACC Cardiovasc. Imaging 7 (7) (2014) 667–675.
[123] V.M. Ferreira, S.K. Piechnik, E. Dall'Armellina, T.D. Karamitsos, J.M. Francis, N. Ntusi, et al., T(1) mapping for the diagnosis of acute myocarditis using CMR: comparison to T2-weighted and late gadolinium enhanced imaging, JACC Cardiovasc. Imaging 6 (10) (2013) 1048–1058.
[124] J.A. Luetkens, J. Doerner, D.K. Thomas, D. Dabir, J. Gieseke, A.M. Sprinkart, et al., Acute myocarditis: multiparametric cardiac MR imaging, Radiology 273 (2) (2014) 383–392.
[125] R. Hinojar, L. Foote, E. Arroyo Ucar, T. Jackson, A. Jabbour, C.Y. Yu, et al., Native T1 in discrimination of acute and convalescent stages in patients with clinical diagnosis of myocarditis: a proposed diagnostic algorithm using CMR, JACC Cardiovasc. Imaging 8 (1) (2015) 37–46.
[126] S. Grun, J. Schumm, S. Greulich, A. Wagner, S. Schneider, O. Bruder, et al., Long-term follow-up of biopsy-proven viral myocarditis: predictors of mortality and incomplete recovery, J. Am. Coll. Cardiol. 59 (18) (2012) 1604–1615.
[127] S. Greulich, I. Kindermann, J. Schumm, A. Perne, S. Birkmeier, S. Grun, et al., Predictors of outcome in patients with parvovirus B19 positive endomyocardial biopsy, Clin. Res. Cardiol. 105 (1) (2016) 37–52.
[128] F. Sanguineti, P. Garot, M. Mana, D. O'H-Ici, T. Hovasse, T. Unterseeh, et al., Cardiovascular magnetic resonance predictors of clinical outcome in patients with suspected acute myocarditis, J. Cardiovasc. Magn. Reson. 17 (1) (2015) 78.
[129] A. Zagrosek, H. Abdel-Aty, P. Boye, R. Wassmuth, D. Messroghli, W. Utz, et al., Cardiac magnetic resonance monitors reversible and irreversible myocardial injury in myocarditis, JACC Cardiovasc. Imaging 2 (2) (2009) 131–138.
[130] P. Paule, N.C. Roche, Y. Chabrillat, J. Quilici, C. Jego, U. Vinsonneau, et al., [Contribution of cardiac MRI in the initial evaluation and follow-up of myocarditis mimicking acute coronary syndrome: a series of 43 patients], Ann. Cardiol. d'angeiologie 63 (5) (2014) 331–338.
[131] D. Klugman, J.T. Berger, C.A. Sable, J. He, S.G. Khandelwal, A.D. Slonim, Pediatric patients hospitalized with myocarditis: a multi-institutional analysis, Pediatr. Cardiol. 31 (2) (2010) 222–228.
[132] S.A. Hunt, W.T. Abraham, M.H. Chin, A.M. Feldman, G.S. Francis, T.G. Ganiats, et al., 2009 focused update incorporated into the ACC/AHA 2005 guidelines for the diagnosis and management of heart failure in adults: a report of the American College of Cardiology Foundation/American Heart Association Task Force on Practice Guidelines: developed in collaboration with the International Society for Heart and Lung Transplantation, Circulation 119 (14) (2009) e391–479.

[133] D.M. McNamara, R.C. Starling, L.T. Cooper, J.P. Boehmer, P.J. Mather, K.M. Janosko, et al., Clinical and demographic predictors of outcomes in recent onset dilated cardiomyopathy: results of the IMAC (intervention in myocarditis and acute cardiomyopathy)-2 study, J. Am. Coll. Cardiol. 58 (11) (2011) 1112–1118.

[134] A. Matsumori, H. Igata, K. Ono, A. Iwasaki, T. Miyamoto, R. Nishio, et al., High doses of digitalis increase the myocardial production of proinflammatory cytokines and worsen myocardial injury in viral myocarditis: a possible mechanism of digitalis toxicity, Jpn. Circ. J. 63 (12) (1999) 934–940.

[135] M.P. Reyes, R. Khatib, G. Khatib, K.L. Ho, F. Smith, R.A. Kloner, Prolonged captopril therapy in murine viral myocarditis, J. Cardiovasc. Pharmacol. Ther. 3 (1) (1998) 43–50.

[136] T.J. Bahk, M.D. Daniels, J.S. Leon, K. Wang, D.M. Engman, Comparison of angiotensin converting enzyme inhibition and angiotensin II receptor blockade for the prevention of experimental autoimmune myocarditis, Int. J. Cardiol. 125 (1) (2008) 85–93.

[137] V. Sukumaran, K. Watanabe, P.T. Veeraveedu, M. Ma, N. Gurusamy, V. Rajavel, et al., Telmisartan ameliorates experimental autoimmune myocarditis associated with inhibition of inflammation and oxidative stress, Eur. J. Pharmacol. 652 (1–3) (2011) 126–135.

[138] Y.Y. Zhang, J.N. Li, H.H. Xia, S.L. Zhang, J. Zhong, Y.Y. Wu, et al., Protective effects of losartan in mice with chronic viral myocarditis induced by coxsackievirus B3, Life Sci. 92 (24–26) (2013) 1186–1194.

[139] J. Xiao, M. Shimada, W. Liu, D. Hu, A. Matsumori, Anti-inflammatory effects of eplerenone on viral myocarditis, Eur. J. Heart Fail. 11 (4) (2009) 349–353.

[140] Y.C. Li, L.S. Ge, P.L. Yang, J.F. Tang, J.F. Lin, P. Chen, et al., Carvedilol treatment ameliorates acute coxsackievirus B3-induced myocarditis associated with oxidative stress reduction, Eur. J. Pharmacol. 640 (1–3) (2010) 112–116.

[141] L. Yue-Chun, G. Li-Sha, R. Jiang-Hua, Y. Peng-Lin, L. Jia-Feng, T. Ji-Fei, et al., Protective effects of carvedilol in murine model with the coxsackievirus B3-induced viral myocarditis, J. Cardiovasc. Pharmacol. 51 (1) (2008) 92–98.

[142] M. Pauschinger, S. Rutschow, K. Chandrasekharan, D. Westermann, A. Weitz, L. Peter Schwimmbeck, et al., Carvedilol improves left ventricular function in murine coxsackievirus-induced acute myocarditis association with reduced myocardial interleukin-1beta and MMP-8 expression and a modulated immune response, Eur. J. Heart Fail. 7 (4) (2005) 444–452.

[143] S. Rezkalla, R.A. Kloner, G. Khatib, F.E. Smith, R. Khatib, Effect of metoprolol in acute coxsackievirus B3 murine myocarditis, J. Am. Coll. Cardiol. 12 (2) (1988) 412–414.

[144] Z. Yuan, C. Kishimoto, K. Shioji, Beneficial effects of low-dose benidipine in acute autoimmune myocarditis: suppressive effects on inflammatory cytokines and inducible nitric oxide synthase, Circ. J. 67 (6) (2003) 545–550.

[145] W.Z. Wang, A. Matsumori, T. Yamada, T. Shioi, I. Okada, S. Matsui, et al., Beneficial effects of amlodipine in a murine model of congestive heart failure induced by viral myocarditis. A possible mechanism through inhibition of nitric oxide production, Circulation 95 (1) (1997) 245–251.

[146] W. Liu, M. Shimada, J. Xiao, D. Hu, A. Matsumori, Nifedipine inhibits the activation of inflammatory and immune reactions in viral myocarditis, Life Sci. 85 (5–6) (2009) 235–240.

[147] H. Ito, K. Ono, R. Nishio, S. Sasayama, A. Matsumori, Amiodarone inhibits interleukin 6 production and attenuates myocardial injury induced by viral myocarditis in mice, Cytokine 17 (4) (2002) 197–202.

[148] B.R. Anderson, E.S. Silver, M.E. Richmond, L. Liberman, Usefulness of arrhythmias as predictors of death and resource utilization in children with myocarditis, Am. J. Cardiol. 114 (9) (2014) 1400–1405.

[149] S. Matsui, Z.P. Zong, J.F. Han, S. Katsuda, N. Yamaguchi, M.L. Fu, Amiodarone minimizes experimental autoimmune myocarditis in rats, Eur. J. Pharmacol. 469 (1–3) (2003) 165–173.

[150] C. Meune, C. Spaulding, I. Mahe, P. Lebon, J.F. Bergmann, Risks versus benefits of NSAIDs including aspirin in myocarditis: a review of the evidence from animal studies, Drug Saf. 26 (13) (2003) 975–981.

[151] H. Nakamura, I. Kunitsugu, K. Fukuda, M. Matsuzaki, M. Sano, Diverse stage-dependent effects of glucocorticoids in a murine model of viral myocarditis, J. Cardiol. 61 (3) (2013) 237–242.

[152] K.Y. Chan, M. Iwahara, L.N. Benson, G.J. Wilson, R.M. Freedom, Immunosuppressive therapy in the management of acute myocarditis in children: a clinical trial, J. Am. Coll. Cardiol. 17 (2) (1991) 458–460.

[153] K.U. Aziz, N. Patel, T. Sadullah, H. Tasneem, H. Thawerani, S. Talpur, Acute viral myocarditis: role of immunosuppression: a prospective randomised study, Cardiol. Young 20 (5) (2010) 509–515.

[154] H.S. Chen, W. Wang, S.N. Wu, J.P. Liu, Corticosteroids for viral myocarditis, Cochrane Database Syst. Rev. 10 (2013) CD004471.

[155] P.R. Camargo, R. Snitcowsky, P.L. da Luz, R. Mazzieri, M.L. Higuchi, M. Rati, et al., Favorable effects of immunosuppressive therapy in children with dilated cardiomyopathy and active myocarditis, Pediatr. Cardiol. 16 (2) (1995) 61–68.

[156] S. Kleinert, R.G. Weintraub, J.L. Wilkinson, C.W. Chow, Myocarditis in children with dilated cardiomyopathy: incidence and outcome after dual therapy immunosuppression, J. Heart Lung Transplant. 16 (12) (1997) 1248–1254.

[157] M.G. Gagliardi, M. Bevilacqua, C. Bassano, B. Leonardi, R. Boldrini, F.D. Camassei, et al., Long term follow up of children with myocarditis treated by immunosuppression and of children with dilated cardiomyopathy, Heart 90 (10) (2004) 1167–1171.

[158] R. Wojnicz, E. Nowalany-Kozielska, C. Wojciechowska, G. Glanowska, P. Wilczewski, T. Niklewski, et al., Randomized, placebo-controlled study for immunosuppressive treatment of inflammatory dilated cardiomyopathy: two-year follow-up results, Circulation 104 (1) (2001) 39–45.

[159] C. Lu, F. Qin, Y. Yan, T. Liu, J. Li, H. Chen, Immunosuppressive treatment for myocarditis: a meta-analysis of randomized controlled trials, J. Cardiovasc. Med. 17 (8) (2016) 631–637.

[160] J.W. Mason, J.B. O'Connell, A. Herskowitz, N.R. Rose, B.M. McManus, M.E. Billingham, et al., A clinical trial of immunosuppressive therapy for myocarditis. The myocarditis treatment trial investigators, N. Engl. J. Med. 333 (5) (1995) 269–275.

[161] C.P. Hia, W.C. Yip, B.C. Tai, S.C. Quek, Immunosuppressive therapy in acute myocarditis: an 18 year systematic review, Arch. Dis. Child. 89 (6) (2004) 580–584.

[162] A. Frustaci, M.A. Russo, C. Chimenti, Randomized study on the efficacy of immunosuppressive therapy in patients with virus-negative inflammatory cardiomyopathy: the TIMIC study, Eur. Heart J. 30 (16) (2009) 1995–2002.

[163] E.W. Gelfand, Intravenous immune globulin in autoimmune and inflammatory diseases, N. Engl. J. Med. 367 (21) (2012) 2015–2025.

[164] A. Haque, S. Bhatti, F.J. Siddiqui, Intravenous immune globulin for severe acute myocarditis in children, Indian Pediatr. 46 (9) (2009) 810–811.

[165] N.A. Drucker, S.D. Colan, A.B. Lewis, A.S. Beiser, D.L. Wessel, M. Takahashi, et al., Gamma-globulin treatment of acute myocarditis in the pediatric population, Circulation 89 (1) (1994) 252–257.

[166] T. Isogai, H. Yasunaga, H. Matsui, H. Tanaka, H. Horiguchi, K. Fushimi, Effect of intravenous immunoglobulin for fulminant myocarditis on in-hospital mortality: propensity score analyses, J. Card. Fail. 21 (5) (2015) 391–397.

[167] D.M. McNamara, R. Holubkov, R.C. Starling, G.W. Dec, E. Loh, G. Torre-Amione, et al., Controlled trial of intravenous immune globulin in recent-onset dilated cardiomyopathy, Circulation 103 (18) (2001) 2254–2259.

[168] L. Gullestad, H. Aass, J.G. Fjeld, L. Wikeby, A.K. Andreassen, H. Ihlen, et al., Immunomodulating therapy with intravenous immunoglobulin in patients with chronic heart failure, Circulation 103 (2) (2001) 220–225.

[169] J. Robinson, L. Hartling, B. Vandermeer, T.P. Klassen, Intravenous immunoglobulin for presumed viral myocarditis in children and adults, Cochrane Database Syst. Rev. 5 (2015) CD004370.

[170] L.R. Herda, C. Trimpert, U. Nauke, M. Landsberger, A. Hummel, D. Beug, et al., Effects of immunoadsorption and subsequent immunoglobulin G substitution on cardiopulmonary exercise capacity in patients with dilated cardiomyopathy, Am. Heart J. 159 (5) (2010) 809–816.

[171] D. Bulut, M. Scheeler, T. Wichmann, J. Borgel, T. Miebach, A. Mugge, Effect of protein A immunoadsorption on T cell activation in patients with inflammatory dilated cardiomyopathy, Clin. Res. Cardiol. 99 (10) (2010) 633–638.

[172] S.B. Felix, A. Staudt, M. Landsberger, Y. Grosse, V. Stangl, T. Spielhagen, et al., Removal of cardiodepressant antibodies in dilated cardiomyopathy by immunoadsorption, J. Am. Coll. Cardiol. 39 (4) (2002) 646–652.

[173] A.O. Doesch, M. Konstandin, S. Celik, A. Kristen, L. Frankenstein, S. Hardt, et al., Effects of protein A immunoadsorption in patients with advanced chronic dilated cardiomyopathy, J. Clin. Apher. 24 (4) (2009) 141–149.

[174] A. Staudt, M. Bohm, F. Knebel, Y. Grosse, C. Bischoff, A. Hummel, et al., Potential role of autoantibodies belonging to the immunoglobulin G-3 subclass in cardiac dysfunction among patients with dilated cardiomyopathy, Circulation 106 (19) (2002) 2448–2453.

[175] A. Staudt, A. Hummel, J. Ruppert, M. Dorr, C. Trimpert, K. Birkenmeier, et al., Immunoadsorption in dilated cardiomyopathy: 6-month results from a randomized study, Am. Heart J. 152(4) (712) (2006) e1–6.

[176] U. Kuhl, M. Pauschinger, B. Seeberg, D. Lassner, M. Noutsias, W. Poller, et al., Viral persistence in the myocardium is associated with progressive cardiac dysfunction, Circulation 112 (13) (2005) 1965–1970.

[177] J.C. Lenzo, G.R. Shellam, C.M. Lawson, Ganciclovir and cidofovir treatment of cytomegalovirus-induced myocarditis in mice, Antimicrob. Agents Chemother. 45 (5) (2001) 1444–1449.

[178] J.G. McCormack, S.D. Bowler, J.E. Donnelly, C. Steadman, Successful treatment of severe cytomegalovirus infection with ganciclovir in an immunocompetent host, Clin. Infect. Dis. 26 (4) (1998) 1007–1008.

[179] N. Dehtiar, M. Eherlichman, E. Picard, D. Kleid, J. Glaser, D. Raveh, et al., Cytomegalovirus myocarditis in a healthy infant: complete recovery after ganciclovir treatment, Pediatr. Crit. Care Med. 2 (3) (2001) 271–273.

[180] D.C. Pevear, T.M. Tull, M.E. Seipel, J.M. Groarke, Activity of pleconaril against enteroviruses, Antimicrob. Agents Chemother. 43 (9) (1999) 2109–2115.

[181] H.A. Rotbart, A.D. Webster, Pleconaril Treatment Registry G. Treatment of potentially life-threatening enterovirus infections with pleconaril, Clin. Infect. Dis. 32 (2) (2001) 228–235.

[182] S. Bauer, G. Gottesman, L. Sirota, I. Litmanovitz, S. Ashkenazi, I. Levi, Severe coxsackie virus B infection in preterm newborns treated with pleconaril, Eur. J. Pediatr. 161 (9) (2002) 491–493.

[183] A. Heim, M. Stille-Seigener, P. Pring-Akerblom, I. Grumbach, C. Brehm, H. Kreuzer, et al., Recombinant Interferons beta and gamma have a higher antiviral activity than interferon-alpha in coxsackievirus B3-infected carrier state cultures of human myocardial fibroblasts, J. Interferon Cytokine Res. 16 (4) (1996) 283–287.

[184] A. Heim, S. Weiss, Interferons in enteroviral heart disease: modulation of cytokine expression and antiviral activity, Med. Microbiol. Immunol. 193 (2–3) (2004) 149–154.

[185] L. Daliento, F. Calabrese, F. Tona, A.L. Caforio, G. Tarsia, A. Angelini, et al., Successful treatment of enterovirus-induced myocarditis with interferon-alpha, J. Heart Lung Transplant. 22 (2) (2003) 214–217.

[186] A. Heim, M. Stille-Siegener, R. Kandolf, H. Kreuzer, H.R. Figulla, Enterovirus-induced myocarditis: hemodynamic deterioration with immunosuppressive therapy and successful application of interferon-alpha, Clin. Cardiol. 17 (10) (1994) 563–565.

[187] U. Kuhl, M. Pauschinger, P.L. Schwimmbeck, B. Seeberg, C. Lober, M. Noutsias, et al., Interferon-beta treatment eliminates cardiotropic viruses and improves left ventricular function in patients with myocardial persistence of viral genomes and left ventricular dysfunction, Circulation 107 (22) (2003) 2793–2798.

[188] S.H. Yun, W.G. Lee, Y.C. Kim, E.S. Ju, B.K. Lim, J.O. Choi, et al., Antiviral activity of coxsackievirus B3 3C protease inhibitor in experimental murine myocarditis, J. Infect. Dis. 205 (3) (2012) 491–497.

[189] B.K. Lim, S.H. Yun, E.S. Ju, B.K. Kim, Y.J. Lee, D.K. Yoo, et al., Soluble coxsackievirus B3 3C protease inhibitor prevents cardiomyopathy in an experimental chronic myocarditis murine model, Virus Res. 199 (2015) 1–8.

[190] R.I. Lala, M. Puschita, D. Darabantiu, L. Pilat, Galectin-3 in heart failure pathology–"another brick in the wall"? Acta Cardiol. 70 (3) (2015) 323–331.
[191] C. Jaquenod De Giusti, A.E. Ure, L. Rivadeneyra, M. Schattner, R.M. Gomez, Macrophages and galectin 3 play critical roles in CVB3-induced murine acute myocarditis and chronic fibrosis, J. Mol. Cell. Cardiol. 85 (2015) 58–70.
[192] P.S. Tavares, R. Rocon-Albuquerque Jr., A.F. Leite-Moreira, Innate immune receptor activation in viral myocarditis: pathophysiologic implications, (Revista portuguesa de cardiologia: orgao oficial da Sociedade Portuguesa de Cardiologia) Port. J. Cardiol. 29 (1) (2010) 57–78.
[193] P. Zhang, C.J. Cox, K.M. Alvarez, M.W. Cunningham, Cutting edge: cardiac myosin activates innate immune responses through TLRs, J. Immunol. 183 (1) (2009) 27–31.
[194] P.A. Gonnella, H. Waldner, P.J. Del Nido, F.X. McGowan, Inhibition of experimental autoimmune myocarditis: peripheral deletion of TcR Vbeta 8.1, 8.2+ CD4+ T cells in TLR-4 deficient mice, J. Autoimmun. 31 (2) (2008) 180–187.
[195] A. Jenke, S. Wilk, W. Poller, U. Eriksson, A. Valaperti, B.H. Rauch, et al., Adiponectin protects against Toll-like receptor 4-mediated cardiac inflammation and injury, Cardiovasc. Res. 99 (3) (2013) 422–431.
[196] S.K. Rajagopal, C.S. Almond, P.C. Laussen, P.T. Rycus, D. Wypij, R.R. Thiagarajan, Extracorporeal membrane oxygenation for the support of infants, children, and young adults with acute myocarditis: a review of the Extracorporeal Life Support Organization registry, Crit. Care Med. 38 (2) (2010) 382–387.
[197] M.L. Paden, S.A. Conrad, P.T. Rycus, R.R. Thiagarajan, E. Registry, Extracorporeal Life Support Organization Registry Report 2012, ASAIO J. 59 (3) (2013) 202–210.
[198] B.W. Duncan, D.J. Bohn, A.M. Atz, J.W. French, P.C. Laussen, D.L. Wessel, Mechanical circulatory support for the treatment of children with acute fulminant myocarditis, J. Thorac. Cardiovasc. Surg. 122 (3) (2001) 440–448.
[199] E. Nahum, O. Dagan, A. Lev, G. Shukrun, G. Amir, G. Frenkel, et al., Favorable outcome of pediatric fulminant myocarditis supported by extracorporeal membranous oxygenation, Pediatr. Cardiol. 31 (7) (2010) 1059–1063.
[200] T. Nakamura, K. Ishida, Y. Taniguchi, T. Nakagawa, M. Seguchi, H. Wada, et al., Prognosis of patients with fulminant myocarditis managed by peripheral venoarterial extracorporeal membranous oxygenation support: a retrospective single-center study, J. Intensive Care 3 (1) (2015) 5.
[201] T.W. Su, Y.H. Tseng, T.I. Wu, P.J. Lin, M.Y. Wu, Extracorporeal life support in adults with hemodynamic collapse from fulminant cardiomyopathies: the chance of bridging to recovery, ASAIO J. 60 (6) (2014) 664–669.
[202] A.G. Cabrera, K.S. Sundareswaran, A.X. Samayoa, A. Jeewa, E.D. McKenzie, J.W. Rossano, et al., Outcomes of pediatric patients supported by the HeartMate II left ventricular assist device in the United States, J. Heart Lung Transplant. 32 (11) (2013) 1107–1113.
[203] D.L. Morales, A.W. Lowry, D.J. Epstein, D.N. Rosenthal, J.M. Chen, C.S. Almond, et al., Outcomes of children implanted with ventricular assist devices in the United States: analysis of the Interagency Registry for Mechanical Circulatory Support (INTERMACS), Circulation 124 (2011) A10088.
[204] C.S. Almond, D.L. Morales, E.H. Blackstone, M.W. Turrentine, M. Imamura, M.P. Massicotte, et al., Berlin Heart EXCOR pediatric ventricular assist device for bridge to heart transplantation in US children, Circulation 127 (16) (2013) 1702–1711.
[205] R.E. McCarthy 3rd, J.P. Boehmer, R.H. Hruban, G.M. Hutchins, E.K. Kasper, J.M. Hare, et al., Long-term outcome of fulminant myocarditis as compared with acute (nonfulminant) myocarditis, N. Engl. J. Med. 342 (10) (2000) 690–695.
[206] A.W. Nugent, P.E. Daubeney, P. Chondros, J.B. Carlin, M. Cheung, L.C. Wilkinson, et al., The epidemiology of childhood cardiomyopathy in Australia, N. Engl. J. Med. 348 (17) (2003) 1639–1646.
[207] T. Bharucha, K.J. Lee, P.E. Daubeney, A.W. Nugent, C. Turner, G.F. Sholler, et al., Sudden death in childhood cardiomyopathy: results from a long-term national population-based study, J. Am. Coll. Cardiol. 65 (21) (2015) 2302–2310.
[208] S. Gupta, D.W. Markham, M.H. Drazner, P.P. Mammen, Fulminant myocarditis, Nat. Clin. Pract. Cardiovasc. Med. 5 (11) (2008) 693–706.
[209] B.A. Pietra, P.F. Kantor, H.L. Bartlett, C. Chin, C.E. Canter, R.L. Larsen, et al., Early predictors of survival to and after heart transplantation in children with dilated cardiomyopathy, Circulation 126 (9) (2012) 1079–1086.
[210] S. Yoshizawa, T.S. Kato, D. Mancini, C.C. Marboe, Outcome of patients having heart transplantation for lymphocytic myocarditis, Am. J. Cardiol. 112 (3) (2013) 405–410.
[211] A.E. Cabinian, R.J. Kiel, F. Smith, K.L. Ho, R. Khatib, M.P. Reyes, Modification of exercise-aggravated coxsackievirus B3 murine myocarditis by T lymphocyte suppression in an inbred model, J. Lab. Clin. Med. 115 (4) (1990) 454–462.
[212] B.J. Maron, D.P. Zipes, R.J. Kovacs, AHA/ACC scientific statement: eligibility and disqualification criteria for athletes with cardiovascular abnormalities, JACC 66 (21) (2015) 2362–2371.

Chapter 17

Dilated Cardiomyopathy

Kimberly Y. Lin[1], Shelley D. Miyamoto[2], Kurt R. Schumacher[3]

[1]*The Perelman School of Medicine at the University of Pennsylvania, Children's Hospital of Philadelphia, Philadelphia, PA, United States;* [2]*University of Colorado School of Medicine, Children's Hospital Colorado, Aurora, CO, United States;* [3]*University of Michigan Medical School, C.S. Mott Children's Hospital, Ann Arbor, MI, United States*

INTRODUCTION

Dilated cardiomyopathy (DCM), characterized by left ventricular (LV) dilation and systolic dysfunction, is the most common form of cardiomyopathy and most common indication for cardiac transplantation in children and adults. The incidence of DCM in adults is about 5.5 per 100,000 people per year, while the incidence in children is between 0.34 and 1.09 per 100,000 people per year [1–3]. While the disease is less common in children, the clinical outcome is similarly poor with 1- and 5-year rates of death or transplantation of approximately 30% and 40%, respectively [2,4]. Even though the incidence, prevalence, and possible etiologies of DCM are different between children and adults, the treatment paradigms remain similar based almost entirely on data derived from adults [5]. Emerging experimental evidence and epidemiologic data suggest that the pediatric DCM population may have distinct differences compared to adult patients and future studies aimed at understanding pediatric heart failure are needed [6].

ETIOLOGY

DCM is a heterogenous form of heart muscle disease that results in a dilated, poorly contracting left ventricle, although the disease process can affect the right ventricle and atria as well. The diagnosis of DCM generally requires exclusion of the presence of hypertension, coronary artery disease, arrhythmias, valve abnormalities, and congenital heart disease. In children, the etiology of DCM is often unknown (idiopathic). Known causes of DCM in children include genetic mutations (e.g., sarcomeric mutations or dystrophinopathies, Chapters 57 and 58), infectious processes (e.g., viral myocarditis, Chapter 16), immunologic abnormalities, metabolic (e.g., malnutrition) or mitochondrial disease, or acquired cases such as toxin-mediated DCM (e.g., anthracyclines, Chapter 33).

PATHOPHYSIOLOGY

The most basic unit of the myocardium is the myofibril. Myofibrils are comprised of many sarcomeres, which are the contractile unit of the heart and are normally arranged in a well-organized longitudinal pattern. Several myofibrils then comprise the cardiac myocyte. The composition of the sarcomere is important to understand as there is increasing evidence that abnormalities within the sarcomere and associated cytoskeletal proteins represent a final common pathway for the development of DCM (Fig. 17.1). Components of the sarcomere include myosin, actin, troponin, and tropomyosin. Genetic mutations in all of these proteins have been identified in association with DCM, especially in those with familial disease [7]. The clinical significance of novel mutations of the sarcomere proteins identified in nonfamilial cases of DCM is less clear (see Chapters 57 and 58 for further discussion on the genetics of DCM). The sarcomere is closely related to cytoskeletal proteins, which have also been implicated in the development of DCM, including dystrophin, desmin, tafazzin, lamin A/C, and titin [8]. Many neuromuscular disorders that are associated with DCM involve mutations in these cytoskeletal proteins. Dystrophin is a large cytoskeletal protein that is important for force transduction and membrane stabilization. Mutations in the dystrophin gene are responsible for Duchenne and Becker muscular dystrophy as well as X-linked forms of isolated DCM [9]. Desmin and lamin A and C are cytoskeletal intermediate filaments also involved in force transduction, while titin is a very large protein that is critical for sarcomere organization as well as mediating the extensibility and elasticity of the sarcomere. Mutations in all of these proteins are associated with DCM. Mitochondrial derangements can also lead to a DCM phenotype. For example, while the function of the mitochondrial phospholipid transacylase tafazzin is poorly understood, mutations in the G4.5 tafazzin gene result in X-linked recessive forms of infantile DCM, Barth Syndrome, and LV noncompaction [10].

Heart Failure in the Child and Young Adult. http://dx.doi.org/10.1016/B978-0-12-802393-8.00017-X

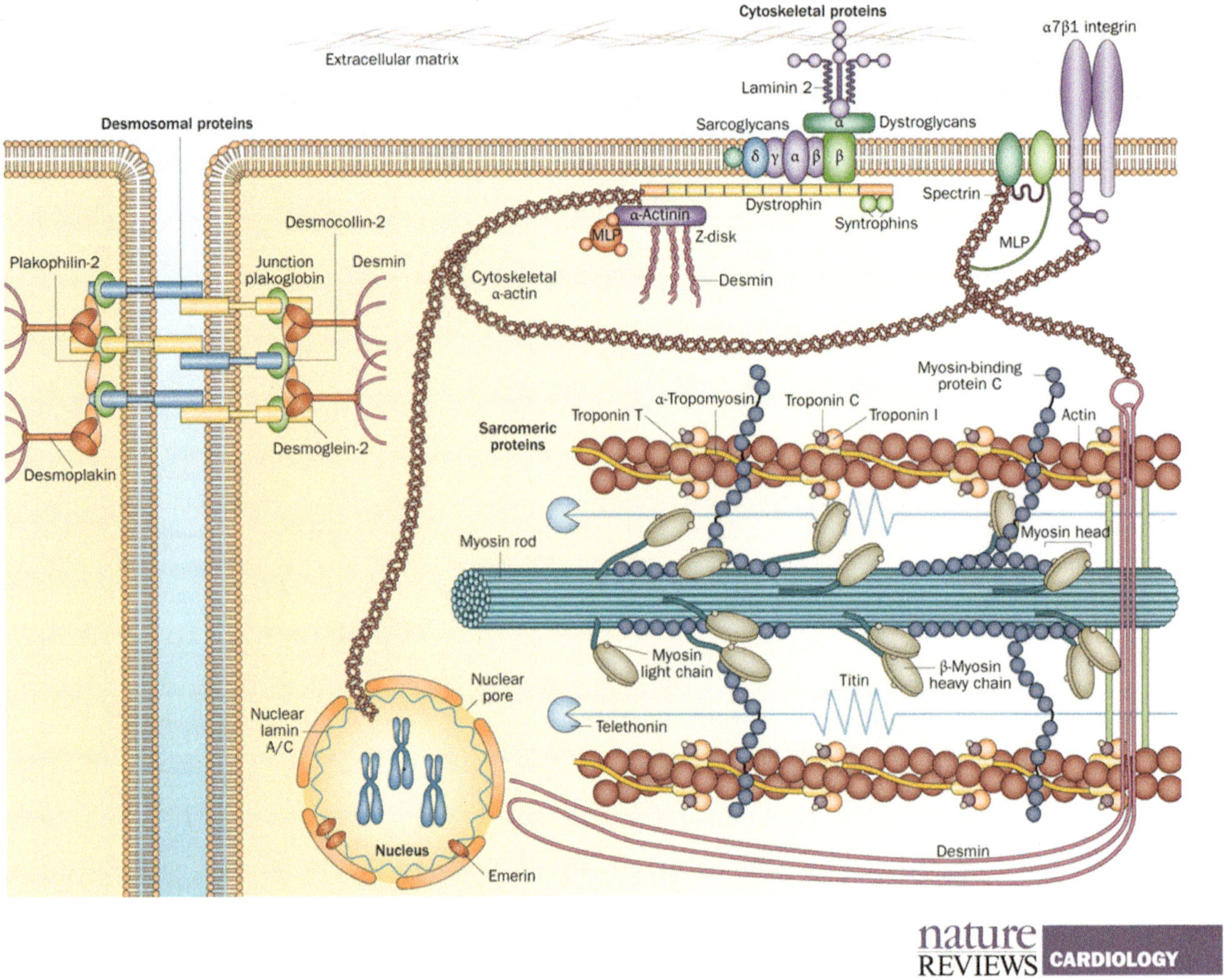

FIGURE 17.1 The main proteins involved in cardiomyopathies. *(A.A.M. Wilde, E.R. Behr, Genetic testing for inherited cardiac disease, Nat. Rev. Cardiol. 10 (10) (2013) 571–583, http://dx.doi.org/10.1038/nrcardio.2013.108.)*

In addition to its reliance on proper protein structure and function, the function of the sarcomere is also dependent on intracellular calcium regulation. Extracellular calcium inflow through the sarcolemma and T-tubules leads to the release of intracellular calcium from the sarcoplasmic reticulum (SR). The SR surrounds the myofibrils, controlling intracellular calcium concentrations thereby stimulating sarcomere contraction. Generation of normal contractile force is dependent on normal electrical conduction, cell depolarization, and calcium signaling. Disruptions in any of these processes can result in contractile failure of the myocardium.

In DCM, an insult such as mechanical strain, circulating catecholamines, inflammatory cytokines, reactive oxygen species, and/or genetic causes trigger myocyte hypertrophy. Associated with myocyte hypertrophy, abnormal microscopic findings such as abnormal structure and number of mitochondria, abnormal glycogen stores, or abnormal lysosomes with vacuolization can be seen. While the myocyte hypertrophy process is initially compensatory, reducing systolic wall stress and limiting cavitary dilation, ultimately myocyte loss (via apoptosis and/or necrosis) along with varying degrees of fibrosis (which can be interstitial, perivascular, or endocardial) occurs. This results in impaired contractile function and decreased cardiac output. Over time, cellular organization begins to deteriorate and cell nuclei enlarge, followed by disruption of the sarcomeric structure (breakdown of the z-band) and ultimately disruption of the usual parallel arrangement of the sarcomeres.

At the macroscopic level, these cellular processes result in ventricular remodeling, which is the process of transition from the usual "bullet-shaped" LV chamber to the more spherical, dilated shape typified by DCM. In the early stages of DCM, through the Frank–Starling mechanism (Fig. 17.2), [11] an increase in preload (ventricular end-diastolic volume)

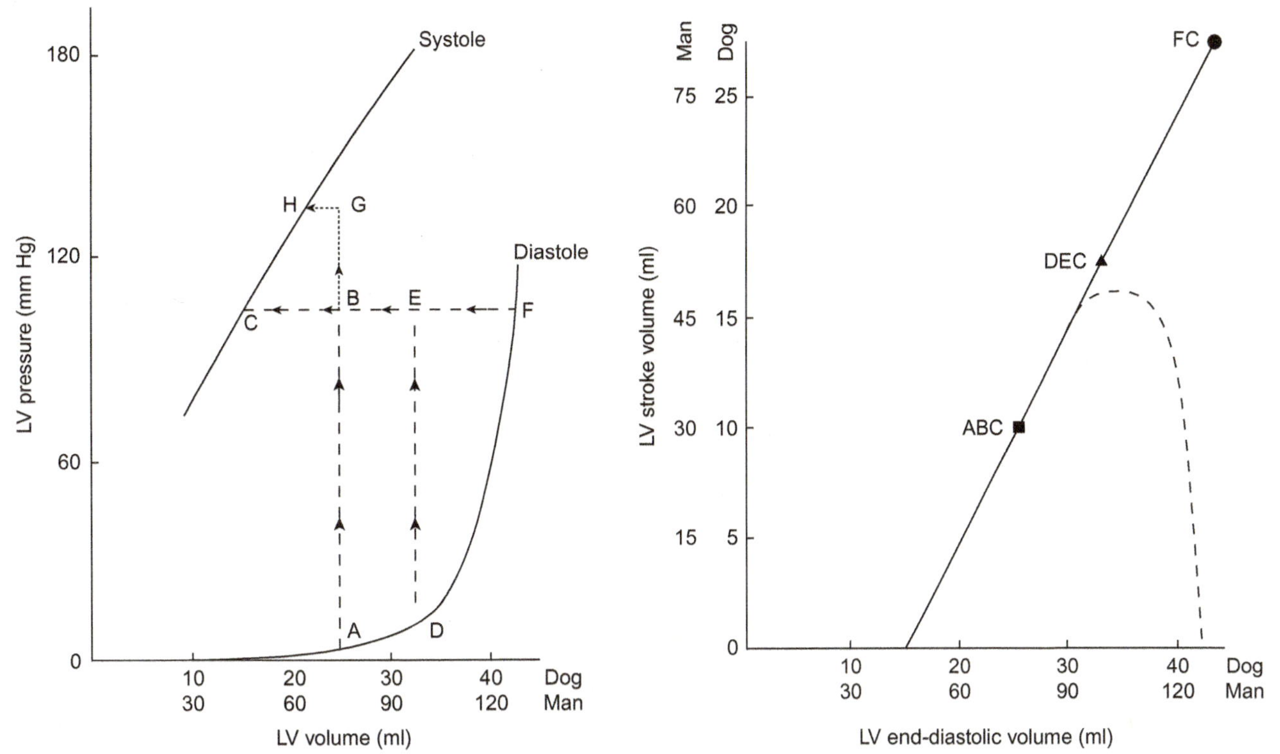

FIGURE 17.2 Frank-Starling diagrams. Left ventricular pressure-volume curve of the dog (left) and stroke volumes in dog and man achieved at increasing left ventricular end diastolic volumes (right). *Broken lines* on the left indicate course of ejecting beat at a systolic pressure of 100 mmHg; *dashed line* on the right indicates actual performance in an overdistended ventricle. Stroke volumes achieved on the right are shown for various contractile performances (ABC, DEC, FC) as demonstrated on the left. *M.I. Noble, The Frank–Starling curve, Clin. Sci. Mol. Med. 54 (1), (1978) 1–7.*

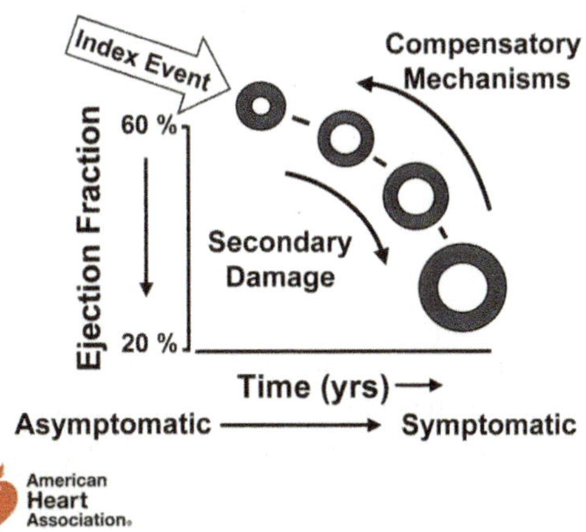

FIGURE 17.3 Pathogenesis of heart failure. *(D.L. Mann, M.R. Bristow, Mechanisms and models in heart failure: the biomechanical model and beyond, Circulation 111 (21) (2005) 2837–2849; Copyright © American Heart Association, Inc. All rights reserved.)*

results in augmentation of ventricular performance and preserved stroke volume despite the limited contractile potential of the myocardium. Other mechanisms including stimulation of the neurohormonal axis through increased activity of the renin–angiotensin–aldosterone system (RAAS) and the sympathetic nervous system allow preservation of vascular resistance, blood pressure, and cardiac output in the short-term. However, unfortunately, DCM is generally a progressive process and ultimately detrimental consequences of these compensatory mechanisms, such as adrenergic receptor downregulation and desensitization, occur and patients develop signs and symptoms of heart failure. These symptoms are a consequence of either decreased cardiac output as further ventricular dilation ensues and stroke volume begins to decrease (Fig. 17.3) [12] or as a result of congestion related to impaired ventricular filling. Additional details regarding the mechanisms involved in the process of cardiac failure can be found in the early chapters of this text.

DIAGNOSTIC EVALUATION

The evaluation of a child with definite or suspected DCM should generally start with the history and physical examination. As the signs and symptoms of heart failure may be quite subtle in a child, specific attention should be given to growth parameters and feeding patterns in addition to the respiratory symptoms and presence of edema, which more commonly manifest in adults. Documentation of the severity and stage of heart failure can facilitate long-term monitoring of disease progression and patient management. The severity of heart failure is typically graded according to the New York Heart Association (NYHA) or Ross classification of symptoms [13,14]. Staging of heart failure, first developed in an effort to describe the development and progression of heart failure in adults, has been modified for infants and children by the International Society for Heart and Lung Transplantation (ISHLT) as well [15,16]. The physical examination may reveal signs of heart failure such as an S3 gallop, a murmur of mitral regurgitation, and lateral displacement of the point of maximal cardiac impulse; jugular venous distension and hepatomegaly; rales or wheezing; pitting edema; and facial swelling. Attention should be given to the vital signs assessment as well, wherein tachycardia, hypotension, decreased oxygen saturation, or poor growth can provide clues as to the severity of cardiac disease.

Laboratory assessment of a child with DCM should include periodic monitoring of end organ function, including renal and liver function tests. While indwelling Swan Ganz catheters are uncommon in the pediatric setting, a central venous line with the tip at the junction of the superior vena cava and the right atrium can provide a sample for a mixed venous saturation to estimate cardiac output. Measurement of B-type natriuretic peptide (BNP), or its more stable relative N-terminal propeptide of BNP (NT-proBNP), can be helpful in distinguishing between cardiac- and noncardiac-related symptoms [17–20]. Furthermore, trends in BNP or NT-BNP may be helpful in the long-term management of a child with DCM with respect to diuretic therapy and prognosis [21]. The utility of newer serum biomarkers such as ST2 in children is a topic of ongoing investigation [22]. Ancillary testing for DCM in children may include chest X-ray, which may show cardiomegaly and pulmonary congestion, and electrocardiogram (ECG), which can provide evidence of underlying etiologies such as ischemia (regional Q waves and ST-T changes) or myocarditis (low voltages).

Other laboratory tests may be helpful in identifying underlying etiologies for DCM in children. Confirmation of newborn screen results and consideration for screening metabolic laboratory tests such as thyroid stimulating hormone, acylcarnitine profile, serum amino acids, urine organic acids, and creatine kinase should be given when an inborn error of metabolism is in the differential diagnosis. In cases of known or suspected myocarditis, markers of myocardial inflammation such as troponin and creatine kinase-MB can be measured and followed serially. Genetic testing for known causes of DCM should be considered, especially in cases where more than one family member is known to be affected, although care should be taken to ensure that proper pre- and posttest genetic counseling is given [23].

The diagnosis of DCM is confirmed by cardiac imaging. The Pediatric Cardiomyopathy Registry (PCMR) defines DCM in children as the presence of LV dilation (Z score$>$2) in the setting of depressed ventricular systolic function (LV shortening fraction or ejection fraction Z score<-2) [24]. In children, such measurements can usually be obtained with relative ease by echocardiography. Cardiac magnetic resonance (CMR) imaging can also provide precise LV volume measurements, although younger or moderately anxious children may have difficulty tolerating a CMR without the inherent risks of sedation. The main advantage of CMR over echocardiogram is its ability to characterize muscle tissue, which can help in some circumstances to identify evidence of fibrosis or underlying etiologies such as myocarditis [25]. Some consider these factors when trying to predict which patients are likely to recover their function and to help decide which interventions to pursue, although the prognostic implications of CMR findings in children with DCM are still a topic of ongoing investigation [26].

Likewise, cardiac catheterization can provide diagnostic and prognostic information in a child with DCM, but only rarely do findings on cardiac catheterization alter the treatment course. Coronary angiography is the gold standard for diagnosis of anomalous left coronary artery from the pulmonary artery (ALCAPA), a congenital heart lesion, which can cause a DCM phenotype but generally warrants surgical intervention, but there are often clues to its presence by ECG and noninvasive methods of cardiac imaging before angiography is performed. The hemodynamic profile of a child with DCM may be helpful in determining whether secondary pulmonary hypertension has developed, whether adequate diuresis has been achieved, and (in severe cases) to confirm heart transplant candidacy.

FAMILY SCREENING

Cardiomyopathy screening with an ECG, echocardiogram, and clinical evaluation should be offered for first degree family members of a child or adult with DCM [23,27]. Cascade genetic testing for potentially affected family members is most helpful when there is a known pathogenic mutation, which tracks with multiple affected family members, as a positive result clearly portends a higher risk for the development of cardiomyopathy, while a negative result may provide a reasonable degree of reassurance.

DISEASE-SPECIFIC THERAPY FOR DILATED CARDIOMYOPATHY

Although the majority of DCM cases are idiopathic, those with identifiable causes may be amenable to disease-specific treatment. ALCAPA may present as DCM in infants through adolescents [28]. Surgical repair with direct coronary reimplantation or intrapulmonary tunnel has been shown to have excellent long-term results, with the majority of patients demonstrating no symptomatic heart failure and long-term normalization of myocardial function [29].

Effective treatment of inborn errors of metabolism may also improve function and symptoms. In individuals afflicted with carnitine deficiency, dietary replacement of carnitine can lead to normalization of ventricular function [30,31]. In propionic acidemia patients who develop DCM, treatment of the disease with liver transplantation has been demonstrated to lead to recovery of myocardial function despite severely depressed function at the time of transplant [32,33]. Correction of nutritional deficiencies with repletion of micronutrients, such as thiamine, selenium, zinc, and copper, and among others, may also lead to improved heart failure in cases where the deficiency is causative [34].

MANAGEMENT OF CHRONIC HEART FAILURE RESULTING FROM DILATED CARDIOMYOPATHY

In the absence of therapies to reverse a known anatomic, metabolic, or nutritional cause of DCM, treatment should be guided by the current pediatric heart failure recommendations from the ISHLT (Table 17.1) [35]. Heart failure in DCM is mediated by neurohormonal stimulation leading to biochemical and molecular mechanisms that cause cardiac remodeling—abnormal

TABLE 17.1 Pediatric Heart Failure Guidelines Summary

Intervention	Which DCM Patients to Consider	Recommendation and Level of Evidence (LOE)
Angiotensin-converting enzyme inhibition	Symptomatic LV dysfunction	Class I (LOE B)
	Asymptomatic LV dysfunction	Class IIa (LOE B)
Angiotensin receptor blockade	Same as above but intolerant of angiotensin-converting enzyme inhibition	Class IIa (LOE C)
Aldosterone antagonism	Systemic ventricular systolic dysfunction	Class I (LOE C)
Beta blockade	Symptomatic and asymptomatic systemic LV dysfunction	Class IIa (LOE B)
Diuretics	Ventricular dysfunction with fluid retention	Class I (LOE C)
Digoxin	Symptomatic heart failure and low ejection fraction	Class IIa (LOE C)
	Recommend against digoxin in asymptomatic LV dysfunction	Class I (LOE C)
Cardiac resynchronization therapy	Systemic LV ejection fraction ≤35%, complete left bundle branch block, QRS > upper limit of normal for age, and NYHA Class II–IV on guideline-determined medical therapy	Class IIa (LOE B)
Implantable cardioverter defibrillator	Secondary prevention after cardiac arrest and exclusion of reversible/treatable cause	Class I (LOE B)
	Secondary prevention after unexplained syncope and at least moderate dysfunction	Class IIa (LOE C)
	Primary prevention consideration in adolescent patient with familial cardiomyopathy with sudden death	Class IIa (LOE C)
Ventricular assist device	Bridge to transplant with early reversible dysfunction of at least one other major organ system	Class I (LOE C)

Class I, evidence and or general agreement that a given procedure or treatment is beneficial, useful or effective; *Class II*, conflicting evidence and/or divergence of opinion that a given procedure or treatment is beneficial, useful, or effective; *Class IIa*—weight of evidence is in favor of usefulness; Level of evidence A, data obtained from multiple randomized trials or metaanalyses; level of evidence B, data derived from a single randomized study or large nonrandomized studies; Level of evidence C, expert consensus opinion, small retrospective studies, or registry data; *DCM*, dilated cardiomyopathy; *LV*, left ventricular. Summarized from R. Kirk, A.I. Dipchand, D.N. Rosenthal, The international society for heart and lung transplantation guidelines for the management of pediatric heart failure (2014); R. Kirk, A.I. Dipchand, D.N. Rosenthal, L. Addonizio , M. Burch, M. Chrisant, et al., The International Society for Heart and Lung Transplantation guidelines for the management of pediatric heart failure: executive summary. [Corrected], J. Heart Lung Transplant. 33 (9) (2014) 888–909.

changes in cardiac structure, myocardial composition, and myocyte deformation. Arrest or reversal of these processes, termed reverse remodeling, is the target of most chronic therapies used in DCM [36]. Thus, neurohormonal blockade has become the goal of treatment in chronic heart failure from DCM.

Neurohormonal Blockade

Renin–Angiotensin System Blockade

Based primarily on the success of angiotensin-converting enzyme inhibitors (ACE-I) in adults with LV dysfunction regardless of etiology [37], the recent pediatric heart failure guidelines designated ACE-I to be a class I recommendation (level of evidence (LOE) B) for symptomatic ventricular dysfunction and a class IIa recommendation (LOE B) for asymptomatic LV dysfunction [35]. Thus, any pediatric patient with DCM presenting with any degree of LV dysfunction should be considered for ACE-I therapy. Although no significant ACE-I trials with outcomes such as death or transplant have been performed in pediatric DCM patients, a number of pediatric studies have demonstrated improvement in LV size and systolic function after ACE-I initiation [38–40].

Similar to ACE-I, angiotensin receptor blockers (ARB) have been demonstrated to reduce morbidity and mortality in adults with chronic heart failure and impaired LV function [41,42]. Although there is minimal published data in children, the current ISHLT heart failure guidelines recommend ARB for any patient in whom RAAS blockade is recommended but is intolerant of ACE-I (Class IIa, LOE C) [35].

Aldosterone Receptor Antagonists

Aldosterone receptor antagonists, including spironolactone and eplerenone, have been shown to promote reverse remodeling and improve mortality in adults with chronic heart failure [43,44]. No studies specific to DCM have been reported. Despite significant clinical experience with these agents in pediatric cardiac patients for their potassium-sparing qualities, studies in pediatric heart failure are not available. Based on data from adults with chronic heart failure of any etiology, it is reasonable to consider aldosterone receptor antagonists in pediatric patients with systemic ventricular dysfunction (recommendation Class I, LOE C) [35].

β-Blockers

β-blockers have been shown to encourage reverse remodeling in adults with impaired LV function via antagonism of the effects of chronic sympathetic activation [45]. Multiple studies in adults with heart failure and LV dysfunction, including studies of nonischemic cardiomyopathy, have demonstrated improvement in hemodynamics, ventricular function, and morbidity and mortality [46–48]. As a result, β-blockade has become a cornerstone of chronic heart failure therapy. In children, a large randomized-controlled trial of carvedilol failed to demonstrate any significant differences in overall outcome due to carvedilol. However, that study's patient cohort was heterogeneous. Subgroup analyses of individuals with systemic ventricle dysfunction indicated a potential benefit, and the study may have been underpowered to adequately assess this effect [49]. Several smaller, nonrandomized studies of β-blockade in children with DCM demonstrated improvements in ventricular systolic function with therapy [50–53]. The ISHLT recommends consideration of β-blockers in symptomatic children with LV dysfunction, particularly those with LV morphology (Class IIa, LOE B) [35].

Neprilysin Inhibitors

Neprilysin, an endopeptidase, degrades several proteins including natriuretic peptides and bradykinin, limiting their ability to counter neurohormonal mechanisms and causing pathologic remodeling. Neprilysin inhibitors block the catabolism of natriuretic peptides, which potentiates their advantageous effects in heart failure, but it also potentiates the renin–angiotensin system [54]. A recent randomized-controlled trial in adults with depressed LV function of ACE-I versus combination neprilysin inhibitor and ARB demonstrated superior survival in the neprilysin–ARB group [55]. As a novel therapeutic that would further enhance neurohormonal blockade to encourage reverse remodeling, this trial has generated significant interest. Pediatric studies of the drug may be forthcoming.

Ivabradine

Ivabradine is a selective inhibitor of cardiac pacemaker cell channels that lowers resting heart rate, thereby potentially lowering myocardial oxygen demand and decreasing arrhythmia risk. In a recent trial of adults with symptomatic heart failure with decreased ejection fraction, a significantly smaller proportion of those on ivabradine therapy met the composite end point of death or hospital admission for heart failure [56]. Pediatric data are extremely limited; one case report demonstrated improvement in LV function and symptoms in two adolescent patients with DCM [57]. There are no formal recommendations regarding ivabradine therapy for adults or children at this time.

Symptomatic Treatment

Although blockade of neurohormonal mechanisms leading to cardiac remodeling is the goal of DCM therapy, several other agents may be of use when ventricular dysfunction results in symptomatic heart failure.

Diuretics are recommended by both the adult and pediatric heart failure guidelines to treat symptomatic fluid overload. Specifically, the pediatric guidelines state that patients with fluid retention associated with ventricular dysfunction should be treated with diuretics to achieve euvolemia (Class I, LOE C) [35]. No data specific to diuretic therapy in pediatric DCM exists. Nonetheless, diuretics should be used in fluid-overloaded DCM patients until symptoms abate and may be continued as maintenance therapy to prevent further symptoms caused by fluid overload.

Digoxin has long been a part of pediatric heart failure treatment as it can be used both for rate control and as an orally available inotropic agent. However, there are no pediatric studies regarding digoxin's efficacy in improving heart failure with depressed ventricular function. Several adult studies have sought to evaluate digoxin's efficacy in improving heart failure outcomes, but results have been negative or mixed [58,59], and it is currently only recommended in patients with atrial fibrillation or NYHA class III or IV heart failure symptoms. Similarly, the ISHLT pediatric heart failure guidelines recommend digoxin only to relieve symptoms in children with symptomatic heart failure and low ejection fraction (Class IIa, LOE C) and specifically do not recommend digoxin for asymptomatic LV dysfunction (Class I, LOE C) [35].

Effect of Chronic Heart Failure Therapy in Pediatric Dilated Cardiomyopathy

Despite the current focus on treating symptoms combined with encouraging cardiac remodeling through neurohormonal blockade of the RAAS and sympathetic overactivation, the overall effect of these therapies remains unclear. A recent single center retrospective cohort study found no lasting advantage for avoidance of death or transplantation in the current treatment era [60]. However, that study was susceptible to selection bias and utilized a composite end point that may not reflect equivalent outcomes by era [61]. Thus, despite no significant data on chronic therapy's effect on outcome in pediatric DCM, the treatments outlined above remain the therapeutic mainstays for the disease.

ADVANCED THERAPY FOR DILATED CARDIOMYOPATHY

Cardiac Resynchronization Therapy

Up to 50% of adults with chronic heart failure symptoms have conduction delay that may impair coordination of ventricular contraction/relaxation and compound the effects of ventricular dysfunction [62]. In reducing conduction delay, multisite biventricular pacing can acutely improve hemodynamics and cardiac output [63]. These changes are accompanied by improvement in NYHA functional class, 6-min walk, and quality of life and may be sustained with permanent pacing [62,64,65]. Initial trials of cardiac resynchronization therapy (CRT) included multiple heart failure etiologies, but studies of CRT in adult DCM patients have demonstrated improvement, including a subset that experiences complete normalization of ventricular function [66,67]. These results have led to specific guidelines for CRT in adults with chronic heart failure [68]. Pediatric studies of CRT are limited and often involve patients with multiple etiologies for heart failure, but similar to adult studies, they have demonstrated significant, sustained improvement in ventricular function with CRT [69,70]. Although a promising therapy, it appears adult guidelines are not necessarily applicable to the pediatric population and optimal selection of pediatric patients needs further definition [71,72]. Current ISHLT recommendations state that CRT can be useful in pediatric patients with a systemic left ventricle, an ejection fraction ≤35%, complete left bundle branch block, QRS duration greater than the upper limit of normal for age, and NYHA class II–IV symptoms (Class IIa, LOE B) [35].

Implantable Cardiac Defibrillator Therapy

Adults with systolic heart failure have increased risk of sudden cardiac death, and implantable cardiac defibrillators (ICDs) have been demonstrated to improve survival in adult patients including those with nonischemic DCM [73,74]. The pediatric incidence of sudden cardiac death (SCD) in children with DCM is lower than reported adult rates, although several risk factors for SCD in children have been identified [75]. However, whether ICD therapy would improve the risk of sudden death from arrhythmia in this group of patients remains unclear, and multiple studies have conflicting results [76,77]. Current ISHLT guidelines recommend ICD for any pediatric survivor of cardiac arrest after evaluation to exclude reversible of treatable causes (Class I, LOE B). In addition, the ISHLT recommends ICD treatment for patients with DCM, at least moderate systolic dysfunction, and unexplained syncope, and for adolescent patients with familial cardiomyopathy with sudden death if the risk/benefit ratio is deemed favorable (Class IIa, LOE C). ICD therapy may be considered in pediatric patients with DCM who have a LV ejection fraction ≤35% who are NYHA class II or III [35].

Ventricular Assist Devices

Ventricular assist device supports, both pulsatile and continuous flow devices, have become increasingly utilized in pediatric patients. Pediatric DCM patients in whom devices are used appear to have good overall outcomes [78,79]. Although not specific to DCM patients, the current ISHLT guidelines recommend consideration of durable ventricular assist device placement as a bridge to transplant for children who are unable to be weaned from inotropic support and are showing early reversible dysfunction of at least one other major organ system (Class I, LOE C) [35].

Pulmonary Artery Banding

Significant dilation of the left ventricle can cause distortion of right ventricular (RV) anatomy, leading to dysfunction and tricuspid regurgitation. RV dysfunction may accelerate heart failure's progression. Patients with atrioventricular discordance after pulmonary artery banding have demonstrated improved tricuspid regurgitation which is thought to be due to conformational changes in the RV architecture [80]. Based on data such as this, pulmonary artery banding has been attempted in DCM patients. In one recent report, pulmonary artery banding in young children with DCM led to an improvement in mitral valve regurgitation and ventricular dysfunction via improved ventricular interaction [81]. This potentially promising therapy needs further evaluation.

PROGNOSIS

In the PCMR of 1803 pediatric DCM patients in North America, the 5-year incidence of SCD was 3%; risk factors for SCD included younger age at diagnosis, higher LV end systolic dimension, and lower LV posterior wall thickness-to-LV end diastolic dimension ratio [75]. A smaller cohort from Australia (the National Australian Childhood Cardiomyopathy Study, or NACCS) showed a 5% 15-year incidence of SCD in children diagnosed with DCM before age 10; risk factors in their cohort included older age at diagnosis, familial cardiomyopathy, and severity of LV dysfunction [82]. As previously discussed, no clear consensus has been reached regarding indications for primary prevention implantation of implantable cardioverter-defibrillators (ICDs) in children with DCM.

With respect to freedom from transplantation and death, both the PCMR and the NACCS have reported similar 1- (69%–74%) and 5- (54%–63%) year outcomes in children with DCM [2,4,83]. Risk factors for death or transplantation in the North American cohort include older age at transplantation, presence of heart failure symptoms, severity of systolic dysfunction, and cause of cardiomyopathy; in the Australian cohort a neonatal diagnosis was also found to predict worse outcome [83]. Conversely, a significant number of children with DCM achieve normalization of LV size and function (20%–69%) [83,84]. Younger age and smaller LV dimension predicted ventricular recovery in the North American cohort [84], while higher baseline and follow-up LV systolic function as well as a diagnosis of myocarditis were positive predictors in the Australian cohort [83]. Further research is needed to better understand the role of serum markers in predicting outcomes and to better demonstrate the role that various interventions play in improving the quality of life and survival of children with DCM.

REFERENCES

[1] A. Arola, E. Jokinen, O. Ruuskanen, M. Saraste, E. Pesonen, A.L. Kuusela, et al., Epidemiology of idiopathic cardiomyopathies in children and adolescents. A nationwide study in Finland, Am. J. Epidemiol. 146 (5) (1997) 385–393.

[2] J.A. Towbin, A.M. Lowe, S.D. Colan, L.A. Sleeper, E.J. Orav, S. Clunie, et al., Incidence, causes, and outcomes of dilated cardiomyopathy in children, JAMA 296 (15) (2006) 1867–1876.

[3] A.W. Nugent, P.E. Daubeney, P. Chondros, J.B. Carlin, M. Cheung, L.C. Wilkinson, et al., The epidemiology of childhood cardiomyopathy in Australia, N. Engl. J. Med. 348 (17) (2003) 1639–1646.

[4] P.E. Daubeney, A.W. Nugent, P. Chondros, J.B. Carlin, S.D. Colan, M. Cheung, et al., Clinical features and outcomes of childhood dilated cardiomyopathy: results from a national population-based study, Circulation 114 (24) (2006) 2671–2678.

[5] R. Kirk, A.I. Dipchand, D.N. Rosenthal, L. Addonizio, M. Burch, M. Chrisant, et al., The International Society for Heart and Lung Transplantation guidelines for the management of pediatric heart failure: executive summary. [Corrected], J. Heart Lung Transplant. 33 (9) (2014) 888–909.

[6] J.W. Rossano, R.E. Shaddy, Update on pharmacological heart failure therapies in children: do adult medications work in children and if not, why not? Circulation 129 (5) (2014) 607–612.

[7] A.A. Wilde, E.R. Behr, Genetic testing for inherited cardiac disease, Nat. Rev. Cardiol. 10 (10) (2013) 571–583.

[8] E.M. McNally, J.R. Golbus, M.J. Puckelwartz, Genetic mutations and mechanisms in dilated cardiomyopathy, J. Clin. Invest. 123 (1) (2013) 19–26.

[9] A. Ferlini, M. Neri, F. Gualandi, The medical genetics of dystrophinopathies: molecular genetic diagnosis and its impact on clinical practice, NMD 23 (1) (2013) 4–14.

[10] J.L. Jefferies, Barth syndrome, Am. J. Med. Genet. C Semin. Med. Genet. 163C (3) (2013) 198–205.

[11] M.I. Noble, The Frank–Starling curve, Clin. Sci. Mol. Med. 54 (1) (1978) 1–7.

[12] D.L. Mann, M.R. Bristow, Mechanisms and models in heart failure: the biomechanical model and beyond, Circulation 111 (21) (2005) 2837–2849.

[13] Association CCotNYH (Ed.), Diseases of the Heart and Blood Vessels; Nomenclature and Criteria for Diagnosis, sixth ed., Little, Brown & Co., Boston, 1964.

[14] R.D. Ross, R.O. Bollinger, W.W. Pinsky, Grading the severity of congestive heart failure in infants, Pediatr. Cardiol. 13 (2) (1992) 72–75.

[15] S.A. Hunt, W.T. Abraham, M.H. Chin, A.M. Feldman, G.S. Francis, T.G. Ganiats, et al., 2009 focused update incorporated into the ACC/AHA 2005 guidelines for the diagnosis and management of heart failure in adults: a report of the American College of Cardiology Foundation/American Heart Association task force on practice guidelines: developed in collaboration with the international society for heart and lung transplantation, Circulation 119 (14) (2009) e391–479.

[16] D. Rosenthal, M.R. Chrisant, E. Edens, L. Mahony, C. Canter, S. Colan, et al., International society for heart and lung transplantation: practice guidelines for management of heart failure in children, J. Heart Lung Transplant. 23 (12) (2004) 1313–1333.

[17] S. Koulouri, R.J. Acherman, P.C. Wong, L.S. Chan, A.B. Lewis, Utility of B-type natriuretic peptide in differentiating congestive heart failure from lung disease in pediatric patients with respiratory distress, Pediatr. Cardiol. 25 (4) (2004) 341–346.

[18] I. Fried, B. Bar-Oz, N. Algur, E. Fried, S. Gavri, I. Yatsiv, et al., Comparison of N-terminal pro-B-type natriuretic peptide levels in critically ill children with sepsis versus acute left ventricular dysfunction, Pediatrics 118 (4) (2006) e1165–e1168.

[19] S. Cohen, C. Springer, A. Avital, Z. Perles, A.J. Rein, Z. Argaman, et al., Amino-terminal pro-brain-type natriuretic peptide: heart or lung disease in pediatric respiratory distress? Pediatrics 115 (5) (2005) 1347–1350.

[20] Y.M. Law, A.W. Hoyer, M.D. Reller, M. Silberbach, Accuracy of plasma B-type natriuretic peptide to diagnose significant cardiovascular disease in children: the Better Not Pout Children! study, J. Am. Coll. Cardiol. 54 (15) (2009) 1467–1475.

[21] S.R. Auerbach, M.E. Richmond, J.M. Lamour, E.D. Blume, L.J. Addonizio, R.E. Shaddy, et al., BNP levels predict outcome in pediatric heart failure patients: post hoc analysis of the Pediatric Carvedilol Trial, Circ. Heart Fail. 3 (5) (2010) 606–611.

[22] J.A. Hauser, S. Demyanets, K. Rusai, C. Goritschan, M. Weber, D. Panesar, et al., Diagnostic performance and reference values of novel biomarkers of paediatric heart failure, Heart **102** (20) (2016) 1633–1639.

[23] R.E. Hershberger, J.D. Siegfried, Update 2011: clinical and genetic issues in familial dilated cardiomyopathy, J. Am. Coll. Cardiol. 57 (16) (2011) 1641–1649.

[24] M.A. Grenier, S.K. Osganian, G.F. Cox, J.A. Towbin, S.D. Colan, P.R. Lurie, et al., Design and implementation of the North American pediatric cardiomyopathy registry, Am. Heart J. 139 (2 Pt 3) (2000) S86–S95.

[25] M.G. Friedrich, U. Sechtem, J. Schulz-Menger, G. Holmvang, P. Alakija, L.T. Cooper, et al., Cardiovascular magnetic resonance in myocarditis: a JACC white paper, J. Am. Coll. Cardiol. 53 (17) (2009) 1475–1487.

[26] H. Latus, K. Gummel, K. Klingel, A. Moysich, M. Khalil, N. Mazhari, et al., Focal myocardial fibrosis assessed by late gadolinium enhancement cardiovascular magnetic resonance in children and adolescents with dilated cardiomyopathy, J. Cardiovasc. Magn. Reson. 17 (2015) 34.

[27] Heart Failure Society of America, J. Lindenfeld, N.M. Albert, J.P. Boehmer, S.P. Collins, J.A. Ezekowitz, et al., HFSA 2010 comprehensive heart failure practice guideline, J. Card. Fail. 16 (6) (2010) e1–194.

[28] R.R. Chang, V. Allada, Electrocardiographic and echocardiographic features that distinguish anomalous origin of the left coronary artery from pulmonary artery from idiopathic dilated cardiomyopathy, Pediatr. Cardiol. 22 (1) (2001) 3–10.

[29] V. Kudumula, C. Mehta, O. Stumper, T. Desai, A. Chikermane, P. Miller, et al., Twenty-year outcome of anomalous origin of left coronary artery from pulmonary artery: management of mitral regurgitation, Ann. Thorac. Surg. 97 (3) (2014) 938–944.

[30] P.L. Magoulas, A.W. El-Hattab, Systemic primary carnitine deficiency: an overview of clinical manifestations, diagnosis, and management, Orphanet J. Rare Dis. 7 (2012) 68.

[31] S.S. Wang, J. Rao, Y.F. Li, Z.W. Zhang, G.H. Zeng, Primary carnitine deficiency cardiomyopathy, Int. J. Cardiol. 174 (1) (2014) 171–173.

[32] F. Charbit-Henrion, F. Lacaille, P. McKiernan, M. Girard, P. de Lonlay, V. Valayannopoulos, et al., Early and late complications after liver transplantation for propionic acidemia in children: a two centers study, Am. J. Transplant. 15 (3) (2015) 786–791.

[33] C. Arrizza, A. De Gottardi, E. Foglia, M. Baumgartner, M. Gautschi, J.M. Nuoffer, Reversal of cardiomyopathy in propionic acidemia after liver transplantation: a 10-year follow-up, Transpl. Int. 28 (12) (2015) 1447–1450.

[34] V. Marinescu, P.A. McCullough, Nutritional and micronutrient determinants of idiopathic dilated cardiomyopathy: diagnostic and therapeutic implications, Expert Rev. Cardiovasc. Ther. 9 (9) (2011) 1161–1170.

[35] R. Kirk, A.I. Dipchand, D.N. Rosenthal, The international society for heart and lung transplantation guidelines for the management of pediatric heart failure, (2014).

[36] N. Koitabashi, D.A. Kass, Reverse remodeling in heart failure–mechanisms and therapeutic opportunities, Nat. Rev. Cardiol. 9 (3) (2012) 147–157.

[37] R. Garg, S. Yusuf, Overview of randomized trials of angiotensin-converting enzyme inhibitors on mortality and morbidity in patients with heart failure. Collaborative Group on ACE Inhibitor Trials, JAMA 273 (18) (1995) 1450–1456.
[38] A.M. Leversha, N.J. Wilson, P.M. Clarkson, A.L. Calder, M.C. Ramage, J.M. Neutze, Efficacy and dosage of enalapril in congenital and acquired heart disease, Arch. Dis. Child. 70 (1) (1994) 35–39.
[39] H. Stern, J. Weil, T. Genz, W. Vogt, K. Buhlmeyer, Captopril in children with dilated cardiomyopathy: acute and long-term effects in a prospective study of hemodynamic and hormonal effects, Pediatr. Cardiol. 11 (1) (1990) 22–28.
[40] A.B. Lewis, M. Chabot, The effect of treatment with angiotensin-converting enzyme inhibitors on survival of pediatric patients with dilated cardiomyopathy, Pediatr. Cardiol. 14 (1) (1993) 9–12.
[41] J.B. Young, M.E. Dunlap, M.A. Pfeffer, J.L. Probstfield, A. Cohen-Solal, R. Dietz, et al., Mortality and morbidity reduction with Candesartan in patients with chronic heart failure and left ventricular systolic dysfunction: results of the CHARM low-left ventricular ejection fraction trials, Circulation 110 (17) (2004) 2618–2626.
[42] B. Pitt, P.A. Poole-Wilson, R. Segal, F.A. Martinez, K. Dickstein, A.J. Camm, et al., Effect of losartan compared with captopril on mortality in patients with symptomatic heart failure: randomised trial–the Losartan heart failure survival study ELITE II, Lancet 355 (9215) (2000) 1582–1587.
[43] F. Zannad, J.J. McMurray, H. Krum, D.J. van Veldhuisen, K. Swedberg, H. Shi, et al., Eplerenone in patients with systolic heart failure and mild symptoms, N. Engl. J. Med. 364 (1) (2011) 11–21.
[44] B. Pitt, F. Zannad, W.J. Remme, R. Cody, A. Castaigne, A. Perez, et al., The effect of spironolactone on morbidity and mortality in patients with severe heart failure. Randomized aldactone evaluation study investigators, N. Engl. J. Med. 341 (10) (1999) 709–717.
[45] M.S. Maurer, J.D. Sackner-Bernstein, L. El-Khoury Rumbarger, M. Yushak, D.L. King, D. Burkhoff, Mechanisms underlying improvements in ejection fraction with carvedilol in heart failure, Circ. Heart Fail. 2 (3) (2009) 189–196.
[46] F. Waagstein, M.R. Bristow, K. Swedberg, F. Camerini, M.B. Fowler, M.A. Silver, et al., Beneficial effects of metoprolol in idiopathic dilated cardiomyopathy. Metoprolol in dilated cardiomyopathy (MDC) trial study group, Lancet 342 (8885) (1993) 1441–1446.
[47] M. Packer, M.B. Fowler, E.B. Roecker, A.J. Coats, H.A. Katus, H. Krum, et al., Effect of carvedilol on the morbidity of patients with severe chronic heart failure: results of the carvedilol prospective randomized cumulative survival (COPERNICUS) study, Circulation 106 (17) (2002) 2194–2199.
[48] Effect of metoprolol CR/XL in chronic heart failure: metoprolol CR/XL randomised intervention trial in congestive heart failure (MERIT-HF), Lancet 353 (9169) (1999) 2001–2007.
[49] R.E. Shaddy, M.M. Boucek, D.T. Hsu, R.J. Boucek, C.E. Canter, L. Mahony, et al., Carvedilol for children and adolescents with heart failure: a randomized controlled trial, JAMA 298 (10) (2007) 1171–1179.
[50] R.E. Shaddy, L.Y. Tani, S.S. Gidding, E. Pahl, G.S. Orsmond, E.M. Gilbert, et al., Beta-blocker treatment of dilated cardiomyopathy with congestive heart failure in children: a multi-institutional experience, J. Heart Lung Transplant. 18 (3) (1999) 269–274.
[51] P. Rusconi, O. Gomez-Marin, M. Rossique-Gonzalez, E. Redha, J.R. Marin, M. Lon-Young, et al., Carvedilol in children with cardiomyopathy: 3-year experience at a single institution, J. Heart Lung Transplant. 23 (7) (2004) 832–838.
[52] M. Bajcetic, A. Kokic Nikolic, M. Djukic, J. Kosutic, J. Mitrovic, D. Mijalkovic, et al., Effects of carvedilol on left ventricular function and oxidative stress in infants and children with idiopathic dilated cardiomyopathy: a 12-month, two-center, open-label study, Clin. Ther. 30 (4) (2008) 702–714.
[53] M. Huang, X. Zhang, S. Chen, Y. Sun, Y. Xiao, J. Sun, et al., The effect of carvedilol treatment on chronic heart failure in pediatric patients with dilated cardiomyopathy: a prospective, randomized-controlled study, Pediatr. Cardiol. 34 (3) (2013) 680–685.
[54] S. Katsanos, V. Bistola, J.T. Parissis, Combining angiotensin II receptor 1 antagonism and neprilysin inhibition for the treatment of heart failure, Expert Rev. Clin. Pharmacol. **9** (4) (2016) 513–523.
[55] J.J. McMurray, M. Packer, A.S. Desai, J. Gong, M.P. Lefkowitz, A.R. Rizkala, et al., Angiotensin-neprilysin inhibition versus enalapril in heart failure, N. Engl. J. Med. 371 (11) (2014) 993–1004.
[56] K. Swedberg, M. Komajda, M. Bohm, J.S. Borer, I. Ford, A. Dubost-Brama, et al., Ivabradine and outcomes in chronic heart failure (SHIFT): a randomised placebo-controlled study, Lancet 376 (9744) (2010) 875–885.
[57] S. Parsons, A.L. Clark, J.G. Cleland, The remarkable effect of ivabradine in two adolescents with dilated cardiomyopathy, Clin. Res. Cardiol. 103 (10) (2014) 847–849.
[58] K.F. Adams Jr., M. Gheorghiade, B.F. Uretsky, J.H. Patterson, T.A. Schwartz, J.B. Young, Clinical benefits of low serum digoxin concentrations in heart failure, J. Am. Coll. Cardiol. 39 (6) (2002) 946–953.
[59] The effect of digoxin on mortality and morbidity in patients with heart failure, N. Engl. J. Med. 336 (8) (1997) 525–533.
[60] P.F. Kantor, J.R. Abraham, A.I. Dipchand, L.N. Benson, A.N. Redington, The impact of changing medical therapy on transplantation-free survival in pediatric dilated cardiomyopathy, J. Am. Coll. Cardiol. 55 (13) (2010) 1377–1384.
[61] T.P. Singh, C. Almond, Are angiotensin-converting enzyme inhibitors and beta-blockers ineffective in children with dilated cardiomyopathy and heart failure? J. Am. Coll. Cardiol. 56 (10) (2010) 823 Author reply-4.
[62] S. Cazeau, C. Leclercq, T. Lavergne, S. Walker, C. Varma, C. Linde, et al., Effects of multisite biventricular pacing in patients with heart failure and intraventricular conduction delay, N. Engl. J. Med. 344 (12) (2001) 873–880.
[63] C. Leclercq, S. Cazeau, H. Le Breton, P. Ritter, P. Mabo, D. Gras, et al., Acute hemodynamic effects of biventricular DDD pacing in patients with end-stage heart failure, J. Am. Coll. Cardiol. 32 (7) (1998) 1825–1831.
[64] W.T. Abraham, Cardiac resynchronization therapy for heart failure: biventricular pacing and beyond, Curr. Opin. Cardiol. 17 (4) (2002) 346–352.
[65] M.R. Bristow, L.A. Saxon, J. Boehmer, S. Krueger, D.A. Kass, T. De Marco, et al., Cardiac-resynchronization therapy with or without an implantable defibrillator in advanced chronic heart failure, N. Engl. J. Med. 350 (21) (2004) 2140–2150.
[66] W.F. Kerwin, E.H. Botvinick, J.W. O'Connell, S.H. Merrick, T. DeMarco, K. Chatterjee, et al., Ventricular contraction abnormalities in dilated cardiomyopathy: effect of biventricular pacing to correct interventricular dyssynchrony, J. Am. Coll. Cardiol. 35 (5) (2000) 1221–1227.

[67] P. Castellant, M. Fatemi, E. Orhan, Y. Etienne, J.J. Blanc, Patients with non-ischaemic dilated cardiomyopathy and hyper-responders to cardiac resynchronization therapy: characteristics and long-term evolution, Europace 11 (3) (2009) 350–355.

[68] A.M. Russo, R.F. Stainback, S.R. Bailey, A.E. Epstein, P.A. Heidenreich, M. Jessup, et al., ACCF/HRS/AHA/ASE/HFSA/SCAI/SCCT/SCMR 2013 appropriate use criteria for implantable cardioverter-defibrillators and cardiac resynchronization therapy: a report of the American College of Cardiology Foundation appropriate use criteria task force, heart rhythm society, American heart association, American society of echocardiography, heart failure society of America, society for cardiovascular angiography and interventions, society of cardiovascular computed tomography, and society for cardiovascular magnetic resonance, Heart Rhythm 10 (4) (2013) e11–58.

[69] A.M. Dubin, J. Janousek, E. Rhee, M.J. Strieper, F. Cecchin, I.H. Law, et al., Resynchronization therapy in pediatric and congenital heart disease patients: an international multicenter study, J. Am. Coll. Cardiol. 46 (12) (2005) 2277–2283.

[70] J. Janousek, R.A. Gebauer, H. Abdul-Khaliq, M. Turner, L. Kornyei, O. Grollmuss, et al., Cardiac resynchronisation therapy in paediatric and congenital heart disease: differential effects in various anatomical and functional substrates, Heart 95 (14) (2009) 1165–1171.

[71] K.S. Motonaga, A.M. Dubin, Cardiac resynchronization therapy for pediatric patients with heart failure and congenital heart disease: a reappraisal of results, Circulation 129 (18) (2014) 1879–1891.

[72] O. Schiller, N. Dham, E.A. Greene, D.M. Heath, M.E. Alexander, C.I. Berul, Pediatric dilated cardiomyopathy patients do not meet traditional cardiac resynchronization criteria, J. Cardiovasc. Electrophysiol. 26 (8) (2015) 885–889.

[73] A. Kadish, A. Dyer, J.P. Daubert, R. Quigg, N.A. Estes, K.P. Anderson, et al., Prophylactic defibrillator implantation in patients with nonischemic dilated cardiomyopathy, N. Engl. J. Med. 350 (21) (2004) 2151–2158.

[74] G.H. Bardy, K.L. Lee, D.B. Mark, J.E. Poole, D.L. Packer, R. Boineau, et al., Amiodarone or an implantable cardioverter-defibrillator for congestive heart failure, N. Engl. J. Med. 352 (3) (2005) 225–237.

[75] E. Pahl, L.A. Sleeper, C.E. Canter, D.T. Hsu, M. Lu, S.A. Webber, et al., Incidence of and risk factors for sudden cardiac death in children with dilated cardiomyopathy: a report from the pediatric cardiomyopathy registry, J. Am. Coll. Cardiol. 59 (6) (2012) 607–615.

[76] A.M. Dubin, C.I. Berul, L.M. Bevilacqua, K.K. Collins, S.P. Etheridge, A.L. Fenrich, et al., The use of implantable cardioverter-defibrillators in pediatric patients awaiting heart transplantation, J. Card. Fail. 9 (5) (2003) 375–379.

[77] E.K. Rhee, C.E. Canter, S. Basile, S.A. Webber, D.C. Naftel, Sudden death prior to pediatric heart transplantation: would implantable defibrillators improve outcome? J. Heart Lung Transplant. 26 (5) (2007) 447–452.

[78] C.D. Fraser Jr., R.D. Jaquiss, D.N. Rosenthal, T. Humpl, C.E. Canter, E.H. Blackstone, et al., Prospective trial of a pediatric ventricular assist device, N. Engl. J. Med. 367 (6) (2012) 532–541.

[79] A.G. Cabrera, K.S. Sundareswaran, A.X. Samayoa, A. Jeewa, E.D. McKenzie, J.W. Rossano, et al., Outcomes of pediatric patients supported by the HeartMate II left ventricular assist device in the United States, J. Heart Lung Transplant. 32 (11) (2013) 1107–1113.

[80] C.A. Kral Kollars, S. Gelehrter, E.L. Bove, G. Ensing, Effects of morphologic left ventricular pressure on right ventricular geometry and tricuspid valve regurgitation in patients with congenitally corrected transposition of the great arteries, Am. J. Cardiol. 105 (5) (2010) 735–739.

[81] D. Schranz, S. Rupp, M. Muller, D. Schmidt, A. Bauer, K. Valeske, et al., Pulmonary artery banding in infants and young children with left ventricular dilated cardiomyopathy: a novel therapeutic strategy before heart transplantation, J. Heart Lung Transplant. 32 (5) (2013) 475–481.

[82] T. Bharucha, K.J. Lee, P.E. Daubeney, A.W. Nugent, C. Turner, G.F. Sholler, et al., Sudden death in childhood cardiomyopathy: results from a long-term national population-based study, J. Am. Coll. Cardiol. 65 (21) (2015) 2302–2310.

[83] P.M. Alexander, P.E. Daubeney, A.W. Nugent, K.J. Lee, C. Turner, S.D. Colan, et al., Long-term outcomes of dilated cardiomyopathy diagnosed during childhood: results from a national population-based study of childhood cardiomyopathy, Circulation 128 (18) (2013) 2039–2046.

[84] M.D. Everitt, L.A. Sleeper, M. Lu, C.E. Canter, E. Pahl, J.D. Wilkinson, et al., Recovery of echocardiographic function in children with idiopathic dilated cardiomyopathy: results from the pediatric cardiomyopathy registry, J. Am. Coll. Cardiol. 63 (14) (2014) 1405–1413.

Chapter 18

Clinical Features of Restrictive Cardiomyopathy and Constrictive Pericarditis

Susan W. Denfield
Texas Children's Hospital, Houston, TX, United States

Restrictive cardiomyopathy (RCM) is a disease of the myocardium or endomyocardium characterized by restrictive filling and reduced diastolic volume of one or both ventricles with normal or near normal wall thickness and systolic function [1]. Restrictive filling results in marked atrial dilation. RCM may be a primary process or secondary to an associated systemic disease.

Pericarditis is an inflammation of the pericardium that may be idiopathic or associated with another disease. Constrictive pericarditis (CP) is a form of cardiac compression resulting from a diseased pericardium that restricts cardiac filling [2].

Although RCM is a disease of the myocardium and CP is a disease of the pericardium, their clinical presentations can be very similar. Both can result in heart failure, due to impaired cardiac filling.

Differentiating RCM from CP is important because the approaches to treatment are distinctly different. This chapter reviews the epidemiology, etiologies, pathology, pathophysiology, clinical presentation, diagnostic evaluation, outcome, and management of pediatric patients with RCM and those with CP.

RESTRICTIVE CARDIOMYOPATHY

Epidemiology

Of the four types of cardiomyopathy categorized by the WHO, RCM is the least common, accounting for 2.5%–5% of the diagnosed cardiomyopathies in children [1,3–7]. Nugent et al., from Australia, reported that RCM accounted for 2.5% of the cardiomyopathies diagnosed in children less than 10 years of age [5]. A US-based study by Lipshultz et al. reported that RCM or other specified types (not dilated or hypertrophic) accounted for 3% of the cardiomyopathies in children less than 18 years of age [6]. The higher 5% estimate was from single institutions and may reflect referral bias [3,4,7].

When considering all types of cardiomyopathy, the incidence is higher in children less than 1 year of age, although RCM may be an exception [5,6]. The incidence of all types of cardiomyopathy, except restrictive, declined rapidly after infancy in the Nugent et al. study [5]. In studies of RCM in children the average age at the time of diagnosis was 6 years with a median of 5 years and a range from 0.1 to 19 years Table 18.1 [3,4,7–32]. The majority, approximately 80%, were diagnosed between the ages of 1 and 11 years.

Gender differences have also been reported in some forms of pediatric cardiomyopathies [5,6]. However, in the Nugent et al. study RCM occurred with equal frequency in boys and girls [5]. Based on literature review the sex distribution is relatively even in RCM with 54% female [3–37] (Table 18.1).

Genetics

Sporadic and familial cases of RCM occur. In published cases, in which family history was reported, 30% of patients had a positive family history [3–37]. Mutations in at least 11 genes have now been identified that may result in a RCM phenotype. Table 18.2 [38–51]. Transmission can be autosomal dominant, autosomal recessive, or X-linked. De novo mutations also occur. A number of systemic diseases with a known genetic basis and several syndromes can also result in a cardiomyopathy with a restrictive phenotype (Table 18.3) [33,52–61].

Heart Failure in the Child and Young Adult. http://dx.doi.org/10.1016/B978-0-12-802393-8.00018-1

TABLE 18.1 Demographics and Clinical Features of Children With Restrictive Cardiomyopathy

Percent of cardiomyopathies	2.5%–5%
Mean/median age at presentation	6/5 year
Female-to-male ratio (%)	54:46
Positive family history	30%
Presenting Complaints	
Respiratory—DOE, "asthma" cough/pneumonia	47%
Abnormal PE—ascites, hepatomegaly, edema, gallop, loud P_2, murmur	21%
Congestive heart failure (not otherwise defined)	10%
Syncope	10%
Other[a]	≤10%

DOE, dyspnea on exertion; *PE*, physical examination.
[a]*Includes sudden death, palpitations, fatigue, embolic events, incidental cardiomegaly on chest X-ray, and positive family history.*

TABLE 18.2 Gene Mutations Reported in Association With Restrictive Cardiomyopathy

Sarcomeric Mutations	Nonsarcomeric Mutations
Troponin I	Desmin
Troponin T	Lamin A/C (Emery–Dreifuss)
Alpha cardiac actin	BAG3
Myosin-binding protein C	
Beta myosin heavy chain	
Myosin light chain	
Titin	
Filamin-C	

TABLE 18.3 Systemic Diseases and Syndromes With Identified Genetic. Mutations in Children and/or Adults Associated With Restrictive Cardiomyopathy

Systemic Diseases	Syndromes
Systemic sclerosis	Alstrom
Pseudoxanthoma elasticum	Coffin Lowry
	Mulibrey nanism
Sarcoidosis	Myhre
Gaucher's disease	
Hurler's disease	
Hereditary amyloidosis	
Hereditary hemochromatosis	
Fabry's disease	
Glycogen storage diseases	

Nonsarcomeric Protein Gene Defects

Desmin is a myofibrillar protein that is the chief intermediate filament of skeletal and cardiac muscle [40]. It maintains the structural and functional integrity of the myofibrils and functions as a cytoskeletal protein linking Z bands to the plasma membrane. Mutations in the desmin gene may cause RCM. This form of RCM may be associated with skeletal myopathy and/or conduction system disease. The inheritance pattern is usually autosomal dominant; however, sporadic mutations also occur [40].

Mutations in genes encoding for BAG3, a Z disc-associated protein with antiapoptotic properties are associated with RCM [50]. Associated noncardiac pathology includes progressive limb and axial muscle weakness, severe respiratory insufficiency, rigid spine, and peripheral neuropathy.

Emery–Dreifuss muscular dystrophy can cause dilated cardiomyopathy, atrial and ventricular arrhythmias, conduction abnormalities, and sudden death. It was first described as an X-linked disorder due to mutations in the gene encoding for emerin on chromosome Xq28 [38]. However, it can also be an autosomal disorder caused by mutations in the gene encoding for lamin A and lamin C (LMNA) on chromosome 1q21.2-q21.3 [38]. Sanna et al. reported on the cardiac features of Emery–Dreifuss caused by LMNA gene mutations, including one adult patient with a restrictive phenotype [38]. The RCM phenotype has not been reported in children with Emery–Dreifuss to date.

Sarcomeric Protein Gene Defects

Mutations in at least 8 genes encoding for sarcomeric proteins have been identified that can cause RCM. RCM and hypertrophic cardiomyopathy (HCM) can both be caused by troponin I mutations [39]. Either phenotype can be expressed in the same family. This suggests that additional genetic or environmental factors or both play a role in disease expression. De novo mutations and autosomal dominant transmission have been documented in RCM patients and their families [39].

In a small pediatric series of 12 patients with RCM, Kaski, et al. reported that 4 had a positive family history of cardiomyopathy, but the phenotypes varied including restrictive, dilated, and left ventricular (LV) noncompaction forms [42]. Gene mutations were found in troponin I (TNNI3), troponin T (TNNT2) and alpha cardiac actin. Peddy et al. reported a de novo mutation in cardiac troponin T in an infant who presented with malignant arrhythmias and RCM [43].

A mutation in the beta myosin heavy chain gene in an infant with RCM was described by Ware and colleagues [44]. Mutations in the beta myosin heavy chain account for approximately 40% of mutations found in HCM in adults [45]. Olson et al. [46] described a child with a myosin light chain mutation resulting in a cardiomyopathy with midcavitary hypertrophy and restrictive physiology that was inherited in an autosomal recessive pattern. Two older siblings had cardiomyopathy with dilated atria, both of whom died related to thrombotic complications. This report also demonstrates overlapping genotype phenotype within the same mutations. Clinically unaffected family members were either heterozygotes or lacked the mutant allele.

Titin is a giant protein that plays a fundamental role in sarcomere structure and regulation of resting tension. A titin mutation was found in a family with RCM in which members in two generations were affected [49].

Filamins are actin cross-linking proteins. They provide scaffolds for a wide range of signaling proteins. Mutations in Filamin-C have been reported to cause familial RCM, with some of the cases presenting in childhood [51]. Additional mutations are likely to be found in the future.

Systemic Diseases With Known Genetic Mutations

The following systemic diseases have one or more identified genetic mutations that are disease causing and can result in the development of RCM, including systemic sclerosis, pseudoxanthoma elasticum, sarcoidosis, hereditary amyloidosis, hereditary hemochromatosis, Gaucher disease, Hurler disease, Fabry disease, and glycogen storage diseases [52].

Genetic Syndromes

Several genetic syndromes have been reported in patients who subsequently developed RCM, including Alstrom, Coffin–Lowry, Mulibrey nanism, and Myhre syndrome.

Alstrom syndrome is characterized by cone-rod dystrophy causing progressive visual impairment, photophobia and nystagmus, obesity, progressive sensorineural hearing impairment, dilated or RCM, insulin resistance, and multiple organ failure [53]. Mutation in the ALMS1 gene is associated with the syndrome and is estimated to be detected in 25%–40% of individuals.

Coffin–Lowry syndrome is characterized by developmental delays, short stature, facial dysmorphisms, and progressive skeletal deformities. About 14% of affected males have cardiac anomalies, with cardiomyopathy being one of the rare but reported cardiac abnormalities, including one patient with a restrictive phenotype [33]. Coffin–Lowry syndrome is caused by mutations in the RSK2 gene on chromosome Xp22.2 and is an X-linked disorder [54].

Mulibrey nanism is characterized by typical craniofacial features including scaphocephaly, facial triangularity, high and broad forehead, and low nasal bridge in over 90% of the patients. Additional findings include a peculiar high-pitched voice (96%), yellowish dots in ocular fundi (79%), cutaneous naevi flammei (65%), hepatomegaly (45%), and fibrous dysplasia of long bones (25%). Mild muscular hypotonicity (68%) is often present. Karlberg et al. reported, congestive heart failure and pericardial constriction were diagnosed during infancy in 12% and 6% of the patients, respectively [55]. While more typically associated with CP, a mixed constrictive/restrictive phenotype has been described. Some patients have not improved after pericardiectomy, and myocardial hypertrophy and fibrosis have been reported [56,57]. It is caused by mutations in the TRIM37 gene on chromosome 17q22-q23 encoding the peroxisomal TRIM37 protein [55].

Myhre syndrome is a connective tissue disorder characterized by deafness, restricted joint movement, compact body habitus, and distinctive craniofacial (short palpebral fissures, short filtrum, maxillary hypoplasia, small mouth, and prognathism) and skeletal features. Myhre syndrome is caused by heterozygous mutations in SMAD4 [58,59]. This results in abnormal TGF beta signaling causing abnormal development of skeletal structures, skeletal and cardiac muscle structure, and the central nervous system. Structural cardiac defects, aortic stenosis, and aortopathies have been described in these patients as well as the development of RCM and a restrictive phenotype in association with left-sided obstructive lesions. Two patients in the Starr et al. study went on to transplant, one cardiac and one bilateral heart lung, both of whom died within approximately 2 months of transplant. They concluded that surgical intervention should be approached with extreme caution due to the potential for exuberant fibrosis/scar tissue development. Both patients had respiratory failure as well [59].

Etiologies

The multiple causes of RCM include myocardial diseases that may be noninfiltrative or infiltrative processes, storage diseases, endomyocardial diseases, myocarditis, and following cardiac transplantation [60], Table 18.4. The pathology and histology vary with the underlying disease process. In adults, outside the tropics, amyloidosis is the most common cause, while endomyocardial fibrosis (EMF), in the tropics, is the most common cause of RCM [61]. Cardiac amyloidosis is nearly unheard of in children with one reported case [7]. In the pediatric population, EMF is likely the most common cause of RCM in the tropics. Outside the tropics, idiopathic RCM is probably the most common cause of RCM in children [3–37].

Endomyocardial Disease

EMF was first described by Davies in 1948 [62]. It occurs most often in children and adolescents and is currently estimated to affect 10 million people worldwide [63,64]. Although EMF is found in tropical and subtropical regions throughout the world, it occurs most frequently in tropical and subtropical Africa, particularly Uganda and Nigeria. When occasionally seen in temperate climates, it is usually in individuals who previously lived in tropical areas. The disease probably affects both sexes equally [65,66]. There may be a genetic predisposition, as there is some familial occurrence and in some countries a higher incidence in some ethnic groups [63,64].

TABLE 18.4 Additional Restrictive Cardiomyopathy Etiologies

Myocardial	Endomyocardial
Scleroderma	Endomyocardial fibrosis
Myocarditis	Hypereosinophilia syndromes (includes Lofflers)
Cardiac transplant	Endocardial fibroelastosis
Diabetic cardiomyopathy	Carcinoid
Fatty infiltration	Metastatic cancers
Acquired hemochromatosis	Radiation
	Drugs

The disease is most commonly biventricular, followed by purely right ventricular (RV) and less commonly isolated LV disease [63,66]. The symptom complex varies with the site or sites of involvement. Symptoms from right-sided disease include signs and symptoms of systemic venous congestion including ascites, while pulmonary venous congestion results from left-sided disease. Involvement of the mitral or tricuspid valve apparatus can result in significant valvular regurgitation. Medical and surgical therapy is palliative. However, surgery including endocardectomy and valve repair/replacement has been reported to increase survival compared to medical therapy, provided patients are not end stage at the time of surgical intervention [66].

The histology of EMF is characterized by fibrosis of the endocardium of variable thickness. Histologic changes occur in predominantly three areas: the LV apex, the mitral valve apparatus, and the RV apex, which may extend to the supporting structures of the tricuspid valve. In severe cases the process may extend to the outflow tracts. Small patches of fibroelastosis may occur in the outflow tracts, but the elastin component is thought to be secondary and not a primary part of the process. Cellular infiltrates are not prominent. Although EMF occurs in areas where parasitic diseases that result in eosinophilia are common, the cause of the process is still unknown. Eosinophilia is not typically a prominent feature in contrast to Loffler endocarditis.

Hypereosinophilic Syndrome/Loffler Endocarditis

One of the hypereosinophilic syndrome (HES)-associated cardiac diseases is Loffler endocarditis. Loffler endocarditis is similar to EMF in many respects; however, there are important differences. Unlike EMF, HES is typically seen in adult males in temperate climates. By definition patients have hypereosinophilia (HE), which is not seen in EMF. HE is defined as >1.5 eosinophils $\times 10^9$/L blood on two tests at least one month apart and/or tissue HE (based on eosinophils on bone marrow biopsy or presence of eosinophilic granule proteins in tissue). A diagnosis of HES requires persistent eosinophilia with evidence of organ involvement due to the HE [67]. Besides the heart, a variety of other organs may be involved, including the lungs, bone marrow, and brain. The cause of the eosinophilia may be leukemic or secondary to parasitic, allergic, granulomatous, hypersensitivity, or neoplastic disorders, but is usually unknown.

Variable degrees of eosinophilic myocarditis (not characteristically seen in EMF) are seen on histologic examination. Inflammatory reaction in the small intramural coronary vessels with thrombosis and fibrinoid change and endocardial mural thrombosis and fibrotic thickening also occur [67].

Symptoms that are frequently seen include weight loss, fever, cough, rash, and heart failure. Systemic embolism is frequent. Death is usually due to cardiac causes. Therapy for the HE includes corticosteroids, and other agents, directed by specialists other than cardiologists. Cardiac therapy has included typical heart failure therapies and anticoagulation. From a surgical perspective, symptoms of intractable heart failure may be addressed by mitral and or tricuspid valve repair or replacement, and excision of fibrotic endocardium. However, pediatric studies of patients with HES and EMF report a relatively high reoperation rate secondary to dysfunction of the mechanical or bioprosthetic valves due to recurrent thrombosis, fibrosis, or tearing despite anticoagulation [68,69]. Not infrequently cardiac symptoms persist (class II–IV) [69].

Infiltrative and Storage Diseases

Sarcoidosis is a granulomatous inflammatory process that can affect the heart and result in RCM. Systolic dysfunction, pericarditis, and conduction system disease and sudden death may also occur. Sarcoidosis is more common in young adults than other age groups. Amyloidosis is a common cause of RCM in adults, with only one reported case in a child [7].

Hemochromatosis may be a primary or secondary disease. The iron overload may result in dysfunction of multiple organs including the heart. Hemochromatosis may result in a restrictive or dilated cardiomyopathy.

Metabolic disorders that have resulted in RCM include lysosomal disorders such as Hurler syndrome, Gaucher disease, Fabry disease, and glycogen storage diseases that can be lysosomal disorders or result from cytoplasmic enzyme deficiencies.

One patient who was diagnosed with nephropathic cystinosis in infancy developed a cardiomyopathy with restrictive features in adulthood [70]. The patient had extremely high cystine levels in the myocardium. It is an autosomal recessive disease that leads to multiorgan failure from intracellular accumulation of cystine. Due to the patient's history of renal failure, renal transplantation, and hypertension the exact etiology of the restrictive physiology is uncertain.

Drugs and Therapeutic Modalities

A number of drugs have been reported to cause RCM including, anthracyclines, serotonin, methysergide, ergotamine, mercurial agents, and busulfan [71–75]. RCM has also developed secondary to mediastinal radiation [76].

Idiopathic

"Idiopathic" RCM is probably the most common form of the disease in children, outside the tropics. However, a genetic basis or predisposition is likely, although the family history is positive in only approximately 30%.

Pathology

The LV cavity size is usually normal with no appreciable LV hypertrophy. The atrial size often dwarfs the ventricular cavity size. Most of the hearts are otherwise structurally normal, although occasional patients who also have atrial septal defects or small hemodynamically insignificant ventricular septal defects are reported [11,30]. The histology in idiopathic RCM is nonspecific revealing varying degrees of fibrosis and myocyte hypertrophy. The histology may reflect the underlying disease process, for example, in amyloidosis or hemochromatosis.

Pathophysiology

Diastolic function is primarily affected by ventricular compliance/stiffness and relaxation. In the normally functioning heart, just after the mitral valve opens, the phase of rapid or early filling occurs as the LV pressure drops below that in the left atrium, accounting for most of ventricular filling [77,78]. The next phase, called diastasis, is variable and heart rate dependent, usually permitting less than 5% of filling. The last phase of diastole is atrial systole, which accounts for approximately 15% of normal ventricular filling. Typically in RCM, ventricular filling is completed in early diastole with little or no filling in late diastole as a result of increased myocardial stiffness with decreased compliance. This results in a marked ventricular pressure rise with small changes in volume.

Isovolumic relaxation is the earliest phase of clinical diastole, which is an active energy-requiring process for the uptake of calcium ions into the sarcoplasmic reticulum. Ischemia and hypertrophy can both result in abnormal relaxation due to changes in calcium uptake.

Abnormal relaxation can also contribute to restrictive physiology as demonstrated by Gewillig et al. in 6 children with RCM who by catheterization and echocardiography had parameters suggesting delayed relaxation as well as restrictive filling. In those patients there was an unusually high contribution of middiastolic filling, accounting for 28% of filling, while early filling contributed relatively less than normal, 56%, and atrial filling 16%. Rather than increased intrinsic stiffness of the ventricular wall, they suggested that the restrictive hemodynamics were caused by dysfunction and delay of active relaxation of the ventricle [12].

It is likely that RCM may result from either abnormal stiffness or abnormal relaxation or both depending on the underlying cause of the disease and disease progression. Studies using skinned muscle fibers reconstituted with troponin mutations are establishing phenotypes consistent with clinical findings, furthering the understanding of diastolic dysfunction [79,80].

Clinical Presentation

Table 18.1 summarizes the presenting complaints of pediatric patients reported in the English literature. In children, RCM frequently masquerades as other diseases. The most common presenting symptoms initially may appear to be pulmonary related. Children with RCM frequently have a history of "recurrent lower respiratory tract infections" or "asthma." Referral to a cardiologist eventually occurs when cardiomegaly is noted on chest X-ray.

The second most common reason for referral is abnormal physical exam findings. Those with ascites, hepatomegaly and edema may be referred to a gastroenterologist first. Earlier referral to a cardiologist occurs when the presenting sign is an abnormal heart sound.

Congestive heart failure, not otherwise defined, and syncope each account for approximately 10% of the presenting complaints. Syncope in this patient population may be related to ischemia, arrhythmias, conduction disturbances, or thromboembolism [11,12]. Ischemia and arrhythmias may be the most common cause of syncope and sudden death in this patient population [11]. Two children had sudden cardiac death as their presentation [14]. Although 30% have a positive family history, this was an infrequent reason for referral.

Physical Examination

Common findings include a gallop rhythm and a loud P2, hepatomegaly, ascites, and edema.

Diagnostic Studies

Electrocardiograms: The electrocardiogram is abnormal in approximately 98%, making it an extremely useful test in screening for RCM [3–12,14–27,30,32,37]. Fig. 18.1 is a representative example. Common abnormalities include right and/or left atrial enlargement, ST segment depression, and ST–T wave abnormalities. RV and/or LV hypertrophy can also be seen in addition to conduction abnormalities.

Holter: Holter evaluations can also be useful for rhythm evaluation and should include ST segment analysis. In one study approximately 67% of children who underwent Holter monitoring had ischemic changes with ST segment depression of at least 3 mm, most evident at higher heart rates [11]. Ventricular tachycardia was reported in a patient who developed chest pain and ST—segment depression. Additional case reports have also demonstrated ischemic or infarct patterns on ECG and autopsy with associated chest pain in some of the children, suggesting this is an important cause of morbidity and mortality in this patient population [8,11,17,18,81]. A myocardial bridge of the left anterior descending coronary artery and stenoses of branches with intimal thickening were reported in an infant with RCM with anginal type symptoms and sudden death [81]. That patient also had ST depression on Holter. It is likely, however, that the most common cause of ischemia in this patient population would be relatively diffuse hypoperfusion of the subendocardial myocardium due to the high diastolic filling pressures impairing coronary perfusion and not isolated coronary anomalies. This type of hypoperfusion, likely diffuse, would also be harder to detect by exercise myocardial perfusion studies. Cardiac MRI with delayed enhancement might be a better tool to further investigate this mechanism. Hayashi et al. did not find coronary abnormalities by catheterization in their RCM patients with ST segment depression nor did they find perfusion defects on exercise testing in the majority of their patients, thus they concluded that arrhythmia is a more common cause of sudden death than ischemia-mediated events [37]. However, ischemia could be the precursor leading to sudden death from an arrhythmia.

Of the pediatric studies reporting arrhythmias, approximately 20% of the patients had arrhythmias and/or conduction disturbances [3,4,9–11,21,25,27,30,82]. Atrial flutter was the most commonly reported arrhythmia. High-grade, second-degree and third-degree heart block were the next most commonly reported disturbances. A relatively high incidence of acute symptomatic heart block and bradycardia was reported by Walsh et al. [82]. They found that a longer PR interval and longer QRS duration were associated with acute cardiac events, resulting in their recommendation to monitor these patients frequently and consider defibrillator/pacemakers [82]. Atrial fibrillation and atrial tachycardias, Wolff–Parkinson–White syndrome with supraventricular tachycardia, symptomatic sinus bradycardia requiring pacing and ventricular tachycardia, and torsade de pointes have also been reported.

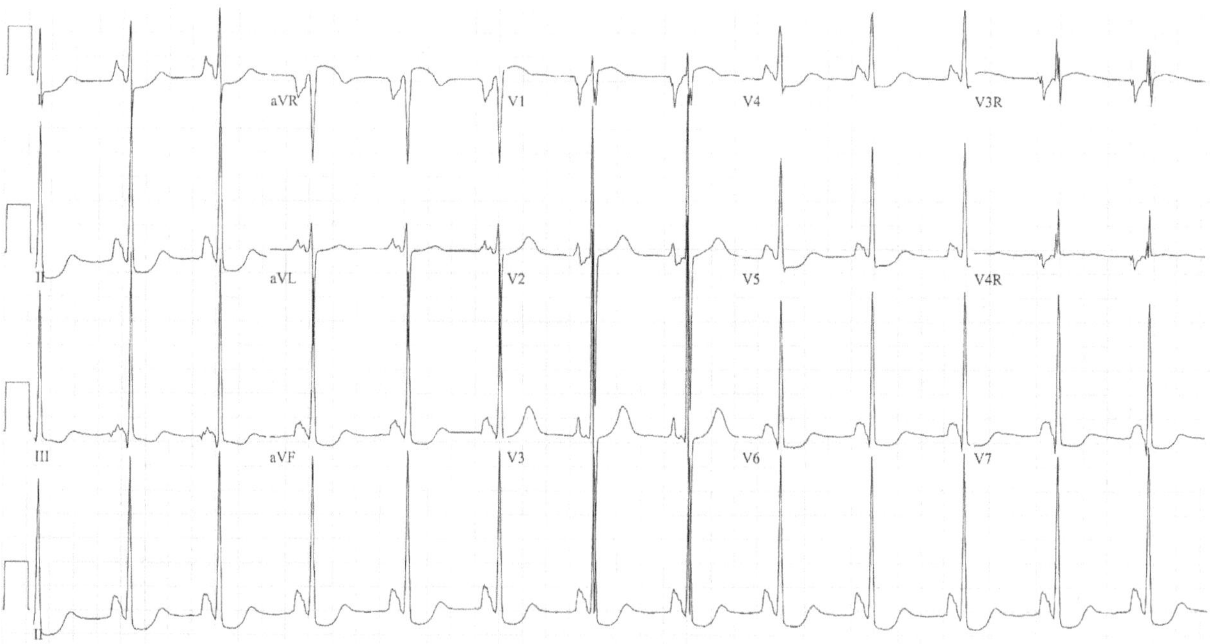

FIGURE 18.1 ECG from a 10-year-old with restrictive cardiomyopathy demonstrating sinus rhythm with biatrial enlargement, left ventricular hypertrophy, probable biventricular hypertrophy, and ST segment depression in the inferior and lateral leads.

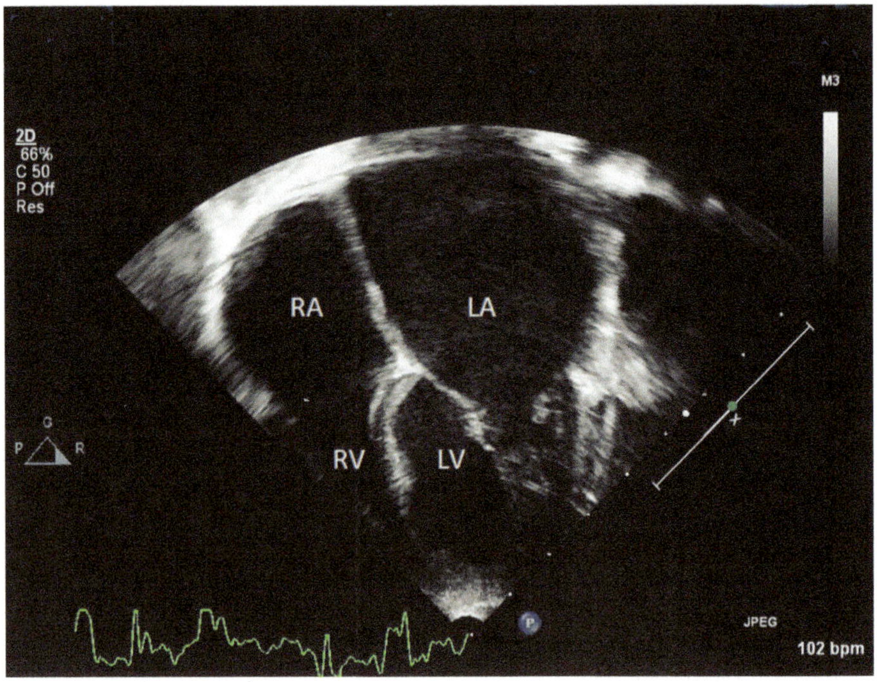

FIGURE 18.2 Apical four chamber view of a child with restrictive cardiomyopathy demonstrating a severely dilated left atrium and moderately dilated right atrium. *LA*, left atrium; *LV*, left ventricle; *RA*, right atrium; *RV*, right ventricle.

Chest radiographs: Approximately 90% of chest X-rays are abnormal, thus it appears to be a useful screening test [3,4,8–12,16–24,30]. The most common abnormalities are cardiomegaly and pulmonary venous congestion.

Echocardiography: The echocardiogram is usually diagnostic Fig. 18.2. On 2D imaging the atria are severely dilated, often making the ventricles appear small. Systolic function is usually normal or nearly normal, and significant hypertrophy or dilatation is typically absent. However, as many as 30% may present with or develop a depressed shortening or ejection fraction, in the moderately depressed range [3,10,12,30]. Subclinical systolic dysfunction in children with RCM was reported by Sasaki et al. [83]. These patients had normal ejection fractions (>55%), but decreased septal S′ and acceleration during isovolumic contraction, when evaluated by tissue Doppler imaging, compared to age- and sex-matched controls.

LV hypertrophy, while classically absent, occurs or develops in as many as 40% and may be progressive [3,4,10,12,30]. Highly variable and eccentric patterns of hypertrophy have been reported. The "mixed restrictive/hypertrophic phenotype" can result in a confusing clinical picture in terms of diagnosis, RCM versus HCM, and optimal therapeutic approaches.

Additionally 2D imaging should evaluate for thrombi, abnormalities of the atrioventricular valves, and the pericardium. Thrombi should be specifically looked for since thrombotic and embolic events have been described in approximately 21% of pediatric patients with idiopathic RCM [3,4,9,12,19,26,30,84–86]. Obliteration of the right and or LV apex by thrombus may occur in HES or EMF. In RCM the atrioventricular valves are typically normal. In HES and EMF the atrioventricular valves are frequently thickened with decreased excursion, particularly of the mitral valve. A thickened pericardium on 2D evaluation would suggest CP.

Doppler patterns of diastolic dysfunction have been well characterized in adults [87]. In the adult, typical Doppler patterns demonstrating restrictive physiology include an E/A ratio >2, mitral valve deceleration time <150 ms, and an isovolumic relaxation time <70 ms. Pulmonary venous Doppler demonstrates a D-wave predominance and increased pulmonary vein atrial reversal velocity and duration [87]. Several pediatric studies have described Doppler findings in children with RCM [9,10,12,27,88–93]. Data sets were frequently incomplete, and findings were not always consistent between studies, nor were parameters measured. In the patients described the findings consistent with restrictive filling and increased LV end-diastolic pressure included elevated E/A ratios, short mitral deceleration times, increased pulmonary vein atrial reversal velocity, and duration and pulmonary vein atrial reversal duration greater than mitral A duration (Figs. 18.3 and 18.4) [9,10,27,88]. However, Sasaki et al. found the mitral valve E/A ratio to be normal in most of their pediatric RCM subjects, and similar to controls [88] Ezon et al. found relatively poor Doppler correlation with LV filling pressures by catheterization in children with cardiomyopathies [91]. In that study the majority of patients with abnormal LV filling pressures had normal mitral E/A ratios, and the majority of patients with normal mitral valve E/A ratios had abnormal LV filling pressures. Although there was a modest statistical correlation of mitral valve E/A ratio with LV filling pressures, MV E/A ratio would make a poor screening tool for elevated LV filling pressures because of its low sensitivity.

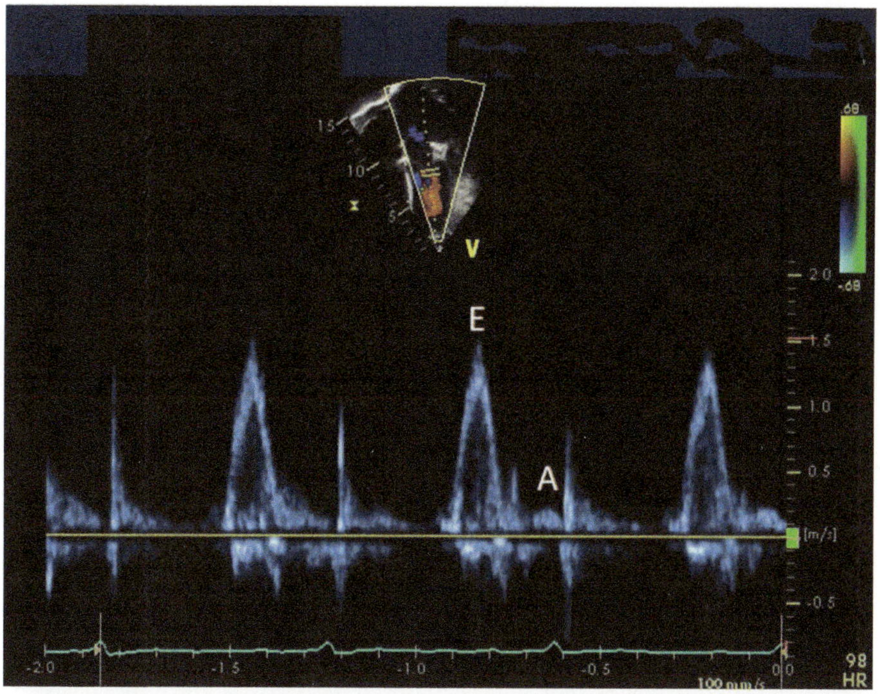

FIGURE 18.3 Mitral valve inflow demonstrates an increased E/A ratio and a shortened deceleration time.

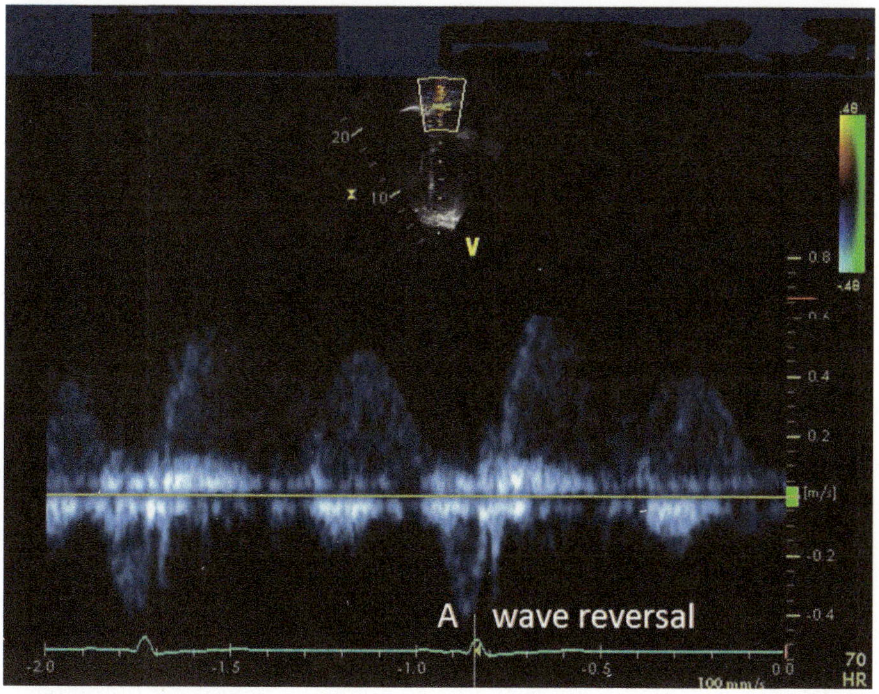

FIGURE 18.4 Pulmonary vein inflow demonstrating prominent A wave reversal with an elevated reversal velocity and duration.

Restrictive hemodynamics are caused by increased ventricular wall stiffness and/or from disorders of delayed active relaxation as evidenced by a triphasic mitral inflow pattern or L wave. Gewillig et al. described six children with idiopathic RCM who had elevated E/A ratios and shortened deceleration times, but they also had prominent mitral L waves with filling during diastasis accounting for approximately 28% of total ventricular filling [12]. On cardiac catheterization the LV pressure curve showed a small, but steady decline during middiastolic filling, implying delayed relaxation and not increased left atrial pressure. The mechanism of delayed relaxation as evidenced by an L wave was proposed by Hatle who described a middiastolic increase in forward mitral flow velocity in an adult patient with marked LV hypertrophy and suggested that prominent middiastolic flow was the result of markedly prolonged relaxation that lowers LV diastolic pressure during middiastole resulting in continued flow during that time [94]. A triphasic pattern has also been described in time velocity curves on cardiac magnetic resonance imaging in a teenager with RCM [92]. A study by Sasaki et al. in children with RCM did not demonstrate an L wave on mitral inflow Doppler, but 7 of 9 RCM patients had an L′ wave on TDI. None of the controls had an L′ wave. They calculated a sensitivity of 78% and specificity of 100% for an L′ at either the lateral or septal wall [88].

In adults, Doppler tissue imaging has been used to help differentiate RCM from CP [95,96]. A mitral E′ of equal to or greater than 8 cm/s was highly sensitive and specific for differentiating CP from RCM [96]. However, in a pediatric study comparing pediatric RCM patients to pediatric controls the mitral E′ in patients with RCM on average was 12.5 cm/s compared to 21.7 cm/s in controls [88]. Therefore the adult cutoff value for differentiating CP from RCM using the mitral E′ of 8 cm/s may not be applicable. Sasaki et al. did find that the average septal E′ was 8.2 cm/s versus controls of 15.5 cm/s, but they concluded that individual cut points for Doppler indices were not very sensitive for identifying restrictive physiology in children [88].

There is a tendency to extrapolate adult data and Doppler patterns of diastolic dysfunction to children. In addition to the Sasaki study two additional pediatric studies provide cautionary notes when diagnosing diastolic dysfunction by echocardiogram in children [88,90,91]. Ezon et al. found relatively poor Doppler correlation with LV filling pressures by catheterization in children with cardiomyopathies [91]. This study included patients with dilated, hypertrophic, and RCM. Of note cardiac catheterization and the echocardiogram studies were not performed at the same time. Sasaki et al. found that a combination of left atrial size, increased septal E/E′, lack of A wave and the presence of a middiastolic L′-wave were the most significant abnormalities in their patients with RCM [88]. Dragulescu et al. found that key echocardiogram parameters to assess diastolic function were not sufficiently discriminatory in the pediatric population, and discrepancies between criteria within individuals prevented consistent classification of diastolic dysfunction [90]. Of the parameters they assessed the septal E′, deceleration time and left atrial volume indexed to body surface area were likely the most useful criteria in evaluating diastolic dysfunction in children with cardiomyopathy (not all of whom were restrictive). The most consistent finding between the Sasaki and Dragulescu studies was the finding of a dilated left atrium in children with significant diastolic dysfunction. A statement by the European Society of Cardiology on heart failure with preserved ejection fraction (HFpEF) in adults in 2012 likely best summarizes echocardiographic criteria for diastolic dysfunction in children as well, and by extrapolation children with RCM [97]. They state, no single echocardiographic parameter is sufficiently accurate and reproducible to be used in isolation to make a diagnosis of LV diastolic dysfunction [97].

Cardiac catheterization and endomyocardial biopsy: Cardiac catheterization is an important part of the evaluation in patients with RCM, primarily to assess the pulmonary vascular resistance. Catheterization can help differentiate between RCM and CP, although virtually all hemodynamic features can overlap [98].

Both diseases typically have an early diastolic dip and subsequent plateau pattern, also called the square root sign [98]. Classically in RCM the LV end-diastolic pressure, left atrial pressure, and pulmonary capillary wedge pressure are markedly elevated and at least 4–5 mmHg (preferably 10 mmHg) greater than the right atrial pressure and RV end-diastolic pressure. A fluid bolus may bring out the differences in pressure between the right and left sides, in cases in which the pressures are essentially equal.

Pulmonary hypertension is frequently present at the time of initial catheterization due to elevated LV end-diastolic pressures [3,10,27,29–31,34–36]. The initial pulmonary vascular resistance index (PVRI) runs the spectrum from normal to prohibitively elevated in regard to orthotopic heart transplant [3,10,27,29–31,34–36]. Studies with follow-up data from 0.3 to 8 years after presentation demonstrated a range of PVRI's from normal to 30 U m^2 [3,30,31]. Frequently, the pulmonary vasculature remains reactive. [31,35,36]. This suggests some pre-as well as postcapillary pulmonary hypertension. Administration of nitric oxide may provide the best response for reactivity testing but needs to be given with caution in this setting [31]. Nonetheless, Weller et al. reported that 40% of their pediatric RCM patients were precluded from orthotopic heart transplant due to an elevated and nonreactive pulmonary vascular resistance, at the time they were evaluated for cardiac transplantation [30]. When and who will develop fixed pulmonary vascular resistance has been unpredictable.

The majority of endomyocardial biopsies are nondiagnostic, revealing varying degrees of fibrosis and hypertrophy, nonspecifically increased numbers of mitochondria, and increased glycogen [3,34,37]. Desmin myopathy can be identified from endomyocardial and/or skeletal muscle biopsy, leading to an etiologic diagnosis [26,40]. When found in the myocardium there should be heightened awareness for impending skeletal myopathy and/or conduction system disease. One case of amyloidosis has been diagnosed by biopsy in a child and rarely eosinophilia-associated myocarditis.

Differential Diagnosis

CP is the disease process that is most commonly confused with RCM and will be discussed further in the chapter. Overlapping phenotypes may occur in cardiomyopathies resulting in confusion as to the type of cardiomyopathy [3,10,12,30]. It is not surprising that phenotypes sometimes overlap since a variety of phenotypes can be seen in the same family with the same gene defect. Some degree of LV hypertrophy may be seen in some children with RCM [3,4,10,12,30] raising the question as to whether the patient has RCM versus HCM, i.e., the "mixed restrictive/hypertrophic phenotype." Some patients with HCM may have relatively mild hypertrophy, but very dilated atria with restrictive physiology. "Pure" HCM in children has a better prognosis than the mixed HCM/RCM phenotype, while children with "pure" RCM have the worst prognosis of the three [99,100]. The Maskatia et al. study reported that children with HCM and restrictive physiology have a long-term survival that is equivalent to average post heart transplant survival in children, therefore listing these patients for transplant may be able to be delayed longer than for those with "pure" RCM [100]. Some patients with noncompaction cardiomyopathy may also have restrictive physiology/phenotype [101–103]. Restrictive physiology may also develop in patients with dilated cardiomyopathy [29]. The presence of mixed physiology worsens the prognosis in cardiomyopathies [104].

Outcome

The prognosis in children with RCM remains poor and is significantly worse than in children with HCM or dilated cardiomyopathy [3,4,6–9,11,12,29,34]. Approximately half the children with RCM die or undergo cardiac transplant within 2–3 years of diagnosis, compared to HCM or dilated cardiomyopathy in whom the 2-year mortality rates are reported to be 12.7% and 13.6%, respectively [6]. Heart failure-related death is the most common mode of death in children with RCM, but sudden death is not uncommon, reportedly occurring in 12%–33% [11,34,37,105]. Rivenes et al. reported that sudden cardiac death occurred in 28% of children with an annual mortality rate of 7% [11]. In comparison, the study by Bharucha et al. reported a cumulative incidence of sudden cardiac death at 15 years of 5% in dilated cardiomyopathy, 6% in HCM, 12% in RCM, and 23% in LV noncompaction [105]. In review of additional literature reports in which data on sudden death were available, including the Rivenes study, approximately 12% of children died suddenly, which is identical to the Bharucha study [8,11,14,19,30,105]. Patients who appear to be at greater risk for sudden death include those who present with signs and symptoms of ischemia, such as syncope and chest pain [11]. Walsh et al. found older age at presentation was associated with sudden cardiac events, which included death, sudden, acute hemodynamic compromise, or syncope likely arrhythmia related [82]. The median PR interval and QRS duration on ECG were longer in children who had an acute cardiac event in that study.

Factors associated with poor prognosis have not been consistent between studies. An increased risk for death from heart failure was found when cardiomegaly and pulmonary venous congestion were seen on chest X-ray, age was less than 5 years, thromboembolic events occurred, or elevated PVRI was present [9,10,30]. Children with heart failure are also at risk from ischemic complications as well [11]. The study by Russo and Webber found higher end-diastolic pressures and larger left atrial:aortic ratios correlated negatively with survival, but age or heart failure symptoms at presentation did not [34]. Based on a report by Weller et al., it is apparent that the majority of children with RCM who undergo cardiac transplant have longer survival than those who do not undergo transplant [30].

Management

There are no known medical therapies that improve outcomes in RCM. None of the standard therapies for systolic heart failure in adults have been shown to improve survival in adults with HFpEF, including RCM, so it is not surprising that pediatric studies have not found any medical therapies to be efficacious given the much smaller number of patients with pure diastolic heart failure in children. There are more recommendations on what not do medically speaking than what to do, all of which are based primarily on expert opinion in children [106,107]. Bengur et al. reported that captopril lowered blood pressure without an increase in cardiac output, when administered during cardiac catheterization to a small number of pediatric patients with RCM, concluding that captopril should not be used in patients with RCM. [106]. However, in pediatric RCM series that reported the use of angiotensin-converting enzyme (ACE) inhibitors neither acute decompensation nor therapeutic benefit was reported [3,4,10,27,30,31,37]. The International Society of Heart and Lung Transplant issued a monograph on the ISHLT guidelines for the management of pediatric heart failure in 2014 [107]. The report states the risks and benefits of ACE inhibitors in pediatric RCM remain to be determined and are not currently recommended unless there are additional factors for which they are indicated, such as hypertension [107]. Drugs that were not recommended (Class III) included calcium channel blockers and digoxin, unless needed for another indication and positive inotropes such as dopamine, dobutamine, and epinephrine and the pulmonary hypertension drug classes of prostaglandins and endothelin receptor antagonists. The only Class 1 recommendation for medical treatment in pediatric diastolic heart failure was to use diuretics to establish euvolemia. When using diuretics, close monitoring of renal function and blood pressure is needed. Overdiuresis should be avoided because these patients are sensitive to alterations in preload.

Tachycardia is poorly tolerated in adults with diastolic dysfunction, therefore beta blockers have been suggested as part of the treatment regimen, although there has been no clear benefit in adults with HFpEF with beta blocker therapy [108,109]. Rivenes et al. suggested the use of beta blocker therapy to blunt rapid heart rates in their pediatric RCM patient population in whom significant ST segment depression was noted at higher heart rates [11]. Subsequently three children less than 5-years old were reported who were begun on propranolol (n = 2) or metoprolol (n = 1) who did not tolerate beta blocker therapy, which was thought to be related to hypoglycemia in two of the cases [110]. The role of beta blocker therapy in RCM remains unclear, therefore their use is not currently recommended in children with RCM unless there is an additional indication [107].

RCM-associated thrombosis has been reported in children ranging in frequency from 0% to 40%. The reported frequency of embolic events ranges from 12% to 33% with approximately 50% being cerebrovascular events [86]. In a compilation of nine pediatric studies, thrombotic and embolic events have been described in approximately 20% of those with idiopathic RCM [3,4,9,10,12,26,30,84,85]. This has resulted in the recommendation that some form of antithrombotic/anticoagulation therapy be prescribed at the time of diagnosis. There are no studies in this patient population to compare the efficacy of aspirin versus warfarin or enoxaparin as prophylaxis. In those without evidence of thrombus formation aspirin is often used as a sole agent, but in those with an identified thrombus more aggressive anticoagulation is necessary and arguably may be agents of choice for prophylaxis.

There has been an increasing focus of attention on pulmonary hypertension secondary to left-sided heart disease, as it is the most common cause of pulmonary hypertension in adults [111]. The development of pulmonary hypertension due to diastolic dysfunction is a significant problem in children with RCM as well. Besides the "fixed" degree of elevation in pulmonary artery pressure that occurs due to elevated diastolic pressures a reactive component may also be present. In some patients a fall in resistance with the administration of 100% oxygen or inhaled nitric oxide occurs. Most classes of drugs used to treat pulmonary hypertension have not been found to be useful in adults with secondary pulmonary hypertension due to left-sided heart disease [111]. Some were felt to be harmful and therefore are not recommended [111]. An older study by Fenton et al. reported that some children may benefit from continuous infusion of prostacyclin while awaiting determination of the best transplant strategy [35], contrary to the current guidelines.

Some smaller adult studies suggested that phosphodiesterase 5 inhibitors (e.g., sildenafil) were beneficial; however, the "RELAX" trial that enrolled adults with HFpEF found no benefit of sildenafil over a 24-week period in regard to clinical status or exercise capacity compared to the placebo group [112]. Currently pulmonary vasodilators used in the treatment of primary pulmonary hypertension are not recommended for routine use in children or adults with left-sided heart disease resulting in pulmonary hypertension.

Cardiac transplantation remains the definitive therapy in children with RCM because current medical therapy is ineffective, the development of pulmonary hypertension is common, and mortality is high. Cardiac transplant outcomes in children with RCM are not significantly different from children undergoing cardiac transplant for other forms of cardiac disease [31,35,36,113–115]. "Early" evaluation and listing for orthotopic heart transplant is prudent, although how early remains controversial in the literature [11,34,35,113]. Some patients with RCM have remained relatively well for over a decade [34], but who will remain well for an extended period of time is unpredictable. At the time of diagnosis cardiac catheterization should be considered, including testing for pulmonary vasoreactivity, particularly if the PVRI is greater the 6 U m^2 or the transpulmonary gradient is greater than 14–15 mmHg. Many patients have a reactive pulmonary vascular bed, and successful orthotopic transplant can be performed. The reactivity of the pulmonary vascular bed may be more important, up to a point. Children with PVRI's above 9 U m^2 have undergone successful orthotopic heart transplant as long as they demonstrated reactivity of the pulmonary vascular bed [35,36]. Two studies by Chiu et al. suggest that the use of a PVRI >6 in children may be too restrictive, suggesting 9 is the threshold over which mortality increased after orthotopic heart transplant [116,117]. Undergoing orthotopic heart transplant is preferable since survival is better than heart–lung transplant, and heterotopic transplant may not be feasible in small children. However, heterotopic heart transplantation has been reported in small children with RCM [35,118]. If pulmonary vasodilator therapies are used, careful monitoring for the development of pulmonary edema is necessary. Some pulmonary vasodilators may cause systemic hypotension that may be poorly tolerated in these patients with limited compensatory mechanisms. Listing these patients prior to their need for these treatment strategies is preferable. Patients not listed at the time of diagnosis require close follow-up to assess for signs of developing pulmonary hypertension.

The outcomes of 145 children with RCM listed for heart transplantation were reviewed by Zangwill et al., with 44% listed UNOS status 1 [113]. In that study, children requiring mechanical support and infants had a significantly higher risk of death while waiting, than other children listed with RCM. An increased wait list mortality has also been reported by Singh et al. for children with nondilated forms of cardiomyopathy (restrictive or hypertrophic) who were on a ventilator at the time of listing [114]. Dipchand et al. reported that children with RCM at the time of listing, when compared to children with dilated cardiomyopathy, were less likely to be listed status 1, ventilated, on inotropes and had fewer arrhythmias [119]. However, they were as likely to die while waiting. This suggests these lower status patients were as vulnerable as the higher status children with dilated cardiomyopathy [119]. These studies support the recommendation of not waiting "too long" to list these patients for heart transplant.

It is much harder to support children on mechanical devices who have RCM. In the Zangwill et al. study wait list mortality was worse for pediatric RCM patients who were on multiple devices including ventilators, extracorporeal membrane oxygenation (ECMO), ventricular assist devices, and intraaortic balloon pumps [113]. In a single center pediatric study there were no long-term ECMO survivors with RCM who were placed on ECMO at the time of cardiac resuscitation (ECPR) [120]. LV assist device support is difficult due to the normal to small ventricular cavity size and generally biventricular nature of the disease. The Berlin EXCOR left ventricular assist device has been used successfully to bridge a small number of children with RCM to transplant [121–124]. Biventricular support was used in one. Most had left atrial cannulation because the LV cavity size was too small to permit the usual LV apical cannulation. There is a 2-year-old with RCM who underwent Berlin support with apical LV cannulation [123]. That patient required resection of the hypertrophied papillary muscles and mitral valve apparatus with placement of a bioprosthetic mitral valve to allow adequate filling of the LV cannula [123].

Medical therapy is supportive and the aim is to reduce symptoms while considering or awaiting cardiac transplantation. Patients should have routine periodic ECG's and Holter monitoring performed, and as symptoms dictate. Evaluating for evidence of ischemia, atrial and ventricular arrhythmias, or developing conduction disturbances is important. For those with significant conduction disturbances pacemakers are indicated. If ventricular tachycardia or evidence of ischemia is seen, implantable defibrillators should be strongly considered. Strenuous physical activity should be avoided. Relatively early listing for cardiac transplantation is prudent.

CONSTRICTIVE PERICARDITIS

CP is very uncommon in pediatric patients in North America and Europe. CP frequently "masquerades" as other cardiac conditions. The clinical presentation and test results of patients with RCM and CP can be very similar. However, if isolated bands of constriction occur CP can "masquerade" as tricuspid or mitral stenosis or subpulmonary or pulmonary stenosis [125–129]. Differentiating CP from another disease state is important, due to differences in treatment and outcome of the underlying disease.

Epidemiology

The incidence and prevalence of CP in children is unknown. In children CP has been reported to account for 0.7%–13% of all cases of pericarditis [130,131]. It is uncommon for CP to present in a child less than 10 years of age [130,132,133]. Male children are reported to be affected more frequently than girls [132–134].

Genetics—Syndromes and Associations

Three syndromes have been described in children that are associated with the development of CP. Both Mulibrey nanism and Myhre syndrome are associated with the development of "pure" CP as well as RCM or restrictive physiology [55,58,59,135]. Another autosomal recessive disorder has been described that includes pericarditis (constrictive), arthritis, and camptodactyly [136–139]. This syndrome has also been called "familial fibrosing serositis" and camptodactyly-arthropathy-coxa vara-pericarditis [136,139]. It is caused by recessive mutations in the PRG4 gene resulting in the lack of the glycoprotein lubricin, which is a lubricant found in joints, tendons, and visceral cavities and inhibits synovial proliferation [139].

Deline and Cable reported a cluster of pericarditis cases that occurred in 2 generations of a family [140]. The phenotype in this family included both effusive and CP. They postulated a possible autosomal dominant inheritance with incomplete penetrance because a familial clustering of common etiologies for pericarditis was not found.

Although a specific syndrome has not been identified there has been an unusually frequent association of atrial septal defects with CP [141]. Ascertainment bias may be a cause for this association.

Etiologies

There are multiple causes of CP (Table 18.5). In prior eras tuberculosis was the leading cause of CP throughout the world and remains a dominant cause in developing countries. In developed countries idiopathic and a combination of other

TABLE 18.5 Reported Associations or Causes of Constrictive Pericarditis in Children and Adults

Idiopathic	Uremia (on dialysis)
Infectious	Hemorrhagic disorders (causing hemopericardium)
Tuberculosis	Atrial septal defect (unrepaired)
Viral	Drugs
Bacterial	Procainamide
Fungal	Methysergide
Parasitic	Practolol
Connective tissue disorders	Hydralazine
Rheumatoid arthritis	Cromolyn sodium
Systemic lupus erythematosus	Penicillins
Dermatomyositis	Isoniazid
Scleroderma (includes CREST syndrome)	Minoxidil
Sarcoidosis	Phenylbutazone
Familial/syndrome/genetic	Porphyria cutanea tarda
Family cluster	Asbestosis
Mulibrey nanism	Whipple syndrome
Familial fibrosing serositis	Chylopericardium
Myhre syndrome	Inflammatory bowel disease
Radiation	Cholesterol pericarditis
Cardiac surgery	ICD patches
Chest trauma (blunt or penetrating)	Epicardial pacemaker
Malignancy	Chemical trauma—sclerotherapy of esophageal varices

CREST, calcinosis, Raynaud phenomenon, esophageal involvement, sclerodactyly, and telangiectasia; *ICD*, implantable cardioverter defibrillator.

infectious agents are common causes. Although the development of CP is not common after cardiac surgery, it has been reported to be one of the most common causes of CP in developed countries. The frequency following cardiac surgery is reported to be 2%–3% in adults [142]. It can occur after any type of cardiac surgery including following cardiac transplantation [143]. Connective tissue diseases/vasculitis, malignancies, and therapeutic radiation are also reported causes.

Pathology

CP results from inflammation of the pericardium with subsequent healing that results in a thick or thin scar that restricts cardiac filling [144]. The thickened pericardium consists of an increased number of fibrous strands with foci of inflammation [145]. Calcification ensues in some cases. An underlying "atrophic myocarditis" may develop and has been suggested as a cause of myocardial dysfunction. There is usually total or near total obliteration of the pericardial space. However, effusive–constrictive pericarditis also occurs in which some effusion is present [146]. Localized bands of constriction can occur, mimicking stenosis of any of the cardiac valves [144,145].

Pathophysiology

The pathophysiologic consequences of CP are due to loss of pericardial compliance resulting in three major effects. (1) Dissociation of intrathoracic and intracardiac pressures with respiration, (2) increased right and LV interdependence, and (3) impaired diastolic filling with increased dependence on heart rate for cardiac output [147].

In CP there is little respiratory variability in the total amount of blood entering the heart [147]. Due to the constriction from the pericardium, the cardiac chambers are isolated from the changes in intrathoracic pressure. However, the pulmonary veins and vena cava flow are affected by changes in intrathoracic pressure. During inspiration there is a reduction in the velocity of diastolic flow in the pulmonary veins and a subsequent reduction in left-sided filling. The ventricles in CP are pathologically coupled (increased RV and LV interdependence). The inspiratory reduction in LV filling is associated with an increase in diastolic filling in the right ventricle, and the ventricular septum shifts to the left. The opposite effects are seen on exhalation, and the septum shifts to the right. This results in the septal bounce seen on echocardiography. These changes also result in an expiratory reduction of flow in the vena cavae, increased hepatic flow reversal, and decreased tricuspid flow velocity.

The fibrotic pericardium results in impaired diastolic filling of all cardiac chambers. Ventricular filling is initially very rapid due to elevated atrial pressures [147]. However, by middiastole the rapid filling abruptly declines due to the noncompliant pericardium. Increasing the heart rate is an effective means of maintaining cardiac output in this condition because filling is severely limited in late diastole. Compared to normal states cardiac output is more dependent on heart rate in CP.

Clinical Presentation

Symptoms are typically present for years before the diagnosis is made, in the chronic form of CP. A specific cause is rarely determined. Ascites and hepatomegaly are the most common presenting complaints, but dyspnea and/or failure to thrive are also common [130,132,148–153]. However, Thompson et al. reported a series of pediatric patients undergoing pericardiectomy for either inflammatory or CP with the most common symptom being chest pain, followed by heart failure symptoms [134]. A relatively higher proportion of inflammatory pericarditis may account for chest pain being the most common presenting symptom in their population. Protein losing enteropathy may also occur [139,154]. CP may also have an acute (days to months) or subacute (arbitrarily defined as 3–12 months) presentation, typically following an infectious illness, or purulent pericarditis [144]. A sterile pericardial effusion associated with meningitis or sepsis may occur in some cases. During the recovery phase of these illnesses CP can develop [131]. Signs and symptoms of CP occur within days to months of the inciting illness, in these cases, and may be transient [155]. In adults the transient form typically takes about 8 weeks to resolve [156].

Physical Examination

In children the most common physical findings in CP are hepatomegaly and ascites. Peripheral edema is usually less striking than the ascites and hepatomegaly. Prominent jugular venous distension is often present. Kussmaul's sign (inspiratory jugular venous distension) may occur. Muffled heart sounds are more frequent in children with this disease than diastolic filling sounds, but a pericardial knock may be present.

Diagnostic Studies

Electrocardiogram: The electrocardiogram is usually nonspecifically abnormal. Relatively low voltage QRS complexes and nonspecific ST–T wave abnormalities are frequent findings. Right atrial enlargement as well as notched P waves were also reported in some patients. Less common findings are ventricular hypertrophy and conduction delays [130,132,149,152–154]. Arrhythmias were uncommon, although atrial flutter was reported in one [150].

Chest radiographs: Chest X-rays are usually abnormal, but nonspecific. Some degree of cardiomegaly is common as well as venous congestion and pleural effusions [132,149,151–153]. Pericardial calcification occurs in up to approximately 21% of children with CP [58].

Echocardiography: A thickened pericardium may be present on transthoracic echocardiogram. However, a thick pericardium alone does not warrant the diagnosis of CP, and the absence of a thickened pericardium does not exclude CP. Transesophageal echocardiography may show the thickened pericardium better in some views. On 2D imaging a septal bounce associated with changes in the respiratory cycle may be present. Dilation of the atria and inferior vena cava may be seen.

Doppler flow patterns are useful for diagnosing CP and differentiating it from RCM. The effects of the respiratory cycle on venous flow patterns and atrioventricular valve inflow patterns help distinguish CP from RCM. With inspiration in CP there is increased hepatic flow with increased diastolic forward flow and decreased flow reversal. During inspiration there is increased RV filling. The peak tricuspid valve E and A waves are increased. During expiration the opposite changes occur.

Pulmonary venous flow reflects diastolic function and left atrial and ventricular filling. In CP, the intrathoracic pulmonary vein flow is dissociated from the encased intracardiac structures and pressure. Peak systolic and diastolic velocities are decreased with inspiration and increased with expiration. LV filling (flow integrals) decreases with inspiration. Isovolumic relaxation time increases. Mitral valve flow velocities decrease with decrease in peak E and A waves. Reciprocal changes occur with expiration.

Doppler tissue imaging and strain rate have also been used to differentiate RCM from CP in adults. Impaired myocardial function distinguishes patients with intrinsic myocardial disease from those with pericardial disease [95,96,157]. In a study of adults, by Welch et al. from the Mayo clinic, the echocardiographic features that best distinguished CP from RCM were the following: (1) respiratory-related ventricular shift, (2) tissue Doppler medial e' velocity ≥9 cm/s, and (3) hepatic vein expiratory diastolic reversal ratio ≥0.79. When septal shift was combined with either of the other two, an 87% sensitivity and a 91% specificity for CP was attained [158]. ASE recommendations for the mitral e' velocity for differentiating CP from RCM in adults is <0.7 cm/s, below that cutoff is more consistent with RCM [159]. As discussed in the RCM section of this chapter the best cutoff value for children is not known.

CT scan and MRI: Pericardial thickening may be detected by computed tomography. In children the pericardium is normally less than 2 mm thick [152]. Secondary-associated findings include a dilated inferior vena cava, acute angulation of the interventricular septum, a deformed ventricular contour, and pericardial calcification. The IVC/aorta ratio should be less than 3.

MRI can also detect a thickened pericardium, but calcification may not be well seen with this modality. Atrial and IVC enlargement may also be seen by this technique as well as abnormal septal configuration and narrowed tubular appearing ventricles [144,160]. Delayed gadolinium enhancement of the pericardium suggests an inflammatory process, particularly if associated with elevated inflammatory markers in adults [161]. These findings suggest a disease process that may be treatable with antiinflammatory agents.

Cardiac catheterization and endomyocardial biopsy: Constrictive hemodynamics closely resemble RCM hemodynamics. In CP right atrial pressure tracings reveal a prominent early diastolic Y descent [145]. The A and V waves have a similar peak pressure, resulting in an "M-configuration." The square root sign is also seen in CP with the LV diastolic pressure tracings demonstrating an early dip and plateau pattern. This reflects the early rapid filling in the first third of diastole. The elevated pressure resulting in the plateau causes an elevation in mean venous pressure. In classic CP there is elevation and equalization of the right atrial, RV, left atrial, and LV end-diastolic pressures to within 4–5 mmHg [145]. Pulmonary hypertension is usually less marked than in RCM. The RV and pulmonary artery systolic pressures do not usually exceed 50 mmHg.

In CP the RV diastolic pressure to RV systolic pressure ratio frequently exceeds 0.33, while in RCM it is usually less than 0.3. In adults, Talreja et al. described an additional catheterization ratio to differentiate between CP and RCM based on the changes in area of the RV and LV pressure curves during inspiration and expiration [162]. During inspiration there is an increase of the area under the RV pressure curve and a decrease in the area of the LV pressure curve relative to expiration. The systolic area index was defined as the ratio of the RV area to the LV area in inspiration versus RV area to LV area in expiration with the CP group having a larger ratio than the group with restrictive disease. Talreja et al. found this ratio or index to have 97% sensitivity and 100% predictive accuracy in identifying adult patients with surgically proven CP. Studies validating this index in children have not been reported.

Occasionally endomyocardial biopsy may be necessary to help distinguish CP from RCM. The absence of myopathic findings support the diagnosis of CP, while the presence of myopathic changes suggests RCM. Children with RCM or CP are hemodynamically fragile. Case series and reports in children with RCM have reported deterioration and death during or shortly after catheterization and biopsy [3,19]. Given the infrequency of finding a specific diagnosis, careful consideration of the risk benefit ratio of the information that is likely to be obtained by the biopsy should be undertaken prior to catheterization.

Exploratory thoracotomy: On rare occasions exploratory thoracotomy is necessary to differentiate CP from RCM. If CP is identified, pericardiectomy at the time may also be curative and is the treatment of choice. However, in patients with RCM exploratory thoracotomy is not a benign procedure and may result in perioperative mortality [30]. Therefore, every effort should be made to diagnose RCM noninvasively.

Outcome

In acute and subacute forms of CP symptom onset typically occurs weeks to several months after a preceding infectious illness or pericarditis [144,155]. Those forms may be transient, resolving with medical therapy. In the chronic form of CP surgical intervention is required with 70%–80% of patients improved or cured [132,163]. In adults predictors of poor outcome include underlying malignancy, previous pericardial surgery, New York Heart Association (NYHA) class IV at presentation, myocardial atrophy, myocardial inflammation and scarring and a Child-Pugh score greater than 7 (Child-Pugh score is a measure for risk stratification of liver function) [147,163]. Predictors of outcome are less well defined in children undergoing pericardiectomy. In a pediatric surgical series reported by Talwar et al. in which 22% died following surgery, the only predictor of nonsurvival was "worse" preoperative NYHA class [164]. In another pediatric series reporting results of pericardiectomy for pericarditis there was only one death (4%); however, over half of their patients (59%) were categorized as inflammatory pericarditis with the other 41% characterized as constrictive [134]. In the Thompson et al. series the majority of patients were categorized as NYHA Class I or II [134]. Both the Thompson et al. and Talwar et al. groups recommended "earlier" consideration of pericardiectomy [134,164].

Management

It may be possible to avoid surgical intervention in the acute and subacute forms as they may be transient. Any identified underlying infectious cause should be treated. Diuretics are used for the management of fluid overload. Some reports have suggested the use of antiinflammatory doses of aspirin or other nonsteroidal antiinflammatory drugs, colchicine or steroids with close observation and follow-up [146,156,165,166]. Steroids have been reported to increase the risk of prolonged or recurrent symptoms in other forms of pericarditis and therefore may not be first line therapy for CP, unless indicated for an associated collagen vascular disorder or the other agents are contraindicated [167]. If symptoms resolve and close follow-up evaluation reveals resolution of the findings of CP then surgery may be avoided. In patients with chronic CP pericardiectomy is the treatment of choice, with as complete resection as possible, preferably before the patient has become severely debilitated.

CURRENT STATUS AND FUTURE DIRECTIONS

In most patients it is possible to distinguish between RCM and CP, without the need for an exploratory thoracotomy Table 18.6. However, there continue to be cases in which the presentation and hemodynamic profile have so much overlap that thoracotomy is required for diagnosis. Henein et al. have suggested that in those cases in which pericardial disease is found that the term restrictive pericarditis should be applied [168]. Wang et al. reported a case of a child with mixed CP and RCM features [169]. Features consistent with CP included pericardial calcification and a lateral mitral annular tissue Doppler velocity of 18 cm/s; however, endomyocardial biopsy showed myocyte hypertrophy and fibrosis, thought to be more consistent with a cardiomyopathic process. Pericardiectomy resulted in symptomatic improvement despite the myopathic features on endomyocardial biopsy and even though the calcified pericardium could not be completely resected. Due to the significant morbidity and mortality associated with thoracotomy in those with RCM, less invasive means of confirming the diagnosis need to continue to be developed. Studies in adults have looked at the utility of B-type natriuretic peptide (BNP) to differentiate between CP and RCM [170,171]. In a small case series of adults by Leya et al., all patients with CP had BNPs that were less than 200 pg/mL and were statistically significantly less than those with RCM [171]. A subsequent study in adults found statistically significant differences in BNP levels between those with CP and those with RCM, but significantly more overlap was seen in the BNPs between groups, particularly if the CP was secondary to prior cardiac surgery or radiation therapy rather than a primary CP, making the BNP less definitive for differentiating between CP and RCM [170]. Another study compared N-terminal proBNP (NT-proBNP) in CP and RCM in relatively younger predominantly adult subjects but did include some children [172]. In that study, patients with RCM had significantly higher NT-proBNPs, than patients with CP, although there was overlap. They found a cutoff value of 459 pg/mL had sensitivity, specificity, and overall accuracy of 90%, 86% and 88%, respectively, for differentiating CP from RCM. In children ongoing assessment and validation of biomarkers, noninvasive echocardiogram and cardiac MRI parameters are needed to help distinguish these diseases.

Improved methods of risk stratification are needed for RCM patients to identify those at greatest risk for rapid progression of elevated pulmonary vascular resistance and sudden death as well as thromboembolism. Better medical therapies are needed for the treatment of RCM since the only definitive therapy, at the present time, is cardiac transplantation.

KEY CONCEPTS

- RCM accounts for 2.5%–5% of pediatric cardiomyopathies.
- Presenting complaints in RCM in children are most commonly respiratory, followed by abnormal physical exam findings, congestive heart failure, and syncope.
- Children with RCM are at increased risk of sudden death.
- The diagnosis of RCM can usually be made noninvasively.

TABLE 18.6 Restrictive Cardiomyopathy (RCM) Versus Constrictive Pericarditis

	RCM	CP[a]
ECG Finding		
Atrial enlargement	Nearly universal	May be present
LVH[b] and/or RVH[c]	Common	Usually absent
Low voltage QRS	Unusual	Common
ST–T wave abnormality	Common	Common
Chest X-ray		
Calcification	Absent	≤21%
Echocardiogram		
Pericardial thickening	Absent	May be thickened
Atrial dilatation	Marked	May be enlarged
Wall thicknesses	Normal to mild hypertrophy	Usually normal
Systolic function	Normal to depressed	Normal
Septal bounce	Absent	Usually present
Doppler: respiratory flow changes	Occasional	Usually marked
Gated MRI/CT		
	Normal pericardium	Usually thickened
Cardiac Catheterization		
	PWP[d] and LVEDP[e] may exceed RAP[f] and RVEDP[g] by >4 mmHg.	RAP = PWP, RVEDP = LVEDP usually within 4 mmHg
	RVSP[h] often >50 mmHg RVEDP/RVESP ≥0.33	RVSP usually <50 mmHg RVEDP/RVESP <0.3
RV[i] endomyocardial biopsy	Usually abnormal (frequently nonspecific)	Usually normal
Thoracotomy	Normal pericardium	Usually abnormal pericardium

[a]*Constrictive pericarditis.*
[b]*Left ventricular hypertrophy.*
[c]*Right ventricular hypertrophy.*
[d]*Pulmonary wedge pressure.*
[e]*Left ventricular end-diastolic pressure.*
[f]*Right atrial pressure.*
[g]*Right ventricular end-diastolic pressure.*
[h]*Right ventricular systolic pressure.*
[i]*Right ventricular.*

- The prognosis in children with RCM remains poor. No medications have been shown to improve survival.
- Medical treatment for RCM is largely supportive with judicious use of diuretics and some form of antiplatelet therapy or anticoagulation.
- Children with RCM are difficult to support mechanically.
- These high-risk patients should be considered early for cardiac transplantation.
- It is important to distinguish between RCM and HCM with restrictive physiology as the prognosis is better in those with HCM than those with pure RCM.
- CP has a better prognosis than RCM, particularly when recognized early.
- Several forms of CP have been described including an acute to subacute form and the chronic type.
- The acute and subacute or transient forms of CP may resolve with treatment of the underlying disease or antiinflammatory agents.
- The treatment for the chronic form of CP is pericardiectomy.

REFERENCES

[1] P. Richardson, W. McKenna, M. Bristow, et al., Report of the 1995 World Health Organization/International Society and Federation of Cardiology Task Force on the definition and classification of cardiomyopathies, Circulation 93 (1996) 841–842.

[2] M.M. LeWinter, W.E. Hopkins, Pericardial diseases, in: tenth ed., in: D.L. Mann, D.P. Zipes, P. Libby, R. Bonow (Eds.), Braunwald's Heart Disease: A Textbook of Cardiovascular Medicine, vol. 71, Elsevier, Philadelphia, PA, 2015, pp. 1636–1657.

[3] S.W. Denfield, G. Rosenthal, R.J. Gajarski, et al., Restrictive cardiomyopathies in childhood etiologies and natural history, Tex. Heart Inst. J. 24 (1997) 38–44.

[4] A.B. Lewis, Clinical profile and outcome of restrictive cardiomyopathy in children, AM. Heart J. 123 (1992) 1589–1593.

[5] A.W. Nugent, P.E.F. Daubeney, P. Chondros, et al., The epidemiology of childhood cardiomyopathy in Australia, N. Engl. J. Med. 348 (2003) 1639–1646.

[6] S.E. Lipshultz, C.A. Sleeper, J.A. Towbin, et al., The incidence of pediatric cardiomyopathy in two regions of the United States, N. Engl. J. Med. 348 (2003) 1647–1655.

[7] I. Malčić, M. Jelušić, H. Kneiwald, N. Barišić, D. Jelašić, J. Boižkov, Epidemiology of cardiomyopathies in children and adolescents: a retrospective study over the last 10 years, Cardiol. Young 12 (2002) 253–259.

[8] L.C. Harris, A.E. Rodin, Q.X. Nghiem, Idiopathic, nonobstructive cardiomyopathy in children, Am. J. Cardiol. 21 (1968) 153–165.

[9] F. Cetta, P.W. O'Leary, J.B. Seward, et al., Idiopathic restrictive cardiomyopathy in childhood: diagnostic features and clinical course, Mayo Clin. Proc. 70 (1995) 634–640.

[10] S. Chen, I.C. Balfour, S. Jureidini, Clinical spectrum of restrictive cardiomyopathy in children, J. Heart Lung Transplant. 20 (2001) 90–92.

[11] S.M. Rivenes, D.L. Kearney, E.O. Smith, et al., Sudden death and cardiovascular collapse in children with restrictive cardiomyopathy, Circulation 102 (2000) 876–882.

[12] M. Gewillig, L. Mertens, P. Moerman, et al., Idiopathic restrictive cardiomyopathy in childhood. A diastolic disorder characterized by delayed relaxation, Eur. Heart J. 17 (1996) 1413–1420.

[13] A.V. Mehta, P.L. Ferrer, A.S. Pickoff, et al., M-mode echocardiographic findings in children with idiopathic restrictive cardiomyopathy, Pediatr. Cardiol. 5 (1984) 273–280.

[14] A.P. Fitzpatrick, L.M. Shapiro, A.F. Rickards, et al., Familial restrictive cardiomyopathy with atrioventricular block and skeletal myopathy, Br. Heart J. 63 (1990) 114–118.

[15] M. Toussaint, C. Planche, E. Villain, et al., Restrictive cardiomyopathy in children. Ultrastructural findings, Virchows Arch. A 412 (1987) 27–29.

[16] D.W. Sapire, A. Casta, L.E. Swischuk, et al., Massive dilatation of the atria and coronary sinus in a child with restrictive cardiomyopathy and persistence of the left superior vena cava, Cathet Cardiovasc. Diagn. 9 (1983) 47–53.

[17] G.H. Erath, T.P. Graham, C.W. Smith, et al., Restrictive cardiomyopathy in an infant with massive biatrial enlargement and normal ventricular size and pump function, Cathet Cardiovasc. Diagn. 4 (1978) 289–296.

[18] M. Ishijima, S. Kawai, R. Okada, et al., An autopsy case of cardiomyopathy with restrictive physiology in a child, Heart Vessel. (Suppl. 5) (1990) 70–73.

[19] T. Maki, I. Niimura, T. Nishikawa, et al., An atypical case of cardiomyopathy in a child: hypertrophic or restrictive, Heart Vessel. (Suppl. 5) (1990) 84–87.

[20] R.A. Schieber, P.R. Lurie, H.B. Neustein, Restrictive cardiomyopathy with pseudotumor formation of the left ventricle, Pediatr. Cardiol. 3 (1982) 153–159.

[21] A. Miyazaki, F. Ichida, Y. Suzuki, et al., Long-term follow-up of a child with idiopathic restrictive cardiomyopathy, Heart Vessel. (Suppl. 5) (1990) 74–76.

[22] T. Nishikawa, Y. Tanaka, Y. Sasaki, et al., A case of pediatric cardiomyopathy with severely restrictive physiology, Heart Vessel. 7 (1992) 206–210.

[23] C. Aroney, N. Bett, D. Radford, Familial restrictive cardiomyopathy, Aust. N.Z. J. Med. 18 (1988) 877–878.

[24] T. Izumi, F. Masani, S. Mitsuma, et al., Juvenile cases of restrictive cardiomyopathy without eosinophilia, Heart Vessel. (Suppl. 5) (1990) 77–79.

[25] C. Rapezzi, P. Ortolani, G. Binetti, et al., Idiopathic restrictive cardiomyopathy in the young: report of two cases, Int. J. Cardiol. 29 (1990) 121–126.

[26] E. Bertini, C. Bosman, M. Bevilacqua, et al., Cardiomyopathy and multicore myopathy with accumulation of intermediate filaments, Eur. J. Pediatr. 149 (1990) 856–858.

[27] U. Neudorf, A. Bolte, D. Lang, et al., Diagnostic findings and outcome in children with primary restrictive cardiomyopathy, Cardiol. Young 6 (1996) 44–47.

[28] A. Angelini, V. Calzolari, G. Thiene, et al., Morphologic spectrum of primary restrictive cardiomyopathy, Am. J. Cardiol. 80 (1997) 1046–1050.

[29] M.L. Hughes, S. Kleinert, A. Keogh, et al., Pulmonary vascular resistance and reactivity in children with end-stage cardiomyopathy, J. Heart Lung Transplant. 19 (2000) 701–794 20.

[30] R.J. Weller, R. Weintraub, L.J. Addonizo, et al., Outcome of idiopathic restrictive cardiomyopathy in children, Am. J. Cardiol. 90 (2002) 501–506.

[31] M.T. Kimberling, D.T. Balzer, R. Hirsch, et al., Cardiac transplantation for pediatric restrictive cardiomyopathy: presentation, evaluation and short term outcome, J. Heart Lung Transplant. 21 (2002) 455–459.

[32] M.L. Schwartz, S.D. Colan, Familial restrictive cardiomyopathy with skeletal abnormalities, Am. J. Cardiol. 92 (2003) 636–639.

[33] J.J. Facher, E.J. Regier, G.H. Jacobs, E. Siwik, J.-P. Delaunoy, N.H. Robin, Cardiomyopathy in Coffin-Lowry syndrome, Am. J. Med. Genet. Part A 128A (2004) 176–178.

[34] L.M. Russo, S.A. Webber, Idiopathic restrictive cardiomyopathy in children, Heart 91 (2005) 1199–1202.

[35] M.J. Fenton, H. Chubb, McMahon, et al., Heart and heart lung transplantation for idiopathic restrictive cardiomyopathy in children, Heart 91 (2005) 185–189.

[36] A.J. Bogard, S. Mital, J.C. Schwarzenberger, et al., Twenty-year experience with heart transplantation infants and children with restrictive cardiomyopathy:1986–2006, Am. J. Transplant. 8 (2008) 201–207.

[37] T. Hayashi, E. Tsuda, K. Kurosaki, et al., Electrocardiographic and clinical characteristics of idiopathic restrictive cardiomyopathy in children, Circ. J. 71 (2007) 1534–1539.

[38] T. Sanna, A. Dello Russo, D. Toniolo, M. Vytopil, G. Pelargonio, G. De Martino, E. Ricci, G. Silvestri, V. Giglio, L. Messano, E. Zachara, F. Bellocci, Cardiac features of Emery-Dreifuss muscular dystrophy caused by lamin A/C gene mutations, Eur. Heart J. 24 (2003) 2227–2236.

[39] J. Mogensen, T. Kubo, M. Duque, et al., Idiopathic restrictive cardiomyopathy is part of the clinical expression of cardiac troponin I mutations, J. Clin. Investig. 111 (2) (2003) 209–216.

[40] M.C. Dalakas, K.-Y. Park, C. Semino-Mora, et al., Desmin myopathy, a skeletal myopathy with cardiomyopathy caused by mutations in the desmin gene, N. Engl. J. Med. 342 (2000) 770–780.

[41] L.G. Goldfarb, K.-Y. Park, L. CerveneKova, et al., Missense mutations in desmin associated with familial cardiac and skeletal myopathy, Nat. Genet. 19 (1998) 402–403.

[42] J.P. Kaski, P. Syrris, M. Burch, et al., Idiopathic restrictive cardiomyopathy in children is caused by gene mutations in cardiac sarcomere protein genes, Heart 94 (2008) 1478–1484.

[43] S.B. Peddy, L.A. Vricella, J.E. Crosson, et al., Infantile restrictive cardiomyopathy resulting from a mutation in the cardiac troponin T gene, Pediatrics 117 (2006) 1830–1833.

[44] S.M. Ware, M.E. Quinn, E.T. Ballard, et al., Pediatric restrictive cardiomyopathy associated with a mutation in beta-myosin heavy chain, Clin. Genet. 73 (2008) 165–170.

[45] P. Richard, P. Charron, L. Carrier, et al., Hypertrophic cardiomyopathy: distribution of disease genes, spectrum of mutations, and implications for molecular diagnosis strategy, Circulation 107 (2003) 2227–2232.

[46] T.M. Olson, M.L. Karst, F.G. Whitby, et al., Myosin light chain mutation causes autosomal recessive cardiomyopathy with mid-cavitary hypertrophy and restrictive physiology, Circulation 105 (2002) 2337–2340.

[47] E. Arbustini, M. Pasotti, A. Pilotto, et al., Desmin accumulation restrictive cardiomyopathy and atrioventricular block associated with desmin gene defects, Eur. J. Heart Fail. 8 (2006) 477–483.

[48] J. Zhang, A. Kumar, H.J. Stalker, et al., Clinical and molecular studies of a large family with desmin-associated restrictive cardiomyopathy, Clin. Genet. 59 (2001) 248–256.

[49] Y. Peled, M. Gramlich, G. Yoskovitz, et al., Titin mutation in familial restrictive cardiomyopathy, Int. J. Cardiol. 171 (1) (January 15, 2014) 24–30.

[50] S. Duygu, F. Muntoni, B.K. Burton, et al., Mutation in BAG3 causes severe dominant childhood muscular dystrophy, Ann. Neurol. 65 (2009) 83–89.

[51] A. Brodehl, R.A. Ferrier, S.J. Hamilton, et al., Mutations in FLNC are associated with familial restrictive cardiomyopathy, Hum. Mutat. 37 (3) (March 2016) 269–279, http://dx.doi.org/10.1002/humu.22942. (Epub January 8, 2016).

[52] S. Sen-Chowdhry, P. Syrris, W.J. McKenna, Genetics of restrictive cardiomyopathy, Heart Fail. Clin. 6 (2) (2010) 179–186.

[53] J.D. Marshall, R.B. Paisey, C. Carey, et al., Alstrom syndrome, in: R.A. Pagan, T.D. Bird, C.R. Dolan, K. Stephens (Eds.), GeneReviews [Internet], University of Washington, Seattle (WA), February 7, 2003, pp. 1993–2014 (Updated May 31, 2012).

[54] J. Delaunoy, F. Abidi, M. Zeniou, S. Jacquot, K. Merienne, S. Pannetier, M. Schmitt, C. Schwartz, A. Hanauer, Mutations in the x-linked RSK 2 gene (RPS6KA3) in patients with Coffin-Lowry Syndrome, Hum. Mutat. 17 (2) (2001) 103–116.

[55] N. Karlberg, H. Jalanko, J. Perheentupa, M. Lipsanen-Nyman, Mulibrey nanism; clinical features and diagnostic criteria, J. Med. Genet. 41 (2004) 92–98.

[56] A. Eerola, J.I. Pihkala, N. Karlberg, M. Lipsanen-Nyman, E. Jokinen, Cardiac dysfunction in children with Mulibrey nanism, Pediatr. Cardiol. 28 (2007) 155–162.

[57] M. Lipsanen-Nyman, J. Preheentupa, J. Rapola, A. Sovijarvi, M. Kupari, Mulibrey heart disease: clinical manifestation, long-term course and results of pericardiectomy in a series of 49 patients born before 1985, Circulation 107 (2003) 2810–2815.

[58] A.E. Lin, C. Michot, V. Cormier-Daire, et al., Gain-of-function mutations in SMAD4 cause a distinctive repertoire of cardiovascular phenotypes in patients with Myhre syndrome, Am. J. Med. Genet. A (June 14, 2016)http://dx.doi.org/10.1002/ajmg.a.37739. (Epub ahead of print).

[59] L.J. Starr, D.K. Grange, J.W. Delaney, et al., Myhre syndrome: clinical features and restrictive cardiopulmonary complications, Am. J. Med. Genet. A 167A (12) (December 2015) 2893–2901, http://dx.doi.org/10.1002/ajmg.a.37273. (Epub September 30, 2015).

[60] E. Pahl, S.A. Miller, B.P. Griffith, et al., Occult restrictive hemodynamics after pediatric heart transplantation, J. Heart Lung Transplant. 14 (1995) 1109–1115.

[61] S.S. Kushwaha, J.T. Fallon, V. Fuster, Restrictive cardiomyopathy, N. Engl. J. Med. 336 (1997) 267–276.

[62] J.N.P. Davies, Endocardial fibrosis in Africans, East Afr. Med. J. 25 (1948) 10.

[63] A.O. Mocumbi, M.B. Ferreira, D. Sidi, et al., A population study of endomyocardial fibrosis in a rural area of Mozambique, N. Engl. J. Med. 359 (2008) 43–49.

[64] A.O. Mocumbi, S. Yacoub, M.H. Yacoub, Neglected tropical cardiomyopthies: II, Heart 94 (2008) 384–390.

[65] R.A. Johnson, I. Palacios, Nondilated cardiomyopathies, Adv. Intern. Med. 30 (1984) 243–274.

[66] A. Grimaldi, A.O. Mocumbi, J. Freers, et al., Tropical endomyocardial fibrosis: natural history, challenges, and perspectives, Circulation 133 (24) (June 14, 2016) 2503–2515.

[67] R. Mankad, C. Bonnichsen, S. Mankad, Hypereosinophilic syndrome: cardiac diagnosis and management, Heart 102 (2) (January 2016) 100–106.
[68] D.J. Radford, R.B. Garlick, P.G. Pohlner, Multiple valvar replacements for hypereosinophilia syndrome, Cardiol. Young 12 (2002) 67–70.
[69] C.L. Santos, C.R. Moraes, F.L. Santos, et al., Endomyocardial fibrosis in children, Cardiol. Young 11 (2001) 205–209.
[70] M.P. Dixit, I. Greifer, Nephropathic cystinosis associated with cardiomyopathy: a 27-year clinical follow-up, BMC Nephrol. 3 (2002) 8–16.
[71] S.A. Mortensen, H.S. Olsen, U. Baandrup, Chronic anthracycline cardiotoxicity: haemodynamic and histopathological manifestations suggesting a restrictive endomyocardial disease, Br. Heart J. 55 (1986) 274–282.
[72] F.A. Bu'Lock, M.G. Mott, A. Oakhill, et al., Left ventricular diastolic function after anthracycline chemotherapy in childhood: relation with systolic function, symptoms and pathophysiology, Br. Heart J. 73 (1995) 340–350.
[73] J.W. Mason, M.E. Billingham, J.P. Friedman, Methysergide-induced heart disease: a case of multivalvular and myocardial fibrosis, Circulation 56 (1977) 889–890.
[74] M.E. Billingham, Pharmacotoxic myocardial disease: an endomyocardial study, Heart Vessel. Suppl. 1 (1985) 278–282.
[75] M. Pieroni, C. Smaldone, A. Camporeale, C. Ierardi, G. Dell'Antonio, F. Bellocci, F. Crea, Chloroquine-Induced transition from dilated to restrictive cardiomyopathy, J. Am. Coll. Cardiol. 57 (2011) 515.
[76] J.S. Gottdiener, M.J. Katin, J.S. Borer, et al., Late cardiac effects of therapeutic mediastinal irradiation: assessment by echocardiography and radionuclide angiography, N. Engl. J. Med. 308 (1983) 569–572.
[77] L.H. Opie, Normal and abnormal cardiac function, in: E. Braunwald, D.P. Zipes, P. Libby (Eds.), Heart Disease a Textbook of Cardiovascular Medicine, sixth ed., W.B. Saunders Company, Philadelphia, 2001, pp. 463–464.
[78] J.S. Child, J.K. Perloff, The restrictive cardiomyopathies, Cardiol. Clin. 6 (1988) 289–316.
[79] M.S. Parvatiyar, J.R. Pinto, D. Dweck, et al., Cardiac troponin mutations and restrictive cardiomyopathy, J. Biomed. Biotechnol. 2010 (2010) 350706, http://dx.doi.org/10.1155/2010/350706. (Epub June 8, 2010).
[80] J.R. Pinto, S.W. Yang, M.-P. Hitz, et al., Fetal cardiac troponin isoforms rescue the increase Ca^{2+} sensitivity produced by a novel double deletion in cardiac troponin T linked to restrictive cardiomyopathy a clinical, genetic and functional approach, J. Biol. Chem. 286 (2011) 20901–20912.
[81] S.C. Greenway, G.J. Wilson, J. Wilson, et al., Sudden death in an infant with angina, restrictive cardiomyopathy, and coronary artery bridging: an unusual phenotype for a β-myosin heavy chain (MYH7) sarcomeric protein mutation, Circ. Heart Fail. 5 (6) (November 2012) e92–e93.
[82] M.A. Walsh, M.A. Grenier, J.L. Jeffries, et al., Conduction abnormalities in pediatric patients with restrictive cardiomyopathy, Circ. Heart Fail. 5 (2012) 267–273.
[83] N. Sasaki, M. Garcia, I. Lytrivi, et al., Utility of Doppler tissue imaging-derived indices in identifying subclinical systolic ventricular dysfunction in children with restrictive cardiomopathy, Pediatr. Cardiol. 32 (2011) 646–651.
[84] H. Turhan, A. Ocal, A.L. Erby, et al., Free-floating left atrial ball thrombus developed in an 11-year old child with restrictive cardiomyopathy during sinus rhythm: manifested as a major embolic event, Int. J. Cardiol. 103 (2005) 111–113.
[85] I.A. Al-Ammouri, Massive intra-atrial thrombosis in an 11 year-old child with restrictive cardiomyopathy, Pediatr. Cardiol. 31 (2010) 735–736.
[86] K. Chen, S. Williams, A.K.C. Chan, et al., Thrombosis and embolism in pediatric cardiomyopathy, Blood Coagul. Fibrinolysis 24 (2013) 221–230.
[87] M.A. Quiñones, Assessment of diastolic function, Prog. Cardiovasc. Dis. 47 (2005) 340–355.
[88] N. Sasaki, M. Garcia, H.H. Ko, et al., Applicability of published guidelines for assessment of left ventricular diastolic dysfunction in adults to children with restrictive cardiomyopathy: an observational study, Pediatr. Cardiol. (September 6, 2014) (Epub ahead of print).
[89] P.W. O'Leary, K. Durongpisitkul, T.M. Cordes, K.R. Bailey, D.J. Hagler, A.J. Tajik, J.B. Seward, Diastolic ventricular function in children: a Doppler echocardiographic study establishing normal values and predictors of increased ventricular end-diastolic pressure, Mayo Clin. Proc. 73 (1998) 616–628.
[90] A. Dragulescu, L. Mertens, M.K. Friedberg, Interpretation of left ventricular diastolic dysfunction in children with cardiomyopathy by echocardiography problems and limitations, Cric. Cardiovasc. Imaging 6 (2013) 254–261.
[91] D.S. Ezon, S.A. Maskatia, K. Sexson-Tejtel, et al., Tissue Doppler imaging measures correlate poorly with left ventricular filling pressures in pediatric cardiomyopathy, Congenit. Heart Dis. 10 (5) (September–October 2015) E203–E209, http://dx.doi.org/10.1111/chd.12267.
[92] M.F. Kozak, M. Alariefy, J.A. Kirsh, Triphasic mitral and tricuspid flows: a sign of diastolic dysfunction in a young patient with severely dilated atria and giant pulmonary veins, Pediatr. Cardiol. 34 (2013) 1979–1981.
[93] M.K. Friedberg, N.H. Silverman, The systolic to diastolic duration ratio in children with heart failure secondary to restrictive cardiomyopathy, J. Am. Soc. Echocardiogr. 19 (2006) 1326–1331.
[94] L. Hatle, Doppler echocardiographic evaluation diastolic function hypertensive cardiomyopathies, Eur. Heart J. 14 (1993) 88–94.
[95] P. Palka, A. Lange, J.E. Donnelly, et al., Differentiation between restrictive cardiomyopathy and constrictive pericarditis by early diastolic Doppler myocardial velocity gradient at the posterior wall, Circulation 102 (2000) 655–662.
[96] N. Rajagopalan, M.J. Garcia, L. Rodriguez, et al., Comparison of new Doppler echocardiographic methods to differentiate constrictive pericardial heart disease and restrictive cardiomyopathy, Am. J. Cardiol. 87 (2001) 86–94.
[97] J.J. McMurray, S. Adamopoulos, S.D. Anker, et al., ESC guidelines for the diagnosis and treatment of acute and chronic heart failure 2012: The task force for the diagnosis and treatment of acute and chronic heart failure 2012 of the European Society of Cardiology. Developed in collaboration with the Heart Failure Association (HFA) of the ESC, Eur. Heart J. 33 (2012) 1787–1847.
[98] M.H. Schoenfeld, The differentiation of restrictive cardiomyopathy from constrictive pericarditis, Cardiol. Clin. 8 (1990) 663–671.
[99] S. Webber, S.E. Lipshultz, L.A. Sleeper, et al., Outcomes of restrictive cardiomyopathy in childhood and the influence of phenotype a report from the pediatric cardiomyopathy registry, Circulation 126 (2012) 1237–1244.

[100] S.A. Maskatia, J.A. Decker, J.A. Spinner, et al., Restrictive physiology is a major predictor of poor outcomes in children with hypertrophic cardiomyopathy, Pediatr. Cardiol. 33 (2012) 141–149.

[101] S. Hook, N.B. Ratliff, E. Rosenkranz, et al., Isolated noncompaction of the ventricular myocardium, Pediatr. Cardiol. 17 (1996) 43–45.

[102] S. Ozkutlu, S. Hascelik, D. Yalnizoglu, et al., Familial isolated non- compaction of myocardium presenting as restrictive cardiomyopathy, Pediatr. Int. 49 (2007) 536–539.

[103] E. Biagini, L. Ragni, M. Ferlito, et al., Different types of cardiomyopathy associated with isolated ventricular noncompaction, Am. J. Cardiol. 98 (2006) 821–824.

[104] S.E. Lipshultz, E.J. Orav, J.D. Wilkinson, et al., Risk stratification at diagnosis for children with hypertrophic cardiomyopathy: an analysis of data from the Pediatric Cardiomyopathy Registry, Lancet 382 (2013) 1889–1897.

[105] T. Bharucha, K.J. Lee, P.E. Daubeney, et al., Sudden death in childhood cardiomyopathy: results from a long-term national population-based study, J. Am. Coll. Cardiol. 65 (21) (June 2, 2015) 2302–2310, http://dx.doi.org/10.1016/j.jacc.2015.03.552.

[106] A.R. Bengur, R.H. Beekman, A.P. Rocchini, et al., Acute hemodynamic effects of Captopril in children with a congestive or restrictive cardiomyopathy, Circulation 83 (1991) 523–527.

[107] D. Rosenthal, R. Weintraub, L. Bannister, et al., Pharmacologic treatment of heart failure with 'preserved EF' (diastolic heart failure), in: R. Kirk, A.I. Dipchand, D.N. Rosenthal, J.K. Kirklin (Eds.), ISHLT Guidelines for the Management of Pediatric Heart Failure, vol. 8, UAB Printing, Birmingham, Alabama, 2014, pp. 142–149.

[108] M.R. Zile, D.L. Brutsaert, New concepts in diastolic dysfunction and diastolic heart failure: part II, Circulation 105 (2002) 1503–1508.

[109] F. Edelmann, L. Musial-Bright, G. Gelbrich, et al., Tolerability and feasibility of beta-blocker titration in HFpEF versus HFrEF: insights from the CIBIS-ELD trial, J. Am. Coll. Cardiol. 4 (2016) 140–149.

[110] S.W. Denfield, Sudden death in children with restrictive cardiomyopathy, CEPR 6 (2002) 163–167.

[111] M. Guazzi, A. Vitelli, V. Labate, et al., Treatment for pulmonary hypertension of left heart disease, Curr. Treat. Options Cardiovasc. Med. 14 (2012) 319–327.

[112] M.M. Redfield, H.H. Chen, B.A. Borlaug, et al., Effect of phosphodiesterase-5 inhibition on exercise capacity and clinical status in heart failure with preserved ejection fraction: a randomized clinical trial, JAMA 309 (2013) 1268–1277.

[113] S.D. Zangwill, D. Naftel, L'Ecuyer, et al., Outcomes of children with restrictive cardiomyopathy listed for heart transplantation: a multi-institutional study, J. Heart Lung Transplant. 28 (2009) 1335–1340.

[114] T.P. Singh, C.S. Almond, G. Piercey, et al., Current outcomes in US children with cardiomyopathy listed for heart transplantation, Circ. Heart Fail. 5 (2012) 594–601.

[115] B. Murtuza, M. Fenton, M. Burch, et al., Pediatric heart transplantation for congenital and restrictive cardiomyopathy, Ann. Thorac. Surg. 95 (2013) 1675–1684.

[116] P. Chiu, M.J. Russo, R.R. Davies, et al., What is high risk? Redefining elevated pulmonary vascular resistance in pediatric heart transplantation, J. Heart Lung Transplant. 31 (2012) 61–66.

[117] P. Chiu, J.M. Schaffer, A.Y. Sheikh, et al., Elevated pretransplant pulmonary vascular resistance index does not predict mortality after isolated orthotopic heart transplantation in children: a retrospective analysis of the UNOS database, Pediatr. Transplant. 19 (6) (September 2015) 623–633, http://dx.doi.org/10.1111/petr.12550. (Epub July 15, 2015). PMID: 26179628.

[118] A. Al-Khaldi, B.A. Reitz, H. Zhu, et al., Heterotopic heart transplant with postoperative sidenafil use for the treatment of restrictive cardiomyopathy, Ann. Thorac. Surg. 81 (2006) 1505–1507.

[119] A.I. Dipchand, D.C. Naftel, B. Feingold, et al., Outcomes of children with cardiomyopathy listed for heart transplant: a multi-institutional study, J. Heart Lung Transplant. 28 (2009) 1312–1321.

[120] J. Philip, C. Burgman, A. Bavare, et al., Nature of the underlying heart disease affects survival in pediatric patients undergoing extracorporeal cardiopulmonary resuscitation, J. Thorac. Cardiovasc. Surg. 148 (5) (November 2014) 2367–2372, http://dx.doi.org/10.1016/j.jtcvs.2014.03.023.

[121] S. Sundararajan, T. Thiruchelvam, T.-Y. Hsia, et al., New 15-ml ventricular assist device in children with restrictive physiology of the left ventricle, J. Thorac. Cardiovasc. Surg. 147 (2014) e79–80.

[122] T.O. Thomas, S. Chandrakasan, M. O'Brien, et al., The use of a Berlin Heart EXCOR LVAD in a child receiving chemotherapy for Castleman's disease, Pediatr. Transplant. 19 (2015) E15–E18.

[123] H. Tunuguntla, S.W. Denfield, E.D. McKenzie, I. Adachi, Mitral valve replacement for inflow obstruction of left ventricular assist device in a child with restrictive cardiomyopathy, J. Thorac. Cardiovasc. Surg. 151 (1) (January 2016) e11–e13.

[124] S.C. Malaisrie, M.P. Pelletier, J.J. Yun, et al., Pneumatic paracorporeal ventricular assist device in infants and children: initial Stanford experience, J. Heart Lung Transplant. 27 (2) (February 2008) 173–177, http://dx.doi.org/10.1016/j.healun.2007.11.567.

[125] J.L. Barros, G.F. Perez, Pulmonary stenosis due to external compression by a pericardial band, Br. Heart J. 29 (1967) 947–949.

[126] E. Chesler, A.S. Mitha, R.E. Matisson, et al., Subpulmonic stenosis as a result of noncalcific constrictive pericarditis, Chest 69 (1976) 425–427.

[127] R.A. Nishimura, F.J. Kazmier, H.C. Smith, et al., Right ventricular outflow obstruction caused by constrictive pericardial disease, AM. J. Cardiol. 55 (1985) 1447–1448.

[128] G.P. Ramdas, T. Ryad, W. Sammy, Constrictive pericarditis causing extrinsic mitral stenosis and a left heart mass, Clin. Cardiol. 19 (1996) 517–519.

[129] J.S. McGinn, D.P. Zipes, Constrictive pericarditis causing tricuspid stenosis, Arch. Intern. Med. 129 (1972) 487–490.

[130] A. Simcha, J.F.N. Taylor, Constrictive pericarditis in childhood, Arch. Dis. Child. 46 (1971) 515–519.

[131] A.W. Strauss, M. Santa-Maria, D. Goldring, Constrictive pericarditis in children, Am. J. Dis. Child. 129 (1975) 822–826.

[132] J. Roshe, H.B. Shumacker, Pericardiectomy for chronic cardiac tamponade in children, Surgery 46 (1959) 1152–1161.

[133] G.G. Griese, Chronic pericarditis in children, Wisc. Med. J. 74 (1975) S21–S24.
[134] J.L. Thompson, H.M. Burkhart, J.A. Dearani, et al., Pericardiectony for pericarditis in the pediatric population, Ann. Thorac. Surg. 88 (5) (November 2009) 1546–1550 PMID: 19853110.
[135] P. Lapunzina, I. Rodriguez, E. de Matteo, et al., Mulibrey Nanism: three additional patients and a review of 39 patients, Am. J. Med. Genet. A 55 (1995) 349–355.
[136] U.N. Verma, R. Misra, S. Radhakrisnan, et al., A syndrome of fibrosing pleuritic, and synovitis with infantile contractures of fingers and toes in 2 sisters: "Familial fibrosing serositis", J. Rheumatol. 22 (1995) 2349–2355.
[137] A. Beundia, F. Attie, M. Martinez-Lavin, The syndrome of pericarditis, arthritis, and camptodactyly: an under-recognized cause of pericardial constriction in children? Cardiol. Young 9 (1999) 526–528.
[138] S.A. Bahabri, W.M. Suwairi, R.M. Laxer, et al., The camptodactyly-arthropathy-cosa vara-pericarditis syndrome, Arthritis Rheum. 41 (1998) 730–735.
[139] B. Peters, J.H. Schuurs-Hoeijmakers, et al., Protein-losing enteropahty in camptodactyly-arthropathy-coxa vara-pericarditis (CAPC) syndrome, Pediatr. Rheumatol. Online J. 14 (1) (May 25, 2016) 32 PMID: 27224999.
[140] J.M. DeLine, D.G. Cable, Clustering of recurrent pericarditis with effusion and constriction in a family, Mayo Clin. Proc. 77 (2002) 39–43.
[141] K. Harada, I. Seki, M. Okuni, Constrictive pericarditis with atrial septal defect in children, Jpn. Heart J. 19 (1978) 531–543.
[142] M. Gaudino, A. Anselmi, N. Pavone, M. Massetti, Constrictive pericarditis after cardiac surgery, Ann. Thorac. Surg. 95 (2) (February 2013) 731–736.
[143] R. Bansal, L. Perez, A. Razzouk, et al., Pericardial constriction after cardiac transplantation, J. Heart Lung Transplant. 29 (3) (2010) 371–377.
[144] D.H. Spodic, Constrictive pericarditis, in: D.H. Spodick (Ed.), The Pericardium: A Comprehensive Textbook, Marcel Dekker, New York, 1997, pp. 214–259.
[145] G.M. Brockington, J. Zebede, N.G. Pandian, Constrictive pericarditis, Cardiol. Clin. 8 (1990) 645–661.
[146] J. Sagrista-Sauleda, J. Angel, A. Sanchez, et al., Effusive-constrictive pericarditis, N. Engl. J. Med. 350 (2004) 469–475.
[147] R.B.H. Myers, D.H. Spodick, Constrictive pericarditis: clinical and pathophysiologic characteristics, Am. Heart J. 138 (1999) 219–232.
[148] D.K. Shea, J.W. Kirklin, J.W. Dushane, Chronic constrictive pericarditis in children, Am. J. Dis. Child. (1957) 93-430-435.
[149] F.S. Idriss, H. Nikaidoh, A. Muster, Constrictive pericarditis simulating liver disease in children, Arch. Surg. 109 (1974) 223–226.
[150] R.D. Greenwood, A. Rosenthal, R. Cassady, et al., Constrictive pericarditis in childhood due to mediastinal irradiation, Circulation 50 (1974) 1033–1039.
[151] G.B. Haycock, S.C. Jordan, Chronic pericardial constriction with effusion in childhood, Arch. Dis. Child. 54 (1979) 890–895.
[152] S.-J. Chen, Y.-W. Li, M.-H. Wu, et al., CT and MRI findings in a child with constrictive pericarditis, Pediatr. Cardiol. 19 (1998) 259–262.
[153] S.M.A.G. Ferreira, A.G. Ferreira, A. de Nascimento Morais, et al., Constrictive chronic pericarditis in children, Cardiol. Young 11 (2001) 210–213.
[154] W.H. Plauth, T.A. Waldmann, D.R. Wochner, et al., Protein-losing enteropathy secondary to constrictive Pericarditis in childhood, Pediatrics 34 (1964) 636–648.
[155] A. Allaria, D. Michelli, H. Capelli, et al., Transient cardiac constriction following purulent pericarditis, Eur. J. Pediatr. 151 (1992) 250–251.
[156] J.H. Haley, A.J. Tajik, G.K. Danielson, et al., Transient constrictive pericarditis: causes and natural history, J. Am. Coll. Cardiol. 43 (2) (January 21, 2004) 271–275.
[157] M. Amaki, J. Savino, D.L. Ain, et al., Diagnostic concordance of echocardiography and cardiac magnetic resonance-based tissue tracking for differentiating constrictive pericarditis from restrictive cardiomyopathy, Circ. Cardiovasc. Imaging 7 (5) (September 2014) 819–827.
[158] T.D. Welch, L.H. Ling, R.E. Espinosa, et al., Echocardiographic diagnosis of constrictive pericarditis: Mayo Clinic criteria, Circ. Cardiovasc. Imaging 7 (3) (2014) 526–534.
[159] A.L. Klein, S. Abbara, D.A. Agler, et al., American Society of Echocardiography clinical recommendations for multimodality cardiovascular imaging of patients with pericardial disease: endorsed by the Society for Cardiovascular Magnetic Resonance and Society of Cardiovascular Computed Tomography, J. Am. Soc. Echocardiogr. 26 (2013) 965.e15–1012 e15.
[160] W.G. Vick, R. Rokey, Cardiovascular magnetic resonance evaluation of the pericardium in health and disease, in: W. Manning, D.J. Pennell (Eds.), Cardiovascular Magnetic Resonance, Churchill Livingstone, Philadelphia, 2002, pp. 355–363.
[161] D. Feng, J. Glockner, K. Kim, et al., Cardiac magnetic resonance imaging pericardial late gadolinium enhancement and elevated inflammatory markers can predict the reversibility of constrictive pericarditis after antiinflammatory medical therapy: a pilot study, Circulation 124 (2011) 1830–1837.
[162] D.R. Talreja, R.A. Nishimura, J.K. Oh, D.R. Holmes, Constrictive pericarditis in the modern era: novel criteria for diagnosis in the cardiac catheterization laboratory, J. Am. Coll. Cardiol. 51 (3) (January 22, 2008) 315–319.
[163] T. Komoda, A. Frumkin, C. Knosalla, R. Hetzer, Child-Pugh score predicts survival after radical pericardiectomy for constrictive pericarditis, Ann. Thorac. Surg. 96 (5) (2013) 1679–1685.
[164] S. Talwar, V.V. Nair, S.K. Choudhary, et al., Pericardiectomy in children <15 years of age, Cardiol. Young 24 (4) (2014) 616–622.
[165] C.T. Hugo-Hamman, H. Scher, M.M.A. De Moor, Tuberculous pericarditis in children: a review of 44 cases, Pediatr. Infect. Dis. J. 13 (1994) 13–18.
[166] Y. Adler, P. Charron, M. Imazio, et al., 2015 ESC guidelines for the diagnosis and management of pericardial diseases: The Task Force for the Diagnosis and Management of Pericardial Diseases of the European Society of Cardiology (ESC)Endorsed by: The European Association for Cardio-Thoracic Surgery (EACTS), Eur. Heart J. 36 (42) (November 7, 2015) 2921–2964, http://dx.doi.org/10.1093/eurheartj/ehv318. (Epub August 29, 2015).
[167] M.M. LeWinter, Acute pericarditis, N. Engl. J. Med. 371 (2014) 2410–2416.

[168] M.Y. Henein, R.D. Rakhit, M.N. Sheppard, et al., Restrictive pericarditis, Heart 82 (1999) 389–392.
[169] A. Wang, R.N. Vincent, G. Johnson, et al., Mixed constrictive pericarditis and restrictive cardiomyopathy in a child: treatment guided by tissue Doppler imaging, Congenit. Heart Dis. 1 (2006) 35–39.
[170] P.P. Sengupta, V.K. Krishnamoorthy, W.P. Abhayaratna, et al., Comparison of usefulness of tissue Doppler imaging versus brain natriuretic peptide for differentiation of constrictive pericardicardial disease from restrictive cardiomyopathy, Am. J. Cardiol. 102 (2008) 876–882.
[171] F.S. Leya, D. Arab, D. Joyal, et al., The efficacy of brain natriuretic peptide levels in differentiating constrictive pericarditis from restrictive cardiomyopathy, J. Am. Coll. Cardiol. 45 (2005) 1900–1902.
[172] N. Parakh, S. Mehrotra, S. Seth, et al., NT pro B type natriuretic peptide levels in constrictive pericarditis and restrictive cardiomyopathy, Indian Heart J. 67 (1) (2015) 40–44.

FURTHER READING

[1] R.L. Van der Horst, Pericardial calcification in childhood, Cardiovasc. Radiol. 1 (1978) 265–267.

Chapter 19

Hypertrophic Cardiomyopathy

Steven D. Colan, Renee Margossian
Boston Children's Hospital, Boston, MA, United States

INTRODUCTION

Hypertrophic cardiomyopathy (HCM) is a rare condition during childhood, representing about 40% of pediatric cardiomyopathy cases with a reported incidence of 0.47/100,000 children [1]. Despite its rarity, it receives considerable attention in part because of an associated risk of sudden death, even in apparently healthy individuals who are not known to have heart disease. HCM in pediatric patients has a more diverse etiologic substrate than that seen in adult cohorts that not only includes familial (sarcomeric) forms but also inborn errors of metabolism, mitochondrial defects, neuromuscular disorders, and malformation syndromes. Although morbidity and mortality are 10-fold higher in the first year of life compared with the rest of childhood, the disease prevalence increases progressively over the course of childhood, particularly during adolescence, and is often associated with an adverse impact on the quality of life for affected children, out of proportion to the risk of sudden death. Despite these risks, most of these patients will have a normal life span. Consequently, the goal of management is to minimize the negative impact of the disease, both from a physical health and a psychosocial perspective.

DEFINITION

The diagnosis of HCM is based on the characteristic phenotype, defined as the presence of a hypertrophied, nondilated ventricle in the absence of a hemodynamic disturbance that can account for the existent magnitude of wall thickening, such as hypertension, aortic valve stenosis, catecholamine-secreting tumors, hyperthyroidism, and other disorders with similar hemodynamic impact. In addition to disease states, physiologic hypertrophy secondary to intense physical activity including sports participation is also excluded from this definition.

DIAGNOSTIC CRITERIA

The American College of Cardiology Foundation(ACCF)/American Heart Association (AHA) criterion for the diagnosis of HCM in adults is a wall thickness ≥15 mm on echocardiography, with wall thickness ≥13 and <15 considered borderline [2]. Because decisions concerning the presence or absence of disease are often not dichotomous, for any given severity of hypertrophy, the probability of disease in any individual should take into consideration those factors predicting a higher prior probability, such as a family history of HCM or confirmed presence of a pathogenic genotype. The European Society of Cardiology (ESC) employs the same diagnostic wall thickness criterion (≥15 mm) for adults but stipulates that wall thickness can be obtained by any imaging technique (echocardiography, cardiac magnetic resonance imaging (CMRI), or computed tomography) and similarly considers wall thicknesses ≥13 and <15 mm to be borderline, but this lesser thickness may be considered definitive in the presence of other features such as family history, myocardial cryps or disarray, or electrocardiographic abnormalities [3]. It is worth noting that isolated or regional hypertrophy is often encountered as the primary manifestation of HCM despite normal total left ventricular (LV) mass [4].

Unfortunately, both organizations recommend that for children the diagnostic criterion should be an LV wall thickness z-score ≥2 (i.e., wall thickness ≥2 standard deviations above the normal mean value for body surface area (BSA)). The error in this criterion relates to a failure to account for prior probability (Bayes Theorem) and is easily detected by calculating the equivalent z-score in adults. The normal LV wall thickness in adults is 6–10 mm, which means for adults the normal mean diastolic wall thickness is 8 mm with a standard deviation of 1 mm. The HCM diagnostic criterion of 15 mm therefore represents a value 7 standard deviations above the normal mean value, that is, z-score = 7, and the borderline

Heart Failure in the Child and Young Adult. http://dx.doi.org/10.1016/B978-0-12-802393-8.00019-3

criterion of 13–14 mm is equivalent to a z-score of 5–6. By setting the threshold for children at a z-score = 2, the AHA and ESC guidelines are using the equivalent of 10 mm in an adult as the diagnostic criterion, guaranteeing marked over-diagnosis of HCM in children. By definition, 2.3% of the normal population has a z-score >2, whereas the prevalence of the sarcomeric (HCM) gene in the general population is 1/500 (0.2%) [5]. However, only a fraction of the gene-positive individuals develop HCM during childhood, with at least one longitudinal study of genotype-positive, phenotype-negative children reporting a conversion rate of only 6% after 12 years of follow-up. The documented incidence of 0.47/100,000 during childhood [1] predicts a cumulative prevalence of 9/10,000 by age 18, which is a disease prior probability of <0.001%. Therefore, use of a z-score ≥2 as the diagnostic criterion for disease presence would result in an estimated false-positive diagnosis of the disease in children of >2000 for each correct diagnosis. This discrepancy in criteria also creates the potential for a teenager who is diagnosed as having HCM based on pediatric criteria requiring reclassification at age 18 years. There are undeniable potential adverse psychological, lifestyle, economic, and career consequences to having a false-positive diagnosis of HCM and very few benefits to early diagnosis of borderline HCM. Based on these observations and the documented low risk associated with mild hypertrophy in HCM, the z-score equivalent of the adult criteria are therefore recommended (z-score ≥7 considered definitive, z-score of ≥5 and <7 considered borderline) as the appropriate diagnostic criteria in children.

ETIOLOGY AND CLASSIFICATION

The etiologic basis for HCM varies markedly depending on age. In contrast to adult series where 85%–90% of cases are believed to be caused by autosomal dominant mutations in sarcomeric proteins, the etiology is far more diverse in pediatrics [6]. During infancy, most cases remain idiopathic, although progress is being made in this regard. The high mortality and lack of effective therapies for many of the nonsarcomeric forms of HCM in combination with the delayed onset of sarcomeric HCM results in familial forms of HCM becoming more prevalent over the course of childhood and by adolescence is by far the dominant cause. The etiology of HCM can be divided into isolated forms, where noncardiac manifestations are absent, and multisystem, where HCM is typically associated with noncardiac abnormalities. Table 19.1 presents a listing of the various types of HCM but should not be considered comprehensive because HCM has been seen in a number of rare diseases for which there are too few observations to know whether this is a chance or real association. Primary HCM accounts for 90% of cases in adults, and sarcomeric mutations are believed to account for the majority of cases of primary HCM in adults [7]. However, in unselected adult populations a pathogenic mutation is identified in only about 50%–60% of cases, with the highest yield in probands with a family history of disease (72% vs. 29% of cases). Thus, although primary HCM has generally been classified as a disease of the sarcomere, this remains to be fully documented, and indeed multiple forms of sarcomeric HCM phenocopies with isolated cardiac involvement have been described that are not sarcomeric in origin, including mitochondrial, storage, and x-linked forms. Furthermore, the yield of genetic testing may actually be lower than that which has been previously reported because misclassification of benign variants as pathogenic has recently been documented to be a significant dilemma when new, genetically distinct populations are studied [8]. The multisystem disorders that have been found to be associated with HCM include metabolic, mitochondrial, neuromuscular, and syndromic forms as listed in Table 19.1 and are discussed further below.

It should be noted that the classification system presented here is standardly used in pediatric cardiology and is aligned with the recommendations of the ESC HCM Guidelines [3]. However, the ACCF/AHA guidelines have taken an alternative approach to the nomenclature of HCM [2]. The ACCF/AHA position is that the multisystem disorders listed above "can mimic clinically diagnosed HCM," but state categorically that "use of the term HCM is not appropriate to describe these and other patients with LV hypertrophy that occurs in the context of a multisystem disorder." This is a recommendation that has been included in the ACCF/AHA guidelines for many years, and no scientific rationale has ever been presented for this recommendation. The multisystem disorders presented in Table 19.1 all meet the definition of HCM as presented above and as presented in the ACCF/AHA guidelines, and the overwhelming majority of publications on these disorders have described the disease as HCM. The alternative terminology recommended by the ACCF/AHA guidelines is "disease with LV hypertrophy" where the name of the systemic disease is substituted. For example, HCM associated with Noonan syndrome would be termed "Noonan syndrome with left ventricular hypertrophy (LVH)." The problem with this alternative nomenclature is that it does not distinguish between a primary disease of the myocardium (i.e., cardiomyopathy) versus ventricular hypertrophy due to hypertension, aortic stenosis, or another hemodynamic cause. The more accurate terminology that is preferred by the pediatric cardiology community is therefore used in this document.

TABLE 19.1 Taxonomy of Hypertrophic Cardiomyopathy

Primary (Isolated)	Disorders of fatty acid metabolism
Sarcomeric (Familial)	Carnitine palmitoyltransferase II deficiency
Mitochondrial	Carnitine-acylcarnitine translocase deficiency
X-linked	Carnitine deficiency
Secondary (Systemic, Syndromic)	Selenium deficiency
Infant of diabetic mother	Fucosidosis type 1
Metabolic	Total lipodystrophy
Glycogenoses	Mucopolysaccharidoses
LAMP2 (Danon disease)	Hurler's syndrome,
Adenosine monophosphate-activated protein kinase (PRKAG2)	Hunter's syndrome
Pompe disease (acid alpha-glucosidase, GAA)	Scheie's syndrome
Glycogen-storage disease III (Forbes disease, amylo-1,6 glucosidase)	Mitochondrial
Glycogen-storage disease IX (phosphorylase kinase deficiency)	MELAS (Mitochondrial encephalopathy, lactic acidosis, and stroke-like episodes)
AMP-activated protein kinase	MERFF (Myoclonic epilepsy with ragged-red fibers)
Lysosoma-storage disease	NADH-Coenzyme Q reductase deficiency
Glycolipid lipidosis (Anderson–Fabry disease)	Cytochrome b Deficiency
Hurler's syndrome	Syndromic
Hunter's syndrome	Friedreich Ataxia
I-Cell disease	Beckwith–Wiedemann syndrome
Mannnosidosis	RASopathies
Infantile sialic acid storage disease	Cardiofacialcutaneous syndrome
Sialidosis	Costello syndrome
Galactosialidosis	Multiple lentinginosis syndrome
Sandhoff disease	Noonan syndrome

LAMP2, lysosome-associated membrane protein 2.

PATHOPHYSIOLOGY AND NATURAL HISTORY

Abnormal myocardial hypertrophy is the essential abnormality of this disease, and the clinical course is largely though not exclusively dominated by this feature. Early descriptions of the disease relied predominantly on studies performed in large, relatively homogeneous cohorts and a typical pattern of new onset hypertrophy in early adolescence that reached a plateau in mid-to-late adolescence was described. Based on this finding, one-time screening of children with a family history of HCM sometime during early-to-midadolescence became the standard practice. With increased availability of imaging of at-risk populations this "typical" scenario has been to some degree confirmed although it has also become clear that the penetrance during childhood is much lower than previously believed [9], and new onset disease expression can occur at any age. Furthermore, a variety of "preclinical" manifestations have been identified on electrocardiography (ECG) and echocardiography in gene-positive family members that can precede the appearance of hypertrophy [10]. The temporal relationship between onset of these preclinical and onset of pathological hypertrophy is currently an area of vigorous investigation, including the issue as to whether some individuals will never progress from preclinical to clinical.

The pathophysiologic relationship between the morphologic manifestations and the genetic abnormalities has been a robust area of controversy. The contemporary mechanistic paradigm for HCM is that pathologic gene mutations trigger a cascade of cardiomyocyte responses including changes in calcium homeostasis, energy use, and gene expression that are associated with alterations in sarcomere function, ultimately culminating in the typical pathological features of myocardial hypertrophy, disarray, and fibrosis [11,12]. The mechanisms by which these gene alterations translate into disease expression have also been a focus of investigation. Although the myosin-binding protein C, cardiac (MYBPC3) mutations appear to reduce the amount of full-length protein, resulting in insufficient protein for normal function [13], most sarcomere mutations associated with HCM are missense alleles that result in single amino acid substitutions, which adversely affect sarcomere function. A substantial body of evidence indicates that HCM mutations in myofilament proteins generally increase Ca^{++} sensitivity and Ca^{++} affinity, and it appears likely that these changes in Ca^{++} sensitivity and the consequent defective intracellular Ca^{++} cycling, sarcoplasmic reticulum Ca^{++} reuptake and protein phosphorylation likely contribute to many aspects of HCM [14]. In contrast, dilated cardiomyopathy has been associated with decreased myofilament Ca^{++} sensitivity [15], leading to a general paradigm of differential effects of sarcomere mutations on integrated tension development compared to normal as a potential explanation for why mutations in the same genes can result in HCM (increased tension index) or dilated cardiomyopathy (decreased tension index) [16], with force development providing a greater predictive capacity than Ca^{++} sensitivity. This paradigm has proven particularly useful in terms of investigations targeting the potential for pharmacologic interventions that might impact this fundamental mechanism.

Myocardial disarray was one of the earliest recognized features of HCM. Myofiber disarray is closely associated with interstitial and subendocardial fibrosis as well as ventricular diastolic dysfunction and risk of arrhythmia [17,18]. Myocardial disarray is not unique to sarcomeric HCM, having been described in association with various forms of congenital heart disease characterized by pressure overload hypertrophy and is also found in some of the nonsarcomeric forms of HCM, including Noonan syndrome and related disorders, thereby indicating that it is not intrinsically linked to sarcomeric disorders. Random and therefore competing myofiber orientation is associated with isometric contraction and would therefore be predicted to result in localized hypertrophy, and indeed the disarray is typically most notable in the areas with the portion of myocardium with the most marked regional hypertrophy. The pattern of myofiber disarray is also seen in animal models of HCM, although it is not clear whether the disarray precedes or accompanies myocardial hypertrophy.

GENETICS OF SARCOMERIC HYPERTROPHIC CARDIOMYOPATHY

The genetic basis for HCM is broadly classified as arising from mutations in contractile (sarcomeric) and noncontractile proteins. Diseases due to mutations in the noncontractile proteins generally have systemic manifestations in addition to nonhemodynamically induced LVH. Examples finclude the GLA gene (encodes the enzyme alpha-galactosidase, responsible for Fabry disease), protein kinase AMP-activated noncatalytic subunit gamma 2 (PRKAG2) and lysosome-associated membrane protein 2 (LAMP2) (related to carbohydrate metabolism), and genes in the RAS MAP kinase pathway involved in Noonan syndrome. These syndromic disorders are discussed in more detail below.

Sarcomeric HCM is inherited in an autosomal dominant pattern; the first-degree relatives of an affected individual each have a 50% chance of sharing the mutation and are thus at risk for developing HCM. The first gene identified was localized to 14q11.2-q12 [19] and since that publication in 1989 more than 1500 mutations have been identified in 15 genes [20]. The majority of these mutations are missense mutations, resulting in a direct amino acid switch, which alters the properties of the protein involved. Frameshift-type mutations, in which a foreshortened form of the protein is generated, are also common. Genetic testing has been commercially available since 2003, and the service is currently provided by several Clinical Laboratory Improvement Amendments approved laboratories, both commercial and institution-based.

Most of the proteins of the sarcomere have disease-causing mutations implicated in HCM, including mutations in MYBPC3, beta myosin heavy chain (MYH7), myosin essential light chains, myosin regulatory light chain 2, cardiac troponin T, cardiac troponin I, alpha tropomyosin, z-disc components, telethonin, and muscle LIM protein, titin and actin. In those patients with a positive family history, 60%–70% of adults and children who undergo genetic testing will have genetic mutations identified, whereas to date only 30%–40% of sporadic cases have a genetic mutation identified [21].

Mutations in MYBPC3 are the most common, accounting for up to half of identified mutations, MYH7 mutations are the second most common, accounting for 25%–40% of patients [22,23], and up to 5% of patients have multiple mutations [24]. Similar results are seen in pediatric-specific investigations. In a study of 79 patients ≤13-years-old, 47 mutations were identified in 42 patients, most commonly MYBPC3 (49% of patients) and MYH7 (36% of patients) [25].

No reliable genotype–phenotype correlations have been established among the identified sarcomeric mutations [26]. However, patients who have an identified mutation are more likely to experience adverse outcomes than those without an identified mutation [27]. Early in the experience of genetic characterization, an expectation developed that genetic testing could be utilized to predict sudden death and symptoms within a familial variant, but this has not been the case [28]. However, it has been established that the 5% of patients who carry multiple mutations develop earlier and more severe forms of the disease [29,30] with compound heterozygotes often manifesting severe neonatal disease [31]. However, there are currently insufficient data to know whether the presence of multiple mutations represents an independent risk factor for sudden death.

Developing guidelines for who should be gene tested has been hampered by the suboptimal diagnostic yield. Another significant issue related to genetic testing is that accurate determination of whether a genetic variant is the cause of disease is complex, and classification of a variant (benign, pathogenic, unknown significance) can change over time as new information becomes available [32]. This derives from the fact that determining the pathogenicity of any identified mutation is probabilistic, rather than binary (yes/no). In other words, the test results are based on the predicted probability that the genetic variant causes disease, based on one or more of the following [33]:

- The mutation cosegregates with the phenotype of HCM in family members or in the database of affected people with HCM
- The mutation has been reported to cause HCM
- The mutation is not present in a control population without HCM
- The mutation causes alterations in protein structure that would be predicted to cause HCM
- The mutation causes a change in a part of the protein that is conservative, as opposed to regions that are known to vary

Mutations that do not meet these criteria are classified as variants of unknown significance and are not useful in family screening to classify phenotype-negative members.

Further issues for genetic testing arise in obtaining coverage by insurers. Declination of coverage has often been based on the premise that the results are unlikely to directly benefit the index case. However, this viewpoint does not take into consideration the costs associated with the repeated, periodic screening of family members that is necessary because phenotypic conversion can occur at any age. Family members who are proven to not carry the familial mutation can avoid decades of phenotypic screening for new onset disease, while those who are positive may then be directed for further clinical evaluation and management. Furthermore, females who carry a known causative mutation can prevent disease transmission to their offspring though assisted reproductive technologies that include embryo preselection.

HYPERTROPHIC CARDIOMYOPATHY DIAGNOSTIC TESTING

The diagnosis of HCM is defined as the presence of a hypertrophied, nondilated LV in the absence of a hemodynamic stimulus that would be expected to cause LVH. In addition to a comprehensive personal history, physical examination and family history, an initial diagnostic evaluation will include an ECG and cardiac imaging to define presence or absence of LVH. In a pediatric population, echocardiography is typically sufficient to establish the diagnosis, although on occasion poor echocardiographic windows will require use of another modality such as CMRI for adequate visualization of LV wall thickness. CMRI is particularly helpful when the apical form of HCM is suspected by family history or when the LV apex is not visualized by echocardiography. Once a diagnosis is made, additional testing including Holter monitor, exercise stress testing, as well as CMRI for evaluation of late gadolinium enhancement (LGE) evidence of myocardial fibrosis should be undertaken for risk stratification purposes.

ECG. An entirely normal ECG is seen in less than 10% of adult HCM patients [34] but is more common in pediatric HCM populations. Abnormalities can include left-axis deviation, repolarization changes (particularly abnormal Q wave patterns), P wave abnormalities consistent with left and/or right atrial enlargement, and/or inverted T waves. The apical form of HCM has a characteristic ECG, with giant (>10 mm) inverted T waves in leads V4–V6 (Fig. 19.1).

Transthoracic echocardiography. Echocardiography is the predominant imaging method to establish the diagnosis of HCM; equally important, it can help distinguish HCM from other conditions in the differential diagnosis, by excluding conditions such as subvalvar, valvar, or supravalvar aortic stenosis. A comprehensive transthoracic echocardiogram including two-dimensional (2D) imaging, color, and spectral Doppler evaluation, and diastolic function assessment including tissue Doppler imaging should be performed on all patients who are undergoing evaluation for HCM or who have a family history of HCM.

The presence of unexplained LVH (LV diastolic wall thickness z-score >7 as diagnostic, and between 5 and 7 as borderline, as noted earlier) confirms the diagnosis of HCM, with measurements primarily performed in parasternal short axis (Fig. 19.2), and parasternal long-axis, apical 2- and 4-chamber views integrate the information. The distribution of hypertrophy can be variable, with the basal anterior septum and adjacent free wall being most commonly affected locations [35,36] (Fig. 19.3). Midseptal hypertrophy with sparing of the basilar septum (Fig. 19.4) and lateral–anterior free wall hypertrophy with relative

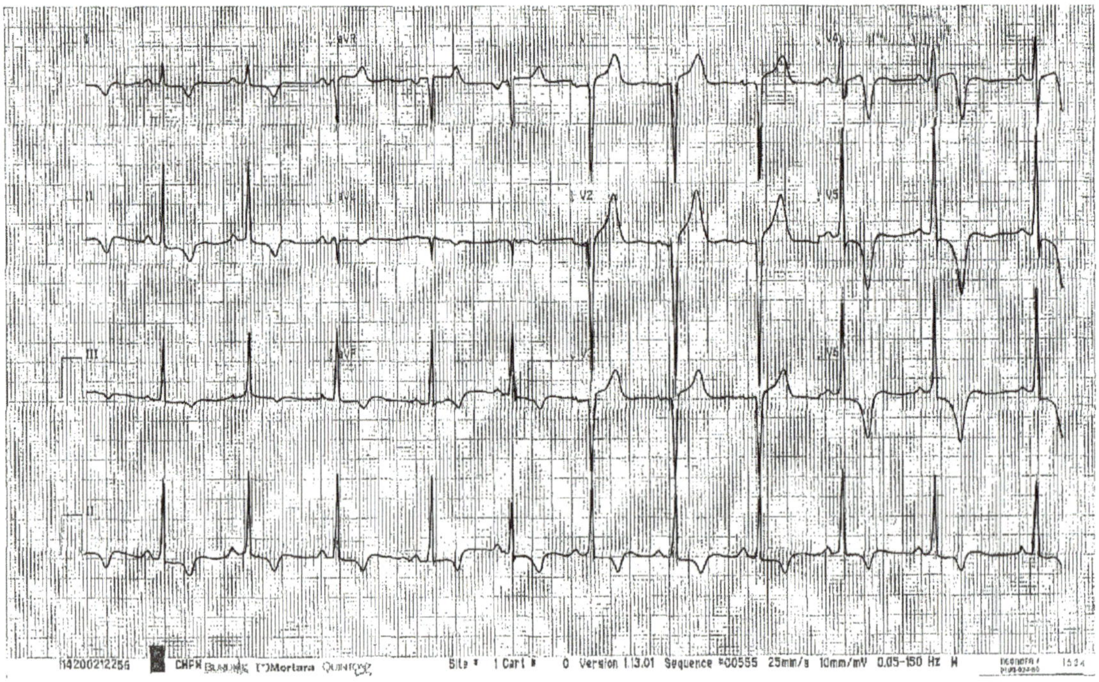

FIGURE 19.1 Electrocardiogram in the apical form of hypertrophic cardiomyopathy. Inverted T waves are present in I, II, III, and aVF, along with giant inverted T waves (>10 mm) in leads V4–V6.

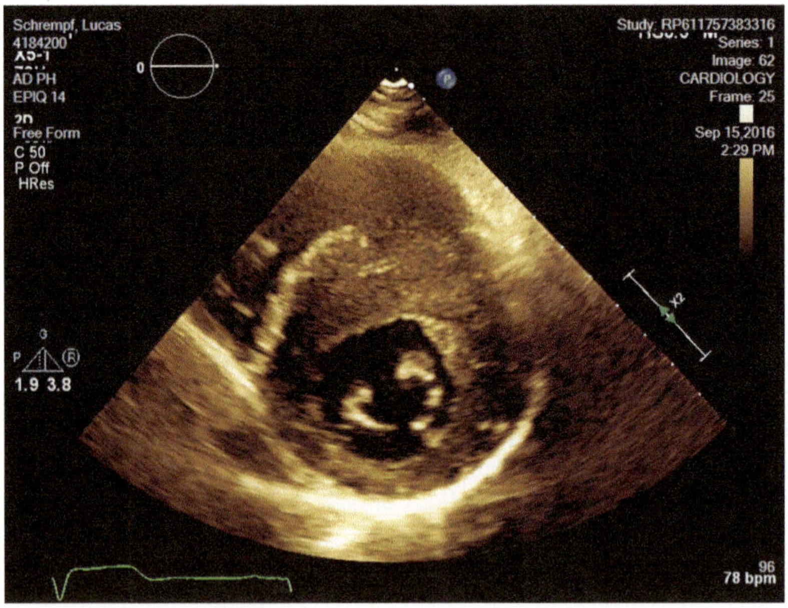

FIGURE 19.2 Asymmetric septal hypertrophy with hypertrophy of the adjacent anterior free wall and sparing of the posterior free wall.

sparing of the ventricular septum (Fig. 19.5) are additional variants. The least common regional variants include isolated hypertrophy of the apex and posterior LV free wall. Wall thickness tends to increase for the first few years after new onset disease and then stabilizes without a tendency to increase thereafter. Continued remodeling does occur in some patients, however. In a series of 106 patients with HCM who had maximum wall thicknesses ≥30 mm, 58% demonstrated wall thinning of > 5 mm over serial evaluations, with length of follow-up a significant predictor of this change [37].

Additional assessments on the echocardiogram should include evaluation of the following: systolic anterior motion (SAM) of the mitral valve; left ventricular outflow tract obstruction (LVOTO); mitral regurgitation (MR); LV diastolic function including left atrial size; and global and regional LV systolic performance.

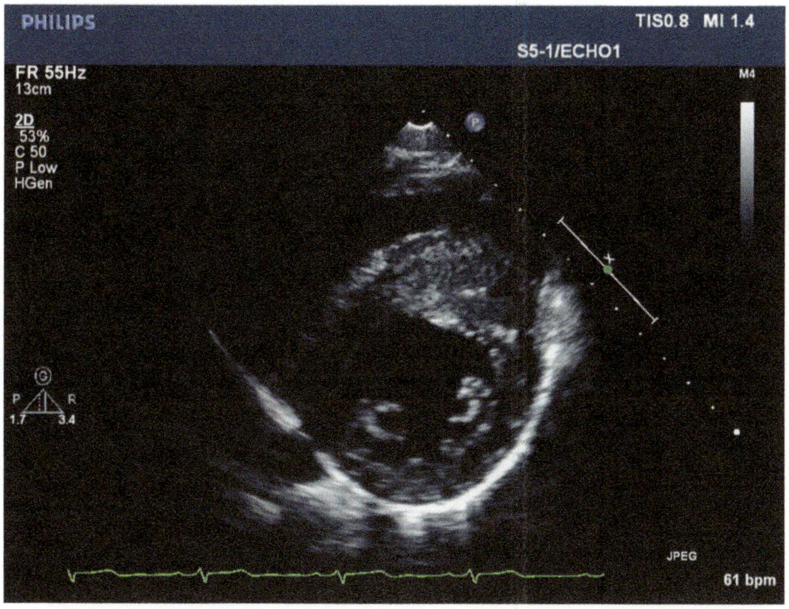

FIGURE 19.3 Anterior wall dominant hypertrophy with sparing of the free wall and most of the interventricular septum.

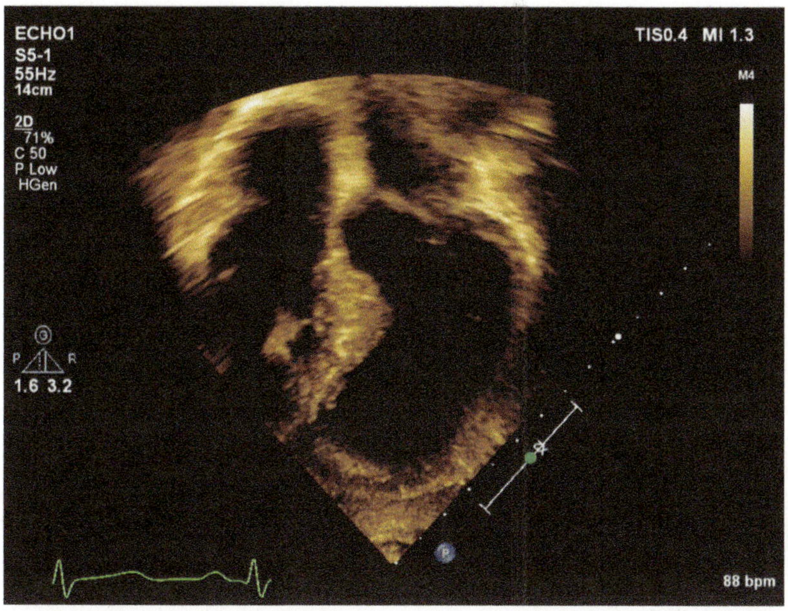

FIGURE 19.4 Severe midseptal hypertrophy with sparing of the basilar and apical septum and no left ventricular outflow tract obstruction.

- SAM of the mitral valve: M-mode across the mitral leaflets in the parasternal long-axis view is particularly helpful in demonstrating SAM, although the presence of SAM is not required for diagnosis. "Buckling" of the anterior mitral leaflet (visible on 2D or 3D imaging) may result in noncoaptation of the mitral valve, resulting in a posteriorly directed jet of MR. There is increasing recognition of the contribution that mitral valve abnormalities make to LVOTO. The anterior papillary muscle is abnormally positioned in the LV, pulling the leaflets into the outflow stream. In addition, the mitral valve leaflets are elongated and redundant resulting in leaflet protrusion into the LV beyond the coaptation point of the leaflets [38]. These abnormalities can be identified in genotypically positive patients even in the absence of hypertrophy [39].
- LVOTO typically results from a combination of hypertrophy of the subaortic septum and anterior displacement of the submitral apparatus. The mechanism of obstruction is often best seen in parasternal long-axis planes, but the magnitude of obstruction is typically assessed in apical 5-chamber views, taking care to avoid contamination of the sample by MR, if present. Outflow obstruction is dynamic in nature, and may not be present at rest. Exercise or dobutamine stress

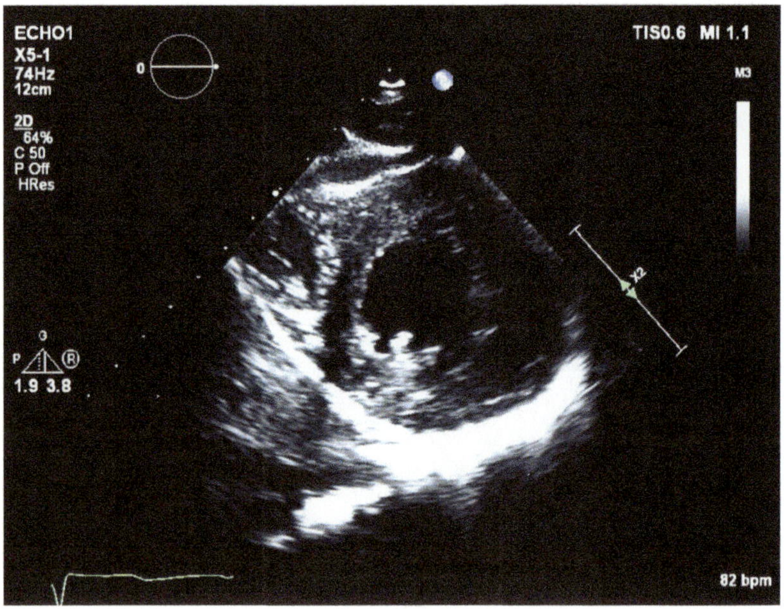

FIGURE 19.5 Lateral and anterior free wall dominant hypertrophy with relative sparing of the septum and posterior wall.

echocardiography may also demonstrate an increase in LVOTO. In a series of 201 patients with HCM and no LVOTO at rest, 106 developed gradients ≥30 mmHg with exercise testing, with 76 of those developing a gradient ≥50 mmHg [40]. This would indicate that symptomatic patients with no resting LVOTO should undergo exercise echocardiography; presence of provocable obstruction may provide a target for medical therapy in symptomatic patients in whom no LVOTO is detected at rest.

- MR: The degree of MR is variable in HCM, from absent to severe. Assessment of the jet velocity is particularly useful when direct measurement of the LV outflow tract gradient is not possible. The modified Bernoulli equation can be applied to the MR jet velocity to give an estimate of LV pressure [41]. Intrinsic mitral valve abnormalities, including elongation and redundancy of the anterior leaflet, with or without mitral valve prolapse, may result in MR in the absence of SAM. It is important to evaluate the mitral valve carefully for such abnormalities prior to planned surgical LVOTO relief, since MR may persist after septal myectomy if additional pathologies are not addressed.
- Diastolic function: Impaired diastolic filling and elevated diastolic pressure in HCM are associated with dyspnea on exertion [42]. Left atrial volume serves as a reflection of chronic LV diastolic dysfunction and/or MR. Left atrial size correlates with degree of exercise intolerance in children and adolescents with HCM [43]. Significant abnormalities of diastolic function can be seen in patients who have relatively mild LVH. Relaxation abnormalities are thought to be related to a variety of influences including LVOTO, subendocardial ischemia, calcium transport abnormalities, and nonuniformity of load [42], whereas abnormalities of compliance occur due to factors such as myocardial fibrosis and cellular disarray [43,44]. As LV filling pressure increases, the early mitral inflow velocity (E) increases and the tissue Doppler early diastolic myocardial velocity (E′) decreases, resulting in an increase in the E/E′ ratio. An increase in the E/E′ ratio has been reported to correlate with sudden cardiac death, arrhythmia, and symptoms in children with HCM [45]. Importantly, abnormal tissue Doppler values are not commonly seen in athlete's heart (see section on Athlete's Heart Syndrome) [46].
- LV systolic function: The typical patient with HCM has an LV cavity size that is below the expected mean value for BSA and a normal or hyperdynamic ejection fraction. Development of systolic dysfunction portends a poor prognosis. Newer modalities such as strain/strain rate imaging have demonstrated the regional nature of myocardial dysfunction in HCM [47,48].

Transesophageal echocardiography. Perioperative imaging by transesophageal echocardiography is important in assessing the patient who is undergoing surgical myectomy for LVOTO relief. Preoperatively, the exam is focused on mitral valve abnormalities and characterization of the location of maximal septal hypertrophy in relation to the aortic valve. Postoperative evaluation is focused on mitral and aortic valve function and evaluation for the presence of an iatrogenic ventricular septal defect [49].

CMRI. CMRI is generally utilized in two HCM-related situations. First, visualization of the myocardium and diagnosis of segmental hypertrophy can be useful for patients who have inadequate echocardiographic images. Once a diagnosis of HCM is confirmed, CMRI with intravenous gadolinium administration to assess LGE can lend additional information for risk stratification. LGE is thought to represent scar formation and can be quantified as a percentage of the total LV mass [50]. The presence and extent of LGE has been associated with heart failure, increased risk of hospitalization, and death [51]. Approximately 50% of adult HCM patients demonstrate LGE, most commonly corresponding to the most hypertrophied sections, and at the junctions of the septum and RV [52]. Development of LGE appears to be age-related [51]. Observational studies have indicated that presence of LGE in HCM patients was associated with a greater risk of ventricular arrhythmias on ambulatory ECG monitor, implying that fibrosis may be the structural substrate for ventricular tachyarrhythmias [53]. Structural abnormalities of the mitral valve and papillary muscles may also be best characterized by CMRI, which may be helpful in planning surgical relief of LVOTO.

CMRI has also been increasingly used to investigate novel parameters to identify genetic mutation carriers before the development of LVH (genotype-positive/phenotype-negative patients). One such parameter, myocardial crypts, has drawn particular attention. Myocardial crypts are discrete, blood filled fissures in otherwise compacted myocardium. While crypts can be seen in control groups, they are noted to be more prevalent in patients referred for screening due to a positive family history of inherited cardiomyopathy (3.6% vs. 23%) [54]. The presence of myocardial crypts appears to be particularly useful in predicting presence of a subclinical HCM phenotype when combined with other CMRI parameters, including elongation of the anterior mitral valve leaflet, abnormal apical LV trabeculae, and the presence of a smaller LV systolic cavity [55].

Exercise testing. An abnormal blood pressure response to exercise is considered a risk factor for sudden death in HCM [56]. Exercise stress testing is preferred over dobutamine stress because it more closely mimics day-to-day physiologic variations in hemodynamics. Beyond blood pressure response, other clinically important findings on exercise testing include development of symptoms with exercise, clinically important arrhythmias at maximum exercise or during recovery, severe ST segment changes. Exercise echocardiography can also be utilized to evaluate development/increase in LVOTO and development/increase in the degree of MR.

Ambulatory ECG. 24- or 48-h ambulatory ECG monitoring should be performed in all patients confirmed to have HCM at the time of diagnosis and repeated periodically for surveillance of ventricular arrhythmias, as part of a risk stratification for sudden death. Surveillance by ambulatory ECG may also reveal atrial fibrillation or flutter, which, while not common in children, may place older adolescents or young adults at risk for embolic complications.

Cardiac catheterization. Invasive evaluation is reserved for those patients for whom there is concern for significant overlap of restrictive phenotype, for those who are planned to undergo septal myectomy, and in the rare patients in whom cardiac transplantation is being considered.

Identification of "preclinical" HCM. Many groups have attempted to identify biomarkers of preclinical HCM (i.e., no LVH present) in family members of index cases who do not have a demonstrable genetic mutation. Candidate predictors have included reduced E' velocities on tissue Doppler evaluation [57,58], and CMRI studies have suggested that increased extracellular myocardial volume [59], LGE [60], or torsion assessment [61] may have discriminatory value. Additional potential biomarkers include impaired myocardial energetics and altered collagen synthesis [23]. However, none of these markers have been able to fully discriminate those who carry genotypic mutations from those who do not even when considered in aggregate [62].

MORPHOLOGIC VARIATIONS IN HYPERTROPHIC CARDIOMYOPATHY

Marked variations exist in the extent and location of LVH in HCM, even within family members who have the same genetic mutation. Most commonly the basal anterior septum and adjacent free wall segments are affected [63]. The LV cavity size is typically reduced for BSA, and systolic function is often supranormal.

"Mixed phenotype" HCM. A mixed morphology of LVH and noncompaction has been described [64], but the difficulty in standardizing the diagnosis of noncompaction has limited the ability to fully characterize this variant [65]. In the Pediatric Cardiomyopathy Registry experience, 6% of the HCM population demonstrated significant LV systolic dysfunction in addition to LVH [66]. Both of these forms demonstrated an increased risk of death or transplant over straightforward HCM morphology. Although infants can present with dilation and dysfunction in conjunction with LVH, transition from classic HCM into a dilated, hypokinetic morphology (so-called "burned-out," or end-stage HCM) is rare in pediatrics.

HCM with restrictive features. There is evidence to suggest that restrictive cardiomyopathy (RCM) may lie along a spectrum with HCM. Pathological evaluation of explanted or postmortem hearts with RCM has demonstrated extensive myocyte and myofibrillar disarray similar to that present in HCM [67]. Additionally, there is phenotypic overlap within some families, with some members demonstrating HCM phenotype and others demonstrating RCM [68]. There is a significant difference in outcomes along this morphologic spectrum, however. Pediatric patients who have a mixed phenotype (HCM and RCM) demonstrate a better transplant-free survival than those with RCM alone [69].

Midcavity LV obstruction. The genesis of midcavity LV obstruction differs from typical LVOTO. The most common variant occurs due to the apposition of the septum and posterior wall in the context of a small LV cavity and hyperdynamic LV systolic function. In this variant, the mid- and apical LV cavity appear nearly or completely obliterated at end-systole, creating mild flow acceleration (Fig. 19.6A and B). Patients are rarely symptomatic in this situation, although beta blockers can be used if necessary. Midcavity obstruction can also occur between hypertrophied papillary muscles and the lateral wall, presenting as an "hour glass" shaped LV. This variant can be associated with apical LV aneurysms of varying sizes, which are associated with a higher incidence of ventricular arrhythmias, thromboembolic events, and heart failure [70]. These aneurysms may be difficult to identify by transthoracic echocardiography, particularly in larger adolescents or adults, and CMRI may be required for diagnosis. Abnormal positioning of the mitral valve papillary muscles can also lead to midcavity obstruction (Fig. 19.7A–C).

Apical HCM. In this form of HCM, hypertrophy is restricted to or predominantly involves the apex of the LV (Fig. 19.8). Some studies have suggested that apical HCM is more common in East Asian populations, others have found similar prevalence in Japanese and European populations [71]. The ECG pattern in apical HCM is characteristic (Fig. 19.1), and patients with this form of HCM tend to have fewer symptoms than those with other forms. Most have no evidence of either LVOTO or midcavity LV obstruction. The apical form of HCM has a better mortality prognosis, but similar event rates for atrial fibrillation and myocardial infarctions [72].

CLINICAL MANIFESTATIONS, COURSE, AND OUTCOMES

The clinical manifestations vary somewhat by etiology. Murmur, chest pain, palpitations, syncope, decrease in exercise capacity, shortness of breath, and heart failure can be the presenting features in all forms of HCM. In patients with actual or potential dynamic LVOTO, it is common to find an outflow murmur that increases in intensity with changes that decrease blood pressure and/or venous return, such as positional changes (squatting) or during a Valsalva. The nonsarcomeric etiologies such as syndromic and metabolic disorders will often have extracardiac manifestations as described below. ECG abnormalities, as described above, are sometimes the initial finding that eventually leads to the diagnosis. Ultimately, the diagnosis rests on cardiac imaging that documents the presence of nonhemodynamically induced myocardial hypertrophy. The clinical course and outcomes are highly dependent on the underlying cause and is therefore considered in more detail in the following sections devoted to the individual forms of HCM.

Severity of hypertrophy. Severity of hypertrophy varies greatly between individuals and among the various causes of the disease and makes a significant contribution to the clinical course. Severe hypertrophy is commonly associated with diastolic dysfunction, outflow tract obstruction, and the presence of symptoms. Severity of hypertrophy has also been reported to represent an important risk factor for sudden death and is one of the findings that has been used to decide when an implantable cardioverter–defibrillator (ICD) should be recommended as primary therapy, including both the ESC [3] and ACCF/AHA [2] guidelines on management of HCM. This finding has more recently been challenged by the observation that the risk of sudden death appears to peak at maximal wall thicknesses between 25 and 30 mm, falling to levels near baseline (i.e., the same risk as those with maximal wall thickness <10) at wall thicknesses >40 mm [73].

LVOTO. The importance of LVOTO to the natural history and pathophysiology of the subgroup of patients with persistent or provocable gradients has been controversial over the years. Although initially believed to be a finding essential to the diagnosis [74], obstruction is now known to be absent in ~30% of patients with HCM. Considerable controversy has surrounded the anatomic and physiologic basis for outflow obstruction, including some observations indicating that it was due to catheter entrapment rather than obstruction to flow. Although catheter entrapment is a source of confusion in a subset of patients with systolic apical obliteration, improved imaging has clarified that the dominant cause is systolic displacement of the anterior mitral leaflet into the outflow steam. The earlier belief that this represented a Venturi effect with diminished lateral pressures secondary to the outflow jet, effectively sucking the anterior mitral leaflet toward the septum [75], has now given way to the recognition that the mitral valve and subvalvar apparatus in HCM is generally abnormally positioned in proximity to the septum [76] and the outflow vector is in fact directed against the free-wall surface of the leaflets, effectively pushing the leaflet(s) toward the septum [77]. The obstruction may be present at rest, provocable (mild at rest but significant with provocation), or latent (not present at rest but evident with provocation). The presence of obstruction significantly worsens ventricular filling and relaxation, may limit cardiac output, and invariably increases myocardial oxygen demand. In addition, the distortion of the mitral valve associated with this physiology often causes or augments MR, further elevating left atrial pressure and thereby exacerbating symptoms of dyspnea.

The contribution of outflow tract obstruction to outcomes in HCM is of considerable interest because although there are therapies that can reduce the severity of obstruction, none are free of risk. There are data in both adults and children that indicate that severe LVOTO creates a risk for heart failure and death, and that intervention to relieve this obstruction is

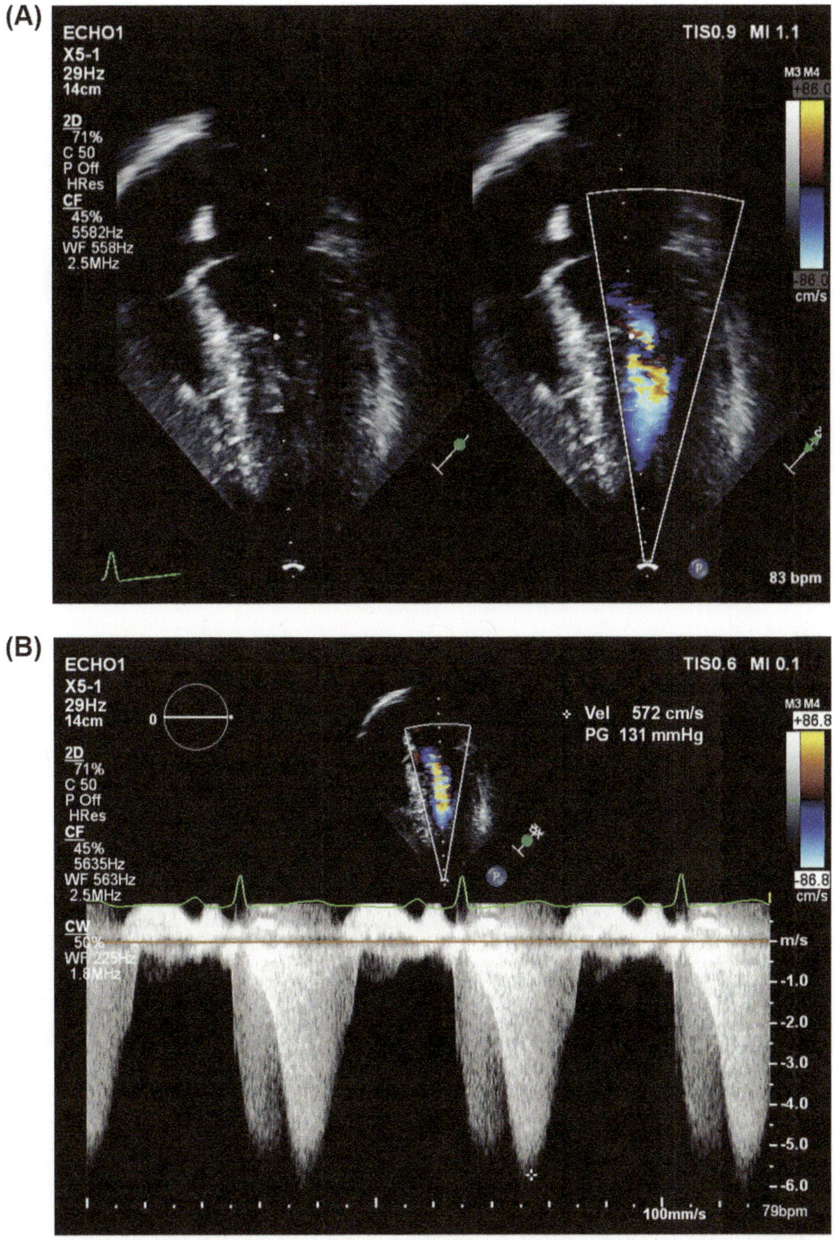

FIGURE 19.6 (A) Midcavity obstruction with apical obliteration with no left ventricular outflow tract obstruction. (B) As a result, continuous wave Doppler shows a late peaking flow jet through the area of midcavity obstruction that is higher velocity than the early peaking mitral regurgitation jet, documenting that the basilar aspect of the left ventricular cavity has normal pressure.

associated with improved outcomes [78]. However, an association with risk of sudden death has proven more controversial. There are some data indicating an increased risk of sudden death associated with LVOTO (defined as an outflow gradient of >30 mm Hg) in adults with HCM [79]. This could be mediated by a number of mechanisms, including the greater risk for MR, left atrial dilation, and atrial fibrillation in patients with obstruction and the decreased survival associated with atrial fibrillation [80]. However, this is a contentious field, indicating primarily that, taken in isolation, the presence or absence of obstruction is unlikely to be a strong risk factor. There have been few studies performed in children but in general the presence or absence of outflow tract obstruction has not been found to be a predictor of survival [81].

Transition to dilated cardiomyopathy. A subset of patients with HCM have been documented to transition to systolic dysfunction and end-stage heart failure. Although occasionally recognized to represent superimposed myocarditis [82], this phenomenon is nearly always a progressive contractile dysfunction that precedes remodeling with cavity dilation and is associated with a progressive fall in the mass-to-volume ratio and onset of atrial fibrillation [83,84]. The transition is

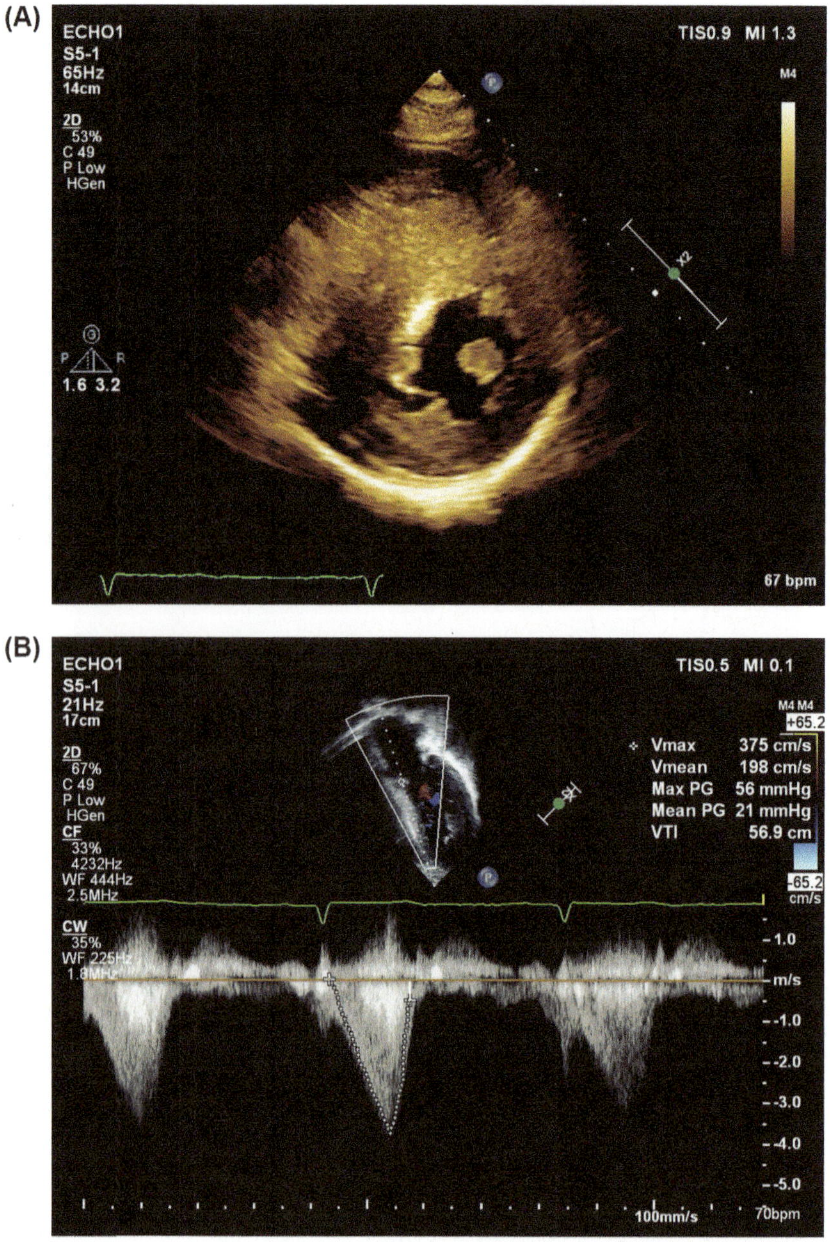

FIGURE 19.7 (A) Mitral valve papillary muscle arising from the septum and attaching to the anterior mitral leaflet. (B) The continuous wave Doppler sample of the midcavity obstruction documents a late peaking jet with a peak velocity of 3.8 m/s.

associated with fibrous replacement of myocardium in a progressive but generally subclinical fashion that becomes clinically manifest at the advanced stages. This can be seen at all ages, including children [84]. Treatment other than cardiac transplantation is generally not efficacious.

Arrhythmias. Although less common in pediatric than adult cohorts, clinically apparent arrhythmias are a challenging aspect of HCM management. Ventricular tachyarrhythmia is the mechanism of sudden death in HCM, arising from the myocyte disarray, fibrosis, and intramyocardial activation and conduction disparities that characterize this disorder. Pharmacologic management has not been found to be effective [85] and has been largely supplanted by the ICD as a prevention strategy. The decision concerning if and when to recommend an ICD is difficult, particularly in children, and this dilemma has therefore led to extensive evaluation of risk factors that might predict which patients are at sufficient risk to outweigh the risk of this therapy. This issue is discussed in more detail in the management section below.

(C)

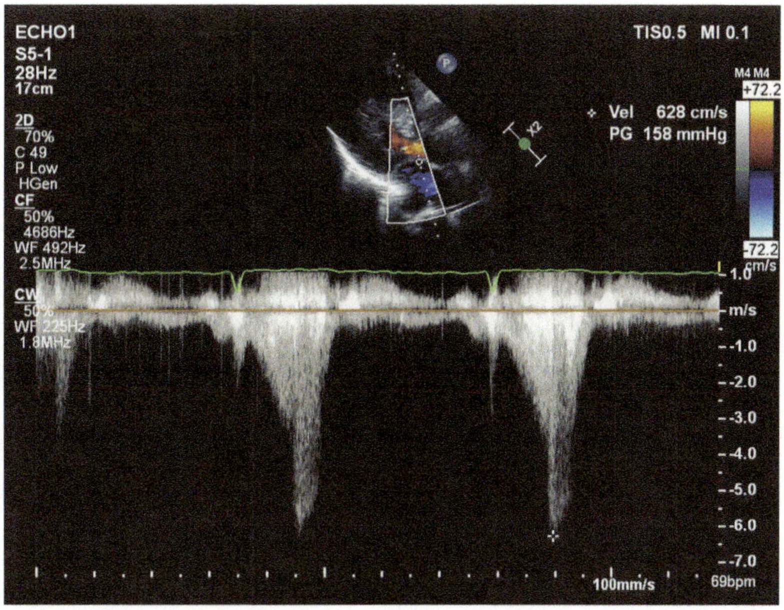

FIGURE 19.7, Cont'd (C) Sampling the mitral valve regurgitant jet with continuous wave Doppler directed orthogonal to the left ventricular outflow tract reveals a peak velocity of 6.3 m/s, verifying that the outflow jet was not contaminated by the mitral valve jet.

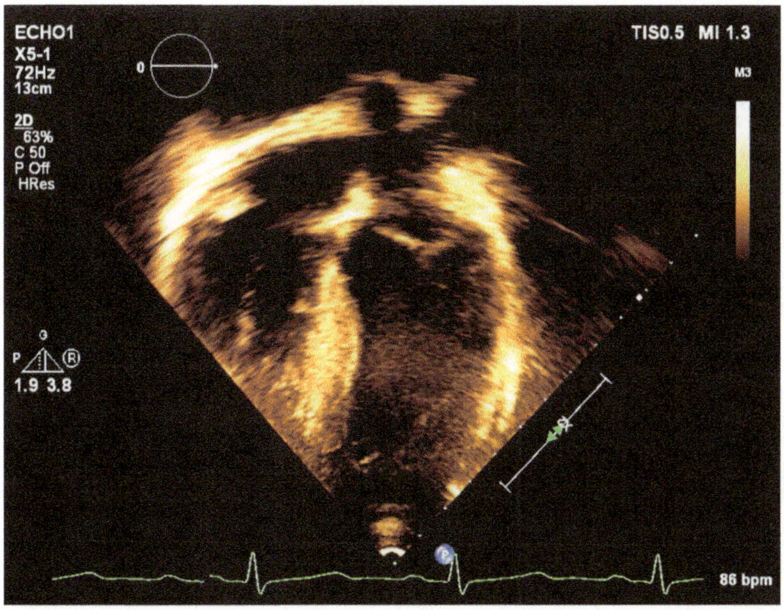

FIGURE 19.8 Apical dominant hypertrophy with normal thickness of the basilar septum and free wall.

Frequent episodes of nonsustained ventricular tachycardia (VT) >10 beats in duration has been reported to represent an increased risk for sudden death in HCM, particularly in young adults [86]. Nonsustained VT on ambulatory monitoring is unusual in pediatric HCM and is generally not found in patients who subsequently experience sudden death [87], but it has been reported to have a greater association with sudden death than in adult cohorts [88]. Thus, it is considered a specific but insensitive risk factor.

Left atrial dilation is uncommon in pediatric HCM and tends to be mostly noted in those with significant MR. This likely accounts for the fact that atrial fibrillation before age 18 is quite unusual, but the prevalence progressively rises thereafter and it is an important predictor of all-cause mortality in adults with HCM [89]. The published experience with ablation of atrial fibrillation in HCM is limited to adult cohorts, where the effectiveness is similar to non-HCM cohorts, although the recurrence rate is twofold higher [90].

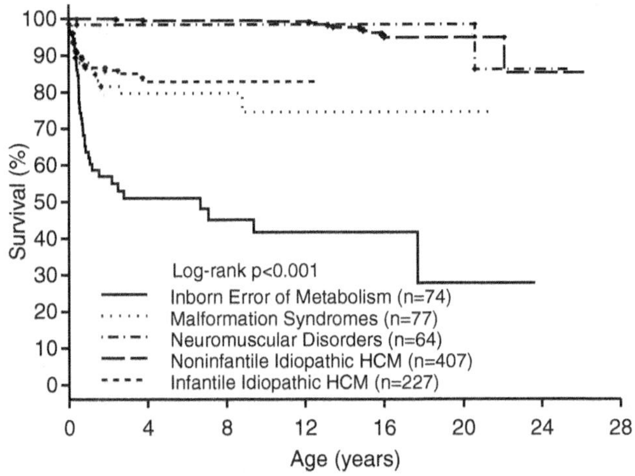

FIGURE 19.9 Survival by age stratified by type of hypertrophic cardiomyopathy (HCM). The impact of etiology and age is dramatic, with the lowest rate of death in the idiopathic forms, which include sarcomeric disease in this cohort that was in large part assembled prior to the wide availability of genetic testing. *Modified from the data in S.D. Colan, S.E. Lipshultz, A.M. Lowe, L.A. Sleeper, J. Messere, G.F. Cox, et al., Epidemiology and cause-specific outcome of hypertrophic cardiomyopathy in children: findings from the Pediatric Cardiomyopathy Registry, Circulation 115 (6) (2007) 773–781.*

Sudden cardiac death. The most feared outcome for HCM is sudden cardiac death. Although previously believed to have a high incidence in HCM, these early reports were primarily based on incident disease in tertiary care centers. As a more representative sample of the patient population with HCM has been acquired, the annual incidence of sudden cardiac death in contemporary reports of unselected adult cohorts with HCM is now reported to be 0.5%–1% [91,92]. The data on sudden cardiac death in children are similar with a 1% annual incidence of death, although the data are somewhat older and are likely to not reflect a comprehensive capture of subclinical disease [6]. The survival rate and cause of death in children is strikingly dependent on age and type of HCM, with familial disease having a higher incidence of sudden death, which occurs less frequently during infancy and early childhood, whereas death in the younger age group is more generally related to progressive congestive heart failure in patients with nonfamilial HCM secondary to syndromic disorders and inborn errors of metabolism (Fig. 19.9) [6].

HYPERTROPHIC CARDIOMYOPATHY SUBTYPES

Sarcomeric and presumed sarcomeric HCM. The familial form of HCM is the most common form of the disorder and is generally inherited in an autosomal dominant fashion. Although the longstanding paradigm concerning age of onset of familial HCM has been that most individuals who eventually develop HCM first manifest LVH during adolescence, the availability of genetic testing has revealed a low conversion rate of gene carriers during childhood (6% over 12 years of follow-up in one study [9]). This has significant implications concerning longitudinal monitoring, as discussed below in the management section.

Preclinical findings. This is a specific issue for the sarcomeric forms of HCM and has not been evaluated in the other forms. Myocardial contraction and relaxation velocities assessed using tissue Doppler imaging are reduced in phenotype-positive HCM patients and also in mutation-positive subjects without LVH [57,93]. Enhanced apical rotation in gene carriers without hypertrophy has been detected using myocardial deformation analysis using speckle-tracking echocardiography [94] and tissue tagging CMRI [61]. Myocardial extracellular volume assessed on T1 mapping (evidence of diffuse or focal myocardial fibrosis or edema) has been noted to be elevated in HCM sarcomere mutation carriers without evidence of LVH [59].

Early reports indicating a very high degree of stratification between carriers and noncarriers led to speculation that noninvasive testing might enable detection of gene carriers, but subsequent studies have reported that LV wall thickness, ventricular size, tissue Doppler parameters, and N-terminal pro b-type natriuretic peptide levels do not reliably differentiate between the HC mutation carriers and normal subjects, failing to facilitate preclinical diagnosis of the disease [58,95]. Patients with subclinical manifestations of the disease are not thought to be at increased risk of sudden death. Nonetheless, there have been isolated reports of mutation-carriers who died suddenly despite wall thickness below the diagnostic threshold [96,97].

Although preclinical findings on noninvasive imaging may not be sufficient to determine genetic status, these findings support the notion that tissue-level changes, including fibrotic remodeling, take place early in disease pathogenesis, prior to the onset of diagnostic levels of hypertrophy. In addition to advancing our understanding of the pathophysiology of the disease, these preclinical findings are now being used as therapeutic end points in interventional trials based on the hypothesis that early intervention can attenuate or prevent disease expression.

Screening of family members. The ACCF/AHA guidelines [2] recommend that all HCM family members undergo cardiac evaluation during adolescence. Because phenotype expression may be delayed to virtually any age, it is also recommended that adult relatives without evidence of disease be screened once every 5 years. This recommendation was supported by a report from the Netherlands documenting a conversion rate of about 4% per year on longitudinal evaluation of adult HCM mutation carriers [98]. The frequency with which screening should be undertaken during childhood is more controversial and is discussed further in the management section below.

Prenatal and infantile hyperinsulinemia. Both congenital hyperinsulinemia [99] and infants of diabetic mothers can manifest reversible HCM with asymmetric septal hypertrophy. The association of marked concentric hypertrophy in newborn infants of mothers with diabetes has been recognized for many years and because gestational diabetes mellitus is the most common medical complication encountered during pregnancy, maternal diabetes is the most common cause of HCM in the newborn period. Although the majority of these infants are asymptomatic, up to 10% have respiratory distress and other evidence of congestive heart failure [100] secondary to reduced stroke volume. With or without symptoms, normalization of plasma insulin levels leads to regression of hypertrophy within 6 to at most 12 months. For those with symptoms, supportive therapy generally permits sufficient reduction in LV mass to eliminate symptoms within 1–3 weeks, although fatal cases have been reported [101].

RASopathies. HCM is associated with several phenotypically distinct developmental disorders caused by mutations in genes that alter the RAS-mediated intracellular signaling and mitogen-activated protein kinases that have been collectively labeled as the RASopathies. These include Noonan syndrome, Noonan syndrome with multiple lentigines, Noonan syndrome with loose anagen hair, Costello syndrome, Cardiofaciocutaneous syndrome, and Neurofibromatosis type 1. Although the extracardiac manifestations are distinguishable from sarcomeric HCM, the cardiac manifestations are similar [102]. Myocardial hypertrophy is usually asymmetric with septal involvement exceeding free wall and is associated with myocardial disarray. Dynamic LVOTO may be present and may progress over time. Congenital valvar pulmonary stenosis can be associated and may be severe. Atrial and/or ventricular septal defects are occasionally seen.

Clinical presentation of HCM in these disorders is nearly always in infancy. It is uncommon for HCM in Noonan syndrome to progress or have new onset beyond early childhood [103], although there are not enough data in the other RASopathies to know whether they follow a similar pattern. Right ventricular outflow tract obstruction is often present in Noonan syndrome and biventricular outflow obstruction related to the combination of valvar and subvalvar pulmonary stenosis with severe HCM-associated dynamic LVOTO, is poorly tolerated, and is associated with poor survival. Presentation during infancy without congestive heart failure is associated with a 70% 3-year survival but when associated with congestive heart failure (21% of cases) the 6-month survival drops to 30% [104]. The diagnosis is generally based on phenotypic characterization with confirmatory genetic testing.

Management of symptomatic HCM in infants with Noonan syndrome is often quite problematic. Biventricular outflow tract obstruction is poorly tolerated and relief of right ventricular obstruction when more than mild is generally advised in the presence of HCM. Septal myectomy is advised when LVOTO is associated with heart failure symptoms, even though recurrence of LVOTO due to muscle regrowth is common when the myectomy is performed at less than 1 year of age. Medical therapies with beta blockers or verapamil rarely result in significant benefit. However, one of the intriguing distinguishing features of the RASopathies is the potential for specific therapy [105]. Based on work in mouse models of Noonan syndrome with multiple lentigines [106], mTOR inhibition using rapamycin and related compounds appears to represent a potential method of interrupting the pathway that ultimately results in HCM in this disorder. These therapies are FDA approved to prevent posttransplant rejection and in-stent stenosis after coronary artery stenting and as such have the potential for near-term testing.

Storage diseases. Major groups of metabolic disorders associated with cardiomyopathy include lysosomal diseases (e.g., Fabry disease), glycogenosis and related disorders (e.g., Pompe disease, LAMP2 (Danon) disease, PRAKAG2 glycogen-storage disease, Anderson–Fabry disease), organic acidurias, and congenital disorders of glycosylation. Most of these rare disorders have extracardiac manifestations that dominate their clinical presentation and lead to a diagnostic metabolic evaluation. However, several of these have variants in which the cardiac manifestations dominate and the systemic manifestations can be subtle or absent.

LAMP2 (Danon) disease is a rare X-linked dominant, lysosomal disease caused by primary deficiency of LAMP2 gene that typically presents with cardiomyopathy, skeletal myopathy, and mental retardation. HCM and electrophysiologic abnormalities are the consequences of glycogen accumulation in the myocardium secondary to the defect in the LAMP2 protein, variably accompanied by systemic manifestations of mental retardation, hepatic involvement, neurological, and/or musculoskeletal deficits. Ventricular preexcitation is encountered at a much higher frequency than in sarcomeric disease [107]. The underlying mechanism is thought to be disrupted autophagy, leading to dramatic increases in cytoplasmic vacuolation, lipid droplets, and cardiomyocyte size, eventually terminating in myocardial degeneration [108]. This sequence corresponds clinically to the natural history of the disorder, with males presenting with HCM in late childhood or early adolescence and subsequently transitioning to dilated cardiomyopathy with progressive heart failure, leading to transplantation or death within 5–10 years [109]. As in other X-linked myocyte disorders, such as the dystrophin disorders, delayed and attenuated presentation in females has been described and is generally attributed to inactivation of nonmutated chromosomes (unfavorable lionization) [110].

Pompe disease (glycogen-storage disorder type II) is an inherited lysosomal-storage disorder caused by mutations in the alpha-glucosidase gene that result in deficiency of the lysosomal enzyme acid alpha-glucosidase. Phenotypic expression is variable, ranging from a rapidly fatal phenotype in infants who typically die from cardiorespiratory failure at less than 1 year of age, to slowly progressive forms in older children and adults, with dominant involvement of skeletal and respiratory muscles. After studies in neonates showed improved survival [111], enzyme replacement therapy with recombinant human acid α-glucosidase was approved for the treatment of Pompe disease. Most patients with infantile-onset disease die in early infancy prior to therapy with enzyme replacement therapy due to delays in diagnosis of the underlying disorder. With early diagnosis, enzyme replacement therapy has been reported to improve survival and protect cognitive development up to at least 24 months of age [112]. Subsequent studies in children and adults have shown beneficial effect on walking distance, pulmonary function, muscle strength, and survival [113]. However, the results also suggest that there is a large variation in the effects of treatment in these patients, possibly related to delays in initiating therapy, with initiation of therapy at <12 days of age yielding more promising results [114].

PRKAG2 syndrome is an autosomal dominant glycogen-storage disease that was previously called HCM with Wolff-Parkinson-White syndrome because of the association with preexcitation and atrial fibrillation followed by later onset of dysfunction of the sinoatrial and atrioventricular nodes [115]. Intracellular glycogen deposition leads to myocyte hypertrophy predominantly involving the LV without evidence of myocyte disarray. Severity of hypertrophy is generally less severe than that seen in Danon disease [116]. Pacemaker implantation is often needed consequent to the conduction system disease and the presence of both atrial fibrillation and preexcitation creates a risk for sudden death [115]. Age of onset varies from prenatal to the fifth decade. Similar to other glycogen-storage disorders, PRKAG2 syndrome creates a high risk for transition from the HCM phenotype to a hypokinetic, dilated cardiomyopathy leading to congestive heart failure. Infantile forms with rapidly progressive hypertrophy and death have been described [117]. No specific therapy is currently available but work in a transgenic, externally modifiable mouse model demonstrated that lowering glycogen content in the heart can reverse cardiomyopathy and electrophysiologic manifestations [118].

Alpha-galactosidase A deficiency (Anderson–Fabry disease) typically has systemic manifestations of acroparesthesia and pain, febrile crises, hypohidrosis, gastrointestinal disturbances, and cutaneous angiokeratomas that begin during childhood, although the cardiac manifestations are more frequently first apparent in adulthood. This X-linked lysosomal-storage disorder is caused by deficiency of the enzyme alpha-galactosidase A and accounts for 1%–3% of HCM cases [119]. The intracellular accumulation of neutral glycosphingolipids results in progressive LVH that is otherwise similar to other HCM phenotypes although it is more frequently characterized by symmetric LVH than are the sarcomeric forms, and dynamic LVOTO is less frequent. Conduction disorders, atrial fibrillation, and sudden death can not only be encountered but also do not distinguish this disease from sarcomeric HCM. Enzyme replacement therapy has been available since 2001, and the results of this therapy have been recently reviewed [120].

Friedreich Ataxia. Friedreich ataxia is a rare (prevalence = 1/50,000) autosomal recessive neurodegenerative disorder associated with progressive HCM and a propensity to transition over time to an end-stage dilated, hypokinetic cardiomyopathy. Genetically, this is one of the "three-peat" disorders in which there is an increased number of repeats of a normal codon. This type of genetic alteration is the basis for a number of otherwise unrelated inherited disorders including Huntington disease, fragile X syndrome, and myotonic dystrophy [121,122]. The affected protein in Friedreich Ataxia is frataxin, a mitochondrial inner membrane protein important to mitochondrial iron homeostasis [123]. In combination with decreased iron chelating capacity in the mitochondria, oxidative damage secondary to iron overload is thought to contribute to the pathogenesis. HCM is seen in about two-third of patients with Friedreich Ataxia, and the severity of cardiomyopathy does not correlate with the severity of the neurologic disease expression [124]. The magnitude of LVH is quite variable and manifests as concentric hypertrophy in the milder forms but asymmetric septal hypertrophy in those with more severe hypertrophy. About a third of pediatric patients with Friedreich Ataxia develop ventricular dysfunction during childhood [125], a transition that is quite rare during childhood with other forms of HCM. Diastolic dysfunction related to concentric myocardial hypertrophy and to interstitial fibrosis is also characteristic of this disorder [126]. Although patients with Friedreich Ataxia generally develop a severe cardiomyopathy leading to death from heart failure in the third to fifth decade of life [127] with heart failure as the primary cause of death in ~60% of cases, symptomatic manifestations of cardiac disease in the first two decades of life are quite rare, perhaps in part because of the limitations in physical activity related to the neurologic manifestations [125]. In general, management of the cardiac disease associated with Friedreich Ataxia is the same as for other forms of HCM. However, idebenone (2,3-dimethoxy-5-methyl-6-(10-hydroxydecyl)-1,4-benzoquinone), a synthetic derivative of coenzyme Q10 that improves electron flux along the electron transport chain, is thought to protect against mitochondrial damage and to enhance respiration and is frequently recommended for this disease. Although several observational reports have described a reduction in the severity of cardiac hypertrophy in patients treated with idebenone, this was not confirmed in a recent double-blind, randomized, placebo-controlled study [128].

Mitochondrial disorders. Disorders of mitochondrial oxidative phosphorylation (OXPHOS) constitute the largest subgroup of inborn errors of metabolism. The mitochondria are both ubiquitous and essential to cellular function. As a consequence, mitochondrial diseases present variably with single or multiorgan involvement and cardiac involvement is seen in 20%–40% [129]. More than 40 different mitochondrial diseases and disorders of mitochondrial function have been associated with HCM [130]. Barth syndrome is among these and although more commonly associated with dilated cardiomyopathy, HCM has also been described. Presentation of many of the mitochondrial forms of HCM is often during infancy when either multisystem manifestations or the combination of HCM and reduced systolic function lead to suspicion of mitochondrial dysfunction. Urine organic acid, acylcarnitine profiles, and plasma and urine carnitine levels are the forms of initial testing most likely to lead to the diagnosis of one of the treatable disorders. Among the many other mitochondrial disorders that are associated with HCM, few have effective therapies other than disorders of mitochondrial fatty acid β-oxidation, coenzyme Q10 deficiency, and thiamine-responsive disorders. Ultimately, biochemical testing of mitochondrial function, although not widely available, is the most effective way to verify the presence of mitochondrial disease. Mitochondrial gene panels with whole exome sequencing have achieved a diagnostic yield as high as 60% [131]. The diagnostic approaches for defining the specific metabolic defect and the genetic basis has been recently reviewed in some detail by Brunel-Guitton et al. [130].

Congenital heart disease. The combination of congenital heart disease in conjunction with asymmetric septal hypertrophy and wall thickness in the range associated with hypertrophy is occasionally observed [132–135]. Complete atrioventricular septal defect, tetralogy of Fallot, and pulmonary stenosis are the most commonly seen disorders. Noonan syndrome is frequently associated both pulmonary stenosis and HCM, both in isolation and in combination, and the natural history of this combination has been well described (see above). In other situations, the combination of the HCM phenotype and congenital heart disease in the same patient creates a diagnostic dilemma because of the uncertainty whether the severe myocardial hypertrophy could be hemodynamically mediated. Documentation of a genetic predisposition to HCM raises the prior probability of HCM but has been rarely reported. In most cases, unless there is temporal resolution of hypertrophy after repair of the congenital defect, the true diagnosis remains uncertain.

HYPERTROPHIC CARDIOMYOPATHY VERSUS ATHLETIC HEART SYNDROME

Exercise-induced physiologic ventricular remodeling, also known as athletic heart syndrome (AHS), is a well-documented adaptive response that has been widely investigated in both animal models and in humans. Physiologic hypertrophy may at times achieve sufficient magnitude to overlap with wall thicknesses that could also represent HCM, creating a diagnostic dilemma. This dilemma has additional importance because HCM is the most common cause of sports-related unexpected sudden death in the United States, accounting for 36% of these deaths overall [136]. The HCM phenotype can usually be differentiated from exercise-induced hypertrophy based on several phenotypical features. It is quite rare, though not impossible, for exercise-associated hypertrophy to result in a wall thickness >15 mm (wall thickness z-score >7), whereas wall thicknesses of 12–14 mm (wall thickness z-score of 4–6) in response to intense athletic training are encountered in up to 2% of athletes. The ventricular dilation that typically accompanies athletic training contrasts with the reduced cavity size that is typical for HCM. The relative wall thickness (thickness-to-dimension ratio) may be mildly elevated in physiologic hypertrophy but rarely to the extent that is typical of HCM. Dynamic outflow obstruction at rest is quite unusual in AHS but exercise-associated dynamic LVOTO is known to occur in the absence of HCM [39].

Other than the absolute wall thickness, there are additional differences in the HCM phenotype, which can generally be used to differentiate HCM from AHS. Most though not all forms of chronic exercise lead to ventricular dilation of some degree, and therefore a ventricular size that is near or above the BSA-adjusted upper-limits of normal is more typical of AHS, whereas ventricular size that is near or below the normal end of normal suggests HCM. Although inducible outflow tract gradients can be seen in AHS, resting gradients are rare. Concentric hypertrophy is more common in AHS and more than mild asymmetry suggests HCM. Abnormal noninvasive indices of diastolic function based on filling patterns and tissue Doppler velocities are common in HCM and are quite unusual in AHS. The ECG findings in AHS have broad overlap with those in HCM and cannot be relied on the two separate conditions. LGE on CMRI, if present, is far more likely due to HCM. Generally, the pattern of findings rather than any single finding in isolation provides the highest discrimination between HCM and AHS. The presence of HCM in a first-degree relative or detection of a probable or definite HCM-associated mutation increases the prior probability of disease but must still be considered in the overall context and cannot be considered a decisive factor in isolation because of the variable age of onset of disease expression.

Ultimately, there are some instances where the distinction between AHS and HCM remains ambiguous. Under these circumstances, the response of the ventricle to deconditioning is generally assessed through a 6- to 12-month period of abstention from athletic participation. Resolution of hypertrophy in response to deconditioning is generally considered the most definitive evidence for AHS, but there are case reports indicating that even this may not be definitive [137].

SCREENING FOR HYPERTROPHIC CARDIOMYOPATHY

Sarcomeric HCM is most commonly transmitted in an autosomal dominant fashion, leading to the general recommendation for screening of family members. There is, however, no agreement on who should be screened and how often. First-degree relatives have a 50% risk of carrying the gene, which drops to 25% in second degree, etc., raising the issue of what level of risk should justify screening. The ACCF/AHA and ESC guidelines recommend periodic echocardiographic screening of first-degree relatives only but provide no justification for this restriction [2,3]. The decision as to how much of the family tree should undergo periodic echocardiographic screening can be avoided if a familial gene can be identified, thereby limiting echocardiographic screening to genetically positive family members, although this option is impeded by combination of the fact that a gene cannot currently be identified in a significant proportion of families who agree to systematic genetic testing and that many family members are unwilling to undergo genetic testing. In contrast to echocardiographic screening, genetic testing can be justifiably limited to a progressive testing of first degree relatives of genetically positive individuals. The decision as to how often to screen at-risk individuals is equally unsettled and is often based on the prior probability of new onset disease but would be more justifiably determined by the anticipated rate of progression. Current screening programs have documented that progression from no evidence of disease to meeting diagnostic criteria can take place in less than a year during the pubertal growth spurt, justifying annual testing during ages 12–18. Studies in adults have documented a slower rate of progression [138–140], leading to the recommendation for repeat screening at 5-year intervals in adults [141].

The situation is more challenging in prepubertal children where the natural history of new onset disease expression is not known. The ACCF/AHA guidelines recommend screening of prepubertal children with a malignant family history or based on clinical suspicion of disease and the ESC guidelines simply indicate that screening at age <10 years "may be considered" for malignant family history. Although systematic longitudinal data concerning rate of progression of new onset disease expression in prepubertal children do not exist, there are data indicating that the risk of sudden death in prepubertal children with HCM is significant and is at least comparable to the risk in adults [6,81,142,143]. We therefore recommend screening every 2–3 years in preadolescent children.

Preparticipation screening of athletes is an even more controversial issue. Undertaking specific testing based on family history, symptoms, and physical exam is already the norm, but this is the standard of care for all children. In contrast, there is considerable controversy as to whether athletes warrant additional specific testing such as ECG or echocardiography. The controversial areas include the cost–benefit analysis, adequacy of current standards, potential harm from false-positive testing, and the issues of equity related to selective testing of athletes rather than general population screening [144,145]. The efficacy of echocardiographic screening in those with no family history of HCM has also been challenged [146]. This controversy is unlikely to be settled until a more accurate, less costly screening method is developed.

HYPERTROPHIC CARDIOMYOPATHY SYMPTOMS AND MANAGEMENT

While it is increasingly common for the diagnosis of HCM to be made in asymptomatic individuals as a result of screening for a positive family history, many are diagnosed following evaluation for symptoms such as palpitations, syncope/presyncope, or appreciation of a new murmur, with or without an abnormal ECG. For the majority of patients with HCM, the diagnosis is compatible with normal longevity, with a reported 1% annual mortality rate among nonreferral-based cohorts [2]. Similar outcomes have also been seen in populations restricted to those presenting at a younger age. Among a cohort of 474 patients <30 (mean 20.2 years) followed for an average of 7.1 years, the annual HCM-related mortality rate was 0.54%, while 1.8% per year had life-threatening events including appropriate ICD therapy, resuscitated sudden cardiac arrest, or heart transplant [147].

Symptoms associated with HCM. The hemodynamic alterations seen with HCM (LVOTO, diastolic dysfunction, myocardial ischemia, and MR) can lead to a variety of symptoms, including fatigue, dyspnea, chest pain, palpitations, presyncope, and syncope. These symptoms can be limited to occurrence with exercise or occur at rest. The severity of symptoms is variable among patients, even between members of the same family, and does not correlate either with the degree of LVOTO or the magnitude of hypertrophy. It is important to keep in mind that development of symptoms can occur at any point, and slow progression of those symptoms over time is common.

Many of the symptoms in HCM have been attributed to LVOTO, as outflow gradients are commonly present, either at rest or with provocation. Physiologic maneuvers to provoke LVOTO during physical examination include squatting to standing and Valsalva maneuvers. Exercise or dobutamine stress echocardiograms may also be performed to elicit LVOTO. Obstruction is dynamic and may vary widely over the course of a day (with activity, altered hydration status, following a heavy meal). The importance and management of LVOTO has been the subject of extensive debate [148]. While significant obstruction may be quite well tolerated for extended periods of time, LVOTO has been associated with progressive symptoms and HCM-related heart failure death. Importantly, the impact of LVOTO on sudden death in adults with HCM remains unclear [2], and the data are even less clear in pediatrics. Therapy targeting reduction of LVOTO is the primary strategy in symptomatic patients; beta blockers and calcium channel blockers are first line choices. Disopyramide can be added to either of these when symptoms are not resolved with beta blocker or calcium channel blocker alone.

Dyspnea and chest pain are the most commonly experienced symptoms, with exertional chest pain occurring in 25%–30% of patients with HCM [149]. These symptoms can result from diastolic dysfunction, LVOTO, MR, or, late in the course of the condition, systolic dysfunction and overt heart failure. Chest pain is thought to be the result of microvascular angina, resulting from increased myocardial oxygen demand and/or reduced myocardial blood flow and oxygen supply [150,151]. An increase in myocardial oxygen demand may result from myocyte hypertrophy and disarray, LVOTO, and increased wall stress associated with elevated diastolic pressures. Reduced myocardial oxygen supply may result from impaired vasodilator reserve, myocardial bridging, and microvascular dysfunction, myocardial fibrosis, and increased capillary separation/inadequate capillary density [152,153]. Medical therapy for these symptoms include beta blockers or L-type calcium channel blockers monotherapy, which prolong diastolic filling time. Disopyramide can be added to either of these when symptoms are not resolved with beta blocker or calcium channel blocker alone.

Both supraventricular and ventricular arrhythmias may occur in HCM, often presenting as palpitations. The most common supraventricular arrhythmias in HCM is atrial fibrillation, although it is uncommon in patients less than 30 years. Predisposing factors for the development of atrial fibrillation include severe hypertrophy, extensive myocardial fibrosis, left atrial dilation, and heart failure symptoms. The risk of thromboembolism is high and anticoagulation is recommended [2]. Therapies include those targeted to rate reduction, with cardioversion restricted to those who are severely symptomatic or hemodynamically unstable. Ventricular arrhythmias can range from isolated ventricular premature beats to nonsustained/sustained VT and ventricular fibrillation. Ventricular arrhythmias are common, with a broad range of severity. As assessed by ambulatory ECG monitoring, ventricular premature beats are highly prevalent, seen in 88%, with nonsustained VT present in 31% in a study of 178 adult patients (age 50 ± 18 years) [154]. Antiarrhythmic agents such as sotalol can be adjunctive therapy in patients with frequent sustained ventricular arrhythmias resulting in ICD shocks or in patients who choose not to have or are not candidates for ICD placement. Amiodarone can also be considered although the long-term side effect profile has more impact in the pediatric age range.

Presyncope or syncope is also commonly experienced symptoms in HCM, with 20% complaining of presyncope and another 15%–25% of patients with HCM have at least one syncopal event [155]. Multiple mechanisms may be responsible, including arrhythmias, LVOTO, or myocardial ischemia. Syncope that is not clearly related to neurocardiogenic causes is considered a marker for risk of sudden death [156]. The patients who experience syncope are more likely to be young (less than 30 years), have smaller LV end-diastolic volumes, and demonstrate nonsustained VT on ambulatory monitoring [155,157].

Progressive heart failure associated with systolic dysfunction is uncommon in adolescents. In the pediatric population, this is most common in infants, particularly those whose HCM is related to inborn errors of metabolism [6].

PHARMACOLOGICAL THERAPY

Beta blockers are the most commonly used medications for relief of symptoms including chest pain and dyspnea as well as palpitations related to ventricular arrhythmias. Beta blockers are negative inotropes. They reduce the heart rate, which prolongs diastole and increases ventricular filling, and therefore reduce LVOTO [158]. While they have not been shown to impact exercise intolerance, chest pain and dyspnea do respond to beta blockade. Side effects are common, with a profile that includes depression, impaired sleep, and decreased school performance, thus limiting their utility in many patients. Beta blockers are used as monotherapy or in combination with disopyramide.

Calcium channel blockers, such as verapamil and diltiazem, improve diastolic relaxation, reducing diastolic pressure and mean left atrial pressure. These actions result in improved exercise tolerance and a reduction in dyspnea. Additionally, they may reduce chest pain symptoms by improving microvascular function and increasing myocardial perfusion [159]. Verapamil has been demonstrated to be well tolerated in children, even neonates [104,160], although it has been associated with increased heart failure in older adults. In fact, side effects from calcium channel blockers are rarely encountered in the pediatric HCM population. Calcium channel blockers are used as monotherapy or in combination with disopyramide.

Disopyramide is an antiarrhythmic agent with negative inotropic properties. It is used as second line therapy (added to either beta blocker or calcium channel blocker) to reduce LVOTO and, secondarily, MR associated with SAM, and improved survival has been reported [161]. It has not been studied in the pediatric HCM population, but the side effect profile when used for neurocardiogenic syncope would suggest a reasonable safety profile [162]. Because it can accelerate atrioventricular nodal conduction and can prolong QTc and can have significant anticholinergic effects, it is not typically used as first line or monotherapy [2].

Angiotensin receptor blockers may have a role in the therapy of HCM based on recent data indicating a role of the renin–angiotensin system in the development of fibrosis and hypertrophy in HCM [163]. While pilot studies have indicated some attenuation of progression of hypertrophy and fibrosis [164], confirmation of the effect awaits larger trials.

Diuretic therapy is typically ineffective as initial therapy for the dyspnea associated with HCM and may exacerbate symptoms by increasing LVOTO, a result of reducing arterial pressure and LV volumes. In patients who do not have LVOTO but have refractory heart failure symptoms with associated volume overload, judicious titration of diuretics may be considered. Angiotensin-converting enzyme inhibitors are rarely used in HCM. Their use results in a further reduction in LV cavity size, increase in dynamic LVOTO, reduced LV compliance, and relaxation [165].

INTERVENTIONAL THERAPY

Medically refractive symptoms in the presence of LVOTO are candidates for septal reduction therapy by either surgical myectomy or alcohol septal ablation. The goal with both therapies is to reduce septal thickness and alter the hemodynamic forces that lead to SAM, LVOTO, and MR.

Septal myomectomy has been performed since the mid-1960s. When performed at an experienced center, obstruction relief is both reliable and durable in adults [166] with near universal improvement in symptoms. Typically performed through an aortotomy, the hypertrophied basal septum is well seen, and resection of this area is readily accomplished (Fig. 19.10A and B). The mitral leaflets and submitral apparatus including chordal structures and attachments can then be addressed as needed [167]. Complications are rare but include aortic regurgitation, ventricular septal defect creation, and conduction abnormalities including left bundle branch block and atrioventricular block, which may require pacemaker therapy. Surgical results in children are similar [168], although recurrence of obstruction occurs more frequently, likely owing to continued somatic growth as well as the intrinsic disease state in infants and children. Mortality rates in adult series are 1%–2% or less [169].

Catheter-based septal ablations are an alternative to surgical myectomy and utilize ethanol injected into a septal perforator branch of the anterior descending coronary artery, which occludes the branch and results in a localized infarction of the basilar septum. The advantage over surgical resection is related to shorter recovery time, although selection of patients is more restrictive since the approach works best in those who have basal septal hypertrophy and no intrinsic mitral valve abnormalities. No clear advantage for either approach has been reported, although incomplete gradient reduction and increased need for permanent pacemaker implantation has been reported in patients undergoing catheter-based ablations [170]. Although commonly offered in adult populations, septal ablation is not widely utilized in pediatrics, in part due to the difficulty in selective cannulation of the very small vessels in children and the concern of the lifelong effect of a large septal infarction. The current ACCF/AHA guidelines advise against routine use of alcohol septal ablations in children and adolescents [2].

It is important to recognize that LVOTO intervention has not been demonstrated to prolong life or decrease the incidence of sudden death. Currently there are no data to indicate that treating asymptomatic obstruction alters the natural history of HCM or improves survival. However, it is possible that prolonged presence of LVOTO-associated ventricular pressure overload may contribute to diastolic dysfunction over the long-term and lending some credence toward an approach that includes earlier intervention.

PREVENTION OF SUDDEN DEATH

Risk of sudden death. Sudden cardiac death may be the initial clinical presentation of HCM [171]. While the annualized risk for the HCM population as a whole is approximately 1%, it is greater in those with multiple risk factors. Observational studies have described the following risk factors for sudden cardiac death:

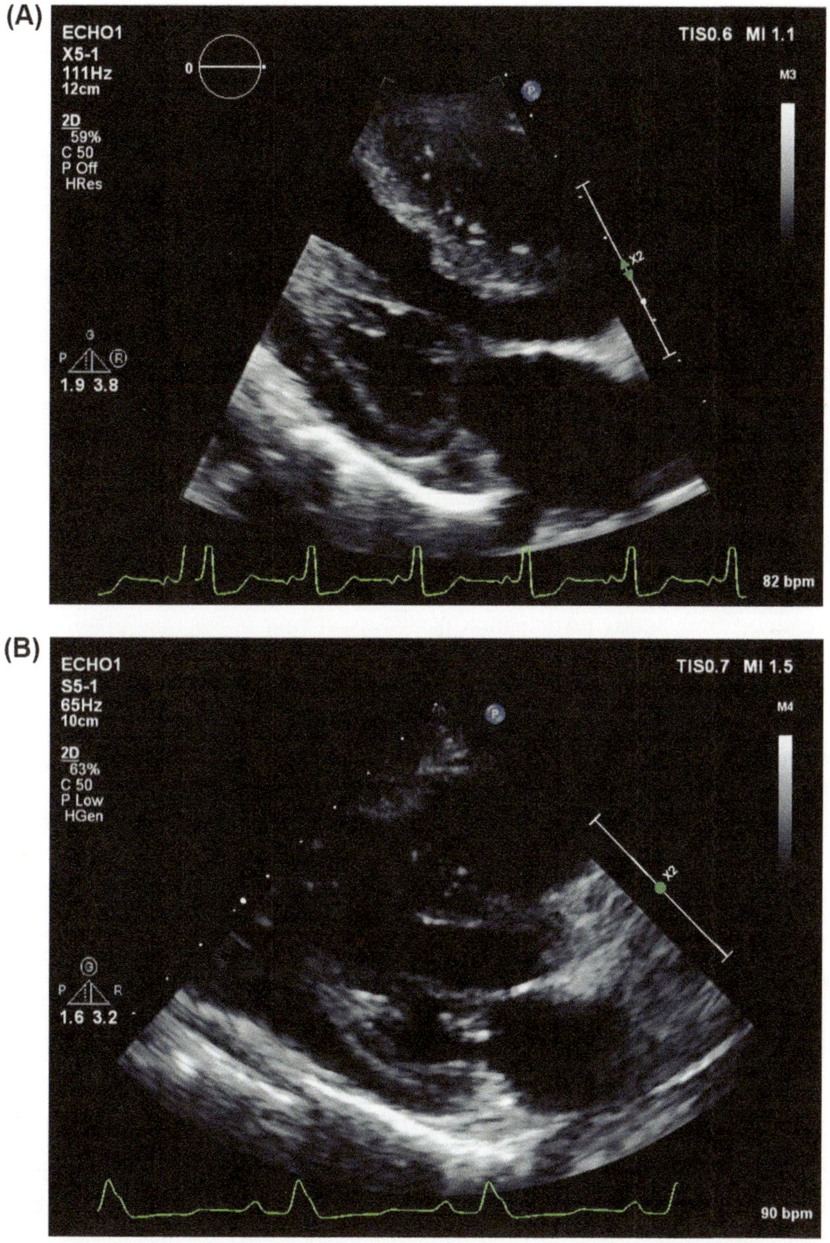

FIGURE 19.10 (A) Left ventricular outflow tract before resection of septal obstruction. (B) Left ventricular outflow tract following resection of septal obstruction.

- Family history of sudden death
- Unexplained syncope
- Nonsustained VT on 24-h ambulatory monitoring
- Severe LVH (maximal LV wall thickness >30 mm)
- Hypotensive blood pressure response during exercise testing

LGE on CMRI has been suggested as an additional potential risk factor, but since most patients with HCM demonstrate LGE, it is unclear whether its presence adds to risk stratification algorithms.

The age range that appears to be at highest risk is adolescence to young adulthood, although sudden death can occur at any age [172]. While medical therapy is not effective in preventing sudden death, ICDs are effective, but carry significant morbidity. In fact, patients are more likely to experience a device-related complication or inappropriate therapy than to receive an appropriate shock [173]. Most instances of sudden death are arrhythmic events, but medical prophylaxis has not been shown to be effective for prevention [174]. With improvement in ICD battery life, decreased device size and increased experience in pediatrics, ICD implantation has become the treatment of choice for those who meet the diagnostic criteria above and are judged to be at high risk for sudden death.

Exercise restriction. While it is clear that some patients with HCM tolerate intense, competitive athletic participation without symptoms or sudden death [175], patients with HCM are commonly advised to avoid intensive competitive sports, particularly those involving burst exertion due to the reported association with sudden death in competitive athletes [176]. The recommendation is based on the presence of a higher than expected association between sudden death and exercise, when adjusted for the amount of time spent exercising [177]. However, the true incidence of sudden death in HCM is not known; genetic confirmation is rarely known and morphologic diagnosis can be confounded by the presence of physiologic hypertrophy in athletes. Population studies have documented the apparent paradox that although there is a transient increase in the risk for sudden death during intense exercise in patients with coronary artery disease who regularly participate in low- and high-level exertion, these individuals experience an overall reduction in the risk for sudden death [178,179]. Additionally, individuals who do not exercise regularly have an exaggerated risk of sudden death during exercise [180]. In fact, it is precisely those individuals with cardiovascular risk factors who derive the largest risk reduction from regular participation in moderate to intense exercise [180]. There are currently no data to indicate improved survival in patients with HCM who are excluded from exercise.

Exclusion from sports participation is especially problematic in older children and adolescents. An adolescent athlete who is suddenly removed from sports participation faces loss of peer interaction, potential social withdrawal, and depression of such severity as to require hospitalization. In patients who have no demonstrable high grade arrhythmias, exercise-induced arrhythmias or hypotension, moderate aerobic activity is unlikely to pose a significant risk and may prove to be psychologically beneficial. In all instances, the risks and benefits of physical activity should be fully individualized, acknowledging the uncertainties on which recommendations are made.

It is important to note here that patients who have been identified as carrying a genetic mutation, through screening of an affected family member, but who do not have LVH on imaging (genotype-positive, phenotype-negative) are not believed to be at increased risk of sudden death [181]. The US consensus guidelines do not recommend formal exercise restriction in these circumstances, although the ESC guidelines do recommend limitations [3,182].

ICD. As discussed above, a number of risk factors have been proposed to assess which patients with HCM would benefit from ICD placement. However, the incidence of sudden death in HCM is less than 1% per year, and because ICDs carry risks as well, determination of the overall risk/benefit is not an easy undertaking. In adult populations, ICDs are more likely to have an inappropriate discharge than a therapeutic discharge, with up to 25% of patients experiencing an inappropriate discharge, 6%–13% experience lead complications, 4%–5% develop device-related infections, and 2%–3% have bleeding or thrombosis-related complications [183,184], with additional, less well-quantified complications including depression, anxiety, and decreased quality of life. The incidences of lead fractures and inappropriate shocks are higher in children, in part due to ongoing somatic growth [185].

Ultimately, decisions regarding ICD implantation must be individualized, with active input from patients and families. Current recommendations for adults indicate ICD implantation in patients with prior cardiac arrest or sustained VT (Class I recommendation), and for those who have 2 or more of the risk factors listed above (Class IIa recommendation). Additionally, for those who do not undergo ICD implantation, periodic risk stratification is indicated, approximately every one to two years [2]. The reports on which these recommendations are based are flawed, with oversampling and overlapping of patient cohorts as well as reports that conflict regarding support for individual risk factors. Risk-predictive models have been independently published by several groups. Maron et al. found that the ESC guidelines, when applied retrospectively to a separate cohort of patients with HCM, identified only 11% of the patients who had experienced sudden death [10]. In addition, the current guidelines do not address potential issues specific to pediatrics, including age-specific stratification guidelines given that children are likely to experience a higher number of ICD-related adverse events. Although defined guidelines for pediatric patients are clearly needed, the rarity of the disease and the low incidence of sudden death within that rare group limit guideline development. The existing data in children suggest that there is no evidence to deviate from the established guidelines in adults. In our institution, resuscitated sudden cardiac arrest is an indication for ICD placement regardless of age. In adolescents, an ICD is recommended for sustained VT, and in those who have two or more risk factors (family history of sudden death, nonsustained VT on 24-h ambulatory monitoring, severe LVH [maximal LV wall thickness > 30 mm], hypotensive blood pressure response during exercise testing, and presence of LGE on CMRI). Decisions for ICD placement in the preadolescent patient are made on a case by case basis, typically requiring additional evidence of risk.

MANAGEMENT OF SPECIAL CIRCUMSTANCES

Pregnancy and delivery. Pregnant HCM patients should be followed by an obstetrician who is experienced with high-risk pregnancies. Vaginal delivery is the preferred method of delivery, and epidural anesthesia should be avoided due to risk of peripheral venous pooling, prolonged labor, and hypovolemia. The delivery team should be prepared for situations of rapid fluid shifts (including hemorrhage) with a large bore venous cannula and access to rapid fluid replacement.

Perioperative considerations. For the majority of low- and medium-risk patients with HCM, the risk of perioperative cardiovascular complications is low, particularly when the procedure is associated with minimal fluid shifts. The hemodynamic fluctuations commonly seen with induction of anesthesia, hemorrhage, or rapid blood pressure shifts may be poorly tolerated [186]. In situations where substantial fluid shifts are likely to occur, invasive monitoring is beneficial.

CONCLUSION

Although the early experience with HCM led to the belief that this is a disabling disease with high incidence of sudden death, extensive epidemiologic and natural history studies in addition to improved diagnostics have led to the recognition that only a small percentage patients experience a substantial diminution in their quality of life, and sudden death is quite rare in nonselected populations. Management options for those who do experience symptoms have steadily improved over time. Newer, gene-specific therapies are under development, and overall the prospects for this disorder are much brighter than previously believed. Screening for family members is also in evolution, with promising advances in genetic testing as well as phenotype characterization through CMRI and biomarkers, thus potentially allowing earlier, preclinical identification of affected individuals.

ABBREVIATIONS

ACCF/AHA American College of Cardiology Foundation/American Heart Association
AHS Athletic heart syndrome
BSA Body surface area
CMRI Cardiac magnetic resonance imaging
ECG Electrocardiography
ESC European Society of Cardiology
HCM Hypertrophic cardiomyopathy
ICD Implantable cardioverter–defibrillator
LGE Late gadolinium enhancement
LV Left ventricular
LVH Left ventricular hypertrophy
LVOTO Left ventricular outflow tract obstruction
MR Mitral regurgitation
MYBPC3 Myosin-binding protein C, cardiac
MYH7 Beta myosin heavy chain
RCM Restrictive cardiomyopathy
SAM Systolic anterior motion
VT Ventricular tachycardia

REFERENCES

[1] S.E. Lipshultz, L.A. Sleeper, J.A. Towbin, A.M. Lowe, E.J. Orav, G.F. Cox, et al., The incidence of pediatric cardiomyopathy in two regions of the United States, N. Engl. J. Med. 348 (17) (2003) 1647–1655.

[2] B.J. Gersh, B.J. Maron, R.O. Bonow, J.A. Dearani, M.A. Fifer, M.S. Link, et al., 2011 ACCF/AHA guideline for the diagnosis and treatment of hypertrophic cardiomyopathy: executive summary: a report of the American College of Cardiology Foundation/American Heart Association task force on practice guidelines, Circulation 124 (24) (2011) 2761–2796.

[3] P.M. Elliott, A. Anastasakis, M.A. Borger, M. Borggrefe, F. Cecchi, P. Charron, et al., 2014 ESC guidelines on diagnosis and management of hypertrophic cardiomyopathy: the task force for the diagnosis and management of hypertrophic cardiomyopathy of the European Society of Cardiology (ESC), Eur. Heart J. 35 (39) (2014) 2733–2779.

[4] I. Olivotto, M.S. Maron, C. Autore, J.R. Lesser, L. Rega, G. Casolo, et al., Assessment and significance of left ventricular mass by cardiovascular magnetic resonance in hypertrophic cardiomyopathy, J. Am. Coll. Cardiol. 52 (7) (2008) 559–566.

[5] C. Semsarian, J. Ingles, M.S. Maron, B.J. Maron, New perspectives on the prevalence of hypertrophic cardiomyopathy, J. Am. Coll. Cardiol. 65 (12) (2015) 1249–1254.

[6] S.D. Colan, S.E. Lipshultz, A.M. Lowe, L.A. Sleeper, J. Messere, G.F. Cox, et al., Epidemiology and cause-specific outcome of hypertrophic cardiomyopathy in children: findings from the Pediatric Cardiomyopathy Registry, Circulation 115 (6) (2007) 773–781.
[7] L.R. Lopes, A. Zekavati, P. Syrris, M. Hubank, C. Giambartolomei, C. Dalageorgou, et al., Genetic complexity in hypertrophic cardiomyopathy revealed by high-throughput sequencing, J. Med. Genet. 50 (4) (2013) 228–239.
[8] A.K. Manrai, B.H. Funke, H.L. Rehm, M.S. Olesen, B.A. Maron, P. Szolovits, et al., Genetic misdiagnoses and the potential for health disparities, N. Engl. J. Med. 375 (7) (2016) 655–665.
[9] M.K. Jensen, O. Havndrup, M. Christiansen, P.S. Andersen, B. Diness, A. Axelsson, et al., Penetrance of hypertrophic cardiomyopathy in children and adolescents: a 12-year follow-up study of clinical screening and predictive genetic testing, Circulation 127 (1) (2013) 48–54.
[10] B.J. Maron, S.A. Casey, R.H. Chan, R.F. Garberich, E.J. Rowin, M.S. Maron, Independent assessment of the European Society of cardiology sudden death risk model for hypertrophic cardiomyopathy, Am. J. Cardiol. 116 (5) (2015) 757–764.
[11] H. Ashrafian, W.J. McKenna, H. Watkins, Disease pathways and novel therapeutic targets in hypertrophic cardiomyopathy, Circ. Res. 109 (1) (2011) 86–96.
[12] C.E. Seidman, J.G. Seidman, Identifying sarcomere gene mutations in hypertrophic cardiomyopathy: a personal history, Circ. Res. 108 (6) (2011) 743–750.
[13] S. Marston, O. Copeland, A. Jacques, K. Livesey, V. Tsang, W.J. McKenna, et al., Evidence from human myectomy samples that MYBPC3 mutations cause hypertrophic cardiomyopathy through haploinsufficiency, Circ. Res. 105 (3) (2009) 219–222.
[14] E.M. Green, H. Wakimoto, R.L. Anderson, M.J. Evanchik, J.M. Gorham, B.C. Harrison, et al., A small-molecule inhibitor of sarcomere contractility suppresses hypertrophic cardiomyopathy in mice, Science 351 (6273) (2016) 617–621.
[15] P. Robinson, P.J. Griffiths, H. Watkins, C.S. Redwood, Dilated and hypertrophic cardiomyopathy mutations in troponin and alpha-tropomyosin have opposing effects on the calcium affinity of cardiac thin filaments, Circ. Res. 101 (12) (2007) 1266–1273.
[16] J. Davis, L.C. Davis, R.N. Correll, C.A. Makarewich, J.A. Schwanekamp, F. Moussavi-Harami, et al., A tension-based model distinguishes hypertrophic versus dilated cardiomyopathy, Cell 165 (5) (2016) 1147–1159.
[17] K.R. Kumar, S.N. Mandleywala, M.S. Link, Atrial and ventricular arrhythmias in hypertrophic cardiomyopathy, Card. Electrophysiol. Clin. 7 (2) (2015) 173–186.
[18] S.C. Menon, B.W. Eidem, J.A. Dearani, S.R. Ommen, M.J. Ackerman, D. Miller, Diastolic dysfunction and its histopathological correlation in obstructive hypertrophic cardiomyopathy in children and adolescents, J. Am. Soc. Echocardiogr. 22 (12) (2009) 1327–1334.
[19] J.A. Jarcho, W. McKenna, J.A. Pare, S.D. Solomon, R.F. Holcombe, S. Dickie, et al., Mapping a gene for familial hypertrophic cardiomyopathy to chromosome 14q1, N. Engl. J. Med. 321 (20) (1989) 1372–1378.
[20] J. Ingles, C. Burns, A. Barratt, C. Semsarian, Application of genetic testing in hypertrophic cardiomyopathy for preclinical disease detection, Circ. Cardiovasc. Genet. 8 (6) (2015) 852–859.
[21] T. Konno, S. Chang, J.G. Seidman, C.E. Seidman, Genetics of hypertrophic cardiomyopathy, Curr. Opin. Cardiol. 25 (3) (2010) 205–209.
[22] S.L. Van Driest, S.R. Ommen, A.J. Tajik, B.J. Gersh, M.J. Ackerman, Sarcomeric genotyping in hypertrophic cardiomyopathy, Mayo Clin. Proc. 80 (4) (2005) 463–469.
[23] C.Y. Ho, Hypertrophic cardiomyopathy in 2012, Circulation 125 (11) (2012) 1432–1438.
[24] P. Richard, P. Charron, L. Carrier, C. Ledeuil, T. Cheav, C. Pichereau, et al., Hypertrophic cardiomyopathy – distribution of disease genes, spectrum of mutations, and implications for a molecular diagnosis strategy, Circulation 107 (17) (2003) 2227–2232.
[25] J.P. Kaski, P. Syrris, M.T. Esteban, S. Jenkins, A. Pantazis, J.E. Deanfield, et al., Prevalence of sarcomere protein gene mutations in preadolescent children with hypertrophic cardiomyopathy, Circ. Cardiovasc. Genet. 2 (5) (2009) 436–441.
[26] A.P. Landstrom, M.J. Ackerman, Mutation type is not clinically useful in predicting prognosis in hypertrophic cardiomyopathy, Circulation 122 (23) (2010) 2441–2449 Discussion 50.
[27] I. Olivotto, F. Girolami, M.J. Ackerman, S. Nistri, J.M. Bos, E. Zachara, et al., Myofilament protein gene mutation screening and outcome of patients with hypertrophic cardiomyopathy, Mayo Clin. Proc. 83 (6) (2008) 630–638.
[28] A.J. Marian, On genetic and phenotypic variability of hypertrophic cardiomyopathy: nature versus nurture, J. Am. Coll. Cardiol. 38 (2) (2001) 331–334.
[29] F. Girolami, C.Y. Ho, C. Semsarian, M. Baldi, M.L. Will, K. Baldini, et al., Clinical features and outcome of hypertrophic cardiomyopathy associated with triple sarcomere protein gene mutations, J. Am. Coll. Cardiol. 55 (14) (2010) 1444–1453.
[30] B.J. Maron, M.S. Maron, C. Semsarian, Double or compound sarcomere mutations in hypertrophic cardiomyopathy: a potential link to sudden death in the absence of conventional risk factors, Heart Rhythm 9 (1) (2012) 57–63.
[31] M.W. Wessels, J.C. Herkert, I.M. Frohn-Mulder, M. Dalinghaus, A. van den Wijngaard, R.R. de Krijger, et al., Compound heterozygous or homozygous truncating MYBPC3 mutations cause lethal cardiomyopathy with features of noncompaction and septal defects, Eur. J. Hum. Genet. 23 (7) (2015) 922–928.
[32] C.Y. Ho, Genetic considerations in hypertrophic cardiomyopathy, Prog. Cardiovasc. Dis. 54 (6) (2012) 456–460.
[33] C.S. Richards, S. Bale, D.B. Bellissimo, S. Das, W.W. Grody, M.R. Hegde, et al., ACMG recommendations for standards for interpretation and reporting of sequence variations: revisions 2007, Genet. Med. 10 (4) (2008) 294–300.
[34] E.J. Rowin, B.J. Maron, E. Appelbaum, M.S. Link, C.M. Gibson, J.R. Lesser, et al., Significance of false negative electrocardiograms in preparticipation screening of athletes for hypertrophic cardiomyopathy, Am. J. Cardiol. 110 (7) (2012) 1027–1032.
[35] M.S. Maron, B.J. Maron, C. Harrigan, J. Buros, C.M. Gibson, I. Olivotto, et al., Hypertrophic cardiomyopathy phenotype revisited after 50 years with cardiovascular magnetic resonance, J. Am. Coll. Cardiol. 54 (3) (2009) 220–228.

[36] A. Florian, P.G. Masci, S. De Buck, G.D. Aquaro, P. Claus, G. Todiere, et al., Geometric assessment of asymmetric septal hypertrophic cardiomyopathy by CMR, JACC Cardiovasc. Imaging 5 (7) (2012) 702–711.
[37] R. Thaman, J.R. Gimeno, S. Reith, M.T. Esteban, G. Limongelli, R.T. Murphy, et al., Progressive left ventricular remodeling in patients with hypertrophic cardiomyopathy and severe left ventricular hypertrophy, J. Am. Coll. Cardiol. 44 (2) (2004) 398–405.
[38] R. Ro, D. Halpern, D.J. Sahn, P. Homel, M. Arabadjian, C. Lopresto, et al., Vector flow mapping in obstructive hypertrophic cardiomyopathy to assess the relationship of early systolic left ventricular flow and the mitral valve, J. Am. Coll. Cardiol. 64 (19) (2014) 1984–1995.
[39] E.K. Alhaj, B. Kim, D. Cantales, S. Uretsky, F.A. Chaudhry, M.V. Sherrid, Symptomatic exercise-induced left ventricular outflow tract obstruction without left ventricular hypertrophy, J. Am. Soc. Echocardiogr. 26 (5) (2013) 556–565.
[40] M.S. Maron, I. Olivotto, A.G. Zenovich, M.S. Link, N.G. Pandian, J.T. Kuvin, et al., Hypertrophic cardiomyopathy is predominantly a disease of left ventricular outflow tract obstruction, Circulation 114 (21) (2006) 2232–2239.
[41] J.A. Panza, R.K. Petrone, L. Fananapazir, B.J. Maron, Utility of continuous wave Doppler echocardiography in the noninvasive assessment of left ventricular outflow tract pressure gradient in patients with hypertrophic cardiomyopathy, J. Am. Coll. Cardiol. 19 (1992) 91–99.
[42] P. Nihoyannopoulos, G. Karatasakis, M. Frenneaux, W.J. McKenna, C.M. Oakley, Diastolic function in hypertrophic cardiomyopathy: relation to exercise capacity, J. Am. Coll. Cardiol. 19 (1992) 536–540.
[43] S.C. Menon, M.J. Ackerman, F. Cetta, P.W. O'Leary, B.W. Eidem, Significance of left atrial volume in patients < 20 years of age with hypertrophic cardiomyopathy, Am. J. Cardiol. 102 (10) (2008) 1390–1393.
[44] S. Betocchi, O.M. Hess, M.A. Losi, H. Nonogi, H.P. Krayenbuehl, Regional left ventricular mechanics in hypertrophic cardiomyopathy, Circulation 88 (1993) 2206–2214.
[45] C.J. McMahon, S.F. Nagueh, R.H. Pignatelli, S.W. Denfield, W.J. Dreyer, J.F. Price, et al., Characterization of left ventricular diastolic function by tissue Doppler imaging and clinical status in children with hypertrophic cardiomyopathy, Circulation 109 (14) (2004) 1756–1762.
[46] D. Vinereanu, N. Florescu, N. Sculthorpe, A.C. Tweddel, M.R. Stephens, A.G. Fraser, Differentiation between pathologic and physiologic left ventricular hypertrophy by tissue Doppler assessment of long-axis function in patients with hypertrophic cardiomyopathy or systemic hypertension and in athletes, Am. J. Cardiol. 88 (1) (2001) 53–58.
[47] K. Serri, P. Reant, M. Lafitte, M. Berhouet, V. Le Bouffos, R. Roudaut, et al., Global and regional myocardial function quantification by two-dimensional strain: application in hypertrophic cardiomyopathy, J. Am. Coll. Cardiol. 47 (6) (2006) 1175–1181.
[48] J. Ganame, L. Mertens, B.W. Eidem, P. Claus, J. D'Hooge, L.M. Havemann, et al., Regional myocardial deformation in children with hypertrophic cardiomyopathy: morphological and clinical correlations, Eur. Heart J. 28 (23) (2007) 2886–2894.
[49] S. Wang, M. Luo, H. Sun, Y. Song, C. Yin, L. Wang, et al., A retrospective clinical study of transaortic extended septal myectomy for obstructive hypertrophic cardiomyopathy in China, Eur. J. Cardiothorac. Surg. 43 (3) (2013) 534–540.
[50] J. Bogaert, I. Olivotto, MR imaging in hypertrophic cardiomyopathy: from magnet to bedside, Radiology 273 (2) (2014) 329–348.
[51] O. Bruder, A. Wagner, C.J. Jensen, S. Schneider, P. Ong, E.M. Kispert, et al., Myocardial scar visualized by cardiovascular magnetic resonance imaging predicts major adverse events in patients with hypertrophic cardiomyopathy, J. Am. Coll. Cardiol. 56 (11) (2010) 875–887.
[52] M.S. Maron, E. Appelbaum, C.J. Harrigan, J. Buros, C.M. Gibson, C. Hanna, et al., Clinical profile and significance of delayed enhancement in hypertrophic cardiomyopathy, Circ. Heart Fail. 1 (3) (2008) 184–191.
[53] A.S. Adabag, B.J. Maron, E. Appelbaum, C.J. Harrigan, J.L. Buros, C.M. Gibson, et al., Occurrence and frequency of arrhythmias in hypertrophic cardiomyopathy in relation to delayed enhancement on cardiovascular magnetic resonance, J. Am. Coll. Cardiol. 51 (14) (2008) 1369–1374.
[54] N. Child, T. Muhr, E. Sammut, D. Dabir, E.A. Ucar, T. Bueser, et al., Prevalence of myocardial crypts in a large retrospective cohort study by cardiovascular magnetic resonance, J. Cardiovasc. Magn. Reson. 16 (2014) 66.
[55] G. Captur, L.R. Lopes, T.J. Mohun, V. Patel, C. Li, P. Bassett, et al., Prediction of sarcomere mutations in subclinical hypertrophic cardiomyopathy, Circ. Cardiovasc. Imaging 7 (6) (2014) 863–871.
[56] P.M. Elliott, J. Poloniecki, S. Dickie, S. Sharma, L. Monserrat, A. Varnava, et al., Sudden death in hypertrophic cardiomyopathy: identification of high risk patients, J. Am. Coll. Cardiol. 36 (7) (2000) 2212–2218.
[57] C.Y. Ho, N.K. Sweitzer, B. McDonough, B.J. Maron, S.A. Casey, J.G. Seidman, et al., Assessment of diastolic function with Doppler tissue imaging to predict genotype in preclinical hypertrophic cardiomyopathy, Circulation 105 (25) (2002) 2992–2997.
[58] M. Michels, O.I. Soliman, M.J. Kofflard, Y.M. Hoedemaekers, D. Dooijes, D. Majoor-Krakauer, et al., Diastolic abnormalities as the first feature of hypertrophic cardiomyopathy in Dutch myosin-binding protein C founder mutations, JACC Cardiovasc. Imaging 2 (1) (2009) 58–64.
[59] C.Y. Ho, S.A. Abbasi, T.G. Neilan, R.V. Shah, Y. Chen, B. Heydari, et al., T1 measurements identify extracellular volume expansion in hypertrophic cardiomyopathy sarcomere mutation carriers with and without left ventricular hypertrophy, Circ. Cardiovasc. Imaging 6 (3) (2013) 415–422.
[60] E.J. Rowin, M.S. Maron, J.R. Lesser, B.J. Maron, CMR with late gadolinium enhancement in genotype positive-phenotype negative hypertrophic cardiomyopathy, JACC Cardiovasc. Imaging 5 (1) (2012) 119–122.
[61] I.K. Russel, W.P. Brouwer, T. Germans, P. Knaapen, J.T. Marcus, V. van d, et al., Increased left ventricular torsion in hypertrophic cardiomyopathy mutation carriers with normal wall thickness, J. Cardiovasc. Magn. Reson. 13 (1) (2011) 3.
[62] T. Germans, I.K. Russel, M.J. Gotte, M.D. Spreeuwenberg, P.A. Doevendans, Y.M. Pinto, et al., How do hypertrophic cardiomyopathy mutations affect myocardial function in carriers with normal wall thickness? Assessment with cardiovascular magnetic resonance, J. Cardiovasc. Magn. Reson. 12 (1) (2010) 13.
[63] L.M. Shapiro, W.J. McKenna, Distribution of left ventricular hypertrophy in hypertrophic cardiomyopathy: a two-dimensional echocardiographic study, J. Am. Coll. Cardiol. 2 (3) (1983) 437–444.

[64] J.L. Jefferies, J.D. Wilkinson, L.A. Sleeper, S.D. Colan, M. Lu, E. Pahl, et al., Cardiomyopathy phenotypes and outcomes for children with left ventricular myocardial noncompaction: results from the pediatric cardiomyopathy registry, J. Card. Fail. 21 (11) (2015) 877–884.

[65] S.F. Saleeb, R. Margossian, C.T. Spencer, M.E. Alexander, L.B. Smoot, A.L. Dorfman, et al., Reproducibility of echocardiographic diagnosis of left ventricular noncompaction, J. Am. Soc. Echocardiogr. 25 (2) (2012) 194–202.

[66] S.E. Lipshultz, E.J. Orav, J.D. Wilkinson, J.A. Towbin, J.E. Messere, A.M. Lowe, et al., Risk stratification at diagnosis for children with hypertrophic cardiomyopathy: an analysis of data from the Pediatric Cardiomyopathy Registry, Lancet 382 (9908) (2013) 1889–1897.

[67] T. Kubo, J.R. Gimeno, A. Bahl, U. Steffensen, M. Steffensen, E. Osman, et al., Prevalence, clinical significance, and genetic basis of hypertrophic cardiomyopathy with restrictive phenotype, J. Am. Coll. Cardiol. 49 (25) (2007) 2419–2426.

[68] A. Angelini, V. Calzolari, G. Thiene, G.M. Boffa, M. Valente, L. Daliento, et al., Morphologic spectrum of primary restrictive cardiomyopathy, Am. J. Cardiol. 80 (8) (1997) 1046–1050.

[69] S.A. Webber, S.E. Lipshultz, L.A. Sleeper, M. Lu, J.D. Wilkinson, L.J. Addonizio, et al., Outcomes of restrictive cardiomyopathy in childhood and the influence of phenotype: a report from the Pediatric Cardiomyopathy Registry, Circulation 126 (10) (2012) 1237–1244.

[70] J.J. Silbiger, Abnormalities of the mitral apparatus in hypertrophic cardiomyopathy: echocardiographic, pathophysiologic, and surgical insights, J. Am. Soc. Echocardiogr. 29 (7) (2016) 622–639.

[71] T. Chikamori, Y.L. Doi, M. Akizawa, Y. Yonezawa, T. Ozawa, W.J. McKenna, Comparison of clinical, morphological, and prognostic features in hypertrophic cardiomyopathy between Japanese and western patients, Clin. Cardiol. 15 (11) (1992) 833–837.

[72] M.J. Eriksson, B. Sonnenberg, A. Woo, P. Rakowski, T.G. Parker, E.D. Wigle, et al., Long-term outcome in patients with apical hypertrophic cardiomyopathy, J. Am. Coll. Cardiol. 39 (4) (2002) 638–645.

[73] C. O'Mahony, F. Jichi, L. Monserrat, M. Ortiz-Genga, A. Anastasakis, C. Rapezzi, et al., Inverted U-shaped relation between the risk of sudden cardiac death and maximal left ventricular wall thickness in hypertrophic cardiomyopathy, Circ. Arrhythm. Electrophysiol. 9 (6) (2016).

[74] E. Braunwald, C.T. Lambrew, S.D. Rockoff, J. Ross Jr., A.G. Morrow, Idiopathic hypertrophic subaortic stenosis. I. A description of the disease based upon an analysis of 64 patients, Circulation 30 (Suppl. 4) (1964) 3–119.

[75] E.D. Wigle, H. Rakowski, B.P. Kimball, W.G. Williams, Hypertrophic cardiomyopathy – clinical spectrum and treatment, Circulation 92 (1995) 1680–1692.

[76] D.H. Kim, M.D. Handschumacher, R.A. Levine, Y.S. Choi, Y.J. Kim, S.C. Yun, et al., In vivo measurement of mitral leaflet surface area and subvalvular geometry in patients with asymmetrical septal hypertrophy: insights into the mechanism of outflow tract obstruction, Circulation 122 (13) (2010) 1298–1307.

[77] M.V. Sherrid, C.K. Chu, E. Delia, A. Mogtader, E.M. Dwyer Jr., An echocardiographic study of the fluid mechanics of obstruction in hypertrophic cardiomyopathy, J. Am. Coll. Cardiol. 22 (1993) 816–825.

[78] P. Sorajja, R.A. Nishimura, B.J. Gersh, J.A. Dearani, D.O. Hodge, H.J. Wiste, et al., Outcome of mildly symptomatic or asymptomatic obstructive hypertrophic cardiomyopathy: a long-term follow-up study, J. Am. Coll. Cardiol. 54 (3) (2009) 234–241.

[79] M.S. Maron, I. Olivotto, S. Betocchi, S.A. Casey, J.R. Lesser, M.A. Losi, et al., Effect of left ventricular outflow tract obstruction on clinical outcome in hypertrophic cardiomyopathy, N. Engl. J. Med. 348 (4) (2003) 295–303.

[80] I. Olivotto, F. Cecchi, S.A. Casey, A. Dolara, J.H. Traverse, B.J. Maron, Impact of atrial fibrillation on the clinical course of hypertrophic cardiomyopathy, Circulation 104 (21) (2001) 2517–2524.

[81] E.J. Hickey, B.W. McCrindle, S.H. Larsen, L. Benson, C. Manlhiot, C.A. Caldarone, et al., Hypertrophic cardiomyopathy in childhood: disease natural history, impact of obstruction, and its influence on survival, Ann. Thorac. Surg. 93 (3) (2012) 840–848.

[82] A. Frustaci, R. Verardo, M. Caldarulo, M.C. Acconcia, M.A. Russo, C. Chimenti, Myocarditis in hypertrophic cardiomyopathy patients presenting acute clinical deterioration, Eur. Heart J. 28 (6) (2007) 733–740.

[83] D. Pasqualucci, A. Fornaro, G. Castelli, A. Rossi, A. Arretini, C. Chiriatti, et al., Clinical spectrum, therapeutic options, and outcome of advanced heart failure in hypertrophic cardiomyopathy, Circ. Heart Fail. 8 (6) (2015) 1014–1021.

[84] K.M. Harris, P. Spirito, M.S. Maron, A.G. Zenovich, F. Formisano, J.R. Lesser, et al., Prevalence, clinical profile, and significance of left ventricular remodeling in the end-stage phase of hypertrophic cardiomyopathy, Circulation 114 (3) (2006) 216–225.

[85] P. Melacini, B.J. Maron, F. Bobbo, C. Basso, B. Tokajuk, M. Zucchetto, et al., Evidence that pharmacological strategies lack efficacy for the prevention of sudden death in hypertrophic cardiomyopathy, Heart 93 (6) (2007) 708–710.

[86] L. Monserrat, P.M. Elliott, J.R. Gimeno, S. Sharma, M. Penas-Lado, W.J. McKenna, Non-sustained ventricular tachycardia in hypertrophic cardiomyopathy: an independent marker of sudden death risk in young patients, J. Am. Coll. Cardiol. 42 (5) (2003) 873–879.

[87] W.J. McKenna, R.C. Franklin, P. Nihoyannopoulos, K.C. Robinson, J.E. Deanfield, Arrhythmia and prognosis in infants, children and adolescents with hypertrophic cardiomyopathy, J. Am. Coll. Cardiol. 11 (1) (1988) 147–153.

[88] L. Ziolkowska, A. Turska-Kmiec, J. Petryka, W. Kawalec, Predictors of long-term outcome in children with hypertrophic cardiomyopathy, Pediatr. Cardiol. 37 (3) (2016) 448–458.

[89] K.C. Siontis, J.B. Geske, K. Ong, R.A. Nishimura, S.R. Ommen, B.J. Gersh, Atrial fibrillation in hypertrophic cardiomyopathy: prevalence, clinical correlations, and mortality in a large high-risk population, J. Am. Heart Assoc. 3 (3) (2014) e001002.

[90] R. Providencia, P. Elliott, K. Patel, J. McCready, G. Babu, N. Srinivasan, et al., Catheter ablation for atrial fibrillation in hypertrophic cardiomyopathy: a systematic review and meta-analysis, Heart 102 (19) (2016) 1533–1543.

[91] P.M. Elliott, J.R. Gimeno, R. Thaman, J. Shah, D. Ward, S. Dickie, et al., Historical trends in reported survival rates in patients with hypertrophic cardiomyopathy, Heart 92 (6) (2006) 785–791.

[92] B.J. Maron, E. Braunwald, Evolution of hypertrophic cardiomyopathy to a contemporary treatable disease, Circulation 126 (13) (2012) 1640–1644.

[93] S.F. Nagueh, L.L. Bachinski, D. Meyer, R. Hill, W.A. Zoghbi, J.W. Tam, et al., Tissue Doppler imaging consistently detects myocardial abnormalities in patients with hypertrophic cardiomyopathy and provides a novel means for an early diagnosis before and independently of hypertrophy, Circulation 104 (2) (2001) 128–130.

[94] J. Forsey, L. Benson, E. Rozenblyum, M.K. Friedberg, L. Mertens, Early changes in apical rotation in genotype positive children with hypertrophic cardiomyopathy mutations without hypertrophic changes on two-dimensional imaging, J. Am. Soc. Echocardiogr. 27 (2) (2014) 215–221.

[95] D. Silva, H. Madeira, A. Almeida, D. Brito, Tissue Doppler imaging and plasma N-terminal probrain natriuretic peptide for the identification of hypertrophic cardiomyopathy mutation carriers, Am. J. Cardiol. 112 (7) (2013) 996–1004.

[96] C.Y. Ho, A.L. Cirino, N.K. Lakdawala, J. Groarke, A.M. Valente, C. Semsarian, et al., Evolution of hypertrophic cardiomyopathy in sarcomere mutation carriers, Heart (2016) (in press). [Epub ahead of print].

[97] C. O'Mahony, F. Jichi, M. Pavlou, L. Monserrat, A. Anastasakis, C. Rapezzi, et al., A novel clinical risk prediction model for sudden cardiac death in hypertrophic cardiomyopathy (HCM risk-SCD), Eur. Heart J. 35 (30) (2014) 2010–2020.

[98] I. Christiaans, E. Birnie, G.J. Bonsel, M.M. Mannens, M. Michels, D. Majoor-Krakauer, et al., Manifest disease, risk factors for sudden cardiac death, and cardiac events in a large nationwide cohort of predictively tested hypertrophic cardiomyopathy mutation carriers: determining the best cardiological screening strategy, Eur. Heart J. 32 (9) (2011) 1161–1170.

[99] T. Huang, A. Kelly, S.A. Becker, M.S. Cohen, C.A. Stanley, Hypertrophic cardiomyopathy in neonates with congenital hyperinsulinism, Arch. Dis. Child Fetal Neonatal Ed. 98 (4) (2013) F351–F354.

[100] G.L. Way, R.R. Wolfe, E. Eshaghpour, R.L. Bender, R.B. Jaffe, H.D. Ruttenberg, The natural history of hypertrophic cardiomyopathy in infants of diabetic mothers, J. Pediatr. 95 (6) (1979) 1020–1025.

[101] J.N. McMahon, P.J. Berry, H.S. Joffe, Fatal hypertrophic cardiomyopathy in an infant of a diabetic mother, Pediatr. Cardiol. 11 (4) (1990) 211–212.

[102] A.E. Lin, M.E. Alexander, S.D. Colan, B. Kerr, K.A. Rauen, J. Noonan, et al., Clinical, pathological, and molecular analyses of cardiovascular abnormalities in Costello syndrome: a Ras/MAPK pathway syndrome, Am. J. Med. Genet. A 155 (3) (2011) 486–507.

[103] J.L. Colquitt, J.A. Noonan, Cardiac findings in Noonan syndrome on long-term follow-up, Congenit. Heart Dis. 9 (2) (2014) 144–150.

[104] J.D. Wilkinson, A.M. Lowe, B.A. Salbert, L.A. Sleeper, S.D. Colan, G.F. Cox, et al., Outcomes in children with Noonan syndrome and hypertrophic cardiomyopathy: a study from the Pediatric Cardiomyopathy Registry, Am. Heart J. 164 (3) (2012) 442–448.

[105] B.D. Gelb, A.E. Roberts, M. Tartaglia, Cardiomyopathies in Noonan syndrome and the other RASopathies, Prog. Pediatr. Cardiol. 39 (1) (2015) 13–19.

[106] T.M. Marin, K. Keith, B. Davies, D.A. Conner, P. Guha, D. Kalaitzidis, et al., Rapamycin reverses hypertrophic cardiomyopathy in a mouse model of LEOPARD syndrome-associated PTPN11 mutation, J. Clin. Investig. 121 (3) (2011) 1026–1043.

[107] M. Arad, B.J. Maron, J.M. Gorham, W.H. Johnson, J.P. Saul, A.R. Perez-Atayde, et al., Glycogen storage diseases presenting as hypertrophic cardiomyopathy, N. Engl. J. Med. 352 (2005) 362–372.

[108] T.J. Rowland, M.E. Sweet, L. Mestroni, M.R. Taylor, Danon disease - dysregulation of autophagy in a multisystem disorder with cardiomyopathy, J. Cell Sci. 129 (11) (2016) 2135–2143.

[109] B.J. Maron, W.C. Roberts, M. Arad, T.S. Haas, P. Spirito, G.B. Wright, et al., Clinical outcome and phenotypic expression in LAMP2 cardiomyopathy, JAMA 301 (12) (2009) 1253–1259.

[110] A. Toib, D.K. Grange, B.A. Kozel, G.A. Ewald, F.V. White, C.E. Canter, Distinct clinical and histopathological presentations of Danon cardiomyopathy in young women, J. Am. Coll. Cardiol. 55 (4) (2010) 408–410.

[111] P.S. Kishnani, D. Corzo, M. Nicolino, B. Byrne, H. Mandel, W.L. Hwu, et al., Recombinant human acid [alpha]-glucosidase: major clinical benefits in infantile-onset Pompe disease, Neurology 68 (2) (2007) 99–109.

[112] C.J. Lai, T.R. Hsu, C.F. Yang, S.J. Chen, Y.C. Chuang, D.M. Niu, Cognitive development in infantile-onset Pompe disease under very early enzyme replacement therapy, J. Child Neurol. 31 (14) (2016) 1617–1621.

[113] A. Toscano, B. Schoser, Enzyme replacement therapy in late-onset Pompe disease: a systematic literature review, J. Neurol. 260 (4) (2013) 951–959.

[114] C.F. Yang, C.C. Yang, H.C. Liao, L.Y. Huang, C.C. Chiang, H.C. Ho, et al., Very early treatment for infantile-onset Pompe disease contributes to better outcomes, J. Pediatr. 169 (2016) 174–180 e1.

[115] M. Arad, D.W. Benson, A.R. Perez-Atayde, W.J. McKenna, E.A. Sparks, R.J. Kanter, et al., Constitutively active AMP kinase mutations cause glycogen storage disease mimicking hypertrophic cardiomyopathy, J. Clin. Investig. 109 (3) (2002) 357–362.

[116] A.G. Porto, F. Brun, G.M. Severini, P. Losurdo, E. Fabris, M.R. Taylor, et al., Clinical spectrum of PRKAG2 syndrome, Circ. Arrhythm. Electrophysiol. 9 (1) (2016) e003121.

[117] H.O. Akman, J.N. Sampayo, F.A. Ross, J.W. Scott, G. Wilson, L. Benson, et al., Fatal infantile cardiac glycogenosis with phosphorylase kinase deficiency and a mutation in the gamma2-subunit of AMP-activated protein kinase, Pediatr. Res. 62 (4) (2007) 499–504.

[118] C.M. Wolf, M. Arad, F. Ahmad, A. Sanbe, S.A. Bernstein, O. Toka, et al., Reversibility of PRKAG2 glycogen-storage cardiomyopathy and electrophysiological manifestations, Circulation 117 (2) (2008) 144–154.

[119] P. Elliott, R. Baker, F. Pasquale, G. Quarta, H. Ebrahim, A.B. Mehta, et al., Prevalence of Anderson-Fabry disease in patients with hypertrophic cardiomyopathy: the European Anderson-Fabry disease survey, Heart 97 (23) (2011) 1957–1960.

[120] C. O'Mahony, P. Elliott, Anderson-Fabry disease and the heart, Prog. Cardiovasc. Dis. 52 (4) (2010) 326–335.

[121] V. Campuzano, L. Montermini, M.D. Molto, L. Pianese, M. Cossee, F. Cavalcanti, et al., Friedreich's ataxia: autosomal recessive disease caused by an intronic GAA triplet repeat expansion, Science 271 (1996) 1423–1427.

[122] A. Linhart, T. Palecek, J. Bultas, J.J. Ferguson, J. Hrudová, D. Karetová, et al., New insights in cardiac structural changes in patients with Fabry's disease, Am. Heart J. 139 (6) (2000) 1101–1108.

[123] M.L. Huang, E.M. Becker, M. Whitnall, Y. Suryo Rahmanto, P. Ponka, D.R. Richardson, Elucidation of the mechanism of mitochondrial iron loading in Friedreich's ataxia by analysis of a mouse mutant, Proc. Natl. Acad. Sci. U.S.A. 106 (38) (2009) 16381–16386.
[124] F. Weidemann, C. Rummey, B. Bijnens, S. Stork, R. Jasaityte, J. Dhooge, et al., The heart in Friedreich ataxia: definition of cardiomyopathy, disease severity, and correlation with neurological symptoms, Circulation 125 (13) (2012) 1626–1634.
[125] A. Kipps, M. Alexander, S.D. Colan, K. Gauvreau, L. Smoot, L. Crawford, et al., The longitudinal course of cardiomyopathy in Friedreich's ataxia during childhood, Pediatr. Cardiol. 30 (3) (2009) 306–310.
[126] A.H. Koeppen, Friedreich's ataxia: pathology, pathogenesis, and molecular genetics, J. Neurol. Sci. 303 (1–2) (2011) 1–12.
[127] P.I. Patel, G. Isaya, Friedreich ataxia: from GAA triplet-repeat expansion to frataxin deficiency, Am. J. Hum. Genet. 69 (1) (2001) 15–24.
[128] S.J. Lagedrost, M.S. Sutton, M.S. Cohen, G.M. Satou, B.D. Kaufman, S.L. Perlman, et al., Idebenone in Friedreich ataxia cardiomyopathy-results from a 6-month phase III study (IONIA), Am. Heart J. 161 (3) (2011) 639–645 e1.
[129] F.G. Debray, M. Lambert, I. Chevalier, Y. Robitaille, J.C. Decarie, E.A. Shoubridge, et al., Long-term outcome and clinical spectrum of 73 pediatric patients with mitochondrial diseases, Pediatrics 119 (4) (2007) 722–733.
[130] C. Brunel-Guitton, A. Levtova, F. Sasarman, Mitochondrial diseases and cardiomyopathies, Can. J. Cardiol. 31 (11) (2015) 1360–1376.
[131] K. Neveling, I. Feenstra, C. Gilissen, L.H. Hoefsloot, E.J. Kamsteeg, A.R. Mensenkamp, et al., A post-hoc comparison of the utility of sanger sequencing and exome sequencing for the diagnosis of heterogeneous diseases, Hum. Mutat. 34 (12) (2013) 1721–1726.
[132] J. Somerville, L. Becu, Congenital heart disease associated with hypertrophic cardiomyopathy, Br. Heart J. 40 (9) (1978) 1034–1039.
[133] A.M. Carvalho, T.C. Diogenes, E.R. Juca, A.F. Carvalho, C.F. Carvalho, J.N. Paes Junior, Tetralogy of Fallot and hypertrophic cardiomyopathy: a rare association, Arq. Bras. Cardiol. 80 (2) (2003) 217–226.
[134] B.J. Maron, J.E. Edwards, J.H. Moller, S.E. Epstein, Prevalence and characteristics of disporportionate ventricular septal thickening in infants with congenital heart disease, Circulation 59 (1) (1979) 126–133.
[135] G. Mahadevaiah, M. Gupta, R. Ashwath, Down syndrome with complete atrioventricular septal defect, hypertrophic cardiomyopathy, and pulmonary vein stenosis, Tex. Heart Inst. J. 42 (5) (2015) 458–461.
[136] B.J. Maron, T.S. Haas, A. Ahluwalia, C.J. Murphy, R.F. Garberich, Demographics and epidemiology of sudden deaths in young competitive athletes: from the United States National Registry, Am. J. Med. 129 (11) (2016) 1170–1177.
[137] K.Y. Kebed, J.M. Bos, N.S. Anavekar, S.L. Mulvagh, M.J. Ackerman, S.R. Ommen, Hypertrophic cardiomyopathy, athlete's heart, or both: a case of hypertrophic cardiomyopathy regression, Circ. Cardiovasc. Imaging 8 (7) (2015) e003312.
[138] H. Niimura, L.L. Bachinski, S. Sangwatanaroj, H. Watkins, A.E. Chudley, W. McKenna, et al., Mutations in the gene for cardiac myosin-binding protein C and late- onset familial hypertrophic cardiomyopathy, N. Engl. J. Med. 338 (18) (1998) 1248–1257.
[139] A.I. Obeid, B.J. Maron, Apical hypertrophic cardiomyopathy developing at a relatively advanced age, Circulation 103 (11) (2001) 1605.
[140] B.J. Maron, H. Niimura, S.A. Casey, M.K. Soper, G.B. Wright, J.G. Seidman, et al., Development of left ventricular hypertrophy in adults with hypertrophic cardiomyopathy caused by cardiac myosin-binding protein C gene mutations, J. Am. Coll. Cardiol. 38 (2) (2001) 315–321.
[141] B.J. Maron, J.G. Seidman, C.E. Seidman, Proposal for contemporary screening strategies in families with hypertrophic cardiomyopathy, J. Am. Coll. Cardiol. 44 (11) (2004) 2125–2132.
[142] I. Ostman-Smith, G. Wettrell, B. Keeton, D. Holmgren, U. Ergander, S. Gould, et al., Age- and gender-specific mortality rates in childhood hypertrophic cardiomyopathy, Eur. Heart J. 29 (9) (2008) 1160–1167.
[143] J.A. Decker, J.W. Rossano, E.O. Smith, B. Cannon, S.K. Clunie, C. Gates, et al., Risk factors and mode of death in isolated hypertrophic cardiomyopathy in children, J. Am. Coll. Cardiol. 54 (3) (2009) 250–254.
[144] M. Brosnan, A. La Gerche, J. Kalman, W. Lo, K. Fallon, A. MacIsaac, et al., The Seattle Criteria increase the specificity of preparticipation ECG screening among elite athletes, Br. J. Sports Med. 48 (15) (2014) 1144–1150.
[145] N. Sheikh, M. Papadakis, S. Ghani, A. Zaidi, S. Gati, P.E. Adami, et al., Comparison of electrocardiographic criteria for the detection of cardiac abnormalities in elite black and white athletes, Circulation 129 (16) (2014) 1637–1649.
[146] N.R. Riding, S. Sharma, O. Salah, N. Khalil, F. Carre, K.P. George, et al., Systematic echocardiography is not efficacious when screening an ethnically diverse cohort of athletes in West Asia, Eur. J. Prev. Cardiol. 22 (2) (2015) 263–270.
[147] B.J. Maron, E.J. Rowin, S.A. Casey, J.R. Lesser, R.F. Garberich, D.M. McGriff, et al., Hypertrophic cardiomyopathy in children, adolescents, and young adults associated with low cardiovascular mortality with contemporary management strategies, Circulation 133 (1) (2016) 62–73.
[148] B.J. Maron, M.S. Maron, E.D. Wigle, E. Braunwald, The 50-year history, controversy, and clinical implications of left ventricular outflow tract obstruction in hypertrophic cardiomyopathy from idiopathic hypertrophic subaortic stenosis to hypertrophic cardiomyopathy: from idiopathic hypertrophic subaortic stenosis to hypertrophic cardiomyopathy, J. Am. Coll. Cardiol. 54 (3) (2009) 191–200.
[149] P.M. Elliott, J.C. Kaski, K. Prasad, H. Seo, A.K. Slade, J.H. Goldman, et al., Chest pain during daily life in patients with hypertrophic cardiomyopathy: an ambulatory electrocardiographic study, Eur. Heart J. 17 (7) (1996) 1056–1064.
[150] A. Pasternac, J. Noble, Y. Streulens, R. Elie, C. Henschke, M.G. Bourassa, Pathophysiology of chest pain in patients with cardiomyopathies and normal coronary arteries, Circulation 65 (1982) 778–789.
[151] I. Olivotto, F. Cecchi, R. Gistri, R. Lorenzoni, G. Chiriatti, F. Girolami, et al., Relevance of coronary microvascular flow impairment to long-term remodeling and systolic dysfunction in hypertrophic cardiomyopathy, J. Am. Coll. Cardiol. 47 (5) (2006) 1043–1048.
[152] R. Krams, M.J.M. Kofflard, D.J. Duncker, C. Von Birgelen, S. Carlier, M. Kliffen, et al., Decreased coronary flow reserve in hypertrophic cardiomyopathy is related to remodeling of the coronary microcirculation, Circulation 97 (3) (1998) 230–233.
[153] P. Camici, G. Chiriatti, R. Lorenzoni, R.C. Bellina, R. Gistri, G. Italiani, et al., Coronary vasodilation is impaired in both hypertrophied and non-hypertrophied myocardium of patients with hypertrophic cardiomyopathy: a study with nitrogen-13 ammonia and positron emission tomography, J. Am. Coll. Cardiol. 17 (1991) 879–886.

[154] A.S. Adabag, S.A. Casey, M.A. Kuskowski, A.G. Zenovich, B.J. Maron, Spectrum and prognostic significance of arrhythmias on ambulatory Holter electrocardiogram in hypertrophic cardiomyopathy, J. Am. Coll. Cardiol. 45 (5) (2005) 697–704.

[155] C.A. Nienaber, S. Hiller, R.P. Spielmann, M. Geiger, K.-H. Kuck, Syncope in hypertrophic cardiomyopathy: multivariate analysis of prognostic determinants, J. Am. Coll. Cardiol. 15 (1990) 948–955.

[156] P. Spirito, C. Autore, C. Rapezzi, P. Bernabo, R. Badagliacca, M.S. Maron, et al., Syncope and risk of sudden death in hypertrophic cardiomyopathy, Circulation 119 (13) (2009) 1703–1710.

[157] F. Manganelli, S. Betocchi, M.A. Losi, C. Briguori, L. Pace, Q. Ciampi, et al., Influence of left ventricular cavity size on clinical presentation in hypertrophic cardiomyopathy, Am. J. Cardiol. 83 (4) (1999) 547–552.

[158] M.V. Sherrid, G. Pearle, D.Z. Gunsburg, Mechanism of benefit of negative inotropes in obstructive hypertrophic cardiomyopathy, Circulation 97 (1) (1998) 41–47.

[159] R. Gistri, F. Cecchi, L. Choudhury, A. Montereggi, O. Sorace, P.A. Salvadori, et al., Effect of verapamil on absolute myocardial blood flow in hypertrophic cardiomyopathy, Am. J. Cardiol. 74 (4) (1994) 363–368.

[160] A.M. Moran, S.D. Colan, Verapamil therapy in infants with hypertrophic cardiomyopathy, Cardiol. Young 8 (3) (1998) 310–319.

[161] M.V. Sherrid, I. Barac, W.J. McKenna, P.M. Elliott, S. Dickie, L. Chojnowska, et al., Multicenter study of the efficacy and safety of disopyramide in obstructive hypertrophic cardiomyopathy, J. Am. Coll. Cardiol. 45 (8) (2005) 1251–1258.

[162] M.C. Sokoloski, Evaluation and treatment of pediatric patients with neurocardiogenic syncope, Prog. Pediatr. Cardiol. 13 (2) (2001) 127–131.

[163] T. Yamazaki, J. Suzuki, R. Shimamoto, T. Tsuji, Y. Ohmoto-Sekine, K. Ohtomo, et al., A new therapeutic strategy for hypertrophic nonobstructive cardiomyopathy in humans. A randomized and prospective study with an Angiotensin II receptor blocker, Int. Heart J. 48 (6) (2007) 715–724.

[164] Y.J. Shimada, J.J. Passeri, A.L. Baggish, C. O'Callaghan, P.A. Lowry, G. Yannekis, et al., Effects of losartan on left ventricular hypertrophy and fibrosis in patients with nonobstructive hypertrophic cardiomyopathy, JACC Heart Fail. 1 (6) (2013) 480–487.

[165] M. Kyriakidis, F. Triposkiadis, J. Dernellis, A.E. Androulakis, P. Mellas, G.A. Kelepeshis, et al., Effects of cardiac versus circulatory angiotensin-converting enzyme inhibition on left ventricular diastolic function and coronary blood flow in hypertrophic obstructive cardiomyopathy, Circulation 97 (14) (1998) 1342–1347.

[166] S.R. Ommen, B.J. Maron, I. Olivotto, M.S. Maron, F. Cecchi, S. Betocchi, et al., Long-term effects of surgical septal myectomy on survival in patients with obstructive hypertrophic cardiomyopathy, J. Am. Coll. Cardiol. 46 (3) (2005) 470–476.

[167] P. Ferrazzi, P. Spirito, A. Iacovoni, A. Calabrese, K. Migliorati, C. Simon, et al., Transaortic chordal cutting: mitral valve repair for obstructive hypertrophic cardiomyopathy with mild septal hypertrophy, J. Am. Coll. Cardiol. 66 (15) (2015) 1687–1696.

[168] K. Minakata, J.A. Dearani, P.W. O'Leary, G.K. Danielson, Septal myectomy for obstructive hypertrophic cardiomyopathy in pediatric patients: early and late results, Ann. Thorac. Surg. 80 (4) (2005) 1424–1429.

[169] J.X. Qin, T. Shiota, H.M. Lever, S.R. Kapadia, M. Sitges, D.N. Rubin, et al., Outcome of patients with hypertrophic obstructive cardiomyopathy after percutaneous transluminal septal myocardial ablation and septal myectomy surgery, J. Am. Coll. Cardiol. 38 (7) (2001) 1994–2000.

[170] R.A. Nishimura, S.R. Ommen, Septal reduction therapy for obstructive hypertrophic cardiomyopathy and sudden death: what statistics cannot tell you, Circ. Cardiovasc. Interv. 3 (2) (2010) 91–93.

[171] B.J. Maron, Hypertrophic cardiomyopathy, Lancet 350 (1997) 127–133.

[172] P. Elliott, P. Spirito, Prevention of hypertrophic cardiomyopathy-related deaths: theory and practice, Heart 94 (10) (2008) 1269–1275.

[173] G. Lin, R.A. Nishimura, B.J. Gersh, D. Phil, S.R. Ommen, M.J. Ackerman, et al., Device complications and inappropriate implantable cardioverter defibrillator shocks in patients with hypertrophic cardiomyopathy, Heart 95 (9) (2009) 709–714.

[174] R. Tung, P. Zimetbaum, M.E. Josephson, A critical appraisal of implantable cardioverter-defibrillator therapy for the prevention of sudden cardiac death, J. Am. Coll. Cardiol. 52 (14) (2008) 1111–1121.

[175] B.J. Maron, H.G. Klues, Surviving competitive athletics with hypertrophic cardiomyopathy, Am. J. Cardiol. 73 (15) (1994) 1098–1104.

[176] B.J. Maron, Sudden death in young athletes, N. Engl. J. Med. 349 (11) (2003) 1064–1075.

[177] C. Semsarian, D.R. Richmond, Sudden cardiac death in familial hypertrophic cardiomyopathy: an Australian experience, Aust. N.Z. J. Med. 29 (3) (1999) 368–370.

[178] V.E. Friedewald Jr., D.W. Spence, Sudden cardiac death associated with exercise: the risk- benefit issue, Am. J. Cardiol. 66 (2) (1990) 183–188.

[179] H.W. Kohl, K.E. Powell, N.F. Gordon, S.N. Blair, R.S. Paffenbarger, Physical activity, physical fitness, and sudden cardiac death, Epidemiol. Rev. 14 (1) (1992) 37–58.

[180] C.R. Richardson, A.M. Kriska, P.M. Lantz, R.A. Hayward, Physical activity and mortality across cardiovascular disease risk groups, Med. Sci. Sports Exerc. 36 (11) (2004) 1923–1929.

[181] B.J. Maron, L. Yeates, C. Semsarian, Clinical challenges of genotype positive (+)-phenotype negative (−) family members in hypertrophic cardiomyopathy, Am. J. Cardiol. 107 (4) (2011) 604–608.

[182] A. Pelliccia, D.P. Zipes, B.J. Maron, Bethesda Conference #36 and the European Society of Cardiology Consensus Recommendations revisited a comparison of U.S. and European criteria for eligibility and disqualification of competitive athletes with cardiovascular abnormalities, J. Am. Coll. Cardiol. 52 (24) (2008) 1990–1996.

[183] A.F. Schinkel, P.A. Vriesendorp, E.J. Sijbrands, L.J. Jordaens, F.J. ten Cate, M. Michels, Outcome and complications after implantable cardioverter defibrillator therapy in hypertrophic cardiomyopathy: systematic review and meta-analysis, Circ. Heart Fail. 5 (5) (2012) 552–559.

[184] P.A. Vriesendorp, A.F. Schinkel, J. Van Cleemput, R. Willems, L.J. Jordaens, D.A. Theuns, et al., Implantable cardioverter-defibrillators in hypertrophic cardiomyopathy: patient outcomes, rate of appropriate and inappropriate interventions, and complications, Am. Heart J. 166 (3) (2013) 496–502.

[185] C.I. Berul, G.F. Van Hare, N.J. Kertesz, A.M. Dubin, F. Cecchin, K.K. Collins, et al., Results of a multicenter retrospective implantable cardioverter-defibrillator registry of pediatric and congenital heart disease patients, J. Am. Coll. Cardiol. 51 (17) (2008) 1685–1691.

[186] L.C. Poliac, M.E. Barron, B.J. Maron, Hypertrophic cardiomyopathy, Anesthesiology 104 (1) (2006) 183–192.

Chapter 20

Left Ventricular Noncompaction Cardiomyopathy

Jeffrey A. Towbin, Jean Ballweg, Jason Johnson
Le Bonheur Children's Hospital, Memphis, TN, United States

Left ventricular noncompaction (LVNC), a classified form of cardiomyopathy, is a genetic disease characterized by excessive and unusual trabeculations within the mature left ventricle (LV). LVNC has been considered to be a developmental failure of the heart to form fully the compact myocardium during the later stages of cardiac development. Clinically and pathologically, LVNC is characterized by a spongy morphological appearance of the myocardium occurring primarily in the LV with the abnormal trabeculations typically being most evident in the apical and midlateral–inferior portions of the LV. The right ventricle (RV) may also be affected alone or in conjunction with the LV. In LVNC, in addition to the regional presence of prominent trabeculae and intertrabecular recesses in the LV, thickening of the myocardium in two distinct layers composed of compacted and noncompacted myocardium is also classically noted. It may be associated with left ventricular dilation or hypertrophy, systolic and/or diastolic dysfunction, atrial enlargement, or various forms of congenital heart disease. The myocardium in LVNC may demonstrate normal or abnormal systolic or diastolic function; and the size, thickness, or function may change unexpectedly ("undulating phenotype"). Affected individuals are at risk of left or right ventricular failure, or both. Heart failure symptoms can be exercise-induced or persistent at rest, but many patients are asymptomatic. Chronically treated patients sometimes present acutely with decompensated heart failure. Other life-threatening risks are ventricular arrhythmias and atrioventricular block, presenting clinically as syncope, and sudden death. Genetic inheritance arises in at least 30%–50% of patients, LVNC is thought to occur in approximately 1 per 7000 live births. It occurs in newborns, young children, and adults, with the worst reported outcomes seen in infants, particularly those with associated systemic disease and metabolic derangement. In some families, a consistent phenotype of LVNC is seen in affected relatives but quite commonly individuals with features of LVNC are found in families where other affected relatives have typical hypertrophic cardiomyopathy (HCM), dilated cardiomyopathy (DCM), or restrictive cardiomyopathy. Mutations in ~15 genes have been implicated and include cytoskeletal, sarcomeric, and ion channel genes, with sarcomere-encoding genes being most common. In the case of LVNC with congenital heart disease, disturbance of the Notch or Wnt signaling pathways appear to be part of a "final common pathway" for this form of the disease. In addition, disrupted mitochondrial function and metabolic abnormalities have a causal role as well. Treatments focus on improvement of cardiac efficiency and reduction of mechanical stress in those with systolic dysfunction. Further, arrhythmia therapy and implantation of an automatic implantable cardioverter–defibrillator (ICD) for prevention of sudden death are mainstays of treatment when deemed necessary and appropriate. Patients with LVNC associated with congenital heart disease commonly require surgical or catheter-based interventions. Despite progress in diagnosis and treatment over the past 10–15 years, understanding of the disorder and outcomes continue to need further improvement.

INTRODUCTION

LVNC, first described by Grant [1] in 1926, is a heterogeneous myocardial disorder characterized by prominent trabeculae, intratrabecular recesses, and left ventricular myocardium having two distinct layers: compacted and noncompacted myocardium [2–4]. Continuity exists between the left ventricular cavity and deep intratrabecular recesses, both of which are filled with blood, and there is no evidence of communication to the epicardial coronary artery system [5,6]. Although LVNC primarily affects the LV, isolated right ventricular and biventricular noncompaction also occurs [7–9]. Imaging and pathology evaluation demonstrates LVNC to be characterized by a spongy morphological appearance of the left ventricular myocardium with abnormal trabeculations typically most evident in the left ventricular apex as we and others have previously reported [3,10]. The LV free wall may also be affected, but the interventricular septum is rarely affected, with the

Heart Failure in the Child and Young Adult. http://dx.doi.org/10.1016/B978-0-12-802393-8.00020-X

exception of the apical portion of the interventricular septum. The American Heart Association "Scientific Statement on Classification of Cardiomyopathies" formally classified LVNC as a distinct cardiomyopathy in 2006 [11].

LVNC has been called by a variety of names including spongy myocardium, fetal myocardium, noncompaction of the left ventricular myocardium, hypertrabeculation syndrome, and left ventricular noncompaction, among others [2,3,6,10–16]. The genesis of LVNC has been speculated to represent arrest of the final stage of myocardial morphogenesis (myocardial compaction) [5,6,17–22]. However, this does not explain the fact that multiple forms of LVNC occur and these include primary myocardial forms of LVNC, a form associated with arrhythmias, and LVNC associated with congenital heart disease, including septal defects, right heart obstructive abnormalities including pulmonic stenosis and Ebstein's anomaly, hypoplastic left heart syndrome, and others [10,12,23–29]. In all forms of LVNC, we and others have shown that metabolic derangements may be notable, particularly in newborns and infants [10,30,31].

PATHOLOGY OF LEFT VENTRICULAR NONCOMPACTION

In the early embryo, the heart is a loose interwoven mesh of muscle fibers [5,6,17,19–21]. The developing myocardium gradually condenses, and the large spaces within the trabecular meshwork disappear, condensing and compacting the ventricular myocardium and solidifying the endocardial surfaces. Trabecular compaction is normally more complete in the left ventricular than in the right ventricular myocardium, and therefore right ventricular trabeculations (albeit small) are normally seen in the mature heart. Hence, this compacting pathway failure is thought to occur due to arrest of endomyocardial morphogenesis, causing postnatal LVNC [5,6,17,19–21]. The gross pathologic appearance of LVNC is characterized by numerous excessively prominent trabeculations with deep intratrabecular recesses resembling the right ventricular endomyocardial morphology. Histologically, the recesses and their troughs are lined with endothelium. Zones of fibrous and elastic tissue may be scattered on the endocardial surfaces with extension into the recesses. The coronary arterial circulation is usually normal; extramural myocardial blood supply is not believed to play a role in these abnormalities [32]. Intramural perfusion, however, could be adversely affected by the prominent trabeculations and intratrabecular recesses, particularly in the subendocardium, causing subendocardial ischemia. Although there is no clear evidence that subendocardial ischemia is causative of LVNC, it is possible that an ischemic insult to critical signaling pathways between the myocardium and the endocardium could impact ventricular trabeculation formation and resorption [33,34]. During cardiogenesis, the cardiac jelly plays an important role in the interaction between these two layers. Whether ischemia could result in a disruption or modification of signaling pathways is not clear [35]. In addition, there is no definitive evidence of subendocardial fibrosis using cardiac MRI and late gadolinium enhancement (LGE). The endomyocardial morphology of LVNC also lends itself to development of mural thrombi within ischemia playing a significant role in the clinical course of patients with LVNC, although in some patients the recesses, which can embolize, causing a stroke or coronary obstruction [3,10,14,36,37]. Arrhythmias may also occur and consists of either tachy- or bradyarrhythmias, and these arrhythmias impact outcome [24,25,38,39].

INCIDENCE OF LEFT VENTRICULAR NONCOMPACTION

Although LVNC has been considered to be rare by some authors, and the incidence and prevalence of LVNC is uncertain, it appears to be the third most commonly diagnosed cardiomyopathy. LVNC is thought to occur in approximately 1 per 7000 live births. It occurs in newborns, young children, and adults, with the worst reported outcomes seen in infants, particularly those with associated systemic disease and metabolic derangement. Ritter et al. [40] reported the prevalence of isolated LVNC to be 0.05% of all adult echocardiographic examinations in a large institution, while Aras et al. [41] reported the prevalence to be <0.14% of adults referred for echocardiograms. In contrast, Sandhu et al. demonstrated a 3.7% prevalence of definite or probable LVNC by echocardiography in adults with left ventricular ejection fractions (LVEFs) ≤45% and 0.26% prevalence for all patients referred for echocardiography [42]. Among heart failure patients, the prevalence of LVNC has been reported as 3%–4% [43,44]. Most recently, Ronderos et al. reported a on a total of 10,857 adult patients who underwent echocardiography [45]. They showed that 2931 (27%) were normal, while LVNC was found in 26 patients (prevalence = 0.24%). In this cohort, 16 patients were women, mean age of 52.6 years. Patients were divided into two groups; group A: EF <50% (n = 20) and group B: normal systolic function (n = 6). Among abnormal studies, 294 (2.7%) were associated with a DCM. In patients with LVNC and EF <50% comprised 6.8% of DCM (20 of 294) and 24% (20 of 75) of patients with idiopathic DC ($P < .0001$). Group A patients were older, and they have less presence of women (both $P < .05$). In conclusion, the prevalence of LVNC in a population assessed for cardiovascular diseases is low. In contrast, it is very high in the subgroup of patients with idiopathic DCM. The group of patients with LVNC and normal LVEF is younger and with a higher presence of women than those with LVNC and depressed LVEF. Coincidence between operators is very good for the identification of echocardiographic criteria.

These wide variations in the reported incidence and prevalence are likely dependent on clinical recognition of the disease, and the diagnosis of LVNC is now becoming more frequent. This is most likely due to an increased awareness of the disease, and the improved imaging technology, as well as recommendations for screening at-risk family members who also have the LVNC phenotype due to its hereditary nature.

CLINICAL FEATURES AND DIAGNOSIS OF LEFT VENTRICULAR NONCOMPACTION

The clinical presentation of LVNC is highly variable. It occurs at any age, can range from asymptomatic to end-stage heart failure, or be associated with lethal arrhythmias, sudden cardiac death, and/or thromboembolic events [2–4,7–10,12–14,46,47]. A high percentage of patients are asymptomatic, being identified serendipitously by echocardiogram after referral due to a murmur or for familial screening. Some patients with LVNC present with clinically significant arrhythmias or conduction system disease as discussed below. Reports regarding outcome in children and adults have been inconsistent, with some demonstrating poor outcomes and others having a low percent of death or transplantation. For instance, Ichida et al. [14] found good survival and limited symptoms in their childhood patients, while Chin et al. [2] reported three deaths in the eight children studied. Our group demonstrated poor outcome in neonates but excellent outcomes in older children, with a 75% five-year survival free of death or transplantation. The neonates that died all had systemic disease (mitochondrial or other metabolic disorders).

Adult clinical studies have consistently described a high risk of ventricular tachyarrhythmias and sudden cardiac death in LVNC, with up to 47% of adults (and 75% of symptomatic patients) dying within 6 years of presentation [4,24,37–39]. More recent reports on an adult cohort, however, have shown a more benign natural history, with lower risk for (malignant) ventricular arrhythmias [48]. Bhatia et al. reviewed published studies of 241 adults with isolated LVNC diagnosed by echocardiographic criteria followed for a mean duration of 39 months [49] and reported an annualized event rate of 4% for cardiovascular deaths, 6.2% for cardiovascular death and its surrogates (transplantation, appropriate ICD shocks), and 8.6% for all cardiovascular events (death, stroke, ICD shocks, transplantation). Familial LVNC was identified in 30% of first-degree relatives of index cases screened by echocardiography [49]. Brescia et al. retrospectively reviewed all children diagnosed with LVNC at a Children's Hospital from January 1990 to January 2009. Patients with congenital cardiac lesions were excluded [50]. Two hundred forty-two children were diagnosed with isolated LVNC over the study period. Thirty-one (12.8%) died, and 13 (5.4%) received a transplant. One hundred fifty (62%) presented with or developed cardiac dysfunction. The presence of cardiac dysfunction was strongly associated with mortality (hazard ratio, 11; $P<.001$). Electrocardiography (ECG) abnormalities were present in 87%, with ventricular hypertrophy and repolarization abnormalities occurring most commonly. Repolarization abnormalities were associated with increased mortality (hazard ratio, 2.1; $P=.02$). Eighty children (33.1%) had an arrhythmia, and those with arrhythmias had increased mortality (hazard ratio, 2.8; $P=.002$). Forty-two (17.4%) had ventricular tachycardia, with 5 presenting with resuscitated sudden cardiac death. In total, there were 15 cases of sudden cardiac death in the cohort (6.2%). Nearly all patients with sudden death (14 of 15) had abnormal cardiac dimensions or cardiac dysfunction. No patient with normal cardiac dimensions and function without preceding arrhythmias died. Preceding cardiac dysfunction or ventricular arrhythmias was associated with increased mortality. The precise substrate for malignant ventricular arrhythmias in LVNC patients remains unknown, however [50].

SUBTYPES OF LEFT VENTRICULAR NONCOMPACTION

Although the diagnosis of LVNC has focused primarily on the identification and description of trabeculations, other features are critical to defining the specific type of LVNC. Most reports of LVNC focus on "isolated LVNC" or LVNC with congenital heart disease. However, both the "isolated" and congenital heart disease–associated forms have a wide spectrum of features [10,51,52]. This "lumping" instead of "splitting" approach has several disadvantages, particularly when considering outcomes and therapies. At least eight different LVNC phenotypes appear to exist, all having different outcomes (Figs. 20.1–20.9). A brief description of the subtypes that we have developed [10] is described below:

1. **"Benign" Form of LVNC:** This subtype is characterized by normal left ventricular size and wall thickness with preserved systolic and diastolic function (Fig. 20.1). This subtype accounts for up to ~35% of LVNC patients and is a predictor of good outcome in the absence of significant arrhythmias [52]. It is this patient population that has led to statements by mostly adult cardiologists that LVNC does not represent a cardiomyopathy and is a benign and normal variant. One possibility for this conclusion is that the more severe forms of LVNC tend to occur in childhood and these patients are either successfully treated, transplanted, or die and, therefore, do not present to adult cardiologists with symptomatic disease. This subtype appears to have the same outcome as the normal population.

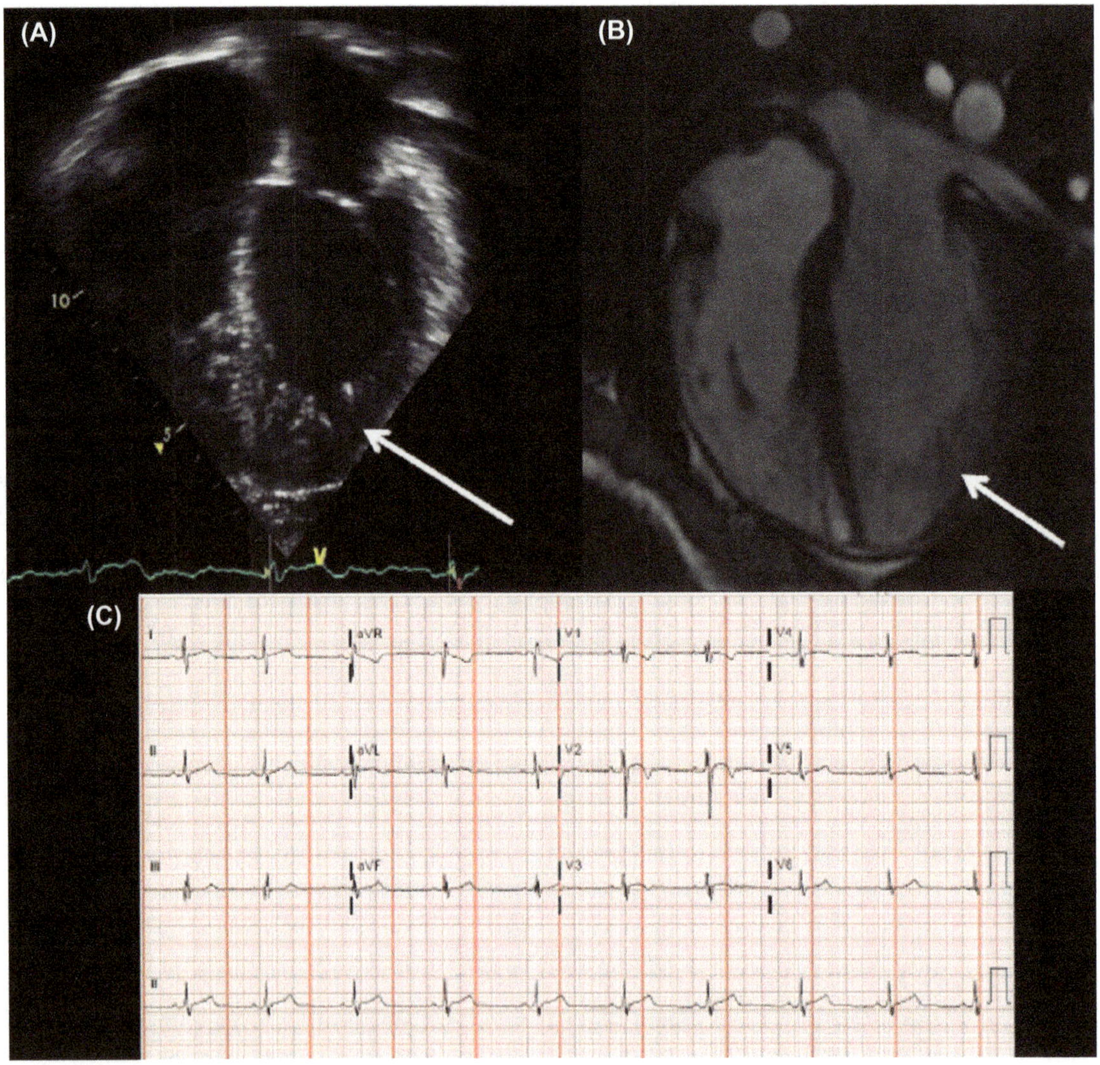

FIGURE 20.1 Benign form of left ventricular noncompaction in a 15-year-old male. (A) Transthoracic echocardiogram and (B) cardiac MRI four chamber views with trabeculations and intratrabecular recesses (*white arrows*) at the apex and apical lateral wall; (C) Twelve lead electrocardiogram with normal sinus rhythm, low QRS voltages, and interventricular conduction delay.

2. **LVNC With Arrhythmias:** This subtype is defined by preserved systolic function with normal left ventricular size and wall thickness but has evidence of underlying arrhythmias, usually identified at the time of diagnosis. We and others have shown that the presence of ventricular arrhythmias is an independent risk factor of mortality, many going unrecognized by current surveillance techniques [10,24,25,37,38,52–56]. This subtype appears to have a worse outcome compared to the normal population or those with similar forms of rhythm disturbance.
3. **Dilated Form of LVNC:** This subtype is characterized by concomitant left ventricular dilation and systolic dysfunction (Fig. 20.2) [3,10,14,42,43,48,52]. During the clinical course of this subtype, an "undulating phenotype" may present in which the LV may become smaller with some wall hypertrophy and improved function before reverting to the dilated subtype [3]. This subtype appears to have a similar outcome compared to those with a similar degree of DCM, except in neonates and infants, who have a worse outcome.
4. **Hypertrophic Form of LVNC:** This subtype is characterized by left ventricular thickening, usually with asymmetric septal hypertrophy, in addition to diastolic dysfunction and hypercontractile systolic function (Fig. 20.3) [10,52]. In some cases left ventricular dilation with systolic dysfunction can occur late in the course of the disease. This subtype appears to have a similar outcome compared to the normal population or those with similar degree of HCM.
5. **Hypertrophic and Dilated Form of LVNC:** This subtype, also known as a mixed phenotype, is characterized by left ventricular thickening, dilation, and depressed systolic function at presentation. This phenotype has increased risk of mortality and, in pediatric patients, is commonly associated with metabolic or mitochondrial disease [3,10,30,52].

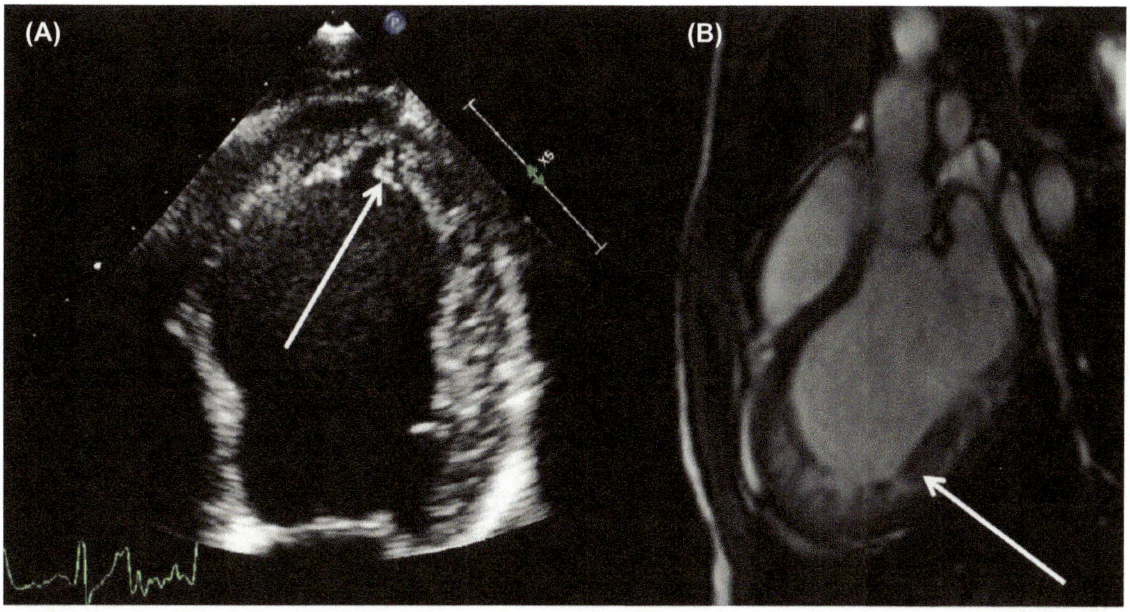

FIGURE 20.2 Dilated form of left ventricular noncompaction in a 17-year-old male. (A) Transthoracic echocardiogram four chamber view zoomed and (B) cardiac MRI left ventricular outflow tract view with trabeculations and intratrabecular recesses (*white arrows*) of the left ventricular basal to apical lateral wall and apex.

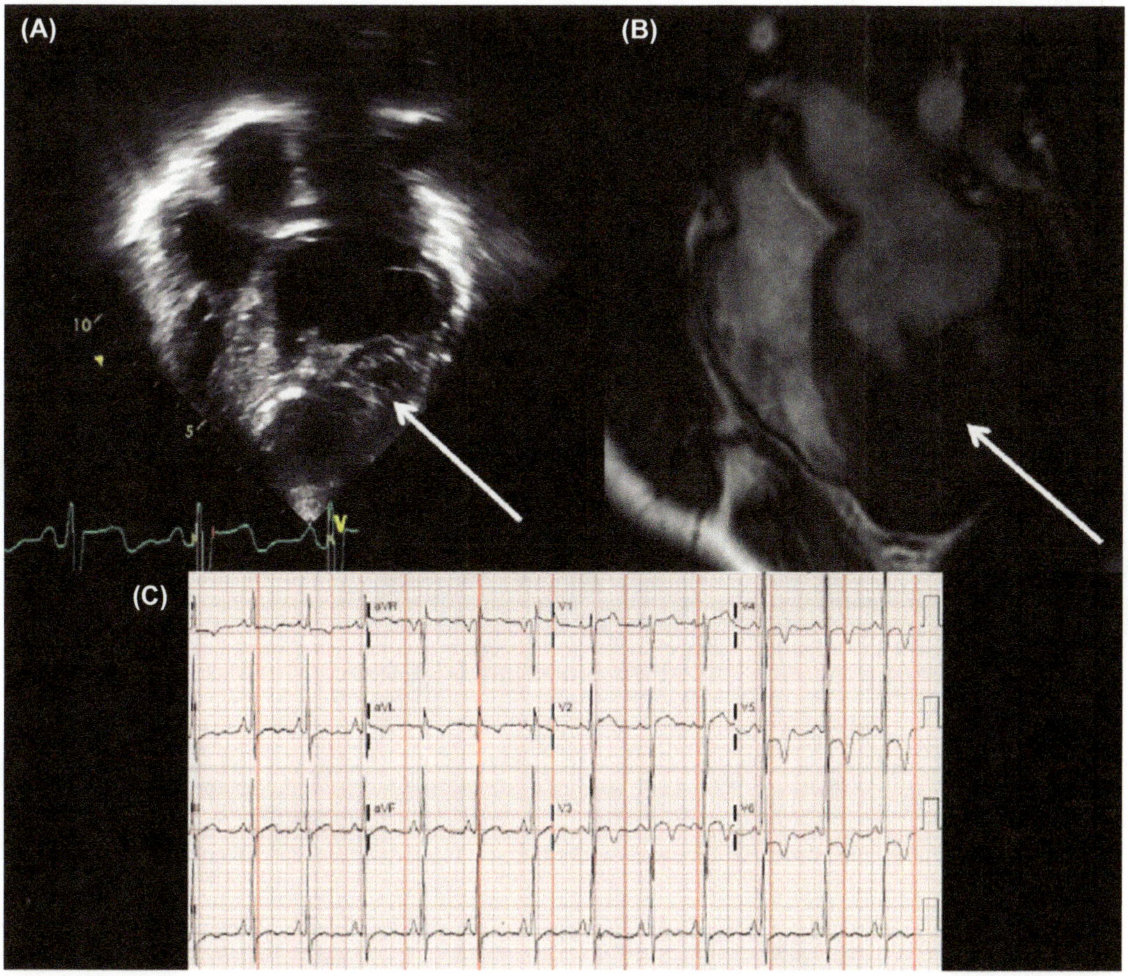

FIGURE 20.3 Hypertrophic form of left ventricular noncompaction in a 19-year-old female. (A) Transthoracic echocardiogram and (B) cardiac MRI four chamber views with hypertrophied trabeculations (*white arrows*) in all apical wall segments obliterating the cavity; (C) Twelve lead electrocardiogram with normal sinus rhythm, left ventricular hypertrophy with strain with ST segment depression, and T wave inversion in lateral leads.

This form is the most common of the "undulating" types and most typically ends as a dilated LV with poor function and heart failure [3,10]. This subtype does worse than patients with mixed phenotypes for other causes, such as "burned out" forms of HCM.

6. **Restrictive Form of LVNC:** This rare form of LVNC is characterized by left atrial or biatrial dilation and diastolic dysfunction (Fig. 20.4). This phenotype mimics the clinical behavior of restrictive cardiomyopathy with a similarly poor outcome, typically due to arrhythmia-related sudden cardiac events or, less commonly, heart failure with preserved ejection fraction [10,52]. This subtype appears to have a similar outcome compared to those with similar forms of restrictive cardiomyopathy.
7. **Right Ventricular or Biventricular Form of LVNC:** This subtype is characterized by hypertrabeculation of both the RV and LV (Fig. 20.5). There are no recognized diagnostic criteria for right ventricular noncompaction. Previous reports have suggested applying left ventricular diagnostic criteria to the RV [57]. We have relied on a finding of very heavy right ventricular trabeculations and a severe spongiform appearance of the RV to make this diagnosis. In these cases, trabeculations are seen in the lateral wall of the RV with hypertrabeculation up to the tricuspid valve, particularly in severe cases [3]. The implications of biventricular involvement remain unknown [7–9,57–59].
8. **LVNC With Congenital Heart Disease:** LVNC has been reported in association with most all congenital heart lesions and may contribute to myocardial dysfunction and/or arrhythmias. Right-sided lesions, especially Ebstein's anomaly, pulmonic stenosis, pulmonary atresia, tricuspid atresia, and double outlet RV, are most common with septal defects and left heart defects less commonly seen (Fig. 20.6) [10,23,26–29,60]. Outcomes are dependent on the specific form of congenital heart disease. However, the inclusion of LVNC with congenital heart disease increases the risk postoperatively and, if ventricular dysfunction occurs at any time, the outcomes also suffer.

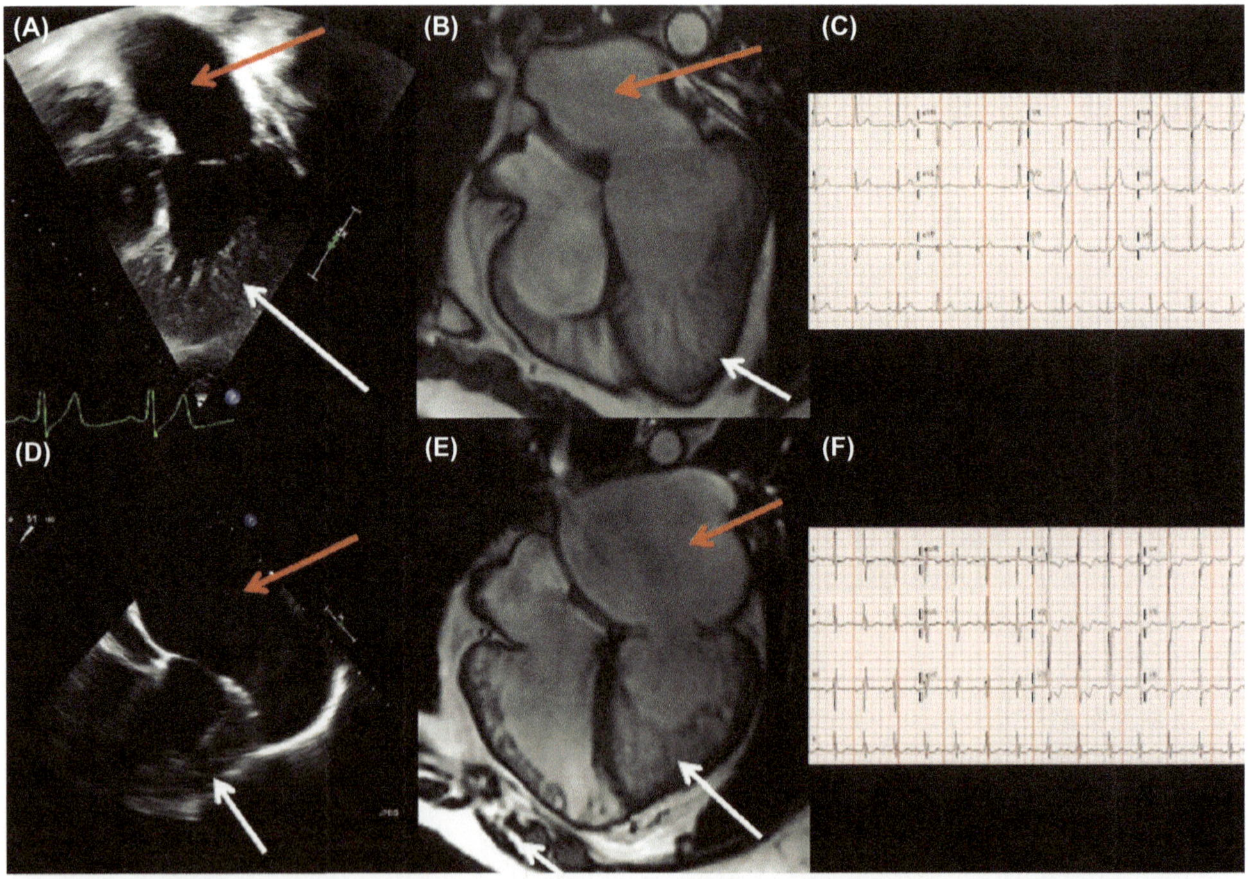

FIGURE 20.4 Restrictive form of left ventricular noncompaction. (A) Transthoracic echocardiogram and (B) cardiac MRI four chamber views in a 44-year-old male with trabeculations (*white arrows*) in all apical wall segments and severe left atrial dilation (*red arrows*), and (C) 12 lead electrocardiogram with normal sinus rhythm and left ventricular hypertrophy; (D) transesophageal echocardiogram and (E) cardiac MRI four chamber views in a 20-year-old female with trabeculations (*white arrows*) in all apical wall segments and severe left atrial dilation (*red arrows*), and (F) 12 lead electrocardiogram with low right atrial rhythm, biventricular hypertrophy with ST segment depression in the precordial leads.

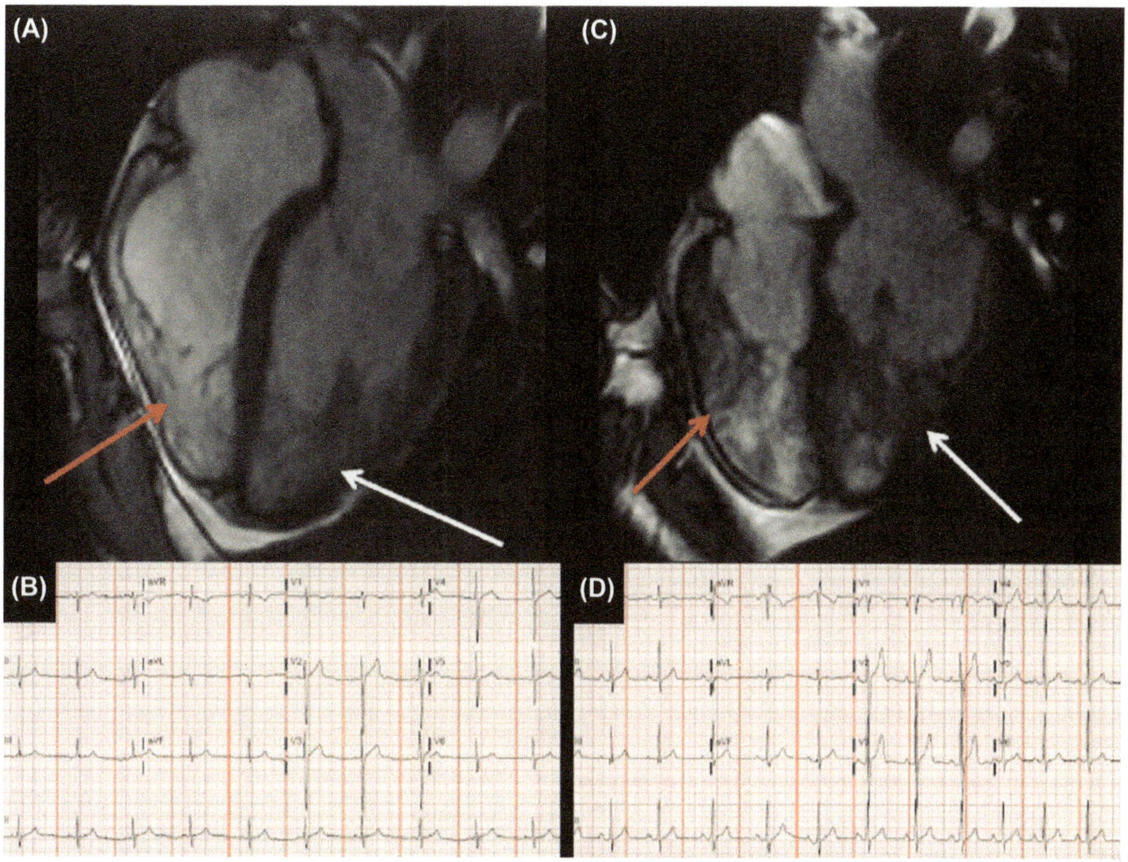

FIGURE 20.5 Biventricular form of noncompaction. (A) Cardiac MRI four chamber view in an 18-year-old male with trabeculations in the left ventricle (*white arrow*) and right ventricle (*red arrow*), and (B) 12 lead electrocardiogram with normal sinus rhythm and right axis deviation; (C) cardiac MRI four chamber view in a 17-year-old male with trabeculations in the left ventricle (*white arrow*) and right ventricle (*red arrow*), and (D) 12 lead electrocardiogram with normal sinus rhythm, sinus arrhythmia, and left atrial dilation.

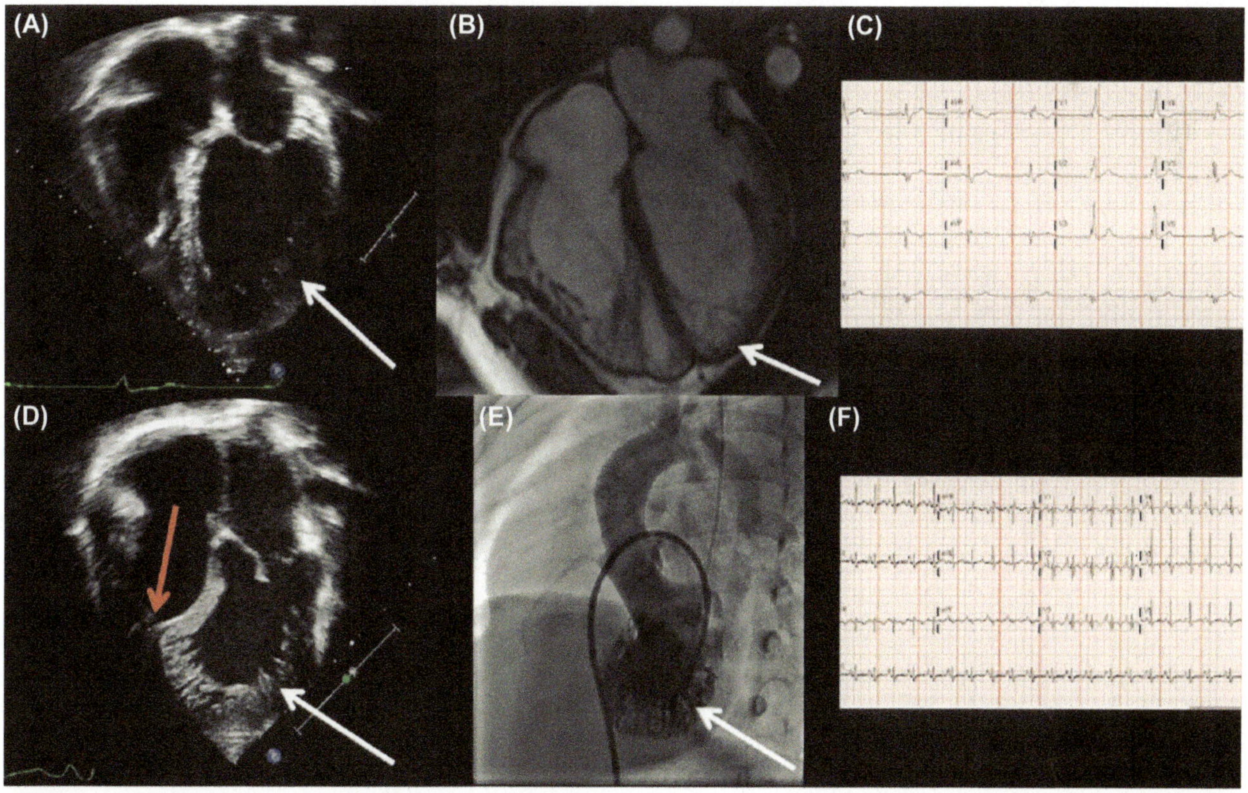

FIGURE 20.6 Congenital form of noncompaction. (A) Transthoracic echocardiogram and (B) cardiac MRI four chamber views in an 18-year-old male with tetralogy of Fallot status post surgical repair and trabeculations (*white arrows*) in the apical left ventricle, and (C) 12 lead electrocardiogram with sinus bradycardia with right bundle branch block and left anterior fascicular block; (D) transthoracic echocardiogram and (E) lateral left ventricular angiogram in a 2-year-old female with Ebstein anomaly of the tricuspid valve (*red arrow*) and trabeculations (*white arrows*) of the apical left ventricle, and (F) 12 lead electrocardiogram with normal sinus rhythm, right atrial enlargement, and left axis deviation.

IMAGING OF LEFT VENTRICULAR NONCOMPACTION

The diagnosis of LVNC relies on noninvasive imaging studies, most typically transthoracic echocardiography and cardiac magnetic resonance imaging (CMR), However, controversy exists regarding the diagnostic criteria used for both modalities. Transthoracic echocardiography remains the most common approach to the diagnosis of LVNC. This is in large part due to widespread availability, interpretability, and cost. The most common criteria for diagnosis uses a ratio of the thickness of the noncompacted layer to the thickness of the compacted layer (T/C) with a ratio >2 at end-diastole being considered diagnostic [61]. Alternative diagnostic criteria have been proposed, including T/C ratios ranging between 2:1 and 3:1, but all require expert assessment to discern between normal variants and LVNC [2,13,62]. One issue that is perplexing is the use of any ratio of noncompact to compact layer thickness or trabecular length. A reasonable question is why would the size of trabeculations or ration of layer thicknesses matter? Another possibility would be that the position of the trabeculations and the density of trabeculations are critical for diagnosis. Some data exist regarding these diagnostic quandaries. Punn and Silverman performed a retrospective analysis of children with LVNC using the 16-segment model described by the American Heart Association and the American Society of Echocardiography [63]. LVEF was inversely related to the number of segments involved and, in younger patients, poor outcomes as defined by death or transplantation were related to the number of segments affected. Advanced echocardiographic techniques such as strain, strain rate, and torsion are now being used as well to assist in the diagnosis of LVNC [64–66]. Authors supporting the ratios of layers support their viewpoints using statistical evidence; however, no gold standard exists to compare these data against. However, due to the lack of definitive diagnostic criteria, concerns have been raised that LVNC has gone from being underrecognized to being overdiagnosed.

Cardiac MRI is becoming increasingly used in the diagnosis and ongoing surveillance of LVNC in both children and adults and the same controversies exist as described for echocardiography. The diagnostic criteria for the LVNC are also based on the T/C ratio, with a ratio >2.3 at end-diastole typically used [67]. However, as with echocardiography, there is a lack of consensus regarding this definition. Thuny et al. [68] evaluated 16 patients with LVNC who underwent both echocardiography and CMR within the same week for comparison. They utilized a standard 17-segment anatomical model and found that the extent of LVNC was better defined by CMR, and that CMR also provided additional morphological characterization of the myocardium. Jacquier et al. [69] proposed diagnostic CMR criteria that assess the amount of left ventricular mass and burden of trabeculations, with trabeculations >20% of the total mass being diagnostic. Cardiac MRI also offers the opportunity to assess for myocardial fibrosis with the presence of delayed/LGE possibly offering prognostic information (Fig. 20.7) [70,71]. Also notable, CMR has shown that the compact layer is commonly abnormally thin, especially at the apex, and can actually be confused with being an apical aneurysm. More recently, cardiac computed tomography (CCT) has been used and is capable of showing the abnormal architecture of the left ventricular wall in noncompaction. CCT enables quantitative and qualitative assessment of global and regional ventricular function and is excellent to exclude coronary artery disease or anomalies, which is usually not feasible with CMR or echocardiography [72]. Since CT is associated with very high radiation doses, while echocardiography and CMR has no radiation exposure, this is an important and limiting concern due to its oncologic potential especially in children or in patients requiring long-term, repeated surveillance [73].

Our group uses a matrix of data to make the diagnosis of LVNC. The criteria used for transthoracic echocardiography include a combination of location of trabeculations, density of trabeculations, and visualization of blood flow into the intertrabecular recesses by color Doppler interrogation on apical four-chamber view (Fig. 20.8). In addition, we measure the T/C ratio for completeness as well as evaluating the thickness of the compact layer compared to normal. We also use the parasternal short axis view to trigger suspicion of the potential diagnosis, facilitating a higher likelihood that attention will be paid to this possible diagnosis. We not only use a similar approach for CMR but also use gadolinium to evaluate for scar burden. In addition, we carefully evaluate left ventricular size, thickness, systolic function and diastolic function, atrial size and volume, as well as analyzing for any associated congenital heart defects. Finally, a careful analysis of the RV and its trabeculation burden should be evaluated.

ELECTROCARDIOGRAPHY IN LEFT VENTRICULAR NONCOMPACTION

The ECG in patients with LVNC is typically abnormal; in up to 87% of patients ECG findings of hypertrophy by voltage criteria (either left ventricular hypertrophy or biventricular hypertrophy), T wave inversion, ST segment abnormalities or strain, left atrial enlargement, left axis deviation, QTc prolongation, or preexcitation will be seen (Figs. 20.3C and 20.4F). In neonates and young children, extreme QRS voltages may be seen [3,14,50,53,74].

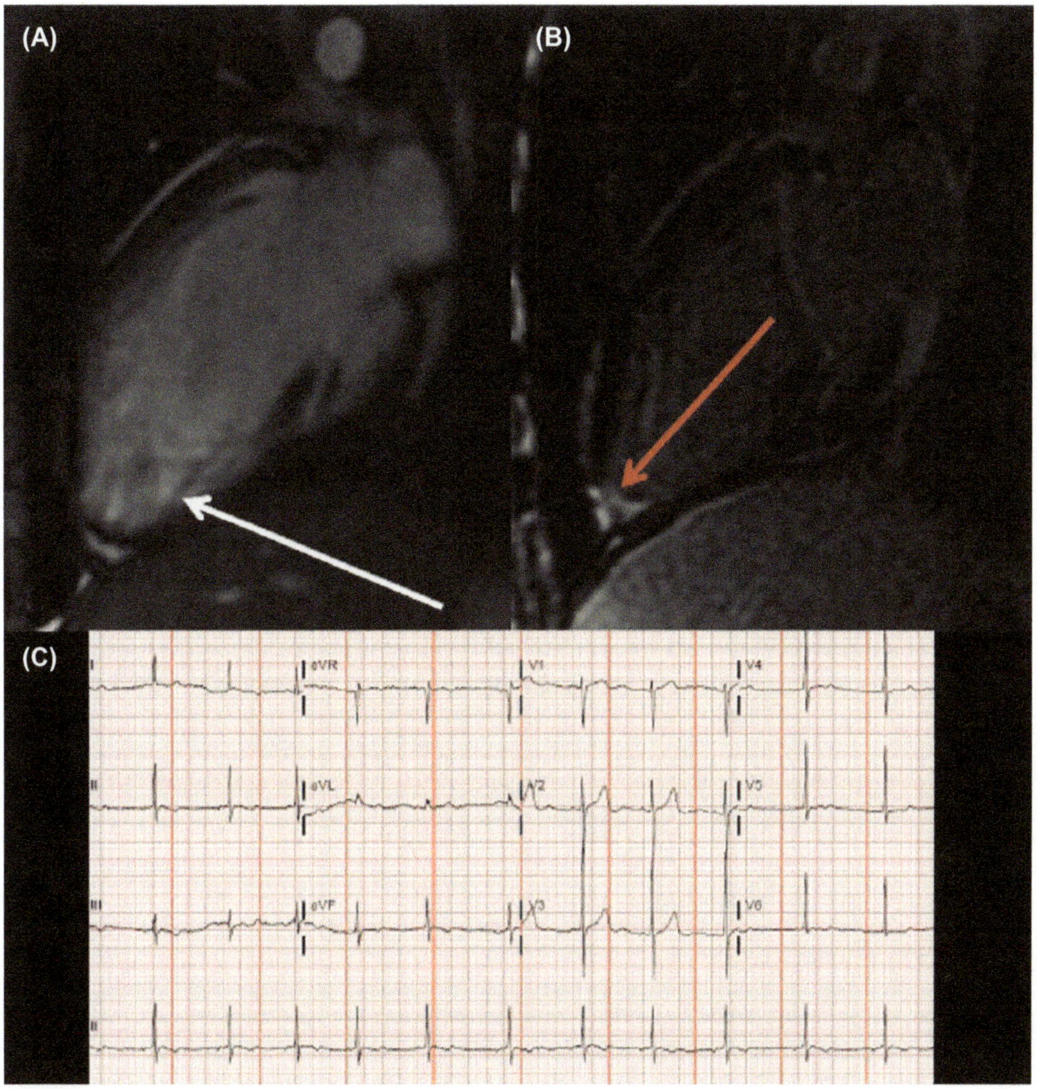

FIGURE 20.7 Cardiac MRI myocardial viability. (A) Cardiac MRI two chamber left ventricle view with trabeculations (*white arrow*) in the apex and (B) late gadolinium enhancement imaging with fibrosis in the apex (*red arrow*); (C) Twelve lead electrocardiogram with low right atrial rhythm and T-wave flattening in the inferior and lateral leads.

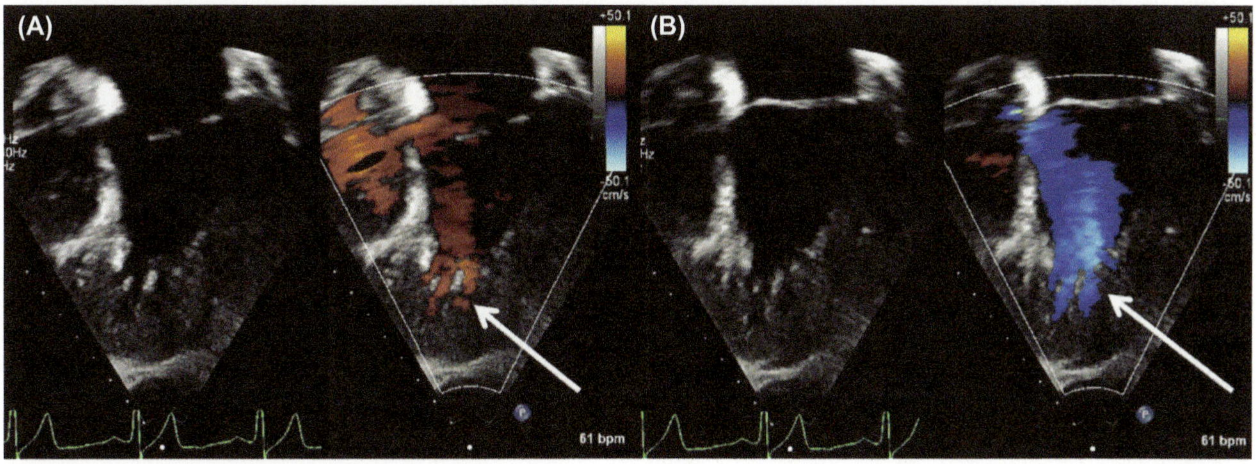

FIGURE 20.8 Color Doppler transthoracic echocardiogram. Transthoracic echocardiogram four chamber view zoomed at the left ventricle with color flow (A) in and (B) out of intratrabecular recesses (*white arrows*).

ARRHYTHMIAS IN LEFT VENTRICULAR NONCOMPACTION

Supraventricular and ventricular arrhythmias, as well as bradyarrhythmias, are frequently observed in LVNC, with many being life-threatening [50]. As noted previously, the LVNC subtype that presents with early-onset rhythm abnormalities generally has significant risk of sudden death. ICDs have been shown to be highly effective for the prevention of sudden arrhythmic death in LVNC patients, including patients with severe left ventricular dysfunction, a prior history of sustained ventricular tachycardia or ventricular fibrillation, recurrent syncope of unknown etiology, or a family history of sudden cardiac death. Ventricular tachyarrhythmias, including those seen in subjects having cardiac arrest due to ventricular fibrillation, has been reported in 38%–47% of adult patients with LVNC and in 13%–18% of subjects experiencing sudden death [18,28,29,41,43]. Caliskan et al. [75] investigated the indications and outcomes of ICD therapy in 77 adult LVNC patients, 57% of whom had an ICD implanted using standard implant guidelines for nonischemic cardiomyopathy. During a mean follow-up of 33 ± 24 months, 8 patients presented with appropriate defibrillator shocks due to sustained ventricular tachycardia after a median of 6.1 (1–16) months, suggesting that LVNC patients could be at high risk for sudden cardiac death. All of the appropriate defibrillator interventions in this patient cohort were due to fast ventricular tachycardias, although it is not certain that the initial rhythm in those patients suffering sudden cardiac death due to ventricular fibrillation was also initiated by a ventricular tachycardia trigger. In LVNC patients presenting with sustained ventricular arrhythmias, there was a 33% risk of recurrent sustained ventricular tachycardia followed by appropriate defibrillator shocks after a median follow-up period of 26 months. Similarly, Kobza et al. reported appropriate shocks in 37% of patients with LVNC and an ICD at a mean follow-up of 40 months [76]. In small children, pharmacologic antiarrhythmia therapies may be indicated prior to consideration of an ICD due to the high rate of lead fractures and inappropriate shocks in this population. In addition, Van Malderen et al. evaluated 101 patients with LVNC to determine the origin of premature ventricular contractions (PVCs) in LVNC and to identify any predominant arrhythmic foci [77]. A total number of 2069 electrocardiograms were studied to determine the origin of PVCs, and echocardiographic data were analyzed in patients with PVCs in all 12 leads. Segments affected by LVNC were compared with the origin of PVCs. PVCs were documented in 250 ECGs from 55 (54%) patients. Thirty-five ECGs recorded PVCs on all 12 leads, and the origin of 20 types of PVCs could be determined. Ninety-five percent of PVCs did not originate from left ventricular noncompact myocardial areas, and two PVCs (10%) had a true myocardial origin. All other PVCs originated from structures such as the outflow tracts (8/20), the fascicles (7/20), especially the posteromedial fascicle (6/20), and the mitral and tricuspid annulus (3/20), suggesting that PVCs in LVNC mainly originate from the conduction system and related myocardium.

OUTCOMES BASED ON PHENOTYPE

The National Heart, Lung, and Blood Institute–funded Pediatric Cardiomyopathy Registry reported on 3219 children with cardiomyopathy, identifying 155 children (4.8%) with definitive LVNC diagnosed from 1990 to 2008 [78]. Each child diagnosed with LVNC patient was classified as having an associated echocardiographically diagnosed cardiomyopathy phenotype including dilated, hypertrophic, restrictive, isolated, or indeterminate. They observed a significant difference among the phenotypic groups in time to death or transplant with isolated LVNC having the best outcomes, followed by those with the HCM-form of LVNC. Children with the DCM-form of LVNC and the indeterminate cardiomyopathy phenotype had the worst outcomes. The hazard ratio for death/transplant (with isolated LVNC as the reference group) was 4.26 (95% confidence interval [CI], 0.78–23.3) for the HCM form of LVNC, 6.35 (95% CI, 1.52–26.6) for the DCM form of LVNC, and 5.66 (95% CI, 1.04–30.9) for the indeterminate phenotype. Time to listing for cardiac transplantation significantly differed by phenotype (P<.001), as did time to transplantation (P=.015). Five-year transplant rates were 0% for isolated LVNC or the HCM form of LVNC, 27% for the DCM form of LVNC, and 27% for the indeterminate phenotype group. Five-year rates for the combined end point of death or transplant (and death or listing) were 33% (35%) for the entire LVNC cohort, phenotype-specific rates were 6% (6%) of isolated LVNC, 43% (45%) for the DCM form of LVNC, 25% (25%) for the HCM form of LVNC, and 33% (42%) for the indeterminate phenotype groups.

Very few isolated LVNC patients developed an associated cardiomyopathy phenotype. Of the 35 cases with isolated LVNC, the 2 deaths observed occurred shortly after diagnosis. One of the deceased patients had an associated DCM phenotype on repeat echocardiogram. Of the remaining 33 isolated LVNC cases, a 2-year repeat echocardiogram was available in 24 subjects, with 2 showing characteristics of HCM. Therefore, they estimated that 12% (3 of 25) progressed to an associated cardiomyopathy phenotype within 2 years. One additional case was reported as RCM at 1 year, but this was done without an associated supporting echocardiogram. This patient was alive at 4 years with an LV wall thickness Z score of <–2, normal LV systolic function, and no evidence of an associated RM phenotype by echocardiogram at that time. The authors concluded that the specific LVNC-associated cardiomyopathy phenotype predicts the risk of death or transplantation and should inform clinical management.

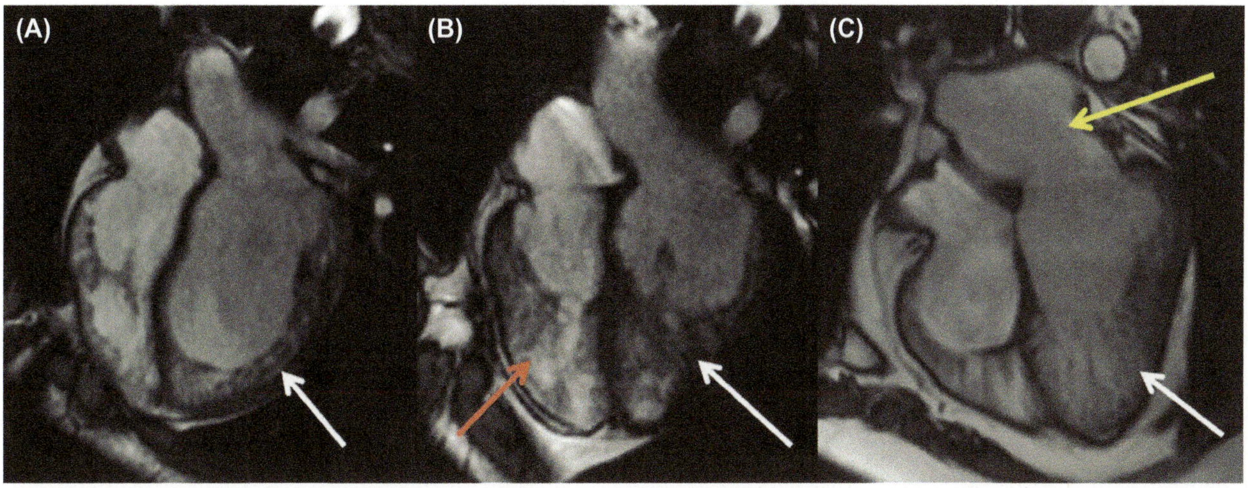

FIGURE 20.9 Familial noncompaction cardiomyopathy. Cardiac MRI four chamber views in a (A) 17-year-old male with dilated form with trabeculations (*white arrow*) in the apex and apical lateral wall of the left ventricle, (B) 17-year-old twin brother with biventricular form with trabeculations in the right ventricle (*red arrow*), and (C) 44-year-old father with restrictive form with severe left atrial dilation (*yellow arrow*).

CLINICAL GENETICS OF LEFT VENTRICULAR NONCOMPACTION

LVNC has been identified in families (Fig. 20.9) with X-linked inheritance, autosomal dominant and autosomal recessive inheritance, as well as maternally inherited (matrilinear) mitochondrial inheritance [3,10,30,79]. In addition, sporadic cases are common, probably involved in 60%–70% of cases. Although several LVNC-susceptibility genes have been identified to date, none predominate, and systematic evaluations of large populations have not been reported. LVNC arising from these genetic causes are associated typically with rare nonsynonymous variants, primarily missense, with occasional nonsense, splice site or small insertion/deletion variants. More than any other form of cardiomyopathy, mitochondrial disease is a prominent feature of infants and young children with LVNC and therefore requires evaluation [30]. When LVNC is associated with congenital heart disease, the congenital cardiac defect may be heterogeneous in families, but this form of LVNC is transmitted as an autosomal dominant trait along with the congenital heart abnormality [10]. In some families with autosomal dominant LVNC associated with congenital heart disease, affected members may be identified in whom no congenital heart disease can be identified at the time of initial evaluation because the cardiac defects include "minor" forms of disease (e.g., small ventricular and atrial septal defects, or patent ductus arteriosus), which have spontaneously closed, while other family members have severe forms of congenital heart disease (e.g., hypoplastic left heart syndrome, Ebstein's anomaly, etc.) [28,29,60]. Penetrance may be reduced in some families. Ichida et al. [14] reported that 44% of her LVNC patients had inherited LVNC, with 70% having autosomal dominant and 30% X-linked inheritance. As noted, chromosomal abnormalities and syndromic patients also have been identified with LVNC [80]. Digilio et al. investigated the prevalence of chromosomal abnormalities in 25 syndromic patients with LVNC using standard cytogenetic, subtelomeric fluorescent in situ hybridization, and array-CGH analysis. Standard chromosome analysis was abnormal in 3 (12%) patients (45,X/46,XX mosaic, 45,X/46,X,i(Y)(p11) mosaic, and de novo Robertsonian 13; 14 translocation), while cryptic chromosome anomalies were found in 6 (24%) cases (1p36 deletion, 7p14.3p14.1 deletion, 18p subtelomeric deletion, 22q11.2 deletion, and distal 22q11.2 deletion) [80]. LVNC and trisomy 18 and with trisomy 13 have also been described [81,82]. LVNC has also been associated with chromosome 8p23.1 deletion [83]. Other syndromes associated with LVNC include Coffin–Lowry syndrome, caused by mutations in the RPS6KA3 gene on chromosome Xp22.2, encoding the ribosomal protein S6 kinase-2 (RSK2) [84], and Sotos syndrome, due to mutations in the nuclear receptor binding SET domain protein 1 (NSD1) gene on chromosome 5q35, encoding a histone methyltransferase implicated in transcriptional regulation via chromatin remodeling [85,86]. Sellars et al. described a newborn with tetrasomy 5q35.2–5q35.3 having LVNC and absent thumbs, possibly consistent with an association with Hunter–McAlpine syndrome [87], while Corrado et al. reported LVNC and Charcot–Marie–Tooth disease type 1A from duplication in PMP22 [88].

Index Cases

A relatively small percentage of patients with LVNC have known genetic mutations, probably on the order of 20%–30%, though larger panels of genes can increase the yield proportionately. For instance, Klassen and colleagues reported a 17% rate of mutation detection when looking at 6 genes among 63 unrelated adult probands [89]. More recently,

Hoedemaekers et al. reported use of a 17-gene panel in which mutations were recognized in 23 of 56 probands (41%) [90]. The clinical diagnosis of LVNC depends on particular expertise and knowledge of disease and imaging modalities, particularly echocardiography and CMR and is supported by electrocardiographic findings. Due to the low rate of a positive genetic test in index cases to date, the utility of genetic testing for the definitive diagnosis and care of the index case is currently of limited use.

Family Relatives

Identification of a definite pathogenic mutation in clinically affected probands should lead to screening of all at-risk (siblings, parents, children) including those individuals with a negative phenotype. One of the important aspects of genetic testing is the ability to confirm mutation-positive or mutation-negative status in family members of clinically affected, genotype-positive subjects. Due to possible X-linked inheritance in some patients, affected male family members may have a pronounced disease expression and females may have milder signs of LVNC (or none at all) and, thus, may serve as transmitters for following generations. Somatic mitochondrial alterations are, in general, not heritable to next generations and require a different clinical and genetic consultation.

Prognostic Role of Genetic Testing for Left Ventricular Noncompaction

No genotype–phenotype correlations have been associated with LVNC to date, and therefore no prognostic implications can be speculated. The only implication of genetic testing at present is confirmation of diagnosis and the potential development of disease in mutation-positive members of the family, if tested. Therapy, therefore, is completely based on phenotypic findings.

Therapeutic Role of Genetic Testing for Left Ventricular Noncompaction

No definitive therapeutic role has been established for LVNC genetic testing. Because associated mitochondrial or metabolic disease (such as Barth syndrome) or syndromes are frequently associated with LVNC, especially in young children, firm diagnosis can lead to improved symptomatic therapy and improved prognostication in affected patients and family members. In addition, identification of mutations in certain genes (such as lamin A/C (LMNA), SCN5A, HCN4) [91–95] can facilitate assessment of arrhythmias and early treatment with medications or ICD.

MOLECULAR GENETICS OF LEFT VENTRICULAR NONCOMPACTION

The genetic cause of LVNC, like the clinical phenotype itself, is heterogeneous. However, like the genetic causes of other forms of cardiomyopathy, LVNC genetics also follows a "final common pathway" (Fig. 20.10) [93,96]. The specific final common pathway, however, depends on the clinical phenotype and mirrors the genetic causes of the clinical subtype in cardiomyopathies devoid of LVNC. For instance, the "final common pathway" of HCM is dysfunction of the sarcomere and, in support of this concept, the vast majority of the genes identified in cases of inherited of HCM either encode for sarcomere proteins (such as β-myosin heavy chain) or encode for proteins that disrupt the function of the sarcomere (such as mitochondrial electron transport chain proteins; see below). However, in LVNC, there appears to be a disturbance of more than a single "final common pathway" and, in most cases, probably disturbs a primary pathway (such as the sarcomere) and a developmental pathway (such as the NOTCH pathway; see section on Animal Models of LVNC, below), commonly via a disturbance of protein–protein binding caused by the primary genetic mutation (Table 20.1).

The first genetic cause of LVNC without evidence of congenital heart disease was initially described by Bleyl et al. [97] who identified mutations in the X-linked TAZ gene in patients and carrier females. TAZ encodes the tafazzin protein, a phospholipid transacylase that is important for membrane function, and when mutated typically causes the multisystem human disorder called Barth syndrome, which is characterized by cardiomyopathy (commonly LVNC), skeletal myopathy, cyclic neutropenia, 3-methylglutaconic aciduria (a marker of mitochondrial dysfunction), and deficiency of a key membrane phospholipid of cardiomyocytes and mitochondria called cardiolipin. It is believed that this defect disturbs mitochondrial function, leading to a combination of an energy production-energy utilization abnormality and because the sarcomere requires energy in the form of adenosine triphosphate, sarcomere dysfunction (see section Animal Models of LVNC, below).

Multiple genes causing autosomal dominant LVNC have since been identified, including mutations in genes causing congenital heart disease with LVNC. Mutations in ~15 genes have been implicated and mostly include

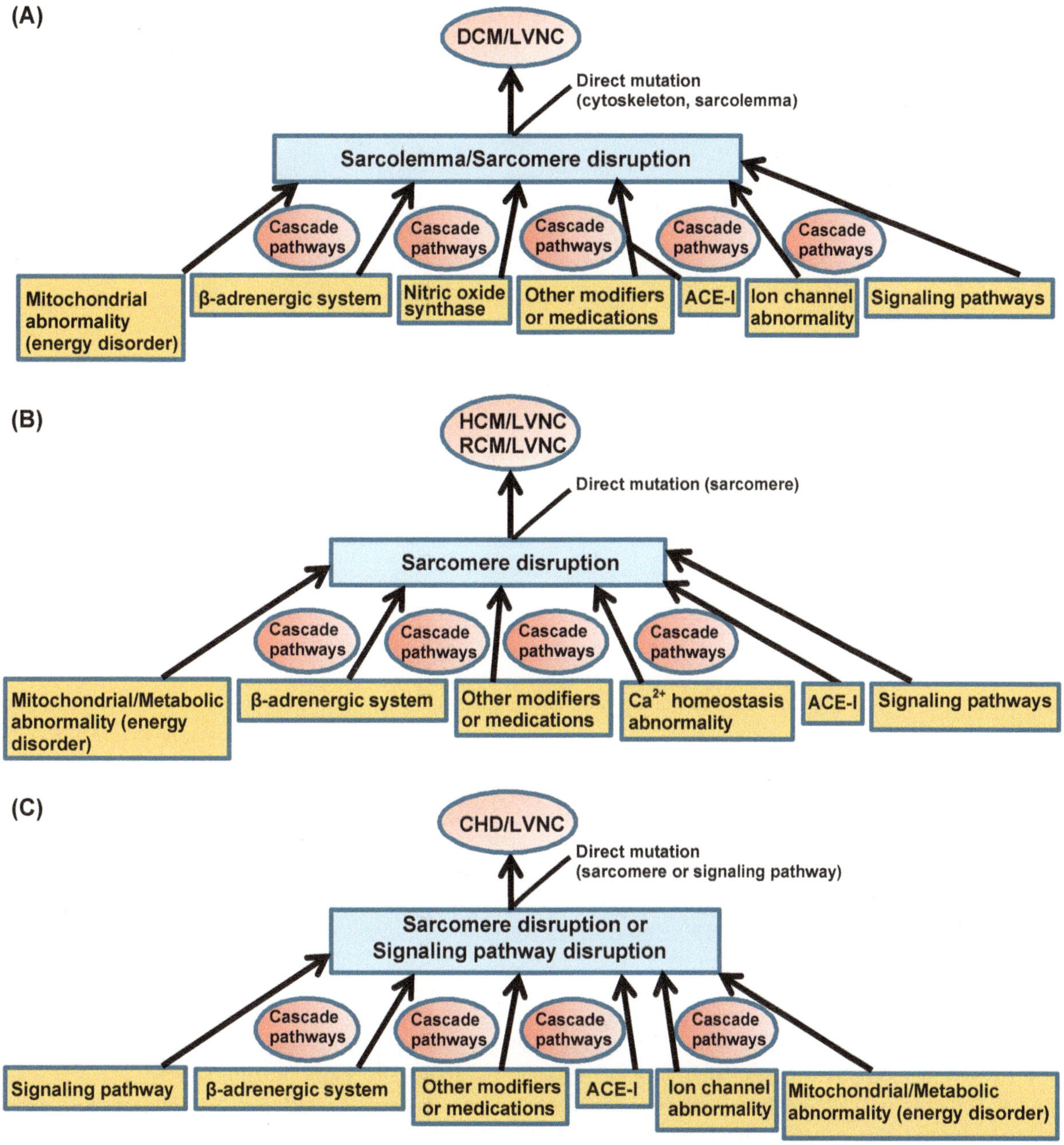

FIGURE 20.10 "Final common pathways" of left ventricular noncompaction (LVNC). (A) Dilated cardiomyopathy occurs due to either direct mutation, most typically in sarcomere protein- or cytoskeletal protein-encoding genes or secondary disruption of the sarcomere–sarcolemmal link through "cascade pathways," including energy production or utilization abnormalities caused by mitochondrial or other metabolic pathway dysfunction, β-adrenergic nervous system dysfunction, or abnormalities in nitric oxide synthase, modifiers (genetic, protein, medications, etc.), angiotensin-converting enzyme inhibitor isoforms, ion channel dysfunction, or signaling pathway disturbance; (B) Final common pathways of the hypertrophic or restrictive cardiomyopathy forms of LVNC. Hypertrophic or restrictive cardiomyopathy forms of LVNC occur due to disruption of sarcomere function that result in structural myocardial abnormalities either via direct mutation in sarcomere protein-encoding genes or secondary disruption of sarcomere function through "cascade pathways," including energy production or utilization abnormalities caused by mitochondrial or other metabolic pathway disturbance, β-adrenergic nervous system dysfunction, modifiers (genetic, protein, medications, etc.), calcium homeostasis abnormalities, angiotensin-converting enzyme inhibitor isoforms, or signaling pathway disturbance; (C) Final common pathways of the congenital heart disease form of LVNC. LVNC with congenital heart disease occurs due to disruption of overlapping pathways that result in structural myocardial abnormalities and in developmental pathways, either direct mutation, most typically in sarcomere protein-encoding genes or developmental signaling pathway genes, or secondary disruption of sarcomere or signaling pathway function through "cascade pathways," including signaling pathway disruption, β-adrenergic nervous system dysfunction, modifiers (genetic, protein, medications, etc.), angiotensin-converting enzyme inhibitor isoforms, ion channel dysfunction, or energy production or utilization abnormalities caused by disturbance of mitochondrial or other metabolic pathways. *ACE-I*, angiotensin-converting enzyme inhibitor; *CHD*, congenital heart disease; *DCM*, dilated cardiomyopathy; *HCM*, hypertrophic cardiomyopathy; *RCM*, restrictive cardiomyopathy. *From Lancet, with permission.*

TABLE 20.1 Genetic Causes of Left Ventricular Noncompaction

Gene	Gene Name	Protein Type
ACTC1	α-Cardiac actin	Sarcomere thin filament
CASQ2	Cardiac calsequestrin 2	Calcium homeostasis
DTNA	α-Dystrobrevin	Cytoskeletal protein
DYS	Dystrophin	Cytoskeletal protein
GLA	α-Galactosidase	Glycoside hydrolase
LDB3	LIM-domain binding 3	Z-disk protein
LMNA	Lamin A/C	Nuclear membrane protein
MIB1	Mindbomb homolog 1	E3 ubiquitin ligase
MYBPC3	Myosin-binding protein C	Sarcomere thick filament
MYH7	β-Myosin heavy chain 7	Sarcomere thick filament
Nkx2-5	Nkx2-5	Transcription factor
TAZ	Tafazzin	Phospholipid transacylase
TNNT2	Cardiac troponin T, type 2	Sarcomere thin filament

cytoskeletal, sarcomeric, and ion channel genes, with sarcomere-encoding genes being most common. In addition, syndromal disorders such as Barth syndrome and muscular dystrophies are known to be associated with LVNC as well. In patients with hypoplastic left heart syndrome and LVNC, we identified α-dystrobrevin causative mutations, while mutations in Nkx-2.5 was identified in children with LVNC and atrial septal defect; and both β-myosin heavy chain (MYH7) mutations and α-tropomyosin (TPM1) have been reported in patients with LVNC and Ebstein's anomaly [98–100].

The most common genes identified include the sarcomere-encoding genes β-myosin heavy chain (*MYH7*), α-cardiac actin (*ACTC1*), cardiac troponin T (*TNNT2*), myosin-binding protein-C (MYBPC3), and *ZASP (also called LIM-domain binding protein 3, LBD3)* [90,100–102]. In addition, mutations in α-tropomyosin (TPM1) and cardiac troponin I (TNNI3) also have been identified. Hoedemaekers et al. [90] additionally demonstrated an association of LVNC with genetic variants in two calcium handling genes, as well as TAZ and LMNA. Probst et al. [101] further showed that sarcomere gene mutations are important in LVNC, showing a prevalence of 29%, with MYH7 and MYBPC3 most frequently mutated (13% and 8%, respectively). Dellefave et al. [102] also identified sarcomere mutations in LVNC, including those presenting with heart failure in infancy. Recently, Hasdtings et al. performed whole genome sequencing, linkage analysis, and functional studies on two families with LVNC and identified missense mutations in titin (TTN), which encodes the giant titin protein found in the Z-disk and sarcomere [103]. Bagnall and colleagues showed an association of LVNC, idiopathic ventricular fibrillation, and sudden death with a mutation in the ACTN2 gene in a family [104].

In addition to sarcomere-encoding and cytoskeleton-encoding genes, we demonstrated that mutations in the sodium channel gene (SCN5A) are associated with LVNC and rhythm disturbance [92]. Another cytoskeletal protein associated with LVNC is dystrophin, the gene causing Duchenne and B ecker muscular dystrophy in boys [105]. In addition, homozygous deletions in desmoplakin (DSP) and plakophilin 2 (PKP2), desmosomal protein-encoding genes known to cause arrhythmogenic cardiomyopathy and DCM, have also been identified in LVNC patients [58,106]. Mitochondrial genome mutations have also been identified to be associated with LVNC [107] and, as noted, chromosomal abnormalities and syndromic patients also have been identified with LVNC [3,80] including 1p36 deletion, 7p14.3p14.1 deletion, 18p subtelomeric deletion, 22q11.2 deletion, distal 22q11.2, trisomies 18 and 13, 8p23.1 deletion, tetrasomy 5q35.2-5q35, Coffin–Lowry syndrome (RPS6KA3 mutation), Sotos syndrome (NSD1 mutation), and Charcot–Marie–Tooth disease type 1A (PMP22 duplication) [80–88,108,109].

Diagnostic testing in patients with LVNC appears to have a detection rate of clinically significant variants in 35%–40% of individuals, with sarcomere-encoding genes most commonly found to be mutated [110].

TABLE 20.2 Mouse Models of Left Ventricular Noncompaction

Mutant Gene	Mutant Type	Clinical Features
Fkbp1a	Fkbp1a-deficient	LVNC, VSD
Bmp10	Bmp10-overexpression	LVNC, VSD
Smad7	Smad7-deficient	LVNC, HF, VSD, RVOTO, Arrhythmia
NF-ATc	NF-ATc-deficient	LVNC, HF, VSD, RVOTO
Jarid2/Jumonji	Jarid2-deficient	LVNC, VSD, DORV
TAZ	TAZ-knockdown	LVNC
MIB1	MIB1-deficient	LVNC, RVNC, DCM, HF
Nkx2–5	Nkx2-5-deficient	LVNC, DCM, HF, AVB

ANIMAL MODELS OF LEFT VENTRICULAR NONCOMPACTION

A number of mouse models with LVNC have been described over the past several years (Table 20.2). These models are being used to discern the underlying mechanism(s) of this form of cardiomyopathy. The most common conclusion reached to date from these studies is that hypertrabeculation results from altered regulation in cell proliferation, differentiation, and maturation during ventricular wall formation, particularly if the NOTCH signaling pathway is altered. Other hypotheses also exist based on some of the models described below.

FKBP12 Null Mutation: FKBP12, also known as Fkbp1a, is a member of the immunophilin protein family that interacts with multiple intracellular protein complexes such as calcium release channels (inositol trisphosphate receptor and ryanodine receptor), BMP/activin/TGFβ type-1 receptors, voltage-gated Na^+ channels, FK506, and rapamycin and inhibits calcineurin and mTOR activity [111–114]. FKBP12-deficient mice develop ventricular hypertrabeculation and noncompaction. Shou et al. reported previously that a mutant mouse model deficient in FKBP12 develops multiple abnormalities in cardiac structure including lack of compaction, thin ventricular wall, deep intertrabecular recesses, increased trabeculae, and ventricular septal defect [115]. Chen et al. showed FKBP12 to be a novel-negative modulator of activated NOTCH1 reporting that overexpression of FKBP12 significantly reduced NOTCH1 stability and direct inhibition of NOTCH signaling significantly reduced hypertrabeculation in FKBP12-deficient mice [116]. These findings suggested that FKBP12-mediated regulation of NOTCH1 plays an important role in intercellular communication between endocardium and myocardium, which is crucial in controlling the formation of the ventricular walls [112].

MIB1 Mutant: Further support for NOTCH1 pathway disturbance as a contributor to LVNC development was shown in families with autosomal dominant LVNC and germ line mutations (V943F and R530X) in human MIB1 (mindbomb homolog 1) [117]. MIB1 encodes for an E3 ubiquitin ligase that is involved in regulation of the endocytosis of the NOTCH ligands DELTA and JAGGED. The patients with MIB1 had reduced NOTCH1 activity, Biventricular noncompaction including LVNC with a dilated phenotype, and heart failure. Functional studies in mice targeting MIB1 inactivation in mouse myocardium resulted in LVNC due to arrest of trabecular maturation and ventricular compaction.

Bmp10 Mutant: BMP10 is a growth factor that is a member of the TGF-β superfamily that has been shown to be upregulated in FKBP12-deficient mice [118]. BMP10 is only expressed briefly in the ventricular myocardium during a critical time when development is shifting from patterning to chamber maturation (E9.0 to E13.5), and its ventricular expression is restricted to the trabecular myocardium during this stage. BMP10-deficient mice typically die in utero at around E10.5 with evidence of very hypoplastic ventricular walls without trabeculae [18]. BMP overexpression leads to LVNC and ventricular septal defect. Upregulation of BMP10 also results in a hypertrabeculation phenotype in Numb/Numblike-deficient and Nkx2.5 knockout mice (see below) [22,118,119]. These findings suggest that BMP10 is an important factor in cardiac trabeculation/compaction.

Tbx20 Mutant: Tbx20 is a member of the Tbx1 subfamily of the T-box family transcription factors. Its expression in mouse embryos can be detected in the cardiac precursor cells at E7.5, persists in the developing myocardium and endocardium at E8.0, and at later developmental stages its expression is more abundant in the atrium compared with the ventricles. In addition, Tbx20 is a key mediator of BMP10 signaling in ventricular wall development and maturation. Overexpression of Tbx20 led to a severe DCM with hypertrabeculation consistent with the DCM form of LVNC [120].

Numb/Numblike Mutant: Numb family proteins, including Numb and numblike, are cell fate determinants for multiple progenitor cell types (hematopoietic stem cells, muscle satellite cells, cancer stem cells, and hemangioblasts), doing so by maintaining neural stem cell fate and regulating its differentiation. In addition, Numb functions as a component of the adherens junction to regulate cell adhesion and migration, complexes with β-catenin to regulate Wnt signaling, and interacts with integrin β subunits to promote their endocytosis for directional cell migration. When Numb and Numblike are deleted in mouse hearts by Nkx2.5$^{Cre/}$, creating a myocardial double knockout of these two genes, LVNC with congenital heart disease occurs [22,119]. The congenital heart defects include atrioventricular septal defects, truncus arteriosus, and double outlet RV. This model demonstrates that Numb family proteins regulate trabecular thickness by inhibiting Notch1 signaling, control cardiac morphogenesis in a Notch1-independent manner, and regulate cardiac progenitor cell differentiation in an endocytosis-dependent manner.

Nkx2-5 Mutant: Mice that harbor a ventricular muscle cell-restricted knockout of Nkx2-5 develop progressive atrioventricular block with progressive conduction system cell dropout and fibrosis with LVNC also being a prominent feature in neonatal mice, with progressive biventricular dilation and heart failure developing early [120]. Nkx2-5, a cardiac homeobox gene, is a transcription factor that regulates heart development in humans, working along with MEF2, HAND1, and HAND2 transcription factors to direct heart looping during early heart development. Nkx2-5 directly activates the MEF2 gene to control cardiomyocyte differentiation and operates in a positive feedback loop with GATA transcription factors to regulate cardiomyocyte formation. Ashraf et al. generated a murine model in a 129/Sv genetic background by knocking-in an Nkx2-5 homeodomain missense mutation previously identified in human, as missense mutations in the Nkx2-5 homeodomain (DNA-binding domain) are the most frequently reported type of human mutation. All heterozygous neonatal Nkx2-5(+/R52G) mice demonstrated a prominent trabecular layer in the ventricular wall along with diverse cardiac anomalies, including atrioventricular septal defects, Ebstein malformation of the tricuspid valve, and perimembranous and muscular ventricular septal defects. These results suggest that heterozygous missense mutation in the murine Nkx2-5 homeodomain (R52G) is highly penetrant and results in pleiotropic cardiac effects. In contrast to heterozygous Nkx2-5 knockout mice, the effects of the heterozygous knockin mice mimic findings in humans with heterozygous missense mutation in Nkx2-5 homeodomain. Heterozygous human mutations of Nkx2-5 are highly penetrant and associated with varied congenital heart defects. The heterozygous knockout of murine Nkx2-5, in contrast, manifests less profound cardiac malformations, with low disease penetrance.

Smad7 Mutant: TGF-β superfamily members exert their biological functions by binding to serine/threonine kinase receptors at the cell surface, followed by signal transduction by the intracellular transducers called Smads [121–123]. Smad proteins can be classified into three functional subclasses, with Smad7 being an inhibitory Smad. Smad7-deficient mutant mice typically die in utero due to multiple defects in cardiovascular development, including ventricular septal defect and LVNC, as well as outflow tract malformations and heart failure [121]. When Smad7 mutant mice live to adulthood, LVNC with impaired cardiac function and severe arrhythmia is notable.

NF-ATc Mutant: The expression of early response genes in lymphocytes is regulated by NF-AT transcription factors. NF-ATc mutant embryos have multiple cardiac abnormalities including myocardial developmental abnormalities, narrowing or occlusion of the ventricular outflow tract, defective septum morphogenesis, and underdevelopment of the semilunar valves with half of the mice dying at day E14.5 from circulatory failure [123]. In 40% of the mutant embryos, ventricular hypertrophy and small chamber size is seen as well as LVNC with hypertrabeculation commonly seen, suggesting that NF-AT signaling pathways are important for valve and septum development as well as development of hypertrabeculation/noncompaction.

Jarid2/Jumonji Mutants: The Jumonji family proteins function as histone demethylases [124]. Jarid2/Jumonji critically regulates developmental processes including cardiovascular development, as demonstrated by Jarid2 knockout mice, which have LVNC associated with a thin compact layer, ventricular septal defects, and double outlet RV [125–127]. Mysliwiec et al. [127] showed that the NOTCH1 pathway is directly controlled by Jarid2 and that failure to regulate NOTCH1 expression, as is the case in Jarid2 knockout mice, leads to proliferation and differentiation defects in the developing heart, which are manifested in the form of LVNC associated with a thin ventricular wall. Deletion of NOTCH1 in the mouse has also been shown to result in impaired trabeculation and myocardial proliferation associated with embryonic lethality due to cardiac insufficiency [128].

Tafazzin (TAZ) Mutant: Barth syndrome, an X-linked, multisystem human disorder characterized by cardiomyopathy (commonly LVNC), skeletal myopathy, cyclic neutropenia, 3-methylglutaconic aciduria, and cardiolipin deficiency, a key membrane phospholipid of cardiomyocytes and mitochondria, is caused by mutations in the X-linked gene tafazzin (TAZ) [10,23,129]. A TAZ knockdown mouse model has been shown to develop LVNC associated with abnormal cardiolipin profiles and mitochondrial structural abnormalities, indicating that mitochondrial function is important for proper myocardial development [130].

THERAPY AND OUTCOME

Therapy in LVNC is predicated on making the correct phenotypic diagnosis given that associated phenotypes require different surveillance and are associated with variable outcomes [5,10,14,27,50,96]. Increasing awareness of the disease is resulting in larger numbers of diagnoses. Furthermore, given the heritability of this disease, at-risk first-degree relatives are recommended for screening resulting in patients being diagnosed that otherwise would have never undergone noninvasive imaging. The role of clinically available genetic testing has also impacted management. Panels that assess for known sarcomeric gene mutations implicated in LVNC are becoming more commonly used and are considered standard of care in many institutions. In those patients with identified pathologic mutation, targeted sequencing can then be performed on first-degree relatives. This has important implications as these sarcomeric genes are known to present as varying cardiac phenotypes within families meaning that a first-degree relative of a known LVNC patient harboring the identical mutation may have an LVNC phenotype or instead have isolated dilated, hypertrophic, or restrictive cardiomyopathy without LVNC. These family members could also have the same mutation as the affected individual and have no phenotype at all. The presence of a pathologic mutation alters ongoing screening recommendations and should result in genetic counseling regarding risk to future offspring.

Therapy for LVNC is largely dictated by concomitant clinical findings associated with myocardial dysfunction and/or significant arrhythmias, or congenital heart disease. Patients with evidence of systolic or diastolic dysfunction should be managed based on existing recommendations [131]. For patients with LVNC and associated systolic dysfunction or DCM phenotype, oral therapies typically include anticongestive medications that help to favorably remodel the LV, including angiotensin-converting enzyme inhibitors and beta blockers, and an aldosterone antagonist. The use of loop diuretics would be considered for patients with evidence of congestion or volume overload, and aspirin is used to reduce the potential for thrombotic complications. Inpatient therapies may consist of intravenous diuretics and/or vasodilatory agents in the setting of acute decompensated heart failure. Inotropes may be used in patients with evidence of low cardiac output and poor end organ perfusion. Patients may be considered for ICDs if they meet criteria for implantation as recommended in published guidelines. Advanced pacing strategies such as cardiac resynchronization may also be employed with improvement being seen in some patients [75,76]. The use of ventricular assist devices and cardiac transplant may also be considered for those patients with end-stage disease. Patients with associated HCM may benefit from symptomatic therapies if left ventricular outflow tract obstruction is present in the form of beta blockers or calcium channel blockers. Internal cardioverter–defibrillator placement may be considered for those patients with increased risk of sudden cardiac death [132].

There are well-known thromboembolic risks associated with LVNC [14,133] although these are largely reported in adults [125]. For this reason, treatment with antiplatelet or systemic anticoagulation may be considered in adults, especially when the LV or atria are dilated. The incidence of stroke or other embolic phenomena in children remains poorly characterized. Antiplatelet therapy may be considered in those with depressed left ventricular systolic dysfunction, evidence of spontaneous echocardiographic contrast, severe left ventricular dilation, and/or dilated atria. The presence of atrial fibrillation may also prompt use of systemic anticoagulation.

In patients with primary diastolic dysfunction, pharmacologic therapy may be instituted but no treatments have proven benefit. In many cases, combination systolic and diastolic dysfunction occurs, causing decompensated heart failure requiring the therapeutic approaches noted above. Some patients develop restrictive physiology, and these patients generally require transplantation. Management strategies for those patients with the diagnosis of mitochondrial disease or metabolic derangements may be managed with additional medical therapies such as coenzyme Q10, L-carnitine, riboflavin, and thiamine in the setting of known mitochondrial disease. However, the benefit of these therapies is unclear.

In patients with associated congenital heart disease, LVNC may alter therapy and confound outcomes. Treatment of congenital heart disease will be dictated by the severity of the lesion and may require percutaneous or surgical intervention. Furthermore, consideration of overarching genetic causes must be considered, which may impact management as well as screening of at-risk family members. The presence of LVNC may complicate management resulting in higher risks of myocardial dysfunction, arrhythmias, and thromboembolic events especially in the perioperative period. Consideration must be given to possible syndromic disease or metabolic diseases, possibly impacting management considerations in patients undergoing catheter-based interventions and/or surgical palliations/corrective surgery. Management will be directed at associated myocardial dysfunction with or without evidence of heart failure as well as significant dysrhythmias.

The outcomes of patients with LVNC are largely associated with the presence of myocardial dysfunction and/or the presence of clinically significant arrhythmias. Brescia et al. [50] reported on our single center experience of 242 children with LVNC. Of these, 150/242 (62%) were noted to have myocardial dysfunction and 80/242 (33.1%) had a significant arrhythmia. The presence of myocardial dysfunction or arrhythmias was strongly associated with mortality ($P<.001$ and $P=.002$, respectively). Similar reports exist in the adult literature citing myocardial dysfunction or ventricular arrhythmias as predictors of mortality.

CONCLUSION

LVNC is a complex, clinically and genetically heterogeneous disorder that with advancement in diagnostic modalities and an increase in awareness has become the third most common cardiomyopathy diagnosed in children and adults. However, controversy remains regarding the diagnostic criteria for LVNC, and this area continues to need improvement. LVNC may be associated with congenital heart disease, systemic disorders of metabolism and energy, dysmorphic syndromes, and chromosomal defects. Due to its heterogeneous clinical phenotype, the propensity for the development of associated arrhythmias, sudden cardiac death, and heart failure that is dependent on the specific clinical phenotype, and its current underrecognition by many clinicians, LVNC is a disorder that requires better clinical identification and pathologic understanding for improved care and new targeted therapies to be developed and for improved outcomes to continue. In addition, because LVNC overlaps with other forms of cardiomyopathy as well as arrhythmias and congenital heart disease, unraveling the underlying developmental and molecular genetic pathophysiology is likely to enhance our understanding of these other disorders as well, making LVNC a paradigm shifting disorder. The genetic causes are beginning to be determined and understood, and animal models are starting to provide insights into the developmental abnormalities that define normal and abnormal development of the compacted and noncompacted myocardium; and together these findings may help define the clinical heterogeneity, differential outcomes, and therapies over the next decade.

RECOMMENDATIONS

1. All patients with LVNC should be assessed with at least a three-generation family history, and first-degree relatives should undergo echocardiographic and electrocardiographic testing to determine if their condition is familial.
2. Genetic counseling should be provided to patients with LVNC; this should include discussion of the risks, benefits, and options available for clinical genetic testing.
3. Genetic testing for patients with LVNC can be useful to confirm the diagnosis, to facilitate cascade screening within the family, and to help with family planning.
4. Genetic testing and counseling should be performed in centers experienced in genetic evaluation and family-based management of cardiomyopathy.
5. Patients with LVNC, particularly infants and young children, should be evaluated for metabolic derangements and neuromuscular abnormalities.

REFERENCES

[1] R.T. Grant, An unusual anomaly of the coronary vessels in the malformed heart of a child, Heart 13 (1926) 273–283.

[2] T.K. Chin, J.K. Perloff, R.G. Williams, K. Jue, R. Mohrmann, Isolated noncompaction of left ventricular myocardium. A study of eight cases, Circulation 82 (1990) 507–513.

[3] R.H. Pignatelli, C.J. McMahon, W.J. Dreyer, et al., Clinical characterization of left ventricular noncompaction in children: a relatively common form of cardiomyopathy, Circulation 108 (2003) 2672–2678.

[4] R. Engberding, T.M. Yelbuz, G. Breithardt, Isolated noncompaction of the left ventricular myocardium – a review of the literature two decades after the initial case description, Clin. Res. Cardiol. 96 (2007) 481–488.

[5] D. Sedmera, T. Pexieder, M. Vuillemin, R.P. Thompson, R.H. Anderson, Developmental patterning of the myocardium, Anat. Rec. 258 (2000) 319–337.

[6] J. Dusek, B. Ostadal, M. Duskova, Postnatal persistence of spongy myocardium with embryonic blood supply, Arch. Pathol. 99 (1975) 312–317.

[7] G. Fazio, M. Lunetta, E. Grassedonio, et al., Noncompaction of the right ventricle, Pediatr. Cardiol. 31 (2010) 576–578.

[8] A. Ranganathan, G. Ganesan, V. Sangareddi, A.P. Pillai, A. Ramasamy, Isolated noncompaction of right ventricle–a case report, Echocardiography 29 (2012) E169–E172.

[9] K. Tigen, T. Karaahmet, E. Gurel, C. Cevik, Y. Basaran, Biventricular noncompaction: a case report, Echocardiography 25 (2008) 993–996.

[10] J.A. Towbin, Left ventricular noncompaction: a new form of heart failure, Heart Fail. Clin. 6 (2010) 453–469.

[11] B.J. Maron, J.A. Towbin, G. Thiene, et al., Contemporary definitions and classification of the cardiomyopathies: an American Heart Association Scientific Statement from the Council on Clinical Cardiology, Heart Failure and Transplantation Committee; Quality of Care and Outcomes Research and Functional Genomics and Translational Biology Interdisciplinary Working Groups; and Council on Epidemiology and Prevention, Circulation 113 (2006) 1807–1816.

[12] C. Stollberger, J. Finsterer, G. Blazek, Left ventricular hypertrabeculation/noncompaction and association with additional cardiac abnormalities and neuromuscular disorders, Am. J. Cardiol. 90 (2002) 899–902.

[13] C. Stollberger, J. Finsterer, Left ventricular hypertrabeculation/noncompaction, J. Am. Soc. Echocardiogr. 17 (2004) 91–100.

[14] F. Ichida, Y. Hamamichi, T. Miyawaki, et al., Clinical features of isolated noncompaction of the ventricular myocardium: long-term clinical course, hemodynamic properties, and genetic background, J. Am. Coll. Cardiol. 34 (1999) 233–240.

[15] D. Cartoni, P. Salvini, R. De Rosa, A. Cortese, M.S. Nazzaro, P. Tanzi, Images in cardiovascular medicine. Multiple coronary artery-left ventricle microfistulae and spongy myocardium: the eagerly awaited link? Circulation 116 (2007) e81–e84.

[16] K. Reynen, K. Bachmann, H. Singer, Spongy myocardium, Cardiology 88 (1997) 601–602.

[17] J.M. Icardo, A. Fernandez-Teran, Morphologic study of ventricular trabeculation in the embryonic chick heart, Acta Anat. 130 (1987) 264–274.

[18] H. Chen, W. Zhang, D. Li, T.M. Cordes, R.M. Payne, W. Shou, Analysis of ventricular hypertrabeculation and noncompaction using genetically engineered mouse models, Pediatr. Cardiol. 30 (2009) 626–634.

[19] R.P. Harvey, Patterning the vertebrate heart, Nat. Rev. Genet. 3 (2002) 544–556.

[20] C.A. Risebro, P.R. Riley, Formation of the ventricles, Sci. World J. 6 (2006) 1862–1880.

[21] D. Sedmera, T. McQuinn, Embryogenesis of the heart muscle, Heart Fail. Clin. 4 (2008) 235–245.

[22] J. Yang, S. Bucker, B. Jungblut, et al., Inhibition of Notch2 by Numb/Numblike controls myocardial compaction in the heart, Cardiovasc. Res. 96 (2012) 276–285.

[23] F. Ichida, S. Tsubata, K.R. Bowles, et al., Novel gene mutations in patients with left ventricular noncompaction or Barth syndrome, Circulation 103 (2001) 1256–1263.

[24] K. Caliskan, B. Ujvari, T. Bauernfeind, et al., The prevalence of early repolarization in patients with noncompaction cardiomyopathy presenting with malignant ventricular arrhythmias, J. Cardiovasc. Electrophysiol. 23 (2012) 938–944.

[25] J. Steffel, F. Duru, Rhythm disorders in isolated left ventricular noncompaction, Ann. Med. 44 (2012) 101–108.

[26] C.H. Attenhofer Jost, H.M. Connolly, C.A. Warnes, et al., Noncompacted myocardium in Ebstein's anomaly: initial description in three patients, J. Am. Soc. Echocardiogr. 17 (2004) 677–680.

[27] W.A. Zuckerman, M.E. Richmond, R.K. Singh, S.J. Carroll, T.J. Starc, L.J. Addonizio, Left-ventricular noncompaction in a pediatric population: predictors of survival, Pediatr. Cardiol. 32 (2011) 406–412.

[28] B.E. Stahli, C. Gebhard, P. Biaggi, et al., Left ventricular non-compaction: prevalence in congenital heart disease, Int. J. Cardiol. 167 (2013) 2477–2481.

[29] S. Madan, S. Mandal, J.E. Bost, et al., Noncompaction cardiomyopathy in children with congenital heart disease: evaluation using cardiovascular magnetic resonance imaging, Pediatr. Cardiol. 33 (2012) 215–221.

[30] F. Scaglia, J.A. Towbin, W.J. Craigen, et al., Clinical spectrum, morbidity, and mortality in 113 pediatric patients with mitochondrial disease, Pediatrics 114 (2004) 925–931.

[31] J. Yaplito-Lee, R. Weintraub, K. Jamsen, C.W. Chow, D.R. Thorburn, A. Boneh, Cardiac manifestations in oxidative phosphorylation disorders of childhood, J. Pediatr. 150 (2007) 407–411.

[32] M.S. Pepper, Transforming growth factor-beta: vasculogenesis, angiogenesis, and vessel wall integrity, Cytokine Growth Factor Rev. 8 (1997) 21–43.

[33] C. Suri, P.F. Jones, S. Patan, et al., Requisite role of angiopoietin-1, a ligand for the TIE2 receptor, during embryonic angiogenesis, Cell 87 (1996) 1171–1180.

[34] N. Ferrara, K. Carver-Moore, H. Chen, et al., Heterozygous embryonic lethality induced by targeted inactivation of the VEGF gene, Nature 380 (1996) 439–442.

[35] W. Zhang, H. Chen, X. Qu, C.P. Chang, W. Shou, Molecular mechanism of ventricular trabeculation/compaction and the pathogenesis of the left ventricular noncompaction cardiomyopathy (LVNC), Am. J. Med. Genet. C Semin. Med. Genet. 163C (2013) 144–156.

[36] C. Stollberger, G. Blazek, C. Dobias, A. Hanafin, C. Wegner, J. Finsterer, Frequency of stroke and embolism in left ventricular hypertrabeculation/noncompaction, Am. J. Cardiol. 108 (2011) 1021–1023.

[37] M. Greutmann, M.L. Mah, C.K. Silversides, et al., Predictors of adverse outcome in adolescents and adults with isolated left ventricular noncompaction, Am. J. Cardiol. 109 (2012) 276–281.

[38] J. Steffel, R. Kobza, E. Oechslin, R. Jenni, F. Duru, Electrocardiographic characteristics at initial diagnosis in patients with isolated left ventricular noncompaction, Am. J. Cardiol. 104 (2009) 984–989.

[39] A. Celiker, S. Ozkutlu, E. Dilber, T. Karagoz, Rhythm abnormalities in children with isolated ventricular noncompaction, Pacing Clin. Electrophysiol. 28 (2005) 1198–1202.

[40] M. Ritter, E. Oechslin, G. Sutsch, C. Attenhofer, J. Schneider, R. Jenni, Isolated noncompaction of the myocardium in adults, Mayo Clin. Proc. 72 (1997) 26–31.

[41] D. Aras, O. Tufekcioglu, K. Ergun, et al., Clinical features of isolated ventricular noncompaction in adults long-term clinical course, echocardiographic properties, and predictors of left ventricular failure, J. Card. Fail. 12 (2006) 726–733.

[42] R. Sandhu, R.S. Finkelhor, D.R. Gunawardena, R.C. Bahler, Prevalence and characteristics of left ventricular noncompaction in a community hospital cohort of patients with systolic dysfunction, Echocardiography 25 (2008) 8–12.

[43] T. Kovacevic-Preradovic, R. Jenni, E.N. Oechslin, G. Noll, B. Seifert, C.H. Attenhofer Jost, Isolated left ventricular noncompaction as a cause for heart failure and heart transplantation: a single center experience, Cardiology 112 (2009) 158–164.

[44] A.P. Patrianakos, F.I. Parthenakis, E.G. Nyktari, P.E. Vardas, Noncompaction myocardium imaging with multiple echocardiographic modalities, Echocardiography 25 (2008) 898–900.

[45] R. Ronderos, G. Avegliano, E. Borelli, P. Kuschnir, F. Castro, G. Sanchez, G. Perea, M. Corneli, M.M. Zanier, S. Andres, A. Aranda, D. Conde, M. Trivi, Estimation of prevalence of the left ventricular noncompaction among adults, 118 (6) (2016) 901–905.

[46] R.J. Sarma, A. Chana, U. Elkayam, Left ventricular noncompaction, Prog. Cardiovasc. Dis. 52 (2010) 264–273.

[47] M. Niemann, S. Stork, F. Weidemann, Left ventricular noncompaction cardiomyopathy: an overdiagnosed disease, Circulation 126 (2012) e240–e243.

[48] R.T. Murphy, R. Thaman, J.G. Blanes, et al., Natural history and familial characteristics of isolated left ventricular non-compaction, Eur. Heart J. 26 (2005) 187–192.
[49] N.L. Bhatia, A.J. Tajik, S. Wilansky, D.E. Steidley, F. Mookadam, Isolated noncompaction of the left ventricular myocardium in adults: a systematic overview, J. Card. Fail. 17 (2011) 771–778.
[50] S.T. Brescia, J.W. Rossano, R. Pignatelli, et al., Mortality and sudden death in pediatric left ventricular noncompaction in a tertiary referral center, Circulation 127 (2013) 2202–2208.
[51] K. Caliskan, A. Kardos, T. Szili-Torok, Empty handed: a call for an international registry of risk stratification to reduce the 'sudden-ness' of death in patients with non-compaction cardiomyopathy, Europace 11 (2009) 1138–1139.
[52] E. Biagini, L. Ragni, M. Ferlito, et al., Different types of cardiomyopathy associated with isolated ventricular noncompaction, Am. J. Cardiol. 98 (2006) 821–824.
[53] Y. Ergul, K. Nisli, M.A. Varkal, et al., Electrocardiographic findings at initial diagnosis in children with isolated left ventricular noncompaction, Ann. Noninvasive Electrocardiol. 16 (2011) 184–191.
[54] O.S. Onay, I. Yildirim, B. Beken, et al., Successful implantation of an intracardiac defibrillator in an infant with long QT syndrome and isolated noncompaction of the ventricular myocardium, Pediatr. Cardiol. 34 (2013) 189–193.
[55] K. Nakashima, I. Kusakawa, T. Yamamoto, et al., A left ventricular noncompaction in a patient with long QT syndrome caused by a KCNQ1 mutation: a case report, Heart Vessel. 28 (2013) 126–129.
[56] B.R. Nascimento, D.F. Vidigal, R.D. Carneiro, et al., Complete atrioventricular block as the first manifestation of noncompaction of the ventricular myocardium, Pacing Clin. Electrophysiol. 36 (2013) e107–e110.
[57] R.E. Ulusoy, N. Kucukarslan, A. Kirilmaz, E. Demiralp, Noncompaction of ventricular myocardium involving both ventricles, Eur. J. Echocardiogr. 7 (2006) 457–460.
[58] T. Williams, W. Machann, L. Kuhler, H. Hamm, J. Müller-Höcker, M. Zimmer, G. Ertl, O. Ritter, M. Beer, J. Schönberger, Novel desmoplakin mutation: juvenile biventricular cardiomyopathy with left ventricular non-compaction and acantholytic palmoplantar keratoderma, Clin. Res. Cardiol. 100 (2011) 1087–1093.
[59] E.K. Wlodarska, O. Wozniak, M. Konka, D. Piotrowska-Kownacka, E. Walczak, P. Hoffman, Isolated ventricular noncompaction mimicking arrhythmogenic right ventricular cardiomyopathy–a study of nine patients, Int. J. Cardiol. 145 (2010) 107–111.
[60] M.L. Hughes, B. Carstensen, J.L. Wilkinson, R.G. Weintraub, Angiographic diagnosis, prevalence and outcomes for left ventricular noncompaction in children with congenital cardiac disease, Cardiol. Young 17 (2007) 56–63.
[61] R. Jenni, E. Oechslin, J. Schneider, C. Attenhofer Jost, P.A. Kaufmann, Echocardiographic and pathoanatomical characteristics of isolated left ventricular non-compaction: a step towards classification as a distinct cardiomyopathy, Heart 86 (2001) 666–671.
[62] E. Oechslin, R. Jenni, Left ventricular non-compaction revisited: a distinct phenotype with genetic heterogeneity? Eur. Heart J. 32 (2011) 1446–1456.
[63] R. Punn, N.H. Silverman, Cardiac segmental analysis in left ventricular noncompaction: experience in a pediatric population, J. Am. Soc. Echocardiogr. 23 (2010) 46–53.
[64] C.J. McMahon, R.H. Pignatelli, S.F. Nagueh, et al., Left ventricular non-compaction cardiomyopathy in children: characterisation of clinical status using tissue Doppler-derived indices of left ventricular diastolic relaxation, Heart 93 (2007) 676–681.
[65] B.W. Eidem, Noninvasive evaluation of left ventricular noncompaction: what's new in 2009? Pediatr. Cardiol. 30 (2009) 682–689.
[66] B.M. van Dalen, K. Caliskan, O.I. Soliman, et al., Left ventricular solid body rotation in non-compaction cardiomyopathy: a potential new objective and quantitative functional diagnostic criterion? Eur. J. Heart Fail. 10 (2008) 1088–1093.
[67] S.E. Petersen, J.B. Selvanayagam, F. Wiesmann, et al., Left ventricular non-compaction: insights from cardiovascular magnetic resonance imaging, J. Am. Coll. Cardiol. 46 (2005) 101–105.
[68] F. Thuny, A. Jacquier, B. Jop, et al., Assessment of left ventricular non-compaction in adults: side-by-side comparison of cardiac magnetic resonance imaging with echocardiography, Arch. Cardiovasc. Dis. 103 (2010) 150–159.
[69] A. Jacquier, F. Thuny, B. Jop, et al., Measurement of trabeculated left ventricular mass using cardiac magnetic resonance imaging in the diagnosis of left ventricular non-compaction, Eur. Heart J. 31 (2010) 1098–1104.
[70] S. Uribe, L. Cadavid, T. Hussain, et al., Cardiovascular magnetic resonance findings in a pediatric population with isolated left ventricular non-compaction, J. Cardiovasc. Magn. Reson. 14 (2012) 9.
[71] T.E. Paterick, A.J. Tajik, Left ventricular noncompaction: a diagnostically challenging cardiomyopathy, Circ. J. 76 (2012) 1556–1562.
[72] G. Melendez-Ramirez, F. Castillo-Castellon, N. Espinola-Zavaleta, A. Meave, E.T. Kimura-Hayama, Left ventricular noncompaction: a proposal of new diagnostic criteria by multidetector computed tomography, J. Cardiovasc. Comput. Tomogr. 6 (2012) 346–354.
[73] C.L. Hollingsworth, T.T. Yoshizumi, D.P. Frush, et al., Pediatric cardiac-gated CT angiography: assessment of radiation dose, Am. J. Roentgenol. 189 (2007) 12–18.
[74] K. Nihei, N. Shinomiya, H. Kabayama, et al., Wolff-Parkinson-White (WPW) syndrome in isolated noncompaction of the ventricular myocardium (INVM), Circ. J. 68 (2004) 82–84.
[75] K. Caliskan, T. Szili-Torok, D.A. Theuns, et al., Indications and outcome of implantable cardioverter-defibrillators for primary and secondary prophylaxis in patients with noncompaction cardiomyopathy, J. Cardiovasc. Electrophysiol. 22 (2011) 898–904.
[76] R. Kobza, J. Steffel, P. Erne, et al., Implantable cardioverter-defibrillator and cardiac resynchronization therapy in patients with left ventricular noncompaction, Heart Rhythm 7 (2010) 1545–1549.
[77] S. Van Malderen, S. Wijchers, F. Akca, K. Caliskan, T. Szili-Torok, Mismatch between the origin of premature ventricular complexes and the noncompacted myocardium in patients with noncompaction cardiomyopathy patients: involvement of the conduction system? Ann. Noninvasive Electrocardiol. (August 29, 2016) http://dx.doi.org/10.1111/anec.12394. [Epub ahead of print].

[78] J.L. Jefferies, J.D. Wilkinson, L.A. Sleeper, S.D. Colan, M. Lu, E. Pahl, P.F. Kantor, M.D. Everitt, S.A. Webber, B.D. Kaufman, J.M. Lamour, C.E. Canter, D.T. Hsu, L.J. Addonizio, S.E. Lipshultz, J.A. Towbin, Pediatric Cardiomyopathy Registry Investigators, Cardiomyopathy phenotypes and outcomes for children with left ventricular myocardial noncompaction: results from the Pediatric Cardiomyopathy Registry, J. Card. Fail. 21 (11) (November 2015) 877–884.

[79] S. Sasse-Klaassen, B. Gerull, E. Oechslin, R. Jenni, L. Thierfelder, Isolated noncompaction of the left ventricular myocardium in the adult is an autosomal dominant disorder in the majority of patients, Am. J. Med. Genet. Part A 119A (2003) 162–167.

[80] M. Digilio, L. Bernardini, M. Gagliardi, et al., Syndromic non-compaction of the left ventricle: associated chromosomal anomalies, Clin. Genet. (2012).

[81] S. Beken, A. Cevik, O. Turan, et al., A neonatal case of left ventricular noncompaction associated with trisomy 18, Genet. Couns. 22 (2) (2011) 161–164.

[82] M. Yukifumi, S. Hirohiko, I. Fukiko, M. Mariko, Trisomy 13 in a 9-year-old girl with left ventricular noncompaction, Pediatr. Cardiol. 32 (2) (2011) 206–207.

[83] J.J. Blinder, H.R. Martinez, W.J. Craigen, J. Belmont, R.H. Pignatelli, J.L. Jefferies, Noncompaction of the left ventricular myocardium in a boy with a novel chromosome 8p23.1 deletion, Am. J. Med. Genet. Part A 155A (9) (2011) 2215–2220.

[84] H.R. Martinez, M.C. Niu, V.R. Sutton, R. Pignatelli, M. Vatta, J.L. Jefferies, Coffin-Lowry syndrome and left ventricular noncompaction cardiomyopathy with a restrictive pattern, Am. J. Med. Genet. Part A 155A (12) (2011) 3030–3034.

[85] H.R. Martinez, J.W. Belmont, W.J. Craigen, M.D. Taylor, J.L. Jefferies, Left ventricular noncompaction in Sotos syndrome, Am. J. Med. Genet. Part A 155A (5) (2011) 1115–1118.

[86] U. Zechner, N. Kohlschmidt, O. Kempf, et al., Familial Sotos syndrome caused by a novel missense mutation, C2175S, in NSD1 and associated with normal intelligence, insulin dependent diabetes, bronchial asthma, and lipedema, Eur. J. Med. Genet. 52 (5) (2009) 306–310.

[87] E.A. Sellars, S.L. Zimmerman, T. Smolarek, R.J. Hopkin, Ventricular noncompaction and absent thumbs in a newborn with tetrasomy 5q35.2-5q35.3: an association with Hunter-McAlpine syndrome? Am. J. Med. Genet. Part A 155A (6) (2011) 1409–1413.

[88] G. Corrado, N. Checcarelli, M. Santarone, C. Stollberger, J. Finsterer, Left ventricular hypertrabeculation/noncompaction with PMP22 duplication-based Charcot-Marie-Tooth disease type 1A, Cardiology 105 (3) (2006) 142–145.

[89] S. Klaassen, S. Probst, E. Oechslin, B. Gerull, G. Krings, P. Schuler, M. Greutmann, D. Hürlimann, M. Yegitbasi, L. Pons, M. Gramlich, J.D. Drenckhahn, A. Heuser, F. Berger, R. Jenni, L. Thierfelder, Mutations in sarcomere protein genes in left ventricular noncompaction, Circulation 117 (2008) 2893–2901.

[90] Y.M. Hoedemaekers, K. Caliskan, M. Michels, et al., The importance of genetic counseling, DNA diagnostics, and cardiologic family screening in left ventricular noncompaction cardiomyopathy, Circ. Cardiovasc. Genet. 3 (2010) 232–239.

[91] J.J. Parent, J.A. Towbin, J.L. Jefferies, Left ventricular noncompaction in a family with lamin A/C gene mutation, Tex. Heart Inst. J. 42 (1) (February 1, 2015) 73–76.

[92] L. Shan, N. Makita, Y. Xing, et al., SCN5A variants in Japanese patients with left ventricular noncompaction and arrhythmia, Mol. Genet. Metab. 93 (2008) 468–474.

[93] J.A. Towbin, Ion channel dysfunction associated with arrhythmia, ventricular noncompaction, and mitral valve prolapse: a new overlapping phenotype, J. Am. Coll. Cardiol. 64 (8) (August 26, 2014) 768–771.

[94] P.A. Schweizer, J. Schröter, S. Greiner, J. Haas, P. Yampolsky, D. Mereles, S.J. Buss, C. Seyler, C. Bruehl, A. Draguhn, M. Koenen, B. Meder, H.A. Katus, D. Thomas, The symptom complex of familial sinus node dysfunction and myocardial noncompaction is associated with mutations in the HCN4 channel, J. Am. Coll. Cardiol. 64 (8) (August 26, 2014) 757–767.

[95] A. Milano, A.M. Vermeer, E.M. Lodder, J. Barc, A.O. Verkerk, A.V. Postma, I.A. van der Bilt, M.J. Baars, P.L. van Haelst, K. Caliskan, Y.M. Hoedemaekers, S. Le Scouarnec, R. Redon, Y.M. Pinto, I. Christiaans, A.A. Wilde, C.R. Bezzina, HCN4 mutations in multiple families with bradycardia and left ventricular noncompaction cardiomyopathy, J. Am. Coll. Cardiol. 64 (8) (August 26, 2014) 745–756.

[96] J.A. Towbin, A. Lorts, J.L. Jefferies, Left ventricular non-compaction cardiomyopathy, Lancet 386 (9995) (August 22, 2015) 813–825.

[97] S.B. Bleyl, B.R. Mumford, M.C. Brown-Harrison, et al., Xq28-linked noncompaction of the left ventricular myocardium: prenatal diagnosis and pathologic analysis of affected individuals, Am. J. Med. Genet. 72 (3) (1997) 257–265.

[98] P. Ouyang, E. Saarel, Y. Bai, et al., A de novo mutation in NKX2.5 associated with atrial septal defects, ventricular noncompaction, syncope and sudden death, Clin. Chim. Acta 412 (2011) 170–175.

[99] A.V. Postma, K. van Engelen, J. van de Meerakker, et al., Mutations in the sarcomere gene MYH7 in Ebstein anomaly, Circ. Cardiovasc. Genet. 4 (2011) 43–50.

[100] A.M. Kelle, S.J. Bentley, L.O. Rohena, A.K. Cabalka, T.M. Olson, Ebstein anomaly, left ventricular non-compaction, and early onset heart failure associated with a de novo α-tropomyosin gene mutation, Am. J. Med. Genet. A 170 (8) (August 2016) 2186–2190.

[101] S. Probst, E. Oechslin, P. Schuler, et al., Sarcomere gene mutations in isolated left ventricular noncompaction cardiomyopathy do not predict clinical phenotype, Circ. Cardiovasc. Genet. 4 (2011) 367–374.

[102] L.M. Dellefave, P. Pytel, S. Mewborn, et al., Sarcomere mutations in cardiomyopathy with left ventricular hypertrabeculation, Circ. Cardiovasc. Genet. 2 (2009) 442–449.

[103] R. Hastings, C.P. de Villiers, C. Hooper, L. Ormondroyd, A. Pagnamenta, S. Lise, S. Salatino, S.J. Knight, J.C. Taylor, K.L. Thomson, L. Arnold, S.D. Chatziefthimiou, P.V. Konarev, M. Wilmanns, E. Ehler, A. Ghisleni, M. Gautel, E. Blair, H. Watkins, K. Gehmlich, Combination of whole genome sequencing, linkage, and functional studies implicates a missense mutation in titin as a cause of autosomal dominant cardiomyopathy with features of left ventricular noncompaction, Circ. Cardiovasc. Genet. 9 (5) (October 2016) 426–435.

[104] R.D. Bagnall, L.K. Molloy, J.M. Kalman, C. Semsarian, Exome sequencing identifies a mutation in the ACTN2 gene in a family with idiopathic ventricular fibrillation, left ventricular noncompaction, and sudden death, BMC Med. Genet. 15 (September 16, 2014) 99.

[105] J. Finsterer, C. Stollberger, Primary myopathies and the heart, Scand. Cardiovasc. J. 42 (2008) 9–24.
[106] F. Ramond, A. Janin, S. Di Filippo, V. Chanavat, L. Chalabreysse, N. Roux-Buisson, D. Sanlaville, R. Touraine, G. Millat, Homozygous PKP2 deletion associated with neonatal left ventricle noncompaction, Clin. Genet. 91 (1) (January 2017) 126–130.
[107] S. Tang, A. Batra, Y. Zhang, E.S. Ebenroth, T. Huang, Left ventricular noncompaction is associated with mutations in the mitochondrial genome, Mitochondrion 10 (2010) 350–357.
[108] A.K. Arndt, S. Schafer, J.D. Drenckhahn, M.K. Sabeh, E.R. Plovie, A. Caliebe, E. Klopocki, G. Musso, A.A. Werdich, H. Kalwa, M. Heinig, R.F. Padera, K. Wassilew, J. Bluhm, C. Harnack, J. Martitz, P.J. Barton, M. Greutmann, F. Berger, N. Hubner, R. Siebert, H.H. Kramer, S.A. Cook, C.A. MacRae, S. Klaassen, Fine mapping of the 1p36 deletion syndrome identifies mutation of PRDM16 as a cause of cardiomyopathy, Am. J. Hum. Genet. 93 (1) (July 11, 2013) 67–77.
[109] F.B. Pearce, S.H. Litovsky, R.J. Dabal, N. Robin, L.J. Dure, J.F. George, J.K. Kirklin, Pathologic features of dilated cardiomyopathy with localized noncompaction in a child with deletion 1p36 syndrome, Congenit. Heart Dis. 7 (1) (January–February 2012) 59–61.
[110] P. Teekakirikul, M.A. Kelly, H.L. Rehm, N.K. Lakdawala, B.H. Funke, Inherited cardiomyopathies: molecular genetics and clinical genetic testing in the postgenomic era, J. Mol. Diagn. 15 (2013) 158–170.
[111] S.L. Schreiber, G.R. Crabtree, Immunophilins, ligands, and the control of signal transduction, Harvey Lect. 91 (1995) 99–114.
[112] T. Wang, P.K. Donahoe, The immunophilin FKBP12: a molecular guardian of the TGF-beta family type I receptors, Front. Biosci. 9 (2004) 619–631.
[113] A.M. Cameron, J.P. Steiner, A.J. Roskams, S.M. Ali, G.V. Ronnett, S.H. Snyder, Calcineurin associated with the inositol 1,4,5-trisphosphate receptor-FKBP12 complex modulates Ca2+ flux, Cell 83 (1995) 463–472.
[114] M. Maruyama, B.Y. Li, H. Chen, et al., FKBP12 is a critical regulator of the heart rhythm and the cardiac voltage-gated sodium current in mice, Circ. Res. 108 (2011) 1042–1052.
[115] W. Shou, B. Aghdasi, D.L. Armstrong, et al., Cardiac defects and altered ryanodine receptor function in mice lacking FKBP12, Nature 391 (1998) 489–492.
[116] H. Chen, W. Zhang, X. Sun, et al., Fkbp1a controls ventricular myocardium trabeculation and compaction by regulating endocardial Notch1 activity, Development 140 (2013) 1946–1957.
[117] G. Luxan, J.C. Casanova, B. Martinez-Poveda, et al., Mutations in the NOTCH pathway regulator MIB1 cause left ventricular noncompaction cardiomyopathy, Nat. Med. 19 (2013) 193–201.
[118] H. Chen, S. Shi, L. Acosta, et al., BMP10 is essential for maintaining cardiac growth during murine cardiogenesis, Development 131 (2004) 2219–2231.
[119] C. Zhao, H. Guo, J. Li, et al., Numb family proteins are essential for cardiac morphogenesis and progenitor differentiation, Development 141 (2014) 281–295.
[120] M. Pashmforoush, J.T. Lu, H. Chen, et al., Nkx2-5 pathways and congenital heart disease; loss of ventricular myocyte lineage specification leads to progressive cardiomyopathy and complete heart block, Cell 117 (2004) 373–386.
[121] Q. Chen, H. Chen, D. Zheng, et al., Smad7 is required for the development and function of the heart, J. Biol. Chem. 284 (2009) 292–300.
[122] J. Liu, J.D. Farmer Jr., W.S. Lane, J. Friedman, I. Weissman, S.L. Schreiber, Calcineurin is a common target of cyclophilin-cyclosporin A and FKBP-FK506 complexes, Cell 66 (1991) 807–815.
[123] J.L. de la Pompa, L.A. Timmerman, H. Takimoto, et al., Role of the NF-ATc transcription factor in morphogenesis of cardiac valves and septum, Nature 392 (1998) 182–186.
[124] J.R. Whetstine, A. Nottke, F. Lan, et al., Reversal of histone lysine trimethylation by the JMJD2 family of histone demethylases, Cell 125 (2006) 467–481.
[125] X. Shen, W. Kim, Y. Fujiwara, et al., Jumonji modulates polycomb activity and self-renewal versus differentiation of stem cells, Cell 139 (2009) 1303–1314.
[126] D. Landeira, S. Sauer, R. Poot, et al., Jarid2 is a PRC2 component in embryonic stem cells required for multi-lineage differentiation and recruitment of PRC1 and RNA Polymerase II to developmental regulators, Nat. Cell Biol. 12 (2010) 618–624.
[127] M.R. Mysliwiec, E.H. Bresnick, Y. Lee, Endothelial Jarid2/Jumonji is required for normal cardiac development and proper Notch1 expression, J. Biol. Chem. 286 (2011) 17193–17204.
[128] J. Grego-Bessa, L. Luna-Zurita, G. del Monte, et al., Notch signaling is essential for ventricular chamber development, Dev. Cell 12 (2007) 415–429.
[129] J.L. Jefferies, Barth syndrome, Am. J. Med. Genet. C Semin. Med. Genet. 163 (2013) 198–205.
[130] C.K. Phoon, D. Acehan, M. Schlame, et al., Tafazzin knockdown in mice leads to a developmental cardiomyopathy with early diastolic dysfunction preceding myocardial noncompaction, J. Am. Heart Assoc. (2012) 1, http://dx.doi.org/10.1161/JAHA.111.000455. pii: jah3-e000455.
[131] C.W. Yancy, M. Jessup, B. Bozkurt, et al., 2013 ACCF/AHA guideline for the management of heart failure: a report of the American College of Cardiology Foundation/American Heart Association Task Force on practice guidelines, J. Am. Coll. Cardiol. 62 (2013) e147–239.
[132] B.J. Gersh, B.J. Maron, R.O. Bonow, et al., American College of Cardiology Foundation/American Heart Association Task Force on practice guidelines. 2011 ACCF/AHA guideline for the diagnosis and treatment of hypertrophic cardiomyopathy: a report of the American College of Cardiology Foundation/American Heart Association Task Force on practice guidelines. Developed in collaboration with the American Association for Thoracic Surgery, American Society of Echocardiography, American Society of Nuclear Cardiology, Heart Failure Society of America, Heart Rhythm Society, Society for Cardiovascular Angiography and Interventions, and Society of Thoracic Surgeons, J. Am. Coll. Cardiol. 58 (2011) e212–e260.
[133] S. Pitta, D. Thatai, L. Afonso, Thromboembolic complications of left ventricular noncompaction: case report and brief review of the literature, J. Clin. Ultrasound 35 (2007) 465–468.

Chapter 21

Arrhythmogenic Right Ventricular Cardiomyopathy

Julia H. Indik, Frank I. Marcus
The University of Arizona, Tucson, AZ, United States

INTRODUCTION

Arrhythmogenic right ventricular cardiomyopathy (ARVC), first clinically described in a cohort of 24 patients in 1982 [1], is a disorder of myocyte cell-to-cell adhesion predominantly affecting the right ventricle (RV) with a prevalence that may be as high as 1 in 1000 people [2]. It is common in the Veneto region of Italy [3] and is a cause of sudden cardiac death in young athletes [4,5]. ARVC rarely manifests prior to puberty [6]. The diagnosis of ARVC requires meeting a combination of criteria based on abnormalities in the categories of (1) ventricular structure and function, (2) tissue characterization, (3) repolarization, (4) depolarization/conduction, (5) arrhythmias, and (6) family history, which is specified in the Task Force Criteria (TFC), revised in 2010 [7].

ARVC is a disease of desmosomal proteins (Fig. 21.1), leading to fibro-fatty infiltration of the myocardium extending from the epicardium to the endocardium. There are three classes of desmosomal proteins. The cadherins include desmoglein and desmocollin, which span the cell membrane to connect cells. The plakin family of proteins includes desmoplakin, which anchors desmosomes to the intermediate filaments. The third class is the armadillo proteins, which include plakoglobin and plakophilin that connect desmoplakin and the cadherins [8,9]. Mutations in five desmosomal proteins have been found in about 60% of patients [10–12], with an autosomal dominant pattern of inheritance. The most common mutation is plakophilin, which accounted for 46% of 439 index patients and 61% of 562 family members from the Johns Hopkins and Dutch registries [11]. Other desmosomal proteins that are affected include desmoplakin, desmocollin, desmoglein, and plakoglobin (Fig. 21.1). Two autosomal recessive forms of ARVC have been described due to mutations in plakoglobin, causing Naxos disease, and in desmoplakin, which causes Carvajal disease that predominantly affects the left ventricle (LV). These disorders also involve abnormalities in desmosomal proteins in the skin and hair. Nondesmosomal mutations involving transforming growth factor β3, the ryanodine receptor, titin, phospholamban, and transmembrane protein 43 have also been described in atypical forms of ARVC [12,13].

In the earliest stages of ARVC, there may be ventricular arrhythmias without overt structural changes, but an almost nonexistent risk of sudden cardiac death in children under the age of 10. Over time, structural changes occur resulting in ventricular wall motion abnormalities and focal aneurysms, with the earliest structural changes occurring in the subtricuspid area. An investigation of cardiac magnetic resonance (CMR) findings in 74 mutation positive ARVC patients showed structural abnormalities in 54 subjects involving the RV in 96%, most commonly affecting the basal inferior (subtricuspid) and basal anterior wall. The most frequent LV abnormality is subepicardial fatty infiltration of the posterolateral wall of the LV. Eventually, biventricular involvement can occur with clinical right heart failure requiring transplant.

For the child with or at risk of developing ARVC, the following key questions should be considered:

- What is the evidence for clinical disease?
- How should a pediatric family member of a proband diagnosed with ARVC be evaluated for their risk of developing the disorder?
- If at risk, how should the child be managed to prevent disease expression or progression of the disease?

WHAT IS THE EVIDENCE FOR CLINICAL DISEASE IN THE CHILD?

Sudden cardiac death in children has been difficult to quantify, with death in early infancy attributed primarily to sudden infant death syndrome [14]. A retrospective analysis of 116 cases of sudden cardiac death in Ontario, Canada, from 2005 to 2009 [14] revealed an incidence of 1.01 per 100,000 person years between the ages of 15 and 19 years. There was a lower

Heart Failure in the Child and Young Adult. http://dx.doi.org/10.1016/B978-0-12-802393-8.00021-1

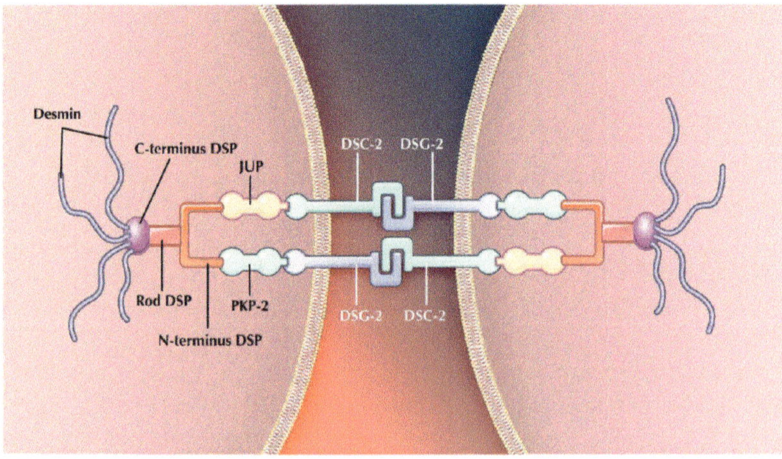

FIGURE 21.1 Desmosomal proteins responsible for cell-to-cell adhesion. There are three families of desmosomal proteins. The cadherins include desmoglein (DSG-2) and desmocollin (DSC-2), which span the cell membrane to connect cells. The plakin family of proteins includes desmoplakin (DSP), which anchors desmosomes to the intermediate filaments. The third class is the armadillo proteins that include plakoglobin (JUP) and plakophilin (PKP-2), which connect desmoplakin and the cadherins. *(From S. Sen-Chowdhry, P. Syrris, W.J. McKenna, Role of genetic analysis in the management of patients with arrhythmogenic right ventricular dysplasia/cardiomyopathy, J. Am. Coll. Cardiol. 50 (2007) 1813–1821, with permission.)*

incidence of sudden cardiac death in children between 10 and 14 years than in the older age-group. Autopsies in 113 of these cases revealed ARVC in 9, with 1 other case of ARVC known prior to death. This study suggests that while sudden cardiac death is rare in children, ARVC accounts for about 8% of cases.

In the Johns Hopkins and Dutch registries of 439 patients with ARVC [11], only 4 patients were under the age of 13 and none were younger than 10 years of age. The rarity of the clinical expression of ARVC in the very young is likely explained by the time needed for the intercalated disk to mature. During early childhood, further development and reorganization of the intercellular junctions in the intercalated disk occurs, with eventual localization to the end of cardiomyocytes [15,16].

The likelihood of clinical expression of ARVC in a child with a known disease causing mutation was analyzed in a cohort of 53 children, mean age 12.3 ± 3.9 years. Of these, 40 patients were classified as family members of a proband [17] with a mean follow-up of 9 ± 7 years. The cohort was further stratified according to age: ≤10 years (16 patients), 11–14 years, and >14–18 years. Of the 53 subjects, 21 met the 2010 TFC [7] for clinical disease, with the youngest subject being 11 years; the mean age at diagnosis was 15 ± 2 years. Another 4 subjects were regarded as borderline, and 28 as unaffected. Ventricular arrhythmias were present in all probands and in 27% of family members. Sustained ventricular tachycardia (VT) was seen in one patient in the 11–14 year group, and in four patients in the 14–18-year group. An additional 12 patients had non-sustained ventricular arrhythmias. One subject, who at age 13 had not met 2010 TFC, died suddenly at age 15 as the first clinical manifestation of the disease. In 21 subjects who had CMR, 9 subjects (43%) had RV abnormalities, and 4 (19%) had LV abnormalities, with gadolinium late enhancement seen in 12 subjects (57%). In the Johns Hopkins and Dutch cohorts, among 577 patients with genetic mutations, the incidence of sudden cardiac death/ventricular fibrillation at first presentation occurred in 36 subjects with a median age of 23 [12].

These studies highlight that while sudden cardiac death in children is rare, ARVC is an important cause of sudden cardiac death in the young. Clinical disease expression generally begins after the age of 10 but can develop with structural abnormalities by adolescence. Thus a strategy for evaluation and management of the child is needed.

HOW SHOULD THE PEDIATRIC FAMILY MEMBER OF A PROBAND DIAGNOSED WITH ARRHYTHMOGENIC RIGHT VENTRICULAR CARDIOMYOPATHY BE EVALUATED FOR THEIR RISK OF DEVELOPING THE DISORDER?

The initial evaluation of family members should be guided according to whether a disease-causing mutation has been identified in the proband. If the proband has been diagnosed with a desmosomal mutation, then cascade screening of the family including children should be performed, and further genetic evaluation, including the children should proceed in those family members of probands who carry the mutation, but not in those family members in whom the proband does not have a desmosomal mutation. In the Johns Hopkins and Dutch registries, the likelihood of diagnosing ARVC in a family member of a proband without a genetic mutation was far less [11]. The likelihood of sustained ventricular arrhythmias or sudden cardiac death occurring in the family member of a proband without a known genetic mutation was much reduced [11]. Nonetheless, family members of an index patient without a known genetic mutation should undergo clinical evaluation and surveillance.

The relationship between the type of genetic mutation and clinical course is an area of active study. In a cohort of 134 desmosomal gene mutation carriers between the ages of 22 and 52 years [18], 78 were considered definite or borderline for

ARVC by the 2010 TFC. There were 21 patients who had a complex genotype: 7 patients with compound heterozygosity (i.e., a single gene with more than one disease causing mutation) and 14 patients with digenic heterozygosity (i.e., two different genes with mutations). Disease penetrance was greater in these 21 patients with multiple mutations compared with the rest of the cohort, while there was no difference in penetrance according to specific mutation type. The presence of multiple mutations as well as male sex were independent predictors of sudden cardiac death or VT. Of the 21 patients with multiple mutations, 8 patients had either aborted sudden cardiac death or sustained VT. In another ARVC cohort, multiple variants in PKP-2 were seen in 38 of 198 probands, with 9 of these subjects showing compound heterozygosity, and 16 with digenic heterozygosity [19]. Among patients with compound or digenic heterozygosity, ventricular fibrillation and exercise-triggered VT was more common and the age of onset of symptoms (ventricular arrhythmias or syncope) was also earlier. Therefore, children who have inherited a complex genotype with compound or digenic heterozygosity may benefit from more frequent evaluation, but this needs further study.

Electrical abnormalities appear to manifest prior to structural abnormalities. In an investigation of 69 patients with ARVC with a known mutation (mean age of 27 ± 15.3 years) but without a history of a sustained ventricular arrhythmia [20], ECG or Holter abnormalities obtained at or closest to initial presentation were seen in 42 patients (61%), while structural abnormalities by CMR were seen in only 20 of those 42 patients. Of the 27 patients without electrical abnormalities at their initial evaluation, only 1 had structural abnormalities by CMR. Over a follow-up of 5.8 ± 4.4 years, 11 patients (16%) had a sustained ventricular arrhythmic event, and all of these patients had both a prior history of electrical abnormalities and an abnormal CMR. Electrical abnormalities were also more prevalent than structural abnormalities in a cohort of 103 ARVC mutation positive patients with both heterozygous and recessive forms, wherein using the 2010 TFC, ECG abnormalities were seen in 96%, and structural abnormalities using echocardiography in 76% [21]. A mouse desmoplakin mutation model [22] also supports a sequence of events in which electrical abnormalities precede structural abnormalities. Therefore, evaluation of the child should focus on a close surveillance for expression of electrical abnormalities.

Nonetheless, children can have structural abnormalities, which were detected in 9 of 21 subjects imaged by CMR in the pediatric cohort studied by Bauce and colleagues [17]. A cohort of 142 pediatric patients (mean age 13.8 ± 3.2 years) evaluated for ARVC using CMR was analyzed by Etoom and colleagues [23]. Using the 2010 TFC, 23 (16%) patients met criteria for definite ARVC and another 32 (23%) were classified as borderline. Regional wall motion abnormalities were present in 83% of the 23 patients with definite disease and 53% of the 32 patients with borderline disease. These authors also noted that 11 of the 23 patients with definite disease would not have been classified as definite without the CMR findings. One limitation of that study was the lack of a second imaging modality such as echocardiography to confirm the imaging findings [24]. Additionally, the 2010 TFC were developed based on the findings of the North American Multidisciplinary Study of Right Ventricular Dysplasia [6], which was a predominantly adult population, with only 9 of 108 probands between the ages of 12 and 18, which may limit the applicability to a pediatric population [24,25].

For the child over the age of 10 who has the genetic mutation of the proband or is a family member of a proband without a known genetic mutation, it is reasonable to perform annual ECGs and Holter monitoring after the age of 8, with CMR to be performed if any abnormalities are detected by ECG or Holter. Exercise testing can also be considered. This evaluation should be performed annually until age 25, and if negative then every 3 years until about age 40–50, and then at every 5 years beyond this age.

IF AT RISK, HOW SHOULD THE CHILD BE MANAGED TO PREVENT DISEASE EXPRESSION OR PROGRESSION?

The goals of management should be to prevent or slow the progression of clinical disease, including risk stratification for sudden cardiac death.

An implantable cardioverter defibrillator (ICD) has an important role for the prevention of sudden cardiac death as shown in the large cohort of adult index patients from the Johns Hopkins and Dutch registries [11]. Over a median follow-up of about 7 years, sudden cardiac death occurred in 16% of patients without an ICD compared to 0.6% in those with an ICD. Family members who met TFC for ARVC also benefited from an ICD, with sudden cardiac death only in family members who did not have an ICD. The mean age at first evaluation among index patients was 36 ± 14 years. In a cohort of 84 patients with ICD implanted for primary prevention from the Johns Hopkins registry [26], the risk factors that were predictive for appropriate ICD therapy over a mean follow-up of 4.7 ± 3.4 years included proband status, inducibility of VT during electrophysiologic study, nonsustained VT, and greater than 1000 PVCs in a 24-h period.

However, studies of the benefit of an ICD for primary prevention of sudden cardiac death in a pediatric population are lacking. Nonetheless, sudden cardiac death does occur in individuals under the age of 18. In the pediatric cohort of 53 patients reported by Bauce and colleagues [17], sudden cardiac death occurred in a 15-year-old. Among a cohort of

116 children with sudden cardiac death in Ontario [14], 14 patients died suddenly with definite or possible ARVC, with 5 of these deaths occurring during moderate or vigorous physical activity. Protection against sudden cardiac death is thus an important consideration in the child, as longevity is otherwise nearly normal in ARVC.

Nonetheless, the decision to implant an ICD in the child must take into account the risk of long-term complications in this age-group. The defibrillator lead may become excessively short relative to body size or even dislodge as the child grows. There is also the risk of inappropriate shocks, for sinus, or supraventricular tachycardia, which can be psychologically harmful. The decision to implant an ICD in an adolescent must consider the risk of sudden cardiac death risk in the individual patient, with the highest risk in patients who have already had sustained ventricular tachyarrhythmia or patients exhibiting frequent ventricular ectopy and nonsustained ventricular tachyarrhythmias.

Medications may be able to prevent the progression of disease. Beta-blockers have a well-proven benefit to prevent sudden cardiac death and improve survival in heart failure patients. It is reasonable to expect that beta-blockers will have a similar beneficial effect in ARVC patients particularly since deaths due to ventricular arrhythmias are more likely to occur during exercise [4,13,14]. Isoproterenol has also been shown to trigger ventricular arrhythmias, lending further support to the probable benefit of beta-blockade. Angiotensin converting enzyme inhibitors may also be of benefit since this medication improves survival in heart failure [13].

Of utmost importance in the management of the child with ARVC or who is at risk of developing the clinical disease is to limit exercise. Several studies have established a relation between exercise and disease expression and progression. It is thought that impaired cell-to-cell adhesion increases RV wall stretch when subjected to the stress of increased cardiac output during exercise. It is hypothesized that abnormal RV wall stretch leads to irreversible myocardial damage, including inflammation, and subsequent fibro-fatty replacement, predisposing to ventricular arrhythmias. In a heterozygous plakoglobin-deficient mouse model, endurance swimming worsened the ARVC phenotype, with larger RV size, lower ejection fraction, and more ventricular arrhythmias compared to wild type mice [27]. Unloading the RV with furosemide and nitrates improved conduction velocity and prevented the inducibility of VT with programmed stimulation in plakoglobin-deficient mice subjected to endurance exercise [28].

The relation between exercise and expression of disease has also been demonstrated in patient cohorts. In a study of 87 subjects with desmosomal mutations [29], endurance exercise was associated with the likelihood of meeting TFC for the diagnosis of ARVC, and developing VT, ventricular fibrillation, or heart failure. Endurance athletes also developed symptoms at an earlier age.

In a cohort of 65 ARVC patients and 45 family members with mutations from Norway and Sweden [30], athletes had worse right and left ventricular function as measured by echo and CMR. A definite ARVC diagnosis by TFC was more likely to be made in athletes compared to nonathletes. Exercise induced ventricular arrhythmias were also more common among athletes. Furthermore, there was a correlation between the amount and intensity of exercise and degree of ventricular dysfunction.

Speculation exists whether exercise alone may create an RV cardiomyopathy, even in the absence of a disease causing mutation. In a cohort of 46 high-level endurance athletes with ventricular arrhythmias [31], 80% had ventricular arrhythmias with a left bundle morphology and 18 athletes had a major arrhythmic event. Sudden cardiac death occurred in nine cyclists, at a median age of 23 years. Of the cohort, 27 met definite criteria for ARVC using the 1994 TFC. In a study of 82 ARVC patients both with and without mutations [32], patients with ARVC who did not have a known mutation and did not have a familial history of ARVC were more likely to have participated in high-intensity exercise, compared to patients with known mutations or familial disease. This suggests that high-intensity exercise adds to the expression of the disease distinct from a disease causing mutation. Among patients younger than 25 years of age, athletic activity was five times more intense among ARVC patients without a known mutation compared to patients with a known mutation. It remains unclear whether ARVC can result solely from high-intensity exercise [32], or if there are as yet still unknown genetic factors, such as genes that encode adherens junction proteins, which contribute to the expression of the disease in these patients [32].

There is evidence to suggest that a safe level of exercise exists. In the North American Multidisciplinary Study, competitive sports was associated with a doubling of the risk of ventricular tachyarrhythmias and death, while risk was similar in patients who engaged in recreational sports or were inactive [33]. A recent study from the Johns Hopkins registry found that family members with desmosomal mutations had a low incidence of meeting TFC if they limited exercise to less than 750 Met-minutes/week [34], which is the minimum amount of exercise recommended for the general public by the American Heart Association to maintain health [35].

The current exercise guidelines in both the United States and Europe are fairly restrictive for patients with ARVC. The 36th Bethesda Conference guidelines recommend that patients with definite or probable ARVC be restricted from participating in competitive sports with the exception of class I-A (low intensity) sports [36]. Examples of low intensity sports are bowling and golf [37]. Whether these restrictions may be further defined in the future to permit limited amounts of moderate intensity sports is unknown. A highly restrictive exercise prescription may be difficult to enforce in adolescents. However, it is important to address exercise habits with patients regularly during follow-up visits.

FUTURE DIRECTIONS

The majority of investigations of patients with ARVC has focused on a predominantly adult population. Studies that specifically evaluate adolescent patients are needed. The implantation of an ICD, which is commonly performed in the adult for primary prevention of sudden cardiac death, can be problematic in the child due to periods of rapid growth. Therefore risk stratification in the adolescent and methods to reduce that risk are needed to obviate the need for ICD implantation. Areas that need further study in children include whether exercise restriction coupled with medical therapy such as beta-blockers may be protective against sudden cardiac death.

CONCLUSION

ARVC is a disorder of cell-to-cell adhesion, with the majority of patients having mutations in desmosomes. Clinical disease can present in adolescent years, and begins with electrical abnormalities on the ECG or Holter, and later with structural abnormalities involving wall motion and focal aneurysms predominantly affecting the RV, particularly the subtricuspid area. Pediatric family members of probands diagnosed with ARVC should be evaluated, beginning with genetic assessment if the proband has an identified disease causing desmosomal mutation. Pediatric family members that have the mutation or family members of a proband without a disease causing mutation should be followed closely. This should include annual assessments for electrical abnormalities, and if present, further imaging evaluation. Treatment for children diagnosed with ARVC needs to be individualized and may require placement of an ICD. It is of utmost importance to restrict exercise in children at risk of developing the disease or who already manifest abnormalities.

REFERENCES

[1] F.I. Marcus, G.H. Fontaine, G. Guiraudon, et al., Right ventricular dysplasia: a report of 24 adult cases, Circulation 65 (1982) 384–398.

[2] S. Peters, M. Trummel, W. Meyners, Prevalence of right ventricular dysplasia-cardiomyopathy in a non-referral hospital, Int. J. Cardiol. 97 (2004) 499–501.

[3] A. Nava, G. Thiene, B. Canciani, et al., Familial occurrence of right ventricular dysplasia: a study involving nine families, J. Am. Coll. Cardiol. 12 (1988) 1222–1228.

[4] G. Thiene, A. Nava, D. Corrado, L. Rossi, N. Pennelli, Right ventricular cardiomyopathy and sudden death in young people, N. Engl. J. Med. 318 (1988) 129–133.

[5] C. Basso, D. Corrado, G. Thiene, Cardiovascular causes of sudden death in young individuals including athletes, Cardiol. Rev. 7 (1999) 127–135.

[6] F.I. Marcus, W. Zareba, H. Calkins, et al., Arrhythmogenic right ventricular cardiomyopathy/dysplasia clinical presentation and diagnostic evaluation: results from the North American Multidisciplinary Study, Heart Rhythm 6 (2009) 984–992.

[7] F.I. Marcus, W.J. McKenna, D. Sherrill, et al., Diagnosis of arrhythmogenic right ventricular cardiomyopathy/dysplasia: proposed modification of the task force criteria, Circulation 121 (2010) 1533–1541.

[8] A.C. Sawant, H. Calkins, Relationship between arrhythmogenic right ventricular dysplasia and exercise, Card. Electrophysiol. Clin. 7 (2015) 195–206.

[9] S. Sen-Chowdhry, P. Syrris, W.J. McKenna, Role of genetic analysis in the management of patients with arrhythmogenic right ventricular dysplasia/cardiomyopathy, J. Am. Coll. Cardiol. 50 (2007) 1813–1821.

[10] A.D. den Haan, B.Y. Tan, M.N. Zikusoka, et al., Comprehensive desmosome mutation analysis in north americans with arrhythmogenic right ventricular dysplasia/cardiomyopathy, Circ. Cardiovasc. Genet. 2 (2009) 428–435.

[11] J.A. Groeneweg, A. Bhonsale, C.A. James, et al., Clinical presentation, long-term follow-up, and outcomes of 1001 arrhythmogenic right ventricular dysplasia/cardiomyopathy patients and family members, Circ. Cardiovasc. Genet. 8 (2015) 437–446.

[12] A. Bhonsale, J.A. Groeneweg, C.A. James, et al., Impact of genotype on clinical course in arrhythmogenic right ventricular dysplasia/cardiomyopathy-associated mutation carriers, Eur. Heart J. 36 (2015) 847–855.

[13] H. Calkins, Arrhythmogenic right ventricular dysplasia/cardiomyopathy-three decades of progress, Circ. J. 79 (2015) 901–913.

[14] C.M. Pilmer, J.A. Kirsh, D. Hildebrandt, A.D. Krahn, R.M. Gow, Sudden cardiac death in children and adolescents between 1 and 19 years of age, Heart Rhythm 11 (2014) 239–245.

[15] Q. Wang, J.L. Lin, S.Y. Chan, J.J. Lin, The Xin repeat-containing protein, mXinbeta, initiates the maturation of the intercalated discs during postnatal heart development, Dev. Biol. 374 (2013) 264–280.

[16] A. Vreeker, L. van Stuijvenberg, T.J. Hund, P.J. Mohler, P.G. Nikkels, T.A. van Veen, Assembly of the cardiac intercalated disk during pre- and postnatal development of the human heart, PLoS One 9 (2014) e94722.

[17] B. Bauce, A. Rampazzo, C. Basso, et al., Clinical phenotype and diagnosis of arrhythmogenic right ventricular cardiomyopathy in pediatric patients carrying desmosomal gene mutations, Heart Rhythm 8 (2011) 1686–1695.

[18] I. Rigato, B. Bauce, A. Rampazzo, et al., Compound and digenic heterozygosity predicts lifetime arrhythmic outcome and sudden cardiac death in desmosomal gene-related arrhythmogenic right ventricular cardiomyopathy, Circ. Cardiovasc. Genet. 6 (2013) 533–542.
[19] T. Xu, Z. Yang, M. Vatta, et al., Compound and digenic heterozygosity contributes to arrhythmogenic right ventricular cardiomyopathy, J. Am. Coll. Cardiol. 55 (2010) 587–597.
[20] A.S. te Riele, A. Bhonsale, C.A. James, et al., Incremental value of cardiac magnetic resonance imaging in arrhythmic risk stratification of arrhythmogenic right ventricular dysplasia/cardiomyopathy-associated desmosomal mutation carriers, J. Am. Coll. Cardiol. 62 (2013) 1761–1769.
[21] N. Protonotarios, A. Anastasakis, L. Antoniades, et al., Arrhythmogenic right ventricular cardiomyopathy/dysplasia on the basis of the revised diagnostic criteria in affected families with desmosomal mutations, Eur. Heart J. 32 (2011) 1097–1104.
[22] J. Gomes, M. Finlay, A.K. Ahmed, et al., Electrophysiological abnormalities precede overt structural changes in arrhythmogenic right ventricular cardiomyopathy due to mutations in desmoplakin-A combined murine and human study, Eur. Heart J. 33 (2012) 1942–1953.
[23] Y. Etoom, S. Govindapillai, R. Hamilton, et al., Importance of CMR within the task force criteria for the diagnosis of ARVC in children and adolescents, J. Am. Coll. Cardiol. 65 (2015) 987–995.
[24] A.S. te Riele, F.I. Marcus, C.A. James, et al., The value of cardiac magnetic resonance imaging in evaluation of pediatric patients for arrhythmogenic right ventricular dysplasia/cardiomyopathy, J. Am. Coll. Cardiol. 66 (2015) 873–874.
[25] T. Geva, Imaging criteria for arrhythmogenic right ventricular cardiomyopathy: an incomplete journey, J. Am. Coll. Cardiol. 65 (2015) 996–998.
[26] A. Bhonsale, C.A. James, C. Tichnell, et al., Incidence and predictors of implantable cardioverter-defibrillator therapy in patients with arrhythmogenic right ventricular dysplasia/cardiomyopathy undergoing implantable cardioverter-defibrillator implantation for primary prevention, J. Am. Coll. Cardiol. 58 (2011) 1485–1496.
[27] P. Kirchhof, L. Fabritz, M. Zwiener, et al., Age- and training-dependent development of arrhythmogenic right ventricular cardiomyopathy in heterozygous plakoglobin-deficient mice, Circulation 114 (2006) 1799–1806.
[28] L. Fabritz, M.G. Hoogendijk, B.P. Scicluna, et al., Load-reducing therapy prevents development of arrhythmogenic right ventricular cardiomyopathy in plakoglobin-deficient mice, J. Am. Coll. Cardiol. 57 (2011) 740–750.
[29] C.A. James, A. Bhonsale, C. Tichnell, et al., Exercise increases age-related penetrance and arrhythmic risk in arrhythmogenic right ventricular dysplasia/cardiomyopathy-associated desmosomal mutation carriers, J. Am. Coll. Cardiol. 62 (2013) 1290–1297.
[30] J. Saberniak, N.E. Hasselberg, R. Borgquist, et al., Vigorous physical activity impairs myocardial function in patients with arrhythmogenic right ventricular cardiomyopathy and in mutation positive family members, Eur. J. Heart Fail. 16 (2014) 1337–1344.
[31] H. Heidbuchel, J. Hoogsteen, R. Fagard, et al., High prevalence of right ventricular involvement in endurance athletes with ventricular arrhythmias. Role of an electrophysiologic study in risk stratification, Eur. Heart J. 24 (2003) 1473–1480.
[32] A.C. Sawant, A. Bhonsale, A.S. te Riele, et al., Exercise has a disproportionate role in the pathogenesis of arrhythmogenic right ventricular dysplasia/cardiomyopathy in patients without desmosomal mutations, J. Am. Heart Assoc. 3 (2014) e001471.
[33] A.C. Ruwald, F. Marcus, N.A. Estes 3rd, et al., Association of competitive and recreational sport participation with cardiac events in patients with arrhythmogenic right ventricular cardiomyopathy: results from the North American multidisciplinary study of arrhythmogenic right ventricular cardiomyopathy, Eur. Heart J. 36 (2015) 1735–1743.
[34] A. Sawant, C. James, A. te Riele, et al., Participation in AHA-recommended minimum weekly exercise is safe for family members with arrhythmogenic right ventricular dysplasia/cardiomyopathy associated desmosomal mutations, Heart Rhythm 12 (2015) S132.
[35] W.L. Haskell, I.M. Lee, R.R. Pate, et al., Physical activity and public health: updated recommendation for adults from the American College of Sports Medicine and the American Heart Association, Circulation 116 (2007) 1081–1093.
[36] B.J. Maron, M.J. Ackerman, R.A. Nishimura, R.E. Pyeritz, J.A. Towbin, J.E. Udelson, Task force 4: HCM and other cardiomyopathies, mitral valve prolapse, myocarditis, and Marfan syndrome, J. Am. Coll. Cardiol. 45 (2005) 1340–1345.
[37] B.J. Maron, B.R. Chaitman, M.J. Ackerman, et al., Recommendations for physical activity and recreational sports participation for young patients with genetic cardiovascular diseases, Circulation 109 (2004) 2807–2816.

Chapter 22

Valvular Insufficiency and Heart Failure

Matthew C. Schwartz[1], Andrew C. Glatz[2], Matthew J. Gillespie[2]
[1]*Arnold Palmer Hospital for Children, Orlando, FL, United States;* [2]*Children's Hospital of Philadelphia, Philadelphia, PA, United States*

INTRODUCTION

Valvular insufficiency is an important cause of heart failure (HF) in children, most commonly occurring in the setting of congenital heart disease [1]. Significant insufficiency less commonly results from acquired causes including endocarditis and rheumatic heart disease or from inherited connective tissue disorders. In general, valvular insufficiency puts a significant volume load on the affected ventricle, which can lead to ventricular deterioration and HF. This chapter focuses on the causes, pathophysiology, evaluation, and treatment of HF associated with valvular insufficiency in children.

AORTIC REGURGITATION AND HEART FAILURE

Etiology

In children, aortic regurgitation (AR) is most typically associated with various types of congenital heart disease. AR can occur following balloon valvuloplasty for congenital aortic stenosis. AR can also develop in those with bicuspid aortic valve with no history of intervention. Patients with aortic valve leaflet prolapse due to an accompanying ventricular septal defect often exhibit AR. Various causes of aortic root dilation can also lead to AR due to annular enlargement including inherited connective tissue disorders such as Marfan syndrome or Ehlers–Danlos syndrome. Aortic root dilation and AR can also result after arterial switch and Ross operations. Acquired etiologies of AR in children are less common and include infectious endocarditis and rheumatic heart disease [2,3].

Pathophysiology

HF can occur in the setting of both acute and chronic severe AR. Chronic AR leads to progressive left ventricular dilation with compensatory ventricular hypertrophy. Eventually, the dilation exceeds the degree of hypertrophy leading to elevated end-systolic wall stress and afterload. These changes cause a decrease in the systolic function of the left ventricle. If severe dilation progresses, intrinsic myocyte function is affected and irreversible injury can occur [2]. HF can ensue because pump function is diminished and because a significant amount of the ventricle's stroke volume leaks back into the ventricle.

The acute development of AR is rare in children but can lead to pronounced HF. In acute AR, the ventricle has not had time to gradually enlarge and, thus, the regurgitant volume causes an abrupt increase in left ventricular end-diastolic pressure. This increase is transmitted to the left atrium and pulmonary veins causing pulmonary edema. Also, the left ventricle is unable to acutely increase stroke volume in the setting of additional regurgitant blood, which causes a decrease in net effective forward blood flow and, thus, a decrease in cardiac output [4].

Presentation and Evaluation

HF symptoms due to severe AR will be due to left-sided cardiac failure and associated pulmonary edema. Infants may develop tachypnea, respiratory insufficiency, and growth failure, while older children and adolescents can develop these symptoms as well as exercise intolerance. In those with severe AR, physical exam will include an early, medium to high frequency diastolic decrescendo murmur at the left sternal border. Because left ventricular stroke volume may be increased in the setting of a dilated ventricle, a systolic ejection murmur may also be present due to increased flow across the aortic valve. An Austin Flint murmur may also be present, a low frequency middiastolic rumble heard near the apex due to limitation in the opening of the mitral valve's anterior leaflet from the AR jet. Pulse pressure will also be widened due to diastolic leakage of blood across the valve, and pulses may be bounding or "water hammer." Patients who have significant HF due to AR may also exhibit tachycardia, tachypnea, and hypoxemia from pulmonary vein desaturation associated with pulmonary edema [2].

Heart Failure in the Child and Young Adult. http://dx.doi.org/10.1016/B978-0-12-802393-8.00022-3

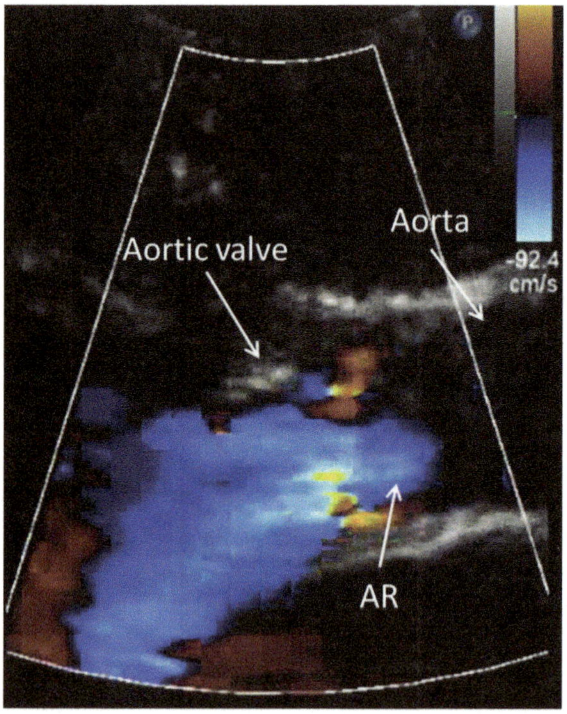

FIGURE 22.1 Transthoracic echocardiogram in the parasternal long-axis view showing severe aortic regurgitation (AR) in a 1-year-old with severe aortic stenosis who underwent balloon valvuloplasty in the neonatal period.

Echocardiography is the cornerstone for evaluating AR in children (Fig. 22.1). The anatomy of the aortic valve, the degree of AR, and the ventricular size and function can all be evaluated [5]. Echocardiographic markers of severe AR include holodiastolic flow reversal in the descending aorta, left ventricular dilation, and/or AI jet width >65% of left ventricular outflow tract diameter [2,6,7]. Magnetic resonance imaging (MRI) can also be helpful in characterizing AR by quantifying ventricular size and function as well as calculating the aortic valve regurgitant fraction [2]. Brain natriuretic peptide (BNP) and N-terminal proBNP levels can reflect the degree of neurohormonal activity in adults with HF, but these findings may not be generalizable to children [5]. Additionally, cardiac catheterization may be used as an adjunct in patient with severe AR and typically will show increased left ventricular end-diastolic pressure. As left ventricular filling pressures rise, left atrial pressure will increase and resultant increase in pulmonary vascular resistance may ensue.

Treatment

Medical

The left ventricle is severely volume overloaded in those patients with severe AR and HF, and diuretics and afterload reduction offer theoretical benefit. In patients who require intensive care unit admission, milrinone can be used to achieve afterload reduction, and intravenous diuretics can improve pulmonary congestion. Intubation with mechanical ventilation can also decrease left ventricular afterload and limit oxygen consumption.

For outpatients with HF, diuretics can improve symptoms of pulmonary congestion, but do not prevent ongoing left ventricular dilation. If hypertension is present, it should be aggressively treated with a vasodilator such as an angiotensin-converting enzyme (ACE) inhibitor [6]. Although afterload reduction with ACE inhibitors offers theoretical benefit, it has not been clearly shown to slow the deterioration of the left ventricle in children [2]. Gisler et al. retrospectively described the course of 18 patients with isolated moderate–severe AR treated with ACE inhibitors. At a median follow-up of 2.3 years, there was no improvement in left ventricular size or shortening fraction or in the degree of AR. Adult studies also have shown variable results and suggest that vasodilator therapy cannot effectively delay need for aortic valve surgery. Evangelista et al. randomized 95 adults with asymptomatic severe AR to vasodilator therapy or placebo. The rate of aortic valve replacement was similar between groups, and there were no differences among groups in regurgitant volume, left ventricular size, or ejection fraction [8].

Invasive

Given the lack of efficacy of medical therapy, aortic valve surgery is the definitive intervention for patients with HF associated with AR. Aortic valve surgery is recommended in symptomatic patients with severe AR and in asymptomatic patients with severe AR and left ventricular ejection fraction <50% or progressive left ventricular dilation [6]. In particular, progressive increase in the left ventricular end-systolic dimension can be an important indication for intervention as children with larger end-systolic dimensions prior to surgery may be less likely to experience recovery in left ventricular size after the operation [9]. Aortic valve surgical options include valve repair or valve replacement. Replacement options include homograft, pulmonary autograft (Ross operation), bioprosthetic valve, or mechanical valve. Choosing the best strategy is dictated by patient age, need for valve growth, risks of anticoagulation, and patient/surgeon preference. Valve repair typically involves pericardial leaflet extension and/or commissuroplasty. This option avoids anticoagulation, but it has limited longevity [10].

The Ross operation includes translocation of the pulmonary valve to the aortic position and offers good durability without the need for anticoagulation. However, the procedure can be technically demanding, and there is modest rate of autograft reintervention and right ventricular outflow tract intervention [11]. Several large series have been recently published describing long-term results of the Ross operation [12,13]. Nelson et al. described 240 patients undergoing Ross operation. Overall survival to discharge was 96%, although infants had significant mortality of 18%. Fifteen-year survival was 87% for the entire cohort and lowest for infants at 72%. At 15 years, overall freedom from left ventricular outflow tract reintervention was 59% and 85% in infants. Overall freedom from right ventricular outflow tract reintervention was 53% at 15 years, but only 19% in infants [13]. In small infants who cannot accommodate a mechanical valve and children and young adolescents wanting to avoid anticoagulation, the Ross operation is a viable option.

Mechanical aortic valve replacement offers excellent longevity and durability, but anticoagulation with warfarin is required. Also, mechanical valve implantation is not an option for infants given aortic valve annular size and annular enlargement can be required in older children to facilitate placement [11]. Shanmugam et al. described 55 children who underwent aortic valve replacement with a mechanical valve. Freedom from reintervention rate was 96% at 5 years and 92% at 20 years with only 1 anticoagulation-related hemorrhage [14].

Bioprosthetic valve replacement does not require ongoing anticoagulation, but durability and longevity are limited, particularly in young children [11,15]. Similarly, replacement with homograft avoids the need for anticoagulation, but durability is very limited as are the number of possible donor grafts [11,15]. Transcatheter aortic valve replacement has become a viable option for adults who are deemed high risk for aortic valve surgery [16]. This technology shows promise, but requires extensive further study prior to its use in younger patients.

Following aortic valve surgery, left ventricular size improves in most children by 6 months. Patients with persistent left ventricular dilation after surgery tend to have larger end-systolic dimension and lower ejection fraction prior to surgery [9]. In patients with severe HF associated with AR, mechanical support using extracorporeal membrane oxygenation (ECMO) or ventricular assist device (VAD) is not typically a viable option as the AR undermines the perfusion strategy. In those with severe AR who fail operative management, cardiac transplantation is also an option.

MITRAL REGURGITATION AND HEART FAILURE

Etiology

Similar to AR, mitral regurgitation (MR) is most commonly associated with congenital heart disease, specifically congenital valve abnormalities such as mitral arcade, parachute mitral valve, or mitral prolapse. MR can also occur in setting of endocardial inflammation from endocarditis, myocarditis, rheumatic fever, or collagen vascular disease. An infiltrative pathology from metabolic disease such as Hurler disease can also lead to insufficiency. In addition, ischemia from any cause can result in papillary muscle infarction and cause valvular leakage. Finally, annular dilation that can occur in connective tissue diseases as well as in the setting of dilated cardiomyopathy can lead to incomplete leaflet coaptation. In children, MR can also follow congenital heart surgery such as repair for congenital mitral stenosis. Patients who undergo complete atrioventricular canal repair also can develop left atrioventricular valve regurgitation after repair.

Pathophysiology

The cardiac pathophysiology of MR is outlined in Fig. 22.2. Patients with severe MR have decreased cardiac output as the regurgitation "steals" blood that should be directed across the aortic valve. In acute insufficiency, left atrial pressure is increased with compromised antegrade flow into the aorta resulting in pulmonary edema and low cardiac output. In chronic MR, the regurgitation leads to increased left atrial and ventricular blood volume and dilation of the left atrium and ventricle. To reduce wall stress associated with the dilation, the ventricle will initially hypertrophy. Similar to chronic AR, progressive dilation will eventually result in irreversible ventricular injury and systolic dysfunction [17].

Presentation and Evaluation

Similar to AR, severe MR can lead to left-sided cardiac failure with respiratory insufficiency and growth failure in infants and exertional issues in older children and adolescents. In severe cases, respiratory failure can occur requiring mechanical

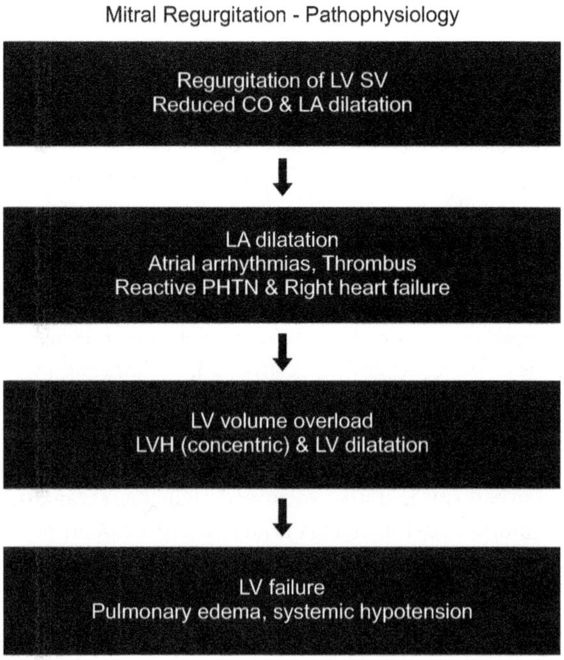

FIGURE 22.2 Flow diagram illustrating the pathophysiology of mitral regurgitation. *CO*, cardiac output; *LA*, left atrial; *LV*, left ventricle; *LVH*, left ventricular hypertrophy; *PHTN*, pulmonary hypertension; *SV*, stroke volume. *(Adapted from Moore, et al., Critical care of patients with paediatric valvar cardiac disease, Cardiol. Young 24 (2014) 1071–1076.)*

ventilation. Physical exam typically includes a holosystolic, blowing murmur best heard at the apex. If left ventricular dilation is present, the apical impulse can be displaced laterally. Patients with severe MR may have a diastolic rumble due to increased flow across the mitral valve. Patients with severe disease may also be tachycardic and tachypneic.

Echocardiography is the most important modality in evaluating a patient with significant MR. Important anatomic detail can be gleaned from the echocardiogram including annular size and leaflet/subvalvar anatomy and function. Markers of severe MR in children include regurgitant jet encompassing >50% of left atrium, left atrial dilation, and left ventricular dilation [6,18,19]. Cardiac MRI can also be used to quantify the mitral valve regurgitant fraction and the left ventricular volume. Cardiac catheterization may also be helpful in the evaluation of patients with severe MR. If the left ventricle is significantly volume overloaded, left ventricular end-diastolic and left atrial pressures will be elevated. Significant elevations in left atrial pressure can cause pulmonary vascular resistance and pulmonary artery pressures to increase also.

Treatment

Medical

In patients with significant HF associated with MR who require intensive care unit admission, left ventricular afterload reduction and improved contractility can be useful. In theory, these measures could encourage forward flow across the aortic valve and decrease regurgitation. Milrinone is a common inotrope as it improves ventricular contractility and vasodilates to decrease afterload. Likewise, mechanical ventilation can lower afterload and decrease oxygen consumption and diuretics are useful to improve pulmonary congestion. In more stable patients, oral afterload reduction with ACE inhibitors can be used as can diuretics. Although some benefit can be seen, medical therapy has limited effectiveness in preventing progressive ventricular dilation and delaying surgery in patients with significant MR [20,21]. Knirsch et al. retrospectively compared 12 children with severe MR who were receiving ACE inhibitors with 12 who were not; left ventricular end-diastolic diameter, shortening fraction, and degree of MR were essentially unchanged between the two groups after 1 year [20].

Invasive

The definitive therapy for patients with HF associated with MR is surgery. In children with severe MR, mitral valve surgery is indicated in the presence of symptoms or in asymptomatic patients with decreased left ventricular systolic function [6]. Surgical options include valve repair or replacement. Repair techniques for congenital mitral valve abnormalities have been reported with success, but repair can be challenging particularly in small infants [22,23]. When repair is not an option or unsuccessful, valve replacement with a mechanical valve is typically preferable given superior durability. With the use of mechanical valve, anticoagulation is required, and reoperation will be necessary in the setting of eventual valve failure or need to upsize the valve to account for somatic growth. Valve replacement can also be challenging in infants and young children due to the small size of the mitral valve annulus, and placement in the supra-annular position may be needed. Brown et al. described mitral valve replacement in nearly 100 pediatric patients with median age of 8 years. Operative mortality was 6%, and freedom from reoperation at 35 years was 63%. Factors associated with increased risk of operative death were age <2 years, presence of an atrioventricular canal defect, univentricular heart, and additional left-sided obstructive lesions [24]. Tierney et al. described mitral valve replacement in 118 children ≤5 years. The valve was placed in the supra-annular position in 32%, and survival was 74% at 1 year. Risk factors for worse survival included age <1 year, presence of an atrioventricular canal defect, and additional procedure coincident with valve replacement [25].

Given the challenges associated with both repair and replacement in young children, use of stented bovine jugular venous valve (Melody valve, Medtronic, Minneapolis, Minnesota) has been employed in this population. Quinonez et al. described 11 patients with median age of 7 months who underwent surgical placement of the Melody valve in the mitral position. This valve can be serially dilated percutaneously as the child grows, a significant potential advantage of this technique [26].

The use of a pulmonary autograft (Ross II technique) in the mitral position has been described in a limited number of patients. This technique can be attractive in women who are interested in having children and in those who have failed previous mechanical valve placement due to thrombotic complications [27]. In patients with severe HF associated with MR who fail surgical intervention, cardiac transplantation can be considered, and mechanical support using ECMO or a VAD could be considered as a bridge to transplantation.

PULMONARY REGURGITATION AND HEART FAILURE

Etiology

In children and adolescents, isolated congenital pulmonary regurgitation (PR) is rare and PR most often results following surgical repair of conotruncal congenital heart lesions. Most commonly, patients with tetralogy of Fallot (TOF) develop chronic PR after transannular patch augmentation of the right ventricular outflow tract during TOF repair. Even patients who undergo a valve-sparing operation may develop significant PR [28]. Other lesions such as TOF with pulmonary atresia, TOF with associated coronary anomaly, or truncus arteriosus may require placement of a right ventricle to pulmonary artery conduit, which typically develops regurgitation. Patients undergoing Ross operation for aortic stenosis and/or regurgitation will also receive a conduit. Additionally, patients who undergo transcatheter pulmonary valvuloplasty can develop PR [29]. Acquired causes of PR such as endocarditis are uncommon.

Pathophysiology

The degree of PR is determined by the regurgitant orifice area, right ventricular compliance, the capacitance of the pulmonary arteries, and duration of diastole. Unlike AR, the diastolic pressure difference between the main pulmonary artery and right ventricle is typically small and, thus, is not a major determinant of the degree of PR. In the case of repaired TOF, the regurgitant orifice is often large immediately after surgery. However, the impact of PR is typically small because the right ventricle is hypertrophied and noncompliant, and the heart rate is fast with shortened diastole. Over time, right ventricular compliance improves. The stroke volume of the ventricle also increases due to ongoing PR and ventricular dilation. Likewise, the heart rate slows with age, increasing length of diastole. These factors encourage a gradual increase in the degree of PR [30].

Significant PR will lead to progressive right ventricular dilation, with similar pathophysiology of left ventricular enlargement due to AR. Initially, as the ventricle dilates, compensatory hypertrophy will occur to maintain a normal mass–volume relationship. However, eventually compensatory hypertrophy will be unable to keep pace with dilation; irreversible myocardial injury can occur with resultant decreased systolic function. Fig. 22.3 depicts the pathophysiology of chronic PR after TOF repair. Also, because the right and left ventricles share myofibers, the interventricular septum, and the pericardial space, right ventricular dilation can negatively influence left ventricular systolic and diastolic function [30,31].

Presentation and Evaluation

Children with chronic, severe PR are initially asymptomatic, often for 10–15 years. With progressive RV dilation and eventual systolic dysfunction, symptoms eventually occur and include exercise intolerance and arrhythmias. Negative ventricular–ventricular interaction can occur and cause left ventricular dysfunction and symptoms of left-sided HF including pulmonary edema [30]. Physical exam will show a soft diastolic, decrescendo murmur at left upper sternal border. There may also be a systolic ejection murmur at the same location due to increased right ventricular stroke volume and flow across the pulmonary valve. If right ventricular dilation is present, parasternal lift may be present.

FIGURE 22.3 Diagram illustrating the pathophysiology of pulmonary regurgitation after tetralogy of Fallot (TOF) repair. *PA*, pulmonary artery; *RV*, right ventricle. *(Adapted from Geva, et al., Repaired tetralogy of Fallot: the roles of cardiovascular magnetic resonance in evaluating pathophysiology and for pulmonary valve replacement decision support. J. Cardiovasc. Magn. Reson. (2011) 13.)*

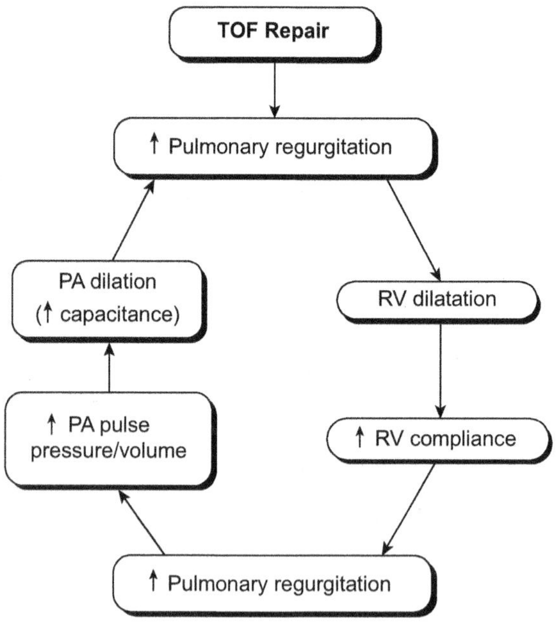

Echocardiography is used to characterize pulmonary valve structure and function and describe the degree of PR. In those with severe PR, the regurgitant color jet fills the right ventricular outflow tract, there is reversal of flow in the branch pulmonary arteries, and there is septal flattening during diastole [6]. However, cardiac MRI is often used to characterize the degree of PR and quantify biventricular size and systolic function. Moderate PR is considered a regurgitant fraction >25% [30]. In fact, MRI results can be very useful in risk stratification of those with repaired TOF and can provide values that are important in clinical decision-making [30,32]. Patients with indexed right ventricular end-diastolic volume >150–170 cc/m^2 may not experience normalization of right ventricular size after valve restoration [33–35].

Serum BNP can also be a useful adjunct to imaging in those with chronic PR. In those with PR related to TOF repair, BNP has been associated with NYHA functional class, right ventricular size, and severity of PR [32].

Treatment

Medical

There are limited data regarding medical therapy for patients with chronic PR and its associated deleterious effects on the right ventricle. The APPROPRIATE study randomized patients with repaired TOF and moderate–severe PR to Ramipril versus placebo. Most patients were asymptomatic, and there was no improvement in right ventricular ejection fraction or right ventricular end-diastolic volume at 6 months [36]. Norozi et al. randomized young adults with repaired TOF and NYHA Class one to two symptoms to bisoprolol versus placebo for 6 months and found no benefit on right ventricular ejection fraction or volume [37]. In patients with significant right-sided HF associated with lower extremity edema and/or ascites, diuretic therapy may offer some short-term symptomatic relief.

Invasive

For patients with HF associated with severe PR, restoration of pulmonary valve competency is the standard of care. This can be accomplished with surgical and transcatheter techniques. Both surgical and transcatheter pulmonary valve replacement have been shown to decrease the degree of PR and right ventricular size and significantly improve HF-associated symptoms [30,38]. While right ventricular size improves including both end-diastolic and end-systolic volumes, right ventricular ejection fraction typically does not change after valve restoration [30].

There are numerous series describing the safety and efficacy of surgical pulmonary valve replacement using bioprosthetic valves, valved conduits, and homografts [11,39]. The procedure is safe with a low rate of major complication and/or early reintervention [39]. Alternatively, some patients are candidates for transcatheter pulmonary valve replacement. The Melody valve (Medtronic Inc., Minneapolis, Minnesota) is available for transcatheter pulmonary valve replacement under a Humanitarian Device Exemption in patients with a right ventricular outflow tract conduit (Fig. 22.4). Thus, patients who have undergone surgical right ventricular outflow tract palliation with homograft conduit, valved conduit, or even bioprosthetic

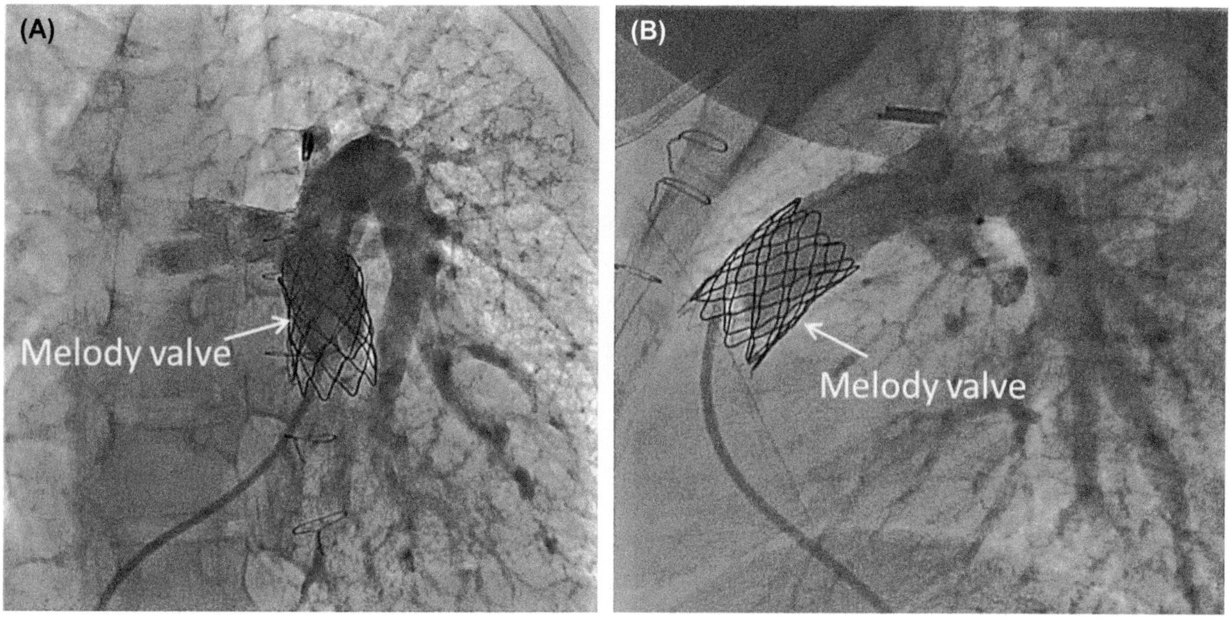

FIGURE 22.4 Anteroposterior (A) and lateral (B) views of angiogram performed in distal right ventricle to pulmonary artery conduit in a 30-year-old female with repaired tetralogy of Fallot and pulmonary atresia after placement of a Melody valve in the conduit to treat severe pulmonary regurgitation. In both projections, there is no regurgitation of contrast into the right ventricle after Melody placement. Will get angio after Melody.

valve can be good candidates for percutaneous Melody valve implantation [38,40]. Patients with a native outflow tract that has not significantly dilated can also be candidates for off-label Melody valve use after outflow tract stenting [41,42]. The Sapien transcatheter valve (Edwards Lifesciences LLC, Irvine, California) has also been used in the pulmonary position and can be used in larger conduits or outflow tracts than the Melody valve, but it is only currently available in the United States as part of an investigational device exemption trial. Similar to surgical pulmonary valve replacement, Melody and Sapien valve implantation is associated with low rate of major complications and good short- and midterm success [43,44].

TRICUSPID REGURGITATION AND HEART FAILURE

Etiology

The most common cause of significant tricuspid regurgitation (TR) in children is Ebstein's anomaly of the tricuspid valve. In this condition, the septal and posterior leaflets fail to delaminate during development and are adherent to the right ventricular myocardium, resulting in apical displacement of the functional tricuspid valve annulus. The anterior leaflet is redundant and "sail-like." Significant TR can result due to abnormal leaflet coaptation [45]. Fig. 22.5 depicts a patient with significant Ebstein's anomaly. Other patients may be born with a dysplastic tricuspid valve that does not meet criteria for Ebstein's anomaly and may also have TR. Acquired causes such as endocarditis are rare.

Pathophysiology

Neonates with severe Ebstein's anomaly may be cyanotic due to right to left shunting at the atrial level with inadequate antegrade pulmonary blood flow due to severe TR. In other patients, ongoing severe TR will lead to right atrial and ventricular dilation. As with severe PR, eventually right ventricular systolic function can become compromised. The combination of TR and right ventricular dysfunction can limit cardiac output, especially with exercise and can lead to symptoms of right HF. Also, as the right ventricle dilates, so does the tricuspid valve annulus, leading to further TR. Right to left shunting may exist at the atrial level causing cyanosis with exertion.

Presentation and Evaluation

Infants with severe Ebstein's anomaly are symptomatic immediately. These patients may have inadequate pulmonary blood flow due to severe TR and elevated pulmonary vascular resistance and even may have "functional" pulmonary atresia requiring prostaglandin infusion. Management of these patients is complex, and a full description is beyond the scope of this chapter

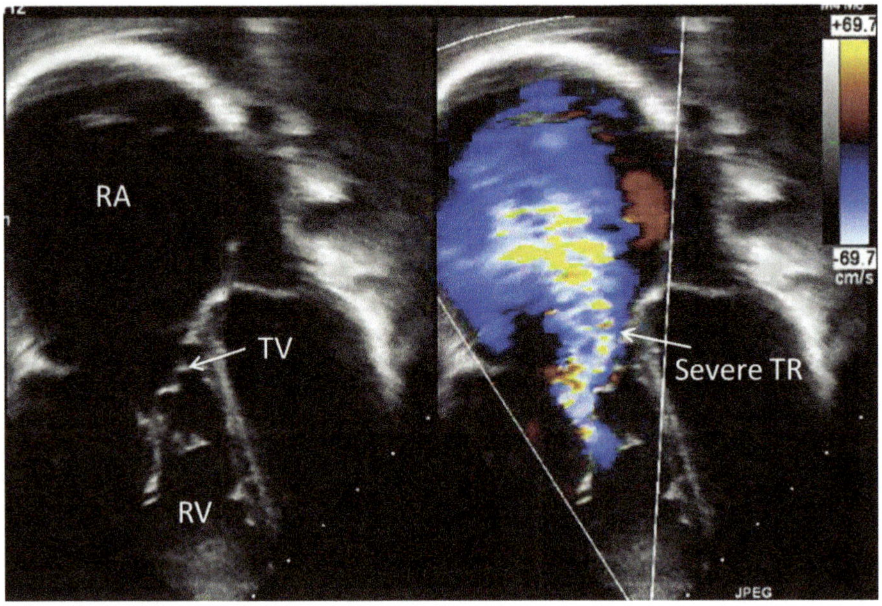

FIGURE 22.5 Transthoracic echocardiogram in the apical view showing severe tricuspid regurgitation in a 3-year-old with Ebstein's anomaly of the tricuspid valve. *RA*, right atrium; *RV*, right ventricle; *TR*, tricuspid regurgitation; *TV*, tricuspid valve.

[46]. Older children and adolescents may develop symptoms from ongoing TR and resultant right atrial and ventricular dilation. These patients will exhibit symptoms of right-sided HF with exercise intolerance, lower extremity edema, and/or ascites. Also, given the chamber dilation and possible presence of preexcitation, arrhythmias often occur and lead to symptoms.

Physical exam often reveals a low frequency holosystolic murmur at the left lower sternal border. Because right ventricular volume is increased, a systolic ejection murmur may be present at the left sternal border due to increased flow across the pulmonary valve. The second heart sound may be normal or widely split if there is significantly increased flow across pulmonary valve.

In terms of evaluation, echocardiogram is the gold standard for characterizing tricuspid valve anatomy and function as well as describing the degree of TR. In those with Ebstein's anomaly or dysplastic tricuspid valve, cardiac MRI is rarely needed [45].

Treatment

Medical

Patients who have significant HF associated with TR can have some symptomatic benefit from diuretics, especially if edema and ascites are present. ACE inhibitors have not been significantly investigated in those with HF associated with TR.

Invasive

Surgery is indicated in those who have symptoms associated with severe TR, in those with significant cyanosis due to atrial level shunting, or in those with significant burden of atrial arrhythmias [6,45]. The nature of the surgery depends on age and size of the patient as well as tricuspid valve anatomy. Typically, tricuspid valve repair is attempted prior to valve replacement with a bioprosthetic valve. For those with Ebstein's anomaly, tricuspid valve annuloplasty, plication of the atrialized portion of the right ventricle and right atrial reduction are often performed, although additional repair options exist including cone reconstruction [47–50]. Hetzer et al. described outcomes after tricuspid valve repair in 67 patients with Ebstein's anomaly. The mean NYHA class improved from 3.4 to 1.3 ($P<.001$), and freedom from reoperation was 98% at 5 years [48]. Dearani et al. reported the Mayo Clinic's experience with cone reconstruction in 89 patients. The series described 1 death and, at last follow-up, 87% had no or mild TR [50]. Also, patients who have only mild-moderate TR, but have significant cyanosis at rest or with exercise, can receive benefit from transcatheter closure of interatrial communication [51].

CONCLUSION

Valvular insufficiency can be an important cause of HF in young children and adolescents. In these patients, insufficiency most often results from congenital valve anomalies, but postoperative regurgitation can also occur following congenital cardiac surgery. Medical therapy is typically ineffective, and surgical or transcatheter valve replacement techniques are typically the treatment of choice for pediatric patients with symptoms of HF associated with any regurgitant valve lesion.

REFERENCES

[1] D.T. Hsu, G.D. Pearson, Heart failure in children: part I: history, etiology, and pathophysiology, Circ. Heart Fail. 2 (1) (January 2009) 63–70 PubMed PMID: 19808316.

[2] J.T. Tretter, A. Langsner, Timing of aortic valve intervention in pediatric chronic aortic insufficiency, Pediatr. Cardiol. 35 (8) (December 2014) 1321–1326 PubMed PMID: 25179463.

[3] H.I. Michelena, S.K. Prakash, A. Della Corte, M.M. Bissell, N. Anavekar, P. Mathieu, et al., Bicuspid aortic valve: identifying knowledge gaps and rising to the challenge from the international bicuspid aortic valve consortium (BAVCon), Circulation 129 (25) (June 24, 2014) 2691–2704 PubMed PMID: 24958752. Pubmed Central PMCID: 4145814.

[4] K.K. Stout, E.D. Verrier, Acute valvular regurgitation, Circulation 119 (25) (June 30, 2009) 3232–3241 PubMed PMID: 19564568.

[5] D.T. Hsu, G.D. Pearson, Heart failure in children: part II: diagnosis, treatment, and future directions, Circ. Heart Fail. 2 (5) (September 2009) 490–498 PubMed PMID: 19808380.

[6] R.O. Bonow, B.A. Carabello, K. Chatterjee, A.C. de Leon Jr., D.P. Faxon, M.D. Freed, et al., 2008 focused update incorporated into the ACC/AHA 2006 guidelines for the management of patients with valvular heart disease: a report of the American College of Cardiology/American Heart Association Task Force on Practice Guidelines (writing committee to revise the 1998 guidelines for the management of patients with valvular heart disease). Endorsed by the Society of cardiovascular Anesthesiologists, Society for cardiovascular Angiography and interventions, and Society of Thoracic surgeons, J. Am. Coll. Cardiol. 52 (13) (September 23, 2008) e1–142 PubMed PMID: 18848134.

[7] L.Y. Tani, L.L. Minich, R.W. Day, G.S. Orsmond, R.E. Shaddy, Doppler evaluation of aortic regurgitation in children, Am. J. Cardiol. 80 (7) (October 1, 1997) 927–931 PubMed PMID: 9382010.

[8] A. Evangelista, P. Tornos, A. Sambola, G. Permanyer-Miralda, J. Soler-Soler, Long-term vasodilator therapy in patients with severe aortic regurgitation, N. Engl. J. Med. 353 (13) (September 29, 2005) 1342–1349 PubMed PMID: 16192479.

[9] D.A. Cox, K. Walton, P.J. Bartz, J.S. Tweddell, P.C. Frommelt, M.G. Earing, Predicting left ventricular recovery after replacement of a regurgitant aortic valve in pediatric and young adult patients: is it ever too late? Pediatr. Cardiol. 34 (3) (March 2013) 694–699 PubMed PMID: 23052669.

[10] T.J. Wilder, C.A. Caldarone, G.S. Van Arsdell, E. Pham-Hung, M. Gritti, M. Al Jughiman, et al., Aortic valve repair for insufficiency in older children offers unpredictable durability that may not be advantageous over a primary Ross operationdagger, Eur. J. Cardiothor. Surg. (June 9, 2015) PubMed PMID: 26059873.

[11] R. Henaine, F. Roubertie, M. Vergnat, J. Ninet, Valve replacement in children: a challenge for a whole life, Arch. Cardiovasc. Dis. 105 (10) (October 2012) 517–528 PubMed PMID: 23062483.

[12] N. Bansal, S.R. Kumar, C.J. Baker, R. Lemus, W.J. Wells, V.A. Starnes, Age-related outcomes of the Ross procedure over 20 years, Ann. Thorac. Surg. 99 (6) (June 2015) 2077–2083 discussion 84–85. PubMed PMID: 25921257.

[13] J.S. Nelson, S.K. Pasquali, C.N. Pratt, S. Yu, J.E. Donohue, E. Loccoh, et al., Long-term survival and reintervention after the Ross procedure across the pediatric age spectrum, Ann. Thorac. Surg. 99 (6) (June 2015) 2086–2094 discussion 94–95. PubMed PMID: 25921260.

[14] G. Shanmugam, K. MacArthur, J. Pollock, Mechanical aortic valve replacement: long-term outcomes in children, J. Heart Valve Dis. 14 (2) (March 2005) 166–171 PubMed PMID: 15792175.

[15] T. Karamlou, K. Jang, W.G. Williams, C.A. Caldarone, G. Van Arsdell, J.G. Coles, et al., Outcomes and associated risk factors for aortic valve replacement in 160 children: a competing-risks analysis, Circulation 112 (22) (November 29, 2005) 3462–3469 PubMed PMID: 16316968.

[16] D.H. Adams, J.J. Popma, M.J. Reardon, Transcatheter aortic-valve replacement with a self-expanding prosthesis, N. Engl. J. Med. 371 (10) (September 4, 2014) 967–968 PubMed PMID: 25184874.

[17] R.A. Moore, S. Flores, D.S. Cooper, Critical care of patients with paediatric valvar cardiac disease, Cardiol. Young 24 (6) (December 2014) 1071–1076 PubMed PMID: 25647381.

[18] H.R. Lee, L.M. Montenegro, S.C. Nicolson, J.W. Gaynor, T.L. Spray, J. Rychik, Usefulness of intraoperative transesophageal echocardiography in predicting the degree of mitral regurgitation secondary to atrioventricular defect in children, Am. J. Cardiol. 83 (5) (March 1, 1999) 750–753 PubMed PMID: 10080431.

[19] Y.T. Wu, A.C. Chang, A.J. Chin, Semiquantitative assessment of mitral regurgitation by Doppler color flow imaging in patients aged <20 years, Am. J. Cardiol. 71 (8) (March 15, 1993) 727–732 PubMed PMID: 8447273.

[20] W. Knirsch, L. Tlach, D. Stambach, U. Bauersfeld, Angiotensin-converting enzyme inhibitors in pediatric patients with mitral valve regurgitation-case-control study and review of the literature, Congenit. Heart Dis. 5 (3) (May–June 2010) 278–284 PubMed PMID: 20576047.

[21] Y. Mori, M. Nakazawa, H. Tomimatsu, K. Momma, Long-term effect of angiotensin-converting enzyme inhibitor in volume overloaded heart during growth: a controlled pilot study, J. Am. Coll. Cardiol. 36 (1) (July 2000) 270–275 PubMed PMID: 10898445.

[22] G. Stellin, M.A. Padalino, V.L. Vida, G. Boccuzzo, E. Orru, R. Biffanti, et al., Surgical repair of congenital mitral valve malformations in infancy and childhood: a single-center 36-year experience, J. Thorac. Cardiovasc. Surg. 140 (6) (December 2010) 1238–1244 PubMed PMID: 20554294.

[23] D. Kalfa, M. Vergnat, M. Ly, B. Stos, V. Lambert, A. Baruteau, et al., A standardized repair-oriented strategy for mitral insufficiency in infants and children: midterm functional outcomes and predictors of adverse events, J. Thorac. Cardiovasc. Surg. 148 (4) (October 2014) 1459–1466 PubMed PMID: 24667029.

[24] J.W. Brown, A.C. Fiore, M. Ruzmetov, O. Eltayeb, M.D. Rodefeld, M.W. Turrentine, Evolution of mitral valve replacement in children: a 40-year experience, Ann. Thorac. Surg. 93 (2) (February 2012) 626–633 discussion 33. PubMed PMID: 22153051.

[25] E.S. Selamet Tierney, F.A. Pigula, C.I. Berul, J.E. Lock, P.J. del Nido, D.B. McElhinney, Mitral valve replacement in infants and children 5 years of age or younger: evolution in practice and outcome over three decades with a focus on supra-annular prosthesis implantation, J. Thorac. Cardiovasc. Surg. 136 (4) (October 2008) 954–961 61 e1-3. PubMed PMID: 18954636. Pubmed Central PMCID: 4230576.

[26] L.G. Quinonez, R. Breitbart, W. Tworetsky, J.E. Lock, A.C. Marshall, S.M. Emani, Stented bovine jugular vein graft (melody valve) for surgical mitral valve replacement in infants and children, J. Thorac. Cardiovasc. Surg. 148 (4) (October 2014) 1443–1449 PubMed PMID: 24332108.

[27] J.W. Brown, M. Ruzmetov, M.D. Rodefeld, M.W. Turrentine, Mitral valve replacement with Ross II technique: initial experience, Ann. Thorac. Surg. 81 (2) (February 2006) 502–507 discussion 7-8. PubMed PMID: 16427839.

[28] V.L. Vida, A. Guariento, B. Castaldi, M. Sambugaro, M.A. Padalino, O. Milanesi, et al., Evolving strategies for preserving the pulmonary valve during early repair of tetralogy of Fallot: mid-term results, J. Thorac. Cardiovasc. Surg. 147 (2) (February 2014) 687–694 discussion 94-6. PubMed PMID: 24314789.

[29] D.M. Harrild, A.J. Powell, T.X. Tran, T. Geva, J.E. Lock, J. Rhodes, et al., Long-term pulmonary regurgitation following balloon valvuloplasty for pulmonary stenosis risk factors and relationship to exercise capacity and ventricular volume and function, J. Am. Coll. Cardiol. 55 (10) (March 9, 2010) 1041–1047 PubMed PMID: 20202522. Pubmed Central PMCID: 4235281.

[30] T. Geva, Repaired tetralogy of Fallot: the roles of cardiovascular magnetic resonance in evaluating pathophysiology and for pulmonary valve replacement decision support, J. Cardiovasc. Magn. Reson. 13 (2011) 9 PubMed PMID: 21251297. Pubmed Central PMCID: 3036629.

[31] M.C. Schwartz, J.J. Rome, M.J. Gillespie, K. Whitehead, M.A. Harris, M.A. Fogel, et al., Relation of left ventricular end diastolic pressure to right ventricular end diastolic volume after operative treatment of tetralogy of fallot, Am. J. Cardiol. 109 (3) (February 1, 2012) 417–422 PubMed PMID: 22078963.

[32] J. Villafane, J.A. Feinstein, K.J. Jenkins, R.N. Vincent, E.P. Walsh, A.M. Dubin, et al., Hot topics in tetralogy of Fallot, J. Am. Coll. Cardiol. 62 (23) (December 10, 2013) 2155–2166 PubMed PMID: 24076489.

[33] E.R. Buechel, H.H. Dave, C.J. Kellenberger, A. Dodge-Khatami, R. Pretre, F. Berger, et al., Remodelling of the right ventricle after early pulmonary valve replacement in children with repaired tetralogy of Fallot: assessment by cardiovascular magnetic resonance, Eur. Heart J. 26 (24) (December 2005) 2721–2727 PubMed PMID: 16214832.

[34] T. Oosterhof, A. van Straten, H.W. Vliegen, F.J. Meijboom, A.P. van Dijk, A.M. Spijkerboer, et al., Preoperative thresholds for pulmonary valve replacement in patients with corrected tetralogy of Fallot using cardiovascular magnetic resonance, Circulation 116 (5) (July 31, 2007) 545–551 PubMed PMID: 17620511.

[35] J. Therrien, Y. Provost, N. Merchant, W. Williams, J. Colman, G. Webb, Optimal timing for pulmonary valve replacement in adults after tetralogy of Fallot repair, Am. J. Cardiol. 95 (6) (March 15, 2005) 779–782 PubMed PMID: 15757612.

[36] S.V. Babu-Narayan, A. Uebing, P.A. Davlouros, M. Kemp, S. Davidson, K. Dimopoulos, et al., Randomised trial of ramipril in repaired tetralogy of Fallot and pulmonary regurgitation: the APPROPRIATE study (Ace inhibitors for Potential PRevention of the deleterious effects of Pulmonary Regurgitation in Adults with repaired TEtralogy of Fallot, Int. J. Cardiol. 154 (3) (February 9, 2012) 299–305 PubMed PMID: 20970202.

[37] K. Norozi, J. Bahlmann, B. Raab, V. Alpers, J.O. Arnhold, T. Kuehne, et al., A prospective, randomized, double-blind, placebo controlled trial of beta-blockade in patients who have undergone surgical correction of tetralogy of Fallot, Cardiol. Young 17 (4) (August 2007) 372–379 PubMed PMID: 17572925.

[38] M.L. O'Byrne, M.J. Gillespie, Will catheter interventions replace surgery for valve abnormalities? Curr. Opin. Cardiol. 29 (1) (January 2014) 83–90 PubMed PMID: 24281347. Pubmed Central PMCID: 4341839.

[39] E.D. McKenzie, M.S. Khan, T.W. Dietzman, F.A. Guzman-Pruneda, A.X. Samayoa, A. Liou, et al., Surgical pulmonary valve replacement: a benchmark for outcomes comparisons, J. Thorac. Cardiovasc. Surg. 148 (4) (October 2014) 1450–1453 PubMed PMID: 24703628.

[40] M.J. Gillespie, J.J. Rome, D.S. Levi, R.J. Williams, J.F. Rhodes, J.P. Cheatham, et al., Melody valve implant within failed bioprosthetic valves in the pulmonary position: a multicenter experience, Circ. Cardiovasc. Interv. 5 (6) (December 2012) 862–870 PubMed PMID: 23212395.

[41] D.E. Boshoff, B.L. Cools, R. Heying, E. Troost, J. Kefer, W. Budts, et al., Off-label use of percutaneous pulmonary valved stents in the right ventricular outflow tract: time to rewrite the label? Catheter. Cardiovasc. Interv. 81 (6) (May 2013) 987–995 PubMed PMID: 22887796.

[42] J.J. Meadows, P.M. Moore, D.P. Berman, J.P. Cheatham, S.L. Cheatham, D. Porras, et al., Use and performance of the melody transcatheter pulmonary valve in native and postsurgical, nonconduit right ventricular outflow tracts, Circ. Cardiovasc. Interv. 7 (3) (June 2014) 374–380 PubMed PMID: 24867892.

[43] J.P. Cheatham, W.E. Hellenbrand, E.M. Zahn, T.K. Jones, D.P. Berman, J.A. Vincent, et al., Clinical and hemodynamic outcomes up to 7 years after transcatheter pulmonary valve replacement in the US melody valve investigational device exemption trial, Circulation 131 (22) (June 2, 2015) 1960–1970 PubMed PMID: 25944758.

[44] D. Kenny, Z.M. Hijazi, S. Kar, J. Rhodes, M. Mullen, R. Makkar, et al., Percutaneous implantation of the Edwards SAPIEN transcatheter heart valve for conduit failure in the pulmonary position: early phase 1 results from an international multicenter clinical trial, J. Am. Coll. Cardiol. 58 (21) (November 15, 2011) 2248–2256 PubMed PMID: 22078433.

[45] C.H. Attenhofer Jost, H.M. Connolly, J.A. Dearani, W.D. Edwards, G.K. Danielson, Ebstein's anomaly, Circulation 115 (2) (January 16, 2007) 277–285 PubMed PMID: 17228014.

[46] U.S. Boston, S.P. Goldberg, K.E. Ward, E.D. Overholt, T. Spentzas, T.K. Chin, et al., Complete repair of Ebstein anomaly in neonates and young infants: a 16-year follow-up, J. Thorac. Cardiovasc. Surg. 141 (5) (May 2011) 1163–1169 PubMed PMID: 21353250.

[47] J.P. da Silva, J.F. Baumgratz, L. da Fonseca, S.M. Franchi, L.M. Lopes, G.M. Tavares, et al., The cone reconstruction of the tricuspid valve in Ebstein's anomaly. The operation: early and midterm results, J. Thorac. Cardiovasc. Surg. 133 (1) (January 2007) 215–223 PubMed PMID: 17198815.

[48] R. Hetzer, P. Hacke, M. Javier, O. Miera, K. Schmitt, Y. Weng, et al., The long-term impact of various techniques for tricuspid repair in Ebstein's anomaly, J. Thorac. Cardiovasc. Surg. (August 14, 2015) PubMed PMID: 26349593.

[49] H.N. Anderson, J.A. Dearani, S.M. Said, M.D. Norris, K.N. Pundi, A.R. Miller, et al., Cone reconstruction in children with Ebstein anomaly: the Mayo Clinic experience, Congenit. Heart Dis. 9 (3) (May–June 2014) 266–271 PubMed PMID: 24373319.

[50] J.A. Dearani, S.M. Said, P.W. O'Leary, H.M. Burkhart, R.D. Barnes, F. Cetta, Anatomic repair of Ebstein's malformation: lessons learned with cone reconstruction, Ann. Thorac. Surg. 95 (1) (January 2013) 220–226 discussion 6-8. PubMed PMID: 23200240.

[51] S.R. Jategaonkar, W. Scholtz, D. Horstkotte, D. Kececioglu, N.A. Haas, Interventional closure of atrial septal defects in adult patients with Ebstein's anomaly, Congenit. Heart Dis. 6 (4) (July–August 2011) 374–381 PubMed PMID: 21435187.

Chapter 23

Valvular Stenosis and Heart Failure

Emily Jean-St.-Michel, Anne I. Dipchand
The Hospital for Sick Children and the University of Toronto, Toronto, ON, Canada

INTRODUCTION

Valvular stenosis can present with congestive heart failure in children and should not be forgotten during the initial assessment. The physiology underlying the heart failure symptoms will differ depending on the specific anatomical lesion. On one hand, there are the pressure overload lesions that lead to systolic and diastolic dysfunction. The most common pressure-overload lesions are aortic and pulmonary stenosis [1,2]. On the other hand, there are lesions that are associated with restriction to ventricular filling such as mitral and tricuspid stenosis. In this chapter, we will discuss these four lesions and describe their prevalence, physiology, symptomatology, and management as etiologies of heart failure in children.

PATHOPHYSIOLOGY OF CHRONIC PRESSURE OVERLOAD

In the setting of abnormal pressure load on the ventricle, myocyte hypertrophy represents the initial response and occurs as a mechanism to reduce wall stress [3]. Animal models of aortic ascending constriction have studied the pressure overload physiology looking at the mechanisms responsible for the transition from myocardial hypertrophy to heart failure [4]. Adverse remodeling can lead to diastolic dysfunction but also pump failure [3]. Accumulation of extracellular matrix [5], increased myocyte apoptosis [6], and altered calcium handling [7,8] have been associated with the development of heart failure in the aortic constriction animal model. The factors that regulate these changes remain unclear, but there is evidence that the mineralocorticoid receptors and the renin angiotensin system are involved in the process [9,10].

Initial stages of disease can be asymptomatic and there is no strong correlation between degree of stenosis and onset of symptoms [11] making the choice for timing of intervention more difficult. Throughout this chapter, we will be referring to the AHA guidelines for valvular disease for management protocols understanding that these guidelines are adult clinical guidelines [12].

AORTIC STENOSIS

Prevalence and Spectrum of Disease

Aortic stenosis is the most common etiology of heart failure secondary to valvular stenosis [2]. The exact prevalence of aortic stenosis is difficult to estimate accurately since mild cases might never be diagnosed; but it is estimated to account for 5% of all congenital heart lesions [13,14]. Congenital aortic stenosis represents a spectrum of diseases from severe aortic stenosis in fetal life that leads to hypoplastic left-heart syndrome [15] to bicuspid aortic valve associated with no significant gradient in older children [16]. Infants with severe stenosis represent most of the pediatric patients presenting with congestive heart failure secondary to aortic stenosis. Anatomically, the stenotic aortic valve can by unicuspid, bicuspid, tricuspid, or multicuspid. The stenosis can also be found at different levels of the outflow tract in the same patient such as subvalvar, valvar, and supravalvar.

Fetal Aortic Stenosis

Presentation

Aortic stenosis is usually well tolerated in utero. Because of the fetal physiology, the right ventricle can handle the entire cardiac output even in the context of aortic atresia [17]. The exception is in the context of a restrictive atrial septum [18] or with subendocardial ischemia and associated myocardial dysfunction, leading to hydrops fetalis [2]. More commonly,

Heart Failure in the Child and Young Adult. http://dx.doi.org/10.1016/B978-0-12-802393-8.00023-5

severe fetal aortic stenosis leads to myocardial hypertrophy, increased ventricular filling pressure, and eventually decreased flow on the left side giving rise to hypoplasia of the left-sided cardiac structure such as coarctation of the aorta, hypoplasia of the transverse aortic arch, mitral stenosis, hypoplastic left ventricle [15].

Diagnosis/Imaging

Improvement in fetal imaging has lead to earlier in utero diagnosis of severe aortic stenosis.

Management

Balloon valvulotomy can now be attempted in utero to stop or slow down this process and maintain adequacy of the left ventricle [19,20] but does not seems to eliminate the need for future postnatal interventions. The current selection criteria for fetal intervention are severe aortic stenosis with a normal or dilated left ventricle and retrograde flow in the transverse aortic arch [15].

Neonatal Aortic Stenosis

Physiology/Mechanisms

As mentioned above, aortic stenosis leads to increased left ventricular pressure and myocyte hypertrophy. This may lead to underdevelopment of the left-sided cardiac structures but can also lead to abnormal coronary perfusion and endomyocardial fibroelastosis (EFE) with or without papillary muscle ischemia [21]. EFE is defined as a thickened endocardium that developed secondary to the accumulation of collagenous and elastic fibers within the layer and can affect both systolic and diastolic ventricular function [22].

Presentation

Symptoms of heart failure or low cardiac output may develop rapidly once the neonate is separated from the placental circulation. The presence of the ductus arteriosus is, in some cases, necessary for sufficient systemic perfusion (ductal-dependent aortic stenosis or critical aortic stenosis) and its closure can lead to circulatory collapse. Undiagnosed infants present within hours or days after birth with decreased perfusion, poor pulses, increased work of breathing, tachypnea, a gallop, and hepatomegaly. A systolic murmur is not always present in those cases. Certain infants might not be immediately symptomatic postductal closure but can rapidly develop signs of ventricular dysfunction or congestive heart failure clinically and on imaging.

Diagnosis/Imaging

Echocardiography is the gold standard to confirm the diagnosis of aortic stenosis and delineate the reminder of the anatomy. Evaluation of the morphologic appearance of the aortic valve and annular size (z-score) is important. Doppler evaluation with associated peak, mean, and peak-to-peak gradients are important for decision-making. These, however can be underestimated in the setting of severe ventricular systolic dysfunction and with the presence of a large ductus arteriosus, thus the 2014 AHA/ACC guidelines [12] recommend intervention without a specific gradient cutoff in the situation of ventricular dysfunction and/or ductal dependency. Evaluation of associated aortic insufficiency and abnormality of the pulmonary valve might also influence the therapeutic options available. The pressure loading on the ventricle, which results in myocyte death and abnormal coronary flow, leads to fibrosis and EFE, contributing to both ventricular systolic and diastolic dysfunction [21,22]. However, the diastolic dysfunction can be seen in isolation and seems to be more common in patients with aortic stenosis present early in gestation and with associated EFE. Ultimately, assessment of ventricular function is of utmost important since it can affect the mortality and morbidity risk associated with the chosen intervention and potentially may even influence the procedure choice in borderline cases.

The other major challenge with these patients is evaluation of the adequacy of the left-heart structures; are the left ventricle and the left ventricular structures sufficient in size to support the systemic circulation? Aortic valve size of 5 mm and mitral size of 9 mm has been described as potential cutoff [23]. Rhodes et al. [24,25] developed an equation to predict success of biventricular repair, and similarly the Congenital Heart Surgeon Society [26] developed a regression equation to predict 5-year-survival postrepair in patients with severe aortic stenosis. In addition, Hammon et al. described the minimal left ventricular volume measured by cardiac catheterization necessary for survival (20 mL/m^2) [27]. This was reproduced using cardiac MRI showing the same cutoff for left ventricular size but also adding 1.0 $mL/min/m^2$ as a minimal measured ascending aorta blood flow [28]. Borderline patients in whom a biventricular path is embarked on can continue to exhibit heart failure symptoms if the left-heart structures (inflow, ventricle, or outflow) do not adapt despite relief of the pressure overload.

Management/Intervention/Outcomes

Ultimately, when the left ventricle is deemed adequate in the context of isolated aortic stenosis in the neonate, balloon valvuloplasty is the first line therapy in most institution. Some advocate for primary surgical valvuloplasty [29,30], but studies have demonstrated similar outcome with the less invasive technique [31,32]. Valve replacement with either bioprosthetic or mechanical valve is not favored in this age group due to size of the patient, the need for multiple future replacements, and the need for anticoagulation in the context of a mechanical valve. Daniel Ross first described using the patient's own pulmonary valve to replace the aortic valve [33]. The "Ross procedure" is the preferred surgical technique for aortic valve replacement in infants, though more technically challenging because of patient size, demonstrating favorable valve life span without the need for anticoagulation. However, the Ross procedure is associated with a higher early (21.7%) and late mortality (27.6%) in this age group compare to older age groups (Fig. 23.1) [34]. In a multivariate analysis, age less than 1 year, prior balloon dilatation of the aortic valve, and an indication for intervention of aortic stenosis were all risk factors for mortality [34,35]. Age less than 1 year was also a risk factor for reintervention both on the left and right-sided outflow tract post-Ross procedure. Overall, all of those procedural choices are palliative interventions since the vast majority of patients will require a reintervention at some point in their lifetime.

With regard to heart failure in these patients, the successful elimination of the obstruction in a candidate for a biventricular circulation will usually allow for recovery of ventricular function. Patients have to be supported in the period surrounding their intervention but usually will not require any long-term heart failure management. The exception will be patients with significant EFE and associated diastolic and systolic dysfunction who might require heart failure management.

Aortic Valve Disease in Older Children

Presentation

Usually, aortic valve stenosis is well tolerated in older children and most cases are asymptomatic. However, in a small portion of patient the stenosis will progress to severe stenosis and lead to ventricular dysfunction. This is more often seen in patients with associated aortic regurgitation. The classic symptoms are exertional angina, syncope, and heart failure [36]. However, even in the context of severe aortic stenosis and associated ventricular dysfunction, patients may be asymptomatic in about 0.4% of cases. The absence of symptoms in this context should not be reassuring since it remains associated with a high mortality [37]. Physical examination of patients with aortic stenosis will change depending on the degree of severity. Mild aortic stenosis with normal ventricular function will usually have a normal physical examination with the

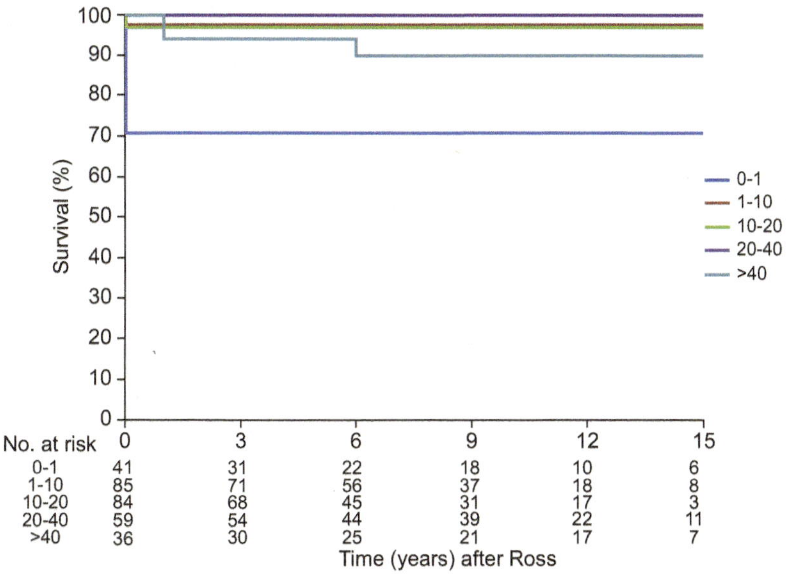

FIGURE 23.1 Kaplan–Meier curve showing survival stratified by age group: 0 to 1 (*dark blue line*), 1 to 10 (*red line*), 10 to 20 (*green line*), 20 to 40 (*purple line*), and older than 40 (*turquoise line*) years after the Ross procedure [30].

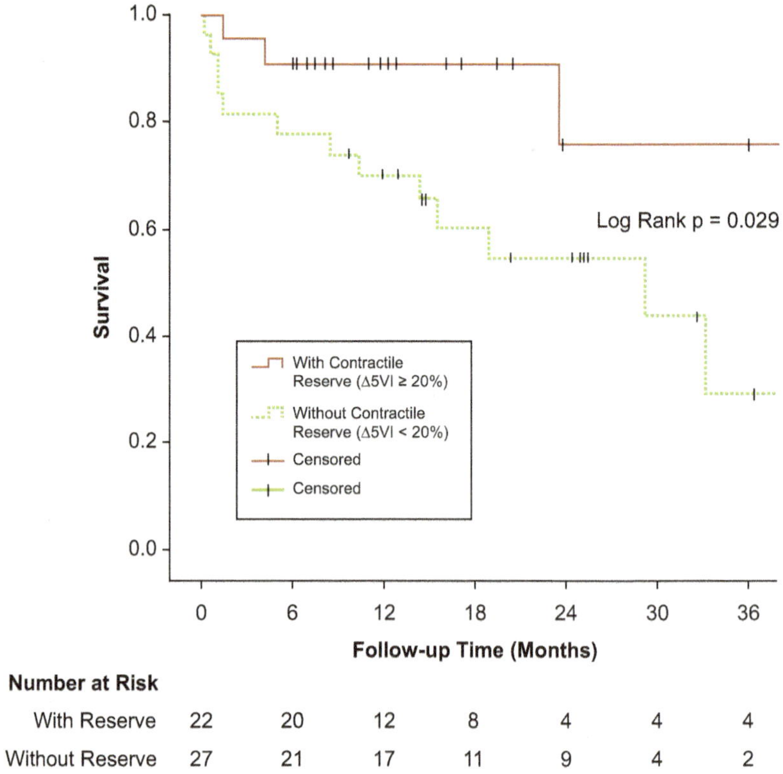

FIGURE 23.2 Kaplan–Meier survival curves of adult patients with severe aortic stenosis stratified by the presence or absence of flow reserve defined as a minimum of 20% increase in stroke volume index with dobutamine infusion [34].

exception of a mild systolic ejection murmur [38]. Moderate and severe stenosis is associated with a strong apical impulse, possible presystolic tap, pericardial or suprasternal notch thrill, split second heart sound, ejection click, systolic crescendo-decrescendo murmur, and possibly a fourth heart sound [38].

Diagnosis/Imaging

According to the 2014 AHA/ACC guidelines [12], echocardiogram and exercise testing are recommended imaging modalities for aortic stenosis. Echocardiogram with Doppler assessment represents the most commonly applied modality. Aortic valve morphology, aortic valve opening, Doppler gradient, and ventricular function should be assessed by echocardiogram in all patients. Exercise testing or dobutamine stress testing can be use to risk stratify adult patients with severe stenosis by assessing the contractile reserve (Fig. 23.2) [39]. Unfortunately, there is no clear evidence in pediatric for the utility of exercise testing in this context. Historically, peak-to-peak pressure gradient measured by cardiac catheterization has been used to guide medical decision-making [38]. Cardiac MRI is not specifically recommended in the current guidelines but can offer information on ventricular volume and function as well as defining the anatomy accurately.

Management/Intervention/Outcomes

According to the 2014 AHA ACC guidelines [12], indications for aortic valve replacement in adults are symptomatic aortic stenosis with mean gradient of 40 mmHg or above. Aortic valve replacement should also be done in the asymptomatic patient with mean gradient above 40 mmHg, only if they also have a below normal ejection fraction (less than 50%), a decreased exercise tolerance on exercise testing, or if another cardiac surgery is indicated. Otherwise, a mean gradient of 60 mmHg is an indication for intervention in the asymptomatic patients.

Determining the optimal time for surgical intervention can be challenging with an overarching attempt to balance expectant observation and early enough surgical intervention to prevent irreversible myocardial damage. Waiting for a decline in ventricular function is not optimal. Decreased ventricular function is a significant procedural risk factor for death [40–42], even in asymptomatic patients [37,43]. A dilated ventricle (end-systolic volume of more than 90 mL/m^2) is also associated with higher mortality and lower ventricular functional recovery postvalve replacement [44]. In addition, animal studies have demonstrated that aortic valve replacement only after onset of symptoms fails to reverse the maladaptive process of the extracellular matrix leading to incomplete recovery in ventricular function [3]. Currently, there is no pediatric data on the impact of ventricular function on outcome. The adult literature certainly demonstrates the benefit of aortic valve intervention even in patients with ventricular dysfunction [40,44].

The simplest but potentially less effective therapeutic option is the balloon aortic valvotomy (BAV). In older children, BAV tends to only give short-term improvement but is used to delay the surgical options [32] allowing for patient growth and therefore allowing the insertion of a bigger size valve. On one hand, prosthetic valves have unfavorable outcomes in children with a freedom from valve failure of 18% at 3 years [45]. Mechanical valves require anticoagulation, which can be challenging in young active children. The Ross procedure has advantages over prosthetic and mechanical valves [35] as discussed above. It eliminates the need for anticoagulation and offers an alternative to aortic valve replacement [34] (Fig. 23.1). In adults, the definitive treatment is either transcatheter or surgical valve replacement. Usually, transcatheter valve replacement is performed in patients that cannot undergo surgical valve replacement and is favored in patients with severely depressed function [46–48]. However, in pediatrics, it only has been reported in one 8-year-old boy [49].

For the management of heart failure in those patients, the elimination of the obstruction leads to immediate or rapid hemodynamic improvement or ventricular function improvement [41,50]. However, complete normalization of the systolic and diastolic function, which happens secondary to the progressive left ventricular remodeling, can take up to few years [51] or in some cases remains unachievable [3]. Certainly, immediate ventricular support postcardiopulmonary bypass with inotropes and phosphodiesterase III inhibitors (e.g., milrinone) is of utmost importance while the acute remodeling is happening. Usually, no long-term heart failure medication is required.

Pulmonary Valve Stenosis

Prevalence and Spectrum of Disease

The most frequent type of congenital obstruction of the right ventricular outflow tract is pulmonary valve stenosis. Pulmonary stenosis is seen in 8%–10% of congenital heart disease [52]. Similarly to aortic stenosis, pulmonary stenosis has a wide spectrum of disease from severe stenosis or atresia in utero to milder disease in older children and in some cases is associated with genetic syndromes such as Noonan syndrome.

Physiology/Mechanism

Pulmonary valve obstruction leads to an increase in right ventricular pressure proportional to the level of obstruction. The obstruction can lead to right ventricular hypertrophy and eventually lead to decreased compliance. The increase in pressure and decrease in compliance lead to right to left shunting in patients with an atrial communication causing cyanosis. Right ventricular failure is uncommon, but progression to severe pulmonary stenosis can cause the right ventricle to dilate and fail especially when it leads to tricuspid regurgitation [53,54]. In utero, severe stenosis causing right ventricular hypertrophy that leads to reduced right ventricular flow can lead to underdevelopment of the right ventricle.

Critical Pulmonary Stenosis

Presentation

Neonates born with either critical or severe pulmonary stenosis at birth are usually asymptomatic with mild cyanosis until the ductus arteriosus starts to close. Then the patient will develop progressive cyanosis, which can lead to circulatory collapse and even death if not treated [55,56]. Symptoms of right-sided heart failure are more often seen in the neonate with associated tricuspid valve anomalies leading to significant tricuspid regurgitation [57]. Pulmonary stenosis has classic signs of physical examination, outside of the cyanosis and poor perfusion. There is a normal first heart sound with a pulmonary ejection click that varies with respiration and severity accompanied with an ejection murmur best heard at the left upper sternal border. The second heart sounds are usually split and a thrill can be felt in severe stenosis cases [56].

Diagnosis/Imaging

Echocardiography is the preferred diagnostic tool and used to define the anatomy of the pulmonary valve, size of the annulus, size of the main pulmonary artery and branch pulmonary arteries, motion of the pulmonary valve leaflets, and the morphology of the right ventricle (unipartite, bipartite, or tripartite). Sometimes the presence of pulmonary insufficiency is the only sign to differentiate pulmonary stenosis versus pulmonary atresia. The assessment of the severity of pulmonary stenosis can be challenging in neonates. Due to the presence of the ductus arteriosus and high pulmonary vascular resistance, the measured pulmonary valve gradient can be underestimated. Assessment of the size (z-score) of the tricuspid valve and pulmonary valve is of utmost importance when assessing adequacy of the right ventricle [58]. It is also important to evaluate for other cardiac lesions such as a dysplastic tricuspid valve. Finally, evaluation for coronary fistula is necessary, however it is mainly seen in the context of pulmonary atresia.

Pulmonary Stenosis in Children and Young Adults

Presentation

Most cases of pulmonary valve stenosis will present during childhood. Symptoms are usually only associated with severe obstruction and adult tends to be more symptomatic than children. More severe cases can present with tricuspid valve regurgitation and right heart failure symptoms. Of note, in symptomatic patients, intervention should be performed at a lower gradient. Cyanosis is not usually part of the presentation of pulmonary stenosis in this age group unless there is an associated atrial septal defect.

Diagnosis/Imaging

Echocardiography is the imaging tool of choice allowing assessment the size of the right outflow tract structures to identify the level of obstruction and also assessing degree of stenosis. Tricuspid valve anatomy and regurgitation are important prognostic factors. Even though right ventricular failure is rare in this population [59], assessment of right ventricular function is essential, but remains challenging [60]. Echocardiography allows an assessment of right ventricular size, qualitative ventricular function, but also offer quantitative methods such as the tricuspid annular plane systolic excursion, tissue Doppler, and right ventricular strain measurement [61]. Magnetic resonance imaging can also be used for right ventricular size and function, allowing for assessment of regional wall motion abnormalities and an evaluation for myocardial fibrosis.

Management/Treatment/Outcomes

Balloon valvuloplasty is the preferred therapy in all age groups except in the presence of severe pulmonary insufficiency or multilevel right ventricular outflow tract obstruction when surgical valvotomy or right ventricular to pulmonary artery conduit insertion may be the preferred option. In the natural history study published in 1977 [54], Nugent et al. demonstrated that out of 565 children included in the study, heart failure symptoms was present on presentation in only 3% of patients and the patients with heart failure symptoms tended to be less than 2 years of age with peak-to-peak gradient above 50 mmHg. Almost half of his cohort was treated medically and there was no association with mortality. There were 184 patients with repeated cardiac catheterization 4–8 years later and the majority of patients had stable pulmonary valve gradient. Only 14% of the cohort had a significant increase in gradient and those patients were less than 4 years old at presentation with gradient above 40 mmHg. The AHA/ACC 2008 [62] adult congenital heart diseases guidelines now recommends balloon valvuloplasty if the peak gradient across the pulmonary valve is above 60 mmHg and mean gradient is above 40 mmHg for asymptomatic patients. For symptomatic patients, intervention maybe considered with mean gradient of 30 mmHg and peak gradient above 50 mmHg. If right ventricular failure is diagnosed, other etiologies of heart failure must be ruled out prior to attributing it to the pulmonary stenosis alone. However, if the diagnosis is confirmed, relief of the obstruction and diuresis are the main management options at our disposal.

RESTRICTION IN PRELOAD AND VENOUS CONGESTION

Tricuspid Stenosis

Isolated congenital tricuspid stenosis is extremely rare. Most cases are acquired tricuspid valve disease secondary to rheumatic heart disease or other forms of obstruction of the right ventricular inflow tract such as cardiac tumors [63]. Much more commonly, newborns are diagnosed with tricuspid atresia with associated hypoplasia of the right ventricle. Similarly, it is not always easy to differentiate stenosis from actual hypoplasia of the tricuspid valve, since both lead to inflow obstruction. The clinical presentation of infants born with congenital tricuspid stenosis will be very similar to patients with tricuspid atresia. Therefore, their pulmonary blood flow will be dependent on the ductus arteriosus and they will present with cyanosis. Patients that develop secondary tricuspid stenosis will present with symptoms of right heart failure such as venous congestion, exertional dyspnea, palpitations, and edema. The 2014 AHA/ACC guidelines [12] define severe tricuspid stenosis as a pressure half time of the tricuspid inflow of more than 190 ms and a valve area of less than 1.0 cm^2. The guidelines also recommend tricuspid valve replacement with severe tricuspid valve stenosis in patients undergoing cardiac surgery for other reasons or in patients who are symptomatic. Ultimately, to treat the heart failure symptoms, the obstruction has to be relieved. In children, the challenge will be patient size, annulus size, and valve choice (bioprosthetic vs. mechanical). In adults, mechanical valves seem to have no real survival advantage but carry a higher rate of thromboembolic complications, whereas bioprosthetic valves have a higher failure rate [64]. There is also a report of percutaneous Melody pulmonary valves implanted in the tricuspid position in children as young as 8 years of age [65], offering a lower profile bioprosthetic valve.

Mitral Stenosis

Isolated congenital mitral stenosis is extremely rare. It is usually associated with other abnormalities such as aortic stenosis, coarctation of the aorta, and Shone complex [66]. The anatomical reasons for the congenital mitral stenosis can be multilevel with supravalvar fibrous rings, valvar etiologies such as leaflet thickening, commissural fusion, and subvalvar causes such as short chordae or fused papillary muscles [67,68]. However, more often mitral stenosis is seen in the context of hypoplastic left-heart syndrome. Acquired mitral stenosis is certainly a more common entity and is more often related to rheumatic heart disease in children [69]. Ultimately, all forms of mitral stenosis causes limitation of the inflow to the left ventricle and causing pulmonary venous congestion, which presents with cough, dyspnea, pulmonary edema, and eventually pulmonary hypertension [67]. Therapeutic options are often limited in very young children due to their size and therefore the intervention is usually delayed until severe symptoms develop, which are not responsive to medical therapy such as diuretics and nutritional supplementation [70]. There is evidence that mitral repair is associated with a higher survival rate than mitral replacement in children [68] and therefore is usually attempted initially. Ultimately, if the obstruction is relieved and there are no other left-sided lesions, the heart failure symptoms will resolve.

CONCLUSION

Overall, valvular stenosis is an important diagnosis to rule out in children presenting with heart failure since symptoms are usually completely reversible after relieving the obstruction. However, having heart failure symptoms at time of surgery or intervention is usually a risk factor for mortality and morbidity, therefore earlier detection of the valvular stenosis is preferable. Echocardiography is the main imaging modality used to make the diagnosis of valvular stenosis and it is part of the usual heart failure work-up.

REFERENCES

[1] S.S. Prabhu, B.V. Dalvi, Treatable cardiomyopathies, Indian J. Pediatr. 67 (4) (April 2000) 279–282.

[2] D.T. Hsu, G.D. Pearson, Heart failure in children: part I: history, etiology, and pathophysiology, Circ. Heart Fail. 2 (1) (January 1, 2009) 63–70.

[3] W.M. Yarbrough, R. Mukherjee, J.S. Ikonomidis, M.R. Zile, F.G. Spinale, Myocardial remodeling with aortic stenosis and after aortic valve replacement: mechanisms and future prognostic implications, J. Thorac. Cardiovasc. Surg. 143 (3) (March 2012) 656–664.

[4] A.C. deAlmeida, R.J. van Oort, X.H.T. Wehrens, Transverse aortic constriction in mice, JoVE (38) (2010).

[5] N. Nishikawa, K. Yamamoto, Y. Sakata, T. Mano, J. Yoshida, T. Miwa, et al., Differential activation of matrix metalloproteinases in heart failure with and without ventricular dilatation, Cardiovasc. Res. 57 (3) (March 2003) 766–774.

[6] G. Condorelli, C. Morisco, G. Stassi, A. Notte, F. Farina, G. Sgaramella, et al., Increased cardiomyocyte apoptosis and changes in proapoptotic and antiapoptotic genes bax and bcl-2 during left ventricular adaptations to chronic pressure overload in the rat, Circulation 99 (23) (June 15, 1999) 3071–3078.

[7] H. Ling, T. Zhang, L. Pereira, C.K. Means, H. Cheng, Y. Gu, et al., Requirement for Ca2+/calmodulin–dependent kinase II in the transition from pressure overload–induced cardiac hypertrophy to heart failure in mice, J. Clin. Invest. 119 (5) (May 1, 2009) 1230–1240.

[8] J. Wang, E. Gao, T.O. Chan, X.-Q. Zhang, J. Song, X. Shang, et al., Induced overexpression of Na(+)/Ca(2+) exchanger does not aggravate myocardial dysfunction induced by transverse aortic constriction, J. Card. Fail. 19 (1) (January 2013) 60–70.

[9] B.J. Morris, J.O. Davis, M.L. Zatzman, G.M. Williams, The renin-angiotensin-aldosterone system in rabbits with congestive heart failure produced by aortic constriction, Circ. Res. 40 (3) (March 1977) 275–282.

[10] G.M. Kuster, E. Kotlyar, M.K. Rude, D.A. Siwik, R. Liao, W.S. Colucci, et al., Mineralocorticoid receptor inhibition ameliorates the transition to myocardial failure and decreases oxidative stress and inflammation in mice with chronic pressure overload, Circulation 111 (4) (February 1, 2005) 420–427.

[11] C.W.L. Chin, A.S.V. Shah, D.A. McAllister, S. Joanna Cowell, S. Alam, J.P. Langrish, et al., High-sensitivity troponin I concentrations are a marker of an advanced hypertrophic response and adverse outcomes in patients with aortic stenosis, Eur. Heart J. 35 (34) (September 7, 2014) 2312–2321.

[12] R.A. Nishimura, C.M. Otto, R.O. Bonow, B.A. Carabello, J.P. Erwin, R.A. Guyton, et al., 2014 AHA/ACC guideline for the management of patients with valvular heart disease: a report of the American College of Cardiology/American Heart Association Task Force on Practice Guidelines, Circulation 129 (23) (June 9, 2014) e521–e643.

[13] E.W. Larson, W.D. Edwards, Risk factors for aortic dissection: a necropsy study of 161 cases, Am. J. Cardiol. 53 (6) (March 1, 1984) 849–855.

[14] W.C. Robert, The congenitally bicuspid aorti valve. A study of 85 autopsy cases, Am. J. Cardiol. 26 (1970) 72–83.
[15] K. Makikallio, Fetal aortic valve stenosis and the evolution of hypoplastic left heart syndrome: patient selection for fetal intervention, Circulation 113 (11) (March 21, 2006) 1401–1405.
[16] H.R. Wagner, R.C. Ellison, J.F. Keane, O.J. Humphries, A.S. Nadas, Clinical course in aortic stenosis, Circulation (December 1, 1977) 1–10.
[17] V. Thakur, J.-C. Fouron, L. Mertens, E.T. Jaeggi, Diagnosis and management of fetal heart failure, Can. J. Cardiol. 29 (7) (July 2013) 759–767.
[18] T. Ide, T. Miyoshi, M. Kitano, K.-I. Kurosaki, J. Yoshimatsu, Fetal critical aortic stenosis with natural improvement of hydrops fetalis due to spontaneous relief of severe restrictive atrial communication, J. Obstet. Gynaecol. Res. 41 (7) (July 2015) 1137–1140.
[19] L.R. Freud, D.B. McElhinney, A.C. Marshall, G.R. Marx, K.G. Friedman, P.J. Del Nido, et al., Fetal aortic valvuloplasty for evolving hypoplastic left heart syndrome: postnatal outcomes of the first 100 patients, Circulation 130 (8) (August 19, 2014) 638–645.
[20] K.G. Friedman, L. Freud, M. Escobar-Diaz, P. Banka, S. Emani, W. Tworetzky, Left ventricular remodeling and function in children with biventricular circulation after fetal aortic valvuloplasty, Pediatr. Cardiol. (May 13, 2015) 1–8 Springer US.
[21] C.R. Cole, P. Eghtesady, The myocardial and coronary histopathology and pathogenesis of hypoplastic left heart syndrome, Cardiol. Young (July 8, 2015) 1–11.
[22] P.R. Lurie, Changing concepts of endocardial fibroelastosis, Cardiol. Young 20 (2) (April 2010) 115–123.
[23] M.P. Leung, R. McKay, A. Smith, R.H. Anderson, R. Arnold, Critical aortic stenosis in early infancy. Anatomic and echocardiographic substrate of successful open valvotomy, J. Thorac. Cardiovasc. Surg. 101 (3) (March 1991) 526–535.
[24] L.A. Rhodes, S.D. Colan, S.B. Perry, R.A. Jonas, S.P. Sanders, Predictors of survival in neonates with critical aortic stenosis, Circulation 84 (6) (1991) 2325–2335.
[25] S.D. Colan, D.B. McElhinney, E.C. Crawford, J.F. Keane, J.E. Lock, Validation and re-evaluation of a discriminant model predicting anatomic suitability for biventricular repair in neonates with aortic stenosis, J. Am. Coll. Cardiol. 47 (9) (May 2006) 1858–1865.
[26] G.K. Lofland, B.W. McCrindle, W.G. Williams, E.H. Blackstone, C.I. Tchervenkov, R. Sittiwangkul, et al., Critical aortic stenosis in the neonate: a multi-institutional study of management, outcomes, and risk factors. Congenital Heart Surgeons Society, J. Thorac. Cardiovasc. Surg. 121 (1) (January 2001) 10–27.
[27] J.W. Hammon Jr., F.M. Lupinetti, M.D. Maples, W.H. Merrill, W.H. Frist, T.P. Graham Jr., H.W. Bender Jr., Predictors of operative mortality in critical valvular aortic stenosis presenting in infancy, Ann. Thorac. Surg. 45 (1988) 537–540.
[28] L. Grosse-Wortmann, T.-J. Yun, O. Al-Radi, S. Kim, M. Nii, K.-J. Lee, et al., Borderline hypoplasia of the left ventricle in neonates: insights for decision-making from functional assessment with magnetic resonance imaging, J. Thorac. Cardiovasc. Surg. 136 (6) (December 2008) 1429–1436.
[29] J.W. Brown, M.D. Rodefeld, M. Ruzmetov, O. Eltayeb, O. Yurdakok, M.W. Turrentine, Surgical valvuloplasty versus balloon aortic dilation for congenital aortic stenosis: are evidence-based outcomes relevant? ATS 94 (1) (July 1, 2012) 146–155 Elsevier Inc.
[30] J. Siddiqui, C.P. Brizard, J.C. Galati, A.J. Iyengar, D. Hutchinson, I.E. Konstantinov, et al., Surgical valvotomy and repair for neonatal and infant congenital aortic stenosis achieves better results than interventional catheterization, J. Am. Coll. Cardiol. 62 (22) (December 3, 2013) 2134–2140.
[31] S. Fratz, H.P. Gildein, G. Balling, W. Sebening, T. Genz, A. Eicken, et al., Aortic valvuloplasty in pediatric patients substantially postpones the need for aortic valve surgery: a single-center experience of 188 patients after up to 17.5 years of follow-up, Circulation 117 (9) (March 4, 2008) 1201–1206.
[32] A. Torres, J.A. Vincent, A. Everett, S. Lim, S.R. Foerster, A.C. Marshall, et al., Balloon valvuloplasty for congenital aortic stenosis: multi-center safety and efficacy outcome assessment, Catheter. Cardiovasc. Interv. 86 (5) (November 2015) 808–820.
[33] D.N. Ross, Replacement of aortic and mitral valve with a pulmonary autograft, Lancet 2 (1967) 959.
[34] N. Bansal, S.R. Kumar, C.J. Baker, R. Lemus, W.J. Wells, V.A. Starnes, Age-related outcomes of the Ross procedure over 20 years, Ann. Thorac. Surg. 99 (6) (June 2015) 2077–2085.
[35] T.J. Wilder, C.A. Caldarone, G.S. Van Arsdell, E. Pham-Hung, M. Gritti, M. Jughiman Al, et al., Aortic valve repair for insufficiency in older children offers unpredictable durability that may not be advantageous over a primary Ross operation†, Eur. J. Cardiothorac. Surg. 49 (3) (March 2016) 883–892.
[36] M.J. Czaynr, J.R. Resar, Diagnosis and management of valvular aortic stenosis, Clin. Med. Insights Cardiol. 8 (Suppl. 1) (October 19, 2014) 15–24.
[37] D.M. Henkel, J.F. Malouf, H.M. Connolly, H.I. Michelena, M.E. Sarano, H.V. Schaff, et al., Asymptomatic left ventricular systolic dysfunction in patients with severe aortic stenosis: characteristics and outcomes, J. Am. Coll. Cardiol. 60 (22) (December 4, 2012) 2325–2329.
[38] H.R. Wagner, R.C. Ellison, J.F. Keane, O.J. Humphries, A.S. Nadas, Clinical course in aortic stenosis, Circulation 56 (1 Suppl.) (August 1977) I47–I56.
[39] S. Hayek, P. Pibarot, A. Harzand, J.-W. Cheng, H. Gay, C. Chrysohoou, et al., Dobutamine stress echocardiography for risk stratification of patients with low-gradient severe aortic stenosis undergoing TAVR, JACC Cardiovasc. Imaging 8 (3) (March 2015) 380–382.
[40] M. Gotzmann, P. Rahlmann, T. Hehnen, P. Müller, M. Lindstaedt, A. Mügge, et al., Heart failure in severe aortic valve stenosis: prognostic impact of left ventricular ejection fraction and mean gradient on outcome after transcatheter aortic valve implantation, Eur. J. Heart Fail. 14 (10) (February 18, 2014) 1155–1162.
[41] T. Pilgrim, P. Wenaweser, F. Meuli, C. Huber, S. Stortecky, C. Seiler, et al., Clinical outcome of high-risk patients with severe aortic stenosis and reduced left ventricular ejection fraction undergoing medical treatment or TAVI, G. Biondi-Zoccai (Ed.), PLoS One 6 (11) (November 10, 2011) e27556.
[42] J.S. Dahl, L. Videbæk, M.K. Poulsen, P.A. Pellikka, K. Veien, L.I. Andersen, et al., Noninvasive assessment of filling pressure and left atrial pressure overload in severe aortic valve stenosis: relation to ventricular remodeling and clinical outcome after aortic valve replacement, J. Thorac. Cardiovasc. Surg. 142 (3) (September 2011) e77–83.
[43] L.E. Miller, V.M. Miller, L.D. Acers, Asymptomatic severe aortic stenosis with left ventricular dysfunction: watchful waiting or valve replacement? Clin. Med. Res. 11 (2) (June 2013) 51–53.

[44] G. Tarantini, P. Buja, R. Scognamiglio, R. Razzolini, G. Gerosa, G. Isabella, et al., Aortic valve replacement in severe aortic stenosis with left ventricular dysfunction: determinants of cardiac mortality and ventricular function recovery, Eur. J. Cardiothorac. Surg. 24 (6) (December 2003) 879–885.

[45] S.F. Saleeb, J.W. Newburger, T. Geva, C.W. Baird, K. Gauvreau, R.F. Padera, et al., Accelerated degeneration of a bovine pericardial bioprosthetic aortic valve in children and young adults, Circulation 130 (1) (July 1, 2014) 51–60.

[46] A. Unbehaun, M. Pasic, S. Buz, S. Dreysse, M. Kukucka, R. Hetzer, et al., Transapical aortic valve implantation in patients with severely depressed left ventricular function, J. Thorac. Cardiovasc. Surg. 143 (6) (June 2012) 1356–1363.

[47] H.W. van der Werf, Y.L. Douglas, A.F.M. van den Heuvel, TAVI in heart failure, how much risk is acceptable? Eur. J. Heart Fail. 14 (10) (February 18, 2014) 1087–1089.

[48] T. Mihaljevic, M. Planinc, S.J. Williams, A.M. Gillinov, J.F. Sabik, L.G. Svensson, et al., Less invasive versus conventional heart valve surgery in patients with severe heart failure, J. Thorac. Cardiovasc. Surg. 148 (1) (July 2014) 161–166.

[49] M.H. Martin, P.J. Gruber, R.G. Gray, Transcatheter neoaortic valve replacement utilizing the melody valve in hypoplastic left heart syndrome, Catheter. Cardiovasc. Interv. 85 (4) (March 2015) 615–619.

[50] B. Villari, G. Vassalli, S. Betocchi, C. Briguori, M. Chiariello, O.M. Hess, Normalization of left ventricular nonuniformity late after valve replacement for aortic stenosis, Am. J. Cardiol. 78 (1) (July 1, 1996) 66–71.

[51] M.M. Elahi, A. Chuang, M.J. Ewing, C.H. Choi, P.W. Grant, B.M. Matata, One problem two issues! Left ventricular systolic and diastolic dysfunction in aortic stenosis, Ann. Transl. Med. 2 (1) (January 2014) 10.

[52] V.C. Pinto Júnior, K.M.P.C. Branco, R.C. Cavalcante, W. Carvalho Junior, J.R.C. Lima, S.M. de Freitas, et al., Epidemiology of congenital heart disease in Brazil, Rev. Bras. Cir. Cardiovasc. 30 (2) (March 2015) 219–224.

[53] L.A. Latson, Critical pulmonary stenosis, J. Interv. Cardiol. 14 (3) (June 2001) 345–350.

[54] E.W. Nugent, R.M. Freedom, J.J. Nora, R.C. Ellison, R.D. Rowe, A.S. Nadas, Clinical course in pulmonary stenosis, Circulation (December 1, 1977) 1–10.

[55] M.D. Freed, A. Rosenthal, W.F. Bernhard, S.B. Litwin, A.S. Nadas, Critical pulmonary stenosis with a diminutive right ventricle in neonates, Circulation 48 (4) (October 1973) 875–881.

[56] W.M. Gersony, W.F. Bernhard, A.S. Nadas, R.E. Gross, Diagnosis and surgical treatment of infants with critical pulmonary outflow obstruction. Study of thirty-four infants with pulmonary stenosis or atresia, and intact ventricular septum, Circulation 35 (4) (April 1967) 765–776.

[57] K.G. Schmidt, J.L. Cloez, N.H. Silverman, Changes of right ventricular size and function in neonates after valvotomy for pulmonary atresia or critical pulmonary stenosis and intact ventricular septum, JAC 19 (5) (April 1992) 1032–1037.

[58] G. Shaath, M. Mutairi Al, O. Tamimi, A. Alakhfash, M. Abolfotouh, F. Alhabshan, Predictors of reintervention in neonates with critical pulmonary stenosis or pulmonary atresia with intact ventricular septum, Catheter. Cardiovasc. Interv. 79 (4) (January 10, 2012) 659–664.

[59] E.W. Nugent, E.W. Nugent, R.M. Freedom, R.M. Freedom, J.J. Nora, J.J. Nora, et al., Clinical course in pulmonary stenosis, Circulation 56 (1 Suppl.) (August 1977) I38–I47.

[60] G.B. Bleeker, Assessing right ventricular function: the role of echocardiography and complementary technologies, Heart 92 (Suppl. 1) (April 1, 2006) i19–i26.

[61] K. Okumura, T. Humpl, A. Dragulescu, L. Mertens, M.K. Friedberg, Longitudinal assessment of right ventricular myocardial strain in relation to transplant-free survival in children with idiopathic pulmonary hypertension, J. Am. Soc. Echocardiogr. 27 (12) (December 1, 2014) 1344–1351 Elsevier Inc.

[62] C.A. Warnes, C.A. Warnes, R.G. Williams, R.G. Williams, T.M. Bashore, T.M. Bashore, et al., ACC/AHA 2008 guidelines for the management of adults with congenital heart disease: a report of the American College of Cardiology/American Heart Association Task Force on Practice Guidelines (writing committee to develop guidelines on the management of adults with congenital heart disease): developed in collaboration with the American Society of echocardiography, Heart Rhythm Society, International Society for Adult Congenital Heart Disease, Society for Cardiovascular Angiography and Interventions, and Society of Thoracic Surgeons, Circulation 118 (23) (December 2, 2008) e714–e833.

[63] Z.-H. Xiao, J. Hu, Da Zhu, Y.-K. Shi, E.-Y. Zhang, Tricuspid valve obstruction and right heart failure due to a giant right atrial myxoma arising from the superior vena cava, J. Cardiothorac. Surg. 8 (1) (October 30, 2013) 200.

[64] F. Filsoufi, A.C. Anyanwu, S.P. Salzberg, T. Frankel, L.H. Cohn, D.H. Adams, Long-term outcomes of tricuspid valve replacement in the current era, Ann. Thorac. Surg. 80 (3) (September 2005) 845–850.

[65] P.A. Roberts, Y. Boudjemline, J.P. Cheatham, A. Eicken, P. Ewert, D.B. McElhinney, et al., Percutaneous tricuspid valve replacement in congenital and acquired heart disease, J. Am. Coll. Cardiol. 58 (2) (July 5, 2011) 117–122.

[66] R.N. Ruckman, R. Van Praagh, Anatomic types of congenital mitral stenosis: report of 49 autopsy cases with consideration of diagnosis and surgical implications, Am. J. Cardiol. 42 (4) (October 1978) 592–601.

[67] M.S. Uva, L. Galletti, F.L. Gayet, D. Piot, A. Serraf, J. Bruniaux, et al., Surgery for congenital mitral valve disease in the first year of life, J. Thorac. Cardiovasc. Surg. 109 (1) (January 1995) 164–174 discussion 174–6.

[68] L.G. Quinonez, P.J. del Nido, Valve reconstruction for congenital mitral valve disease, Multimed. Man. Cardiothorac. Surg. 2015 (0) (January 5, 2015) mmv007–7.

[69] N.D. Hillman, L.Y. Tani, L.G. Veasy, L.L. Lambert, G.B. Di Russo, D.B. Doty, et al., Current status of surgery for rheumatic carditis in children, Ann. Thorac. Surg. 78 (4) (October 2004) 1403–1408.

[70] P.J. del Nido, C. Baird, Congenital mitral valve stenosis: anatomic variants and surgical reconstruction, Semin. Thorac. Cardiovasc. Surg. Pediatr. Card. Surg. Annu. 15 (1) (2012) 69–74 Elsevier Inc.

Chapter 24

Ischemic Coronary Artery Disease

James C. Fang, Weining David Xu
University of Utah School of Medicine, Salt Lake City, UT, United States

INTRODUCTION

Ischemic disease and heart failure in the adolescent and young adult is a special topic due to the low incidence of overall ischemic disease in this population. Unlike ischemic disease in the middle-aged adult, which is overwhelmingly due to atherosclerosis, the cause of coronary artery disease and subsequent myocardial ischemia in adolescents may be attributed to multiple uncommon disease etiologies. Broadly speaking, these rare diseases can be grouped into the categories of metabolic, autoimmune, congenital or cryptogenic.

Unlike the typical presentations of angina in adults, younger children may not be present with chest pain. Ischemia in children may be present as irritability or failure to thrive, or even sudden cardiac death. Contrarily, chest pain in the emergency room is rarely ischemic in nature. Of the 650,000 emergency visits for chest pain by patients between ages 10 and 21, less than 5% of these encounters are attributed to primarily cardiac causes [1,2]. The commonest cause of chest pain continues to be musculoskeletal in nature, but this chapter will focus on disruptions in the normal supply of oxygenated blood through coronary arteries to myocardium.

The commonest reported cause of ischemic cardiomyopathy in children is Kawasaki disease, which is an acquired form of coronary disease from an autoimmune reaction as well as direct myocardial damage [3]. Other autoimmune diseases can also disrupt coronary blood flow such as systemic lupus erythematous [4].

Aside from autoimmune etiologies, causes of coronary artery disease in the young include anatomic disruptions such as spontaneous coronary dissection, coronary artery embolism, and anomalous origin of the coronary arteries. These anatomic disruptions can be present in sudden and acute ways.

Finally, familial hypercholesterolemia is a metabolic dysregulation of low-density lipoprotein (LDL) that accelerates atherosclerotic disease progression in adolescents. Generally, there is strong family history of early onset coronary disease, and children have been identified and treated early in their lives to reduce their exposure to elevated serum LDL.

The varied causes of ischemic coronary disease in the adolescent and young adult require early diagnosis and tailored treatment as early as possible to prevent irreversible myocardial damage, which can lead to segmental wall motion abnormality and congestive heart failure. The treatment of chronic heart failure in adolescents is not well studied as the incidence of this clinical syndrome is rare and, therefore, extrapolated from robust data from randomized clinical trials of adults. These treatment modalities will not be reviewed in detail; rather the focus of this chapter will be in the acute presentation for each etiology of ischemia.

KAWASAKI DISEASE

Kawasaki disease, also known as mucocutaneous lymph node syndrome named for the organs that it affects, was first described in 1957 by Dr. Tomisaku Kawasaki in Japan [5]. The exact pathogenesis is still not completely elucidated, but due to a dysregulation of the immune system, the disease acutely attacks medium-sized blood vessels as well as myocardium, skin, mucous membranes, and lymph nodes, which produces the characteristic strawberry tongue [6,7]. A recent study suggests that airborne toxin originating from croplands in northeastern China and carried by winds toward Japan and the western American seaboard may be the culprit [8].

The disease cycle can be split into three phases: acute, subacute, and the convalescent phase. During the acute phase, the primary symptoms are a high fever, mucocutaneous erythema, and coronary arteritis [9]. If diagnosis and treatment is not initiated quickly, this phase can last from 1 to 2 weeks. Sequelae from cardiac involvement can manifest during the subacute phase, which follows for up to 4 weeks after the completion of the untreated acute phase. These sequelae include coronary artery aneurysms, myocarditis, and pericarditis during which the risk of sudden cardiac death is the highest. With

Heart Failure in the Child and Young Adult. http://dx.doi.org/10.1016/B978-0-12-802393-8.00024-7

early diagnosis and treatment of Kawasaki disease during the acute phase, up to 5% of children develop transient coronary artery dysfunction and dilatation and 1% develop giant aneurysms [10]. Acute coronary artery thrombosis can occur as well as rupture of the aneurysmal segment of the artery leading to sudden cardiac death.

Since Kawasaki disease is a systemic autoimmune disease, treatment is not targeted only to coronary arteritis. The treatment is often dual fold in stopping the autoimmune process and decreasing the inflammation associated. Intravenous immunoglobulin (IVIG) is a mainstay of treatment and should be initiated immediately after the diagnosis is made [11,12]. Response to therapy should be seen within 24 h from the start of therapy with defervescence.

Salicylic acid is another mainstay of therapy in addition to IVIG that must be initiated for its antiplatelet, anti-inflammatory, and antipyretic effects [13]. High dose salicylic acid is the initial treatment during the acute phase, with slow tapering to long-term low dose salicylic acid for several months after the initial presentation.

Although systemic heparin or novel anticoagulants have not been tested or are first-line therapies to prevent coronary thrombosis, if there is documented evidence of coronary thrombosis on diagnostic testing despite optimal first-line therapy, adjunctive systemic anticoagulation is a reasonable consideration to treat life-threatening thrombosis [14].

Patients with no response to the standard of care will generally have worse prognosis with large aneurysms and late complications with coronary arterial stenosis. Depending on the extent of coronary artery disease and myocardial damage, percutaneous coronary intervention or primary surgical intervention may be needed in the short term and even orthotopic cardiac transplantation may be necessary in the longer term [15,16].

ANOMALOUS ORIGIN OF THE CORONARY ARTERY

Anomalous origin of the coronary artery is a rare but serious disease of the adolescent and young adult as it typically presents in sudden cardiac death. A higher incidence of coronary artery anomalies is observed in young adults who are victims of sudden cardiac death than in middle-aged adults. In normal coronary anatomy, the left main coronary artery takes off from the left coronary cusp and the right coronary artery takes off from the right coronary cusp. The commonest anomaly is the origin of the left circumflex coronary artery originating from the right coronary artery [17]. With the variations of differing origins, the takeoff of the coronary artery can be oblique or have the artery course between the main pulmonary artery and aorta making it susceptible to compression during activity [18,19].

Patients are often asymptomatic early in their clinical course, during which the origin of the oblique takeoff develops atherosclerotic plaque likely due to turbulent blood flow. Once the stenosis reaches a critical threshold in a young adult, angina, syncope, and dyspnea can develop in a previously healthy subject during intense exercise. Similarly younger children who have a coronary artery that courses between the trunks of the great artery can also develop these symptoms during exercise. In infants, angina may be manifested by irritability, poor feeding, pallor or failure to thrive in the setting of a low cardiac output state. Laboratory studies must be utilized to distinguish this clinical entity from more common causes such as sepsis in infants as they can present in the same manner.

Diagnosis can be achieved through multiple modalities of imaging. Stress testing with transthoracic echocardiogram is useful in the initial assessment of a patient with functional intolerance as segmental wall motion abnormalities in a specific coronary artery distribution may be seen. Even without stress testing, resting transthoracic echocardiogram may show globally decreased and poorly functioning left ventricle consistent with significant congenital abnormalities of the coronaries. In the child with good imaging windows, transthoracic echocardiogram with color flow Doppler signal can even be used to identify anomalous origins of coronary arteries [20].

Once there is suspicion of a congenital coronary artery abnormality, computed tomography of the coronary artery is also useful in reconstructing the full anatomy of the patient especially with multiple anomalous origins or fistulas of the coronary arterial system. However in the pediatric population, resting tachycardia can be a technical challenge.

Treatment often focuses on stabilizing and optimizing the patient initially as a bridge to more definitive therapy. Medication such as loop diuretics in the acute setting may be required to relieve symptoms of congestive heart failure. Other intensive care therapies include inotropes if the patient is in a persistently low cardiac output state.

The definitive treatment once the patient is stabilized then becomes surgical revascularizatoin. This includes unroofing the coronary artery and reanastomosis to a more favorable location on the aorta [21–23].

CORONARY ARTERY EMBOLISM

Coronary artery embolization is another rare clinical event that can lead to permanent myocardial damage depending on the time of presentation to diagnosis and treatment. Although atrial fibrillation is overall the commonest cause of coronary artery embolism, this arrhythmia is a fairly uncommon entity in the pediatric population. In the younger population intracardiac shunts such as patent foramen ovale or atrial septal defect may allow a clot to pass into the systemic circulation and cause an embolic event such as cerebral strokes or coronary embolisms [24,25].

Diagnosis of an acute myocardial infarction due to this phenomenon can be difficult and be delayed owing to the rare nature and further hinder treatment. The patient would present with angina, diaphoresis, and possibly cardiogenic shock depending on the extent and duration of ischemia. The initial screening tool should be a rapid assessment by electrocardiogram, which can show ST segment elevation, depression, or hyperacute T waves. Cardiac biomarkers with creatine kinase MB would be the earliest sign of myocardial injury followed by cardiac troponins [26].

A bedside transthoracic echocardiogram that shows segmental wall motion abnormality in a coronary artery distribution is highly suggestive of a coronary arterial event. When there are multiple vascular territories of embolic injury such as cerebral stroke, early treatment within the appropriate window using thrombolytics is a reasonable approach.

Often there is diagnostic uncertainty owing to the rare nature of this disease. Therefore the patient should be transferred to a center that has the ability to perform coronary angiography, which would be diagnostic and therapeutic [27]. If the normal vascular architecture of the intima is not disrupted, thrombectomy or targeted thrombolysis may be the only intervention required.

Once the acute insult is resolved, the clinical workup includes evaluation for a hypercoagulable state. If there is a primary hypercoagulable state, lifelong systemic anticoagulation therapy should be initiated. If the hypercoagulable state is secondary to another process, treatment should be tailored to that disease process.

An echocardiogram with bubble study to evaluate for intracardiac shunt should also be done if the source of the embolism is from the venous circulation. Closure of the intracardiac shunt can be discussed with the patient's doctor as this can be done surgically or percutaneously in the cardiac catheterization laboratory [26].

TRAUMATIC CORONARY ARTERY DISSECTION

Traumatic coronary artery dissection is a rare event in previously healthy young adults that have been reported following direct blows to the chest during sports or motor vehicle accidents. Patients may present with chest pain, and initial evaluation with electrocardiogram may have ST segment changes consistent with ischemia or infarction. Cardiac biomarkers may also be abnormally elevated [28,29].

To clinically distinguish a coronary artery dissection from an embolic event, one would need advanced diagnostic capabilities during coronary angiography [30]. During the catheterization if no obvious dissection flap is seen, further interrogation with intravascular ultrasound or optical coherence tomography can offer better spatial resolution in a suspicious segment of the coronary artery, often revealing a dissection flap in the intimal layer of the coronary artery [31,32].

Treatment of coronary artery dissection should correlate with the extent of the dissection. Conservative treatment for dissections with antiplatelet agents such as aspirin and systemic heparinization is the first-line therapy [33,34]. Over time, the intima will heal and no further treatment is required. Response to treatment should be monitored in the patient's anginal symptoms, electrocardiogram, and serial cardiac biomarkers.

For a small portion of patients with refractory chest pain despite medical therapy and also have large areas of myocardial ischemia percutaneous coronary intervention or urgent surgical revascularization can be considered to improve symptoms and minimize myocardial damage [33,34].

SPONTANEOUS CORONARY ARTERY DISSECTION

Spontaneous coronary artery dissection is another disease process that can be caused by distinctly separate disease modalities. The patient population disproportionately linked to spontaneous coronary artery dissection is the female gender. 80% of cases occur during the perinatal period or while taking hormonal oral contraceptives. It is unknown if the hormones of pregnancy such as oxytocin or prolactin may contribute to changes in the connective tissues of medium-sized arteries [35,36].

Vasculitis has also been noted in some cases with the presence of eosinophilic infiltrates and degraded collagen [37]. Other conditions that are associated with spontaneous coronary artery dissection include fibromuscular dysplasia, sarcoidosis, illicit drug use primarily cocaine, and copper deficiency.

Unlike other causes of coronary artery dissection, spontaneous coronary artery dissections occur in the media or between the media and adventitia. The left anterior descending artery is affected in 75% of cases, particularly predominant in females. The right coronary artery is affected in 20% of cases, typically in males. Sudden cardiac death may occur in up to 50% of cases, especially with left main coronary artery involvement [38].

Diagnostic testing begins with electrocardiogram, which may show ischemic changes in the ST segment or T waves and laboratory testing, which may show elevations in cardiac biomarkers such as creatine kinase MB as well as troponins.

A transthoracic echocardiogram that shows segmental wall motion abnormalities in a specific coronary distribution would be further evidence of coronary artery dysfunction.

Definitive diagnosis of coronary artery dissection would require coronary angiography, which would show the presence of extraluminal contrast dye. Advanced imaging techniques used in conjunction with coronary angiography such as intravascular ultrasound or optical coherence tomography would provide further evidence of dissection in the media flap from a primary atherosclerotic process [31,32].

Treatment with medical therapy using antiplatelet agents, systemic heparinization, nitrates, and beta blockers to reduce symptoms of angina is first-line therapy. This strategy is reasonable in stable patients with limited myocardium at risk for infarction [33,34].

Patients with proximal dissection of major coronary arteries, refractory chest pain, or other evidence of ongoing ischemia, percutaneous coronary intervention may be indicated but oftentimes technically challenging. If multiple coronary arteries are affected or the left main coronary artery is involved, coronary artery bypass surgery is another option but again can be difficult with long, spiral dissections. Rarely myocardial dysfunction from large areas of persistent and prolonged ischemia leads to congestive heart failure that does not improve with medical therapy and may necessitate orthotopic heart transplantation [34].

FIBROMUSCULAR DYSPLASIA

Fibromuscular dysplasia is a noninflammatory, nonatherosclerotic vascular disease that overall affects more females than males, but can be seen in either sexes in the younger population. The disease is likely underdiagnosed as certain individuals may be asymptomatic. The exact etiology is unknown but there seems to be a genetic predisposition to this disease [39].

The commonest vascular bed affected is the renal artery but fibromuscular dysplasia can also affect the coronaries, carotids, splanchnics, and peripheral vessels. Presentation of coronary vasculopathy due to fibromuscular dysplasia can include progressive stenosis, dissection with or without complete occlusion, as well as aneurysms. Since fibromuscular dysplasia can cause spontaneous coronary artery dissections, this disease has been postulated to contribute to the sudden death in the younger population.

Patients typically do not present with angina or laboratory findings consistent with ischemia unless a coronary artery occlusion is present. Since the renal arteries are affected most commonly, fibromuscular dysplasia is usually diagnosed during the workup for causes of secondary hypertension [40]. Markers of chronic inflammation such as erythrocyte sedimentation rate and C-reactive protein would also be unremarkable.

If there is a strong suspicion of fibromuscular dysplasia, diagnostic imaging should be tailored to the vascular bed most affected by the disease. This often includes initial noninvasive testing such as renal artery duplex ultrasound and carotid artery duplex ultrasound, along with Doppler flow velocities [41]. Computed tomography angiography is a higher sensitivity and specificity test that can evaluate coronary, mesenteric, renal, and cerebral vessels, which can show the typical "string of beads" sign [42]. Magnetic resonance angiography is not the test of choice due to the low spatial resolution and decreased specificity for fibromuscular dysplasia [43].

Treatment of this disease is dependent of the vascular bed. In the setting of coronary disease, it may be reasonable to perform selective coronary angiography to establish a baseline as well percutaneous coronary intervention in the setting of occlusive disease from a significant dissection. If there is no significant stenosis or occlusion, conservative management may be utilized.

FAMILIAL HYPERCHOLESTEROLEMIA

Familial hypercholesterolemia is a rare metabolic disease that advances the progression of atherosclerotic disease in the young adult. The commonest mutations affect the LDL receptor and apolipoprotein B, which normally regulates serum levels of LDL. Loss-of-function mutations in these two proteins cause dysregulation of the LDL to many folds the normal levels and therefore accelerate cholesterol plaque deposition in arteries. These mutations are transmitted in an autosomal dominant fashion to cause heterozygous familial hypercholesterolemia [44].

Patients with heterozygous familial hypercholesterolemia typically have early onset atherosclerosis between the ages of 30 and 40 and have an prevalence of 1 in 500 patients in the North American population, but the prevalence can vary geographically [45]. Presentation is typical of atherosclerotic disease with unstable angina, non-ST segment elevation myocardial infarction, or ST segment elevation myocardial infarction.

Patients with loss of function in both copies of the same gene are extremely rare and result in homozygous familial hypercholesterolemia. This disease occurs only once in a million live births. These patients will present with atheromas and lipid-rich depositions in various organ tissues such as tendons and eye lids [46]. They will present even earlier in life with atherosclerotic coronary artery disease, typically between the ages of 20 and 30.

Treatment of acute coronary syndrome is similar to the adult population. Early recognition with diagnostic testing such as electrocardiogram and cardiac biomarkers would be consistent with ischemia or infarction. Initial medical treatment includes aspirin and heparinization. If laboratory or diagnostic testing is consistent with non-ST segment elevation or ST segment elevation myocardial infarction, additional antiplatelet agents such as clopidogrel or ticagrelor is indicated. Prompt revascularization with percutaneous coronary intervention or coronary artery bypass grafting is indicated.

Prevention and delay of coronary atherosclerotic disease are the mainstay of therapy in these patients. Patients typically do not respond to routine LDL therapy with low intensity statins [47]. Even with maximal titration of high intensity statin medications, their LDL levels remain above the upper limit of normal [48]. Adjunctive therapy invariably is needed for homozygous patient, which includes addition of ezetimibe, lipopheresis, and surgical intervention. Liver transplantation from a donor that can produce LDL receptors normally can normalize circulating levels of LDL in the recipient. PCSK9 inhibitors have also shown promise in their ability to drastically reduced LDL but currently are not well studied.

REFERENCES

[1] B.H. Rowe, C.S. Dulberg, R.G. Peterson, P. Vlad, M.M. Li, Characteristics of children presenting with chest pain to a pediatric emergency department, CMAJ 143 (5) (1990) 388–394.

[2] S.E. Epstein, L.H. Gerber, J.S. Borer, Chest wall syndrome. A common cause of unexplained cardiac pain, JAMA 241 (26) (1979) 2793–2797.

[3] J.C. Burns, M.P. Glode, Kawasaki syndrome, Lancet 364 (9433) (2004) 533–544.

[4] Y. Asanuma, A. Oeser, A.K. Shintani, E. Turner, N. Olsen, S. Fazio, et al., Premature coronary-artery atherosclerosis in systemic lupus erythematosus, N. Engl. J. Med. 349 (25) (2003) 2407–2415.

[5] T. Kawasaki, Acute febrile mucocutaneous syndrome with lymphoid involvement with specific desquamation of the fingers and toes in children, Arerugi 16 (3) (1967) 178–222.

[6] C.L. Wang, Y.T. Wu, C.A. Liu, H.C. Kuo, K.D. Yang, Kawasaki disease: infection, immunity and genetics, Pediatr. Infect. Dis. J. 24 (11) (2005) 998–1004.

[7] J.W. Newburger, M. Takahashi, M.A. Gerber, M.H. Gewitz, L.Y. Tani, J.C. Burns, et al., Diagnosis, treatment, and long-term management of Kawasaki disease: a statement for health professionals from the committee on rheumatic fever, endocarditis, and Kawasaki disease, council on cardiovascular disease in the young, American heart association, Pediatrics 114 (6) (2004) 1708–1733.

[8] X. Rodo, R. Curcoll, M. Robinson, J. Ballester, J.C. Burns, D.R. Cayan, et al., Tropospheric winds from northeastern China carry the etiologic agent of Kawasaki disease from its source to Japan, Proc. Natl. Acad. Sci. U.S.A. 111 (22) (2014) 7952–7957.

[9] H. Fujiwara, Y. Hamashima, Pathology of the heart in Kawasaki disease, Pediatrics 61 (1) (1978) 100–107.

[10] H. Nakano, K. Ueda, A. Saito, K. Nojima, Repeated quantitative angiograms in coronary arterial aneurysm in Kawasaki disease, Am. J. Cardiol. 56 (13) (1985) 846–851.

[11] M. Terai, S.T. Shulman, Prevalence of coronary artery abnormalities in Kawasaki disease is highly dependent on gamma globulin dose but independent of salicylate dose, J. Pediatr. 131 (6) (1997) 888–893.

[12] M. Miura, H. Ohki, T. Tsuchihashi, H. Yamagishi, Y. Katada, K. Yamada, et al., Coronary risk factors in Kawasaki disease treated with additional gammaglobulin, Arch. Dis. Child. 89 (8) (2004) 776–780.

[13] K.S. Hsieh, K.P. Weng, C.C. Lin, T.C. Huang, C.L. Lee, S.M. Huang, Treatment of acute Kawasaki disease: aspirin's role in the febrile stage revisited, Pediatrics 114 (6) (2004) e689–e693.

[14] C. Manlhiot, L.R. Brandao, Z. Somji, A.L. Chesney, C. MacDonald, R.C. Gurofsky, et al., Long-term anticoagulation in Kawasaki disease: initial use of low molecular weight heparin is a viable option for patients with severe coronary artery abnormalities, Pediatr. Cardiol. 31 (6) (2010) 834–842.

[15] M. Ishii, T. Ueno, T. Akagi, K. Baba, K. Harada, K. Hamaoka, et al., Guidelines for catheter intervention in coronary artery lesion in Kawasaki disease, Pediatr. Int. 43 (5) (2001) 558–562.

[16] H. Muta, M. Ishii, Percutaneous coronary intervention versus coronary artery bypass grafting for stenotic lesions after Kawasaki disease, J. Pediatr. 157 (1) (2010) 120–126.

[17] R.L. Click, D.R. Holmes Jr., R.E. Vlietstra, A.S. Kosinski, R.A. Kronmal, Anomalous coronary arteries: location, degree of atherosclerosis and effect on survival–a report from the coronary artery surgery study, J. Am. Coll. Cardiol. 13 (3) (1989) 531–537.

[18] R.M. Donaldson, M.J. Raphael, M.H. Yacoub, D.N. Ross, Hemodynamically significant anomalies of the coronary arteries. Surgical aspects, Thorac. Cardiovasc. Surg. 30 (1) (1982) 7–13.

[19] W.C. Roberts, Major anomalies of coronary arterial origin seen in adulthood, Am. Heart J. 111 (5) (1986) 941–963.

[20] D.H. King, D.A. Danford, J.C. Huhta, H.P. Gutgesell, Noninvasive detection of anomalous origin of the left main coronary artery from the pulmonary trunk by pulsed Doppler echocardiography, Am. J. Cardiol. 55 (5) (1985) 608–609.

[21] R.R. Grace, P. Angelini, D.A. Cooley, Aortic implantation of anomalous left coronary artery arising from pulmonary artery, Am. J. Cardiol. 39 (4) (1977) 609–613.

[22] Z. Jin, F. Berger, F. Uhlemann, C. Schroder, R. Hetzer, V. Alexi-Meskhishvili, et al., Improvement in left ventricular dysfunction after aortic reimplantation in 11 consecutive paediatric patients with anomalous origin of the left coronary artery from the pulmonary artery. Early results of a serial echocardiographic follow-up, Eur. Heart J. 15 (8) (1994) 1044–1049.

[23] M.L. Schwartz, R.A. Jonas, S.D. Colan, Anomalous origin of left coronary artery from pulmonary artery: recovery of left ventricular function after dual coronary repair, J. Am. Coll. Cardiol. 30 (2) (1997) 547–553.
[24] T. Shibata, S. Kawakami, T. Noguchi, T. Tanaka, Y. Asaumi, T. Kanaya, et al., Prevalence, clinical features, and prognosis of acute myocardial infarction attributable to coronary artery embolism, Circulation 132 (4) (2015) 241–250.
[25] A. Jungbluth, R. Erbel, H. Darius, H.J. Rumpelt, J. Meyer, Paradoxical coronary embolism: case report and review of the literature, Am. Heart J. 116 (3) (1988) 879–885.
[26] N. Carano, A. Agnetti, D.J. Hagler, B. Tchana, U. Squarcia, S. Bernasconi, Acute myocardial infarction in a child: possible pathogenic role of patent foramen ovale associated with heritable thrombophilia, Pediatrics 114 (2) (2004) e255–e258.
[27] R. Crump, A.H. Shandling, B. Van Natta, M. Ellestad, Prevalence of patent foramen ovale in patients with acute myocardial infarction and angiographically normal coronary arteries, Am. J. Cardiol. 85 (11) (2000) 1368–1370.
[28] J.H. Chun, S.C. Lee, H.C. Gwon, S.H. Lee, K.P. Hong, J.D. Seo, et al., Left main coronary artery dissection after blunt chest trauma presented as acute anterior myocardial infarction: assessment by intravascular ultrasound: a case report, J. Korean Med. Sci. 13 (3) (1998) 325–327.
[29] D. Leong, M. Brown, Blunt traumatic dissection of the proximal left anterior descending artery, Emerg. Med. J. 23 (12) (2006) e67.
[30] Y. Sato, N. Matsumoto, S. Komatsu, S. Matsuo, T. Kunimasa, S. Yoda, et al., Coronary artery dissection after blunt chest trauma: depiction at multidetector-row computed tomography, Int. J. Cardiol. 118 (1) (2007) 108–110.
[31] F. Alfonso, E. Canales, G. Aleong, Spontaneous coronary artery dissection: diagnosis by optical coherence tomography, Eur. Heart J. 30 (3) (2009) 385.
[32] J.R. Arnold, N.E. West, W.J. van Gaal, T.D. Karamitsos, A.P. Banning, The role of intravascular ultrasound in the management of spontaneous coronary artery dissection, Cardiovasc. Ultrasound 6 (2008) 24.
[33] R. Sarmento-Leite, P.R. Machado, S.L. Garcia, Spontaneous coronary artery dissection: stent it or wait for healing? Heart 89 (2) (2003) 164.
[34] G. Vanzetto, E. Berger-Coz, G. Barone-Rochette, O. Chavanon, H. Bouvaist, R. Hacini, et al., Prevalence, therapeutic management and medium-term prognosis of spontaneous coronary artery dissection: results from a database of 11,605 patients, Eur. J. Cardiothorac. Surg. 35 (2) (2009) 250–254.
[35] C.J. Vrints, Spontaneous coronary artery dissection, Heart 96 (10) (2010) 801–808.
[36] A. Roth, U. Elkayam, Acute myocardial infarction associated with pregnancy, J. Am. Coll. Cardiol. 52 (3) (2008) 171–180.
[37] A.C. Borczuk, K.H. van Hoeven, S.M. Factor, Review and hypothesis: the eosinophil and peripartum heart disease (myocarditis and coronary artery dissection)–coincidence or pathogenetic significance? Cardiovasc. Res. 33 (3) (1997) 527–532.
[38] F.Q. Almeda, S. Barkatullah, C.J. Kavinsky, Spontaneous coronary artery dissection, Clin. Cardiol. 27 (7) (2004) 377–380.
[39] J.W. Olin, B.A. Sealove, Diagnosis, management, and future developments of fibromuscular dysplasia, J. Vasc. Surg. 53 (3) (2011) 826–836 e1.
[40] R. Estepa, N. Gallego, L. Orte, E. Puras, E. Aracil, J. Ortuno, Renovascular hypertension in children, Scand. J. Urol. Nephrol. 35 (5) (2001) 388–392.
[41] J.W. Olin, M.R. Piedmonte, J.R. Young, S. DeAnna, M. Grubb, M.B. Childs, The utility of duplex ultrasound scanning of the renal arteries for diagnosing significant renal artery stenosis, Ann. Intern. Med. 122 (11) (1995) 833–838.
[42] R. Sabharwal, P. Vladica, P. Coleman, Multidetector spiral CT renal angiography in the diagnosis of renal artery fibromuscular dysplasia, Eur. J. Radiol. 61 (3) (2007) 520–527.
[43] G.B. Vasbinder, P.J. Nelemans, A.G. Kessels, A.A. Kroon, J.H. Maki, T. Leiner, et al., Accuracy of computed tomographic angiography and magnetic resonance angiography for diagnosing renal artery stenosis, Ann. Intern. Med. 141 (9) (2004) 674–682 Discussion 82.
[44] A. van der Graaf, H.J. Avis, D.M. Kusters, M.N. Vissers, B.A. Hutten, J.C. Defesche, et al., Molecular basis of autosomal dominant hypercholesterolemia: assessment in a large cohort of hypercholesterolemic children, Circulation 123 (11) (2011) 1167–1173.
[45] R. Minhas, S.E. Humphries, N. Qureshi, H.A. Neil, N.G.D. Group, Controversies in familial hypercholesterolaemia: recommendations of the NICE guideline development group for the identification and management of familial hypercholesterolaemia, Heart 95 (7) (2009) 584–587 Discussion 7–91.
[46] D.J. Rader, J. Cohen, H.H. Hobbs, Monogenic hypercholesterolemia: new insights in pathogenesis and treatment, J. Clin. Investig. 111 (12) (2003) 1795–1803.
[47] P. Jones, S. Kafonek, I. Laurora, D. Hunninghake, Comparative dose efficacy study of atorvastatin versus simvastatin, pravastatin, lovastatin, and fluvastatin in patients with hypercholesterolemia (the CURVES study), Am. J. Cardiol. 81 (5) (1998) 582–587.
[48] T.J. Smilde, S. van Wissen, H. Wollersheim, M.D. Trip, J.J. Kastelein, A.F. Stalenhoef, Effect of aggressive versus conventional lipid lowering on atherosclerosis progression in familial hypercholesterolaemia (ASAP): a prospective, randomised, double-blind trial, Lancet 357 (9256) (2001) 577–581.

Chapter 25

Chronic Heart Failure in Congenital Heart Disease Including Single Ventricle Circulation

David N. Rosenthal
Stanford University, Palo Alto, CA, United States

INTRODUCTION

Mortality associated with surgical repair of congenital heart disease has improved remarkably over the past 75 years. In the current era, surgical mortality in pediatric cardiovascular centers approaches 4.1%, and virtually all forms of congenital heart disease have a defined surgical approach [1]. As there are approximately 32,000 infants with congenital heart disease born annually in the United States, there is now a large and expanding population of children and adults with repaired congenital cardiac lesions [2]. However, because of complexities of the initial cardiac anatomy, residual pathology, and multiple derangements in cardiac physiology, up to 50% of this population suffers from chronic heart failure [3]. Heart failure, in turn, is responsible for up to 40% of observed mortality attributable to congenital heart disease [4,5]. Treatment for heart failure associated with congenital heart disease remains challenging, with few validated therapies. Further investigation into this area is of great importance.

For patients with biventricular forms of congenital heart disease, the general clinical picture of heart failure bears many similarities to heart failure, because it is commonly manifested in adults with ischemic and dilated cardiomyopathy. Given that 75 million US adults have Stage A heart failure, our understanding of heart failure naturally stems from this population [6]. From this vantage point, heart failure can be understood as a clinical syndrome that typically arises from myocardial dysfunction and manifests with venous congestion of either the pulmonary or systemic circulation, or both, and reduced systemic cardiac output [7]. In children with biventricular congenital heart disease, the etiologies of heart failure are extremely heterogeneous and differ greatly from the typical adult heart failure patient, but the end-stage physiology is fairly similar between these populations.

For patients with univentricular forms of heart disease, on the other hand, the circulatory abnormalities are so profound as to complicate even the use of the term "heart failure." It can reasonably be argued that all patients who have completed the Fontan palliation for univentricular anatomy (total cavopulmonary connection) are in chronic heart failure. In this chapter, the term "Fontan circulatory syndrome" will be used to describe the circulatory physiology that accompanies the Fontan operation, and the term "heart failure" is used to describe the components of this physiology that arise from the heart itself. This is by no means a standard or widely accepted terminology, and there is no consistent usage in the relevant literature. Whatever the terminology, it is important to distinguish the circulatory abnormalities from those that arise more directly from the heart, as there are important implications for both treatment and prognosis.

BIVENTRICULAR CONGENITAL HEART DISEASE

Etiology of Heart Failure

Chronic heart failure associated with congenital heart disease may have features of either congestion (systemic venous, pulmonary venous, or both) or low cardiac output. The large number of possible specific anatomic diagnoses may be consolidated into a small number of underlying pathophysiologic categories, as shown in Table 25.1. These include lesions associated with volume and pressure overload. In both circumstances, heart failure may develop from the volume or pressure overload, whereas the underlying myocardium remains normal, or there may be secondary myocardial dysfunction resulting from the pressure/volume abnormalities, contributing further to heart failure. It is important to note that a given anatomic lesion may present with features of more than one of the pathophysiologic variants, such as an atrioventricular

Heart Failure in the Child and Young Adult. http://dx.doi.org/10.1016/B978-0-12-802393-8.00025-9

TABLE 25.1 Common Heart Failure Etiologies in Congenital Heart Disease

Volume Overload
Left-to-right Shunt
Atrial septal defect
Atrioventricular canal defect
Patent ductus arteriosus
Ventricular septal defect
Valvular Insufficiency
Aortic
Mitral
Pulmonary
Tricuspid
Pressure Overload
Left sided
Aortic stenosis
Coarctation of the aorta
Right sided
Pulmonic stenosis

canal defect, which may have volume loading from left-to-right shunting in combination with volume loading from atrioventricular valve regurgitation.

Volume overload due to left-to-right shunting lesions increases blood return from the lungs, which leads to distension of the left ventricle. Early on, intrinsic myocardial contractility is maintained, and because of the Frank–Starling principle, the net ejection fraction is often increased. This is accomplished via elevation in left ventricular filling pressure, and in left atrial pressure, which leads to pulmonary edema and altered respiratory mechanics. With modest degrees of shunting, cardiac output is maintained, but with more severe lesions, or if there is a superimposed myocardial disease, there may be compromise in the cardiac output, as only a fraction of the left ventricular output is actually delivered to the systemic circulation. Right-to-left shunting is neither typically associated with volume overload, nor with heart failure as a direct consequence of shunting. Rather, the manifestation of right-to-left shunting is cyanosis.

Volume overload may also result from valvular insufficiency. In the case of mitral or aortic insufficiency, the volume load is delivered to the left ventricle, with manifestations similar to those of left-to-right shunting. When the tricuspid or pulmonary valve is involved, the volume load influences the right-sided structures, leading to increased systemic venous pressure, with congestive findings in the hepatic, intestinal, and renal systems. Additionally, with any valvular insufficiency, a low cardiac output may ensue in severe cases.

Pressure overload may be found in either the right or left side of the circulation due to obstruction of blood flow at any of several levels in the circulation. Depending on the level of obstruction, heart failure symptoms may develop as a direct consequence of the lesion (e.g., mitral stenosis resulting in elevated left atrial pressure) or via an altered myocardial ejection (e.g., coarctation of the aorta).

In addition to these lesions, there are also congenital lesions associated with heart failure due to primary systolic or diastolic dysfunction of the myocardium, in the absence of shunt lesions or pressure overload. These include restrictive cardiomyopathy, in which diastolic function is impaired, or hypertrophic cardiomyopathy, also primarily a lesion of diastolic dysfunction, but occasionally of systolic failure [8]. Additionally, dilated cardiomyopathy is found in children as in adults. These lesions are discussed elsewhere.

Lesions in which the right ventricle functions in the systemic circulation are particularly prone to myocardial dysfunction, particularly systolic dysfunction. These lesions include congenitally corrected transposition of the great arteries or transposition of the great arteries that was surgically repaired by atrial switch. The incidence of heart failure following the atrial switch procedure is approximately 20% [9–11]. Heart failure with a systemic right ventricle is frequently due to a combination of myocardial dysfunction and tricuspid valve regurgitation leading to superimposed volume load.

Clinical Features

The features of heart failure are shaped by both underlying etiology and age. With respect to etiology, the specific lesion will determine whether there is elevation of right atrial pressure, left atrial pressure, or both. This determines the symptoms of heart failure, because left atrial hypertension will lead to tachypnea and limited oral intake leading to failure to thrive, whereas right atrial hypertension is more likely to lead to an impaired appetite and abdominal pain (and thereby to failure to thrive as well), but will not have tachypnea as a dominant feature.

Tachypnea is particularly common in infants with heart failure, occurring in 62% of one series of infants [12]. Tachypnea is seen in more than half of infants with left-to-right shunts, regardless of heart failure, as a result of reduced tidal volume, reduced pulmonary compliance, and increased airway resistance [13].

In older children, heart failure is more commonly associated with gastrointestinal symptoms such as abdominal pain, nausea, vomiting, or a diminished appetite [12]. In a significant minority of children, gastrointestinal symptoms are the only recognized finding at the time of diagnosis of heart failure. Surprisingly, in all age groups, fluid overload is seldom recognized.

Failure to thrive is frequently the most important morbidity from heart failure in children, whether the heart failure is from congenital heart disease or some other etiology. Heart failure is associated with reduced oral intake mediated through both respiratory and gastrointestinal symptoms. This results in a calorie deficit that impairs growth [14]. Failure to thrive due to heart failure is a frequent indication for surgical repair in congenital heart disease.

Diagnostic Assessment of Heart Failure

The initial assessment of heart failure in children with congenital heart disease consists of a detailed medical history to characterize the specific symptoms, coupled with a physical examination focused on peripheral perfusion, and findings of congestion. Although it was developed for adults, the use of heart failure hemodynamic profiles can be readily applied to children as well [15]. In this approach, patients are evaluated with respect to the presence or absence of perfusion, and for adequacy of peripheral perfusion. This results in a 2×2 grid in which patients can be classified into four groups: Cold/Wet, Cold/Dry, Warm/Wet, and Warm/Dry.

The severity of heart failure due to congenital heart disease can be graded using several scales, including the Ross Heart Failure Classification [16]. The Ross score is analogous to the New York Heart Failure score, ranging from I (no symptoms) to IV (symptoms present at rest).

For heart failure due to congenital heart disease, assessment of heart failure, as described previously, should be accompanied by an investigation into the specific anatomy and pathophysiology of the congenital lesion. This is most readily accomplished by echocardiography, which provides both anatomic and functional information. At times, invasive measurements of hemodynamics may be required to delineate the cardiac lesion more completely. This is more likely to be needed when there are specific questions concerning pulmonary vascular resistance or diastolic filling pressures, which can be difficult to estimate using echocardiography.

Treatment Options

The treatment of heart failure associated with congenital heart disease is lesion-specific, and a complete description of the options for each lesion is beyond the scope of this section. However, some general principles can be elucidated. Treatment options typically include medical therapies, nonsurgical interventions such as transcatheter devices, and cardiac surgery.

For unrepaired congenital heart lesions for which a definitive surgical procedure exists, medical therapy is most commonly employed as a temporary measure to improve surgical candidacy. For example, an infant with atrioventricular canal defect can undergo surgical repair with good results, but delaying surgery for several months probably reduces surgical risk. Diuretics and nutritional support may help to achieve this delay while maintaining adequate muscle mass and overall strength to facilitate good convalescence from surgery. For lesions where surgical outcomes are less satisfactory, there may be a balance between medical management and surgical repair for which disease severity, surgical outcome, and efficacy of medical therapy all factor into decision making. Finally, surgical therapy and transcatheter therapy are an ever-evolving area, in which the two approaches ideally complement each other to broaden the range of available options while optimizing procedure outcomes. Transcatheter closure of atrial septal defect is an example of this, where a progressively large proportion of atrial septal defects is amenable to transcatheter closure as the field matures.

Medical therapy of heart failure in congenital heart disease may be the sole option remaining, should there be significant residual disease after surgical repair. There is a severe deficit of knowledge regarding efficacy of heart failure medication in this circumstance, and extrapolation from adult clinical trial results is fraught with uncertainty, although it is commonly performed in clinical practice. For lesions with volume overload but presumably normal myocardium, diuretic therapy to reduce congestive symptoms is thought to be useful. Neurohumoral blockade of the adrenergic and renin–angiotensin systems is often used to treat failing left ventricles in children, with equivocal results from clinical trials [17,18]. A recent multicenter guideline document provides detailed recommendations of medication use in children with heart failure, including those with congenital heart disease [19]. For the failing systemic right ventricle, the optimal approach is not known. For the failing systemic left ventricle, medications useful to adults with heart failure (angiotensin-converting enzyme inhibitors, beta blockers, and aldosterone blockers) are thought to have a reasonable likelihood of efficacy.

UNIVENTRICULAR CONGENITAL HEART DISEASE

Introduction

Heart failure in the patient with a univentricular heart is not a singular entity. Inasmuch as the fundamental circulation is altered radically by the surgical palliation at each stage, so too is the form of heart failure dependent on the stage of palliation. For this reason, each surgical stage will be discussed separately.

Shunted Stage

Clinical Features

Before surgery, the patient with a univentricular heart may have a reasonable balance of pulmonary and systemic blood flow or may have excessive flow to one compartment at the expense of the other. The initial palliation of the univentricular heart aims to provide a balanced degree of left-to-right shunt, so as to permit tolerable levels of cyanosis coupled with adequate systemic blood flow. This goal may be difficult to achieve and most neonates with shunt physiology have some degree of heart failure associated with the volume load of a left-to-right shunt. As with volume loading in the biventricular congenital heart lesion, this is frequently associated with elevated left atrial pressure, respiratory symptoms, and failure to thrive. Complicating factors may include atrioventricular valve insufficiency that exacerbates the volume load or myocardial dysfunction associated with coronary hypoperfusion.

Treatment Options

Management options for heart failure in these circumstances are limited. Appropriate balancing of systemic and pulmonary circulation is critical to controlling heart failure. Diuretics are an important tool in managing the severity of left atrial hypertension and nutritional support with enteral tube feeding may help the patient to overcome some of the consequences of volume loading to achieve adequate caloric intake despite respiratory insufficiency. In the end, the "definitive" management of heart failure associated with shunt physiology consists of altering the underlying physiology by advancing to the next stage of palliation.

Bidirectional Cavopulmonary Connection Stage

Clinical Features

The Glenn operation, or the bidirectional cavopulmonary connection, is performed to remove the volume load from the circulation. Following the bidirectional cavopulmonary connection, there is no longer a significant left-to-right volume overload, and therefore the primary source of heart failure in the univentricular shunted circulation is resolved. In most instances, heart failure is therefore not a prominent feature of the patient with the bidirectional cavopulmonary connection. However, in a subset of patients who undergo this operation, there may be persistent atrioventricular or semilunar valve insufficiency or myocardial dysfunction even after the circulatory revision. In such cases, there will also be persistent findings of heart failure, with respiratory symptoms and failure to thrive as the most common manifestations of heart failure. As with biventricular heart failure, the severity of symptoms is variable. The obligatory cyanosis that arises from the bidirectional cavopulmonary connection often limits exertional capability for patients at this stage, which may confound the assessment of heart failure severity. Distinguishing the relative contribution of heart failure and cyanosis is a matter of clinical judgment.

Treatment Options

The treatment of heart failure associated with the Glenn shunt is largely derived from the underlying cause of the heart failure, although it should be emphasized that there are minimal data to support any particular approach. If heart failure symptoms arise from volume load due to valvular insufficiency, diuretic therapy is a reasonable option to consider. If there is systolic dysfunction of a systemic left ventricle, then consideration may be given to neurohumoral blockade using angiotensin-converting enzyme inhibitors, beta blockers, and aldosterone blockers. The efficacy of this approach is unknown.

Total Cavopulmonary Connection Stage

Clinical Features

Following the bidirectional cavopulmonary connection, the Fontan operation, or total cavopulmonary connection, is the next planned palliative step for patients with a univentricular heart. The physiology following the total cavopulmonary connection is unlike any other circulatory derangement and is markedly different from that which prevails after the bidirectional Glenn [20]. In brief, the Fontan circulation is characterized by a circulatory bottleneck at the level of the pulmonary vasculature due to the absence of a right heart pump. This leads to an obligatory elevation in systemic venous pressure, to drive blood through the pulmonary bed and to a reduction in the cardiac output due to an inability to fully compensate for the absence of a right heart pump.

This combination of elevated systemic venous pressure and reduced cardiac output leads to a Fontan circulatory syndrome that bears a strong similarity to heart failure. Whether it should be termed heart failure is currently an unresolved definitional issue, but for the purposes of this section, the distinction will be made between the Fontan circulatory syndrome, which is a nearly obligatory feature of the Fontan circulation, and heart failure, which is the result of altered heart function (including systolic dysfunction, diastolic dysfunction, and abnormal valvular function). As heart failure in a Fontan patient may serve to amplify the consequences of the Fontan circulatory syndrome, this may seem to be a distinction without a difference. However, when one considers the approach to treatment, the distinction becomes important.

The Fontan circulatory syndrome has been thoroughly described even if it remains imperfectly understood [21]. Among the most important consequences are the injuries to which the liver is subjected, which include both ischemic damage and fibrosis. Involvement of the liver is extremely common and increases with the passage of time, although the injuries are often subclinical for a prolonged interval. Ascites is common, whereas synthetic function is typically preserved until the disease is very severe. Hepatic fibrosis is found in nearly all Fontan survivors [21,22].

The lymphatic system is frequently impaired by the Fontan circulation, with consequences of luminal protein loss. In the intestines, this is manifest as protein-losing enteropathy and carries a very high burden of morbidity and mortality [23,24]. Lymphatic overflow into the bronchial tree produces plastic bronchitis, also a highly morbid condition. Knowledge of these conditions is limited by a deficiency in diagnostic approaches to the lymphatic system, which has, to some degree, been improved recently with novel MRI techniques.

These toxicities are by no means the only consequences of the Fontan circulation, but they represent the most important and best-understood entities. Lymphopenia, bone demineralization, and thromboembolic events have also been described, although their relationship to the circulatory abnormalities of the total cavopulmonary connection is not clearly defined [21].

Patients who have undergone the total cavopulmonary connection are also at risk of developing heart failure as defined previously. This may stem from intrinsic anatomic risk factors and prior cardiovascular surgery that may entail residual anatomic disease. Heart failure may serve to worsen the Fontan circulatory syndrome, bring a subclinical problem to view, or produce independent heart failure problems such as renal dysfunction, poor oral intake, fluid overload, etc. Because of the obligatory elevation in systemic venous pressure above pulmonary venous pressure, it is less common to have primary respiratory congestive symptoms in a total cavopulmonary connection patient with heart failure, although it is occasionally seen, particularly in conjunction with systemic venous congestive symptoms.

Treatment Options

Specific complications related to the Fontan circulatory syndrome rarely have definitive treatments, but occasionally can be improved with targeted therapies. Recent data suggest that plastic bronchitis can be improved by interventional techniques that occlude specific lymphatic channels that drain into the bronchi [25,26]. Long-term results of this approach are unknown. Protein-losing enteropathy has been treated with a number of medications, with occasional success [23].

General treatment options to counteract the Fontan circulatory syndrome are limited. Although one might expect diuresis to reduce the systemic venous pressure and provide benefit, there are no clinical data to support this approach. From a theoretical perspective, diuresis might be as likely to exacerbate low output symptoms as to improve congestive symptoms. Likewise, afterload reduction is unproven, despite several small studies that have attempted to show physiologic benefits from the use of enalapril or sildenafil [27,28]. Fenestration of the total cavopulmonary connection to permit a controlled right-to-left shunt is fairly well studied in acute settings and does lead to improved cardiac output. In chronic settings, fenestration may lead to resolution of plastic bronchitis and protein-losing enteropathy, with the limiting factor being the ability to tolerate the cyanosis produced by this approach.

The most drastic remedy for the Fontan circulatory syndrome is to remove the Fontan circulation. This can be done by a surgical takedown of the total cavopulmonary connection to a shunted circulation or to a bidirectional cavopulmonary shunt [29]. These solutions are limited in applicability by the intrinsic drawbacks of the alternative circulations. Transition to a truly biventricular circulation can be achieved via heart transplantation. This is anatomically feasible in most patients but is technically complex and carries a higher perioperative risk than heart transplantation in a cardiomyopathy patient. Survival after heart transplantation in this circumstance is 70% at 3 years [30,31]. Use of transplantation is limited by donor availability.

SUMMARY

Heart failure is a common occurrence in many different forms of congenital heart disease and is an important contributor to both morbidity and mortality. Heart failure in this setting is characterized by a very broad range of anatomic substrate and diverse etiologies. Conventional treatment for heart failure in dilated cardiomyopathy is unproven in this situation and frequently seems to target a different pathophysiology, particularly for the problem of heart and circulatory failure in the Fontan patient.

REFERENCES

[1] J.P. Jacobs, et al., Variation in outcomes for risk-stratified pediatric cardiac surgical operations: an analysis of the STS congenital heart surgery database, ATS 94 (2012) 564–572.

[2] R.M. Simeone, et al., CDC grand rounds: understanding the causes of major birth defects — steps to prevention, Morb. Mortal. Wkly. Rep. 64 (2015) 1104–1107.

[3] K.K. Stout, et al., Chronic heart failure in congenital heart disease: a scientific statement from the American Heart Association, Circulation 133 (2016) 770–801.

[4] H.P. Nieminen, E.V. Jokinen, H.I. Sairanen, Causes of late deaths after pediatric cardiac surgery. A population-based study, J. Am. Coll. Cardiol. 50 (2007) 1263–1271.

[5] E.N. Oechslin, D.A. Harrison, M.S. Connelly, G.D. Webb, S.C. Siu, Mode of death in adults with congenital heart disease, Am. J. Cardiol. 86 (2000) 1111–1116.

[6] L.C. Kovell, S.P. Juraschek, S.D. Russell, A.M. Chamberlain, Stage a heart failure is not adequately recognized in US adults: analysis of the national health and nutrition examination surveys, 2007–2010, PLoS One 10 (2015) 2007–2010.

[7] K.F. Adams, et al., Executive summary: HFSA 2006 comprehensive heart failure practice guideline, J. Card. Fail. 12 (2006) 10–38.

[8] B.J. Maron, et al., Hypertrophic cardiomyopathy in children, adolescents, and young adults associated with low cardiovascular mortality with contemporary management strategies, Circulation 133 (2016) 62–73.

[9] S. Piran, G. Veldtman, S. Siu, G.D. Webb, P.P. Liu, Heart failure and ventricular dysfunction in patients with single or systemic right ventricles, Circulation 105 (2002) 1189–1194.

[10] D. Sarkar, et al., Comparison of long-term outcomes of atrial repair of simple transposition with implications for a late arterial switch strategy, Circulation 100 (1999) II176–II181.

[11] N.J. Wilson, et al., Long-term outcome after the mustard repair for simple transposition of the great arteries: 28-year follow-up, J. Am. Coll. Cardiol. 32 (1998) 758–765.

[12] S.A. Hollander, et al., Abdominal complaints as a common first presentation of heart failure in adolescents with dilated cardiomyopathy, Am. J. Emerg. Med. 31 (2013) 684–686.

[13] R. Buchhorn, A. Hammersen, D. Bartmus, J. Bursch, The pathogenesis of heart failure in infants with congenital heart disease, Cardiol. Young 11 (2001) 498–504.

[14] A. Mehrizi, A. Drash, Growth disturbance in congenital heart disease, J. Pediatr. 61 (1962) 418–429.

[15] A. Nohria, et al., Clinical assessment identifies hemodynamic profiles that predict outcomes in patients admitted with heart failure, J. Am. Coll. Cardiol. 41 (2003) 1797–1804.

[16] R.D. Ross, et al., Plasma norepinephrine levels in infants and children with congestive heart failure, Am. J. Cardiol. 59 (1987) 911–914.

[17] A.B. Lewis, M. Chabot, The effect of treatment with angiotensin-converting enzyme inhibitors on survival of pediatric patients with dilated cardiomyopathy, Pediatr. Cardiol. 14 (1993) 9–12.

[18] R. Shaddy, et al., Carvedilol for children and adolescents with heart failure, JAMA 298 (2007) 1171–1179.

[19] R. Kirk, et al., The International Society for Heart and Lung Transplantation Guidelines for the management of pediatric heart failure: executive summary, J. Hear. Lung Transplant. 33 (2014) 888–909.

[20] M. Gewillig, S.C. Brown, The Fontan circulation after 45 years: update in physiology, Heart (2016). http://dx.doi.org/10.1136/heartjnl-2015-307467.

[21] J. Rychik, The relentless effects of the fontan paradox, Semin. Thorac. Cardiovasc. Surg. 19 (2016) 37–43.

[22] J. Rychik, et al., End-organ consequences of the Fontan operation: liver fibrosis, protein-losing enteropathy and plastic bronchitis, Cardiol. Young 23 (2013) 831–840.

[23] A.S. John, et al., Clinical outcomes and improved survival in patients with protein-losing enteropathy after the fontan operation, J. Am. Coll. Cardiol. 64 (2014) 54–62.

[24] L. Mertens, D.J. Hagler, U. Sauer, J. Somerville, M. Gewillig, Protein-losing enteropathy after the Fontan operation: an international multicenter study, J. Thorac. Cardiovasc. Surg. 115 (1998) 1063–1073.

[25] Y. Dori, M.S. Keller, J. Rychik, M. Itkin, Successful treatment of plastic bronchitis by selective lymphatic embolization in a Fontan patient, Pediatrics 134 (2014) e590–e595.

[26] Y. Dori, et al., Percutaneous lymphatic embolization of abnormal pulmonary lymphatic flow as treatment of plastic bronchitis in patients with congenital heart disease, Circulation 133 (2016) 1160–1170.

[27] A.A. Kouatli, J.A. Garcia, T.M. Zellers, E.M. Weinstein, L. Mahony, Enalapril does not enhance exercise capacity in patients after Fontan procedure, 96 (1997) 1507–1512.

[28] A. Van De Bruaene, et al., Sildenafil improves exercise hemodynamics in fontan patients, Circ. Cardiovasc. Imaging 7 (2014) 265–273.

[29] J.P. van Melle, et al., Surgical options after Fontan failure, Heart (2016) 1127–1133, http://dx.doi.org/10.1136/heartjnl-2015-309235.

[30] D. Bernstein, et al., Outcome of listing for cardiac transplantation for failed Fontan: a multi-institutional study, Circulation 114 (2006) 273–280.

[31] K.R. Schumacher, et al., Fontan-associated protein-losing enteropathy and heart transplant: a Pediatric Heart Transplant Study analysis, J. Hear. Lung Transplant. 34 (2015) 1–8.

Chapter 26

Heart Failure in Adults With Congenital Heart Disease

Luke J. Burchill[1], Heather J. Ross[2], Alexander R. Opotowsky[3,4]

[1]Oregon Health and Science University, Portland, OR, United States; [2]University Health Network, Toronto, ON, Canada; [3]Boston Children's Hospital, Boston, MA, United States; [4]Brigham and Women's Hospital, Boston, MA, United States

INTRODUCTION

The number of adults living with congenital heart disease (CHD) is growing and this growing population is aging. The incidence of heart failure (HF) increases with age and constitutes the most common cause of death in these patients. Some adults with CHD present with typical findings for HF, while others exhibit disease-specific manifestations. As such, it is not a trivial task to define exactly what constitutes HF in adults with CHD. This challenge, along with the marked heterogeneity in both underlying disease and management, has served to limit progress in understanding the epidemiology and optimal treatment. This chapter reviews the current understanding of HF in adults with CHD, with specific comment on diagnoses most strongly associated with premature HF.

EPIDEMIOLOGY

Lower infant mortality and improved survival throughout childhood and adolescence have led to a rapidly growing population of adults with congenital heart disease (CHD). There are more than 1 million adults with CHD in the United States, growing by an estimated 50,000 people per year [1–3]. Adults now outnumber children living with CHD [2], placing the onus of care on clinicians with expertise in diagnosing and managing adult onset complications including heart failure (HF). Determining the prevalence of HF in adult congenital heart disease (ACHD) is a challenge in the absence of a consensus definition for HF in this population and also because many younger patients do not exhibit overt clinical HF until late in their disease trajectory. Yet adverse myocardial remodeling [4] and neurohormonal activation [5] are common and frequently progress over time. In parallel with a rapid rise in all types of ACHD hospitalizations, there has been an 80% increase in the number of ACHD-related HF hospitalizations over the last decade [6]. Among those with ACHD who require hospitalization, 20% have a diagnosis of HF [7]. Once hospitalized for HF ACHD patients are at increased risk of dying, with an in-hospital mortality of 4% [7].

The rapid rise in ACHD-related HF hospitalizations reflects not only an expanded ACHD population but also an increasing number of patients with more complex or severe forms of CHD surviving to adulthood. Over the last decade, the prevalence of severe CHD increased by 62% in adults [8]. Compared to adults with other forms of heart disease in whom HF hospitalizations peak after age 70, the burden of HF hospitalizations in ACHD is spread evenly across all age groups (Fig. 26.1). ACHD subgroups at highest risk of HF are those with systemic right or single ventricles [9], with clinical evidence of HF in 20%–40% [10]. Further, ACHD HF patients are often medically complex with a high prevalence of pulmonary hypertension and arrhythmias both of which further increase HF hospitalization and mortality risk [7].

Cardiovascular events are the most common mode of death in ACHD, and these events are often secondary to HF [12,13]. Cross-sectional studies from large referral centers have been important for understanding ACHD HF mortality. In a study of 2600 patients followed at the Toronto Congenital Cardiac Center for Adults between 1981 and 1996, there were 199 deaths occurring at a mean age of 37±15 years. Mortality was highest in patients with complex CHD including single or systemic right ventricle or Eisenmenger syndrome [12]. HF was the primary cause of death in 21%. Among 1000 patients followed at the Mayo Clinic between 1987 and 1995, 53 died at a mean age of 40.6±14 years. In this series, HF was the cause of death in 13% of patients [14]. More recently, the Royal Brompton Hospital reported the cause of death in 6969 ACHD patients followed between 1991 and 2014 [15]. The median age of death was 47 years, somewhat older than the Toronto and Mayo Clinic patient cohorts. HF accounted for 42% of deaths, the cumulative incidence of HF deaths rising

Heart Failure in the Child and Young Adult. http://dx.doi.org/10.1016/B978-0-12-802393-8.00026-0

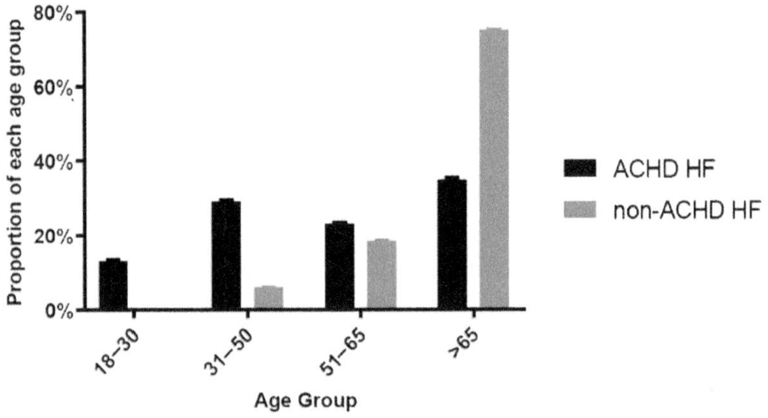

FIGURE 26.1 Age distribution of heart failure hospitalizations in non-ACHD versus ACHD patients admitted to United States acute care hospitals 1998–2011 [11]. *ACHD*, adult congenital heart disease; *HF*, heart failure.

sharply after age 40. Taken together, these studies identify HF as a common cause of death in ACHD and indicate that HF mortality is increasing in parallel with an aging ACHD population.

Evaluating circumstances of death in ACHD, the CONCOR Dutch National Registry Population reported one-quarter of patients dying secondary to HF [9]. An important insight from CONCOR was the identification of two distinct clinical profiles or HF subgroups within the ACHD population; the first comprises younger patients with complex CHD presenting with HF in early adulthood and the second includes older (age >75 years) patients with "simple" CHD such as atrial septal defects (ASD) presenting with HF associated with coronary and valvular heart disease [9]. The clinical profile of this second group is akin to HF seen in acquired heart disease populations. Just as the ACHD population incorporates anatomic and surgical subgroups it is becoming clearer that HF subgroups exist with clinical profiles that differ according to age, comorbidities, and underlying etiologies.

Further research is needed to better define the epidemiology of HF in ACHD although the emerging clinical picture is that of a condition that impacts ACHD patients across the life span with a mortality risk that rises with age and defect complexity.

GENERAL CONCEPTS, DEFINITION, AND CLASSIFICATION

The diagnosis of HF in the adult is usually considered in the context of a previously asymptomatic patient with a structurally normal heart. The American College of Cardiology/American Heart Association guidelines define HF as a clinical syndrome characterized by symptoms of dyspnea and fatigue, and signs of congestion (e.g., peripheral edema, rales), resulting from any structural or functional cardiac disorder [16]. This definition includes a broad array of clinical presentations such as systolic and diastolic ventricular dysfunction, left and right HF, as well as ischemic, nonischemic, and valvular HF syndromes. Despite this broad scope of patients with HF, the management recommendations for patients diagnosed with HF are most applicable to patients with acquired left heart disease, and almost entirely those with systolic dysfunction.

The manifestation of circulatory failure in ACHD patients is often quite different than standard HF symptoms and signs. ACHD patients are younger and remain asymptomatic despite severe ventricular dysfunction and reduced aerobic capacity. In single ventricle Fontan patients, diarrhea (protein-losing enteropathy) or coughing up casts (plastic bronchitis) may be the first manifestation of a failing circulation. The presentation in transposition patients seen after an atrial switch operation may be presyncope or worsening atrial arrhythmia.

The American College of Cardiology/American Heart Association further classifies HF into Stages A to D [16]. Stage A refers to patients at risk for HF but without apparent structural abnormalities (e.g., patients with hypertension). Stage B refers to those without symptoms but with some structural manifestation associated with HF (e.g., left ventricular (LV) hypertrophy). Stages C and D focus on patients with symptomatic HF. ACHD patients all have apparent structural disease, and therefore all have Stage B/C/D HF. According to guidelines, clinicians are encouraged to initiate and up-titrate angiotensin-converting enzyme inhibitors, beta blockers, and aldosterone antagonists in a stepwise manner leading to consideration of advanced therapies (inotropes, ventricular assist devices, heart transplant) in patients with refractory HF. Unfortunately, there are few data to support this recommendation, or any of these therapies, in ACHD patients and best practices must be cautiously extrapolated [17,18].

Neurohormonal modulation is a cornerstone of acquired HF. Invasive hemodynamic assessment is largely reserved for patients with progressive HF despite medical therapy or those who pose a diagnostic dilemma. The converse is the approach

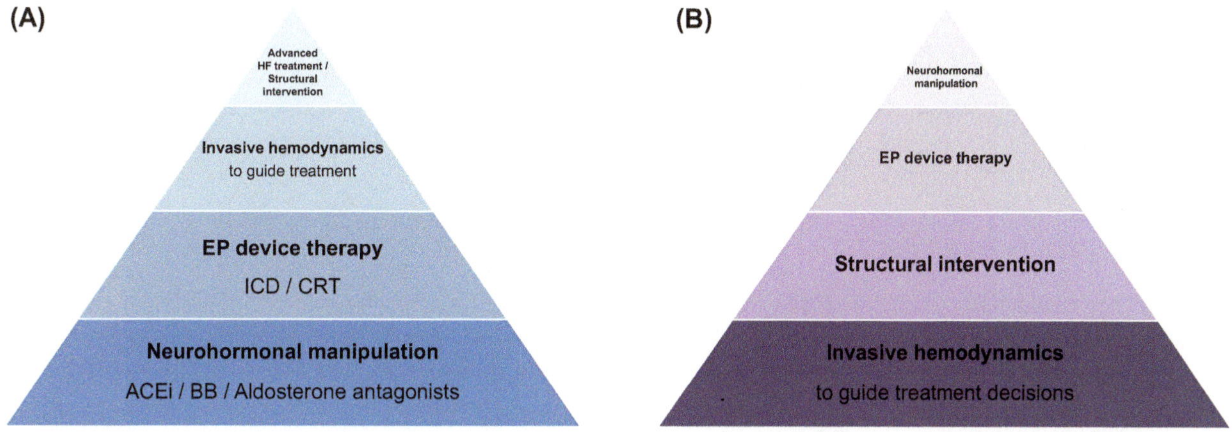

FIGURE 26.2 General paradigms of approach to heart failure in adults with (A) acquired heart disease and those with (B) congenital heart disease. *ACEi*, angiotensin-converting enzyme inhibitors; *ACHD*, adult congenital heart disease; *BB*, beta blockers; *CRT*, cardiac resynchronization therapy; *EP*, electrophysiology; *ICD*, implantable cardioverter defibrillator. *(With permission, J. McLarry, C. Broberg, A.R. Opotowsky, T. Kaufman, K. Stout, L.J. Burchill, Defining heart failure in adult congenital heart disease, Prog. Pediatr. Cardiol. 38 (1) (2014) 3–7.)*

to most ACHD diagnoses, with management focusing first on invasive hemodynamic assessment and structural (percutaneous or surgical) intervention to address apparent anatomic causes for symptoms (Fig. 26.2).

Much of the challenge in systematically studying, understanding, and caring for HF in ACHD rests in defining just who has HF and what that means. It is tempting to apply the impressive advances in medical and device therapy in acquired adult HF to ACHD patients. The diagnostic approach to and data for the care of symptomatic older adults with recent onset systolic LV dysfunction may, however, be applicable only to a small minority of ACHD patients.

HIGH-RISK GROUPS AND LESION-SPECIFIC FACTORS

ACHD subgroups at highest risk for developing HF are those with either tetralogy of Fallot (TOF), a systemic right ventricle, a single ventricle Fontan circulation, and those or Eisenmenger syndrome. While complex disease without repair or only palliated by systemic-to-pulmonary artery shunts are also at high risk of developing HF, these situations are increasingly rare and not discussed below.

TETRALOGY OF FALLOT

Corrective surgery in infants with TOF is associated with low operative mortality [20]. While early outcomes are excellent, HF risk steadily rises in adulthood. Several factors establish the foundations for late-onset HF including cyanosis, residual shunts from incomplete closure of ASD and ventricular septal defects (VSD), myocardial injury at the time of cardiopulmonary bypass or related to coronary injury, and adverse ventricular mechanics from patching of the right ventricular (RV) outflow tract. Additional factors associated with RV systolic dysfunction include RV pressure overload, conduction disturbances, subendocardial ischemia, and diffuse myocardial fibrosis. While all of these factors contribute to HF pathophysiology, in most patients it is pulmonary regurgitation that drives ventricular remodeling and HF. By promoting progressive RV dilation, pulmonary regurgitation can initiate a cycle in which tricuspid annular dilation leads to worsening tricuspid regurgitation, which exacerbates RV volume overload leading to RV systolic dysfunction, HF, tachyarrhythmias, and, in some cases, death. Among 137 adults with TOF seen 25 years after repair, features of HF were common including worse functional class [New York Heart Association (NYHA) Class II, III or IV] 2 (16%), orthopnea (15%), need for diuretics (15%), and echocardiogram with more than mild RV dilation (34%), tricuspid regurgitation of at least moderate severity (32%), and moderate-to-severe pulmonary regurgitation (55%) [21]. Atrial fibrillation or flutter was appreciated in 19% of patients, while ventricular tachycardia and sudden cardiac death (SCD) each affected 9% of the study cohort.

TOF patients are also at increased risk for LV dysfunction. Various mechanisms may contribute to LV dysfunction including interactions (reflecting ventricular interdependence, septal shift, and shared coronary perfusion and myocardial fibers), electrical dyssynchrony [22], historical cyanosis, aortic regurgitation [23], and fibrosis. LV systolic dysfunction can be present in children soon after TOF repair with abnormal LV excitation–contraction coupling commonly seen despite preserved ejection fraction [24]. By adulthood, gross LV systolic dysfunction is present in up to 21% of patients. Moderate-to-severe LV systolic dysfunction has been reported in 6% [25] to 12% [21]. Once detected, LV systolic dysfunction is an independent predictor of mortality in adults with repaired TOF. Mortality is highest in patients with severely reduced EF and QRS duration >180 ms [21,26,27]. Elevated LV end-diastolic pressure is also an independent predictor of SCD [28], the leading cause of death in younger adults with TOF with an estimated incidence of ~0.3% per year [29].

SYSTEMIC RIGHT VENTRICLE

Adults with a systemic RV account for a significant number of ACHD patients presenting with HF. This population includes patients born with d-transposition of the great arteries (d-TGA) post-atrial switch (Mustard/Senning) surgery, and those with l-TGA or congenitally corrected transposition of the great arteries (ccTGA). In d-TGA, the position of the great vessels is switched—the aorta arises from the right ventricle and the pulmonary artery from the left ventricle. Associated cardiac defects are common and include VSD (45%), LV outflow tract obstruction (25%), and aortic coarctation (5%) [30]. Until the 1980s–90s, with timing depending on center, the most common surgical approach for infants born with d-TGA was an atrial switch procedure, either a Mustard or Senning operation. These involve surgically created atrial "baffles" or channels, which create a physiological correction in blood flow. Deoxygenated blood is redirected toward the lungs and oxygenated blood to the brain and body. Despite this physiologic correction, a fundamental drawback of the Mustard and Senning procedures is that the morphologic RV functions as the systemic ventricle. Early after the Mustard/Senning, the right ventricle engages adaptive mechanisms to maintain cardiac output including hypertrophy and increased ventricular mass to augment wall stress. However, by the third to fourth decade of life these compensatory mechanisms commonly fail leaving the majority of adult Mustard/Senning survivors with significant systemic RV systolic dysfunction [31]. The deterioration of systemic RV function with advancing age is related to a variety of causes, which vary between patients. These include the combined effects of RV remodeling (hypertrophy and dilation), subendocardial ischemia arising from increased myocardial oxygen demand, and inadequate coronary blood flow from a single right coronary artery [32]. Tricuspid regurgitation contributing to systemic RV volume overload is also important (especially since it may be surgically repaired if identified early) along with sinus node dysfunction, atrial arrhythmias, chronotropic incompetence, ventricular dyssynchrony, and pacemaker-related complications.

As opposed to Mustard/Senning patients, those with l-TGA, also referred to as physiologically or ccTGA, are born with unmatched atria and ventricles (right atrium to left ventricle, left atrium to right ventricle). The ventricles are also unmatched to the great arteries (left ventricle to PA, right ventricle to aorta). Hence there is a physiologic "correction" of venous blood flow despite discordant atrioventricular (AV) and ventriculoarterial connections. Case reports of ccTGA patients presenting only late in life do exist [33]. This, however, is rare. More than half of patients with ccTGA develop clinical signs of HF with moderate-to-severe systemic RV dysfunction by their mid-40s [30]. As in the Mustard/Senning population, ccTGA patients have abnormal systemic RV myocardial perfusion [34] and increased myocardial fibrosis [35]. Associated defects are common and include VSD (60%–80%), pulmonary (LV outflow tract) stenosis (30%–50%), and tricuspid valve abnormalities including Ebstein-like malformation (14%–56%) [30]. Additional cardiac defects in ccTGA are associated with increased HF risk, particularly systemic AV valve regurgitation, which is recognized as an important cause of progressive ventricular dysfunction and increased mortality [36]. Abnormal AV conduction anatomy is seen in patients with L-looped ventricles, and this predisposes to complete heart block, with an annual incidence of 2% per year [37]. Atrial arrhythmias increase over time and the onset of atrial flutter or fibrillation often coincides with symptoms and signs of congestive HF.

SINGLE VENTRICLE CIRCULATION

The term single ventricle circulation encompasses a range of complex CHD subtypes, which share the common feature of having only one ventricle capable of supporting the pulmonary and systemic circulations. Whereas one ventricle is dominant, a second smaller ventricle is either too small or cannot function independently due to complex anatomical arrangements; these are not static concepts, but rather have shifted over time with increasing experience. Most patients with a single ventricle circulation undergo palliation with the Fontan operation in which systemic venous return is diverted to the pulmonary circulation without an interposed subpulmonary ventricle [38]. Over time the Fontan connections have evolved from anastomosis of the right atrium to the pulmonary artery (atriopulmonary Fontan) to a synthetic conduit sutured within the wall of the right atrium that connects the inferior vena cava (IVC) to the pulmonary artery (lateral tunnel Fontan) to an extracardiac conduit, which bypasses the heart altogether to direct caval flow to the pulmonary arteries (extracardiac

Fontan). A principal advantage of the Fontan circulation is the separation of systemic and pulmonary venous circulations so as to normalize systemic arterial oxygen saturation and spare the systemic ventricle additional volume loading. However, a number of disadvantages are present and contribute to late-onset HF and a clinical "failing Fontan" phenotype.

In the absence of a subpulmonary ventricle, systemic venous return from the superior vena cava (SVC) and IVC to the pulmonary circulation is passive. The venous (muscle) pump and postcapillary energy and systemic venous pressure are the driving forces for pulmonary blood flow, augmented by respirophasic changes in intrathoracic pressure and ventricular diastolic function [39–42]. This leads to chronic volume unloading of the systemic ventricle, which limits cardiac output augmentation, most notably during exercise. Ventricular deconditioning is also present with older Fontan patients having significantly lower ventricular mass compared to younger Fontan patients and healthy controls [43].

Among CHD specialists, the term "failing Fontan" is the most widely accepted term to describe HF in Fontan patients and refers to an array of multisystem disorders presenting as some combination of systemic venous congestion, protein-losing enteropathy (PLE), and arrhythmias, usually in the setting of preserved ventricular systolic function [44]. Advanced systolic dysfunction and pulmonary edema are infrequent, whereas diastolic dysfunction and complications of elevated systemic venous pressures, including venous insufficiency, liver congestion, cirrhosis, and ascites, are common. HF in younger Fontan patients may be concealed until early adulthood when an acute trigger, such as arrhythmia, thromboembolism, or sepsis, tips the delicate physiologic balance toward a decompensated state. While the manifestations of HF may differ enormously from more typical adult HF presentations, many physiologic findings such as impaired aerobic capacity and exercise oscillatory ventilation may be present [45]. The incidence of HF increases with age with up to 40% of adult Fontan patients meeting Framingham criteria for a diagnosis of HF [10]. Predictors of HF include elevated right atrial/Fontan pathway pressure, PLE, and, in some but not all studies, a dominant ventricle of RV morphology. Mortality after HF diagnosis is high [46] and frequently coincides with worsening arrhythmias and multiorgan dysfunction.

EISENMENGER SYNDROME

Atrial, ventricular, or aortopulmonary shunts expose the pulmonary vascular bed to excessive blood flow and, for the latter defects, systemic pressures. Without repair, this appears to activate a range of signaling pathways that promote pulmonary arteriolar vasoconstriction, inflammation, thickening, and obliteration, culminating in pulmonary hypertension in a subset of patients. Eisenmenger syndrome is the most extreme manifestation of this condition and is defined as pulmonary hypertension due to high pulmonary vascular resistance with reversed or bidirectional shunting leading to cyanosis [47]. The penetrance and age at presentation differ according to the level of the shunt. When arising secondary to large aortopulmonary and interventricular shunts, Eisenmenger syndrome is very common and usually presents in childhood. By comparison, Eisenmenger syndrome due to atrial level shunts most commonly presents in adulthood and only affects 10%–20% of patients with very large shunts [48].

In Eisenmenger syndrome, chronic cyanosis leads to erythrocytosis, hyperviscosity, thrombocytopenia, and coagulation defects, all of which predispose to thrombosis and hemorrhage. Iron deficiency is common along with a range of complications that impact morbidity and survival including gout, cholelithiasis, cerebrovascular events (stroke and cerebral abscess), kidney dysfunction, arrhythmias, HF, and SCD [12,48]. Many adults with Eisenmenger syndrome do well until the onset of cardiovascular complications in the third to fourth decade of life. Some survive until the seventh or eighth decade of life, but this is rare. Common mechanisms of death include progressive right HF, arrhythmia, SCD, pulmonary hypertensive crisis, and/or hemorrhage. Depending on institution and duration of follow-up, HF is the cause of death in 20% [49] to 50% [15]. There has been a shift towards heart failure as an increasingly common cause of death in Eisenmenger syndrome over the past several decades [49a]. RV systolic dysfunction and right atrial dilation are strongly associated with increased mortality in Eisenmenger patients [50] along with elevations in serum B-type natriuretic peptide (BNP) [51,52]. The factors leading to transition from a compensated state to progressive RV failure, decreased cardiac output, and elevated central venous pressure are poorly understood. Although myocardial fibrosis is common in Eisenmenger syndrome the burden of fibrosis is low and does not correlate strongly with ventricular dysfunction or survival [53]. Further research is needed to understand the interaction of the LV and RV in various forms of Eisenmenger syndrome, the relations between RV and pulmonary function and the cellular changes that accompany decompensated HF including the impact of myocyte apoptosis and cytokine expression [54].

DIAGNOSIS OF HEART FAILURE IN ADULT CONGENITAL HEART DISEASE

Symptoms and idiosyncratic presentations: As outlined above, it is difficult to define HF in ACHD, and the manifestations of circulatory failure vary widely. Some exhibit classical findings of HF with reduced systemic ventricular function in a two-ventricle circulation. Symptoms and physical findings would usually be expected, in such cases, to be equivalent

TABLE 26.1 Examples of Atypical Presentations of Heart Failure in Adults With Congenital Heart Disease

Diagnostic Category	Presentation	Reason
Fontan	Diarrhea, hypoalbuminemia	Protein-losing enteropathy
	Cough with bronchial casts	Plastic bronchitis
	Ascites (less commonly pleural effusions)	Unknown, combination elevated right atrial pressure, cirrhosis, lymphatic obstruction
d-transposition of the great arteries with atrial switch repair	Fatigue, superior vena cava syndrome	Superior baffle limb obstruction
Simple shunt lesion, Eisenmenger syndrome	Worsening cyanosis, erythrocytosis	Pulmonary arterial hypertension with right-to-left shunt

to those with acquired causes of HF. Many diagnoses have a set of idiosyncratic presentations (Table 26.1). Atypical nonspecific symptoms are also common, with fatigue or abdominal pain often reflecting low output. Even more commonly, the severity of symptoms often seems unrelated to the severity of underlying cardiovascular dysfunction, with little warning before presentation with advanced disease.

Because of the issues in diagnosis based on presenting symptoms and signs alone, noninvasive testing is important to estimate clinical and functional status in ACHD. Because there is no way to confidently diagnose a distinct HF syndrome per se in many patients with CHD, the focus is on grading the degree and stability of structural abnormalities and functional limitations.

Imaging: Imaging plays a large role in the assessment and management of ACHD and is optimally suited to defining anatomic and structural reasons underlying deterioration. Imaging has limited ability, however, to make a diagnosis of HF. This assertion follows obviously from the high prevalence, near ubiquity, of notable anatomic and structural abnormalities in the population. The same is true for the diagnosis of HF in acquired ventricular dysfunction: the presence of low LV ejection fraction does not constitute a diagnosis of clinical HF. But because low LV ejection fraction is very uncommon in the general population, the imaging finding alone is important and reasonably specific. With the exception of major changes over time between tests, few isolated imaging findings are similarly specific in ACHD patients. It may be that dynamic imaging or invasive testing, whether with exercise, volume loading, or pharmacologic stress [55–57], may provide more useful data, but such testing is not yet standard for regular follow-up in any group of adults with CHD.

Biomarkers: Circulating biomarkers are also appealing, in that changes in such markers would be expected to reflect fundamental pathophysiology rather than idiosyncratic anatomy. One would expect BNP to be elevated from increased ventricular wall tension whatever type of ventricle. Indeed, BNP is elevated in a subset of ACHD patients and such elevation does generally correlate with worse physical quality of life, functional class, and outcomes [58–61]. One challenge is that the vast majority of patients have BNP levels considered normal for a given assay based on the more common older adult population norms. Levels at the higher end of the normal range may, therefore, be informative as may serial BNP assessment. Overall, BNP is mainly helpful to identify patients with more typical types of HF, especially those with reduced ventricular function or pulmonary arterial hypertension [51,52]. Since a subset of ACHD HF is not related directly to elevated filling pressures and many adverse outcomes are unrelated to HF per se, BNP is not as widely applicable to this group of patients as it is in acquired HF.

Many other biomarkers tend to correspond to overall illness, such as serum sodium, albumin, bilirubin, or creatinine. Uric acid is a strong predictor of adverse outcomes in some type of CHD [62], but this does not point to a unique pathophysiology. A few studies have explored more recently introduced biomarkers of HF and myocardial injury, including high sensitivity troponin, growth/differentiation factor 15, and galectin-3, which correspond to alternative mechanisms of disease in cardiovascular failure [63–68]. The role of such markers in ACHD care remains to be defined.

Exercise testing: Cardiopulmonary exercise testing (CPET) is perhaps, with the exception of the ECG and chest radiograph, the most broadly applicable noninvasive test in ACHD. Its strength is in precise definition of aerobic functional capacity (peak VO_2). CPET is also very useful to differentiate between alternative causes of dyspnea. While there is a subset of ACHD patients with underappreciated restrictive, or less commonly obstructive, lung disease, this is a less common question in ACHD. More often, CPET is used to provide objective confirmation of a patient's subjective report of functional capacity. Many young ACHD patients do not complain of symptoms despite markedly reduced objective functional capacity, and CPET can identify important changes before a patient may identify an issue. While CPET can provide a precise measure of aerobic capacity, it has limited specificity for identifying the cause of cardiovascular limitation. The dynamic functional information provided by CPET is therefore synergistic with structural and anatomic imaging data. Invasive CPET provides further data but is reserved for situations where noninvasive or more common invasive testing fails to identify a cause [69–71].

COMORBIDITIES AND COMPLICATIONS ASSOCIATED WITH HEART FAILURE IN ADULT CONGENITAL HEART DISEASE

Comorbidities associated with ACHD-related HF overlap with those seen patients with acquired forms of HF. However, there are also important differences because of starkly different epidemiology (e.g., younger age), causes of underlying disease (e.g., genetic syndromes), and prior management (e.g., multiple operations). Some specific considerations applicable to ACHD HF are discussed below.

Arrhythmia/sudden cardiac death: Both supraventricular and ventricular arrhythmias play an important role in the pathophysiology of HF in ACHD [72]. Arrhythmia can be either cause or effect of progressive HF, as is the case in acquired heart disease. The epidemiology of arrhythmia mechanism differs from those with acquired heart disease, however, with scar-based macroreentrant circuits being much more common in ACHD. A detailed discussion is beyond the scope of this chapter, but it is important to highlight the challenges of risk stratification for sudden death in ACHD, which informs the difficulties faced by the clinician in identifying patients who may benefit from primary prevention implantable cardioverter defibrillators. Adults with CHD are at lower absolute risk of sudden death compared with acquired HF patients. Monomorphic ventricular tachycardia may be hemodynamically stable for prolonged periods in some types of ACHD, making it difficult to equate appropriate shocks with prevention of sudden death. They also have a notably higher rate of inappropriate discharges because of younger age (higher sinus rates), T-wave oversensing and higher prevalence of concomitant supraventricular tachycardia. Thoughtful device programming may partly address this issue. The incidence of device complications, such as lead fracture, is also greater in this younger, more active group of patients with convoluted vascular access [28,46,73]. Device implantation requires surgical epicardial lead placement in some of the patients at highest risk (e.g., Eisenmenger syndrome) since intracardiac leads are associated with thromboembolism. Subcutaneous defibrillators may be very useful for ACHD patients, though structural constraints may limit broad application.

Liver disease: Few comorbidities are more frequently discussed, with as little certainty regarding clinical importance or optimal approach, as liver disease in ACHD-related HF [74]. This reflects a clinical disparity between the severity of structural and functional findings [75]. Moderate or severe liver fibrosis is very common almost ubiquitous in some diagnostic groups [76–78] (while most research has focused on the single ventricle Fontan circulation, it is clear that liver fibrosis may be an issue for other patient groups) [79]. However, liver synthetic function is usually normal and findings of advanced cirrhosis such as variceal bleeding, asterixis, and hepatic encephalopathy are quite rare [77,80]. While there is a real risk of hepatocellular carcinoma [81], severity and pattern of fibrosis do not appear to predict outcomes [77]. Other findings, such as ascites or splenomegaly or low platelet count or elevated MELD score, may relate to elevated systemic venous pressure or lymphatic disease. The main importance of this distinction comes in transplant or other surgical deliberations. Programs vary widely in approach to such patients.

Kidney disease: Reduced glomerular filtration rate (GFR) is common in ACHD patients, especially those with HF [82]. About half of patients who had creatinine measured in a referral center in the United Kingdom were found to have an estimated GFR $<90\,mL/min/1.72\,m^2$, with almost 10% having GFR <60. These latter patients were threefold more likely to die during follow-up. It is unclear if serum creatinine is a reliable marker of GFR in these patients with often abnormal body composition, and alternative methods (e.g., cystatin C, nuclear GFR estimation) may be useful when precise estimates of GFR are critical. Important risk factors were older age, cyanosis, and diuretic use. Reasons for the high prevalence of kidney dysfunction may also relate to historical cyanosis, genetic predisposition or developmental renal abnormalities, chronic inflammation, and prior procedures, especially repeated surgeries requiring prolonged bypass/aortic cross-clamping and repeated catheterization and other procedures using iodinated contrast. The relationship between cyanosis, secondary erythrocytosis, uric acid metabolism, and kidney dysfunction has been explored in more mechanistic detail [83–85]. There is also preliminary evidence that other aspects of kidney function can be affected. For example, there seems to be a high prevalence of microalbuminuria in young patients with cyanosis or single ventricle Fontan circulation [86–88].

Lung disease: ACHD patients have a high burden of restrictive lung disease. This partly relates to multiple prior thoracic surgeries and the known association between scoliosis and cyanotic heart disease [89]. Other contributors may include impaired lung growth during development and iatrogenic diaphragmatic dysfunction or more general muscle weakness [90,91]. Specific diagnoses (i.e., TOF with pulmonary atresia) are also associated with reactive airway disease. In specific subsets of patients low forced vital capacity is associated with worse aerobic exercise capacity [92], and in an all-comer ACHD population moderate-to-severely reduced forced vital capacity was an independent predictor of mortality [89]. The presence of parenchymal lung disease and diaphragmatic dysfunction has direct implications on consideration of transplant options.

Thromboembolism: Because of many of the comorbidities listed above, as well as the presence of foreign material in the heart and vessels, coagulation abnormalities, venous obstruction, chronic venous insufficiency, and otherwise stagnant flow among other mechanisms, many ACHD patients have a propensity to thrombosis [93–96]. The frequent presence of intracardiac or vascular communications provides an opportunity for paradoxical embolism. Diagnostic categories associated with especially high risk of such events include patients with Eisenmenger syndrome, D-looped transposition of the great arteries with atrial switch repair, and Fontan circulation. Unfortunately, many of these patients are also at increased risk for bleeding complications. Any patient with an atrial arrhythmia or a patent shunt and transvenous leads are also at increased risk [97]. Thromboembolism is an important cause of adverse outcomes [95,98]. But while anticoagulation is often unquestionably indicated, there is little evidence to guide the clinician on how best to approach anticoagulation in ACHD patients [99,100].

Psychological and neurodevelopmental: Genetic, developmental, and experiential factors all can result in cognitive and neuropsychiatric problems [101]. Genetic syndromes associated with CHD, such as 22q11 deletion, are often associated with developmental delay and psychiatric disease, and there is preliminary evidence that in a small subset of nonsyndromic CHD there is a genetic predisposition to impaired neurodevelopmental outcomes [102]. Some diagnoses, such as d-TGA and some single ventricles, are also associated with abnormal in utero cerebral flow and thereby may cause subclinical but importantly abnormal neurodevelopment [103,104]. Repeated cardiac bypass runs and circulatory arrest, multiple stressful procedures, parental overprotection [105], and abnormal early nutrition and social exposure may also influence early development [101,105]. While CHD does not preclude superior intelligence, normal psychological function and extraordinary achievement [106], there is a high prevalence of developmental delay, depression, anxiety and posttraumatic stress disorder [107,108]. These issues can complicate care for HF and the ability for self-care. Therefore, they often play a role in decisions regarding device support or transplant for HF.

MANAGEMENT OF HEART FAILURE IN ADULT CONGENITAL HEART DISEASE

Given the limited data and diverse clinical presentations, it is difficult to identify a pathway for optimal therapy applicable to ACHD HF. Fig. 26.3 provides a broad conceptual approach to evaluation and treatment of HF ACHD patients. As depicted in the figure, care for these patients is necessarily iterative and reiterative. The following sections aim to provide further context for possible specific clinical interventions.

Pharmacologic

There is currently no systematic evidence to support the use of the standard pharmacologic strategies for treating HF in patients with ACHD. This does not imply that HF medications such as diuretics, beta blockers, and renin–angiotensin–aldosterone system (RAAS) antagonists are of no value in select individuals but rather highlights clinical trials in HF ACHD patients as being inadequate for determining their clinical efficacy. ACHD HF trials have been hampered by heterogeneity within the ACHD population, inclusion of patients with and without clinical HF, short study duration, imperfect surrogate outcomes, and small cohort size. Consequently, studies have been inadequately powered to evaluate the effects of HF medications on HF outcomes and clinical surrogates such as ventricular ejection fraction. In one of the few randomized controlled HF trials in CHD, carvedilol treatment in children and adolescents (76/161 with CHD and 43 with a systemic right ventricle) did not influence a complex composite outcome of clinical HF worsening or a combined outcome of death or HF hospitalization. A possible detrimental effect of carvedilol on systemic RV function was observed but could not be confirmed [109]. In the largest study of HF in ACHD to date, 88 patients with TGA (both d-TGA and ccTGA) were randomized to placebo or the angiotensin receptor blocker (ARB) valsartan. Followed over 3.2 years, ARB was well tolerated but had no impact on RV ejection fraction (RVEF), tricuspid regurgitation severity, neurohormonal activation, or quality of life [110]. Like other studies that failed to show improved outcomes in systemic RV patients treated with RAAS antagonists [111–114], this study was underpowered to demonstrate improvements in RVEF with treatment. Hence, the question of whether RAAS blockers improve systemic RV function remains unanswered. Despite the lack of evidence for efficacy, in clinical practice therapy for the systemic right ventricular or other forms of HF in ACHD often parallels what would be standard for other forms of HF [17].

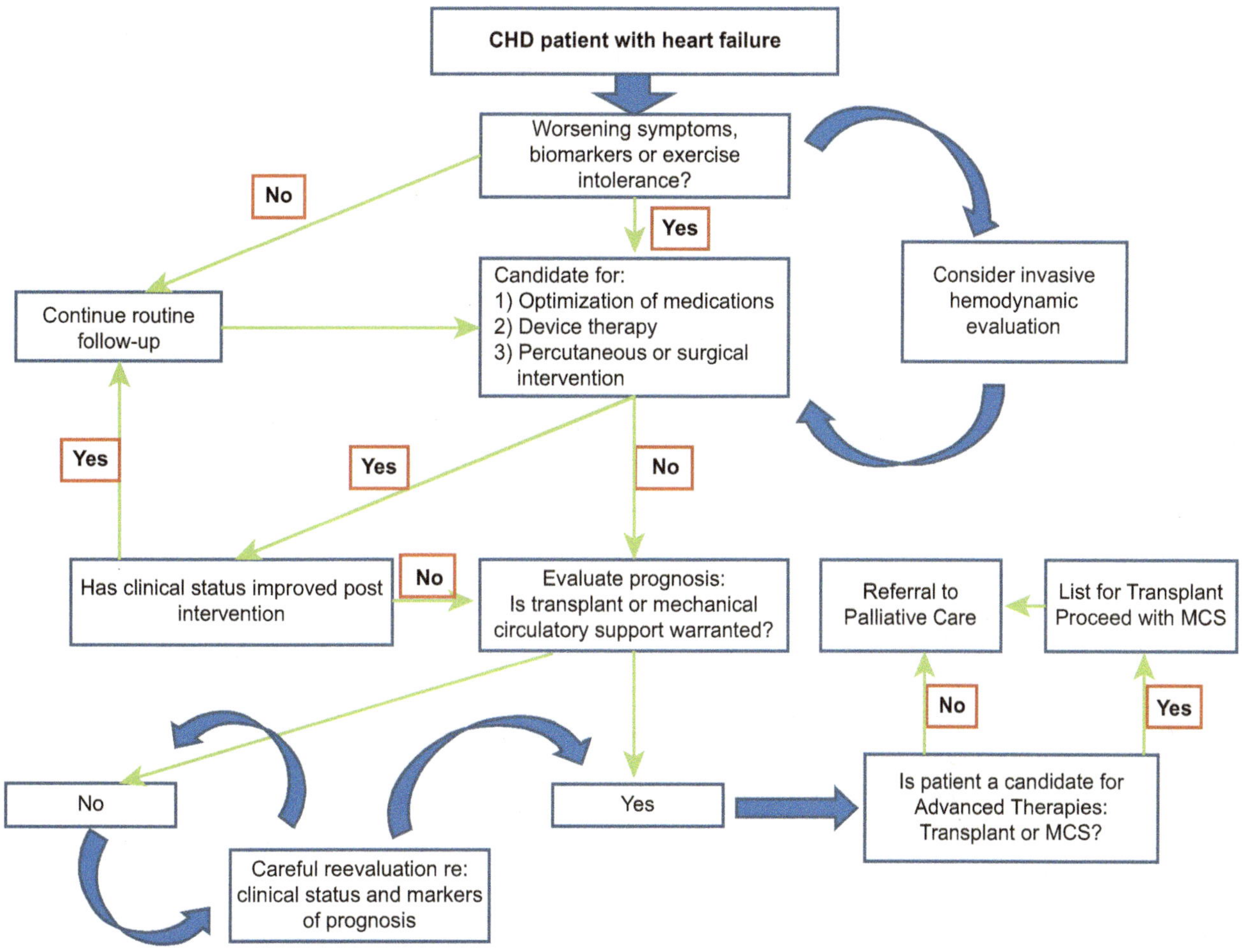

FIGURE 26.3 Overview of an approach to advanced heart failure in congenital heart disease. *CHD*, congenital heart disease; *MCS*, mechanical circulatory support. *(With permission H.J. Ross, Y. Law, W.M. Book, C.S. Broberg, L. Burchill, F. Cecchin, et al., Transplantation and mechanical circulatory support in congenital heart disease: a scientific statement from the American heart association, Circulation 133 (8) (2016) 802–820.)*

In contrast to standard HF medications, there is evidence to support the use of pulmonary vasodilator therapy in ACHD patients with Eisenmenger syndrome. Endothelin receptor antagonists [115,116], phosphodiesterase inhibitors [117,118], and prostanoids [119] have each been shown to improve symptoms and exercise capacity. In a 16-week randomized double-blind placebo-controlled study in Eisenmenger patients, treatment with the endothelin receptor antagonist bosentan led to significantly lower pulmonary vascular resistance and pulmonary artery pressure and improved exercise capacity [116]. Although bosentan has been most extensively studied in randomized trials and the European Society of Cardiology guidelines recommend its use (class I) [120], no evidence suggests that other agents are less safe or effective. Combination therapy (e.g., endothelin receptor antagonist and phosphodiesterase inhibitor) is reasonable in patients who experience a functional decline on a single agent [121]. There is now specific data to support starting combination therapy in pulmonary arterial hypertension overall [122]. Whether this approach will be similarly effective in Eisenmenger syndrome is unknown. A summary of pharmacologic strategies in CHD groups vulnerable to HF is provided in Table 26.2 [123]. A better understanding of pharmacologic approaches in ACHD has been identified as a high priority clinical research topic [124].

Nonpharmacologic

Consideration of nonpharmacologic strategies for treating ACHD-related HF and its complications is important when caring for this growing patient population. This approach relies heavily on collaboration between ACHD cardiologists, advanced HF specialists, structural interventional cardiologists, electrophysiologists, and congenital heart surgeons.

TABLE 26.2 Summary of Selected Studies of Pharmacological Interventions for Heart Failure in Congenital Heart Disease

Reference	Study Type	Drug	Number of Patients	Mean Age of Patients	Follow-Up	Key Findings
Studies in Patients With Subaortic Right Ventricle in a Biventricular Circulation						
van der Bom et al. [110]	Multicenter randomized double-blind placebo-controlled trial	Valsartan	44	33 years	3 years	No effect of treatment on exercise capacity or quality of life
Therrien et al. [114]	Single-center double-blind randomized placebo-controlled trial	Ramipril	17	26 years	1 years	No effect of treatment on RVEF, RVEDV, or RVESV
Dore et al. [111]	Multicenter randomized double-blind placebo-controlled crossover trial	Losartan	29	30 years	15 weeks	No improvement in exercise capacity or reduction in NT-proBNP levels
Giardini et al. [125]	Prospective nonrandomized, no control group	Carvedilol	8	26 years	12 months	RVEF increased (34% vs. 42%; $P=.004$); LVEF increased (44% vs. 49%; $P=.01$); No change in peak oxygen uptake
Lester et al. [113]	Prospective randomized controlled crossover trial	Losartan	7	Not provided (all > 7 years)	8 weeks	During active treatment: systolic BP decreased, tricuspid regurgitation decreased, duration of exercise increased
Hechter et al. [112]	Retrospective comparison of MRI and exercise test results before and after ACE inhibitors	ACE inhibitors	14	31 years	18 months	No significant differences
Robinson et al. [126]	Prospective study of patients before and after enalapril	Enalapril	9	14 years	1 year	No significant differences in measures of exercise performance; BP decreased compared with baseline; no change in tricuspid regurgitation
Shaddy et al. [109]	Multicenter randomized double-blind placebo-controlled trial	Carvedilol	43 with "nonleft" systemic ventricle	22–43 months	6 months	Patients whose systemic ventricle was not a left ventricle appeared to have a trend to "nonbenefit" or possible worsening during treatment with carvedilol
Yehya et al. [127]	Retrospective chart review	Advanced therapies for PHT	6	29 years	6 months	After 6-months treatment all had improvement in functional class; no change in RVEF

Doughan et al. [128]	Retrospective chart review	Beta blockers (metoprolol succinate or carvedilol)	60 (31 on beta blocker)	28 years	4 months	Patients treated with beta blocker had improvement in NYHA functional class, no significant change in RVEF or degree of tricuspid regurgitation
Studies in Patients With Repaired Tetralogy of Fallot						
Norozi et al. [129]	Prospective double-blind placebo controlled	Bisoprolol	34	30 years	6 months	Bisoprolol, in patients with repaired TOF and BNP > 100 pg/mL and peak VO_2 < 25 mL/kg/min had no effect on peak VO_2 or ventricular function
Babu Narayan et al. [130]	Prospective double-blind placebo controlled	Ramipril in patients with moderate-to-severe pulmonary regurgitation	64	30 years	6 months	No improvement in RVEF
Studies in Patients With Eisenmenger Syndrome						
D'Alto et al. [131]	Prospective nonrandomized, no control group	Addition of sildenafil treatment in patients already taking bosentan	32	37 years	6 months	Addition of sildenafil to baseline bosentan was safe and well tolerated at 6 months and resulted in improved clinical status, O_2 saturation on exertion, and hemodynamic characteristics
Dimopoulos et al. [132]	Retrospective chart review	Advanced therapies for PHT	229	35 years	4 years	Patients taking advanced medical therapy for PHT were at lower risk of death during follow-up than those who are not; most of these patients were on bosentan consistent with early use of advanced therapies. Of note, a later study from a largely overlapping patient sample did not confirm these earlier findings [133]
Mukhopadhyay et al. [134]	Prospective nonrandomized, no control group	Tadalafil	16	25 years	12 weeks	PVR and O_2 saturation improved acutely and at 12 week functional class and 6-min walk distance improved at 12 week
Mukhopadhyay et al. [117]	Prospective randomized crossover trial	Tadalafil	28	29 years	6 weeks	Tadalafil was associated with increase in 6-min walk distance and O_2 saturation, decrease in PVR and improvement in NYHA functional class
Galie et al. [116]	Multicenter randomized double-blind placebo-controlled trial	Bosentan	54	37 years	16 weeks	Compared with placebo bosentan reduced pulmonary vascular resistance index and improved 6-min walk test
Studies in Patients With a Single Ventricle Circulation						
Hsu et al. [135]	Multicenter randomized double-blind placebo-controlled trial	Enalapril	230	20 days	14 months	Death, transplantation, adverse events, BNP levels, functional class, ejection fraction, and weight gain did not differ between the groups

Continued

TABLE 26.2 Summary of Selected Studies of Pharmacological Interventions for Heart Failure in Congenital Heart Disease—cont'd

Reference	Study Type	Drug	Number of Patients	Mean Age of Patients	Follow-Up	Key Findings
Kouatli et al. [136]	Randomized double-blind placebo-controlled cross-over trial	Enalapril	18	15 years	10 weeks	Treatment did not change heart rate, BP, diastolic filling patterns or exercise duration. The ability to increase cardiac index during exercise decreased during enalapril treatment
Hebert et al. [137]	Randomized double-blind placebo-controlled cross-over trial	Bosentan	75	20 years	14 weeks	Bosentan was associated with modest increase in peak VO_2 and trend toward improved NYHA functional class
Schuuring et al. [138]	Randomized open label placebo-controlled trial with crossover of placebo arm	Bosentan	42 (32 completed study)	28 years	6 months	Bosentan was not associated with any effect on exercise capacity or functional class or any other marker of disease severity (e.g., BNP)
Goldberg et al. [139]	Randomized double-blind placebo-controlled cross-over trial	Sildenafil	28 (27 completed study)	15 years	6 weeks	Sildenafil was associated with lower V_E:VCO_2 but did not affect peak VO_2 or peak work rate

ACE, angiotensin-converting enzyme; *BNP*, B-type natriuretic peptide; *LVEF*, left ventricular ejection fraction; *NT*-proBNP, N-terminal proBNP; *NYHA*, New York Heart Association; *PHT*, pulmonary hypertension; *PVR*, pulmonary vascular resistance; *RVEDV*, right ventricular end-diastolic volume; *RVEF*, right ventricular ejection fraction; *RVESV*, right ventricular end-systolic volume.
Adapted From S.L. Roche, A.N. Redington, The failing right ventricle in congenital heart disease, Can. J. Cardiol. 29 (7) (2013) 768–778 With Permission.

Exercise and Cardiac Rehabilitation

Exercise is an appealing therapy for adults with CHD and HF for a number of reasons. As outlined above, ACHD HF patients not only have residual cardiovascular lesions but they also have a high prevalence of an array of pulmonary, neurodevelopmental, psychiatric, orthopedic, and other comorbidities that may adversely affect quality and length of life [108,140–142]. Medical and interventional therapies may successfully address the active primary cardiovascular issue, but the results are often disappointing because of other important limits. Thoughtful exercise training has diverse effects on cardiopulmonary–cardiovascular performance and may also independently address limitations related to additional comorbidities. Further, ACHD patients tend to be sedentary, a factor contributing to poor outcomes [143,144]. This learned behavior is in part a result of how health providers counseled these patients during childhood. Restricting participation in sports and other forms of exercise has been standard management of many forms of CHD, resulting in a sedentary, obese population [145]. Unlike many other problems these patients face, sedentary lifestyle is modifiable.

Increasing aerobic physical activity, formal exercise training, and comprehensive cardiac rehabilitation programs have all been explored as therapy to increase physical capacity and improve effort tolerance. A number of investigators have reported positive effects of varied interventions in specific groups of patients [146–150].

In the absence of a strong contraindication, ACHD HF patients should be counseled to engage frequently in moderately strenuous aerobic conditioning. More active patients tend to maintain aerobic capacity over time and peak VO_2 tends to increase for those who increase their aerobic conditioning regimen compared with those who maintain or decrease the frequency of moderate aerobic activity [151]. Even a simple, short intervention to encourage regular gentle walking at home has been shown to improve quality of life in ACHD patients [147]. There are few data to support an optimal regimen or precise frequency or duration or intensity of such aerobic activity; within the normal range of activity reported in this population one would expect greater benefit with higher frequency and intensity as is seen for acquired forms of HF [152]. Some types of directed exercise have been questioned as potentially harmful, including intense static/isometric exercise and extremely prolonged, intense, aerobic exercise. There is little research on the impact of intense static/isometric exercise in ACHD patients, though maximally intense static/isometric activity (single repetition weight lifting) is considered contraindicated in many patients, such as those with aortic dilation, based mainly on expert consensus. Unlike aerobic conditioning, findings in acquired heart disease suggest one would expect less substantial improvements in cardiovascular outcomes with this type of exercise and it is unclear if expected improvements in quality of life and mobility would be equivalent in a cohort of much younger patients. While some express concern that overly intense aerobic activity may have adverse effects on specific subsets of patients [153], this is an essentially hypothetical concern; very few patients come near a level that would merit any concern.

Cardiac rehabilitation programs have been widely studied in adults with acquired heart disease. These programs involve exercise training as well as counseling on behavioral change (e.g., tobacco cessation, healthy diet) [154,155]. Cardiac rehabilitation improves exercise capacity and pVO_2, improves quality of life, and decreases mortality [156,157]. It is difficult to identify a specific "mechanism" for the benefit since exercise and behavioral interventions have pleiotropic effects. Cardiac rehabilitation is less well studied in children and adults with CHD; while the existing data support safety and do suggest a benefit [148,158,159], insurance programs often decline coverage for CHD patients with chronic HF. There is little reason to doubt that formal cardiac rehabilitation would benefit many ACHD HF patients and the risks are minimal, though it remains unknown if such formal programs are superior to intensive counseling, exercise prescription, or exercise training.

INVASIVE HEMODYNAMIC EVALUATION AND TRANSCATHETER INTERVENTIONS IN ADULT CONGENITAL HEART DISEASE–RELATED HEART FAILURE

Cardiac catheterization enables HF therapy to be tailored according to an individual's hemodynamic profile. In ACHD, invasive hemodynamic assessment assumes even greater importance due to the high prevalence of residual defects that may contribute to HF pathophysiology. When present, these are commonly pressure or volume overload lesions arising secondary to valvular disease or shunts. Lesion-specific interventions may be important for certain ACHD subgroups, including Mustard/Senning patients, those with failing Fontan physiology and adults with repaired TOF.

Baffle leaks are found in up to 25% of Mustard/Senning patients [160] and varying degrees of baffle stenosis (SVC more often than IVC or pulmonary venous) may be seen in 5%–15% [161,162]. Baffle leaks are usually small but may contribute to ventricular volume overload, systemic arterial desaturation, or systemic embolic events. SVC baffle stenosis is often asymptomatic due to venous collaterals and azygous flow reversal developing as an alternative route for venous return to the heart. IVC baffle stenosis or obstruction is less well tolerated and may lead to hepatic venous congestion, hepatomegaly, and ascites. Pulmonary venous baffle obstruction is a potentially reversible cause of pulmonary edema and hypertension that should be considered in Mustard/Senning patients presenting with acute onset HF. Intervention to address these issues can translate to significant improvements in functional class and hemodynamics [163]. Percutaneous interventions include balloon angioplasty for baffle stenosis with or without stent placement. Transcatheter interventions may be considered in Fontan patients with or without HF. Indications for transcatheter interventions in Fontan patients include relief of pulmonary artery stenosis in an effort to lower Fontan pressures, coil embolization of collateral vessels to reduce systemic desaturation and/or ventricular volume load, and angioplasty/stenting of aortic coarctation to reduce ventricular afterload. Transcatheter fenestration creation may be used in patients with PLE but is an uncommon strategy in patients with other types of failing Fontan physiology as a bridge to heart transplantation [164,165]. Unfortunately, new cyanosis may be poorly tolerated by older patients and fenestrations often close after being created; in such cases, PLE recurrence is the norm [166].

Arguably, the greatest advance in percutaneous intervention for ACHD within the past decade has been catheter-based (primarily Melody, a bovine jugular valve sutured within a platinum iridium stent) valve implantation in right ventricle to pulmonary artery conduits or bioprosthetic pulmonary valves in adults with residual pulmonary regurgitation or stenosis following surgical TOF repair. Melody valve implantation is widely accepted as an alternative to surgery and is associated with excellent procedural outcomes. Relief of RV outflow tract obstruction leads to early improvements in biventricular performance (stroke volume and ejection fraction), symptom burden, and exercise tolerance [167]. Similar improvements in ventricular function are seen in patients who undergo percutaneous pulmonary valve implant for pulmonary regurgitation although measures of exercise capacity are usually unchanged suggesting volume overload may have a differential effect on myocardial contractile reserve [168]. Primary valve failure is rare after Melody valve implant although reintervention is necessary in ~20% of patients, most commonly due to recurrent RV outflow tract obstruction [169]. Endocarditis and endarteritis have also emerged as important late complications after Melody valve implant.

ARRHYTHMIA INTERVENTIONS IN ADULT CONGENITAL HEART DISEASE–RELATED HEART FAILURE

Arrhythmias are common in ACHD-related HF, both as a cause and consequence of impaired hemodynamics. Tachyarrhythmias such as intraatrial reentrant tachycardia (IART) and atrial fibrillation are common and frequently trigger HF. Conversely, decompensated HF with increased atrial and ventricular filling pressures, oxygen desaturation, low cardiac output, and tachycardia may precipitate arrhythmias. Regardless of whether arrhythmia or progressive HF is the trigger for clinical decompensation, treatment of both conditions is required. Optimization of fluid status and ventricular function is necessary for antiarrhythmic therapies to be effective, while elimination of arrhythmias helps to reverse the hemodynamic derangements. Reflecting the increasing complexity of the arrhythmia substrate in ACHD patients, arrhythmia management relies on pharmacologic, device-based, catheter-based, and surgical treatment strategies, either alone or in combination.

Of the atrial arrhythmias occurring in ACHD patients, IART caused by a macroreentrant loop arising from fibrosis from suture lines or patches is the most common [170,171]. IART usually has an atrial rate of 150–250 bpm, which may enable 1:1 conduction leading to hemodynamic compromise, HF and SCD [46]. Initial success rate for IART ablation in CHD patients is above 80% but recurrence can be up to 40% within 2 years of ablation for Fontan patients [172].

Cardiac resynchronization therapy (CRT) is being increasingly used in ACHD patients. Most commonly CRT is considered in ACHD patients with HF who meet indications for pacemaker due to serious conduction abnormalities. CRT has been used successfully to restore ventricular function and in some cases enabled ACHD patients to be removed from the heart transplant list [173,174]. The benefits of CRT appear to be greatest in those with biventricular anatomy and reduced left ventricular ejection fraction [175] such as adults with repaired TOF. The presence of a systemic left ventricle is an independent predictor of a greater improvement in ventricular function and remodeling after CRT [173]. In contrast, standard CRT criteria apply to a small fraction (5%) of patients with a systemic right ventricle. Despite the lack of data, improvements in NYHA Functional Class, RVEF, and peak oxygen uptake are seen leading to a Class IIb recommendation for CRT in systemic RV patients from the Heart Rhythm Society [176]. Whether CRT is useful for patients with single ventricle circulation is less clear with mixed results to date [177,178].

SURGICAL INTERVENTIONS IN ADULT CONGENITAL HEART DISEASE–RELATED HEART FAILURE

Surgical intervention for significant cardiac residua before the onset of progressive ventricular dysfunction and clinical HF is recommended across the ACHD spectrum. The challenge for clinicians is identifying when ventricular dysfunction is likely to improve or progress after cardiac surgery. Large cohort studies from tertiary ACHD centers have reported high perioperative mortality in patients with significant (>moderate) ventricular dysfunction [12], inferring that cardiac surgical risk may be prohibitive in those with advanced ACHD-related HF.

Systemic RV failure and severe tricuspid (systemic AV valve) regurgitation often coexist in patients with ccTGA. In up to 70% of ccTGA patients, the systemic AV valve is abnormal and inferiorly displaced with an Ebstein-like appearance [179]. Discerning whether TR is the cause or consequence of RV dilation and dysfunction remains a challenge. Survival with ccTGA is closely linked to the degree of systemic AV valve regurgitation and systemic RV function. An RVEF >40% is associated with improved survival [180], and the benefits of preserved ventricular function [36] have been used to argue for earlier surgical intervention of systemic AV valve regurgitation.

Fontan conversion improves hemodynamics and arrhythmia burden although perioperative mortality is as high as 11% in some centers and a subgroup of patients (~5%) will still proceed to heart transplantation [181]. A recent publication has questioned the traditional indications for the conversion procedure, citing a high (86%) 8-year transplant-free survival among patients undergoing "early conversion" [182]. Early Fontan conversion improved NYHA class and reduced arrhythmia burden, although these findings need to be confirmed prospectively before this approach can be recommended as standard of care. Risk factors for transplant or death after Fontan conversion surgery include a dominant right ventricle, ascites, and PLE. There is now general agreement that the presence of ascites or PLE denotes advanced failing Fontan physiology, and heart transplantation is often a better alternative to high-risk Fontan conversion [183].

CONCLUSION

The increasing number of adults with complex forms of CHD presenting with HF highlights the pressing need to better understand ACHD-related HF. Reducing ACHD-related HF complications and improving survival is essential if we are to improve outcomes in those who are entrusted to our care. Currently little is known about who is caring for these patients, the relevance of mainstream HF programs, or the relative importance of care by ACHD specialists versus non-ACHD HF specialists. Much of our current "knowledge base" is extrapolated from acquired HF. The very few studies that have been conducted among adults with CHD provide little useful information for treating HF in this unique context. This knowledge gap compounded by the challenges associated with identifying HF in this heterogeneous population requires that clinicians caring for these patients take a flexible but consistent and comprehensive approach to HF diagnosis and treatment. Worsening symptoms, unexplained exercise intolerance, or elevated biomarkers should prompt further investigation and consideration of HF as an underlying cause. By necessity HF diagnosis and treatment must be highly individualized and often begins with invasive hemodynamic assessment to identify residual defects contributing to HF pathophysiology. Comprehensive treatment of ACHD-related HF relies not only on standard HF medications but also tailored exercise/cardiac rehabilitation programs, transcatheter interventions, arrhythmia management, and, in some patients, cardiac surgery. While much remains opaque about this emerging epidemic, there is consensus about its importance and hope that growing collaboration between committed clinical investigators from diverse specialties will soon advance our understanding of and management of HF in adults with CHD.

REFERENCES

[1] J.I. Hoffman, S. Kaplan, R.R. Liberthson, Prevalence of congenital heart disease, Am. Heart J. 147 (3) (2004) 425–439.

[2] A.J. Marelli, A.S. Mackie, R. Ionescu-Ittu, E. Rahme, L. Pilote, Congenital heart disease in the general population: changing prevalence and age distribution, Circulation 115 (2) (2007) 163–172.

[3] P. Moons, P. Engelfriet, H. Kaemmerer, F.J. Meijboom, E. Oechslin, B.J. Mulder, et al., Delivery of care for adult patients with congenital heart disease in Europe: results from the Euro heart survey, Eur. Heart J. 27 (11) (2006) 1324–1330.

[4] C.S. Broberg, L.J. Burchill, Myocardial factor revisited: the importance of myocardial fibrosis in adults with congenital heart disease, Int. J. Cardiol. 189 (2015) 204–210.

[5] A.P. Bolger, R. Sharma, W. Li, M. Leenarts, P.R. Kalra, M. Kemp, et al., Neurohormonal activation and the chronic heart failure syndrome in adults with congenital heart disease, Circulation 106 (1) (2002) 92–99.

[6] A.R. Opotowsky, O.K. Siddiqi, G.D. Webb, Trends in hospitalizations for adults with congenital heart disease in the U.S., J. Am. Coll. Cardiol. 54 (5) (2009) 460–467.

[7] F.H. Rodriguez 3rd, D.S. Moodie, D.R. Parekh, W.J. Franklin, D.L. Morales, F. Zafar, et al., Outcomes of heart failure-related hospitalization in adults with congenital heart disease in the United States, Congenit. Heart Dis. 8 (6) (2013) 513–519.

[8] A.J. Marelli, R. Ionescu-Ittu, A.S. Mackie, L. Guo, N. Dendukuri, M. Kaouache, Lifetime prevalence of congenital heart disease in the general population from 2000 to 2010, Circulation 130 (9) (2014) 749–756.

[9] A.C. Zomer, I. Vaartjes, C.S. Uiterwaal, E.T. van der Velde, L.F. van den Merkhof, L.H. Baur, et al., Circumstances of death in adult congenital heart disease, Int. J. Cardiol. 154 (2) (2012) 168–172.

[10] S. Piran, G. Veldtman, S. Siu, G.D. Webb, P.P. Liu, Heart failure and ventricular dysfunction in patients with single or systemic right ventricles, Circulation 105 (10) (2002) 1189–1194.
[11] L. Burchill, A.S. Saidi, Heart Failure in Congenital Heart Disease: Age of Uncertainty, April 30, 2016. 2017. Available from: http://professional.heart.org/professional/ScienceNews/UCM_480697_Heart-Failure-in-Congenital-Heart-Disease-Age-of-Uncertainty.jsp.
[12] E.N. Oechslin, D.A. Harrison, M.S. Connelly, G.D. Webb, S.C. Siu, Mode of death in adults with congenital heart disease, Am. J. Cardiol. 86 (10) (2000) 1111–1116.
[13] C.L. Verheugt, C.S. Uiterwaal, E.T. van der Velde, F.J. Meijboom, P.G. Pieper, A.P. van Dijk, et al., Mortality in adult congenital heart disease, Eur. Heart J. 31 (10) (2010) 1220–1229.
[14] H.A.N. Connolly, C. Warnes, One thousand patients with adult congenital heart disease: causes of death and lessons learned, J. Am. Coll. Cardiol. 29A (1997).
[15] G.P. Diller, A. Kempny, R. Alonso-Gonzalez, L. Swan, A. Uebing, W. Li, et al., Survival prospects and circumstances of death in contemporary adult congenital heart disease patients under follow-up at a large tertiary centre, Circulation 132 (22) (December 1, 2015) 2118–2125. doi:10.1161/CIRCULATIONAHA.115.017202. Epub 2015 Sep 14. PMID: 26369353.
[16] S.A. Hunt, W.T. Abraham, M.H. Chin, A.M. Feldman, G.S. Francis, T.G. Ganiats, et al., ACC/AHA 2005 guideline update for the diagnosis and management of chronic heart failure in the adult: a report of the American college of cardiology/American heart association task force on practice guidelines (writing committee to update the 2001 guidelines for the evaluation and management of heart failure): developed in collaboration with the American college of chest physicians and the international society for heart and lung transplantation: endorsed by the heart rhythm society, Circulation 112 (12) (2005) e154–235.
[17] K.K. Stout, C.S. Broberg, W.M. Book, F. Cecchin, J.M. Chen, K. Dimopoulos, et al., Chronic heart failure in congenital heart disease: a scientific statement from the American heart association, Circulation 133 (8) (2016) 770–801.
[18] H.J. Ross, Y. Law, W.M. Book, C.S. Broberg, L. Burchill, F. Cecchin, et al., Transplantation and mechanical circulatory support in congenital heart disease: a scientific statement from the American heart association, Circulation 133 (8) (2016) 802–820.
[19] J. McLarry, C. Broberg, A.R. Opotowsky, T. Kaufman, K. Stout, L.J. Burchill, Defining heart failure in adult congenital heart disease, Prog. Pediatr. Cardiol. 38 (1) (2014) 3–7.
[20] V.M. Reddy, J.R. Liddicoat, D.B. McElhinney, M.M. Brook, P. Stanger, F.L. Hanley, Routine primary repair of tetralogy of fallot in neonates and infants less than three months of age, Ann. Thorac. Surg. 60 (6 Suppl.) (1995) S592–S596.
[21] A. Ghai, L. Harris, D.A. Harrison, G.D. Webb, S.C. Siu, Outcomes of late atrial tachyarrhythmias in adults after the fontan operation, J. Am. Coll. Cardiol. 37 (2) (2001) 585–592.
[22] K. Nanthakumar, S. Masse, K. Poku, C.K. Silversides, V.S. Chauhan, J.A. Mariani, et al., Intraoperative high-density global mapping in adult-repaired tetralogy of fallot altered left ventricular and right ventricular activation and implications for resynchronization strategies, J. Am. Coll. Cardiol. 55 (21) (2010) 2409–2411.
[23] F.P. Mongeon, M.Z. Gurvitz, C.S. Broberg, J. Aboulhosn, A.R. Opotowsky, J.D. Kay, et al., Aortic root dilatation in adults with surgically repaired tetralogy of fallot: a multicenter cross-sectional study, Circulation 127 (2) (2013) 172–179.
[24] S.L. Roche, L. Grosse-Wortmann, M.K. Friedberg, A.N. Redington, D. Stephens, P.F. Kantor, Exercise echocardiography demonstrates biventricular systolic dysfunction and reveals decreased left ventricular contractile reserve in children after tetralogy of fallot repair, J. Am. Soc. Echocardiogr. 28 (3) (2015) 294–301.
[25] C.S. Broberg, J. Aboulhosn, F.P. Mongeon, J. Kay, A.M. Valente, P. Khairy, et al., Prevalence of left ventricular systolic dysfunction in adults with repaired tetralogy of fallot, Am. J. Cardiol. 107 (8) (2011) 1215–1220.
[26] T. Geva, B.M. Sandweiss, K. Gauvreau, J.E. Lock, A.J. Powell, Factors associated with impaired clinical status in long-term survivors of tetralogy of fallot repair evaluated by magnetic resonance imaging, J. Am. Coll. Cardiol. 43 (6) (2004) 1068–1074.
[27] A.L. Knauth, K. Gauvreau, A.J. Powell, M.J. Landzberg, E.P. Walsh, J.E. Lock, et al., Ventricular size and function assessed by cardiac MRI predict major adverse clinical outcomes late after tetralogy of fallot repair, Heart 94 (2) (2008) 211–216.
[28] P. Khairy, L. Harris, M.J. Landzberg, S. Viswanathan, A. Barlow, M.A. Gatzoulis, et al., Implantable cardioverter-defibrillators in tetralogy of fallot, Circulation 117 (3) (2008) 363–370.
[29] M.A. Gatzoulis, S. Balaji, S.A. Webber, S.C. Siu, J.S. Hokanson, C. Poile, et al., Risk factors for arrhythmia and sudden cardiac death late after repair of tetralogy of fallot: a multicentre study, Lancet 356 (9234) (2000) 975–981.
[30] T.P. Graham Jr., Y.D. Bernard, B.G. Mellen, D. Celermajer, H. Baumgartner, F. Cetta, et al., Long-term outcome in congenitally corrected transposition of the great arteries: a multi-institutional study, J. Am. Coll. Cardiol. 36 (1) (2000) 255–261.
[31] J.W. Roos-Hesselink, F.J. Meijboom, S.E. Spitaels, R. van Domburg, E.H. van Rijen, E.M. Utens, et al., Decline in ventricular function and clinical condition after Mustard repair for transposition of the great arteries (a prospective study of 22-29 years), Eur. Heart J. 25 (14) (2004) 1264–1270.
[32] T. Millane, E.J. Bernard, E. Jaeggi, R.B. Howman-Giles, R.F. Uren, T.B. Cartmill, et al., Role of ischemia and infarction in late right ventricular dysfunction after atrial repair of transposition of the great arteries, J. Am. Coll. Cardiol. 35 (6) (2000) 1661–1668.
[33] L. Wissocque, B. Mondesert, A.E. Dubart, Late diagnosis of isolated congenitally corrected transposition of the great arteries in a 92-year old woman, Eur. J. Cardiothorac. Surg. 49 (5) (2016) 1524–1525.
[34] T.S. Hornung, E.J. Bernard, D.S. Celermajer, E. Jaeggi, R.B. Howman-Giles, R.B. Chard, et al., Right ventricular dysfunction in congenitally corrected transposition of the great arteries, Am. J. Cardiol. 84 (9) (1999) 1116–1119 A10.
[35] A.M. Valente, S.F. Idriss, P. Cawley, J. Heitner, I. Klem, J. Kay, A.M. Nawrocki, M. Parker, J.R. Herlong, R. Kim, Myocardial fibrosis patterns correlate with adverse right ventricular morphology and function in patients with repaired conotruncal heart defects, J. Am. Coll. Cardiol. 43 (2004).

[36] F.P. Mongeon, H.M. Connolly, J.A. Dearani, Z. Li, C.A. Warnes, Congenitally corrected transposition of the great arteries ventricular function at the time of systemic atrioventricular valve replacement predicts long-term ventricular function, J. Am. Coll. Cardiol. 57 (20) (2011) 2008–2017.
[37] J.C. Huhta, J.D. Maloney, D.G. Ritter, D.M. Ilstrup, R.H. Feldt, Complete atrioventricular block in patients with atrioventricular discordance, Circulation 67 (6) (1983) 1374–1377.
[38] F. Fontan, E. Baudet, Surgical repair of tricuspid atresia, Thorax 26 (3) (1971) 240–248.
[39] M.H. Gewillig, U.R. Lundstrom, J.E. Deanfield, C. Bull, R.C. Franklin, T.P. Graham Jr., et al., Impact of fontan operation on left ventricular size and contractility in tricuspid atresia, Circulation 81 (1) (1990) 118–127.
[40] D.J. Penny, A.N. Redington, Diastolic ventricular function after the fontan operation, Am. J. Cardiol. 69 (9) (1992) 974–975.
[41] D.J. Penny, M.L. Rigby, A.N. Redington, Abnormal patterns of intraventricular flow and diastolic filling after the fontan operation: evidence for incoordinate ventricular wall motion, Br. Heart J. 66 (5) (1991) 375–378.
[42] K.M. Shafer, J.A. Garcia, T.G. Babb, D.E. Fixler, C.R. Ayers, B.D. Levine, The importance of the muscle and ventilatory blood pumps during exercise in patients without a subpulmonary ventricle (fontan operation), J. Am. Coll. Cardiol. 60 (20) (2012) 2115–2121.
[43] L.J. Burchill, A.N. Redington, C.K. Silversides, H.J. Ross, L. Jimenez-Juan, S. Mital, et al., Renin-angiotensin-aldosterone system genotype and serum BNP in a contemporary cohort of adults late after fontan palliation, Int. J. Cardiol. 197 (2015) 209–215.
[44] K.A. Jayakumar, L.J. Addonizio, M.R. Kichuk-Chrisant, M.E. Galantowicz, J.M. Lamour, J.M. Quaegebeur, et al., Cardiac transplantation after the fontan or glenn procedure, J. Am. Coll. Cardiol. 44 (10) (2004) 2065–2072.
[45] A.S. Nathan, B. Loukas, L. Moko, F. Wu, J. Rhodes, R.H. Rathod, et al., Exercise oscillatory ventilation in patients with fontan physiology, Circ. Heart Fail. 8 (2) (2015) 304–311.
[46] P. Khairy, L. Harris, M.J. Landzberg, S.M. Fernandes, A. Barlow, L.A. Mercier, et al., Sudden death and defibrillators in transposition of the great arteries with intra-atrial baffles: a multicenter study, Circ. Arrhythm. Electrophysiol. 1 (4) (2008) 250–257.
[47] P. Wood, The eisenmenger syndrome or pulmonary hypertension with reversed central shunt, Br. Med. J. 2 (5099) (1958) 755–762.
[48] A.R. Opotowsky, M.J. Landzberg, M. Beghetti, The exceptional and far-flung manifestations of heart failure in eisenmenger syndrome, Heart Fail. Clin. 10 (1) (2014) 91–104.
[49] L. Daliento, J. Somerville, P. Presbitero, L. Menti, S. Brach-Prever, G. Rizzoli, et al., Eisenmenger syndrome. Factors relating to deterioration and death, Eur. Heart J. 19 (12) (1998) 1845–1855.
[49a] C.M. Hjortshøj, A. Kempny, A.S. Jensen, K. Sørensen, E. Nagy, M. Dellborg, B. Johansson, V. Rudiene, G. Hong, A.R. Opotowsky, W. Budts, et al., Past and current cause-specific mortality in Eisenmenger syndrome, Eur. Heart J. (April 18, 2017) ehx201.
[50] P. Moceri, K. Dimopoulos, E. Liodakis, I. Germanakis, A. Kempny, G.P. Diller, et al., Echocardiographic predictors of outcome in eisenmenger syndrome, Circulation 126 (12) (2012) 1461–1468.
[51] G.P. Diller, R. Alonso-Gonzalez, A. Kempny, K. Dimopoulos, R. Inuzuka, G. Giannakoulas, et al., B-type natriuretic peptide concentrations in contemporary eisenmenger syndrome patients: predictive value and response to disease targeting therapy, Heart 98 (9) (2012) 736–742.
[52] L.C. Reardon, R.J. Williams, L.S. Houser, P.D. Miner, J.S. Child, J.A. Aboulhosn, Usefulness of serum brain natriuretic peptide to predict adverse events in patients with the eisenmenger syndrome, Am. J. Cardiol. 110 (10) (2012) 1523–1526.
[53] C.S. Broberg, S.K. Prasad, C. Carr, S.V. Babu-Narayan, K. Dimopoulos, M.A. Gatzoulis, Myocardial fibrosis in eisenmenger syndrome: a descriptive cohort study exploring associations of late gadolinium enhancement with clinical status and survival, J. Cardiovasc. Magn. Reson. 16 (2014) 32.
[54] N.F. Voelkel, R.A. Quaife, L.A. Leinwand, R.J. Barst, M.D. McGoon, D.R. Meldrum, et al., Right ventricular function and failure: report of a national heart, lung, and blood institute working group on cellular and molecular mechanisms of right heart failure, Circulation 114 (17) (2006) 1883–1891.
[55] K. Pushparajah, J.K. Wong, H.R. Bellsham-Revell, T. Hussain, I. Valverde, A. Bell, et al., Magnetic resonance imaging catheter stress haemodynamics post-fontan in hypoplastic left heart syndrome, Eur. Heart J. Cardiovasc. Imaging 17 (6) (2016) 644–651.
[56] W. De Mey, B. Cools, R. Heying, W. Budts, J.J. Louw, D.E. Boshoff, et al., Can a volume challenge pinpoint the limiting factor in a fontan circulation? Acta Cardiol. 70 (5) (2015) 536–542.
[57] R.J. Butts, S.M. Chowdhury, G.H. Baker, V. Bandisode, A.J. Savage, A.M. Atz, Effect of sildenafil on pressure-volume loop measures of ventricular function in fontan patients, Pediatr. Cardiol. 37 (1) (2016) 184–191.
[58] J.A. Eindhoven, A.E. van den Bosch, E. Boersma, J.W. Roos-Hesselink, The usefulness of brain natriuretic peptide in simple congenital heart disease – a systematic review, Cardiol. Young 23 (3) (2013) 315–324.
[59] J.A. Eindhoven, A.E. van den Bosch, P.R. Jansen, E. Boersma, J.W. Roos-Hesselink, The usefulness of brain natriuretic peptide in complex congenital heart disease: a systematic review, J. Am. Coll. Cardiol. 60 (21) (2012) 2140–2149.
[60] J.A. Eindhoven, A.E. van den Bosch, T.P. Ruys, P. Opic, J.A. Cuypers, J.S. McGhie, et al., N-terminal pro-B-type natriuretic peptide and its relationship with cardiac function in adults with congenital heart disease, J. Am. Coll. Cardiol. 62 (13) (2013) 1203–1212.
[61] J.O. Younge, J.A. Eindhoven, E.W. Utens, P. Opic, J.A. Cuypers, A.E. van den Bosch, et al., Association between N-terminal pro-brain natriuretic peptide and quality of life in adult patients with congenital heart disease, Cardiol. Young 25 (2) (2015) 288–294.
[62] H. Oya, N. Nagaya, T. Satoh, F. Sakamaki, S. Kyotani, M. Fujita, et al., Haemodynamic correlates and prognostic significance of serum uric acid in adult patients with eisenmenger syndrome, Heart 84 (1) (2000) 53–58.
[63] J.A. Eindhoven, A.E. van den Bosch, R.M. Oemrawsingh, V.J. Baggen, I. Kardys, J.A. Cuypers, et al., Release of growth-differentiation factor 15 and associations with cardiac function in adult patients with congenital heart disease, Int. J. Cardiol. 202 (2016) 246–251.
[64] J.A. Eindhoven, J.W. Roos-Hesselink, A.E. van den Bosch, I. Kardys, J.M. Cheng, J.F. Veenis, et al., High-sensitive troponin-T in adult congenital heart disease, Int. J. Cardiol. 184 (2015) 405–411.

[65] M.J. Schuuring, A.C. van Riel, J.C. Vis, M.G. Duffels, J.P. van Straalen, S.M. Boekholdt, et al., High-sensitivity troponin T is associated with poor outcome in adults with pulmonary arterial hypertension due to congenital heart disease, Congenit. Heart Dis. 8 (6) (December 2012) 520–526.

[66] A.R. Opotowsky, F.R. Baraona, J. Owumi, B. Loukas, M.N. Singh, A.M. Valente, et al., Galectin-3 is elevated and associated with adverse outcomes in patients with single ventricle fontan circulation, J. Am. Heart Assoc. 5 (1) (2016).

[67] V.J. Baggen, A.E. van den Bosch, J.A. Eindhoven, A.W. Schut, J.A. Cuypers, M. Witsenburg, et al., Prognostic value of N-terminal pro-B-type natriuretic peptide, troponin-T, and growth-differentiation factor 15 in adult congenital heart disease, Circulation 135 (3) (2017) 264–279.

[68] S. Rajpal, L. Alshawabkeh, A.R. Opotowsky, Current role of blood and urine biomarkers in the clinical care of adults with congenital heart disease, Curr. Cardiol. Rep. 19 (6) (2017) 50.

[69] F. Rischard, R. Vanderpool, I. Jenkins, M. Dalabih, J. Colombo, D. Lax, et al., Selective pulmonary vasodilation improves ventriculovascular coupling and gas exchange in a patient with unrepaired single-ventricle physiology, Pulm. Circ. 5 (2) (2015) 407–411.

[70] A.R. Opotowsky, D. Halpern, T.J. Kulik, D.M. Systrom, F. Wu, Inadequate venous return as a primary cause for fontan circulatory limitation, J. Heart Lung Transplant. 33 (11) (2014) 1194–1196.

[71] N.C. Berry, A. Manyoo, W.M. Oldham, T.E. Stephens, R.H. Goldstein, A.B. Waxman, et al., Protocol for exercise hemodynamic assessment: performing an invasive cardiopulmonary exercise test in clinical practice, Pulm. Circ. 5 (4) (2015) 610–618.

[72] P. Khairy, G.F. Van Hare, S. Balaji, C.I. Berul, F. Cecchin, M.I. Cohen, et al., PACES/HRS expert consensus statement on the recognition and management of arrhythmias in adult congenital heart disease: developed in partnership between the pediatric and congenital electrophysiology society (PACES) and the heart rhythm society (HRS). Endorsed by the governing bodies of PACES, HRS, the American college of cardiology (ACC), the American heart association (AHA), the European heart rhythm association (EHRA), the Canadian heart rhythm society (CHRS), and the international society for adult congenital heart disease (ISACHD), Can. J. Cardiol. 30 (10) (2014) e1–e63.

[73] C.C. Benson, A.M. Valente, K.E. Economy, Y. Hoffman-Sage, L.M. Bevilacqua, M. Podovei, et al., Discovery and management of diaphragmatic hernia related to abandoned epicardial pacemaker wires in a pregnant woman with {S,L,L} transposition of the great arteries, Congenit. Heart Dis. 7 (2) (2012) 183–188.

[74] J. Rychik, G. Veldtman, E. Rand, P. Russo, J.J. Rome, K. Krok, et al., The precarious state of the liver after a fontan operation: summary of a multidisciplinary symposium, Pediatr. Cardiol. 33 (7) (2012) 1001–1012.

[75] I.N. Guha, S. Bokhandi, Z. Ahmad, N. Sheron, R. Cope, C. Marshall, et al., Structural and functional uncoupling of liver performance in the fontan circulation, Int. J. Cardiol. 164 (1) (2013) 77–81.

[76] T.J. Kendall, B. Stedman, N. Hacking, M. Haw, J.J. Vettukattill, A.P. Salmon, et al., Hepatic fibrosis and cirrhosis in the fontan circulation: a detailed morphological study, J. Clin. Pathol. 61 (4) (2008) 504–508.

[77] F.M. Wu, M.M. Jonas, A.R. Opotowsky, A. Harmon, R. Raza, C. Ukomadu, et al., Portal and centrilobular hepatic fibrosis in fontan circulation and clinical outcomes, J. Heart Lung transplant. 34 (7) (2015) 883–891.

[78] A.A. Ghaferi, G.M. Hutchins, Progression of liver pathology in patients undergoing the fontan procedure: chronic passive congestion, cardiac cirrhosis, hepatic adenoma, and hepatocellular carcinoma, J. Thorac. Cardiovasc. Surg. 129 (6) (2005) 1348–1352.

[79] E.V. Krieger, L.E. Moko, F. Wu, M.J. Landzberg, A.M. Valente, G.E. Assenza, et al., Single ventricle anatomy is associated with increased frequency of nonalcoholic cirrhosis, Int. J. Cardiol. 167 (5) (2013) 1918–1923.

[80] C.H. Kiesewetter, N. Sheron, J.J. Vettukattill, N. Hacking, B. Stedman, H. Millward-Sadler, et al., Hepatic changes in the failing fontan circulation, Heart 93 (5) (2007) 579–584.

[81] T. Saliba, S. Dorkhom, E.M. O'Reilly, E. Ludwig, B. Gansukh, G.K. Abou-Alfa, Hepatocellular carcinoma in two patients with cardiac cirrhosis, Eur. J. Gastroenterol. Hepatol. 22 (7) (2010) 889–891.

[82] K. Dimopoulos, G.P. Diller, E. Koltsida, A. Pijuan-Domenech, S.A. Papadopoulou, S.V. Babu-Narayan, et al., Prevalence, predictors, and prognostic value of renal dysfunction in adults with congenital heart disease, Circulation 117 (18) (2008) 2320–2328.

[83] S. Dittrich, N.A. Haas, C. Buhrer, C. Muller, I. Dahnert, P.E. Lange, Renal impairment in patients with long-standing cyanotic congenital heart disease, Acta Paediatr. 87 (9) (1998) 949–954.

[84] J.R. Burke, E.F. Glasgow, D.A. McCredie, H.R. Powell, Nephropathy in cyanotic congenital heart disease, Clin. Nephrol. 7 (1) (1977) 38–42.

[85] E.A. Ross, J.K. Perloff, G.M. Danovitch, J.S. Child, M.M. Canobbio, Renal function and urate metabolism in late survivors with cyanotic congenital heart disease, Circulation 73 (3) (1986) 396–400.

[86] E. Martinez-Quintana, F. Rodriguez-Gonzalez, M. Fabregas-Brouard, V. Nieto-Lago, Serum and 24-hour urine analysis in adult cyanotic and noncyanotic congenital heart disease patients, Congenit. Heart Dis. 4 (3) (2009) 147–152.

[87] P. Anne, W. Du, T.K. Mattoo, M.V. Zilberman, Nephropathy in patients after fontan palliation, Int. J. Cardiol. 132 (2) (2009) 244–247.

[88] A.R. Opotowsky, F.R. Baraona, F.R. Mc Causland, B. Loukas, E. Landzberg, M.J. Landzberg, et al., Estimated glomerular filtration rate and urine biomarkers in patients with single-ventricle fontan circulation, Heart 103 (6) (2017) 434–442.

[89] R. Alonso-Gonzalez, F. Borgia, G.P. Diller, R. Inuzuka, A. Kempny, A. Martinez-Naharro, et al., Abnormal lung function in adults with congenital heart disease: prevalence, relation to cardiac anatomy, and association with survival, Circulation 127 (8) (2013) 882–890.

[90] A.R. Opotowsky, Abnormal spirometry in congenital heart disease: where do we go from here? Circulation 127 (8) (2013) 865–867.

[91] M. Greutmann, T.L. Le, D. Tobler, P. Biaggi, E.N. Oechslin, C.K. Silversides, et al., Generalised muscle weakness in young adults with congenital heart disease, Heart 97 (14) (2011) 1164–1168.

[92] A.R. Opotowsky, M.J. Landzberg, M.G. Earing, F.M. Wu, J.K. Triedman, A. Casey, et al., Abnormal spirometry after the fontan procedure is common and associated with impaired aerobic capacity, Am. J. Physiol. Heart Circ. Physiol. 307 (1) (2014) H110–H117.

[93] P. Monagle, M. Andrew, Coagulation abnormalities after fontan procedures, J. Thorac. Cardiovasc. Surg. 115 (3) (1998) 732–733.

[94] A.M. Valente, A.B. Bhatt, S. Cook, M.G. Earing, D.R. Gersony, J. Aboulhosn, et al., The CALF (congenital heart disease in adults lower extremity systemic venous health in fontan patients) study, J. Am. Coll. Cardiol. 56 (2) (2010) 144–150.

[95] P. Khairy, S.M. Fernandes, J.E. Mayer Jr., J.K. Triedman, E.P. Walsh, J.E. Lock, et al., Long-term survival, modes of death, and predictors of mortality in patients with fontan surgery, Circulation 117 (1) (2008) 85–92.

[96] C.K. Silversides, J.T. Granton, E. Konen, M.A. Hart, G.D. Webb, J. Therrien, Pulmonary thrombosis in adults with eisenmenger syndrome, J. Am. Coll. Cardiol. 42 (11) (2003) 1982–1987.

[97] P. Khairy, M.J. Landzberg, M.A. Gatzoulis, L.A. Mercier, S.M. Fernandes, J.M. Cote, et al., Transvenous pacing leads and systemic thromboemboli in patients with intracardiac shunts: a multicenter study, Circulation 113 (20) (2006) 2391–2397.

[98] C.S. Broberg, M. Ujita, S. Prasad, W. Li, M. Rubens, B.E. Bax, et al., Pulmonary arterial thrombosis in eisenmenger syndrome is associated with biventricular dysfunction and decreased pulmonary flow velocity, J. Am. Coll. Cardiol. 50 (7) (2007) 634–642.

[99] J. Sandoval, L.E. Santos, J. Cordova, T. Pulido, G. Gutierrez, E. Bautista, et al., Does anticoagulation in eisenmenger syndrome impact long-term survival? Congenit. Heart Dis. 7 (3) (2012) 268–276.

[100] P. Monagle, A. Cochrane, R. Roberts, C. Manlhiot, R. Weintraub, B. Szechtman, et al., A multicenter, randomized trial comparing heparin/warfarin and acetylsalicylic acid as primary thromboprophylaxis for 2 years after the fontan procedure in children, J. Am. Coll. Cardiol. 58 (6) (2011) 645–651.

[101] B.S. Marino, P.H. Lipkin, J.W. Newburger, G. Peacock, M. Gerdes, J.W. Gaynor, et al., Neurodevelopmental outcomes in children with congenital heart disease: evaluation and management: a scientific statement from the American heart association, Circulation 126 (9) (2012) 1143–1172.

[102] J. Homsy, S. Zaidi, Y. Shen, J.S. Ware, K.E. Samocha, K.J. Karczewski, et al., De novo mutations in congenital heart disease with neurodevelopmental and other congenital anomalies, Science 350 (6265) (2015) 1262–1266.

[103] S.P. Miller, P.S. McQuillen, S. Hamrick, D. Xu, D.V. Glidden, N. Charlton, et al., Abnormal brain development in newborns with congenital heart disease, N. Engl. J. Med. 357 (19) (2007) 1928–1938.

[104] J.R. Kaltman, H. Di, Z. Tian, J. Rychik, Impact of congenital heart disease on cerebrovascular blood flow dynamics in the fetus, Ultrasound Obstet. Gynecol. 25 (1) (2005) 32–36.

[105] L. Ong, R.P. Nolan, J. Irvine, A.H. Kovacs, Parental overprotection and heart-focused anxiety in adults with congenital heart disease, Int. J. Behav. Med. 18 (3) (2011) 260–267.

[106] H.B. Sprague, P.D. White, The tetralogy of fallot, J. Am. Med. Assoc. 92 (10) (1929) 787–791.

[107] L.X. Deng, A.M. Khan, D. Drajpuch, S. Fuller, J. Ludmir, C.E. Mascio, et al., Prevalence and correlates of post-traumatic stress disorder in adults with congenital heart disease, Am. J. Cardiol. 117 (5) (2015) 853–857.

[108] A.H. Kovacs, A.S. Saidi, E.A. Kuhl, S.F. Sears, C. Silversides, J.L. Harrison, et al., Depression and anxiety in adult congenital heart disease: predictors and prevalence, Int. J. Cardiol. 137 (2) (2009) 158–164.

[109] R.E. Shaddy, M.M. Boucek, D.T. Hsu, R.J. Boucek, C.E. Canter, L. Mahony, et al., Carvedilol for children and adolescents with heart failure: a randomized controlled trial, JAMA 298 (10) (2007) 1171–1179.

[110] T. van der Bom, M.M. Winter, B.J. Bouma, M. Groenink, H.W. Vliegen, P.G. Pieper, et al., Effect of valsartan on systemic right ventricular function: a double-blind, randomized, placebo-controlled pilot trial, Circulation 127 (3) (2013) 322–330.

[111] A. Dore, C. Houde, K.L. Chan, A. Ducharme, P. Khairy, M. Juneau, et al., Angiotensin receptor blockade and exercise capacity in adults with systemic right ventricles: a multicenter, randomized, placebo-controlled clinical trial, Circulation 112 (16) (2005) 2411–2416.

[112] S.J. Hechter, P.M. Fredriksen, P. Liu, G. Veldtman, N. Merchant, M. Freeman, et al., Angiotensin-converting enzyme inhibitors in adults after the Mustard procedure, Am. J. Cardiol. 87 (5) (2001) 660–663 A11.

[113] S.J. Lester, D.B. McElhinney, E. Viloria, G.P. Reddy, E. Ryan, W. Tworetzky, et al., Effects of losartan in patients with a systemically functioning morphologic right ventricle after atrial repair of transposition of the great arteries, Am. J. Cardiol. 88 (11) (2001) 1314–1316.

[114] J. Therrien, Y. Provost, J. Harrison, M. Connelly, H. Kaemmerer, G.D. Webb, Effect of angiotensin receptor blockade on systemic right ventricular function and size: a small, randomized, placebo-controlled study, Int. J. Cardiol. 129 (2) (2008) 187–192.

[115] G.P. Diller, K. Dimopoulos, M.G. Kaya, C. Harries, A. Uebing, W. Li, et al., Long-term safety, tolerability and efficacy of bosentan in adults with pulmonary arterial hypertension associated with congenital heart disease, Heart 93 (8) (2007) 974–976.

[116] N. Galie, M. Beghetti, M.A. Gatzoulis, J. Granton, R.M. Berger, A. Lauer, et al., Bosentan therapy in patients with eisenmenger syndrome: a multicenter, double-blind, randomized, placebo-controlled study, Circulation 114 (1) (2006) 48–54.

[117] S. Mukhopadhyay, S. Nathani, J. Yusuf, D. Shrimal, S. Tyagi, Clinical efficacy of phosphodiesterase-5 inhibitor tadalafil in eisenmenger syndrome–a randomized, placebo-controlled, double-blind crossover study, Congenit. Heart Dis. 6 (5) (2011) 424–431.

[118] E.L. Tay, M. Papaphylactou, G.P. Diller, R. Alonso-Gonzalez, R. Inuzuka, G. Giannakoulas, et al., Quality of life and functional capacity can be improved in patients with eisenmenger syndrome with oral sildenafil therapy, Int. J. Cardiol. 149 (3) (2011) 372–376.

[119] S.M. Fernandes, J.W. Newburger, P. Lang, D.D. Pearson, J.A. Feinstein, K. Gauvreau, et al., Usefulness of epoprostenol therapy in the severely ill adolescent/adult with eisenmenger physiology, Am. J. Cardiol. 91 (5) (2003) 632–635.

[120] H. Baumgartner, P. Bonhoeffer, N.M. De Groot, F. de Haan, J.E. Deanfield, N. Galie, et al., ESC guidelines for the management of grown-up congenital heart disease (new version 2010), Eur. Heart J. 31 (23) (2010) 2915–2957.

[121] K. Iversen, A.S. Jensen, T.V. Jensen, N.G. Vejlstrup, L. Sondergaard, Combination therapy with bosentan and sildenafil in eisenmenger syndrome: a randomized, placebo-controlled, double-blinded trial, Eur. Heart J. 31 (9) (2010) 1124–1131.

[122] N. Galie, J.A. Barbera, A.E. Frost, H.A. Ghofrani, M.M. Hoeper, V.V. McLaughlin, et al., Initial use of ambrisentan plus tadalafil in pulmonary arterial hypertension, N. Engl. J. Med. 373 (9) (2015) 834–844.

[123] S.L. Roche, A.N. Redington, The failing right ventricle in congenital heart disease, Can. J. Cardiol. 29 (7) (2013) 768–778.

[124] T. Cotts, P. Khairy, A.R. Opotowsky, A.S. John, A.M. Valente, A.N. Zaidi, et al., Clinical research priorities in adult congenital heart disease, Int. J. Cardiol. 171 (3) (2014) 351–360.

[125] A. Giardini, L. Lovato, A. Donti, R. Formigari, G. Gargiulo, F.M. Picchio, et al., A pilot study on the effects of carvedilol on right ventricular remodelling and exercise tolerance in patients with systemic right ventricle, Int. J. Cardiol. 114 (2) (2007) 241–246.

[126] B. Robinson, C.T. Heise, J.W. Moore, J. Anella, M. Sokoloski, E. Eshaghpour, Afterload reduction therapy in patients following intraatrial baffle operation for transposition of the great arteries, Pediatr. Cardiol. 23 (6) (2002) 618–623.

[127] A. Yehya, T. Lyle, M.A. Pernetz, M.E. McConnell, B. Kogon, W.M. Book, Pulmonary arterial hypertension in patients with prior atrial switch procedure for d-transposition of great arteries (dTGA), Int. J. Cardiol. 143 (3) (2010) 271–275.

[128] A.R. Doughan, M.E. McConnell, W.M. Book, Effect of beta blockers (carvedilol or metoprolol XL) in patients with transposition of great arteries and dysfunction of the systemic right ventricle, Am. J. Cardiol. 99 (5) (2007) 704–706.

[129] K. Norozi, J. Bahlmann, B. Raab, V. Alpers, J.O. Arnhold, T. Kuehne, et al., A prospective, randomized, double-blind, placebo controlled trial of beta-blockade in patients who have undergone surgical correction of tetralogy of fallot, Cardiol. Young 17 (4) (2007) 372–379.

[130] S.V. Babu-Narayan, A. Uebing, P.A. Davlouros, M. Kemp, S. Davidson, K. Dimopoulos, et al., Randomised trial of ramipril in repaired tetralogy of fallot and pulmonary regurgitation: the APPROPRIATE study (Ace inhibitors for Potential PRevention of the deleterious effects of pulmonary regurgitation in adults with repaired TEtralogy of fallot, Int. J. Cardiol. 154 (3) (2012) 299–305.

[131] M. D'Alto, E. Romeo, P. Argiento, B. Sarubbi, G. Santoro, N. Grimaldi, et al., Bosentan-sildenafil association in patients with congenital heart disease-related pulmonary arterial hypertension and eisenmenger physiology, Int. J. Cardiol. 155 (3) (2012) 378–382.

[132] K. Dimopoulos, R. Inuzuka, S. Goletto, G. Giannakoulas, L. Swan, S.J. Wort, et al., Improved survival among patients with eisenmenger syndrome receiving advanced therapy for pulmonary arterial hypertension, Circulation 121 (1) (2010) 20–25.

[133] A. Kempny, K. Dimopoulos, R. Alonso-Gonzalez, M. Alvarez-Barredo, O. Tutarel, A. Uebing, et al., Six-minute walk test distance and resting oxygen saturations but not functional class predict outcome in adult patients with eisenmenger syndrome, Int. J. Cardiol. 168 (5) (2013) 4784–4789.

[134] S. Mukhopadhyay, M. Sharma, S. Ramakrishnan, J. Yusuf, M.D. Gupta, N. Bhamri, et al., Phosphodiesterase-5 inhibitor in eisenmenger syndrome: a preliminary observational study, Circulation 114 (17) (2006) 1807–1810.

[135] D.T. Hsu, V. Zak, L. Mahony, L.A. Sleeper, A.M. Atz, J.C. Levine, et al., Enalapril in infants with single ventricle: results of a multicenter randomized trial, Circulation 122 (4) (2010) 333–340.

[136] A.A. Kouatli, J.A. Garcia, T.M. Zellers, E.M. Weinstein, L. Mahony, Enalapril does not enhance exercise capacity in patients after fontan procedure, Circulation 96 (5) (1997) 1507–1512.

[137] A. Hebert, U.R. Mikkelsen, U. Thilen, L. Idorn, A.S. Jensen, E. Nagy, et al., Bosentan improves exercise capacity in adolescents and adults after fontan operation: the TEMPO (treatment with endothelin receptor antagonist in fontan patients, a randomized, placebo-controlled, double-blind study measuring peak oxygen consumption) study, Circulation 130 (23) (2014) 2021–2030.

[138] M.J. Schuuring, J.C. Vis, A.P. van Dijk, J.P. van Melle, H.W. Vliegen, P.G. Pieper, et al., Impact of bosentan on exercise capacity in adults after the fontan procedure: a randomized controlled trial, Eur. J. Heart Fail. 15 (6) (2013) 690–698.

[139] D.J. Goldberg, B. French, M.G. McBride, B.S. Marino, N. Mirarchi, B.D. Hanna, et al., Impact of oral sildenafil on exercise performance in children and young adults after the fontan operation: a randomized, double-blind, placebo-controlled, crossover trial, Circulation 123 (11) (2011) 1185–1193.

[140] M.M. Massin, I. Astadicko, H. Dessy, Noncardiac comorbidities of congenital heart disease in children, Acta Paediatr. 96 (5) (2007) 753–755.

[141] J. Deanfield, E. Thaulow, C. Warnes, G. Webb, F. Kolbel, A. Hoffman, et al., Management of grown up congenital heart disease, Eur. Heart J. 24 (11) (2003) 1035–1084.

[142] S. Tabbutt, J.W. Gaynor, J.W. Newburger, Neurodevelopmental outcomes after congenital heart surgery and strategies for improvement, Curr. Opin. Cardiol. 27 (2) (2012) 82–91.

[143] N.M. Pinto, B.S. Marino, G. Wernovsky, S.D. de Ferranti, A.Z. Walsh, M. Laronde, et al., Obesity is a common comorbidity in children with congenital and acquired heart disease, Pediatrics 120 (5) (2007) e1157–e1164.

[144] J.S. Dua, A.R. Cooper, K.R. Fox, A. Graham Stuart, Physical activity levels in adults with congenital heart disease, Eur. J. Cardiovasc. Prev. Rehabil. 14 (2) (2007) 287–293.

[145] M.A. Stefan, W.M. Hopman, J.F. Smythe, Effect of activity restriction owing to heart disease on obesity, Arch. Pediatr. Adolesc. Med. 159 (5) (2005) 477–481.

[146] T. Becker-Grunig, H. Klose, N. Ehlken, M. Lichtblau, C. Nagel, C. Fischer, et al., Efficacy of exercise training in pulmonary arterial hypertension associated with congenital heart disease, Int. J. Cardiol. 168 (1) (2013) 375–381.

[147] J.S. Dua, A.R. Cooper, K.R. Fox, G. Stuart, Exercise training in adults with congenital heart disease: feasibility and benefits, Int. J. Cardiol. 138 (2) (2010) 196–205.

[148] J. Rhodes, T.J. Curran, L. Camil, N. Rabideau, D.R. Fulton, N.S. Gauthier, et al., Impact of cardiac rehabilitation on the exercise function of children with serious congenital heart disease, Pediatrics 116 (6) (2005) 1339–1345.

[149] N. Duppen, T. Takken, M.T. Hopman, A.D. ten Harkel, K. Dulfer, E.M. Utens, et al., Systematic review of the effects of physical exercise training programmes in children and young adults with congenital heart disease, Int. J. Cardiol. 168 (3) (2013) 1779–1787.

[150] M.M. Winter, T. van der Bom, L.C. de Vries, A. Balducci, B.J. Bouma, P.G. Pieper, et al., Exercise training improves exercise capacity in adult patients with a systemic right ventricle: a randomized clinical trial, Eur. Heart J. 33 (11) (2012) 1378–1385.

[151] A. Ubeda Tikkanen, A.R. Opotowsky, A.B. Bhatt, M.J. Landzberg, J. Rhodes, Physical activity is associated with improved aerobic exercise capacity over time in adults with congenital heart disease, Int. J. Cardiol. 168 (5) (2013) 4685–4691.

[152] H. Ismail, J.R. McFarlane, A.H. Nojoumian, G. Dieberg, N.A. Smart, Clinical outcomes and cardiovascular responses to different exercise training intensities in patients with heart failure: a systematic review and meta-analysis, JACC 1 (6) (2013) 514–522.
[153] J.H. O'Keefe, H.R. Patil, C.J. Lavie, A. Magalski, R.A. Vogel, P.A. McCullough, Potential adverse cardiovascular effects from excessive endurance exercise, Mayo Clin. Proc. 87 (6) (2012) 587–595.
[154] N.K. Wenger, Current status of cardiac rehabilitation, J. Am. Coll. Cardiol. 51 (17) (2008) 1619–1631.
[155] G.J. Balady, M.A. Williams, P.A. Ades, V. Bittner, P. Comoss, J.M. Foody, et al., Core components of cardiac rehabilitation/secondary prevention programs: 2007 update: a scientific statement from the American heart association exercise, cardiac rehabilitation, and prevention committee, the council on clinical cardiology; the councils on cardiovascular nursing, epidemiology and prevention, and nutrition, physical activity, and metabolism; and the American association of cardiovascular and pulmonary rehabilitation, Circulation 115 (20) (2007) 2675–2682.
[156] R.S. McKelvie, K.K. Teo, R. Roberts, N. McCartney, D. Humen, T. Montague, et al., Effects of exercise training in patients with heart failure: the exercise rehabilitation trial (EXERT), Am. Heart J. 144 (1) (2002) 23–30.
[157] B.S. Heran, J.M. Chen, S. Ebrahim, T. Moxham, N. Oldridge, K. Rees, et al., Exercise-based cardiac rehabilitation for coronary heart disease, Cochrane Database Syst. Rev. (7) (2011) CD001800.
[158] J. Rhodes, T.J. Curran, L. Camil, N. Rabideau, D.R. Fulton, N.S. Gauthier, et al., Sustained effects of cardiac rehabilitation in children with serious congenital heart disease, Pediatrics 118 (3) (2006) e586–e593.
[159] A.U. Tikkanen, A.R. Oyaga, O.A. Riano, E.M. Alvaro, J. Rhodes, Paediatric cardiac rehabilitation in congenital heart disease: a systematic review, Cardiol. Young (2012) 1–10.
[160] S.C. Park, W.H. Neches, R.A. Mathews, F.J. Fricker, L.B. Beerman, D.R. Fischer, et al., Hemodynamic function after the mustard operation for transposition of the great arteries, Am. J. Cardiol. 51 (9) (1983) 1514–1519.
[161] A.R. Castaneda, G.A. Trusler, M.H. Paul, E.H. Blackstone, J.W. Kirklin, The early results of treatment of simple transposition in the current era, J. Thorac. Cardiovasc. Surg. 95 (1) (1988) 14–28.
[162] P. Moons, M. Gewillig, T. Sluysmans, H. Verhaaren, P. Viart, M. Massin, et al., Long term outcome up to 30 years after the mustard or senning operation: a nationwide multicentre study in Belgium, Heart 90 (3) (2004) 307–313.
[163] K.D. Hill, G. Fleming, J. Curt Fudge, E.L. Albers, T.P. Doyle, J.F. Rhodes, Percutaneous interventions in high-risk patients following mustard repair of transposition of the great arteries, Catheter. Cardiovasc. Interv. 80 (6) (2012) 905–914.
[164] N.D. Bridges, J.E. Lock, A.R. Castaneda, Baffle fenestration with subsequent transcatheter closure. Modification of the fontan operation for patients at increased risk, Circulation 82 (5) (1990) 1681–1689.
[165] H. Laks, J.M. Pearl, G.S. Haas, D.C. Drinkwater, E. Milgalter, J.M. Jarmakani, et al., Partial fontan: advantages of an adjustable interatrial communication, Ann. Thorac. Surg. 52 (5) (1991) 1084–1094 discussion 94–95.
[166] H. Vyas, D.J. Driscoll, A.K. Cabalka, F. Cetta, D.J. Hagler, Results of transcatheter fontan fenestration to treat protein losing enteropathy, Catheter. Cardiovasc. Interv. 69 (4) (2007) 584–589.
[167] L. Coats, S. Khambadkone, G. Derrick, S. Sridharan, S. Schievano, B. Mist, et al., Physiological and clinical consequences of relief of right ventricular outflow tract obstruction late after repair of congenital heart defects, Circulation 113 (17) (2006) 2037–2044.
[168] L. Coats, S. Khambadkone, G. Derrick, M. Hughes, R. Jones, B. Mist, et al., Physiological consequences of percutaneous pulmonary valve implantation: the different behaviour of volume- and pressure-overloaded ventricles, Eur. Heart J. 28 (15) (2007) 1886–1893.
[169] J.P. Cheatham, W.E. Hellenbrand, E.M. Zahn, T.K. Jones, D.P. Berman, J.A. Vincent, et al., Clinical and hemodynamic outcomes up to 7 Years after transcatheter pulmonary valve replacement in the US Melody valve investigational device exemption trial, Circulation 131 (22) (2015) 1960–1970.
[170] J. Bouchardy, J. Therrien, L. Pilote, R. Ionescu-Ittu, G. Martucci, N. Bottega, et al., Atrial arrhythmias in adults with congenital heart disease, Circulation 120 (17) (2009) 1679–1686.
[171] E.P. Walsh, F. Cecchin, Arrhythmias in adult patients with congenital heart disease, Circulation 115 (4) (2007) 534–545.
[172] J.K. Triedman, D.M. Bergau, J.P. Saul, M.R. Epstein, E.P. Walsh, Efficacy of radiofrequency ablation for control of intraatrial reentrant tachycardia in patients with congenital heart disease, J. Am. Coll. Cardiol. 30 (4) (1997) 1032–1038.
[173] J. Janousek, R.A. Gebauer, H. Abdul-Khaliq, M. Turner, L. Kornyei, O. Grollmuss, et al., Cardiac resynchronisation therapy in paediatric and congenital heart disease: differential effects in various anatomical and functional substrates, Heart 95 (14) (2009) 1165–1171.
[174] J.A. Kirsh, E.A. Stephenson, A.N. Redington, Images in cardiovascular medicine. Recovery of left ventricular systolic function after biventricular resynchronization pacing in a child with repaired tetralogy of fallot and severe biventricular dysfunction, Circulation 113 (14) (2006) e691–e692.
[175] J.B. Thambo, M. De Guillebon, O. Xhaet, P. Dos Santos, F. Roubertie, L. Labrousse, et al., Biventricular pacing in patients with tetralogy of fallot: non-invasive epicardial mapping and clinical impact, Int. J. Cardiol. 163 (2) (2013) 170–174.
[176] P. Khairy, G.F. Van Hare, S. Balaji, C.I. Berul, F. Cecchin, M.I. Cohen, et al., PACES/HRS expert consensus statement on the recognition and management of arrhythmias in adult congenital heart disease: developed in partnership between the pediatric and congenital electrophysiology society (PACES) and the heart rhythm society (HRS). Endorsed by the governing bodies of PACES, HRS, the American college of cardiology (ACC), the American heart association (AHA), the European heart Rhythm association (EHRA), the Canadian heart rhythm society (CHRS), and the international society for adult congenital heart disease (ISACHD), Heart Rhythm 11 (10) (2014) e102–e165.
[177] F. Cecchin, P.A. Frangini, D.W. Brown, F. Fynn-Thompson, M.E. Alexander, J.K. Triedman, et al., Cardiac resynchronization therapy (and multisite pacing) in pediatrics and congenital heart disease: five years experience in a single institution, J. Cardiovasc. Electrophysiol. 20 (1) (2009) 58–65.
[178] A.M. Dubin, J. Janousek, E. Rhee, M.J. Strieper, F. Cecchin, I.H. Law, et al., Resynchronization therapy in pediatric and congenital heart disease patients: an international multicenter study, J. Am. Coll. Cardiol. 46 (12) (2005) 2277–2283.
[179] L.R. Prieto, A.J. Hordof, M. Secic, M.S. Rosenbaum, W.M. Gersony, Progressive tricuspid valve disease in patients with congenitally corrected transposition of the great arteries, Circulation 98 (10) (1998) 997–1005.

[180] J.A. van Son, G.K. Danielson, J.C. Huhta, C.A. Warnes, W.D. Edwards, H.V. Schaff, et al., Late results of systemic atrioventricular valve replacement in corrected transposition, J. Thorac. Cardiovasc. Surg. 109 (4) (1995) 642–652 discussion 52–53.
[181] C. Mavroudis, B.J. Deal, C.L. Backer, R.D. Stewart, W.H. Franklin, S. Tsao, et al., J. maxwell chamberlain memorial paper for congenital heart surgery. 111 fontan conversions with arrhythmia surgery: surgical lessons and outcomes, Ann. Thorac. Surg. 84 (5) (2007) 1457–1465 discussion 65–66.
[182] C.L. Poh, A. Cochrane, J.C. Galati, A. Bullock, D.S. Celermajer, T. Gentles, et al., Ten-year outcomes of fontan conversion in Australia and New Zealand demonstrate the superiority of a strategy of early conversiondagger, Eur. J. Cardiothorac. Surg. 49 (2) (2016) 530–535.
[183] C.L. Backer, J.M. Costello, B.J. Deal, Fontan conversion: guidelines from down under, Eur. J. Cardiothorac. Surg. 49 (2) (2016) 536–537.

Chapter 27

Dysrhythmias and Ventricular Dysfunction and Heart Failure

Jeffrey J. Kim[1], Maully J. Shah[2]
[1]Texas Children's Hospital, Houston, TX, United States; [2]Children's Hospital of Philadelphia, Philadelphia, PA, United States

INTRODUCTION

Heart failure (HF) affects millions of Americans and remains a serious problem in children, not only in terms of lives lost but also in terms of morbidities and its effect on society [1]. Arrhythmias are intricately intertwined in the pathophysiology of HF, and its implications in pediatrics are far reaching. Currently, it is estimated that as much as 50% of deaths in HF may be due to malignant arrhythmias [2]. The mechanisms of these arrhythmias can be diverse and are dependent on the underlying electrophysiological changes caused not only by HF itself but also by the processes that led to the final pathway. In a population where etiologies of HF are varied, including primary or acquired cardiomyopathy and structural heart disease, this interplay can be quite complex. Indeed, both the acute and chronic treatments of HF itself are known to have proarrhythmic proclivity [3]. Additionally, chronic sustained tachyarrhythmias can lead to myocardial ischemia secondary to prolonged periods of decreased diastolic filling, resulting in the progression of ventricular dysfunction (tachycardia-induced cardiomyopathy) [4]. As such, understanding of the implications of arrhythmias and their management strategies in the different paradigms of HF in children remains essential.

In this chapter, we aim to review the interplay of dysrhythmias and ventricular dysfunction and HF from several perspectives. First, we hope to gain a better understanding of the molecular mechanisms for arrhythmogenesis in HF. We will then focus from a clinical perspective on both rhythm abnormalities implicated in causing HF as well as cardiomyopathy and their consequent arrhythmias. Lastly, we will discuss current concepts in the treatment of these arrhythmias.

MOLECULAR MECHANISMS FOR ARRHYTHMIAS IN HEART FAILURE

The mechanism for arrhythmogenesis in any clinical scenario is dependent on both the presence of electrophysiologic substrate and a trigger. Cardiac arrhythmias in HF are no different. Although some of the electrophysiologic perturbations may be dependent on the cause of HF and the underlying disease, data consistently display several common molecular denominators in HF-induced arrhythmias. These include ion channel remodeling, cellular uncoupling, altered calcium homeostasis, and extracellular matrix changes. In nearly all experimental models of HF, ventricular action potential prolongation is prominently seen [5,6]. Indeed, from a clinical standpoint, QT prolongation and T-wave abnormalities are commonly noted. It has been postulated that this action potential prolongation may be a compensatory response for the loss of myocardial contractility. From a molecular standpoint, the primary causes of AP prolongation are likely related to a reduction in repolarizing currents I_{to}, I_{Ks}, and I_{K1}, as well as an increase in late inward current carried by sodium [7]. These changes may predispose patients to ventricular arrhythmias due to several resultant factors. First, it results in decreased stability of the resting membrane, which allows the myocardium to be more susceptible to spontaneous afterdepolarizations (EADs). These EADs can act as a trigger for arrhythmias, which may induce Torsade de Pointes or ventricular fibrillation (VF). Myocardium excised from human hearts with HF has indeed demonstrated a propensity for EADs [8]. Additionally, increased dispersion of repolarization and heterogeneity across myocardium, which has also been demonstrated in patients with HF, favors the initiation and propagation of reentrant ventricular arrhythmias [9,10].

Cellular coupling is essential for conduction of the cardiac impulse and is dependent on major gap junction proteins, such as connexin43 (Cx43). Another generally accepted molecular feature of HF is the decreased expression of Cx43, which in some models can be reduced by up to 50% [11]. Additionally, connexins are noted to redistribute in HF into a more disorganized pattern [12]. These changes theoretically result in inhibited electrical cell to cell communication (uncoupling) and in combination with sodium channel dysfunction could lead to conduction slowing. Although experiments have

Heart Failure in the Child and Young Adult. http://dx.doi.org/10.1016/B978-0-12-802393-8.00027-2

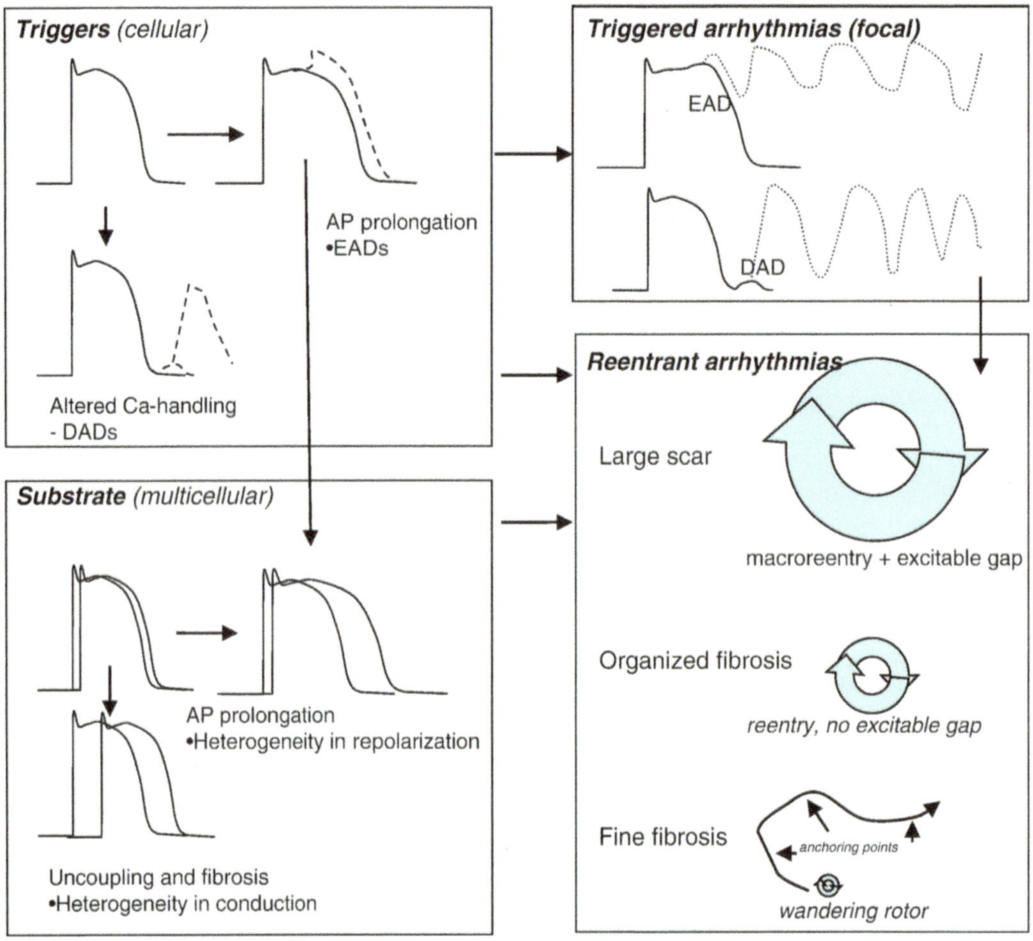

FIGURE 27.1 Diagram of the cellular and molecular mechanisms leading to arrhythmogenesis in heart failure. *DAD*, delayed afterdepolarization; *EAD*, spontaneous afterdepolarization. *Reproduced with permission from R. Coronel, R. Wilders, A.O. Verkerk, R.F. Wiegerinck, D. Benoist, O. Bernus, Electrophysiological changes in heart failure and their implications for arrhythmogenesis, Biochim. Biophys. Acta 1832 (2013) 2432–2441.*

not universally corroborated in vivo effects, simulations consistently show an increase in transmural activation times and heterogeneity in repolarization, which are hallmarks of arrhythmogenesis [13].

HF is also associated with altered calcium homeostasis. This is manifest primarily by increased intracellular diastolic Ca^{2+} concentration, decreased sarcoplasmic reticulum (SR) Ca^{2+} content, and downregulation of the SR Ca^{2+} ATPase. There is also reversed frequency dependence of the amplitude of Ca^{2+} transients. These maladaptations result in a setup for spontaneous Ca^{2+} release from the SR ("calcium sparks") [14]. In addition, the sarcolemmal Na^+/Ca^{2+} exchanged (NCX) is upregulated allowing for removal of excess Ca^{2+} out of the cell. This results in a net inward current of Na^+ in the presence of intracellular Ca^{2+} overload, which can lead to delayed afterdepolarizations (DADs) and triggered activity [14]. Myocardial stretch and dilation in itself has also been associated with opening of stretch-sensitive ion channels and spontaneous membrane depolarization [15].

Lastly, HF leads to structural changes in the myocardium that can result in fibrosis and changes in the extracellular matrix [16]. Although this has been shown to be true in primary cardiomyopathic processes in themselves, in the pediatric population, where congenital heart disease (CHD) is often implicated in etiology, this may be even more relevant. Fibrosis and alterations in the matrix not only affect the diastolic function of the heart but they can also impede cardiac impulse propagation leading to conduction delay and block [17]. Indeed electrogram fractionation in humans has been shown to be associated with significant activation delay [18]. This has implications for arrhythmogenesis as these structural alterations can facilitate the genesis of both focal arrhythmias based on increased anisotropy as well as the propagation of reentrant arrhythmias [19].

In sum, the combination of molecular changes in association with known cellular and extracellular remodeling described, provide the framework for both the "trigger" (EADs/DADs) and the electrophysiologic substrate for reentry (repolarization heterogeneity, fibrosis, conduction delay) (Fig. 27.1) [20]. From a clinical standpoint, the overlay of modulatory factors such as pharmacological treatment, autonomic regulation/dysregulation, genetic variation, and mechanical interactions add to the complexity of the paradigm. Clinical manifestations and implications are further reviewed below.

RHYTHM ABNORMALITIES CAUSING HEART FAILURE

When the heart rate is elevated beyond physiologic rates for a significant period of time, or atrioventricular (AV) synchrony is disrupted, hemodynamic consequences can eventually result in ventricular dysfunction. Although children with cardiac dysfunction are more prone to developing arrhythmias, occasionally, the primary cause of ventricular dysfunction is the tachyarrhythmia itself [21]. As it is often difficult to delineate which abnormality is primary at presentation (chicken or the egg), it is critical that tachycardiomyopathies are diagnosed correctly to avoid unnecessary treatment and even transplantation [22]. Generally, tachyarrhythmias resulting in cardiomyopathy are incessant, and in the pediatric population, usually associated with ectopic atrial tachycardia (EAT), junctional ectopic tachycardia (JET), permanent junctional reciprocating tachycardia (PJRT), or forms of unrecognized supraventricular tachycardia (SVT). In CHD, prolonged episodes of intraatrial reentrant tachycardia (IART) or atrial flutter are also implicated. Although there is no "minimal heart rate necessary" to develop tachycardiomyopathy (TCM), in children, studies suggest ventricular rates in excess of 140 bpm are typically seen [23].

EAT has been well described in association with TCM, with a predilection toward the pediatric age group [24]. Recent reports estimate an incidence of TCM in approximately 10% of patients with EAT, particularly in incessant or frequent forms [25]. While incompletely understood, the mechanism of EAT is likely related to abnormal automaticity with spontaneous atrial depolarization. Distinct P waves with abnormal axis and morphology are thus frequently visible. Treatment of EAT can be challenging in these scenarios as complete pharmacologic control may be difficult to achieve. However, multiple medications have been utilized to reasonable effect, including beta blockers, flecainide, sotalol, and amiodarone [26–28]. Several reports also point to the safety and potential efficacy of combination therapy, particularly amiodarone and beta blockers in this setting [28,29]. Although in infants, a high incidence of spontaneous resolution exists and only limited treatment may be necessary; in children older than 3 years, resolution is uncommon [30]. In these children, or in those where medical control is inadequate, catheter ablation should be considered. Radiofrequency ablation of EAT in young patients appears to be safe and effective with acute success rates of ~90%, potentially making it the preferred therapeutic approach in older children, particularly in the setting of cardiac dysfunction [25,31]. With adequate control of tachycardia or after successful ablation, recovery of cardiac function is expected, although this may take weeks to months dependent on the duration of the dysrhythmia [32,33].

Congenital JET is a rare arrhythmia that can be seen in young children, particularly infants, and can also be associated with TCM [34]. JET is a narrow complex tachyarrhythmia thought to be due to an automatic or ectopic focus originating at the AV junction and is often manifest with AV dissociation. Therapeutic options include medications such as beta blockers, propafenone, or amiodarone, although amiodarone appears to be superior [34,35]. In recalcitrant cases and patients with cardiac dysfunction, ablation of the focus can be attempted, although there is risk of AV nodal damage and need for permanent pacing [34].

PJRT is a form of accessory pathway–mediated tachycardia and is perhaps considered the most classic mechanism for TCM in children [36,37]. PJRT is typically an incessant form of SVT, which utilizes a slowly conducting accessory pathway in the posterior septum as the retrograde limb. This results in a long RP tachycardia with deeply negative P waves in the inferior ECG leads (Fig. 27.2). Tachycardia rates are usually in the range of 120–200 beats/min, and due to the relatively slow rate may not be recognized until cardiac dysfunction is present. In a recent multicenter evaluation, the incidence of TCM in this population was nearly 20% [37]. Antiarrhythmic medications, such as beta blockers, flecainide, sotalol, and amiodarone, were commonly employed, but rarely achieved complete control [37]. As such, in children older than 3–4 years of age with recalcitrant PJRT and associated cardiac dysfunction, catheter ablation can be considered the preferred method of treatment [37,38]. In infants and smaller children, due to higher risks associated with ablation, medical treatment with rate control and close monitoring remains reasonable. As with other forms of TCM, adequate control of tachycardia or successful ablation should result in recovery of cardiac function [37,39].

Although likely less common as a cause of TCM than supraventricular arrhythmias, ventricular arrhythmias have also been implicated as a cause of cardiac dysfunction. This can be secondary to rapid and prolonged episodes of sustained monomorphic ventricular tachycardia (VT) or even frequent isolated ventricular ectopy [40–42]. Early historical studies reported a 36% incidence of left ventricular (LV) dysfunction in children with incessant VT [41]. Pharmacologic control is somewhat variable dependent on substrate; however, even control of rate and frequency may be beneficial in ameliorating resultant HF. Beta blockers, calcium channel blockers, sotalol, and amiodarone have all been described as therapeutic options [41,42]. Also, in the current era, novel technologies such as three-dimensional (3D) mapping and noncontact

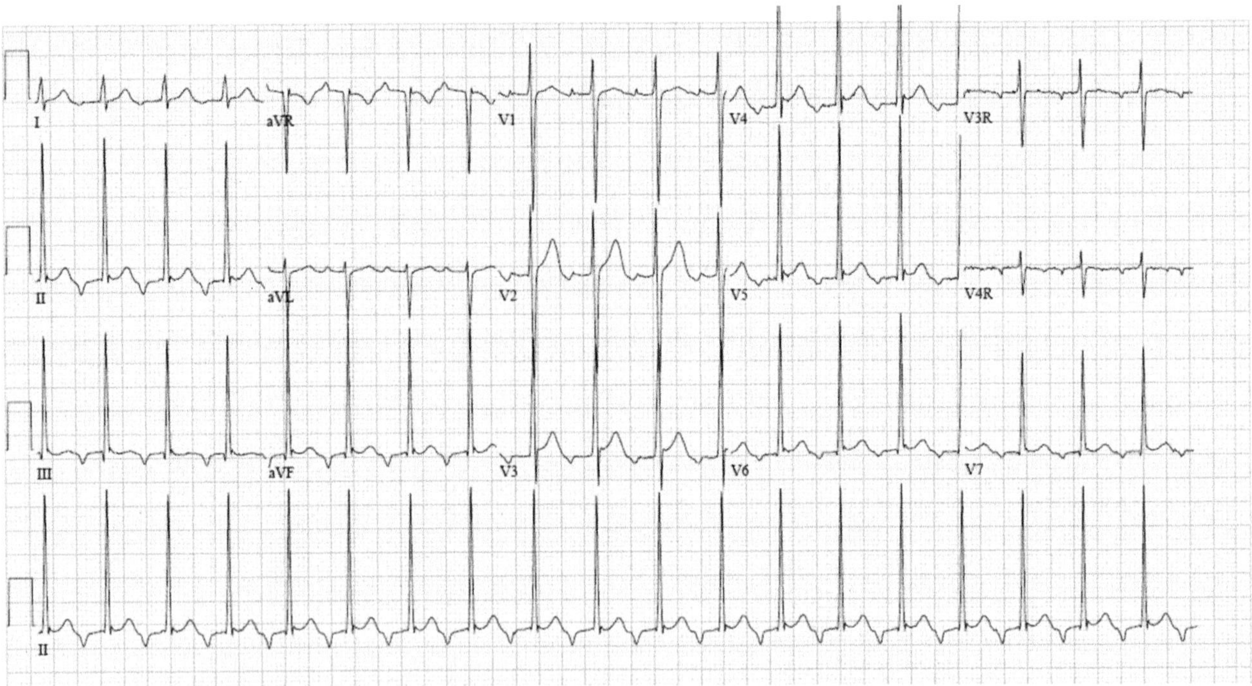

FIGURE 27.2 Fifteen lead ECG of child with incessant permanent junctional reciprocating tachycardia. Note long RP is in relationship with deeply negative P waves in the inferior leads.

mapping have increased the efficacy of transcatheter ablation techniques for VT in children, with acute success rates of ~90%, making it an additional treatment option [43–45]. More recently, even in the absence of sustained arrhythmias, frequent isolated premature ventricular contractions (PVCs), defined as >20% of beats, have been associated with the presence or development of LV dysfunction in adults [46]. This novel association suggests that assessment for symptoms and associated cardiomyopathy is warranted in patients presenting with a high burden of PVCs [46]. Although evaluation of comparable associations in children remains incomplete, limited studies do suggest that there is a higher prevalence of cardiomyopathy in children with higher PVC burden [47,48]. In such cases, treatment to decrease the burden of PVCs with either medical treatment or ablation is recommended. Multiple reports demonstrate recovery and often normalization of LV dysfunction after ablation of frequent ventricular ectopy [49–51].

In addition to tachyarrhythmias, there is mounting evidence regarding AV block, AV dyssynchrony, and pacing-induced cardiomyopathy. This will be covered later in the text (Chapter 46).

HEART FAILURE AND CONSEQUENT ARRHYTHMIAS

Although arrhythmias can indeed in themselves be the primary cause of cardiac dysfunction, the more classic association is that of arrhythmias as a consequent development of existing HF or cardiomyopathy.

Myocarditis

Acute viral myocarditis has variable clinical manifestations and may present as a self-limiting condition that runs a benign course or may result in myocardial dysfunction, malignant VT, or unheralded VF. Myocarditis is thought to account for a large proportion of sudden cardiac deaths (SCDs) in young people without prior structural heart disease [52]. The precise mechanism or more likely mechanisms by which ventricular arrhythmias result from acute myocarditis are unclear, although several hypotheses have been postulated. The formation of reentry circuits consequent on the regional slowing of action potentials due to viral-induced myocardial fibrosis and secondary hypertrophy has been proposed. The development of focal areas of inflammation in electrically sensitive regions of myocardium may also invoke ventricular arrhythmia. The inflammatory process itself seems proarrhythmic, and resolution of this may also lessen the proarrhythmic substrate [53]. Acute fulminant myocarditis (AFM) is rare but life-threatening in children because of its rapid and aggressive progression to congestive HF or cardiogenic shock. AFM is commonly associated with hemodynamic compromise dysrhythmias such as complete AV block or VT, which present with severe symptoms (Fig. 27.3A and B). Intensive cardiovascular support

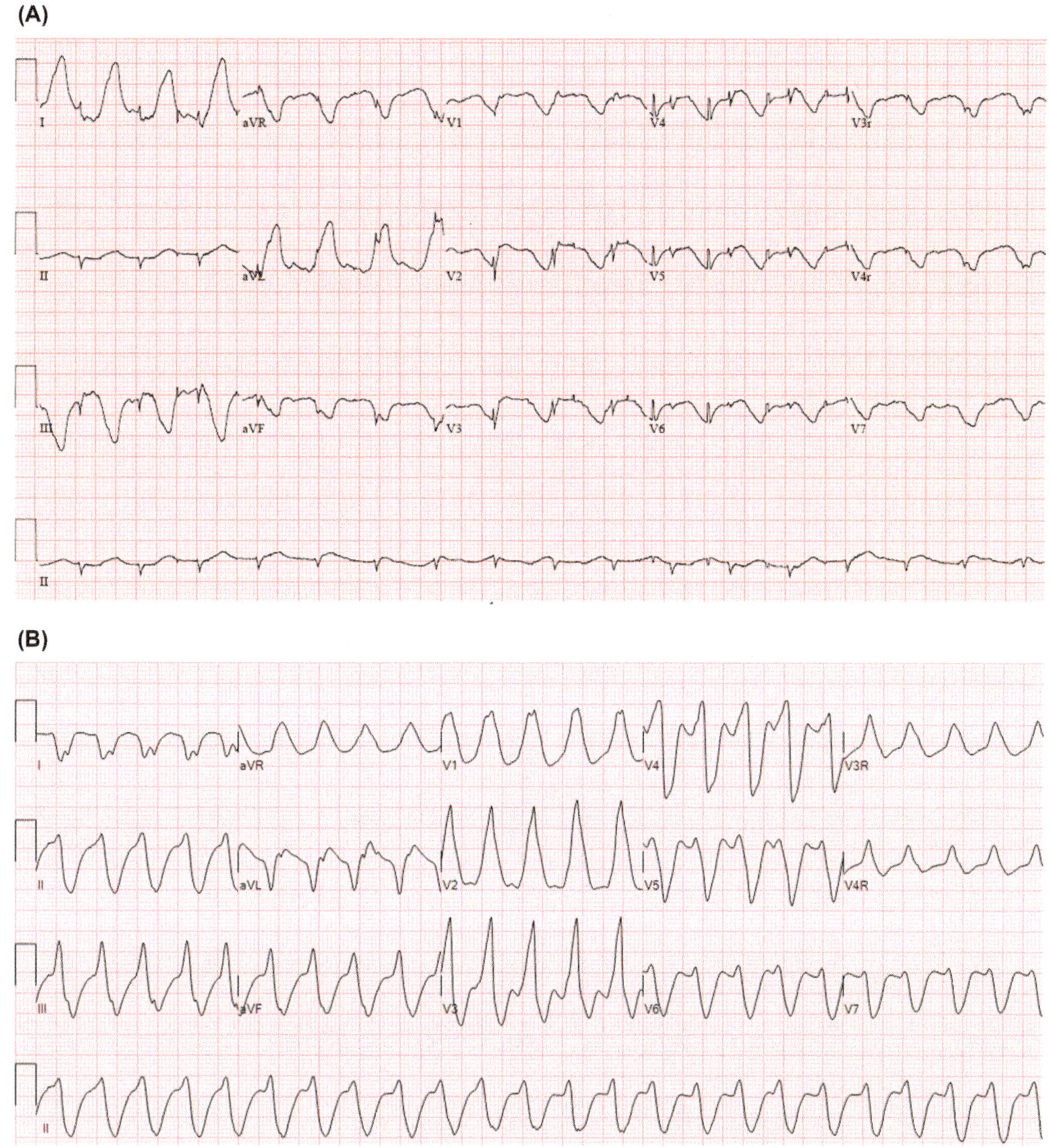

FIGURE 27.3 (A) ECG showing sinus rhythm with significant diffuse ST segment elevation and very small QRS voltages in a 12-year-old with a 2-days history of fever and lethargy, progressing rapidly to acute cardiogenic shock. (B) ECG showing sustained monomorphic VT (ventricular rate: 155 bpm) with right bundle branch block morphology and inferiorly directed QRS axis in the same patient with acute fulminant myocarditis on extracorporeal membrane oxygenation for circulatory support. *Provided with courtesy by Dr. Maully Shah.*

may be required [54], and antiarrhythmic medications should be administered judiciously due to potential for negative inotropic and proarrhythmic effects.

Giant cell myocarditis (GCM) is a rare cause of HF and arrhythmias in children. As in adults, GCM can often be distinguished clinically by a failure to respond to usual care and the frequent occurrence of ventricular arrhythmias or heart block in the setting of acute cardiomyopathy. The pathologic criteria for GCM are a diffuse or multifocal inflammatory infiltrate consisting of lymphocytes with multinucleated giant cells. GCM usually results in death or heart transplantation, and in some cases, mechanical circulatory support is necessary as a bridge to transplantation. Treatment with immunosuppression has been associated with prolonged transplant-free survival [55].

Recent publications in the literature have reported the association of acute myocarditis and ventricular arrhythmia with cardiac channelopathies, notably Brugada syndrome, short QT syndrome, and early repolarization. The precise mechanisms that link myocarditis, ventricular arrhythmia, and channelopathy remain to be defined but may be secondary to temperature-dependent modifications of ion channel properties [56,57].

Dilated Cardiomyopathy

In children with dilated cardiomyopathy (DCM), the reported 5-year mortality rate is 14%–50% from either SCD or pump failure [58–60]. Some reports indicate that mortality from SCD in DCM is much lower in children than in adults. In a single institutional study of 85 children with DCM, the incidence of documented ventricular arrhythmias was 13% and the incidence of SCD was 1% [59]. In another pediatric study, symptomatic events from either VT or VF occurred in 12% of children with DCM [61]. Unlike the adult HF population, wherein a persistently reduced ejection fraction of ≤35% has been identified as the single most important risk marker for SCD, a unifying risk factor has not been identified in pediatric DCM. Some studies have identified demographics, ECG, and echocardiographic characteristics, such as age, LV end-diastolic dimension, QRS duration, and QTc intervals as risk factors for life-threatening arrhythmic events, but these results have not been validated in large populations [61–63].

Atrial fibrillation (AF) is the most common atrial arrhythmia complicating DCM and HF in adult patients. Long-term registry-based reports from adult HF cohorts indicate that 35%–45% of HF patients have documented AF [64,65]. AF is less commonly encountered in the pediatric HF population, especially in the absence of structural heart disease. However, atrial arrhythmias may be present in patients with certain familial dilated cardiomyopathies, most commonly associated with mutations in the SCN5A, lamin A/C, TNNI3K, and desmosomal genes. In these types of cardiomyopathy there may be coexistence of atrial arrhythmias, ventricular arrhythmias, and conduction disease [66–69].

The DEFINITE trial (Defibrillators in Non-Ischemic Cardiomyopathy Treatment Evaluation) and the Sudden Cardiac Death in Heart Failure Trial (SCD-HeFT) demonstrated that the implantation of an implantable cardioverter–defibrillator (ICD) in addition to standard medical therapy significantly reduced the risk of SCD from arrhythmias in the adult population [64,65]. The current recommendations for implantation of an ICD for primary prevention of SCD in adults with DCM are the presence of New York Heart Association class II and III HF and a measured ejection fraction of ≤35% [70]. In absence of large randomized trials in the pediatric population, current risk stratification and treatment strategies for primary prevention of SCD in DCM are primarily extrapolated from the adult population [71]. Pharmacologic treatment of VA in pediatric DCM mimics that of the adult cohorts, and beta blockers remain the cornerstone in therapy with well-documented ability to reduce SCD by 40%–45% [72,73]. Amiodarone seems to be a reasonable antiarrhythmic therapy for VT and prevention of appropriate ICD shocks, but there is a lack of documentation of effects and risk of toxicity [73–75].

Left Ventricular Noncompaction Cardiomyopathy

The clinical manifestations of left ventricular noncompaction cardiomyopathy (LVNC) are highly variable, ranging from asymptomatic to progressive HF and/or life-threatening arrhythmias. Both ventricular and supraventricular arrhythmias are now well described as prominent clinical components of LVNC and have been shown to be associated with prognosis and outcome. The major clinical manifestations of LVNC are HF, embolic events, and arrhythmias [76–80]. VT has been considered the hallmark arrhythmia of the disease; however, there is considerable variability in the reported incidence of VT [77,78]. SCD accounts for a significant proportion of reported mortality [77].

Brescia et al. reported a 17% incidence of VT in 242 children with LVNC in a tertiary care single center institutional study. Presence of cardiac dysfunction and presence of arrhythmias were associated with higher mortality [79]. A recent systematic metaanalysis by Bhatia et al., which included over 200 adults, reported a 38% incidence of VT [76]. The primary type of VA reported in LVNC is monomorphic VT, but different morphologies and mechanism have been described, including outflow tract VT, bundle branch reentry, fascicular VT, bidirectional VT, polymorphic VT, and VF [81]. The precise mechanism for VA in LVNC is not clearly delineated. However, it is postulated that presence of intratrabecular crypts and ischemia-related fibrosis at the subendocardial noncompacted regions can cause electrical inhomogeneity and act as a substrate for reentry [80]. Rates of SCD have also varied significantly, ranging from 0% to 18% [76–79]. In the largest tertiary center pediatric study of isolated LVNC, SCD was reported to be 6% [79]. Unfortunately, risk factors for SCD have not been well defined making it difficult to identify patients who would benefit from primary prevention strategies. However, several risk factors for SCD have been cited: age at presentation, decreased LV systolic function, abnormal

LV dimensions, presence of clinical VA, and inducible VA with programmed electrical stimulation [78–82]. In children, dysmorphic features and the presence of Wolff–Parkinson–White (WPW) have also been associated with an increased risk of SCD [79,83,84].

Supraventricular arrhythmias are also implicated in LVNC. In adult studies, AF seems to be the primary manifestation [84]. In children, the mechanism of supraventricular arrhythmias seems to be related to AV reentrant SVT and focal tachycardia with AF having a low prevalence [79,83]. The higher incidence of SVT in children may be due to the common association with WPW syndrome [85]. In some instances, SVT can trigger life-threatening VA.

Therapeutic approaches for arrhythmias in LVNC include standard treatment for AF if present, risk stratification and catheter ablation of WPW bypass tracts, antiarrhythmic medications, catheter ablation of VT, and ICD implantation for secondary and perhaps primary prevention of SCD. Arrhythmia surveillance with heart rhythm monitoring should be conducted in LVNC patients to monitor ongoing arrhythmias and to detect development of new arrhythmias [79,80].

Arrhythmogenic Right Ventricular Cardiomyopathy

Arrhythmogenic right ventricular cardiomyopathy (ARVC) is an inherited desmosomal cardiomyopathy characterized pathologically by fibrofatty replacement of the right ventricular (RV) myocardium and clinically by electrical instability resulting in ventricular arrhythmias [86]. Unlike other cardiomyopathies, VA and SCD often are presenting symptoms before the development of any overt myocardial dysfunction. Frequent ventricular ectopy and exercise-induced VT are common manifestations of ARVC that are likely catecholamine facilitated [86–89].

The primary type of VT reported in ARVC is a left bundle branch block VT with an inferior axis, which may mimic a typical of focal RV outflow tract tachycardia (Fig. 27.4A and B). In patients with ARVC, VT usually coexists with anterior T-wave inversion and ventricular arrhythmias of multiple morphologies [89,90]. Other distinguishing VT morphology markers that imply the presence of ARVC are QRS duration in lead I of ≥120 ms, QRS transition at V_6, presence of notching on any QRS complex, and earliest onset QRS in lead V_1 [90]. Atrial arrhythmias are also encountered in patients with ARVC, particularly AF and atrial flutter necessitating ablative or pharmacologic treatment [69,91]. Chu et al. demonstrated that atrial arrhythmias were more common in patients with RV enlargement and moderate/severe tricuspid regurgitation [91].

Management of ARVC is directed toward symptom reduction, delay of disease progression, and prevention of SCD. Mainstay therapies consist of lifestyle modification (exercise restriction), beta-blocking and antiarrhythmic agents (class III agents such as amiodarone), and ICD implantation [89,92,93]. ICD implantation is recommended in all individuals with prior sustained VT or resuscitated SCD [70]. The use of ICDs for primary prevention of SCD is much more controversial although several risk factors are recognized including syncope, young age, male gender, athletic history, nonsustained VT, severe RV dysfunction, and LV involvement [70,89]. In addition, radiofrequency ablation results have been encouraging in recent years in reducing the burden of VT and ICD shocks [94].

Congenital Heart Disease

The relationship of ventricular dysfunction, HF, and arrhythmias is increasingly appreciated in the CHD population. CHD patients with HF have substrates for atrial and ventricular arrhythmias, such as myocardial scarring, chronic ventricular volume and pressure load, prosthetic material, and intrinsic myocardial disease [95–97].

Atrial arrhythmias that are exacerbated due to HF in CHD patients include AF, atrial flutter, IART, and focal atrial tachycardia [97,98] IART typically has a slower atrial rate (150–200 bpm) than typical isthmus-dependent flutter, which may favor 1:1 AV conduction that can lead to hemodynamic instability due to a rapid ventricular response [95–98] (Fig. 27.5A and B). It is most often seen in older Fontan patients with atriopulmonary connections (50%–60%) or lateral and extracardiac tunnels (10%–30%), patients with Mustard or Senning atrial baffles for d-transposition of the great arteries (30%), or patients with tetralogy of Fallot (33%), but can also occur with repair of simple cardiac defects such as atrial septal defects [95–102]. Prevalence of atrial flutter/IART is more common in the presence of diminished ventricular function, and increasing attention should also be paid to diastolic dysfunction as rapid heart rate may limit ventricular filling, compromising cardiac output [103–105].

Management principles of AF are similar to those encountered in other forms of adult heart disease, beginning with anticoagulation and ventricular rate control, and typically followed by electrical or medical cardioversion. Acute treatment of IART and AF by electrical means (DC cardioversion or overdrive pacing) or chemical means (class I or III antiarrhythmics) is effective, but maintenance of sinus rhythm in the long term is challenging. Therapeutic options for recurrent atrial arrhythmias include antiarrhythmic drugs, catheter ablation, pacemaker implantation for tachy-brady syndrome or to

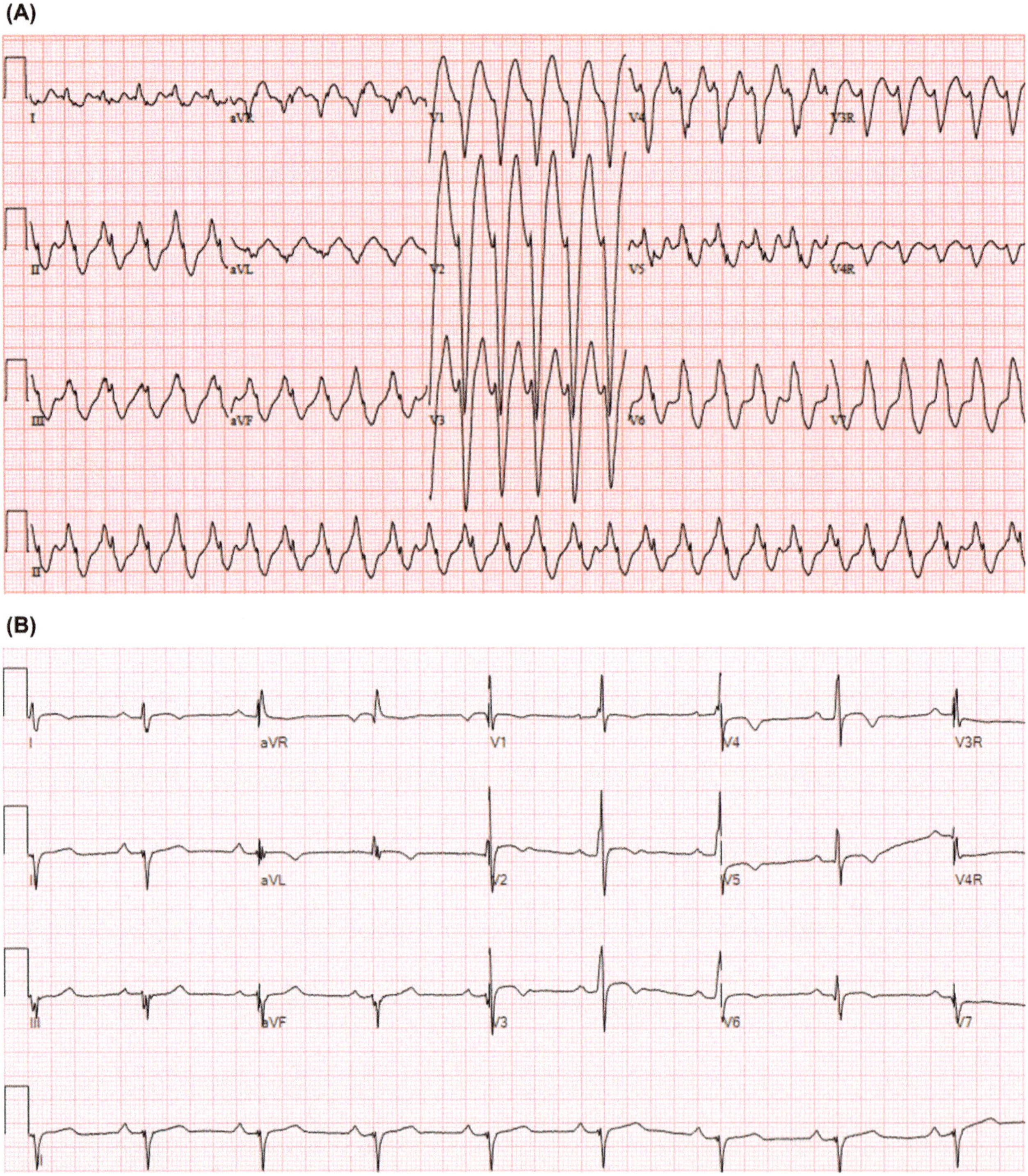

FIGURE 27.4 (A) ECG showing sustained monomorphic VT (ventricular rate: 170 bpm) with a left bundle branch block morphology, inferiorly directed QRS axis, and late R/S precordial transition in a 14-year-old boy with arrhythmogenic right ventricular cardiomyopathy (ARVC) with a pathogenic desmosomal mutation and right ventricular (RV) wall motion abnormalities on echocardiogram and cardiac MRI. (B) Baseline ECG in the same patient with ARVC showing sinus rhythm, RV conduction delay, superior QRS axis, and T-wave inversion in all the precordial leads. *Provided with courtesy by Dr. Maully Shah.*

provide antitachycardia pacing, and surgical intervention with a modified atrial maze or Cox's Maze operation. The treatment choice must be tailored to the hemodynamic and electrophysiological status of the individual patient. Selecting an appropriate antiarrhythmic therapy requires careful consideration of several factors in the HF patient because of undesirable side effects such as concomitant bradyarrhythmia, negative inotropic effects, and proarrhythmia that may be enhanced in the setting of HF [95–97].

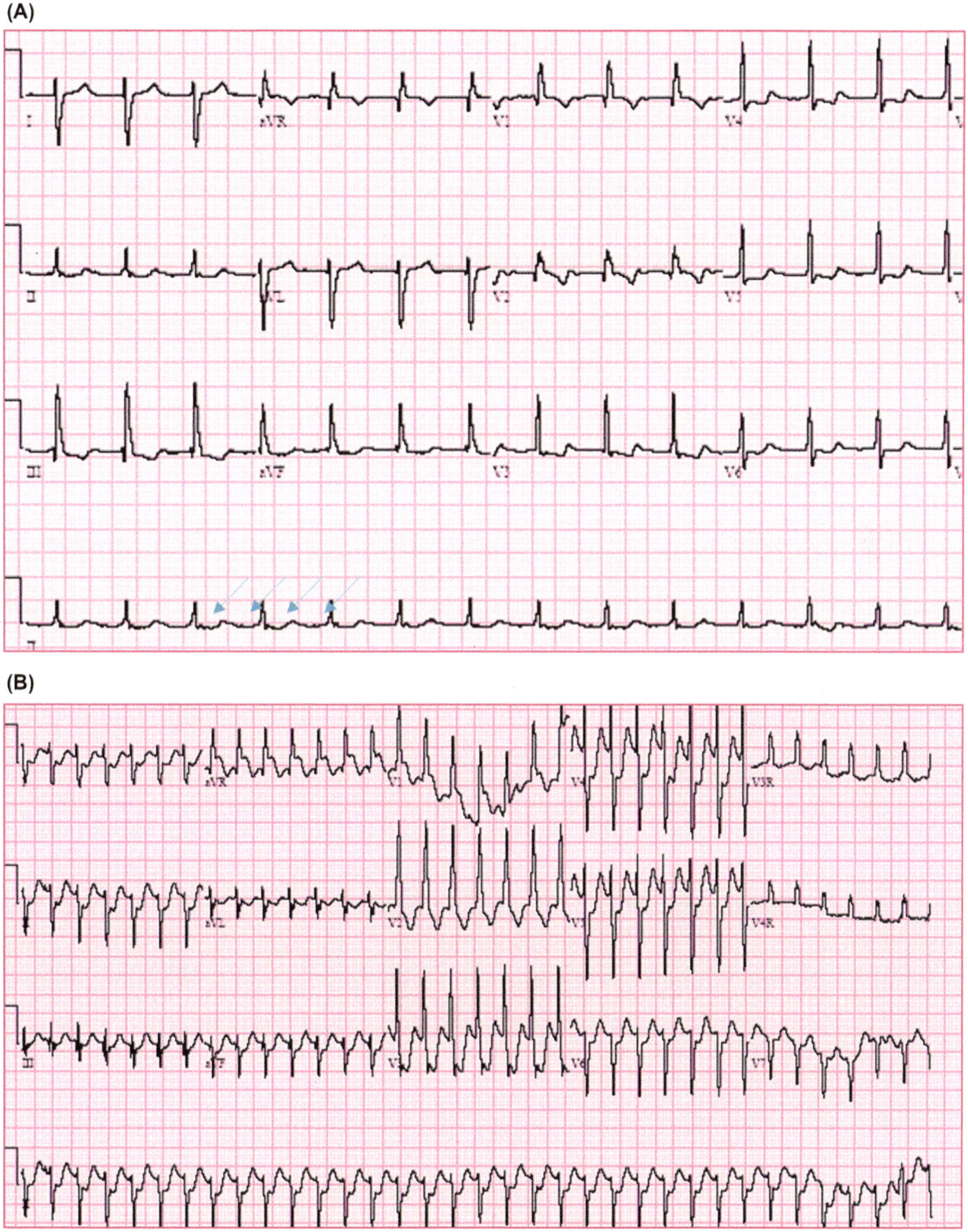

FIGURE 27.5 (A) ECG showing intraatrial reentrant tachycardia with 2:1 atrioventricular (AV) conduction in a 30-year-old patient with d-transposition of the great arteries (d-TGA) s/p Mustard procedure. The P waves are typically small and indistinct and are indicated by *arrows* on bottom rhythm strip (lead II). The atrial rate is 215 bpm (cycle length 280 ms). The ventricular rate is 107 bpm (cycle length 560 ms). (B) ECG showing intraatrial reentrant tachycardia in the same 30-year-old patient with d-TGA s/p Mustard procedure with abrupt change in ventricular rate to 215 bpm. (cycle length 280 ms) due to 1:1 AV conduction of intraatrial reentrant tachycardia. Note that QRS axis and morphology is similar in (A) and (B) indicating an atrially derived tachycardia. *Provided with courtesy by Dr. Maully Shah.*

VA and SCD are widely appreciated as a sequela of systemic ventricular dysfunction in complex CHD [98,101–104]. Additionally, RV–LV interactions are increasingly acknowledged, and subpulmonary RV failure itself contributes to the complex interplay of factors associated with sudden death [104]. VA and SCD are reported in 2%–9% patients with univentricular physiology s/p Fontan procedure, in the presence of ventricular dysfunction [95,106–109].

Despite the heterogeneous nature of HF and ventricular dysfunction in CHD, and lack of randomized-controlled trials, consensus guidelines for management of VA and SCD prevention have outlined reasonable strategies [70,97]. Class I indications for ICD implantation in a patient with CHD includes aborted sudden cardiac arrest without a reversible cause and sustained VT after hemodynamic and electrophysiologic evaluation. Class IIa indications include syncope of undetermined origin in the presence of either ventricular dysfunction or inducible ventricular arrhythmias. Antiarrhythmic drugs are generally not considered first-line stand-alone therapy for VA in patients with CHD and HF. Nevertheless, they have an important role in decreasing the recurrence of VT and risk of shocks in ICD recipients. Beta blockers as well as amiodarone are often used for this purpose. Several recent case series have addressed the role of catheter ablation in the treatment of VT in patients with CHD [110,111]. Another alternative is surgical ablation of VT, which has primarily been reported in patients with TOF who require reoperations for pulmonary regurgitation and/or tricuspid regurgitation [112,113].

TREATMENT OF ARRHYTHMIAS IN HEART FAILURE

Antiarrhythmic medications are commonly employed in the treatment algorithm of children with HF and arrhythmias. Beta blockers remain important antiarrhythmic drugs in these patients and may serve a twofold purpose in associated with reverse remodeling. Alternatively, the class I sodium channel-blocking drugs (mexiletine, procainamide, flecainide, and propafenone) should be avoided due to negative inotropic effects and a potential for proarrhythmic activity. Amiodarone remains a good choice for antiarrhythmic therapy for ventricular and supraventricular arrhythmias in patients with HF, largely, because it is relatively safe from a cardiac standpoint. Ventricular proarrhythmic activity is unusual with amiodarone, although bradycardia, due to sinus and AV node depression as well as noncardiac toxicity remain problems [114,115]. Another class III antiarrhythmic drug that has been approved for therapy of AF is dofetilide. The Danish Investigations of Arrhythmia and Mortality on Dofetilide (DIAMOND) study demonstrated that the dofetilide-treated patients were less likely to be rehospitalized for exacerbation of HF than the placebo arm. The major toxicity is torsade de pointes, and dofetilide is contraindicated in patients with impaired renal function [116]. The class III drug sotalol blocks the same potassium current that is blocked by dofetilide (IKr). Unlike dofetilide, sotalol is also a potent nonselective adrenergic blocker. Sotalol has not been specifically evaluated in HF patients. It causes torsade de pointes at an incidence similar to that of dofetilide and can also aggravate bradyarrhythmias. Small retrospective studies in CHD patients suggest that sotalol is associated with reasonable safety and efficacy [97].

Catheter ablation is commonly used for early treatment of tachyarrhythmias particularly when antiarrhythmic drugs fail or are poorly tolerated. Advances in 3D mapping techniques and catheter technologies have provided new optimism for arrhythmia management in patients with and without structural heart disease. Combining 3D electroanatomic mapping with good anatomic imaging, new catheter technologies, and a thorough understanding of underlying structural disease, most arrhythmias can be safely and successfully ablated, even in individuals with HF. The procedure remains challenging in patients with complex CHD due to issues related to venous access, surgical baffles and patches, difficulty creating transmural lesions, and multiple arrhythmia mechanisms [117–121]. Another significant challenge, particularly in the presence of systemic ventricular dysfunction, is maintaining hemodynamic stability during electrophysiologic mapping of arrhythmias. Catheter ablation can be performed with circulatory support provided by extracorporeal membrane oxygenation or percutaneous ventricular assist devices (VADs) such as the Impella devices (Abiomed, Danvers, Massachusetts) and TandemHeart (CardiacAssist, Pittsburgh, Pennsylvania, United States) [122,123]. In some cases, catheter ablation can also be performed using substrate mapping, pace mapping, and transection of critical isthmuses without induction of a tachyarrhythmia thus avoiding hemodynamic instability [110].

In the current era, the ICD is the mainstay therapy for primary and secondary prevention of SCD in patients with HF. In children, high rates of inappropriate shocks have consistently been reported as a result of coexisting supraventricular tachyarrhythmias and lead failures [70,71,97,124]. ICDs should thus be programmed carefully, bearing in mind the potential hemodynamic and psychological sequelae of inappropriate discharges. Strategies may include activation of antitachycardia pacing, programming higher defibrillation detection thresholds and/or prolonging time to detection, and the use of tailored SVT discrimination and therapy algorithms. An entirely subcutaneous ICD (S-ICD, Boston Scientific, Massachusetts) is available for patients who do not require bradycardia or antitachycardia pacing [125].

VADs have also been employed to treat arrhythmias that are refractory to medical therapy in both adults and children. These include case reports of patients with AF, VT, and recalcitrant EAT. The temporary use of an LVAD can maintain hemodynamic stability during the treatment of pharmacological refractory tachycardia and may allow a successful bridge to recover from tachycardia-induced cardiomyopathy, myocarditis, and other acute cardiomyopathies [126–128]. Unloading the myocardium in its decompensated state may also serve to decrease arrhythmia burden.

KEY POINTS

- Arrhythmias are intricately intertwined in the pathophysiology of HF.
- There are several common molecular denominators in HF-induced arrhythmias, including ion channel remodeling, cellular uncoupling, altered calcium homeostasis, and extracellular matrix changes.
- Tachyarrhythmias resulting in cardiomyopathy are typically incessant, and in the pediatric population, usually associated with EAT, JET, PJRT, or forms of unrecognized SVT.
- In tachycardia-induced cardiomyopathy, adequate control of tachycardia or successful ablation generally results in recovery of cardiac function, although this may take weeks to months dependent on the duration of the dysrhythmia.
- Both ventricular and supraventricular arrhythmias are well-described clinical sequelae of HF and cardiomyopathies (myocarditis, DCM, LVNC, ARVC) as well as in the presence of CHD.
- SCD remains an important cause of mortality, although unlike in adults, unifying risk factors have not been consistently identified.
- Proven therapeutic approaches include antiarrhythmics, ablations, VADs, and implantable defibrillators. The treatment choice must be tailored to the hemodynamic and electrophysiological status of the individual patient, including consideration undesirable side effects such as concomitant bradyarrhythmia, negative inotropic effects, and proarrhythmia that may be enhanced in the setting of HF.

REFERENCES

[1] J.W. Rossano, J.J. Kim, J.A. Decker, J.F. Price, F. Zafar, D.E. Graves, D.L. Morales, J.S. Heinle, B. Bozkurt, J.A. Towbin, S.W. Denfield, W.J. Dreyer, J.L. Jefferies, Prevalence, morbidity, and mortality of heart failure-related hospitalizations in children in the United States: a population-based study, J. Card. Fail. 18 (2012) 459–470.
[2] G.F. Tomaselli, D.P. Zipes, What causes sudden death in heart failure? Circ. Res. 95 (2004) 754–763.
[3] G.L. Stump, A.A. Wallace, D.B. Gilberto, J.R. Gehret, J.J. Lynch Jr., Arrhythmogenic potential of positive inotropic agents, Basic Res. Cardiol. 95 (3) (2000) 186–198.
[4] G. Fenelon, W. Wijns, E. Andries, P. Brugada, Tachycardiomyopathy: mechanisms and clinical implications, Pacing Clin. Electrophysiol. 19 (1996) 95–106.
[5] T. Aiba, G. Tomaselli, Electrical remodeling in dyssynchrony and resynchronization, J. Cardiovasc. Trans. Res. 5 (2012) 170–179.
[6] S. Nattel, A. Maguy, S. Le Bouter, Y.H. Yeh, Arrhythmogenic ion-channel remodeling in the heart: heart failure, myocardial infarction, and atrial fibrillation, Physiol. Rev. 87 (2007) 425–456.
[7] G. Michael, L. Xiao, X.Y. Qi, D. Dobrev, S. Nattel, Remodeling of cardiac repolarization: how homeostatic responses can lead to arrhythmogenesis, Cardiovasc. Res. 81 (2009) 491–499.
[8] J.T. Vermeulen, M.A. McGuire, T. Opthof, R. Coronel, J.M.T. De Bakker, C. Kloepping, M.J. Janse, Triggered activity and automaticity in ventricular trabeculae of failing human and rabbit hearts, Cardiovasc. Res. 28 (1994) 1547–1554.
[9] D.J. Pinsky, E.S. Sciacca, J.S. Steinberg, QT dispersion as a marker of risk in patients awaiting heart transplantation, J. Am. Coll. Cardiol. 29 (1997) 1576–1584.
[10] R. Coronel, F.J.G. Wilms-Schopman, T. Opthof, M.J. Janse, Dispersion of repolarization and arrhythmogenesis, Heart Rhythm 6 (2009) 537–543.
[11] R.F. Wiegerinck, A.A. van Veen, C.N. Belterman, C.A. Schumacher, M. Noorman, J.M. de Bakker, R. Coronel, Transmural dispersion of refractoriness and conduction velocity is associated with heterogeneously reduced connexin43 in a rabbit model of heart failure, Heart Rhythm 5 (2008) 1178–1185.
[12] N.J. Severs, A.F. Bruce, E. Dupont, S. Rothery, Remodelling of gap junctions and connexin expression in diseased myocardium, Cardiovasc. Res. 80 (2008) 9–19.
[13] K. Gima, Y. Rudy, Ionic current basis of electrocardiographic waveforms: a model study, Circ. Res. 90 (2002) 889–896.
[14] A. Baartscheer, C.A. Schumacher, C.N.W. Belterman, R. Coronel, J.W.T. Fiolet, SR calcium handling and calcium after-transients in a rabbit model of heart failure, Cardiovasc. Res. 58 (2003) 99–108.
[15] Z. Wang, K. Taylor, W.D. Denney, D.E. Hansen, Initiation of ventricular extrasystoles by myocardial stretch in chronically dilated and failing canine left ventricle, Circulation 90 (1994) 2022–2031.
[16] K.T. Weber, C.G. Brill, J.S. Janicki, Myocardial fibrosis: functional significance and regulatory factors, Cardiovasc. Res. 27 (1993) 341–348.
[17] M.G. Hoogendijk, M. Potse, A. Vinet, J.M. de Bakker, R. Coronel, ST segment elevation by current-to-load mismatch: an experimental and computational study, Heart Rhythm 8 (2011) 111–118.
[18] J.M. deBakker, F.J. van Capelle, M.J. Janse, S. Tasseron, J.T. Vermeulen, N. de Jonge, J.R. Lahpor, Slow conductin in the infarcted human heart. "Zigzag" course of activation, Circulation 88 (1993) 915–926.

[19] R. Wilder, M.B. Wagner, D. Golod, R. Kumar, Y.G. Wang, W.N. Goolsby, R.W. Joyner, H.J. Jongsma, Effects of anisotropy on the development of cardiac arrhythmias associated with focal activity, Pfluegers Arch. 441 (2000) 301–312.
[20] R. Coronel, R. Wilders, A.O. Verkerk, R.F. Wiegerinck, D. Benoist, O. Bernus, Electrophysiological changes in heart failure and their implications for arrhythmogenesis, Biochim. Biophys. Acta 1832 (2013) 2432–2441.
[21] F. Arunjo, J.L. Ducla-Aoares, Tachycardiomyopathies, Rev. Port. Cardiol. 21 (2002) 585–592.
[22] N.L. Walker, S.M. Cobbe, D.H. Birnie, Tachycardiomyopathy: a diagnosis not to be missed, Heart 90 (2004) e7.
[23] B.D. Gelb, A. Garson Jr., Noninvasive discrimination of right atrial ectopic tachycardia from sinus tachycardia in "dilated cardiomyopathy", Am. Heart J. 120 (1990) 886–891.
[24] P.C. Gillette, R.T. Smith, A. Garson, C.R. Mullins, H.P. Gutgesell, T.H. Goh, D.A. Cooley, D.G. McNamara, Chronic supraventricular tachycardia: a curable cause of congestive cardiomyopathy, JAMA 253 (1985) 391–392.
[25] C. Medi, J.M. Kalman, H. Haggani, J.K. Vohra, J.B. Morton, P.B. Sparks, P.M. Kistler, Tachycardia-mediated cardiomyopathy secondary to focal atrial tachycardia: long-term outcome after catheter ablation, J. Am. Coll. Cardiol. 53 (2009) 1791–1797.
[26] A.V. Mehta, G.R. Sanchez, E.J. Sacks, A. Casta, J.M. Dunn, R.M. Donner, Ectopic automatic atrial tachycardia in children: clinical characteristics, management and follow-up, J. Am. Coll. Cardiol. 11 (1988) 379–385.
[27] S.A. Luedtke, R.J. Kuhn, F.M. McCaffrey, Pharmacologic management of supraventricular tachycardia in children, Ann. Pharmacother. 31 (1997) 1227–1243.
[28] Z.J. Naheed, J.F. Strasburger, D.W.J.R. Benson, B.J. Deal, Natural history and management strategies of automatic atrial tachycardia in children, Am. J. Cardiol. 75 (1995) 405–407.
[29] R. Juneja, S. Shah, N. Naik, S.S. Kothari, A. Saxena, K.K. Talwar, Management of cardiomyopathy resulting from incessant supraventricular tachycardia in infants and children, Indian Heart J. 54 (2002) 176–180.
[30] J.C. Salerno, N.J. Kertesz, R.A. Friedman, A.L. Fenrich Jr., Clinical course of atrial ectopic tachycardia is age-dependent: results and treatment in children <3 or > or =3 years of age, J. Am. Coll. Cardiol. 43 (2004) 438–444.
[31] E.P. Walsh, J.P. Saul, J.E. Hulse, L.A. Rhodes, A.J. Hordof, J.E. Mayer, J.E. Lock, Transcatheter ablation of ectopic atrial tachycardia in young patients using radiofrequency current, Circulation 86 (1992) 1138–1146.
[32] S. Berger, A.M. Dubin, Arrhythmogenic forms of heart failure in children, Heart Fail. Clin. 6 (2010) 471–481.
[33] L.E. Rabbani, P.J. Wang, G.L. Couper, P.L. Friedman, Time course of improvement in ventricular function after ablation of incessant automatic atrial tachycardia, Am. Heart J. 121 (1991) 816–819.
[34] E. Villain, V.L. Vetter, J.M. Garcia, J. Herre, A. Cifarelli, A. Garson Jr., Evolving concepts in the management of congenital junctional ectopic tachycardia: a multicenter study, Circulation 81 (1990) 1544–1549.
[35] T. Paul, A. Reimer, J. Janousek, H.C. Kallfelz, Efficacy and safety of propafenone in congenital junctional ectopic tachycardia, J. Am. Coll. Cardiol. 20 (1992) 911–914.
[36] M.A. McGuire, K.C. Lau, L.M. Davis, P. Knight, J.B. Uther, D.L. Ross, Permanent junctional reciprocating tachycardia misdiagnosed as 'cardiomyopathy', Aust. N.Z. J. Med. 21 (1991) 239–241.
[37] K.T. Kang, J.E. Potts, A.E. Radbill, M.J. LaPage, J. Papagiannis, J.M. Garnreiter, P. Kubus, M.J. Kantoch, N.H. Von Bergen, A. Fournier, J.M. Cote, T. Paul, C.C. Anderson, B.C. Cannon, C.Y. Miyake, A.D. Blaufox, S.P. Etheridge, S. Sanatani, Permanent junctional reciprocating tachycardia in children: a multicenter experience, Heart Rhythm 11 (2014) 1426–1432.
[38] E. Semizel, C. Ayabakan, N. Ceviz, A. Celiker, Permanent form of junctional reciprocating tachycardia and tachycardia-induced cardiomyopathy treated by catheter ablation: a case report, Turk. J. Pediatr. 45 (2003) 338–341.
[39] P. Noe, V. Van Driel, F. Wittkampf, N. Sreeram, Rapid recovery of cardiac function after catheter ablation of persistent junctional reciprocating tachycardia in children, Pacing Clin. Electrophysiol. 25 (2002) 191–194.
[40] A. Tsuji, M. Nagashima, S. Hasegawa, N. Nagai, K. Nishibata, M. Goto, M. Matsushima, Long-term follow-up of idiopathic ventricular arrhythmias in otherwise normal children, Jpn. Circ. J. 59 (1995) 654–662.
[41] J.P. Pfammetter, T. Paul, Idiopathic ventricular tachycardia in infancy and childhood: a multicenter study on clinical profile and outcome, J. Am. Coll. Cardiol. 33 (1999) 2067–2072.
[42] M.E. Alexander, C.I. Berul, Ventricular arrhythmias: when to worry, Pediatr. Cardiol. 21 (2000) 532–541.
[43] S.B. Fishberger, M.M. Olen, N.L. Rollinson, A.F. Rossi, Creation of partial fascicular block: an approach to ablation of idiopathic left ventricular tachycardia in the pediatric population, Pacing Clin. Electrophysiol. 38 (2015) 209–215.
[44] K.K. Collins, M.S. Schaffer, L. Liberman, E. Saarel, M. Knecht, R.E. Tanel, D. Bradley, A.M. Dubin, T. Paul, J. Salerno, Y. Bar-Cohen, N. Sreeram, S. Sanatani, I.H. Law, A. Blaufox, A. Batra, J.M. Moltedo, G.F. van Hare, J. Reed, P.S. Ro, J. Kugler, C. Anderson, J.K. Triedman, Pediatric and Congenital Electrophysiology Society, Fascicular and nonfascicular left ventricular tachycardias in the young: an international multicenter study, J. Cardiovasc. Electrophysiol. 24 (2013) 640–648.
[45] H.E. Schneider, T. Kriebel, K. Jung, V.D. Gravenhorst, T. Paul, Catheter ablation of idiopathic left and right ventricular tachycardias in the pediatric population using noncontact mapping, Heart Rhythm 7 (2010) 731–739.
[46] P.L. Eugenio, Frequent premature ventricular contractions: an electrical link to cardiomyopathy, Cardiol. Rev. 23 (2015) 168–172.
[47] B. Kakavand, H.O. Ballard, T.G. Disessa, Frequent ventricular premature beats in children with a structurally normal heart: a cause for reversible left ventricular dysfunction? Pediatr. Cardiol. 31 (2010) 986–990.
[48] Z.Z. Spector, S.P. Seslar, Premature ventricular contraction-induced cardiomyopathy in children, Cardiol. Young (June 17, 2015) 1–7 (Epub ahead of print).

[49] R.K. Yarlagadda, S. Iwai, K.M. Stein, S.M. Markowitz, B.K. Shah, J.W. Cheung, V. Tan, B.B. Lerman, S. Mittal, Reversal of cardiomyopathy in patients with repetitive monomorphic ventricular ectopy originating from the right ventricular outflow tract, Circulation 112 (2005) 1092–1097.

[50] M. Yokokawa, E. Good, T. Crawford, A. Chugh, F. Pelosi Jr., R. Latchamsetty, K. Jongnarangsin, W. Armstrong, H. Ghanbari, H. Oral, F. Morady, F. Bogun, Recovery from left ventricular dysfunction after ablation of frequent premature ventricular complexes, Heart Rhythm 10 (2013) 172–175.

[51] M. Zang, T. Zhang, J. Mao, S. Zhou, B. He, Beneficial effects of catheter ablation of frequent premature ventricular complexes on left ventricular function, Heart 100 (2014) 787–793.

[52] S. Sagar, P.P. Liu, L.T. Cooper Jr., Myocarditis, Lancet 379 (2012) 738–747.

[53] K.M. Lin, M.H. Li, K.S. Hsieh, H.C. Kuo, M.C. Cheng, J.J. Sheu, Y.J. Lin, Impact of extracorporeal membrane oxygenation on acute fulminant myocarditis-related hemodynamic compromise arrhythmia in children, Pediatr. Neonatol. 57 (6) (March 16, 2016) 480–487.

[54] A.J. Baksi, G.S. Kanaganayagam, S.K. Prasad, Arrhythmias in viral myocarditis and pericarditis, Card. Electrophysiol. Clin. 7 (2) (June 2015) 269–281.

[55] F. Salerno, N. Girerd, L. Chalabreysse, et al., Myocarditis and cardiac channelopathies: a deadly association? Int. J. Cardiol. 147 (3) (2011) 468–470.

[56] Buob, S. Siaplaouras, I. Janzen, et al., Focal parvovirus B19 myocarditis in a patient with Brugada syndrome, Cardiol. Rev. 11 (1) (2003) 45–49.

[57] L.T. Cooper, Giant cell myocarditis in children, Prog. Pediatr. Cardiol. 24 (1) (November 2007) 47–49.

[58] S.E. Lipshultz, L.A. Sleeper, J.A. Towbin, A.M. Lowe, E.J. Orav, G.F. Cox, P.R. Lurie, K.L. McCoy, M.A. McDonald, J.E. Messere, S.D. Colan, The incidence of pediatric cardiomyopathy in two regions of the United States, N. Engl. J. Med. 348 (2003) 1647–1655.

[59] R.A. Friedman, J.P. Moak, A. Garson, Clinical course of idiopathic dilated cardiomyopathy in children, J. Am. Coll. Cardiol. 18 (1991) 152–156.

[60] V.V. Dimas, S.W. Denfield, R.A. Friedman, B.C. Cannon, J.J. Kim, E.O. Smith, S.K. Clunie, J.A. Price, W.J. Dreyer, N.J. Kertesz, Frequency of cardiac death in children with idiopathic dilated cardiomyopathy, Am. J. Cardiol. 104 (2009) 1574–1577.

[61] S. Chen, K.S. Motonaga, S.A. Hollander, C.S. Almond, D.N. Rosenthal, B.D. Kaufman, L.J. May, K. Avasarala, D.T. Dao, A.M. Dubin, S.R. Ceresnak, Electrocardiographic repolarization abnormalities and increased risk of life-threatening arrhythmias in children with dilated cardiomyopathy, Heart Rhythm 13 (6) (June 2016) 1289–1296.

[62] K.M. Molina, P. Shrader, S.D. Colan, S. Mital, R. Margossian, L.A. Sleeper, G. Shirali, P. Barker, C.E. Canter, K. Altmann, E. Radojewski, E.S. Tierney, J. Rychik, L.Y. Tani, Pediatric heart network investigators. predictors of disease progression in pediatric dilated cardiomyopathy, Circ. Heart Fail. 6 (2013) 1214–1222.

[63] D.T. Dao, S.A. Hollander, D.N. Rosenthal, A.M. Dubin, QRS prolongation is strongly associated with life-threatening ventricular arrhythmias in children with dilated cardiomyopathy, J. Heart Lung Transpl. 32 (2013) 1013–1019.

[64] Kadish, A. Dyer, J.P. Daubert, R. Quigg, N.A. Estes, K.P. Anderson, H. Calkins, D. Hoch, J. Goldberger, A. Shalaby, W.E. Sanders, A. Schaechter, J.H. Levine, Prophylactic defibrillator implantation in patients with nonischemic dilated cardiomyopathy, N. Engl. J. Med. 350 (2004) 2151–2158.

[65] G. Bardy, K.L. Lee, D.B. Mark, J.E. Poole, D.L. Packer, R. Boineau, M. Domanski, C. Troutman, J. Anderson, G. Johnson, S.E. McNulty, N. Clapp-Channing, L.D. Davidson-Ray, E.S. Fraulo, D.P. Fishbein, R.M. Luceri, J.H. Ip, Amiodarone or an implantable cardioverter-defibrillator for congestive heart failure, N. Engl. J. Med. 352 (2005) 225–237.

[66] W.P. McNair, G. Sinagra, M.R. Taylor, A. Di Lenarda, D.A. Ferguson, E.E. Salcedo, D. Slavov, X. Zhu, J.H. Caldwell, L. Mestroni, Familial Cardiomyopathy Registry Research Group, SCN5A mutations associate with arrhythmic dilated cardiomyopathy and commonly localize to the voltage-sensing mechanism, J. Am. Coll. Cardiol. 57 (21) (May 24, 2011) 2160–2168.

[67] A.E. Emery, Emery Dreifuss muscular dystrophy-a 40 year retrospective, Neuromuscul. Disord. 10 (2000) 228–232.

[68] J.L. Theis, M.T. Zimmermann, B.T. Larsen, I.N. Rybakova, P.A. Long, J.M. Evans, S. Middha, M. de Andrade, R.L. Moss, E.D. Wieben, V.V. Michels, T.M. Olson, TNNI3K mutation in familial syndrome of conduction system disease, atrial tachyarrhythmia and dilated cardiomyopathy, Hum. Mol. Genet. 23 (21) (November 1, 2014) 5793–5804.

[69] C.F. Camm, C.A. James, C. Tichnell, B. Murray, A. Bhonsale, A.S. Riele, D.P. Judge, H. Tandri, H. Calkins, Prevalence of atrial arrhythmias in arrhythmogenic right ventricular dysplasia/cardiomyopathy, Heart Rhythm 10 (11) (November 2013) 1661–1668.

[70] A.E. Epstein, J.P. DiMarco, K.A. Ellenbogen, N.A. Estes 3rd, R.A. Freedman, L.S. Gettes, A.M. Gillinov, G. Gregoratos, S.C. Hammill, D.L. Hayes, M.A. Hlatky, L.K. Newby, R.L. Page, M.H. Schoenfeld, M.J. Silka, L.W. Stevenson, M.O. Sweeney, C.M. Tracy, A.E. Epstein, D. Darbar, J.P. DiMarco, S.B. Dunbar, N.A. Estes 3rd, T.B. Ferguson Jr., S.C. Hammill, P.E. Karasik, M.S. Link, J.E. Marine, M.H. Schoenfeld, A.J. Shanker, M.J. Silka, L.W. Stevenson, W.G. Stevenson, P.D. Varosy, American college of cardiology foundation; American heart association task force on practice guidelines; heart rhythm society. 2012 ACCF/AHA/HRS focused update incorporated into the ACCF/AHA/HRS 2008 guidelines for device-based therapy of cardiac rhythm abnormalities: a report of the American college of cardiology foundation/American heart association task force on practice guidelines and the heart rhythm society, J. Am. Coll. Cardiol. 61 (3) (January 22, 2013) e6–75.

[71] A.M. Dubin, C.I. Berul, L.M. Bevilacqua, K.K. Collins, S.P. Etheridge, A.L. Fenrich, R.A. Friedman, R.M. Hamilton, M.S. Schaffer, M. Shah, M.J. Silka, G.F. Van Hare, N.J. Kertesz, The use of implantable cardioverter-defibrillators in pediatric patients awaiting heart transplantation, J. Card. Fail. 9 (5) (October 2003) 375–379.

[72] The cardiac insufficiency bisoprolol study II (CIBIS-II): A randomized trial, Lancet 353 (1999) 9–13.

[73] J.P. Piccini, J.S. Berger, C.M. O'Connor, Amiodarone for the prevention of sudden cardiac death: a meta-analysis of randomized controlled trials, Eur. Heart J. 30 (10) (May 2009) 1245–1253.

[74] D.G. Katritsis, W. Zareba, A.J. Camm, Nonsustained ventricular tachycardia, J. Am. Coll. Cardiol. 60 (20) (November 13, 2012) 1993–2004.

[75] P. Ponikowski, A.A. Voors, S.D. Anker, H. Bueno, J.G. Cleland, A.J. Coats, V. Falk, J.R. González-Juanatey, V.P. Harjola, E.A. Jankowska, M. Jessup, C. Linde, P. Nihoyannopoulos, J.T. Parissis, B. Pieske, J.P. Riley, G.M. Rosano, L.M. Ruilope, F. Ruschitzka, F.H. Rutten, P. van der Meer, 2016 ESC guidelines for the diagnosis and treatment of acute and chronic heart failure: the task force for the diagnosis and treatment of acute and chronic heart failure of the European society of cardiology (ESC)developed with the special contribution of the heart failure association (HFA) of the ESC, Eur. Heart J. 37 (27) (May 20, 2016) 2129–2200.

[76] J. Steffel, F. Duru, Rhythm disorders in isolated left ventricular noncompaction, Ann. Med. 44 (2012) 101–108.

[77] G. Fazio, G. Corrado, E. Zachara, C. Rapezzi, A.K. Sulafa, L. Sutera, C. Pizzuto, C. Stollberger, L. Sormani, J. Finsterer, A. Benatar, G. Di Gesaro, C. Cascio, D. Cangemi, Y. Cavusoglu, M. Baumhakel, F. Drago, S. Carerj, S. Pipitone, S. Novo, Ventricular tachycardia in non-compaction of left ventricle: is this a frequent complication? Pacing Clin. Electrophysiol. 30 (4) (April 2007) 544–546.

[78] N.L. Bhatia, A.J. Tajik, S. Wilansky, D.E. Steidley, F. Mookadam, Isolated noncompaction of the left ventricular myocardium in adults: a systematic overview, J. Card. Fail. 17 (9) (September 2011) 771–778.

[79] S.T. Brescia, J.W. Rossano, R. Pignatelli, J.L. Jefferies, J.F. Price, J.A. Decker, S.W. Denfield, W.J. Dreyer, O. Smith, J.A. Towbin, J.J. Kim, Mortality and sudden death in pediatric left ventricular noncompaction in a tertiary referral center, Circulation 127 (22) (June 4, 2013) 2202–2208.

[80] F. Ichida, Y. Hamamichi, T. Miyawaki, Y. Ono, T. Kamiya, T. Akagi, H. Hamada, O. Hirose, T. Isobe, K. Yamada, S. Kurotobi, H. Mito, T. Miyake, Y. Murakami, T. Nishi, M. Shinohara, M. Seguchi, S. Tashiro, H. Tomimatsu, Clinical features of isolated noncompaction of the ventricular myocardium: long-term clinical course, hemodynamic properties, and genetic background, J. Am. Coll. Cardiol. 34 (1) (July 1999) 233–240.

[81] F. Santoro, V. Manuppelli, N.D. Brunetti, Multiple morphology ventricular tachycardia in non-compaction cardiomyopathy: multi-modal imaging, Europace 15 (2) (February 2013) 304.

[82] G. Junga, S. Kneifel, A. Von Smekal, H. Steinert, U. Bauersfeld, Myocardial ischaemia in children with isolated ventricular non-compaction, Eur. Heart J. 20 (12) (June 1999) 910–916.

[83] B.C. Weiford, V.D. Subbarao, K.M. Mulhern, Noncompaction of the ventricular myocardium, Circulation 109 (24) (June 22, 2004) 2965–2971.

[84] G. Fazio, G. Corrado, C. Pizzuto, E. Zachara, C. Rapezzi, A.K. Sulafa, L. Sutera, C. Stollberger, L. Sormani, J. Finsterer, A. Benatar, G. Di Gesaro, G. Novo, Y. Cavusoglu, M. Baumhakel, F. Drago, S. Carerj, S. Pipitone, S. Novo, Supraventricular arrhythmias in noncompaction of left ventricle: is this a frequent complication? Int. J. Cardiol. 127 (2) (July 4, 2008) 255–256.

[85] J. Fichet, A. Legras, A. Bernard, D. Babuty, Aborted sudden cardiac death revealing isolated noncompaction of the left ventricle in a patient with wolff-Parkinson-white syndrome, Pacing Clin. Electrophysiol. 30 (3) (March 2007) 444–447.

[86] F.I. Marcus, G.H. Fontaine, G. Guiraudon, et al., Right ventricular dysplasia: a report of 24 adult cases, Circulation 65 (1982) 384–398.

[87] B. Philips, S. Madhavan, C. James, et al., High prevalence of catecholamine-facilitated focal ventricular tachycardia in patients with arrhythmogenic right ventricular dysplasia/cardiomyopathy, Circ. Arrhythm. Electrophysiol. 6 (2013) 160–166.

[88] D. Corrado, G. Thiene, Arrhythmogenic right ventricular cardiomyopathy/dysplasia: clinical impact of molecular genetic studies, Circulation 113 (2006) 1634–1637.

[89] F.I. Marcus, W.J. McKenna, D. Sherrill, et al., Diagnosis of arrhythmogenic right ventricular cardiomyopathy/dysplasia: proposed modification of the task force criteria, Circulation 121 (2010) 1533–1541.

[90] K.S. Hoffmayer, O.N. Machado, G.M. Marcus, Y. Yang, C.J. Johnson, S. Ermakov, E. Vittinghoff, U. Pandurangi, H. Calkins, D. Cannom, K.C. Gear, C. Tichnell, Y. Park, W. Zareba, F.I. Marcus, M.M. Scheinman, Electrocardiographic comparison of ventricular arrhythmias in patients with arrhythmogenic right ventricular cardiomyopathy and right ventricular outflow tract tachycardia, J. Am. Coll. Cardiol. 58 (2011) 831–838.

[91] A.F. Chu, E. Zado, F.E. Marchlinski, Atrial arrhythmias in patients with arrhythmogenic right ventricular cardiomyopathy/dysplasia and ventricular tachycardia, Am. J. Cardiol. 106 (5) (September 1, 2010) 720–722.

[92] C.A. James, A. Bhonsale, C. Tichnell, B. Murray, S.D. Russell, H. Tandri, et al., Exercise increases age-related penetrance and arrhythmic risk in arrhythmogenic right ventricular dysplasia/cardiomyopathy-associated desmosomal mutation carriers, J. Am. Coll. Cardiol. 62 (2013) 1290–1297.

[93] G.M. Marcus, D.V. Glidden, B. Polonsky, W. Zareba, L.M. Smith, D.S. Cannom, et al., Efficacy of antiarrhythmic drugs in arrhythmogenic right ventricular cardiomyopathy: a report from the North American ARVC Registry, J. Am. Coll. Cardiol. 54 (2009) 609–615.

[94] F.C. Garcia, V. Bazan, E.S. Zado, J.F. Ren, F.E. Marchlinski, Epicardial substrate and outcome with epicardial ablation of ventricular tachycardia in arrhythmogenic right ventricular cardiomyopathy/dysplasia, Circulation 120 (2009) 366–375.

[95] E.P. Walsh, F. Cecchin, Arrhythmias in adult patients with congenital heart disease, Circulation 115 (4) (January 30, 2007) 534–545.

[96] K.S. Motonaga, P. Khairy, A.M. Dubin, Electrophysiologic therapeutics in heart failure in adult congenital heart disease, Heart Fail. Clin. 10 (1) (January 2014) 69–89.

[97] P. Khairy, G.F. Van Hare, S. Balaji, C.I. Berul, F. Cecchin, M.I. Cohen, C.J. Daniels, B.J. Deal, J.A. Dearani, Nd Groot, A.M. Dubin, L. Harris, J. Janousek, R.J. Kanter, P.P. Karpawich, J.C. Perry, S.P. Seslar, M.J. Shah, M.J. Silka, J.K. Triedman, E.P. Walsh, C.A. Warnes, PACES/HRS expert consensus statement on the recognition and management of arrhythmias in adult congenital heart disease: developed in partnership between the pediatric and congenital electrophysiology society (PACES) and the heart rhythm society (HRS). Endorsed by the governing bodies of PACES, HRS, the American college of cardiology (ACC), the American heart association (AHA), the European heart rhythm association (EHRA), the Canadian heart rhythm society (CHRS), and the international society for adult congenital heart disease (ISACHD), Heart Rhythm 11 (10) (October 2014) e102–e165.

[98] J.A. Kirsh, E.P. Walsh, J.K. Triedman, Prevalence of and risk factors for atrial fibrillation and intra-atrial reentrant tachycardia among patients with congenital heart disease, Am. J. Cardiol. 90 (2002) 338–340.

[99] S. Balaji, A. Daga, D.J. Bradley, S.P. Etheridge, I.H. Law, A.S. Batra, S. Sanatani, A.K. Singh, K.K. Gajewski, S. Tsao, H.R. Singh, S. Tisma-Dupanovic, S. Tateno, M. Takamuro, H. Nakajima, J.W. Roos-Hesselink, M. Shah, An international multicenter study comparing arrhythmia prevalence between the intracardiac lateral tunnel and the extracardiac conduit type of Fontan operations, J. Thorac. Cardiovasc. Surg. 148 (2) (August 2014) 576–581.

[100] E.A. Stephenson, M. Lu, C.I. Berul, S.P. Etheridge, S.F. Idriss, R. Margossian, J.H. Reed, A. Prakash, L.A. Sleeper, V.L. Vetter, A.D. Blaufox, Pediatric Heart Network Investigators, Arrhythmias in a contemporary fontan cohort: prevalence and clinical associations in a multicenter cross-sectional study, J. Am. Coll. Cardiol. 56 (11) (September 7, 2010) 890–896.

[101] W. Li, J. Somerville, Atrial flutter in grown-up congenital heart (GUCH) patients. Clinical characteristics of affected population, Int. J. Cardiol. 75 (2000) 129–213.

[102] J. Roos-Hesselink, M.G. Perlroth, J. McGhie, S. Spitaels, Atrial arrhythmias in adults after repair of tetralogy of Fallot: correlations with clinical, exercise, and echocardiographic findings, Circulation 91 (1995) 2214–2219.

[103] M. Gelatt, R.M. Hamilton, B.W. McCrindle, M. Connelly, A. Davis, L. Harris, R.M. Gow, W.G. Williams, G.A. Trusler, R.M. Freedom, Arrhythmia and mortality after the Mustard procedure: a 30-year single-center experience, J. Am. Coll. Cardiol. 29 (1) (January 1997) 194–201.

[104] P. Khairy, L. Harris, M. Landzberg, S.M. Fernandes, A. Barlow, L. Mercier, S. Viswanathan, P. Chetaille, E. Gordon, A. Dore, F. Cecchin, Sudden death and defibrillators in transposition of the great arteries with intra-atrial baffles: a multicenter study, Circ. Arrhythm. Electrophysiol. 1 (2008) 250–257.

[105] C.J. Flinn, G.S. Wolff, M. Dick II, R.M. Campbell, G. Borkat, A. Casta, A. Hordof, T.J. Hougen, R.-E. Kavey, M.D. John Kugler, M.D. Jerome Liebman, J. Greenhouse, B.S. Paul Hees, Cardiac rhythm after the mustard operation for complete transposition of the great arteries, N. Engl. J. Med. 310 (1984) 1635–1638.

[106] M.J. Silka, B.G. Hardy, V.D. Menashe, C.D. Morris, A population-based prospective evaluation of risk of sudden cardiac death after operation for common congenital heart defects, J. Am. Coll. Cardiol. 32 (1) (July 1998) 245–251.

[107] L. Dos, L. Teruel, I. J Ferreira, J. Rodriguez-Larrea, L. Miro, J. Girona, D. C Albert, A. Gonçalves, M. Murtra, J. Casaldaliga, Late outcome of senning and mustard procedures for correction of transposition of the great arteries, Heart 91 (5) (2005) 652–656.

[108] M. Schwerzmann, O. Salehian, L. Harris, S.C. Siu, W.G. Williams, G.D. Webb, J.M. Colman, A. Redington, C.K. Silversides, Ventricular arrhythmias and sudden death in adults after a Mustard operation for transposition of the great arteries, Eur. Heart J. 30 (15) (August 2009) 1873–1879.

[109] J. Villafañe, J.A. Feinstein, K.J. Jenkins, R.N. Vincent, E.P. Walsh, A.M. Dubin, T. Geva, J.A. Towbin, M.S. Cohen, C. Fraser, J. Dearani, D. Rosenthal, B. Kaufman, T.P. Graham Jr., A. Congenital, Pediatric cardiology section, American college of cardiology. Hot topics in tetralogy of fallot, J. Am. Coll. Cardiol. 62 (23) (December 10, 2013) 2155–2166.

[110] K. Zeppenfeld, M.J. Schalij, M.M. Bartelings, U.B. Tedrow, B.A. Koplan, K. Soejima, W.G. Stevenson, Catheter ablation of ventricular tachycardia after repair of congenital heart disease: electroanatomic identification of the critical right ventricular isthmus, Circulation 116 (20) (November 13, 2007) 2241–2252.

[111] J.G. Morwood, J.K. Triedman, C.I. Berul, P. Khairy, M.E. Alexander, F. Cecchin, E.P. Walsh, Radiofrequency catheter ablation of ventricular tachycardia in children and young adults with congenital heart disease, Heart Rhythm 1 (3) (September 2004) 301–308.

[112] J. Therrien, S.C. Siu, L. Harris, A. Dore, K. Niwa, J. Janousek, W.G. Williams, G. Webb, M.A. Gatzoulis, Impact of pulmonary valve replacement on arrhythmia propensity late after repair of tetralogy of fallot, Circulation 103 (20) (May 22, 2001) 2489–2494.

[113] B.J. Deal, C. Mavroudis, C.L. Backer, Beyond Fontan conversion: surgical therapy of arrhythmias including patients with associated complex congenital heart disease, Ann. Thorac. Surg. 76 (2003) 542–553.

[114] G.Y.H. Lip, F.R. Heinzel, F. Gaita, J.R. Gonzalez Juanatey, J.Y. Le Heuzey, T. Potpara, J.H. Svendsen, M.A. Vos, S.D. Anker, A.J. Coats, W. Haverkamp, A.S. Manolis, M.K. Chung, P. Sanders, B. Pieske, B. Gorenek, D. Lane, G. Boriani, C. Linde, G. Hindricks, H. Tsutsui, S. Homma, S. Brownstein, J.C. Nielsen, M. Lainscak, M. Crespo-Leiro, M. Piepoli, P. Seferovic, Irene Savelieva on behalf of (EP-Europace), European heart rhythm association/heart failure association joint consensus document on arrhythmias in heart failure, endorsed by the heart rhythm society and the Asia Pacific heart rhythm society, Europace 18 (1) (August 2015) 12–36.

[115] S.N. Singh, R.D. Fletcher, S.G. Fisher, et al., Amiodarone in patients with congestive heart failure and asymptomatic ventricular arrhythmia. Survival trial of antiarrhythmic therapy in congestive heart failure, N. Engl. J. Med. 333 (1995) 77–82.

[116] B. Brendorp, H. Elming, L. Jun, L. Køber, M. Malik, G.B. Jensen, C. Torp-Pedersen, DIAMOND Study Group, Qtc interval as a guide to select those patients with congestive heart failure and reduced left ventricular systolic function who will benefit from antiarrhythmic treatment with dofetilide, Circulation 103 (10) (March 13, 2001) 1422–1427.

[117] R. Correa, E.D. Sherwin, J. Kovach, D.Y. Mah, M.E. Alexander, F. Cecchin, E.P. Walsh, J.K. Triedman, D.J. Abrams, Mechanism and ablation of arrhythmia following total cavopulmonary connection, Circ. Arrhythm. Electrophysiol. 8 (2) (April 2015) 318–325.

[118] J.K. Triedman, M.E. Alexander, B.A. Love, K.K. Collins, C.I. Berul, L.M. Bevilacqua, E.P. Walsh, Influence of patient factors and ablative technologies on outcomes of radiofrequency ablation of intra-atrial re-entrant tachycardia in patients with congenital heart disease, J. Am. Coll. Cardiol. 39 (2002) 1827–1835.

[119] E.P. Walsh, Interventional electrophysiology in patients with congenital heart disease, Circulation 115 (25) (June 26, 2007) 3224–3234.

[120] J.K. Triedman, D.M. Bergau, J.P. Saul, M.R. Epstein, E.P. Walsh, Efficacy of radiofrequency ablation for control of intraatrial reentrant tachycardia in patients with congenital heart disease, J. Am. Coll. Cardiol. 30 (1997) 1032–1038.

[121] D.S. Frankel, M.J. Shah, P.F. Aziz, M.D. Hutchinson, Catheter ablation of atrial fibrillation in transposition of the great arteries treated with mustard atrial baffle, Circ. Arrhythm Electrophysiol. 5 (2) (April 2012) e41–e43.

[122] F. SB, J.D. Asnes, N.L. Rollinson, M.W. Cleman, Percutaneous right ventricular support during catheter ablation of intra-atrial reentrant tachycardia in an adult with a mustard baffle–a novel use of the Impella device, J. Interv. Card. Electrophysiol. 29 (1) (October 2010) 69–72.

[123] J.N. Silva, C.C. Erickson, C.D. Carter, E.A. Greene, M. Kantoch, K.K. Collins, C.Y. Miyake, M.P. Carboni, E.K. Rhee, A. Papez, V. Anand, T.M. Bowman, G.F. Van Hare, Participating members of pediatric and congenital electrophysiology society (PACES). Management of pediatric tachyarrhythmias on mechanical support, Circ. Arrhythm. Electrophysiol. 7 (4) (August 2014) 658–663.

[124] P. Khairy, L. Harris, M.J. Landzberg, S. Viswanathan, A. Barlow, M.A. Gatzoulis, S.M. Fernandes, L. Beauchesne, J. Therrien, P. Chetaille, E. Gordon, I. Vonder Muhll, F. Cecchin, Implantable cardioverter-defibrillators in tetralogy of fallot, Circulation 117 (3) (January 22, 2008) 363–370.

[125] B. D'Souza, A.E. Epstein, F.C. Garcia, Y.Y. Kim, S.C. Agarwal, P.H. Belott, M.C. Burke, A.R. Leon, J.M. Morgan, K.K. Patton, M.J. Shah, Patients with congenital heart disease receiving the subcutaneous implantable-cardioverter defibrillator: results from a pooled analysis from the IDE study and EFFORTLESS S-ICD registry, JACCCEP 2 (5) (May 18, 2016) 615–622.

[126] P. Fasseas, S.P. Kutalek, F.L. Samuels, E.C. Holmes, L.E. Samuels, Ventricular assist device support for management of sustained ventricular arrhythmias, Tex. Heart Inst. J. 29 (2002) 33–36.

[127] H. Tatewaki, M. Masuda, T. Nishida, et al., Successful treatment of tachycardia-induced cardiomyopathy with LVAD in a 12-year- old boy, Ann. Thorac. Surg. 80 (2005) e5–e7.

[128] P. Fasseas, S.P. Kutalek, B.K. Kantharia, Prolonged sustained ventricular fibrillation without loss of consciousness in patients supported by a left ventricular assist device, Cardiology 97 (4) (2002) 210–213.

Chapter 28

Fetal Heart Failure

Edgar T. Jaeggi[1], Mary T. Donofrio[2]

[1]University of Toronto, Toronto, ON, Canada; [2]National Children's Health System, Washington, DC, United States

INTRODUCTION

Congestive fetal heart failure (HF), defined as inadequate blood supply to meet the needs of the developing fetus, is a common final pathway of many disease states and may lead to end-organ failure and in-utero demise. While some of the underlying conditions are unique to the intrauterine environment, others may occur at any patient age. This chapter will review the pathophysiology of fetal HF and provide a practical approach to the diagnosis, management, and the prognosis of the more common causes.

FETAL CIRCULATION AND CARDIAC FUNCTION

Fetal Versus Postnatal Circulation

There are clinically important differences in cardiac function and the circulation before and after birth. In the postnatal circulation, with the closure of the arterial duct, desaturated systemic venous blood from the caval veins enters the right heart and is forwarded into the low pressure and low resistant pulmonary vasculature with no significant admixture with oxygenated blood. Highly oxygenated pulmonary venous blood passes through the left heart and the aorta to supply the body. Thus, the left (LV) and right (RV) ventricles work in series and are pumping similar stroke volumes during each cardiac cycle. In this arrangement of functionally separated systemic and pulmonary circulations, severe dysfunction of one of the two ventricles is sufficient to result in circulatory failure.

In contrast, the prenatal presence of three physiological pathways (ductus venosus (DV), ductus arteriosus, and foramen ovale) enables the two ventricles of the fetus to work in parallel rather than in series. In this arrangement, the stroke volume of each ventricle is determined by its individual preload, afterload, myocardial properties, ventricular–ventricular interactions, and the constraint that is exerted on the heart by surrounding tissues and the amniotic fluid. Right and left atrial pressures are similar due to the widely patent interatrial communication, and right and left ventricular pressures are equal due to the patency of the arterial duct.

Fetal Cardiac Function

As with the mature heart, an increase in afterload leads to an increase in the amount of tension exerted on the heart muscle during contraction and lowers the ventricular stroke volume. An increase in preload, which reflects how "filled" the heart is, leads to an increased stretch of the ventricular myocardium before it begins to contract and results in increased contractility with a larger stroke volume according to the Frank–Starling mechanism. This allows prompt adjustments to circulatory hemodynamic changes on a beat-to-beat basis. Nonetheless, due to maturational differences in the structure of the contractile apparatus, in the excitation–contraction coupling mechanisms, and in the nervous control of the heart, the fetal myocardium is significantly less contractile and less compliant compared to the mature heart [1–3]. While the Frank–Starling mechanism does also operate in the fetal heart, the capacity to augment stroke volume by increasing end-diastolic pressure is very limited as the ventricles are already operating close to the top of their function curves [4]. Liquid-filled lungs and amniotic fluid exert a positive pressure on fetal cardiac chambers, which further limits the diastolic ventricular filling reserve. Due to the physiologically fast resting heart rate, the cardiac reserve of the fetus to augment cardiac output (CO) by simply increasing the heart rate is also minimal [5].

Finally, related to intrinsic differences in the geometry and myofiber architecture of the RV and LV there are also significant interventricular differences in the ability to deform and develop contractile force [1,6]. The normal architecture of the ellipsoid-shaped LV comprises an array of longitudinal, circumferential, and oblique/spiraling muscle layers that

Heart Failure in the Child and Young Adult. http://dx.doi.org/10.1016/B978-0-12-802393-8.00028-4

allow a homogenous transmural workload and stiffness in all directions parallel to the plane in which the fibers lie. [7] The trapezoid-shaped RV mainly contains longitudinal myofibers [8]. The mechanical consequences are that the RV in comparison to the LV is more compliant but generates less force, does not twist in systole to store energy and recoil in diastole to release energy and, in consequence, is significantly less resistant to increased cardiac loading [9,10]. Compared to the LV, RV dysfunction occurs earlier and is more severe in response to high afterload.

Fetal Cardiac Output and Its Distribution

Given that the circulation functions in parallel rather than in series, in the human fetus under normal physiological loading conditions, the RV handles about 60% and the LV about 40% of the combined CO of about 450–500 mL/kg/min [11]. The placenta is the source of fetal oxygenation and nutrient delivery. The DV, a narrowed short vessel that connects the intraabdominal umbilical vein (UV) with the inferior vena cava at its inlet to the right atrium and bypassing the liver, is an important regulator of the oxygenated blood flow from the placenta to the left heart. In response to hypoxemia the DV is able to distend over its entire length to increase ductal flow [12,13]. In midgestation about 30% of well-oxygenated blood from the placenta is shunted across the DV [14]. Venous blood that passes the DV is accelerated from a peak flow velocity of 10–20 cm/s at its entrance to velocities >60 cm/s at its exit. The flow from the DV is preferentially directed through the foramen ovale to the left heart where it is ejected into the aorta and upper body including the brain [15]. Deoxygenated blood from the inferior vena cava, the right hepatic veins, and the superior vena cava is mainly directed to the RV and then pumped to the pulmonary arteries and via the arterial duct to the lower body and the placenta. Given that the branch pulmonary arteries have a high vascular resistance, the fetal lungs are only perfused by about 15% of the combined CO [11], while the low resistance placental circulation receives about 30% of the total output [11,16,17]. The aortic isthmus serves as an arterial watershed between the circulation of the upper body and that of the lower body including the placenta [18]. The aortic isthmus flow pattern provides important information about the differences in impedance between the cerebral circulation and that of the placenta and lower fetal body. In addition, flow through the isthmus is influenced by LV output. In late gestation, approximately 10%–15% of the combined CO passes from the ascending aorta through the isthmus and to the lower body [11]. The aortic isthmus and aortic arch may be perfused in the opposite direction by blood from the RV and arterial duct if the LV output is low (e.g., due to severe aortic stenosis), the downstream impedance is increased (due to placental compromise) and/or the impedance of the cerebral vasculature is decreased (e.g., cerebral vasodilation in response to hypoxemia) [19–21].

MECHANISMS AND MANIFESTATION OF FETAL HEART FAILURE

Univentricular Heart Failure

Despite the functional limitations of the immature heart, the parallel fetal circulation is a remarkably flexible and adaptive arrangement that permits a shift in flow from one part of the circulation to another in response to functional or anatomical cardiovascular anomalies. This includes conditions in which the stroke volume of one ventricle is reduced and the contralateral ventricle is able to increase its work in a compensatory manner [10,22]. This allows in-utero survival to birth with only one functional ventricle, although the overall delivery of CO may be insufficient to entirely meet the needs of the developing fetus [10,22,23]. Using quantitative MRI techniques to assess fetal blood flow and oxygenation, compared to age-matched healthy controls, fetuses with univentricular congenital heart disease (CHD) showed significant reductions in the combined CO (mean 365 vs. 460 mL/kg/min (controls)) and in umbilical venous flow from the placenta (92 vs. 129 mL/kg/min). This was accompanied by lower ascending aorta saturation (44% vs. 58%), lower cerebral O_2 delivery (14.5 vs. 20.4 mL/min/kg) and O_2 consumption (3.3 vs. 4.0 mL/min/kg), and smaller overall brain volumes (281 vs. 319 mL). Subnormal CO and oxygen delivery may contribute to the widespread neurodevelopmental anomalies of children with CHD, specifically those with hypoplastic left heart syndrome that show abnormalities even before they undergo surgery, including smaller weight-adjusted brain volumes, white matter injury, and metabolic changes compatible with delayed brain maturation [24,25].

Biventricular Heart Failure

Circulatory failure in the fetus typically results from the inability of both ventricles to fill and eject enough blood to meet the needs of the developing fetus. Conditions associated with biventricular dysfunction are numerous and include myocardial disease, abnormal loading conditions, arrhythmias, hypoxia, ischemia, and cardiac compression among the etiologies. Some of the conditions are unique to the in-utero environment and may resolve after birth. Others are transient and may improve spontaneously or with treatment prior to delivery.

Irrespective of the nature of the primary cardiac insult, severe cardiac dysfunction leads to a cascade of adaptive cardiovascular responses to improve forward flow and perfusion of those organs that are critical for immediate survival. At a compensated stage of reduced output, the fetus will react by lowering cerebral vascular resistance to preferentially redirect blood flow to the brain to avoid hypoxemic brain injury [26]. The coronary circulation is equally responsive to a drop in PO_2. This brain/heart-sparing circulation occurs at the expense of lower body perfusion. Reduced renal perfusion activates the renin–angiotensin system causing water and salt retention [27]. Increased wall stress due to abnormal loading triggers ventricular hypertrophy, which increases myocardial oxygen consumption and may induce myocardial fibrosis, thus worsening myocardial performance [28]. To overcome the reduction in ventricular compliance, the end-diastolic ventricular filling pressure and central venous pressure increase.

As previously noted, the immature fetal heart is physiologically less compliant and has a very limited preload reserve to increase CO by increasing end-diastolic filling pressure [4]. In addition, even a small increase in the hydrostatic venous pressure will greatly affect the fetal fluid balance. Related to a physiologically low tissue turgor and low plasma albumin concentration (low colloid osmotic pressure), body water content and the proportion of extracellular fluid are physiologically much larger in the fetus compared to children and adults. Moreover, fetal extracellular fluid clearance relies on high-rate lymph drainage via the thoracic duct [29]. In this situation, an increase in hydrostatic venous pressure of 2–3 mmHg enhances the extravascular fluid shift and critically reduces lymphatic drainage leading to progressive fluid accumulation in the fetal pericardial and pleural space, abdomen, and skin (fetal hydrops). It is, however, important to recognize that fetal hydrops is a typical but nonspecific finding of advanced HF. Fetal cavity effusions are also commonly seen in association with extracardiac pathology such as fetal systemic infections, lung masses and chromosomal disorders, and, unless the heart is compressed, in the absence of other signs of HF [30]. At a terminal stage of HF, low CO, and hypoxia will eventually evolve to multiorgan failure culminating in fetal demise.

PRENATAL ASSESSMENT

Introduction

Assessments of the fetal well-being and cardiac function and identification of a likely disease mechanism are important diagnostic steps in the clinical evaluation of the fetus with cardiac compromise. Table 28.1 summarizes the echocardiographic features of the main conditions associated with in-utero HF. The prenatal diagnosis of HF primarily relies on the ultrasound-based documentation of systolic and/or diastolic cardiac dysfunction and the circulatory consequences [31].

Measures of the Cardiovascular Status

In early stages of HF, disease manifestations that are readily detectable by echocardiography may be subtle. At more advanced stages (Fig. 28.1), findings include ascites, pleural effusion, pericardial effusion, or a combination of these findings, in addition to cardiomegaly, valvar regurgitation, poly- or oligohydramnios, preferential shunting of blood flow to the brain and heart, absence or reversal of the end-diastolic umbilical artery (UA) flow, and reduced or absent fetal movements. In end-stage HF, generalized skin edema is seen easily over the scalp and abdominal wall.

Measures of Cardiac Function

M-mode is useful to quantify the fetal systolic ventricular function by measurements of the changes in ventricular dimensions at the end of diastole (EDD) and of systole (ESD), respectively. *Ventricular shortening fraction* is calculated as SF (%) = (EDD-ESD)/EDD × 100. An LV or RV SF <28% suggests impaired ventricular systolic function. A low SF is most commonly related to myocardial disease or high afterload [32] and is usually seen in association with other functional consequences such as diastolic dysfunction, cardiomegaly, and atrioventricular (AV) valvar regurgitation [33,34].

Measurement of the *peak velocity* (v_{max}) *of the AV regurgitation* jet, if present, is a geometry-independent indirect measure of the ventricular contractile force. The peak pressure a ventricle is able to generate in the setting of AV regurgitation is estimated as pressure = $4 \times (v_{max})^2$ + atrial pressure. A normal fetal atrial pressure is about 3–4 mmHg and a normal mid- to late-gestational AV valvar pressure gradient is typically in the range of 40–60 mmHg [29]. A lower pressure gradient in the setting of moderate/severe AV regurgitation and reduced/absent forward flow across the pulmonary or aortic valve indicates subnormal pressure-generating capacity of the related ventricle.

CO (mL/min/kg) is a crude estimate of the global cardiac function and can be calculated as $CO = VTI \times \pi \times (D^2/4) \times HR/$ estimated fetal weight [35]. VTI relates to the velocity–time integral of the systolic aortic or pulmonary flow, D to the

TABLE 28.1 Echocardiographic Features of Conditions Associated With Fetal Heart Failure

Condition	Hypertrophy	Heart Size	Function		Cardiac Output	Other Frequent Findings/Associations
			Diastolic	Systolic		
Myocarditis • Viral • Anti-Ro/SSA antibodies	–	N or ↑	↓	↓	N or ↓	Pericardial effusion Anemia; ischemia; hypoalbuminemia Myocardial echogenicity; CHB
Nonhypertrophic CM	–	N or ↑	↓	↓	↓	EFE; calcifications; NC; other anomalies
Hypertrophic CM	Global	N	↓	N	↓	Other anomalies
Diabetic hypertrophy	IVS > free wall	N	N or ↓	N	N	Macrosomia
TTTS (recipient)	RV > LV	↑	RV > LV	RV > LV	↓ RV > LV	Polyhydramnios
Vascular tumors; TRAP	–	↑	N	↑	↑	Dilated systemic vein(s)
Agenesis of the DV	–	↑	N	↑	↑	Dilated umbilical vein
Constriction of the DA	–	↑ RV	↓ RV	↓ RV	↓ RV	Tricuspid regurgitation
Fetal anemia	–	↑	N	↑	↑	↑ peak MCA Doppler flow
Fetal hypoxemia ± acidosis	–	↑	N or ↓	N or ↓	N or ↓	Brain sparing
CCAM	–	↓	↓	N or ↓	↓	Chest mass
Large pericardial effusion	–	↓	↓	N or ↓	↓	Pericardial teratoma

CCAM, congenital cystic adenomatoid malformations of the lung; *CHB*, complete heart block; *CM*, cardiomyopathy; *DA*, ductus arteriosus; *DV*, ductus venosus; *EFE*, endocardial fibroelastosis; *MCA*, middle cerebral artery; *N*, normal; *NC*, ventricular noncompaction; *RV > LV*, right ventricle more severely affected than the left ventricle; *TRAP*, twin reversed arterial perfusion sequence; *TTTS*, twin–twin transfusion syndrome; ↑, increased; ↓, decreased; –, absent.

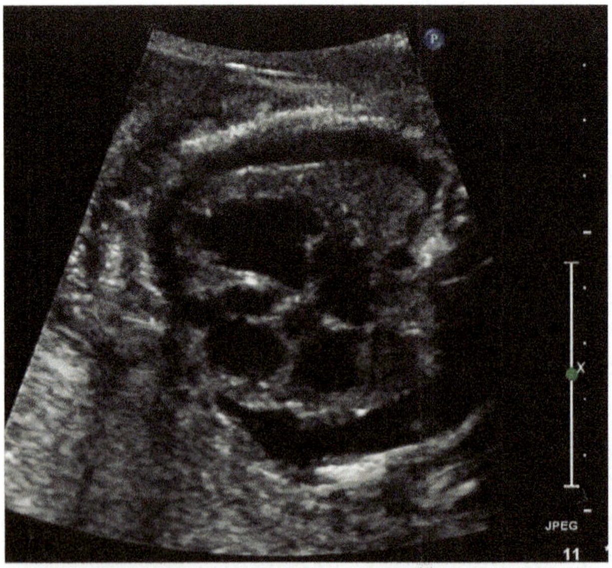

FIGURE 28.1 Cardiac four-chamber view of a fetus diagnosed at 30 gestational weeks with a severe form of nonhypertrophic cardiomyopathy of unknown etiology. Findings included massive cardiomegaly, severe biventricular dilatation and dysfunction, and fetal hydrops.

annulus diameter of the corresponding valve, and HR to the fetal heart rate. CO is not routinely measured but is useful to detect and monitor conditions associated with high-output failure such as AV malformations or vascular tumors [36–41].

Doppler flow profiles of the ventricular inflow, the systemic veins, and the DV provide crucial information on ventricular relaxation and compliance during diastole [42–44]. Normal fetal ventricular filling across the AV valves consists of three phases: (1) isovolumetric relaxation preceding ventricular inflow (IVR); (2) early passive filling (E-wave); and (3) late active filling during atrial contraction (A-wave). At a normal fetal heart rate, the duration of the IVR is <43 ms, and the Doppler inflow pattern is biphasic with a dominant A-wave as diastolic ventricular filling mainly results from atrial contraction [42,45]. Venous forward flow is initiated with the opening of the AV valves in early diastole, which causes an immediate drop in atrial pressure. Forward flow then slowly decreases with increasing ventricular pressure as the ventricles fill. With the onset of atrial contraction in late diastole there is a sudden increase in atrial pressure, which briefly slows the forward flow in the DV and briefly reverses the flow in the hepatic and caval veins away from the heart (a-waves). Doppler flows compatible with normal diastolic ventricular function include the following: (1) antegrade DV flow throughout the entire cardiac cycle; (2) a-wave flow reversal of <20 cm/s in the inferior vena cava; and (3) the absence of UV pulsations [46,47]. Biventricular diastolic dysfunction is very poorly tolerated by the fetus. The diagnosis of compromised diastolic filling is made on the detection of abnormal Doppler flows across the AV valves (monophasic, short inflow, or low E/A ratio; prolonged IVR interval), the DV (absent or reversed a-wave), and the inferior vena cava (a-wave reversal >20 cm/s) (Fig. 28.2). The presence of umbilical venous pulsations is a most useful predictor of imminent perinatal death in fetal hydrops.

The *myocardial performance index (MPI)* is a combined measure of systolic and diastolic ventricular function and is calculated as the sum of the mitral or tricuspid isovolumetric relaxation and contraction times divided by the aortic or pulmonary ejection time, for the LV or RV, respectively. Doppler-derived MPI values above 0.48 are considered abnormal [48].

Heart Failure Score

The *cardiovascular profile score* (CVPS) is a composite scoring system that is used to grade the severity of fetal HF [49–51]. The score is based on the result of five ultrasound parameters that have been correlated with poor fetal outcome (Table 28.2): (1) cavity effusions; (2) venous Doppler; (3) cardiothoracic area ratio (CTR); (4) cardiac function; and (5) UA Doppler. Severity of HF is rated on a 10 point scale, and 1 or 2 points are deducted for abnormalities of each component marker. The degree of failure is graded as being absent (10 points), mild (8 or 9 points), moderate (6 or 7 points), or severe (<5 points). One point is deducted from the score at the detection of each of the following findings: (1) isolated effusion; (2) DV a-wave flow reversal; (3) CTR of 35%–50%; (4) holosystolic tricuspid regurgitation *or* SF <28%; and (5)

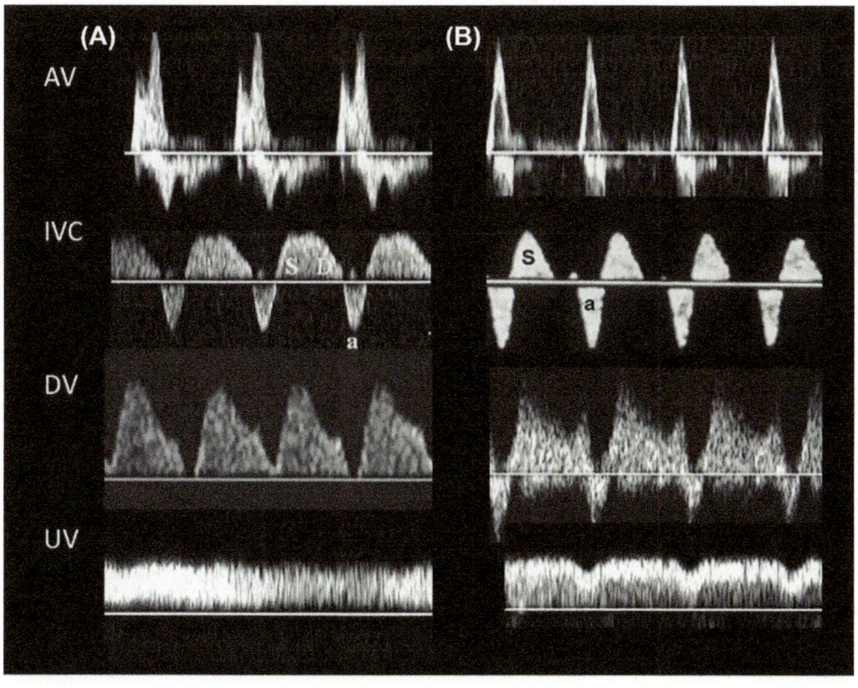

FIGURE 28.2 Atrioventricular (AV), inferior vena cava (IVC), venous duct (DV), and umbilical vein (UV) Doppler flow pattern in a fetus with progression from mild (A) to severe (B) diastolic dysfunction. (A) In mild diastolic dysfunction, the AV flow is still biphasic, while there is mildly increased reversal of flow in the IVC (>20 cm/s) and in the DV (to baseline) during atrial contraction (a-wave). The UV flow is nonpulsatile. (B) In severe diastolic dysfunction, the AV flow is monophasic and the inflow duration short. Related to the decreased relaxation and compliance and the increase in ventricular filling pressures, there is no early diastolic (D) forward flow in the IVC, a-wave reversal in DV, and pulsatile UV flow. *a*, late diastolic flow; *D*, early diastolic flow; *S*, systolic flow.

TABLE 28.2 Cardiovascular Profile to Assess the Severity of Heart Failure Based on the Combined Result of Five Echocardiographic Variables. The Heart Failure Score is 10 if There Are no Abnormal Signs and Reflects Two Points for Each of Five Categories: Hydrops; Venous Doppler; Heart Size; Cardiac Function; and Arterial Doppler

	Normal	−1 Point	−2 Points
Hydrops	None (2 pts)	Ascites *or* pleural effusion *or* pericardial effusion	Skin edema
Venous Doppler (umbilical vein and ductus venosus)	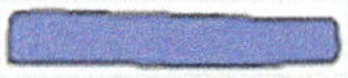 UV 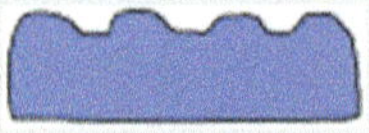 DV (2 pts)	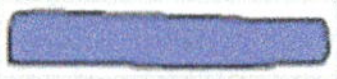 UV 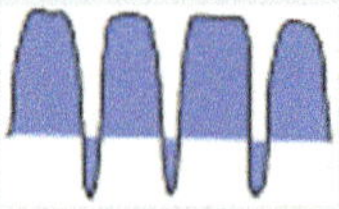 DV	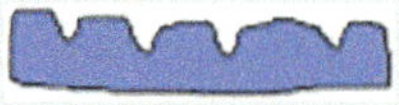 UV pulsations
Heart size (heart area/chest area)	>0.20 and <0.35 (2 pts)	0.35–0.50	>0.50 or <0.20
Cardiac function	Normal TV and MV RV/LV SF >0.28 biphasic diastolic filling (2 pts)	Holosystolic TR *or* RV/LV SF <0.28	Holosystolic MR *or* TR *dP/dt* 400 *or* monophasic filling
Arterial Doppler (umbilical artery)	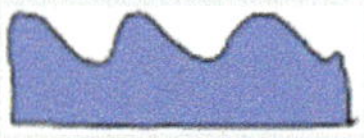 UA (2 pts)	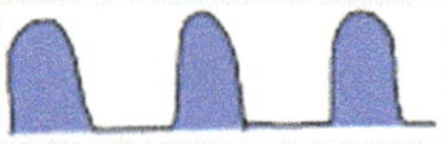 UA (AEDV)	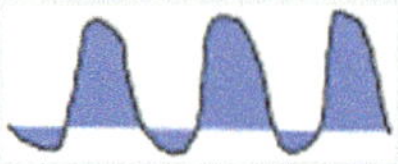 UA (REDV)

AEDV, absent end-diastolic velocity; *dP/dt*, change in pressure over time of TR jet; *DV*, ductus venosus; *LV*, left ventricle; *MR*, mitral valve regurgitation; *MV*, mitral valve; *pts*, points; *REDV*, reversed end-diastolic velocity; *RV*, right ventricle; *SF*, ventricular shortening fraction; *TR*, tricuspid valve regurgitation; *TV*, tricuspid valve; *UV*, umbilical vein.

absent end-diastolic UA flow. Two points are deducted with each of these findings: (1) skin edema; (2) pulsatile UV flow; (3) CTR >50%; (4) holosystolic mitral regurgitation *or* monophasic AV inflow; and (5) end-diastolic UA flow reversal.

Using a modified CVPS from the original scoring system (replacement of "skin edema" with "fetal hydrops" and elimination of "tricuspid valve dP/dt" as 2-point criteria) in a study of fetal patients with primary forms of cardiomyopathy (CM), a lower score at the baseline exam was already significantly associated with mortality (hazard ratio: 1.45 per point decrease; 95% confidence interval: 1.16–1.79; P=.001) despite the potential of disease progression later in gestation or after birth: 1-year survival on diagnosis was 24% with a score ≤6 but 79% with a score of 7 or higher [51]. While this supports that the modified CVPS is a useful prognostic marker for fetal CM, it is important to recognize that its predictive value depends on the HF cause and whether treatment is available. For example, HF in an anemic fetus with acute parvovirus infection can be treated with blood transfusions and is expected to have a better outcome compared with a fetus with CM and the same low CVPS.

CAUSES, MANAGEMENT, AND PROGNOSIS OF CONDITIONS ASSOCIATED WITH FETAL HEART FAILURE

Introduction

The prognosis and management of in-utero HF depends on the etiology, the severity, and the rate of progression of the disease. In addition, the gestational age at diagnosis is important, given that in some instances, the best option is likely early delivery and initiation of postnatal therapy. For this reason, close follow-up with frequent assessment of fetal cardiovascular status and well-being is imperative to assess the severity and course of the disease. For some fetuses and conditions, prenatal treatment will either not be required or not be available. If hydrops develops, there are no good in-utero treatment options other than expectant care with early delivery for most babies with an intrinsic form of myocardial disease, though transplacental digoxin has been attempted [33,52–54]. If HF is secondary, treatment of the primary cause is the best strategy if it is possible. This includes HF secondary to a fetal tachyarrhythmia, anemia, twin–twin transfusion syndrome (TTTS), or cardiac compression by a chest effusion or a large mass [41,55–60]. It is also important to understand the wishes of the family when considering treatment options, given that some of the in-utero interventions may impose significant risks to both fetus and mother with uncertain promise of benefit. In these cases, termination of pregnancy, expectant management, or delivery with palliative care may be the best option.

Myocardial Disease

Myocarditis

Viruses that may invade the fetal heart following an *intrauterine infection* include parvovirus B19, adenovirus, enterovirus, coxsackievirus, and cytomegaly virus [61–65]. The frequency of viral transmission-related myocarditis damage is unknown, but it is likely that many infections go unnoticed and resolve spontaneously. Prenatal management of symptomatic viral infections is usually expectant and for parvovirus infections may include life-saving blood transfusions if fetal anemia develops. Progression to therapy-resistant dilated CM following intrauterine viral infections has rarely been reported [66].

Transplacental passage of *maternal anti-Ro/SSA* may cause inflammation, necrosis, and fibrosis of the AV conduction system and endomyocardium in 1%–5% of exposed fetuses [67]. Complete heart block (CHB), cardiac dysfunction, and pericardial effusion are the main echocardiographic findings at the time of fetal diagnosis. In antibody-mediated myocarditis there has been experience with using transplacental therapy with dexamethasone, β-sympathomimetic agents, and/or intravenous immunoglobulin (IVIG) to temper the cardiac inflammation and to improve the fetal CO. While CHB represents an irreversible state of AV nodal damage, improved outcomes, resolution of effusions, and normalization of the cardiac function have been reported with the use of transplacental antiinflammatory treatment [57,68]. In a Canadian multicenter experience [57], 37 fetuses were studied; 21 were treated with dexamethasone at a dosage of 4 or 8 mg/day for 2 weeks, followed by 4 mg/day and when possible maintained for the duration of the pregnancy, tapering at times to 2 mg/day in the third trimester. Nine were treated with a β-sympathomimetic agent, added in pregnancies with CHB when the fetal heart rate fell below 55 bpm. The 21 patients treated with dexamethasone had a 1-year survival rate of 90%, compared to 46% without glucocorticoid therapy ($P=.02$). Immune-mediated conditions (myocarditis, hepatitis, CM) resulting in postnatal death or heart transplantation were more common in untreated pregnancies compared to those treated with steroids (0/18 vs. 4/9 live births; $P=.007$).

Cardiomyopathy

CM originates from a broad spectrum of postinflammatory, genetic-metabolic, chromosomal, familial, and unknown etiologies that may present phenotypically very similar and often involve other organs, further impacting the prognosis. Moreover, conditions of the same etiology may present and evolve very differently, which makes parental counseling a challenge. Finally, the diagnostic workup for CM is relatively invasive and may not be obtainable during pregnancy. In a recent retrospective study from Ontario [51], the incidence of prenatally diagnosed CM was 6.2 of 100,000 fetuses, which is comparable to that reported in children younger than 1 year of age in Finland (4.1/100,000), Australia (7.8/100,000), and the United States (8.3/100,000) [69–71]. The CVPS and a simple classification on the basis of a hypertrophic phenotype correlated well with the prognosis. The chance of survival of a fetus with a CVPS ≤6 was poor, irrespective of the underlying cause [51]. For survivors to birth, freedom from death or cardiac transplantation was significantly worse for those with a hypertrophic form of CM when compared with the nonhypertrophic phenotype (20% vs. 75% at 5 year) (Fig. 28.3) [51].

While no prenatal treatment is available for genetic, metabolic, familial, and postinfectious causes of CM, perinatal antiinflammatory medication has been used to treat *anti-Ro antibody-mediated CM including endocardial fibroelastosis* (EFE). In a study [72] that evaluated 19 fetuses with EFE, 17 were given transplacental high-dose dexamethasone and 9 at least one dose of maternal IVIG at a dose of 70 g (1 g/kg) before birth. Multiple IVIG doses were used in the setting of widespread EFE and ventricular dysfunction. Of 9 cases treated with IVIG and steroids, 6 demonstrated improved ventricular function within 1–3 weeks of treatment. In three hydropic fetuses, the improvement was only transient, with 1 in-utero death. Three without hydrops had improved function at birth, and in 1, the severity of fibrosis had lessened.

A significantly better outcome than with primary hypertrophic CM can be expected for the fetus with myocardial hypertrophy secondary to *pregestational and gestational maternal diabetes* [52]. The myocardial hypertrophy, which is secondary to fetal hyperinsulinism, predominantly involves the ventricular septum rather than the free walls. The ventricular myocardium and diastolic function of diabetic fetuses are already abnormal from early pregnancy, as evidenced by abnormal ventricular inflow patterns and prolonged IRT [73]. Still, the prenatal course is generally relatively benign and the hypertrophy resolves completely after birth [52]. Severe hypertrophy leading to fetal hydrops and death or needing neonatal mechanical support has been reported even with well-controlled diabetes [74–76].

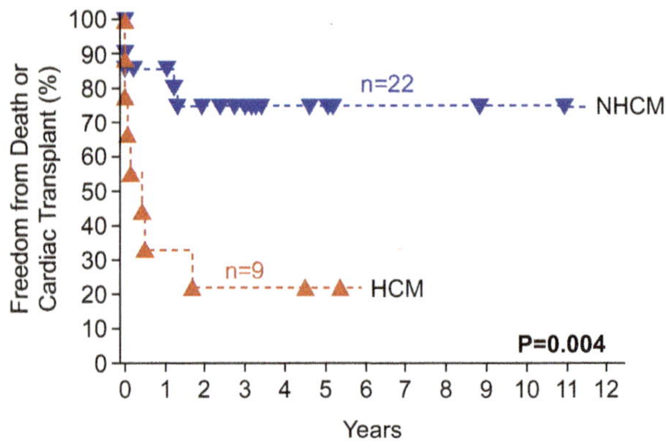

FIGURE 28.3 Kaplan–Meier estimates for freedom from death or transplantation from birth for fetuses with hypertrophic cardiomyopathy (HCM) versus nonhypertrophic cardiomyopathy (NHCM). Included are cases with myocardial disease unrelated to structural heart disease, tachyarrhythmia, abnormal cardiac loading, ischemia, or maternal diabetes.

Abnormal Cardiac Loading

Twin–Twin Transfusion Syndrome

TTTS affects about 20% of the monochorionic twin pregnancies with an overall prevalence of 1–3/10,000 pregnancies. The condition originates from an imbalance of placental flow due to abnormal placental vascular connections between the twins. The recipient of the transplacental shunt is exposed to significantly increased preload and afterload due to hypervolemia and arterial hypertension leading to progressive ventricular hypertrophy, diastolic dysfunction, and HF. The five-stage Quintero system based on ultrasound findings is the most common nomenclature to describe the severity of TTTS in the recipient twin [77]. Quintero stage III is defined by the appearance of abnormal Doppler flow waveforms of the UV, UA, and DV secondary to cardiac dysfunction and stage IV by fetal hydrops of one or both twins. The natural history of advanced TTTS ≥III is bleak, with a reported perinatal loss rate of 70%–100% [78]. Laser or radiofrequency ablation of the intertwin anastomosis has become the treatment of choice to reverse HF and fetal hydrops in the recipient twin [56,79,80]. Unfortunately, laser-treated TTTS remains associated with a significant perinatal mortality of 30%–50% and a 5%–20% chance of long-term neurologic handicap [78].

Vascular Tumors and Twin Reversed Arterial Perfusion

Vascular fetal or placental tumors such as sacrococcygeal teratomas, cavernous hemangiomas, or chorioangiomas are rare. The masses can function as large arteriovenous anastomoses, leading to high-output HF and death [59,60,81]. A similar situation is encountered in the twin reversed arterial perfusion (TRAP) sequence whereby a healthy fetus perfuses a malformed, acardiac sibling. TRAP sequence occurs in 1% of monochorionic twin pregnancies. The typical echocardiographic findings [82] of the pump twin include preserved cardiac function despite the increased CO, cardiomegaly, and a widely dilated inferior vena cava, draining the blood from the vascularized mass to the heart. In more advanced disease states, however, HF develops, leading to polyhydramnios, hydrops, and placentomegaly. Close surveillance for signs of fast tumor growth and cardiac decompensation is warranted as this predicts a worse fetal outcome [82,83]. In the presence of fetal circulatory failure, delivery should be considered. If the fetus is not viable, in-utero therapy may be the only option aiming at interrupting the blood flow to the vascularized mass. In TRAP, this can be done by radiofrequency ablation of the vessels entering the acardiac fetus or occlusion of its umbilical cord, which results in survival of the pump twin in 80%–92% [84,85]. Prenatal treatment options for sacrococcygeal teratomas include open fetal surgery to remove the tumor or closed invasive procedures to occlude the vascular supply to the tumor with laser, radiofrequency, sclerotherapy, cautery, or vascular coiling. A multicenter review [59] found 32 cases, 20 of which were hydropic that underwent a closed invasive procedure. Perinatal survival was 44% overall, 30% in fetuses with HF and 67% in those without. Prematurity was common (mean age at delivery: 29.7 gestational weeks) and mostly due to premature rupture of membranes. Additionally, 12 fetuses were identified in this review that underwent open fetal surgery, including 11 with hydrops. Perinatal survival was 50%, and prematurity again was common (mean age: 29.8 weeks).

Congenital Heart Disease With Severe Atrioventricular Valvar Regurgitation

CHD with valvar regurgitation results in an increased ventricular preload. This typically does not lead to cardiac decompensation unless both ventricles are dysfunctional. Critical aortic stenosis with severe mitral regurgitation and closed atrial septum may result in low CO and fetal hydrops likely due to RV compression by the massively dilated left heart [86].

To decompress the RV, options as salvage rescue therapy may include fetal aortic valvuloplasty to improve aortic forward flow thus reducing the amount of mitral regurgitation and the LV size [86,87].

Agenesis of the Ductus Venosus

Congenital absence of the DV is most commonly associated with aberrant extrahepatic drainage of the UV into an internal iliac vein, the inferior vena cava, or directly into the heart. Since the liver is entirely bypassed, the umbilical venous blood flow to the heart becomes "unrestricted," which occasionally results in high-output HF and demise [88].

Constriction of the Ductus Arteriosus

Acute in-utero constriction of the arterial duct usually in late gestation may occur due to the ingestion of nonsteroidal medication or a diet rich in polyphenols [89,90]. In a retrospective single center experience [91] of 45 fetuses with ductal constriction (n=41) or closure (n=4), RV dilatation was present in 82%, tricuspid insufficiency in 87%, and HF in 22%. Removal of the inciting agent usually reversed the constriction but neonatal pulmonary hypertension occurred in 18%. Late follow-up showed all 43 survivors alive and healthy with only two deaths from unrelated causes.

Fetal Anemia

Fetal anemia caused by parvovirus infection or a hemoglobinopathy such as α-thalassemia may lead to hyperdynamic circulation that attempts to recirculate the available hemoglobin more rapidly to maintain adequate tissue perfusion. This, in combination with less viscous blood due to the lack of erythrocytes, leads to increased SF% and higher blood flow peak velocities unless the anemia is severe enough to lead to myocardial ischemia and low output. Doppler assessment of the middle cerebral artery peak velocity is helpful to determine the severity of the anemia [26]. Cardiac dysfunction and hydrops secondary to fetal anemia can be treated with single or repeated fetal blood transfusions through the UV [92].

Brady- and Tachyarrhythmias

Fetal arrhythmias that present with sustained slow (<45 bpm) or fast (>200 bpm) ventricular rates are common causes of fetal venous congestion and low output failure. The need and choice of in-utero therapy depends on the arrhythmia mechanism, the hemodynamic consequences, and the gestational age of the fetus as well as the potential risk of the mother and her baby from the fetal therapy when compared to a premature surgical delivery.

For tachyarrhythmia, including supraventricular tachycardia (SVT) and atrial flutter (AF) as the most common conditions, the primary aim of prenatal treatment is cardioversion to a normal rhythm or, if this is not achievable, to slow the tachycardia to a near normal rate to improve cardiac dysfunction and to allow resolution of hydrops. Transplacental antiarrhythmic medication is available to treat all forms of the fetal tachyarrhythmia although there may be differences in efficacy among agents. A recent review found that fetal SVT may be best treated with digoxin or flecainide, while sotalol appeared superior to control AF [55]. Moreover, digoxin and flecainide had the best effect on decreasing the tachycardia rate if cardioversion was not obtained within 5 days of treatment. SVT and AF associated with fetal hydrops carries a 20%–30% risk of in-utero mortality. To achieve more rapid cardioversion to a normal rhythm, primary treatment with two antiarrhythmic agents or direct fetal therapy as rescue therapy via intramuscular, intravascular, intraperitoneal, or intracardiac route should be considered [93,94].

Fetal sinus tachycardia resulting in HF has been described in the presence of fetal hyperthyroidism from maternal Graves' disease and elevated thyroid stimulating hormone. Maternal treatment with propylthiouracil and β-blocker therapy may be used to control the fetal thyrotoxicosis, to lower the fetal heart rate, and to improve heart function [95].

Fetal bradycardia due to anti-Ro antibody-mediated CHB may be treated with dexamethasone and a β-sympathomimetic agent to minimize myocardial damage, improve CO, and thus improve the chances of survival [57]. Maternal β-agonists including terbutaline and salbutamol have been used to increase the fetal heart rate, decrease systemic resistance, and improve cardiac function [96,97]. One study showed that CHB with ventricular rates <50 bpm responded to high-dose salbutamol (10 mg q8) or terbutaline (2.5–7.5 mg q6) with a heart rate increase up to 5–10 bpm [98]. CHB in association with left atrial isomerism usually results in progressive HF and intrauterine demise, while the prognosis is better with congenital corrected transposition. Treatment with β-agonists to improve the outcome of left isomerism complicated by CHB has been largely ineffective [99,100].

Effusions and Space Occupying Lesions

Intrathoracic effusions and masses such as large *congenital cystic adenomatoid malformations of the lung (CCAMs)* can extrinsically compress the heart, restrict ventricular filling, and decrease the venous return to the heart. This may lead to a lower CO, venous congestion, and hydrops. Cardiac tamponade from a large pericardial effusion occurs most commonly in the presence of a pericardial teratoma. Pericardiocentesis, insertion of pericardio-amniotic shunts, and fetal surgery have been attempted as salvage procedures. A review of the literature found 31 cases with pericardial tumors (77% with hydrops), of which 11 underwent pericardial drainage [101]. Of 9 fetal survivors, 7 had hydrops at delivery. Fetal surgery to remove a pericardial tumor in the presence of severe hydrops has also been described [102]. Though the surgery was considered successful, the hydrops did not resolve and the baby did not survive.

The most common chest mass affecting cardiac function is a CCAM. Measurement of the CCAM volume to head circumference ratio (CVR) has been used to quantify the size of the mass and to predict the need for perinatal therapy [103,104]. A CVR >1.6 or masses containing large cysts are considered highest risk [103]. Growth of CCAMs typically occurs during midgestation. After 32 weeks, delivery is usually recommended. If there is hydrops, an EXIT (ex-utero intrapartum treatment) procedure may allow stabilization of the newborn prior to surgery [105]. There has also been success using maternal betamethasone: survival was improved when used in cases with a CVR >1.6, despite no significant change in the size of the tumor [106]. Prior to 32 weeks, intervention to treat HF may include a thoracoamniotic shunt or open fetal surgery to debulk the mass [107,108].

CONCLUSION

Fetal HF is an important cause of intrauterine and postnatal morbidity and mortality. Echocardiography is the modality of choice to noninvasively detect systolic and, even more importantly, diastolic dysfunction, to quantify the severity of fetal HF, and to determine or exclude possible etiologies. Significant advances have been made in the management of some causes of cardiac failure over the last decades. This includes blood transfusions for fetal anemia, antiarrhythmic drug therapy for SVT and AF, antiinflammatory treatment for antibody-mediated myocarditis or CM, and in-utero interventions for TTTS and parasitic masses. For many other conditions efficient in-utero treatment of fetal HF remains unavailable. In this situation, close surveillance of the fetal state with early delivery for postnatal HF management may be the only chance of survival for the hemodynamically compromised fetus.

REFERENCES

[1] T. Romero, J. Covell, W.F. Friedman, A comparison of pressure-volume relations of the fetal, newborn, and adult heart, Am. J. Physiol. 222 (5) (1972) 1285–1290.

[2] R.D. Gilbert, Control of fetal cardiac output during changes in blood volume, Am. J. Physiol. 238 (1) (1980) H80–H86.

[3] W.F. Friedman, The intrinsic physiologic properties of the developing heart, Prog. Cardiovasc. Dis. 15 (1) (1972) 87–111.

[4] J. Rychik, Fetal cardiovascular physiology, Pediatr. Cardiol. 25 (3) (2004) 201–209.

[5] A.M. Rudolph, M.A. Heymann, Cardiac output in the fetal lamb: the effects of spontaneous and induced changes of heart rate on right and left ventricular output, Am. J. Obstet. Gynecol. 124 (2) (1976) 183–192.

[6] M.D. Reller, M.J. Morton, D.L. Reid, K.L. Thornburg, Fetal lamb ventricles respond differently to filling and arterial pressures and to in utero ventilation, Pediatr. Res. 22 (6) (1987) 621–626.

[7] P.P. Sengupta, J. Korinek, M. Belohlavek, J. Narula, M.A. Vannan, A. Jahangir, et al., Left ventricular structure and function: basic science for cardiac imaging, J. Am. Coll. Cardiol. 48 (10) (2006) 1988–2001.

[8] F. Sheehan, A. Redington, The right ventricle: anatomy, physiology and clinical imaging, Heart 94 (11) (2008) 1510–1515.

[9] J.C. Huhta, Right ventricular function in the human fetus, J. Perinat. Med. 29 (5) (2001) 381–389.

[10] J. Rasanen, R.H. Debbs, D.C. Wood, S. Weiner, S.R. Weil, J.C. Huhta, Human fetal right ventricular ejection force under abnormal loading conditions during the second half of pregnancy, Ultrasound Obstet. Gynecol. 10 (5) (1997) 325–332.

[11] M. Prsa, L. Sun, J. van Amerom, S.J. Yoo, L. Grosse-Wortmann, E. Jaeggi, et al., Reference ranges of blood flow in the major vessels of the normal human fetal circulation at term by phase-contrast magnetic resonance imaging, Circ. Cardiovasc. Imaging 7 (4) (2014) 663–670.

[12] M. Tchirikov, C. Rybakowski, B. Huneke, H.J. Schroder, Blood flow through the ductus venosus in singleton and multifetal pregnancies and in fetuses with intrauterine growth retardation, Am. J. Obstet. Gynecol. 178 (5) (1998) 943–949.

[13] T. Kiserud, S.H. Eik-Nes, H.G. Blaas, L.R. Hellevik, Ultrasonographic velocimetry of the fetal ductus venosus, Lancet 338 (8780) (1991) 1412–1414.

[14] T. Kiserud, S. Rasmussen, S. Skulstad, Blood flow and the degree of shunting through the ductus venosus in the human fetus, Am. J. Obstet. Gynecol. 182 (1 Pt 1) (2000) 147–153.

[15] D.I. Edelstone, A.M. Rudolph, Preferential streaming of ductus venosus blood to the brain and heart in fetal lambs, Am. J. Physiol. 237 (6) (1979) H724–H729.

[16] M. Van Lierde, D. Oberweis, K. Thomas, Ultrasonic measurement of aortic and umbilical blood flow in the human fetus, Obstet. Gynecol. 63 (6) (1984) 801–805.

[17] M.G. Sutton, T. Plappert, P. Doubilet, Relationship between placental blood flow and combined ventricular output with gestational age in normal human fetus, Cardiovasc. Res. 25 (7) (1991) 603–608.

[18] J.C. Fouron, M. Zarelli, P. Drblik, M. Lessard, Flow velocity profile of the fetal aortic isthmus through normal gestation, Am. J. Cardiol. 74 (5) (1994) 483–486.

[19] S.E. Sonesson, J.C. Fouron, Doppler velocimetry of the aortic isthmus in human fetuses with abnormal velocity waveforms in the umbilical artery, Ultrasound Obstet. Gynecol. 10 (2) (1997) 107–111.

[20] M.T. Donofrio, Y.A. Bremer, R.M. Schieken, C. Gennings, L.D. Morton, B.W. Eidem, et al., Autoregulation of cerebral blood flow in fetuses with congenital heart disease: the brain sparing effect, Pediatr. Cardiol. 24 (5) (2003) 436–443.

[21] K. Makikallio, P. Jouppila, J. Rasanen, Retrograde net blood flow in the aortic isthmus in relation to human fetal arterial and venous circulations, Ultrasound Obstet. Gynecol. 19 (2) (2002) 147–152.

[22] A. Szwast, Z. Tian, M. McCann, D. Donaghue, J. Rychik, Right ventricular performance in the fetus with hypoplastic left heart syndrome, Ann. Thorac. Surg. 87 (4) (2009) 1214–1219.

[23] L. Sun, C.K. Macgowan, J.G. Sled, S.J. Yoo, C. Manlhiot, P. Porayette, et al., Reduced fetal cerebral oxygen consumption is associated with smaller brain size in fetuses with congenital heart disease, Circulation 131 (15) (2015) 1313–1323.

[24] S.P. Miller, P.S. McQuillen, S. Hamrick, D. Xu, D.V. Glidden, N. Charlton, et al., Abnormal brain development in newborns with congenital heart disease, N. Engl. J. Med 357 (19) (2007) 1928–1938.

[25] C. Limperopoulos, W. Tworetzky, D.B. McElhinney, J.W. Newburger, D.W. Brown, R.L. Robertson Jr., et al., Brain volume and metabolism in fetuses with congenital heart disease: evaluation with quantitative magnetic resonance imaging and spectroscopy, Circulation 121 (1) (2010) 26–33.

[26] G. Mari, R.L. Deter, R.L. Carpenter, F. Rahman, R. Zimmerman, K.J. Moise Jr., et al., Noninvasive diagnosis by doppler ultrasonography of fetal anemia due to maternal red-cell alloimmunization. Collaborative Group for Doppler Assessment of the Blood Velocity in Anemic Fetuses, N. Engl. J. Med. 342 (1) (2000) 9–14.

[27] D. Mahieu-Caputo, M. Dommergues, A.L. Delezoide, M. Lacoste, Y. Cai, F. Narcy, et al., Twin-to-twin transfusion syndrome. Role of the fetal renin-angiotensin system, Am. J. Pathol. 156 (2) (2000) 629–636.

[28] H.M. Gardiner, Response of the fetal heart to changes in load: from hyperplasia to heart failure, Heart 91 (7) (2005) 871–873.

[29] A. Rudolph, Congenital Diseases of the Heart: Clinical-Physiological Considerations, third ed., Wiley-Blackwell, 2009.

[30] G.A. Machin, Hydrops revisited: literature review of 1,414 cases published in the 1980s, Am. J. Med. Genet. 34 (3) (1989) 366–390.

[31] C.S. Kleinman, R.L. Donnerstein, G.R. DeVore, C.C. Jaffe, D.C. Lynch, R.L. Berkowitz, et al., Fetal echocardiography for evaluation of in utero congestive heart failure, N. Engl. J. Med. 306 (10) (1982) 568–575.

[32] L.D. Allan, M.C. Joseph, E.G. Boyd, S. Campbell, M. Tynan, M-mode echocardiography in the developing human fetus, Br. Heart J. 47 (6) (1982) 573–583.

[33] L.K. Hornberger, D.J. Sahn, C.S. Kleinman, J.A. Copel, K.L. Reed, Tricuspid valve disease with significant tricuspid insufficiency in the fetus: diagnosis and outcome, J. Am. Coll. Cardiol. 17 (1) (1991) 167–173.

[34] K. Hecher, Y. Ville, R. Snijders, K. Nicolaides, Doppler studies of the fetal circulation in twin-twin transfusion syndrome, Ultrasound Obstet. Gynecol. 5 (5) (1995) 318–324.

[35] G. Mielke, N. Benda, Cardiac output and central distribution of blood flow in the human fetus, Circulation 103 (12) (2001) 1662–1668.

[36] J.C. Huhta, J.J. Paul, Doppler in fetal heart failure, Clin. Obstet. Gynecol. 53 (4) (2010) 915–929.

[37] K.G. Schmidt, N.H. Silverman, M.R. Harison, P.W. Callen, High-output cardiac failure in fetuses with large sacrococcygeal teratoma: diagnosis by echocardiography and Doppler ultrasound, J. Pediatr. 114 (6) (1989) 1023–1028.

[38] D.N. Alter, K.L. Reed, G.R. Marx, C.F. Anderson, L. Shenker, Prenatal diagnosis of congestive heart failure in a fetus with a sacrococcygeal teratoma, Obstet. Gynecol. 71 (6 Pt 2) (1988) 978–981.

[39] D. Oepkes, R. Devlieger, E. Lopriore, F.J. Klumper, Successful ultrasound-guided laser treatment of fetal hydrops caused by pulmonary sequestration, Ultrasound Obstet. Gynecol. 29 (4) (2007) 457–459.

[40] A. Sau, G. Sharland, J. Simpson, Agenesis of the ductus venosus associated with direct umbilical venous return into the heart–case series and review of literature, Prenat. Diagn. 24 (6) (2004) 418–423.

[41] R.F. Lamont, J.D. Sobel, E. Vaisbuch, J.P. Kusanovic, S. Mazaki-Tovi, S.K. Kim, et al., Parvovirus B19 infection in human pregnancy, BJOG 118 (2) (2011) 175–186.

[42] K.L. Reed, D.J. Sahn, S. Scagnelli, C.F. Anderson, L. Shenker, Doppler echocardiographic studies of diastolic function in the human fetal heart: changes during gestation, J. Am. Coll. Cardiol. 8 (2) (1986) 391–395.

[43] A.M. Carceller-Blanchard, J.C. Fouron, Determinants of the Doppler flow velocity profile through the mitral valve of the human fetus, Br. Heart J. 70 (5) (1993) 457–460.

[44] T. Van Mieghem, L. Gucciardo, E. Done, D. Van Schoubroeck, E.M. Graatsma, G.H. Visser, et al., Left ventricular cardiac function in fetuses with congenital diaphragmatic hernia and the effect of fetal endoscopic tracheal occlusion, Ultrasound Obstet. Gynecol. 34 (4) (2009) 424–429.

[45] G. Tulzer, P. Khowsathit, S. Gudmundsson, D.C. Wood, Z.Y. Tian, K. Schmitt, et al., Diastolic function of the fetal heart during second and third trimester: a prospective longitudinal Doppler-echocardiographic study, Eur. J. Pediatr. 153 (3) (1994) 151–154.

[46] R. Axt-Fliedner, S. Diler, T. Georg, M. Friedrich, K. Diedrich, Reference values of ductus venosus blood flow velocities and waveform indices from 10 to 20 weeks of gestation, Arch. Gynecol. Obstet. 269 (3) (2004) 199–204.

[47] J.C. Huhta, Fetal congestive heart failure, Semin. Fetal Neonat. Med. 10 (6) (2005) 542–552.

[48] B.W. Eidem, J.M. Edwards, F. Cetta, Quantitative assessment of fetal ventricular function: establishing normal values of the myocardial performance index in the fetus, Echocardiography 18 (1) (2001) 9–13.
[49] C. Hofstaetter, M. Hansmann, S.H. Eik-Nes, J.C. Huhta, S.L. Luther, A cardiovascular profile score in the surveillance of fetal hydrops, J. Matern. Fetal Neonat. Med. 19 (7) (2006) 407–413.
[50] A. Wieczorek, J. Hernandez-Robles, L. Ewing, J. Leshko, S. Luther, J. Huhta, Prediction of outcome of fetal congenital heart disease using a cardiovascular profile score, Ultrasound Obstet. Gynecol. 31 (3) (2008) 284–288.
[51] R. Weber, P. Kantor, D. Chitayat, M.K. Friedberg, F. Golding, L. Mertens, et al., Spectrum and outcome of primary cardiomyopathies diagnosed during fetal life, JACC Heart Fail. 2 (4) (2014) 403–411.
[52] S.R. Pedra, J.F. Smallhorn, G. Ryan, D. Chitayat, G.P. Taylor, R. Khan, et al., Fetal cardiomyopathies: pathogenic mechanisms, hemodynamic findings, and clinical outcome, Circulation 106 (5) (2002) 585–591.
[53] A. Arunamata, R. Punn, B. Cuneo, S. Bharati, N.H. Silverman, Echocardiographic diagnosis and prognosis of fetal left ventricular noncompaction, J. Am. Soc. Echocardiogr. 25 (1) (2012) 112–120.
[54] S.R. Deshpande, D.A. Fyfe, Aorto-right atrial tunnel: fetal heart failure, diagnosis, and treatment, Pediatr. Cardiol. 31 (2) (2010) 299–300.
[55] E.T. Jaeggi, J.S. Carvalho, E. De Groot, O. Api, S.A. Clur, L. Rammeloo, et al., Comparison of transplacental treatment of fetal supraventricular tachyarrhythmias with digoxin, flecainide, and sotalol: results of a nonrandomized multicenter study, Circulation 124 (16) (2011) 1747–1754.
[56] M.V. Senat, J. Deprest, M. Boulvain, A. Paupe, N. Winer, Y. Ville, Endoscopic laser surgery versus serial amnioreduction for severe twin-to-twin transfusion syndrome, N. Engl. J. Med. 351 (2) (2004) 136–144.
[57] E.T. Jaeggi, J.C. Fouron, E.D. Silverman, G. Ryan, J. Smallhorn, L.K. Hornberger, Transplacental fetal treatment improves the outcome of prenatally diagnosed complete atrioventricular block without structural heart disease, Circulation 110 (12) (2004) 1542–1548.
[58] F. Alkazaleh, M. Saleem, E. Badran, Intrathoracic displacement of pleuroamniotic shunt after successful in utero treatment of fetal hydrops secondary to hydrothorax. Case report and review of the literature, Fetal Diagn. Ther. 25 (1) (2009) 40–43.
[59] T. Van Mieghem, A. Al-Ibrahim, J. Deprest, L. Lewi, J.C. Langer, D. Baud, et al., Minimally invasive therapy for fetal sacrococcygeal teratoma: case series and systematic review of the literature, Ultrasound Obstet. Gynecol. 43 (6) (2014) 611–619.
[60] D. Baud, R. Windrim, J.R. Kachura, A. Jefferies, S. Pantazi, P. Shah, et al., Minimally invasive fetal therapy for hydropic lung masses: three different approaches and review of the literature, Ultrasound Obstet. Gynecol. 42 (4) (2013) 440–448.
[61] J.M. Faure, P.L. Giacalone, F. Deschamps, P. Boulot, Nonimmune hydrops fetalis caused by intrauterine human parvovirus B19 infection: a case of spontaneous reversal in utero, Fetal Diagn. Ther. 12 (2) (1997) 66–67.
[62] J.A. Towbin, L.D. Griffin, A.B. Martin, S. Nelson, B. Siu, N.A. Ayres, et al., Intrauterine adenoviral myocarditis presenting as nonimmune hydrops fetalis: diagnosis by polymerase chain reaction, Pediatr. Infect. Dis. J. 13 (2) (1994) 144–150.
[63] A. Bonnin, M. Tassin, C. Vauloup-Fellous, E. Letamendia, B. Stos, D. Bonnet, et al., Case of a healthy infant born following antenatal enterovirus myocarditis and hydrops, J. Clin. Virol. 61 (3) (2014) 459–462.
[64] J.F. Modlin, Perinatal echovirus and group B coxsackievirus infections, Clin. Perinat. 15 (2) (1988) 233–246.
[65] C.P. Barnett, E. Jaeggi, R.K. Han, O. Nevo, S. Keating, P. Shannon, et al., Unusual cardiac presentation of congenital cytomegalovirus infection, Ultrasound Obstet. Gynecol. 35 (1) (2010) 119–120.
[66] C.S. von Kaisenberg, G. Bender, J. Scheewe, S.W. Hirt, M. Lange, J. Stieh, et al., A case of fetal parvovirus B19 myocarditis, terminal cardiac heart failure, and perinatal heart transplantation, Fetal Diagn. Ther. 16 (6) (2001) 427–432.
[67] E. Jaeggi, C. Laskin, R. Hamilton, J. Kingdom, E. Silverman, The importance of the level of maternal anti-Ro/SSA antibodies as a prognostic marker of the development of cardiac neonatal lupus erythematosus a prospective study of 186 antibody-exposed fetuses and infants, J. Am. Coll. Cardiol. 55 (24) (2010) 2778–2784.
[68] S. Saleeb, J. Copel, D. Friedman, J.P. Buyon, Comparison of treatment with fluorinated glucocorticoids to the natural history of autoantibody-associated congenital heart block: retrospective review of the research registry for neonatal lupus, Arthritis Rheum. 42 (11) (1999) 2335–2345.
[69] A. Arola, E. Jokinen, O. Ruuskanen, M. Saraste, E. Pesonen, A.L. Kuusela, et al., Epidemiology of idiopathic cardiomyopathies in children and adolescents. A nationwide study in Finland, Am. J. Epidemiol. 146 (5) (1997) 385–393.
[70] A.W. Nugent, P.E. Daubeney, P. Chondros, J.B. Carlin, M. Cheung, L.C. Wilkinson, et al., The epidemiology of childhood cardiomyopathy in Australia, N. Engl. J. Med 348 (17) (2003) 1639–1646.
[71] S.E. Lipshultz, L.A. Sleeper, J.A. Towbin, A.M. Lowe, E.J. Orav, G.F. Cox, et al., The incidence of pediatric cardiomyopathy in two regions of the United States, N. Engl. J. Med 348 (17) (2003) 1647–1655.
[72] S.M. Trucco, E. Jaeggi, B. Cuneo, A.J. Moon-Grady, E. Silverman, N. Silverman, et al., Use of intravenous gamma globulin and corticosteroids in the treatment of maternal autoantibody-mediated cardiomyopathy, J. Am. Coll. Cardiol. 57 (6) (2011) 715–723.
[73] S. Turan, O.M. Turan, J. Miller, C. Harman, E.A. Reece, A.A. Baschat, Decreased fetal cardiac performance in the first trimester correlates with hyperglycemia in pregestational maternal diabetes, Ultrasound Obstet. Gynecol. 38 (3) (2011) 325–331.
[74] B.H. Arzuaga, A. Groner, Utilization of extracorporeal membrane oxygenation in congenital hypertrophic cardiomyopathy caused by maternal diabetes, J. Neonat. Perinat. Med. 6 (4) (2013) 345–348.
[75] J.F. Goldberg, C.M. Mery, P.S. Griffiths, D.R. Parekh, S.E. Welty, R.A. Bronicki, et al., Extracorporeal membrane oxygenation support in severe hypertrophic obstructive cardiomyopathy associated with persistent pulmonary hypertension in an infant of a diabetic mother, Circulation 130 (21) (2014) 1923–1925.
[76] M.G. Sardesai, A.A. Gray, M.M. McGrath, S.E. Ford, Fatal hypertrophic cardiomyopathy in the fetus of a woman with diabetes, Obstet. Gynecol. 98 (5 Pt 2) (2001) 925–927.

[77] R.A. Quintero, W.J. Morales, M.H. Allen, P.W. Bornick, P.K. Johnson, M. Kruger, Staging of twin-twin transfusion syndrome, J. Perinatol. 19 (8 Pt 1) (1999) 550–555.

[78] Society for Maternal-Fetal Medicine, L.L. Simpson, Twin-twin transfusion syndrome, Am. J. Obstet. Gynecol. 208 (1) (2013) 3–18.

[79] R.H. Chmait, E.V. Kontopoulos, L.M. Korst, A. Llanes, I. Petisco, R.A. Quintero, Stage-based outcomes of 682 consecutive cases of twin-twin transfusion syndrome treated with laser surgery: the USFetus experience, Am. J. Obstet. Gynecol. 204(5) (393) (2011) e1–6.

[80] T. Van Mieghem, A.M. Martin, R. Weber, C. Barrea, R. Windrim, L.K. Hornberger, et al., Fetal cardiac function in recipient twins undergoing fetoscopic laser ablation of placental anastomoses for Stage IV twin-twin transfusion syndrome, Ultrasound Obstet. Gynecol. 42 (1) (2013) 64–69.

[81] J. Ding, Q. Chen, P. Stone, Percutaneous laser photocoagulation of tumour vessels for the treatment of a rapidly growing sacrococcygeal teratoma in an extremely premature fetus, J. Matern. Fetal Neonat. Med. 23 (12) (2010) 1516–1518.

[82] F.A. Byrne, H. Lee, A.K. Kipps, M.M. Brook, A.J. Moon-Grady, Echocardiographic risk stratification of fetuses with sacrococcygeal teratoma and twin-reversed arterial perfusion, Fetal Diagn. Ther. 30 (4) (2011) 280–288.

[83] R.D. Wilson, H. Hedrick, A.W. Flake, M.P. Johnson, M.W. Bebbington, S. Mann, et al., Sacrococcygeal teratomas: prenatal surveillance, growth and pregnancy outcome, Fetal Diagn. Ther. 25 (1) (2009) 15–20.

[84] H. Lee, A.J. Wagner, E. Sy, R. Ball, V.A. Feldstein, R.B. Goldstein, et al., Efficacy of radiofrequency ablation for twin-reversed arterial perfusion sequence, Am. J. Obstet. Gynecol. 196 (5) (2007) 459.e1–459.e4.

[85] R.A. Quintero, R.H. Chmait, T. Murakoshi, Z. Pankrac, M. Swiatkowska, P.W. Bornick, et al., Surgical management of twin reversed arterial perfusion sequence, Am. J. Obstet. Gynecol. 194 (4) (2006) 982–991.

[86] M. Vogel, D.B. McElhinney, L.E. Wilkins-Haug, A.C. Marshall, C.B. Benson, A.L. Juraszek, et al., Aortic stenosis and severe mitral regurgitation in the fetus resulting in giant left atrium and hydrops: pathophysiology, outcomes, and preliminary experience with pre-natal cardiac intervention, J. Am. Coll. Cardiol. 57 (3) (2011) 348–355.

[87] W. Arzt, D. Wertaschnigg, I. Veit, F. Klement, R. Gitter, G. Tulzer, Intrauterine aortic valvuloplasty in fetuses with critical aortic stenosis: experience and results of 24 procedures, Ultrasound Obstet. Gynecol. 37 (6) (2011) 689–695.

[88] E.T. Jaeggi, J.C. Fouron, L.K. Hornberger, F. Proulx, I. Oberhansli, S.J. Yoo, et al., Agenesis of the ductus venosus that is associated with extrahepatic umbilical vein drainage: prenatal features and clinical outcome, Am. J. Obstet. Gynecol. 187 (4) (2002) 1031–1037.

[89] G. Koren, A. Florescu, A.M. Costei, R. Boskovic, M.E. Moretti, Nonsteroidal antiinflammatory drugs during third trimester and the risk of premature closure of the ductus arteriosus: a meta-analysis, Ann. Pharmacother. 40 (5) (2006) 824–829.

[90] P. Zielinsky, A.L. Piccoli Jr., I. Vian, A.M. Zilio, A.A. Naujorks, L.H. Nicoloso, et al., Maternal restriction of polyphenols and fetal ductal dynamics in normal pregnancy: an open clinical trial, Arq. Bras. Cardiol. 101 (3) (2013) 217–225.

[91] L.M. Lopes, M.C. Carrilho, R.P. Francisco, M.A. Lopes, V.L. Krebs, M. Zugaib, Fetal ductus arteriosus constriction and closure: analysis of the causes and perinatal outcome related to 45 consecutive cases, J. Matern. Fetal Neonat. Med. 29 (4) (2016) 638–645.

[92] A. Chauvet, A. Dewilde, D. Thomas, S. Joriot, P. Vaast, V. Houfflin-Debarge, et al., Ultrasound diagnosis, management and prognosis in a consecutive series of 27 cases of fetal hydrops following maternal parvovirus B19 infection, Fetal Diagn. Ther. 30 (1) (2011) 41–47.

[93] M. Hansmann, U. Gembruch, R. Bald, M. Manz, D.A. Redel, Fetal tachyarrhythmias: transplacental and direct treatment of the fetus-a report of 60 cases, Ultrasound Obstet. Gynecol. 1 (3) (1991) 162–168.

[94] B.V. Parilla, J.F. Strasburger, M.L. Socol, Fetal supraventricular tachycardia complicated by hydrops fetalis: a role for direct fetal intramuscular therapy, Am. J. Perinat. 13 (8) (1996) 483–486.

[95] T. Matsumoto, K. Miyakoshi, Y. Saisho, T. Ishii, S. Ikenoue, Y. Kasuga, et al., Antenatal management of recurrent fetal goitrous hyperthyroidism associated with fetal cardiac failure in a pregnant woman with persistent high levels of thyroid-stimulating hormone receptor antibody after ablative therapy, Endocr. J. 60 (12) (2013) 1281–1287.

[96] J. Finley, M. Katz, M. Rojas-Perez, J.M. Roberts, R.K. Creasy, N.B. Schiller, Cardiovascular consequences of beta-agonist tocolysis: an echocardiographic study, Obstet. Gynecol. 64 (6) (1984) 787–791.

[97] J. Rasanen, The effects of ritodrine infusion on fetal myocardial function and fetal hemodynamics, Acta Obstet. Gynecol. Scand. 69 (6) (1990) 487–492.

[98] B.F. Cuneo, H. Zhao, J.F. Strasburger, M. Ovadia, J.C. Huhta, R.T. Wakai, Atrial and ventricular rate response and patterns of heart rate acceleration during maternal-fetal terbutaline treatment of fetal complete heart block, Am. J. Cardiol. 100 (4) (2007) 661–665.

[99] E.T. Jaeggi, L.K. Hornberger, J.F. Smallhorn, J.C. Fouron, Prenatal diagnosis of complete atrioventricular block associated with structural heart disease: combined experience of two tertiary care centers and review of the literature, Ultrasound Obstet. Gynecol. 26 (1) (2005) 16–21.

[100] C. Berg, A. Geipel, T. Kohl, J. Breuer, U. Germer, M. Krapp, et al., Atrioventricular block detected in fetal life: associated anomalies and potential prognostic markers, Ultrasound Obstet. Gynecol. 26 (1) (2005) 4–15.

[101] R. Bader, L.K. Hornberger, L.J. Nijmeh, F. Al-Kazaleh, G. Ryan, A. Toi, et al., Fetal pericardial teratoma: presentation of two cases and review of literature, Am. J. Perinat. 23 (1) (2006) 53–58.

[102] R.M. Sydorak, T. Kelly, V.A. Feldstein, P.L. Sandberg, N.H. Silverman, M.R. Harrison, et al., Prenatal resection of a fetal pericardial teratoma, Fetal Diagn. Ther. 17 (5) (2002) 281–285.

[103] T.M. Crombleholme, B. Coleman, H. Hedrick, K. Liechty, L. Howell, A.W. Flake, et al., Cystic adenomatoid malformation volume ratio predicts outcome in prenatally diagnosed cystic adenomatoid malformation of the lung, J. Pediatr. Surg. 37 (3) (2002) 331–338.

[104] S. Ehrenberg-Buchner, A.M. Stapf, D.R. Berman, R.A. Drongowski, G.B. Mychaliska, M.C. Treadwell, et al., Fetal lung lesions: can we start to breathe easier? Am. J. Obstet. Gynecol. 208 (2) (2013) 151.e1–151.e7.

[105] H.L. Hedrick, A.W. Flake, T.M. Crombleholme, L.J. Howell, M.P. Johnson, R.D. Wilson, et al., The ex utero intrapartum therapy procedure for high-risk fetal lung lesions, J. Pediatr. Surg. 40 (6) (2005) 1038–1043.
[106] P.F. Curran, E.B. Jelin, L. Rand, S. Hirose, V.A. Feldstein, R.B. Goldstein, et al., Prenatal steroids for microcystic congenital cystic adenomatoid malformations, J. Pediatr. Surg. 45 (1) (2010) 145–150.
[107] S. Schrey, E.N. Kelly, J.C. Langer, G.A. Davies, R. Windrim, P.G. Seaward, et al., Fetal thoracoamniotic shunting for large macrocystic congenital cystic adenomatoid malformations of the lung, Ultrasound Obstet. Gynecol. 39 (5) (2012) 515–520.
[108] N.S. Adzick, Open fetal surgery for life-threatening fetal anomalies, Semin. Fetal Neonat. Med. 15 (1) (2010) 1–8.

Chapter 29

Heart Failure in the Neonate

Thomas D. Ryan[1], Steven J. Kindel[2], Matthew J. O'Connor[3]
[1]Cincinnati Children's Hospital Medical Center, Cincinnati, OH, United States; [2]Children's Hospital of Wisconsin, Milwaukee, WI, United States; [3]Children's Hospital of Philadelphia, Philadelphia, PA, United States

INTRODUCTION

Heart failure can most simply be defined as the clinical syndrome produced by the inability of the heart to meet the metabolic demands of the body. Etiologic, mechanistic, and symptomatic descriptions include systolic and/or diastolic dysfunction, ventricular volume and/or pressure overload, right ventricle (RV) and/or left ventricle (LV) failure, and low cardiac output and/or congestive symptoms. Hsu and Pearson elegantly described heart failure in the pediatric patient as "a progressive clinical and pathophysiological syndrome caused by cardiovascular and non-cardiovascular abnormalities that results in characteristic signs and symptoms including edema, respiratory distress, growth failure, and exercise intolerance, and accompanied by circulatory, neurohormonal, and molecular derangements" [1]. Neonatal patients represent a significant proportion of children diagnosed with heart failure. Their pathophysiology, diagnosis, and care are made more complex by the anatomic and physiologic changes that accompany transition from fetal to postnatal life.

EPIDEMIOLOGY AND ETIOLOGY OF HEART FAILURE IN THE NEONATE

While the incidence and impact of heart failure in adult patients is well defined, the epidemiology of pediatric, and particularly neonatal, heart failure has been more elusive. Recent analyses of two national inpatient databases from the United States have begun to analyze the issue. Webster et al. identified 5610 patients out of nearly 2 million hospital admissions in 1997 who were 18 years old or younger with a primary or secondary diagnosis of heart failure. Of those, 57% were infants (younger than 1 year old), with a diagnosis of congenital heart disease in 83% [2]. In a separate study utilizing the Healthcare Cost and Utilization Project Kids' Inpatient Database, Rossano, and Jefferies et al. reported an annual rate of 11,153–13,892 pediatric heart failure admissions from 1997 to 2006, of which 55%–64% were infants. Cardiomyopathy diagnosis accounted for 13%–15% and congenital heart disease 61%–69% in the cohort [3]. In both studies, the neonatal (less than 30 day) group was not further defined beyond that of infant. These data are limited only to patients in need of admission to the hospital and likely skew toward the critically ill and those with congenital heart disease.

Inherited Cardiomyopathy

Cardiomyopathy can be segregated by gross cardiac phenotype into five general classifications: dilated cardiomyopathy (DCM), hypertrophic cardiomyopathy (HCM), restrictive cardiomyopathy, arrhythmogenic ventricular cardiomyopathy, and left ventricular noncompaction cardiomyopathy (LVNC) (Fig. 29.1) [4]. Notably these morphologic categories may overlap and as such do not clearly define etiology. While all forms of cardiomyopathy may present in childhood or infancy, phenotypic restrictive, and arrhythmogenic cardiomyopathy are exceptionally rare in neonates and will not be discussed further in detail.

Data from four national cardiomyopathy registries have furthered our understanding of the incidence of these forms of heart disease. A retrospective review of Finnish national health records for patients less than 21 years old demonstrated an overall rate of 0.74 new cases per 100,000 children per year when including autopsy only diagnoses, and 0.65 new cases per 100,000/year when looking at clinical diagnoses; DCM and HCM occurred at nearly equal rates [5]. The Pediatric Cardiomyopathy Registry (PCMR) in the United States and National Australian Childhood Cardiomyopathy Study collected data prospectively and retrospectively, respectively. The overall incidence of discovered cardiomyopathy (with or without heart failure symptoms) was 1.13/100,000 in PCMR and 1.24/100,000 in the Australian study. These numbers were significantly higher for the neonatal group, at 8.34/100,000 and 7.84/100,000, respectively [6,7]. The distribution between the DCM and HCM phenotypes in PCMR was nearly even, at 0.57/100,000 and 0.47/100,000, however, in neonates DCM

Heart Failure in the Child and Young Adult. http://dx.doi.org/10.1016/B978-0-12-802393-8.00029-6

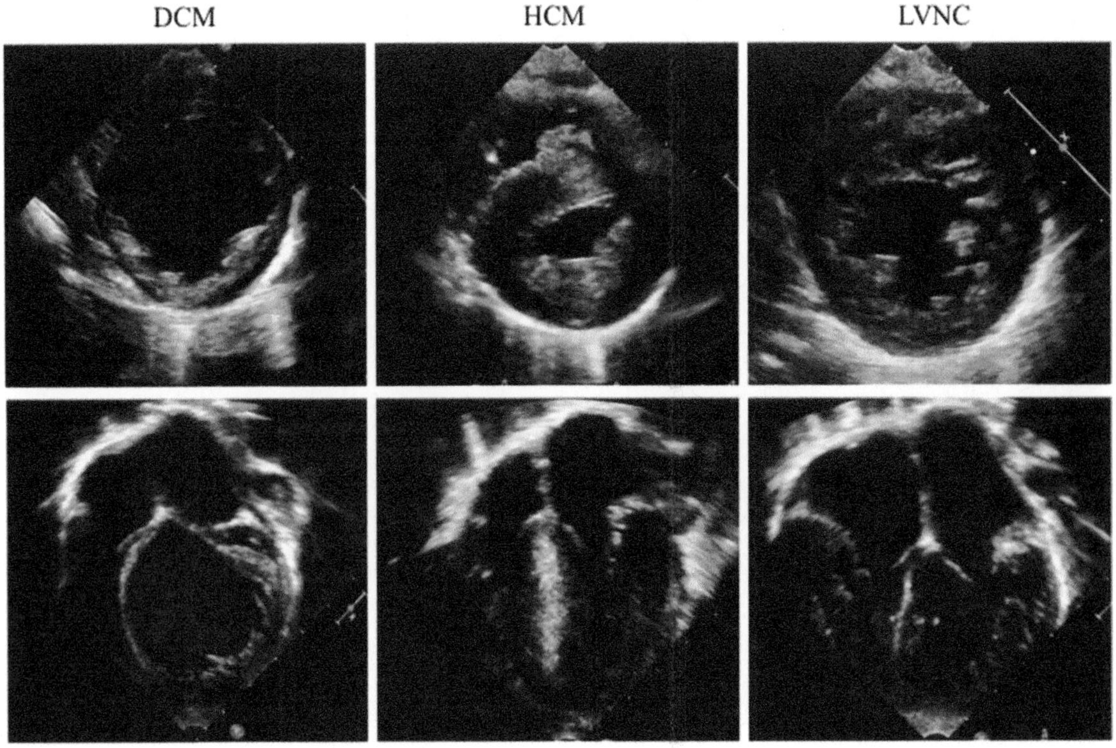

FIGURE 29.1 **Common presentations of congenital cardiomyopathy.** Still images from echocardiography in the parasternal short axis (top row) and inverted apical-four chamber (bottom row) views. Dilated cardiomyopathy (DCM) with a dilated left ventricular chamber and relatively thin walls. Hypertrophic cardiomyopathy (HCM) demonstrates increased left ventricular wall dimension and relatively small chamber diameter. Left ventricular noncompaction (LVNC) is notable for deep intertrabecular recesses.

was nearly 1.5 times more common at 4.4/100,000 [8,9]. Most recently data from 17 pediatric programs in the United Kingdom and Ireland were reported detailing children presenting with heart failure symptoms in the setting of cardiomyopathy. Seventy-seven percent of patients were diagnosed with DCM, with likely myocarditis representing nearly 25% of all diagnoses, familial DCM 7%, arrhythmogenic 7%, metabolic 4%, neuromuscular 2%, and the remainder idiopathic. Of these children, 48% were diagnosed in infancy. From these data the authors calculated an overall incidence of new onset heart failure from heart muscle disease at 0.87/100,000 children [10].

DCM is phenotypically described as the presence of a dilated LV chamber, relatively decreased LV wall thickness, and systolic and/or diastolic dysfunction (Fig. 29.1) [11–13]. In the PCMR data set, the most common age of presentation was less than 1 year old (41%), and 71% of all patients presented with symptomatic heart failure [6]. Although myocarditis was the most common cause of DCM reported in the PCMR, some question the accuracy of this rate as myocarditis is challenging to diagnose (particularly in infants where biopsy is rare) and the clinically available genetic testing at the time of the PCMR study was quite limited. In fact, data would suggest that up to 20% of children with newly diagnosed DCM have family members with positive genetic or clinical screening results [14,15]. Recently, familial DCM has been shown to occur in 30%–40% of cases with autosomal dominant inheritance being the predominant pattern of transmission although X-linked, autosomal recessive, and mitochondrial inheritance have all been reported [16]. Currently greater than 75 genes have been associated with DCM, the majority coding for either cytoskeletal or sarcomeric proteins. Metabolic and dysmorphic syndromes can also cause DCM, including Barth syndrome, which is an X-linked syndrome associated with short stature, cyclic neutropenia, and 3-methylglutaconic aciduria, and mitochondrial diseases such as Alstrom syndrome and Kearns–Sayre [15–18]. Neuromuscular diseases will frequently cause significant DCM, and while Duchenne and Becker muscular dystrophy rarely if ever affect infants, myofibrillar myopathy, eye–brain–muscle disease, and other rare neuromuscular diseases are reported in infants.

HCM is morphologically characterized by hypertrophy of the left (and occasionally right) ventricle with histologic features of myocyte hypertrophy, myofibrillar disarray, and interstitial fibrosis. Ventricular hypertrophy occurs most commonly in an asymmetric pattern, although in pediatric forms of disease concentric, apical, or multisegmental disease are all described (Fig. 29.1) [9,19,20]. In the PCMR cohort, survival was significantly lower in patients presenting as infants, and the vast majority of patients presented with congestive heart failure symptoms [9]. Molecular genetic studies provide insight into the pathogenesis of HCM with current studies demonstrating a genetic cause is responsible for half of presumed

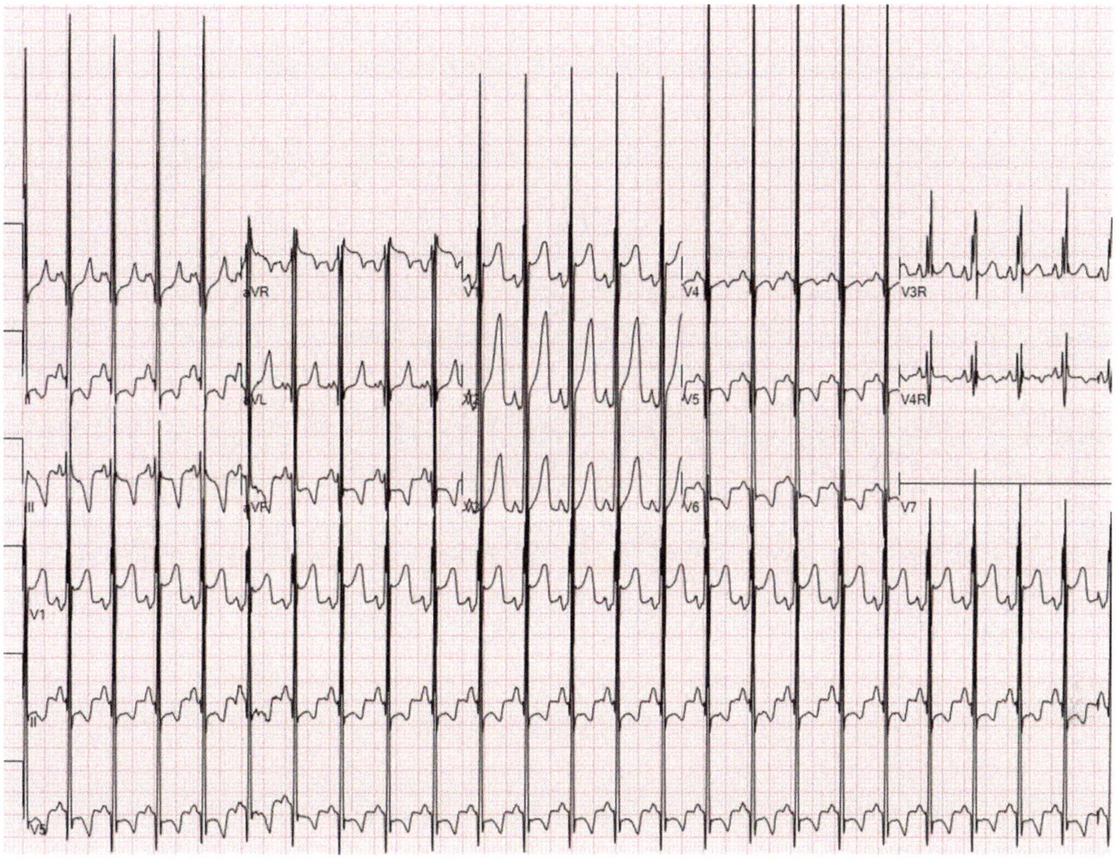

FIGURE 29.2 **Electrocardiogram in Pompe disease.** This neonatal study demonstrates biatrial enlargement and massive biventricular hypertrophy with strain. Study performed at full standard.

sporadic, and two-thirds of familial cases of pediatric HCM in both adults and older children [21,22]. The majority of the disease-causing genes identified to date code for proteins that are part of the sarcomere and are inherited in an autosomal dominant fashion. However, sporadic mutations are relatively common and genetic characterization has been somewhat challenged by high rates of novel mutations. While the vast majority of adult diagnoses of HCM relate to the sarcomeric form of the disease, pediatric HCM is more diverse with genetic-syndromic and metabolic abnormalities contributing up to 43% of diagnoses in one study [15]. Important nonsarcomeric causes in infants include glycogen storage disorders (GSD) (e.g., Pompe disease, Fig. 29.2), lysosomal storage disease (e.g., sialidosis and Fabry disease), disorders of the RAS-MAPK pathway (e.g., Noonan syndrome), and mitochondrial disorders.

Left ventricular noncompaction, also known as persistent fetal myocardium, is a genetically and clinically heterogeneous disorder that was classified as a distinct form of cardiomyopathy in 2006 [4]. The primary characteristics are the presence of prominent trabeculae, intertrabecular recesses, and thickening of the myocardium in two distinct layers composed of compacted and noncompacted tissue (Fig. 29.1) [23]. Pignatelli et al. reported median age at presentation of 90 days (range 1 day–17 years) [24]. In this study, 40% of the children presented with low cardiac output or congestive heart failure. In a single-center review, Brescia et al. found 25% mortality in infantile LVNC [25]. The typical modes of inheritance in pediatric LVNC are either autosomal dominant (70%) or X-linked recessive (30%) [26–28]. The first gene described as causative of isolated LVNC was TAZ, which is responsible for Barth syndrome [29]. Genetic determinants remain largely undiscovered but multiple publications have noted sarcomeric, cytoskeletal, and mitochondrial genes in patients with isolated LVNC.

ACQUIRED CARDIOMYOPATHIES

The identifiable etiologies of acquired cardiomyopathy in neonates are numerous and are similar to those encountered in older children. A proposed list of etiologies is presented in Table 29.1 and can be categorized as inflammatory, infectious, metabolic, toxic, vascular, and arrhythmia-induced, although overlap exists between categories. Determination of cause is of paramount importance, and in some cases may even be lifesaving, e.g., metabolic etiologies [30].

TABLE 29.1 Etiologies of Neonatal Heart Failure

Primary Cardiomyopathies	**Vascular**
Dilated cardiomyopathy	Extracardiac arteriovenous malformations
Hypertrophic cardiomyopathy	Congenital cutaneous hemangiomas
Left ventricular noncompaction cardiomyopathy	Hypertension
Restrictive cardiomyopathy	**Arrhythmia-Induced**
Arrhythmogenic right ventricular dysplasia	Supraventricular tachycardias
Inflammatory	Complete heart block
Myocarditis	**Congenital Heart Disease**
Rheumatic heart disease	Obstructive left heart lesions
Kawasaki disease	Aortic regurgitation
Small-vessel vasculitides	Mitral regurgitation
Infectious	Obstructed pulmonary venous return
Endocarditis	Overcirculation heart failure
Sepsis (viral, bacterial)	**Other**
Metabolic	Twin–twin transfusion syndrome
Disorders of fatty acid oxidation	Sacrococcygeal teratoma
Disorders of carnitine-dependent fatty acid transport	Myocardial ischemia
Disorders of mitochondrial metabolism	Perinatal hypoxemic-ischemic injury
Glycogen storage disorders (Pompe)	Coronary thrombosis
Mucopolysaccharidoses	Anomalous origin of the left coronary artery from the pulmonary artery
Mucolipidoses	Pulmonary hypertension
Infants of diabetic mothers	
Disorders of thyroid function	
Toxic	
Calcium-channel blockers	
Anthracycline chemotherapy	
Ionizing radiation	

Inflammatory and Infectious Cardiomyopathies

Myocarditis, defined as lymphocytic infiltration of the myocardium with associated myocyte damage [31], may affect the neonate either following transplacental infection during the third trimester or as a postnatally acquired disease. With transplacental acquisition, a maternal history of a nonspecific upper respiratory tract infection may be present. Common causative agents mirror those found in older children and adults including adenovirus, parvovirus, enterovirus, herpes virus, and cytomegalovirus infections among many others. Fulminant presentation with rapid clinical deterioration can mimic overwhelming sepsis and necessitate mechanical ventilator and/or circulatory support [32,33]. Clinically, the presence of a pericardial effusion or evidence of cardiac edema points toward the diagnosis and serum testing positive for the above viruses can indicate current or recent infection.

Rheumatic heart disease is a rare entity in developed countries, although sporadic outbreaks continue to occur. While rare in neonates, likely owing to the low level of infection with group A streptococci in this age-group, primary rheumatic heart disease should be considered in the differential diagnosis of a myocarditis-like clinical picture with valvular involvement in patients where the disease is endemic [34].

Kawasaki disease (KD) is a systemic inflammatory process manifesting as prolonged fever, rash, conjunctivitis, lymphadenopathy, and mucosal erythema, typically in children <5 years of age [35]. The etiologic agent of has yet to be identified. KD is less common in neonates and infants; when it manifests in children <6 months of age, it is referred to as atypical or incomplete and may manifest with fever alone [36]. The most prominent and concerning complication in children with KD is the development of coronary artery aneurysms, which may develop in ~25% of untreated patients. Even in the absence of coronary changes one can see an inflammatory myocarditis with significant deficits in systolic and/or diastolic function. Treatment entails supportive therapies, intravenous immunoglobulin administration, and antiplatelet medications [37,38].

Endocarditis is a cardiac infection of the heart lining (endocardium) and/or cardiac valves. Risk is significantly increased in hospital-bound neonates with indwelling central catheters, but overall incidence is low [39–42]. Endocarditis can lead to significant rapidly progressive valve disease or to a sepsis syndrome. In the latter the host response, including activation of the complement cascade and release of inflammatory cytokines, can manifest as low cardiac output syndrome. The focus of therapy is supportive while simultaneously treating the inciting organism [43].

Metabolic and Toxic Cardiomyopathies

Cardiomyopathies secondary to inborn errors of metabolism can present in neonates. Disorders in the oxidation of fatty acids or their transport within the myocyte frequently result in cardiac dysfunction [44]. A classic example of such a defect is very-long-chain acyl-coA dehydrogenase deficiency, in which neonates present with non- or hypoketotic hypoglycemia. Without a constant source of glucose, cardiac energy utilization is disrupted with consequent dysfunction and ultimately fatal hypoglycemia. Carnitine is a compound necessary for transport of fatty acids across the inner mitochondrial membrane; carnitine deficiency is another important and potentially treatable cause of metabolic cardiomyopathy. Until a diagnosis is established, some advocate carnitine supplementation for all neonates and infants with a suspected cardiomyopathy, although this remains controversial [45,46].

Disorders of mitochondrial metabolism can present with cardiomyopathy as a primary feature or as part of a constellation of multisystem disease. Cardiomyopathy in neonates may present in any form, but most common is HCM [24,47]. Barth syndrome (X-linked DCM/LVNC with cyclic neutropenia and skeletal myopathy) is held up as a classic example, however, many other disorders exist [48–50].

GSD also represent an important cause of neonatal cardiomyopathy. The infantile form of Pompe disease is the prototypical GSD with symptoms occurring early in life. Pompe disease results from decreased activity of α-1,4-glucosidase and manifests as cardiomegaly, HCM, macroglossia, and hypotonia (Fig. 29.2) [51,52]. Early consultation of a metabolic specialist is essential to aid in the prompt diagnosis as recombinant enzyme therapy is available for many patients [53,54].

To a variable degree, infants of diabetic mothers (IDM) can also be considered to have a metabolic cardiomyopathy, although the associated cardiomyopathy in IDM is a result of an adverse intrauterine environment rather than an intrinsically abnormal metabolic process. The natural history of cardiomyopathy in IDM has been well described and includes biventricular hypertrophy proportional to the severity of maternal hyperglycemia particularly late in pregnancy [55–57]. Many of these patients will see regression of the hypertrophy over several months and some case reports support the use of beta-blockade to promote reverse-remodeling and improve cardiac hemodynamics during recovery [58].

Toxic exposures are usually less of a concern in the neonate than older children; however, certain situations warrant comment. Neonatal myocardium is particularly sensitive to perturbations in calcium transport, with hypocalcemia frequently leading to clinically significant depression of cardiac contractility [59]. As such, administration of calcium-channel blockers, particularly nondihydroperidine class (e.g., verapamil) should be done with extreme caution. Chemotherapeutic agents, notably anthracycline agents, have a well-known cardiotoxicity profile that is dose-dependent, with toxicity typically developing months to years following exposure and more rarely in the acute phase of therapy [60]. However, acute and subacute toxicity can occur and studies have demonstrated that there is no "safe dose" that will avoid cardiac injury.

Arrhythmogenic Cardiomyopathies

Neonatal tachyarrhythmias and bradyarrhythmias may result in clinically important decreases in cardiac function [61]. The mechanisms by which arrhythmias perturb cardiac function are unknown, however, disruption of atrioventricular synchrony and loss of heart rate variability may be key [62]. In support of this theory, prolonged periods of sinus tachycardia alone typically do not result in ventricular dysfunction. Supraventricular tachycardias, including ectopic atrial tachycardias, orthodromic, or antidromic atrioventricular reentrant tachycardias, the permanent form of reciprocating junctional tachycardia and atrial flutter are the most commonly described neonatal arrhythmias associated with cardiac dilation and systolic dysfunction. When initiated in utero, and if sustained, incessant tachycardia can induce hydrops fetalis. The degree of ventricular dysfunction is proportional to the cumulative time spent in tachycardia and these arrhythmias may go unnoticed for extended periods of times such that at diagnosis the degree of ventricular dysfunction can be profound. In most cases, termination of the dysrhythmia results in normalization of ventricular function over a period of weeks to months [63]. Congenital complete heart block is often present as sequelae of transplacental passage of maternal anti-SSA (Sjögren's-syndrome-related antigen A) or anti-SSB (Sjögren's-syndrome-related antigen B) antibodies, or as an associated feature of certain complex congenital heart defects such as heterotaxy syndrome. Persistent heart block can induce ventricular dilation and dysfunction. Many patients will see recovery of function with atrioventricular sequential pacing [64].

Arteriovenous Malformations and Other Vascular Lesions

With large intracardiac left-to-right shunts, the LV may pump as much as three times its normal systemic output, which is achieved by increased heart rate and stroke volume. Ventricular dilation is initially adaptive to increase stroke volume, but eventually reaches an unfavorable point on the Frank–Starling curve, and decreases in cardiac contractility ensue. Extracardiac left-to-right shunts (e.g., patent ductus arteriosus or aortopulomary collaterals) share the same physiologic effects as their intracardiac counterparts. Arteriovenous malformations such as those seen in the liver or brain are extracardiac left-to-right shunts that may manifest as a cardiomyopathy and can present with physical findings of a loud continuous bruit over the liver or fontanelle, respectively [65,66].

Large congenital cutaneous hemangiomas do not impose a left-to-right shunt on the heart but may cause a "high-output" state by virtue of their demand for blood flow. Treatment is varied and may include corticosteroids, surgical excision, interventional radiology techniques, or propranolol [67].

Hypertension

Hypertension is a critically important, and underrecognized, cause of acquired cardiomyopathy in neonates [68–70]. In the fetal circulation the LV ejects mainly into the low-resistance cerebral circulation. Separation from the placenta and clamping of the umbilical cord at birth acutely increases afterload and transitions the LV to being the systemic ventricle, and thus early hypertension may not be well tolerated. Important extracardiac causes of hypertension in neonates include renal vein thrombosis, renal parenchymal vasculitis, and medications such as corticosteroids [71,72].

Other

Twin–twin transfusion syndrome includes abnormal and unbalanced vascular connections establishing a scenario in which one twin becomes a "donor" to the "recipient" twin. The donor twin becomes oligemic and exhibits oligohydramnios, while the recipient twin exhibits increases in preload and afterload that result in polyhydramnios and a predictable set of cardiovascular consequences [73]. The donor twin is frequently small, but with normal cardiac structure and function. The recipient twin, on the other hand, will often exhibit variable degrees of ventricular hypertrophy [74,75]. Regression after birth may occur, however, more recently fetal therapy with laser photocoagulation of the interplacental connections has shown success in resolving these cardiac abnormalities [76,77].

Acquired ischemic cardiomyopathy is rare in neonates; however, coronary artery thrombosis with associated regional ventricular dysfunction has been [78,79]. In the absence of preexisting risk factors such as indwelling central venous catheters, hematology consultation and investigation for inherited predisposition for thrombosis are warranted [80].

An important cause of RV dysfunction in neonates is pulmonary hypertension. Outside of its association with congenital diaphragmatic hernia, pulmonary hypertension in neonates and infants may be seen in two broad categories: persistent pulmonary hypertension of the newborn, which can be observed acutely in preterm or term infants; and pulmonary hypertension observed in the setting of chronic lung disease, which is a disease of premature infants [81].

CARDIOMYOPATHY IN CONGENITAL HEART DISEASE

The signs and symptoms of cardiomyopathy in the neonate can overlap with those of congenital heart disease. To better understand the etiology, it is helpful to consider whether the cause of symptoms is pump dysfunction, low cardiac output, or pulmonary overcirculation. Congenital heart disease may induce low cardiac output via obstructive lesions of left-sided heart structures (e.g., critical aortic stenosis, hypoplastic left heart syndrome, critical coarctation), regurgitant lesions (e.g., severe mitral or aortic regurgitation), or lesions with obstruction to pulmonary venous return and inadequate atrial level shunting.

While timing of discovery of these entities is variable, the persistence of a low cardiac output state will inevitably lead to poor oxygen delivery and metabolic acidosis. Often the patient appears clinically well prior to developing significant restriction or closure of the ductus arteriosus, at which point systemic blood flow is significantly compromised. Clinically these patients manifest shock with multisystem organ dysfunction, a clinical state with high morbidity and mortality that can present from hours to weeks following birth [82].

The term "heart failure" is widely applied to neonates and infants with large left-to-right shunt lesions that result in increased pulmonary blood flow including large ventricular septal defects, atrioventricular canal defects, truncus arteriosus, aortopulmonary window, and patent ductus arteriosus. In this setting the cardiac output is maintained and the symptomatology in these lesions is due to pulmonary overcirculation determined by the net shunt, which is in turn determined by the relative resistances between the pulmonary and systemic vascular beds. As the pulmonary vascular resistance falls within the first several weeks of life to normal adult levels, the degree of left-to-right shunt increases significantly. The LV is then ejecting several times its normal output, requiring the circulating blood volume to increase and the LV and atria to dilate. Volume expansion leads to hepatomegaly and pulmonary venous congestion, clinically manifested by tachypnea, tachycardia, intolerance of feeds, and poor weight gain. The American Heart Association has recently classified this condition as "overcirculation heart failure" to help distinguish it from the traditional definition of heart failure.

Anomalous origin of the left coronary artery from the pulmonary artery (ALCAPA) is an important but rare cause of ischemic cardiomyopathy in young infants. Correct establishment of this diagnosis in an infant with a dilated, dysfunctional LV is critical because corrective surgery is available with excellent short- and long-term results. The onset of symptoms typically occurs within the first 1–3 months of life, when the pulmonary vascular resistance drops and is manifested by irritability, poor feeding, and tachypnea. However, in some patients, sufficient collateralization may occur to mitigate or prevent early symptoms. The ECG will show ST segment abnormalities and prominent Q waves; the echocardiogram shows a dilated, dysfunctional LV, frequently with mitral regurgitation. Reimplantation of the left main coronary artery is the surgical treatment of choice, with excellent long-term results, although myocardial dysfunction and dilation may persist for several months postoperatively [83,84].

DIAGNOSTIC APPROACH

A careful history is essential in the evaluation of a neonate with a suspected diagnosis of cardiomyopathy. The birth and perinatal histories, as well as any need for resuscitation, should be examined in detail. The mother's prenatal history should be reviewed, with attention paid to any illnesses or toxic exposures, particularly during the last trimester of pregnancy. A family history, extending at least three generations if possible, is essential to screen for recessive genetic conditions. Deaths that are sudden, unexplained, or occurring under unusual circumstances should be ascertained, as should any history of stillbirths.

A complete physical examination of the baby should be performed, with careful attention to the baby's weight, comparison to birth weight (if applicable), and comparison to normal values. Assessment of blood pressure and saturations in the right upper and a lower extremity is critical to exclude coarctation and assess for hypertension. The cardiac examination should focus on the presence of abnormal murmurs, a gallop rhythm, thrills, and the intensity of the heart sounds.

Initial studies should include examination of the chest radiograph and an electrocardiogram. The chest radiograph may yield important information about heart size and semiquantification of pulmonary blood flow or vascular congestion. An electrocardiogram should be reviewed to assess rhythm, ventricular hypertrophy, Q waves, and ST and T wave changes that may suggest myocardial inflammation and/or ischemia (Fig. 29.2).

At a minimum, laboratory studies should include a serum chemistry panel, hepatic function panel, complete blood count with differential, thyroid function studies, a B-type natriuretic peptide, and serum troponin level. Troponin I is preferred generally due to being a primary cardiac isoform where as troponin T can be elevated in states of skeletal muscle injury. If myocarditis is suspected, serum inflammatory markers such as a C-reactive protein and erythrocyte sedimentation rate should be obtained, as should blood PCR for adenovirus, parvovirus B19, human herpes virus 6, enterovirus, cytomegalovirus, human immunodeficiency virus, and additional viral studies as is appropriate for the local epidemiology. Metabolic consultation and basic metabolic labs, including urine organic acids, serum amino acids, and a serum carnitine level, should be considered in all neonates with newly discovered cardiomyopathy or heart failure. Commercially available testing for gene mutations associated with cardiomyopathy can be considered but are more helpful to confirm rather than exclude a diagnosis, as currently only ~30%–35% of familial cardiomyopathies have an identifiable genetic etiology [85]. Genetic investigations are best pursued with a multidisciplinary team including a medical geneticist and genetic counselors to help ensure a complete and thorough three generation pedigree and to help explain testing and results. Whole exome sequencing can be considered for the identification of mitochondrial disorders but remains expensive and should be performed in consultation with appropriately trained team members.

Echocardiography is the primary diagnostic modality for evaluation of heart failure in children and infants due to reliable imaging quality, noninvasive and nontoxic nature, portability, and availability. Neonates typically have excellent echocardiographic windows, allowing for clear visualization of cardiac structures. A full anatomic study is necessary in neonates with suspected cardiomyopathy to evaluate for congenital and acquired conditions. Echocardiography can provide accurate assessments of LV systolic function including shortening fraction and ejection fraction. Assessment of RV systolic function is more limited although tricuspid annular plane systolic excursion provides some quantitative data [86]. Echocardiography allows semiquantification of atrioventricular and semilunar valve regurgitation and estimates of physiologic variables such as the RV systolic pressure and gradients across stenotic valves.

Assessment of diastolic function via tissue Doppler imaging has been the subject of much interest. Tissue Doppler measurements of myocardial velocities at the mitral valve annulus correlate with LV filling pressures at catheterization in adult populations. Normative values for tissue Doppler measurements in children have recently been published [87,88]; however, their correlation with catheterization-derived data in children and particularly neonates is uncertain, as studies have shown varying results [89,90]. Strain rate imaging and 3-D volumetric measures of right and left ventricular systolic function are currently under investigation but have not gained wide use in the evaluation of children and infants due to technical challenges and lack of easy reproducibility [91].

Cardiac magnetic resonance imaging (MRI) is assuming an increasingly important role in the assessment of cardiomyopathies in all age groups [92]. In children, cardiac MRI application is challenged by the need for sedation and/or general anesthesia. Higher heart rates in children (especially neonates) further hamper ECG gating. Cardiac MRI is superior to echocardiography in image quality of both the LV and RV and allows for accurate volumetric calculation of ejection fraction of both ventricles. In addition, cardiac MRI provides information regarding tissue characteristics, such as assessment for myocardial scarring via the presence of late gadolinium enhancement and T1 mapping when gating can be achieved. Unlike older patients, sedation is required for cardiac MRI in the neonate.

Cardiac catheterization continues to have a role in evaluation of selected groups of neonates with new onset heart failure. Confirmation of coronary anatomy is best accomplished with selective coronary injection or aortic root angiography and should be considered if there is persistent suspicion of ALCAPA following other imaging evaluation. While endomyocardial biopsy is the gold standard diagnostic test for myocarditis, the decision to biopsy in an infant has to be weighed against a higher risk of vascular or myocardial injury [93]. When severe valvar congenital heart disease (e.g., critical aortic stenosis) is the etiology for acute heart failure catheterization can offer an interventional modality in addition to its diagnostic utility. Similarly, in cases of refractory arrhythmias invasive intracardiac electrophysiologic procedures can be considered for diagnosis confirmation or very rarely for intervention. Finally, despite the progress made in noninvasive monitoring, diagnostic right heart catheterization still provides direct hemodynamic assessment of the right atrial pressures as well as estimates of left atrial pressure (via pulmonary capillary wedge pressure), cardiac output (via the Fick equation), and pulmonary vascular resistance.

MANAGEMENT STRATEGIES

Management of the infant with new onset heart failure begins with assessment of clinical stability and, when necessary, provision of support. Determining whether the patient is "wet or dry" to assess congestion and "warm or cold" to determine cardiac output may be useful in making a treatment plan [94]. Cautious monitoring should be instituted to assess for progression of disease and careful consideration should be given to placement in an intensive care unit.

Once hemodynamic stability is obtained, imaging to determine etiology of heart failure becomes a critical decision point to drive the next steps of care. In the setting of a left-to-right shunt with pulmonary overcirculation, the primary medical modality is volume contraction through diuretics. By reducing the circulating volume some children will regain a compensated state where feeding and growth can resume for some period of time. Ultimately the essential therapy is closure of the shunt, be that spontaneous via intrinsic growth or by intervention in the operating room or cardiac catheterization suite. Critical outflow tract obstruction, atrioventricular valve regurgitation, hypoplasia of left-sided structures, ALCAPA, and other critical forms of heart disease may be palliated to some extent via medications but definitive therapies generally require corrective or durable surgical palliation.

In the case of heart failure due to inherited or acquired cardiomyopathies, therapy in many cases is supportive, particularly in infants. Of note, medical therapies in neonates with heart failure have not been studied in large, randomized control trials and the concepts presented herein stem primarily from large adult trials, a few small clinical drug trials in children, and single-center studies that are mostly retrospective and uncontrolled.

TABLE 29.2 Modified Ross Criteria for Classification of Heart Failure in Children

Class I Heart Failure
Asymptomatic
Class II Heart Failure
Mild tachypnea or diaphoresis with feeding in infants; dyspnea on exertion in older children
Class III Heart Failure
Marked tachypnea or diaphoresis with feeding in infants; prolonged feeding times with growth failure resulting from HF; marked dyspnea on exertion in older children
Class IV Heart Failure
Symptoms such as tachypnea, retractions, grunting, or diaphoresis at rest

Adapted from P.F. Kantor, et al., Presentation, diagnosis, and medical management of heart failure in children: Canadian cardiovascular society guidelines, Can. J. Cardiol. 29 (2013) 1535–1552.

Initial Stabilization

Assessment of severity of heart failure in children, and particularly neonates, can be challenging. In many cases the presenting symptoms (feeding intolerance, vomiting, poor weight gain, tachypnea, tachycardia, pallor, and fatigue) may not be noted at initial evaluation or may be attributed to noncardiac causes, and many children pass through primary care and emergency room assessments in the days prior to the recognition of the true diagnosis [95]. The Ross Clinical Score, initially designed to assess pulmonary overcirculation, is used in modified form as a pediatric equivalent to the New York Heart Failure Association clinical score and is summarized in Table 29.2 [96]. This score primarily relies on tachypnea and exam findings relative to activity rather than reported symptoms. Attempts to use laboratory and imaging data to understand the severity of heart failure at presentation have had mixed success and are not yet in wide clinical use. What such scores and laboratory studies lack is the ability to predict recovery, which must be considered when choosing treatment modalities. Infants with DCM in particular have a significant potential for recovery, especially in cases of proven or suspected myocarditis [97]. Even in those with familial or idiopathic cardiomyopathy, 10%–30% will have stabilization or improvement of echocardiographic abnormalities either spontaneously or with introduction of heart failure medications [98,99].

In the neonate with inadequate cardiac output due to systolic or diastolic dysfunction, the goals of early therapy are appropriate hemodynamics, maintenance of oxygen delivery, and prevention of end organ injury. Medical and mechanical support options need to be considered and close monitoring of the effects of interventions through both invasive (central venous pressures, direct mixed-venous saturation measurement, and laboratory monitoring of end-organ perfusion) and noninvasive (continuous heart rate monitoring, frequent vital signs, and measures of oxygen delivery such as near infrared spectroscopy) measures should be utilized.

Medical management is the first-line treatment for newly discovered systolic dysfunction in neonates. In more stable infants with congestive symptoms, diuresis may be adequate to restore homeostasis without additional intervention. Loop diuretics such as furosemide and bumetandie and thiazides such as chlorothiazide are safe in infants at standard dosing and provide excellent augmentation of diuresis in most cases, although monitoring for hypotension is necessary due to rapid fluid shifts or significant electrolyte wasting.

When diuresis is inadequate to stabilize the patient a number of inotropic and vasoactive agents are available. Milrinone is a phosphodiesterase inhibitor that acts downstream from the beta-receptor to inhibit the breakdown of cyclic adenosine monophosphate in the heart and vascular smooth muscle cells to increase inotropy and vasodilation. As calcium reuptake in the myocyte is dependent on cAMP, milrinone is also thought to enhance cardiac relaxation, so-called lusitropy. While no randomized controlled trials have been performed in children with acute systolic dysfunction utilizing milrinone, adult data have shown improvement in hemodynamic measures and symptoms, although there is a risk of increased dysrhythmias. Milrinone has been studied in the setting of low cardiac output syndrome in children following heart surgery, with patients placed on milrinone showing decreased utilization of additional inotrope or mechanical support, and demonstrated safety at doses up to 0.75 μg/kg/min [100].

Commonly utilized inotropic agents in the treatment of infants with acute heart failure include the catecholamines dopamine, dobutamine, and epinephrine, with choice of medication dependent on region and practitioner. Dopamine is the immediate precursor for norepinephrine in the endogenous catecholamine biosynthetic pathway, and a central neurotransmitter in sympathetic nerve terminals and the adrenal medulla. At low doses (<5 μg/kg/min), dopamine stimulates receptors located in the brain, kidney, mesentery, and coronary arteries, promoting vasodilatation and blood flow to these organs. At moderate doses (5–10 μg/kg/min) dopamine provides direct beta-receptor stimulation increasing heart rate and inotropy although at the expense of increased cardiac oxygen consumption. At high doses (>10 μg/kg/min) alpha-adrenergic effects begin to predominate increasing vascular tone and systemic vascular resistance, changes that are not generally considered beneficial in acute decompensated heart failure. Dobutamine is a synthetic catecholamine with strong beta agonism and mild to moderate alpha antagonism resulting in increased inotropy, vasodilation, and a modest effect on heart rate. The net effect in children has been shown to be improved myocardial function, increased cardiac index, and stroke volume with less dramatic increase in heart rate. Epinephrine is an endogenous catecholamine derived from the N-methylation of norepinephrine, which activates alpha, $beta_1$, and $beta_2$ receptors in a dose-dependent manner. Similar to dobutamine, beta agonism predominates at lower doses increasing stroke volume and heart rate and lowering systemic vascular resistance via peripheral vasodilation.

Calcium chloride is a commonly used medication both following cardiac arrest and in the management of neonates after heart surgery experiencing low cardiac output syndrome. While no randomized controlled trials have been conducted to study the agent directly, the medication profile would suggest a potential role in managing children and particularly infants with significant decompensated heart failure. Increase of the calcium concentration within the myocyte directly increases troponin C binding allowing increased actin–myosin activity and thereby increasing contractility. In neonates, the myocardial calcium stores are generally inadequate for the stresses induced by acute heart failure, and the less mature sarcoplasmic reticulum is less reactive to calcium-induced calcium release. For this reason, neonates can be particularly sensitive to increased calcium concentrations with significant improvements in cardiac contractility being directly tied to serum calcium levels [59]. Calcium additionally has the benefit of not increasing heart rate or cardiac oxygen demand, in contrast to the effects of catecholamine medications.

Vasodilators (nipride, nitroglycerine, and nicardipine) have demonstrated survival benefit in adults with heart failure. These drugs are particularly helpful in those patients with low cardiac output accompanied by high systemic vascular resistance, typically driven by increased catecholamines in response to low organ perfusion pressures. Data on these medications in children are sorely lacking and concerns with use are often raised in neonates. Nitroprusside is a commonly used vasodilatory with rapid onset and effect that can be used in neonates although utility is limited by cyanide toxicity from metabolic byproducts and should be monitored particularly in small infants. Nicardipine is a dihydropyridine calcium-channel blocker that has vasodilatory effects on the vascular system without intrinsic myocardial inhibition. However, caution has been recommended in its use in neonates due to their low calcium stores and stereotypic calcium sensitivity especially in the setting of myocardial dysfunction due to concerns for contractility effects. Nesiritide, the recombinant form of brain natriuretic peptide, has been used in adults and children as an infusion for patients with acute decompensated heart failure and in adults was shown to improve outcomes although not clearly better than other vasodilators. Small studies in infants and children have shown benefits in urine output and decreased filling pressures without significant hypotension, although no survival benefit was demonstrated [101,102].

Chronic Therapy

Most of the data regarding chronic treatment of pediatric heart failure are extrapolated from adult studies. The goals of treatment are reducing fluid overload (with diuretics), reducing afterload (with vasodilators), and downregulating neurohormonal responses through blockade of angiotensin, renin, aldosterone, and catecholamines. Afterload reduction in chronic heart failure is mainly achieved by blockade of the conversion of angiotensin I to angiotensin II via angiotensin conversion enzyme inhibitors (ACEi). Decreased angiotensin II yields less vasoconstriction and aldosterone production, as well as inhibiting the reuptake of sodium, potassium, and water in the tubules and collecting duct. Several large adult randomized trials on ACEi in heart failure have shown that they provide symptomatic relief, reduce hospitalization, and decrease mortality. There are limited pediatric data available regarding the use of ACEi; however, due to the conserved physiologic and pathologic sequences in heart failure in adults and children these drugs remain a mainstay of treatment in pediatric patients. In general, formulations with shorter half-life (captopril, enalapril) are chosen over those with once daily dosing (lisinopril) in neonates to allow for better control of dosing. Use of angiotensin receptor blockers is often indicated by intolerance of ACEi in the form of a chronic cough and is generally not a concern in neonatal patients.

Adrenergic blockade with beta antagonists has been shown to provide additive survival benefits for adults with chronic heart failure especially when combined with ACEi. While several beta-blockers have been used in adult trials with positive survival benefit these data have not been replicated in children. Carvedilol, a nonselective beta-blocker with additional alpha-1 antagonism and antioxidative properties, has shown mild morbidity and mortality improvements in adult studies.

A randomized controlled trial in children failed to show therapeutic benefit over placebo, however, this study was challenged by low enrollment and ultimately was underpowered to detect a survival benefit due to the high rate of spontaneous recovery in the placebo group [98]. Subanalyses of this patient population did demonstrate improved echocardiographic parameters in the patients treated with carvedilol [103].

Use of digoxin, a cardiac glycoside that increases sarcoplasmic calcium concentrations via inhibition of the Na/K-ATPase, is much less common in adult patients now than in years past. This medication continues to be common in some pediatric centers in part because of use in dysrhythmias, but it is no longer considered frontline for management of heart failure [104].

Mechanical Ventilatory Support

Certain patients will continue to deteriorate despite maximal medical therapy and ultimately may require mechanical support. Mechanical ventilation is a reasonable first-line strategy in infants that may stabilize and even improve hemodynamics and allow for more aggressive medical intervention. Positive intrathoracic pressure typically benefits patients with LV systolic and diastolic dysfunction by reducing afterload and wall tension. Positive pressure ventilation has an added benefit of helping ameliorate the effects of pulmonary edema and recruit atelectatic lung, further improving the symptoms of heart failure. While mechanical ventilation and increased airway pressures tend to improve the left heart function they can have mixed effects on the right heart. Increases in pulmonary distension beyond functional residual capacity will increase pulmonary vascular resistance and therefore RV afterload. Additionally high intrathoracic pressures increase systemic venous pressures and can worsen systemic edema, inhibit ventricular filling, and worsen secondary organ injury due to elevation of central venous pressure thus effectively decreasing perfusion pressure gradients.

Mechanical Circulatory Support

For decades the mainstay of neonatal mechanical circulatory support has been extracorporeal membrane oxygenation (ECMO). This modality provides full heart support combined with oxygenation of systemic blood, allowing for cardiopulmonary support of critically ill infants and children. While neonatal ECMO has been considered a low yield option in prior decades, it is now a readily available and often-successful means of short-term support in children of all ages. Limitations of ECMO include the need for systemic anticoagulation, the need for large-bore cannulae often with central placement through the chest in infants, and risk of both embolic and hemorrhagic complications. Successful duration of ECMO support has increased over time with improved circuits, hospital experience, and antithrombotic strategies.

Despite these improvements, outcomes are still generally poor particularly for those patients who undergo transplantation [105].

In the last two decades mechanical circulatory support has become a mainstay of adult advanced heart failure programs with the majority of patients undergoing device implantation prior to transplantation and a growing number having support devices placed as "destination therapy." Similarly in pediatrics there has been growing utilization of various devices, but in small children the primary option outside of ECMO has been the Berlin EXCOR pulsatile ventricular assist device. This pneumatically driven extracorporeal device is the only one approved in the United States by the Federal Drug Administration for use in children as a bridge to transplantation. The Berlin EXCOR comes in multiple pump sizes and is capable of supporting children as small as 3–4 kg. The device was first utilized in Europe but has now been placed in greater than 1500 patients and has been utilized throughout the international community. The device allows for reliable support of either or both ventricles although in the current era the primary placement is as LV support alone. Overall success rate for bridge to transplant or explant and recovery is roughly 75%, with superior survival after heart transplant when compared to ECMO [106,107]. It should be noted, however, that in children under 10 kg at implantation survival was lower than that of the entire group, at 57%. This was predominantly due to patients with congenital heart disease, weight <5 kg, and evidence of biventricular failure through elevated bilirubin. In fact none of the patients with congenital heart disease and weighing less than 5 kg survived. However, in patients greater than 5 kg but less than 10 kg, survival similar to other age and size groups can be achieved [108].

Heart Transplantation

Ultimately, infants with end-stage heart failure due to congenital, acquired, or myopathic causes face cardiac transplantation as their last palliative option. The first cardiac transplant in an infant, and the second ever in a human, was performed in December 1967 by Adrian Kantrowitz, just days following Dr. Christian Barnard's initial historic procedure. It was not until the approval of cyclosporine in 1981 that infant heart transplantation began to gain a more solid foothold as a legitimate therapeutic option. Through the 1980s the use of transplantation in infants, particularly those with severe forms of congenital heart disease (e.g., hypoplastic left heart syndrome), grew steadily until now roughly 500–600 pediatric heart transplants are performed annually worldwide, with infant recipients accounting for roughly 25% of these cases [109]. The primary indication for heart transplantation in infants remains congenital heart disease, however, in the last 3 decades, the number of cardiomyopathy cases has increased so that now only 55% of recipients have congenital disease to 41% cardiomyopathy, compared to approximately 75% congenital heart disease in the 1980s [109].

For those patients who successfully make it to transplantation, long-term outcomes are relatively good. Infants suffer from the highest rates of early graft loss with 1-year survival rates close to 85%–90% at most centers. However, due to their relatively immature immune systems they seem to have greater graft accommodation allowing for a less severe mortality rate than their older counterparts. Current data show a median survival of approximately 20 years, which has been steadily improving over time. For those patients who survive the first year the median survival stretches out to greater than 25 years. For those patients surviving 5 years posttransplant, greater than 60% will survive to 25 years [109].

CONCLUSION

Heart failure in the neonate is a complex syndrome representing a constellation of symptoms and signs. The causes are varied and include congenital heart disease, inherited or acquired myopathy, and systemic disease. Defining the problem is made even more difficult by patient size and the physiology unique to a patient making the transition from fetal to postnatal life. Accurate diagnosis of etiology is key for appropriate therapy and is comprised of thorough evaluation including family history, focused physical exam, radiography, electrocardiography, noninvasive cardiac imaging, laboratory testing, and in appropriate cases invasive testing including endomyocardial biopsy. Treatment options include diuretic therapy, afterload reduction, beta-blockade, inotropic and vasoactive medications, mechanical ventilatory support, mechanical circulatory support, and ultimately heart transplantation in cases of intractable disease. In the majority of instances, however, these treatment modalities have been described in adult or older pediatric populations, and can only be extrapolated to the neonatal age-group. Ongoing studies and advances in support technology should improve overall outcomes and allow for increased survival.

REFERENCES

[1] D.T. Hsu, G.D. Pearson, Heart failure in children: part I: history, etiology, and pathophysiology, Circ. Heart Fail. 2 (1) (2009) 63–70.

[2] G. Webster, J. Zhang, D. Rosenthal, Comparison of the epidemiology and co-morbidities of heart failure in the pediatric and adult populations: a retrospective, cross-sectional study, BMC Cardiovasc. Disord. 6 (2006) 23.

[3] J.W. Rossano, J.J. Kim, J.A. Decker, J.F. Price, F. Zafar, D.E. Graves, et al., Prevalence, morbidity, and mortality of heart failure-related hospitalizations in children in the United States: a population-based study, J. Card. Fail. 18 (6) (2012) 459–470.

[4] B.J. Maron, J.A. Towbin, G. Thiene, C. Antzelevitch, D. Corrado, D. Arnett, et al., Contemporary definitions and classification of the cardiomyopathies: an American Heart Association scientific statement from the council on clinical cardiology, heart failure and transplantation committee; quality of care and outcomes research and functional genomics and translational biology interdisciplinary working groups; and council on epidemiology and prevention, Circulation 113 (14) (2006) 1807–1816.

[5] A. Arola, E. Jokinen, O. Ruuskanen, M. Saraste, E. Pesonen, A.L. Kuusela, et al., Epidemiology of idiopathic cardiomyopathies in children and adolescents. A nationwide study in Finland, Am. J. Epidemiol. 146 (5) (1997) 385–393.

[6] J.D. Wilkinson, D.C. Landy, S.D. Colan, J.A. Towbin, L.A. Sleeper, E.J. Orav, et al., The pediatric cardiomyopathy registry and heart failure: key results from the first 15 years, Heart Fail. Clin. 6 (4) (2010) 401–413 vii.

[7] A.W. Nugent, P.E. Daubeney, P. Chondros, J.B. Carlin, M. Cheung, L.C. Wilkinson, et al., The epidemiology of childhood cardiomyopathy in Australia, N. Engl. J. Med. 348 (17) (2003) 1639–1646.

[8] J.A. Towbin, A.M. Lowe, S.D. Colan, L.A. Sleeper, E.J. Orav, S. Clunie, et al., Incidence, causes, and outcomes of dilated cardiomyopathy in children, JAMA 296 (15) (2006) 1867–1876.

[9] S.D. Colan, S.E. Lipshultz, A.M. Lowe, L.A. Sleeper, J. Messere, G.F. Cox, et al., Epidemiology and cause-specific outcome of hypertrophic cardiomyopathy in children: findings from the pediatric cardiomyopathy registry, Circulation 115 (6) (2007) 773–781.

[10] R.E. Andrews, M.J. Fenton, D.A. Ridout, M. Burch, British Congenital Cardiac Association, New-onset heart failure due to heart muscle disease in childhood: a prospective study in the United Kingdom and Ireland, Circulation 117 (1) (2008) 79–84.

[11] P. Elliott, B. Andersson, E. Arbustini, Z. Bilinska, F. Cecchi, P. Charron, et al., Classification of the cardiomyopathies: a position statement from the European society of cardiology working group on myocardial and pericardial diseases, Eur. Heart J. 29 (2) (2008) 270–276.

[12] J.L. Jefferies, J.A. Towbin, Dilated cardiomyopathy, Lancet 375 (9716) (2010) 752–762.

[13] J.N. Silva, C.E. Canter, Current management of pediatric dilated cardiomyopathy, Curr. Opin. Cardiol. 25 (2) (2010) 80–87.

[14] V.V. Michels, P.P. Moll, F.A. Miller, A.J. Tajik, J.S. Chu, D.J. Driscoll, et al., The frequency of familial dilated cardiomyopathy in a series of patients with idiopathic dilated cardiomyopathy, N. Engl. J. Med. 326 (2) (1992) 77–82.

[15] S.J. Kindel, E.M. Miller, R. Gupta, L.H. Cripe, R.B. Hinton, R.L. Spicer, et al., Pediatric cardiomyopathy: importance of genetic and metabolic evaluation, J. Card. Fail. 18 (5) (2012) 396–403.

[16] J.A. Towbin, N.E. Bowles, The failing heart, Nature 415 (6868) (2002) 227–233.

[17] R.I. Kelley, J.P. Cheatham, B.J. Clark, M.A. Nigro, B.R. Powell, G.W. Sherwood, et al., X-linked dilated cardiomyopathy with neutropenia, growth retardation, and 3-methylglutaconic aciduria, J. Pediatr. 119 (5) (1991) 738–747.

[18] A.E. Roberts, C. Nixon, C.G. Steward, K. Gauvreau, M. Maisenbacher, M. Fletcher, et al., The barth syndrome registry: distinguishing disease characteristics and growth data from a longitudinal study, Am. J. Med. Genet. A 158A (11) (2012) 2726–2732.

[19] B.J. Maron, Hypertrophic cardiomyopathy: a systematic review, JAMA 287 (10) (2002) 1308–1320.

[20] P. Elliott, W.J. McKenna, Hypertrophic cardiomyopathy, Lancet 363 (9424) (2004) 1881–1891.

[21] H. Watkins, Genetic clues to disease pathways in hypertrophic and dilated cardiomyopathies, Circulation 107 (10) (2003) 1344–1346.

[22] H. Morita, H.L. Rehm, A. Menesses, B. McDonough, A.E. Roberts, R. Kucherlapati, et al., Shared genetic causes of cardiac hypertrophy in children and adults, N. Engl. J. Med. 358 (18) (2008) 1899–1908.

[23] R. Engberding, T.M. Yelbuz, G. Breithardt, Isolated noncompaction of the left ventricular myocardium – a review of the literature two decades after the initial case description, Clin. Res. Cardiol. 96 (7) (2007) 481–488.

[24] R.H. Pignatelli, C.J. McMahon, W.J. Dreyer, S.W. Denfield, J. Price, J.W. Belmont, et al., Clinical characterization of left ventricular noncompaction in children: a relatively common form of cardiomyopathy, Circulation 108 (21) (2003) 2672–2678.

[25] S.T. Brescia, J.W. Rossano, R. Pignatelli, J.L. Jefferies, J.F. Price, J.A. Decker, et al., Mortality and sudden death in pediatric left ventricular noncompaction in a tertiary referral center, Circulation 127 (22) (2013) 2202–2208.

[26] F. Ichida, Y. Hamamichi, T. Miyawaki, Y. Ono, T. Kamiya, T. Akagi, et al., Clinical features of isolated noncompaction of the ventricular myocardium: long-term clinical course, hemodynamic properties, and genetic background, J. Am. Coll. Cardiol. 34 (1) (1999) 233–240.

[27] J.A. Towbin, Left ventricular noncompaction: a new form of heart failure, Heart Fail. Clin. 6 (4) (2010) 453–469 viii.

[28] S. Sasse-Klaassen, B. Gerull, E. Oechslin, R. Jenni, L. Thierfelder, Isolated noncompaction of the left ventricular myocardium in the adult is an autosomal dominant disorder in the majority of patients, Am. J. Med. Genet. A 119A (2) (2003) 162–167.

[29] S.B. Bleyl, B.R. Mumford, M.C. Brown-Harrison, L.T. Pagotto, J.C. Carey, T.J. Pysher, et al., Xq28-linked noncompaction of the left ventricular myocardium: prenatal diagnosis and pathologic analysis of affected individuals, Am. J. Med. Genet. 72 (3) (1997) 257–265.

[30] M. Tariq, S.M. Ware, Importance of genetic evaluation and testing in pediatric cardiomyopathy, World J. Cardiol. 6 (11) (2014) 1156–1165.

[31] C.E. Canter, K.P. Simpson, Diagnosis and treatment of myocarditis in children in the current era, Circulation 129 (1) (2014) 115–128.

[32] K. Madden, R.R. Thiagarajan, P.T. Rycus, S.K. Rajagopal, Survival of neonates with enteroviral myocarditis requiring extracorporeal membrane oxygenation, Pediatr. Crit. Care Med. 12 (3) (2011) 314–318.

[33] S.A. Teele, C.K. Allan, P.C. Laussen, J.W. Newburger, K. Gauvreau, R.R. Thiagarajan, Management and outcomes in pediatric patients presenting with acute fulminant myocarditis, J. Pediatr. 158 (4) (2011) 638–643 e1.

[34] J.G. Lawrence, J.R. Carapetis, K. Griffiths, K. Edwards, J.R. Condon, Acute rheumatic fever and rheumatic heart disease: incidence and progression in the Northern Territory of Australia, 1997 to 2010, Circulation 128 (5) (2013) 492–501.

[35] J.W. Newburger, M. Takahashi, M.A. Gerber, M.H. Gewitz, L.Y. Tani, J.C. Burns, et al., Diagnosis, treatment, and long-term management of Kawasaki disease: a statement for health professionals from the Committee on Rheumatic Fever, Endocarditis and Kawasaki Disease, Council on Cardiovascular Disease in the Young, American Heart Association, Circulation 110 (17) (2004) 2747–2771.

[36] M. Hangai, Y. Kubota, J. Kagawa, M. Yashiro, R. Uehara, Y. Nakamura, et al., Neonatal Kawasaki disease: case report and data from nationwide survey in Japan, Eur. J. Pediatr. 173 (11) (2014) 1533–1536.

[37] H. Yoshikawa, Y. Nomura, K. Masuda, D. Hazeki, K. Yotsumoto, M. Arata, et al., Four cases of Kawasaki syndrome complicated with myocarditis, Circ. J. 70 (2) (2006) 202–205.

[38] J.T. Kanegaye, M.S. Wilder, D. Molkara, J.R. Frazer, J. Pancheri, A.H. Tremoulet, et al., Recognition of a Kawasaki disease shock syndrome, Pediatrics 123 (5) (2009) e783–e789.

[39] J.A. Johnson, T.G. Boyce, F. Cetta, J.M. Steckelberg, J.N. Johnson, Infective endocarditis in the pediatric patient: a 60-year single-institution review, Mayo Clin. Proc. 87 (7) (2012) 629–635.

[40] M.D. Day, K. Gauvreau, S. Shulman, J.W. Newburger, Characteristics of children hospitalized with infective endocarditis, Circulation 119 (6) (2009) 865–870.

[41] D. Marom, I. Levy, O. Gutwein, E. Birk, S. Ashkenazi, Healthcare-associated versus community-associated infective endocarditis in children, Pediatr. Infect. Dis. J. 30 (7) (2011) 585–588.

[42] Y.T. Lin, K.S. Hsieh, Y.S. Chen, I.F. Huang, M.F. Cheng, Infective endocarditis in children without underlying heart disease, J. Microbiol. Immunol. Infect. (Wei mian yu gan ran za zhi) 46 (2) (2013) 121–128.

[43] S. Raj, J.S. Killinger, J.A. Gonzalez, L. Lopez, Myocardial dysfunction in pediatric septic shock, J. Pediatr. 164 (1) (2014) 72–77 e2.

[44] J. Baruteau, P. Sachs, P. Broue, M. Brivet, H. Abdoul, C. Vianey-Saban, et al., Clinical and biological features at diagnosis in mitochondrial fatty acid beta-oxidation defects: a French pediatric study of 187 patients, J. Inherit. Metab. Dis. 36 (5) (2013) 795–803.

[45] E. Helton, R. Darragh, P. Francis, F.J. Fricker, K. Jue, G. Koch, et al., Metabolic aspects of myocardial disease and a role for L-carnitine in the treatment of childhood cardiomyopathy, Pediatrics 105 (6) (2000) 1260–1270.

[46] S.C. Winter, N.R. Buist, Cardiomyopathy in childhood, mitochondrial dysfunction, and the role of L-carnitine, Am. Heart J. 139 (2 Pt 3) (2000) S63–S69.

[47] F. Scaglia, J.A. Towbin, W.J. Craigen, J.W. Belmont, E.O. Smith, S.R. Neish, et al., Clinical spectrum, morbidity, and mortality in 113 pediatric patients with mitochondrial disease, Pediatrics 114 (4) (2004) 925–931.

[48] J.L. Jefferies, Barth syndrome. American journal of medical genetics Part C, Semin. Med. Genet. 163C (3) (2013) 198–205.

[49] S.B. Wortmann, M. Duran, Y. Anikster, P.G. Barth, W. Sperl, J. Zschocke, et al., Inborn errors of metabolism with 3-methylglutaconic aciduria as discriminative feature: proper classification and nomenclature, J. Inherit. Metab. Dis. 36 (6) (2013) 923–928.

[50] E.A. Dominic, A. Ramezani, S.D. Anker, M. Verma, N. Mehta, M. Rao, Mitochondrial cytopathies and cardiovascular disease, Heart 100 (8) (2014) 611–618.

[51] P.S. Kishnani, H.M. Amartino, C. Lindberg, T.M. Miller, A. Wilson, J. Keutzer, et al., Timing of diagnosis of patients with Pompe disease: data from the Pompe registry, Am. J. Med. Genet. A 161A (10) (2013) 2431–2443.

[52] B.J. Byrne, P.S. Kishnani, L.E. Case, L. Merlini, W. Muller-Felber, S. Prasad, et al., Pompe disease: design, methodology, and early findings from the Pompe Registry, Mol. Genet. Metab. 103 (1) (2011) 1–11.

[53] J.C. Levine, P.S. Kishnani, Y.T. Chen, J.R. Herlong, J.S. Li, Cardiac remodeling after enzyme replacement therapy with acid alpha-glucosidase for infants with Pompe disease, Pediatr. Cardiol. 29 (6) (2008) 1033–1042.

[54] P.S. Kishnani, D. Corzo, N.D. Leslie, D. Gruskin, A. Van der Ploeg, J.P. Clancy, et al., Early treatment with alglucosidase alpha prolongs long-term survival of infants with Pompe disease, Pediatr. Res. 66 (3) (2009) 329–335.

[55] H.P. Gutgesell, M.E. Speer, H.S. Rosenberg, Characterization of the cardiomyopathy in infants of diabetic mothers, Circulation 61 (2) (1980) 441–450.

[56] H.P. Gutgesell, C.E. Mullins, P.C. Gillette, M. Speer, A.J. Rudolph, D.G. McNamara, Transient hypertrophic subaortic stenosis in infants of diabetic mothers, J. Pediatr. 89 (1) (1976) 120–125.

[57] T. Huang, A. Kelly, S.A. Becker, M.S. Cohen, C.A. Stanley, Hypertrophic cardiomyopathy in neonates with congenital hyperinsulinism, Arch. Dis. Child. Fetal Neonatal Ed. 98 (4) (2013) F351–F354.

[58] M.C. Vaillant, A. Chantepie, A. Casasoprana, C. Chamboux, A.L. Suc, F. Gold, et al., Transient hypertrophic cardiomyopathy in neonates after acute fetal distress, Pediatr. Cardiol. 18 (1) (1997) 52–56.

[59] J.F. Price, Unique aspects of heart failure in the neonate, in: R.E. Shaddy (Ed.), Heart Failure in Congenital Heart Disease: From Fetus to Adult, Springer-Verlag London, London, UK, 2011, pp. 21–42.

[60] S.E. Lipshultz, M.J. Adams, S.D. Colan, L.S. Constine, E.H. Herman, D.T. Hsu, et al., Long-term cardiovascular toxicity in children, adolescents, and young adults who receive cancer therapy: pathophysiology, course, monitoring, management, prevention, and research directions: a scientific statement from the American Heart Association, Circulation 128 (17) (2013) 1927–1995.

[61] N. Sekarski, E.J. Meijboom, S. Di Bernardo, T.B. Ksontini, Y. Mivelaz, Perinatal arrhythmias, Eur. J. Pediatr. 173 (8) (2014) 983–996.

[62] E.R. Ellis, M.E. Josephson, Heart failure and tachycardia-induced cardiomyopathy, Curr. Heart Fail. Rep. 10 (4) (2013) 296–306.

[63] J.P. Moore, P.A. Patel, K.M. Shannon, E.L. Albers, J.C. Salerno, M.A. Stein, et al., Predictors of myocardial recovery in pediatric tachycardia-induced cardiomyopathy, Heart Rhythm 11 (7) (2014) 1163–1169.

[64] M.S. Silvetti, F. Drago, L. Rava, Determinants of early dilated cardiomyopathy in neonates with congenital complete atrioventricular block, Europace 12 (9) (2010) 1316–1321.

[65] D. Khullar, A.M. Andeejani, K.R. Bulsara, Evolution of treatment options for vein of Galen malformations, J. Neurosurg. Pediatr. 6 (5) (2010) 444–451.

[66] A. Berenstein, J.T. Fifi, Y. Niimi, S. Presti, R. Ortiz, S. Ghatan, et al., Vein of Galen malformations in neonates: new management paradigms for improving outcomes, Neurosurgery 70 (5) (2012) 1207–1213 discussion 13–14.

[67] N.A. Weitz, C.T. Lauren, T.J. Starc, J.J. Kandel, D.A. Bateman, K.D. Morel, et al., Congenital cutaneous hemangioma causing cardiac failure: a case report and review of the literature, Pediatr. Dermatol. 30 (6) (2013) e180–e190.

[68] N. Xiao, A. Tandon, S. Goldstein, A. Lorts, Cardiogenic shock as the initial presentation of neonatal systemic hypertension, J. Neonatal Perinatal Med. 6 (3) (2013) 267–272.

[69] J. Louw, S. Brown, L. Thewissen, A. Smits, B. Eyskens, R. Heying, et al., Neonatal circulatory failure due to acute hypertensive crisis: clinical and echocardiographic clues, Cardiovasc. J. Afr. 24 (3) (2013) 72–75.

[70] A.L. Peterson, P.C. Frommelt, K. Mussatto, Presentation and echocardiographic markers of neonatal hypertensive cardiomyopathy, Pediatrics 118 (3) (2006) e782–e785.

[71] J.M. Dionne, C.L. Abitbol, J.T. Flynn, Hypertension in infancy: diagnosis, management and outcome, Pediatr. Nephrol. 27 (1) (2012) 17–32.

[72] D.L. Batisky, Neonatal hypertension, Clin. Perinatol. 41 (3) (2014) 529–542.

[73] J. Rychik, The twin-twin transfusion syndrome: evolving concepts, in: C.S. Kleinman, I. Seri (Eds.), Hemodnynamics and Cardiology: Neonatology Questions and Controversies, Saunders, 2008, pp. 387–402.

[74] J. Rychik, Z. Tian, M. Bebbington, F. Xu, M. McCann, S. Mann, et al., The twin-twin transfusion syndrome: spectrum of cardiovascular abnormality and development of a cardiovascular score to assess severity of disease, Am. J. Obstet. Gynecol. 197 (4) (2007) 392 e1–8.

[75] T. Van Mieghem, A.M. Martin, R. Weber, C. Barrea, R. Windrim, L.K. Hornberger, et al., Fetal cardiac function in recipient twins undergoing fetoscopic laser ablation of placental anastomoses for Stage IV twin-twin transfusion syndrome, Ultrasound Obstet. Gynecol. 42 (1) (2013) 64–69.

[76] D. Roberts, J.P. Neilson, M.D. Kilby, S. Gates, Interventions for the treatment of twin-twin transfusion syndrome, Cochrane Database Syst. Rev. 1 (2014) CD002073.

[77] C. Barrea, C. Debauche, O. Williams, S. Jasienski, P. Steenhaut, T. Sluysmans, et al., Twin-to-twin transfusion syndrome: perinatal outcome and recipient heart disease according to treatment strategy, J. Paediatr. Child Health 49 (1) (2013) E28–E34.

[78] L. Abdurrahman, S.M. Schwartz, R.H. Beekman 3rd, Thrombotic occlusion of the main stem of the left coronary artery in a neonate, Cardiol. Young 9 (2) (1999) 189–191.

[79] G. Giralt, F. Gran, P. Betrian, Q. Ferrer, Acute myocardial infarction in a neonate caused by a coronary thrombosis: a considerable diagnostic and therapeutic challenge, Rev. Esp. Cardiol. 68 (10) (2015) 903–904.

[80] A.B. Clark, T.A. Stokes, H.F. Krous, D.N. Carbine, Myocardial infarction in a newborn heterozygous for the MTHFR C677T mutation, Pediatr. Dev. Pathol. 15 (3) (2012) 232–236.

[81] D.D. Ivy, S.H. Abman, R.J. Barst, R.M. Berger, D. Bonnet, T.R. Fleming, et al., Pediatric pulmonary hypertension, J. Am. Coll. Cardiol. 62 (25 Suppl.) (2013) D117–D126.

[82] A.R. Kemper, W.T. Mahle, G.R. Martin, W.C. Cooley, P. Kumar, W.R. Morrow, et al., Strategies for implementing screening for critical congenital heart disease, Pediatrics 128 (5) (2011) e1259–e1267.

[83] K. Ma, L. Wang, Z. Hua, K. Yang, S. Hu, J. Yan, et al., Outcomes of coronary transfer for anomalous origin of the left coronary artery from the pulmonary artery, Eur. J. Cardio Thorac. Surg. 47 (4) (2015) 659–664.

[84] J. Weigand, C.D. Marshall, E.A. Bacha, J.M. Chen, M.E. Richmond, Repair of anomalous left coronary artery from the pulmonary artery in the modern era: preoperative predictors of immediate postoperative outcomes and long term cardiac follow-up, Pediatr. Cardiol. 36 (3) (2015) 489–497.

[85] R.E. Hershberger, J.D. Siegfried, Update 2011: clinical and genetic issues in familial dilated cardiomyopathy, J. Am. Coll. Cardiol. 57 (16) (2011) 1641–1649.

[86] M. Koestenberger, B. Nagel, W. Ravekes, A. Gamillscheg, G. Pichler, A. Avian, et al., Right ventricular performance in preterm and term neonates: reference values of the tricuspid annular peak systolic velocity measured by tissue Doppler imaging, Neonatology 103 (4) (2013) 281–286.

[87] F. Dallaire, C. Slorach, W. Hui, T. Sarkola, M.K. Friedberg, T.J. Bradley, et al., Reference values for pulse wave Doppler and tissue Doppler imaging in pediatric echocardiography, Circ. Cardiovasc. Imaging 8 (2) (2015) e002167.

[88] M. Cantinotti, L. Lopez, Nomograms for blood flow and tissue Doppler velocities to evaluate diastolic function in children: a critical review, J. Am. Soc. Echocardiogr. 26 (2) (2013) 126–141.

[89] F.I. Lunze, S.D. Colan, K. Gauvreau, A.R. Perez-Atayde, R.N. Smith, E.D. Blume, et al., Tissue Doppler imaging for rejection surveillance in pediatric heart transplant recipients, J. Heart Lung Transplant. 32 (10) (2013) 1027–1033.

[90] D.J. Goldberg, M.D. Quartermain, A.C. Glatz, E.K. Hall, E. Davis, S.A. Kren, et al., Doppler tissue imaging in children following cardiac transplantation: a comparison to catheter derived hemodynamics, Pediatr. Transplant. 15 (5) (2011) 488–494.

[91] S. Kutty, A. Padiyath, L. Li, Q. Peng, S. Rangamani, A. Schuster, et al., Functional maturation of left and right atrial systolic and diastolic performance in infants, children, and adolescents, J. Am. Soc. Echocardiogr. 26 (4) (2013) 398–409 e2.

[92] American College of Cardiology Foundation Task Force on Expert Consensus Documents, W.G. Hundley, D.A. Bluemke, J.P. Finn, S.D. Flamm, M.A. Fogel, et al., ACCF/ACR/AHA/NASCI/SCMR 2010 expert consensus document on cardiovascular magnetic resonance: a report of the American College of Cardiology Foundation Task Force on Expert Consensus Documents, Circulation 121 (22) (2010) 2462–2508.

[93] S.G. Pophal, G. Sigfusson, K.L. Booth, S.A. Bacanu, S.A. Webber, J.A. Ettedgui, et al., Complications of endomyocardial biopsy in children, J. Am. Coll. Cardiol. 34 (7) (1999) 2105–2110.

[94] L.W. Stevenson, Tailored therapy to hemodynamic goals for advanced heart failure, Eur. J. Heart Fail. 1 (3) (1999) 251–257.

[95] S.M. Macicek, C.G. Macias, J.L. Jefferies, J.J. Kim, J.F. Price, Acute heart failure syndromes in the pediatric emergency department, Pediatrics 124 (5) (2009) e898–904.

[96] P.F. Kantor, J. Lougheed, A. Dancea, M. McGillion, N. Barbosa, C. Chan, et al., Presentation, diagnosis, and medical management of heart failure in children: Canadian cardiovascular society guidelines, Can. J. Cardiol. 29 (12) (2013) 1535–1552.

[97] S.R. Foerster, C.E. Canter, A. Cinar, L.A. Sleeper, S.A. Webber, E. Pahl, et al., Ventricular remodeling and survival are more favorable for myocarditis than for idiopathic dilated cardiomyopathy in childhood: an outcomes study from the pediatric cardiomyopathy registry, Circ. Heart Fail. 3 (6) (2010) 689–697.

[98] R.E. Shaddy, M.M. Boucek, D.T. Hsu, R.J. Boucek, C.E. Canter, L. Mahony, et al., Carvedilol for children and adolescents with heart failure: a randomized controlled trial, JAMA 298 (10) (2007) 1171–1179.

[99] M.D. Everitt, L.A. Sleeper, M. Lu, C.E. Canter, E. Pahl, J.D. Wilkinson, et al., Recovery of echocardiographic function in children with idiopathic dilated cardiomyopathy: results from the pediatric cardiomyopathy registry, J. Am. Coll. Cardiol. 63 (14) (2014) 1405–1413.

[100] T.M. Hoffman, G. Wernovsky, A.M. Atz, T.J. Kulik, D.P. Nelson, A.C. Chang, et al., Efficacy and safety of milrinone in preventing low cardiac output syndrome in infants and children after corrective surgery for congenital heart disease, Circulation 107 (7) (2003) 996–1002.

[101] B.S. Moffett, J.L. Jefferies, J. Rossano, J.A. Towbin, Nesiritide therapy in a term neonate with renal disease, Pharmacotherapy 26 (2) (2006) 281–284.

[102] J.L. Jefferies, J.F. Price, S.W. Denfield, A.C. Chang, W.J. Dreyer, C.J. McMahon, et al., Safety and efficacy of nesiritide in pediatric heart failure, J. Card. Fail. 13 (7) (2007) 541–548.

[103] C. Petko, L.L. Minich, M.D. Everitt, R. Holubkov, R.E. Shaddy, L.Y. Tani, Echocardiographic evaluation of children with systemic ventricular dysfunction treated with carvedilol, Pediatr. Cardiol. 31 (6) (2010) 780–784.

[104] M.J. O'Connor, D.N. Rosenthal, R.E. Shaddy, Outpatient management of pediatric heart failure, Heart Fail. Clin. 6 (4) (2010) 515–529 ix.

[105] A.I. Dipchand, W.T. Mahle, M. Tresler, D.C. Naftel, C. Almond, J.K. Kirklin, et al., Extracorporeal membrane oxygenation as a bridge to pediatric heart transplantation: effect on post-listing and post-transplantation outcomes, Circ. Heart Fail. 8 (5) (2015) 960–969.

[106] P. Eghtesady, C.S. Almond, C. Tjossem, D. Epstein, M. Imamura, M. Turrentine, et al., Post-transplant outcomes of children bridged to transplant with the Berlin Heart EXCOR pediatric ventricular assist device, Circulation 128 (11 Suppl. 1) (2013) S24–S31.

[107] C.S. Almond, D.L. Morales, E.H. Blackstone, M.W. Turrentine, M. Imamura, M.P. Massicotte, et al., Berlin Heart EXCOR pediatric ventricular assist device for bridge to heart transplantation in US children, Circulation 127 (16) (2013) 1702–1711.

[108] J. Conway, J. St Louis, D.L. Morales, S. Law, C. Tjossem, T. Humpl, Delineating survival outcomes in children <10 kg bridged to transplant or recovery with the Berlin Heart EXCOR ventricular assist device, JACC Heart Fail. 3 (1) (2015) 70–77.

[109] A.I. Dipchand, L.B. Edwards, A.Y. Kucheryavaya, C. Benden, F. Dobbels, B.J. Levvey, et al., The registry of the international society for heart and lung transplantation: seventeenth official pediatric heart transplantation report–2014; focus theme: retransplantation, J. Heart Lung Transplant. 33 (10) (2014) 985–995.

Chapter 30

Right Heart Failure in Pediatric Pulmonary Hypertension

Dunbar Ivy
University of Colorado School of Medicine, Aurora, CO, United States

INTRODUCTION

Pulmonary hypertension (PH) is an important cause of morbidity and mortality in pediatric patients of diverse causes. Although advances in the understanding of pathology of pulmonary arterial hypertension (PAH) have led to novel therapies, there is no cure for many forms of PH. Right ventricular function is a major determinant of prognosis in severe PH. The diagnosis of right heart failure is a clinical one but is supported by imaging and catheterization modalities. This chapter will discuss diagnosis of right ventricular failure in children, imaging of the right ventricle, and acute and chronic therapeutic options.

DEFINITION

PH is defined as a mean pulmonary arterial pressure greater of 25 mmHg [1]. PAH, a subtype of PH, is also defined as a mean pulmonary arterial pressure greater of 25 mmHg and with a normal pulmonary artery wedge pressure less than 15 mmHg and an increase in pulmonary vascular resistance index (PVRI) greater than 3 wood units × m^2. This definition is appropriate for children and adults [2]. However, in children younger than 3 months of age, the mean pulmonary artery pressure is typically referenced to the systemic pressure with an abnormal value greater than half the systemic blood pressure.

PH is caused by various diseases leading to vascular remodeling of the small pulmonary arteries with abnormal proliferation of vascular smooth muscle, endothelial cells, and adventitia. PAH is characterized by inflammation, fibrosis, and a proproliferative state with apoptosis resistance [3]. The most common causes in children are idiopathic, previously known as primary pulmonary hypertension, or PH associated with congenital heart disease [2]. There are five categories of PH that are organized based on similar pathology, etiology, and treatment (Table 30.1). Therapy for PH will be briefly discussed later in this chapter [1].

The normal pulmonary circulation is a low pressure low resistance system with a large reserve of low perfused pulmonary capillaries [4,5]. The right ventricle is thin walled and is able to accommodate large changes in volume or preload; however, there is limited contractile reserve to compensate for an increase in impedance or afterload. An increase in afterload will lead to a decrease in right ventricle stroke volume and output. This leads to bulging of the interventricular septum into the left ventricle leading to decrease left ventricular filling and to further decrease left ventricular output [6,7]. An elevation of right ventricular pressure and volume also leads to dilation and thus may cause tricuspid regurgitation, which further reduces forward cardiac output and ultimately end organ perfusion. Right ventricular failure can occur both acutely and chronically. In many patients with chronic PH, the increase in pulmonary vascular resistance occurs gradually in the right ventricle initially hypertrophies (adaptive response). At a later stage the right ventricle begins to fail and dilate with reduced cardiac output and elevated filling pressure (maladaptive response) [8]. The right ventricle is perfused both during diastole and systole because of low wall tension. When pulmonary artery pressure becomes systemic the perfusion of the right ventricle is markedly diminished leading to a spiral decrease in overall cardiac output (Fig. 30.1).

Right heart failure is a clinical syndrome that is characterized by elevated venous pressure and/or decreased delivery of blood to the pulmonary circulation [5]. Right ventricular failure is a major component of right heart failure and occurs when cardiac output and blood pressure drop despite an increase in right ventricular end diastolic pressure. A surrogate for this is an elevation of right atrial pressure leading to an increase central venous pressure.

Heart Failure in the Child and Young Adult. http://dx.doi.org/10.1016/B978-0-12-802393-8.00030-2

TABLE 30.1 Updated Clinical Classification of Pulmonary Hypertension

1. Pulmonary arterial hypertension
   - 1.1 Idiopathic
   - 1.2 Heritable (1.2.1 BMPR2, 1.2.2 ALK-1, ENG, SMAD9, CAV1, KCNK3, 1.2.3 unknown)
   - 1.3 Drug and toxin induced
   - 1.4 Associated (1.4.1 Connective tissue disease, 1.4.2 HIV infection, 1.4.3 Portal hypertension, 1.4.4 Congenital heart diseases, 1.4.5 Schistosomiasis)
   - 1′ Pulmonary veno-occlusive disease/pulmonary capillary hemangiomatosis
   - 1″ Persistent pulmonary hypertension of the newborn
2. Pulmonary hypertension due to left heart disease
   - 2.1 Left ventricular systolic dysfunction
   - 2.2 Left ventricular diastolic dysfunction
   - 2.3 Valvular disease
   - 2.4 Congenital/acquired left heart inflow/outflow tract obstruction, congenital cardiomyopathies
3. Pulmonary hypertension due to lung disease and/or hypoxia
   - 3.1 Chronic obstructive pulmonary disease
   - 3.2 Interstitial lung disease
   - 3.3 Other pulmonary diseases with mixed restrictive and obstructive pattern
   - 3.4 Sleep-disordered breathing
   - 3.5 Alveolar hypoventilation disorders
   - 3.6 Chronic exposure to high altitude
   - 3.7 Developmental lung diseases
4. Chronic thromboembolic pulmonary hypertension
5. Pulmonary hypertension due to unclear multifactorial mechanisms
   - 5.1 Hematologic disorders: chronic hemolytic anemia, myeloproliferative disorders, splenectomy
   - 5.2 Systemic disorders: sarcoidosis, pulmonary histiocytosis, lymphangioleiomyomatosis
   - 5.3 Metabolic disorders: glycogen storage disease, Gaucher disease, thyroid disorders
   - 5.4 Other: tumoral obstruction, fibrosing mediastinitis, chronic renal failure, segmental PH

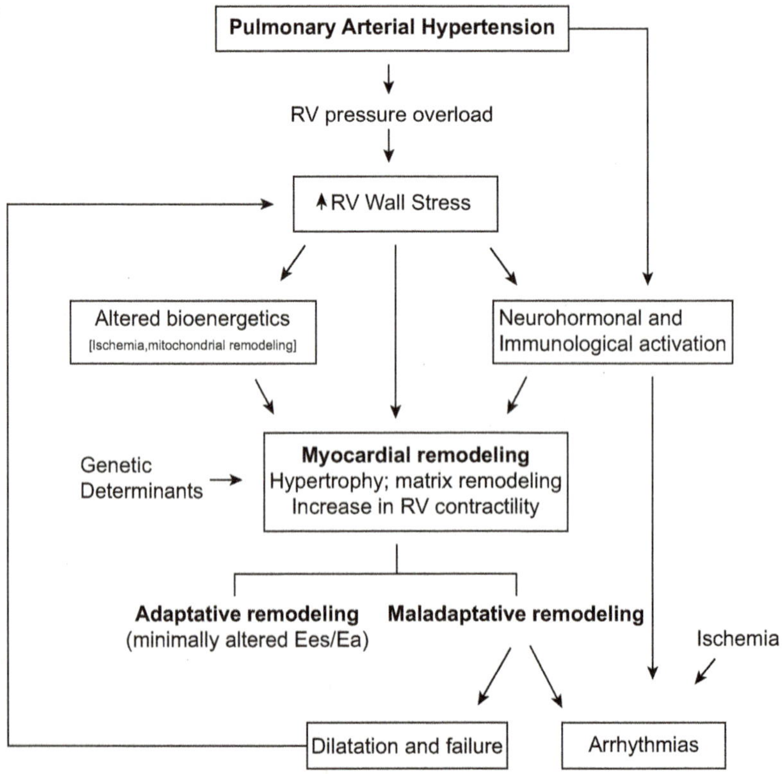

FIGURE 30.1 Pathophysiology of right ventricular (RV) dysfunction in pulmonary arterial hypertension (PAH). Increased (RV) wall stress, neurohormonal activation, inflammation, and altered bioenergetics contribute to RV remodeling in PAH. Adaptive remodeling is associated with minimally altered ventriculoarterial coupling. Progressive RV dilation with maladaptive remodeling further contributes to RV stress. *(From A. Vonk-Noordegraaf, et al., J. Am. Coll. Cardiol. 62 (25 Suppl.) (2013) D22–D33.)*

Right ventricular afterload is measured by the pulmonary input impedance, a sum of pulmonary arterial compliance and pulmonary vascular resistance [9–13]. Normally in pediatric cardiology, pulmonary vascular resistance has been used as the sole measure of right ventricular afterload. Pulmonary vascular resistance (PVR) measures the static component of impedance and compliance measures the dynamic component. It has been increasingly shown that pulmonary artery compliance is crucial to the success of the right ventricle in maintaining cardiac output [14,15]. Compliance of the pulmonary vasculature is determined by the dynamic components of afterload and determines how the blood volume is ejected and can be estimated by the ratio of the stroke volume to pulse pressure. Recent measures of pulmonary vascular input impedance have been shown to have added value in the measure of right ventricular afterload; however, these measures are not frequently used in clinical practice at this time [16–19].

DIAGNOSIS

The classic findings of right heart failure include elevated jugular venous distention with a prominent v wave. Frequently facial, hand, or foot edema is associated. Hepatomegaly and/or splenomegaly is frequently present. Auscultation may reveal a holosystolic murmur of tricuspid regurgitation in addition to a loud pulmonary component of the second heart sound. A right ventricular heave is frequently present. An S3 or S4 gallop may be present. A palpable second heart sound is occasionally present.

The electrocardiogram in PH shows signs of right ventricular hypertrophy but is not present in all cases of PH. Right axis deviation, an R:S wave of greater than 1 in V_1, a deep S wave in V_6 and electrocardiographic signs of right atrial enlargement (P pulmonale) with P wave amplitude greater than 3 mm in leads II, III, and aVF are commonly present. A qR pattern in lead V_1 is pathognomonic of right ventricular hypertrophy.

Many different modalities may aid the clinician in determination of right ventricular function and therefore the cause of right heart failure. These include cardiac catheterization, echocardiography, and cardiac MRI. Cardiac catheterization is mandatory for the diagnosis of PH. Evaluation shows clues of right heart failure by evaluation of cardiac output, right atrial pressure, PVRI, and pulmonary artery pressure. All of the measures are predictors of adverse outcome. In particular, cardiac output and right atrial pressure are better predictors of outcome in PH than pulmonary artery pressure (PAP) alone (Fig. 30.2).

Echocardiography is an important noninvasive technique, which allows for easy and repeatable evaluation of right heart function [20,21]. The difficulty in echocardiographic evaluation of the right ventricle is the crescent/glove shape of the right ventricle, whereas the conical shape of the left ventricle makes evaluation of left ventricular function much easier. Several measures are available to attempt to quantify the degree of RV dysfunction including the Tei index (myocardial performance

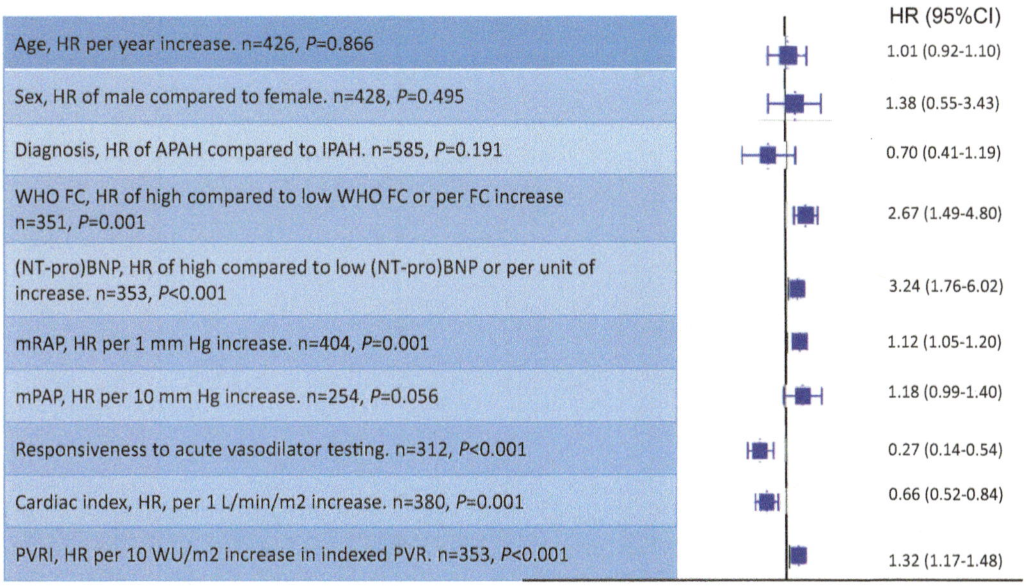

FIGURE 30.2 Metaanalysis of prognostic factors in pediatric PAH. Data are presented as hazard ratio (95% confidence interval). *(NT-pro)BNP*, (N-terminal-pro) brain natriuretic peptide; *APAH*, associated pulmonary arterial hypertension; *CI*, 95% confidence interval; *HR*, hazard ratio; *IPAH*, idiopathic pulmonary arterial hypertension; *mPAP*, mean pulmonary arterial pressure; *mRAP*, mean right atrial pressure; *PVRi*, (indexed) pulmonary vascular resistance; *WHO-FC*, WHO functional class; *WU*, wood units. *(Adapted from M.J. Ploegstra, et al., Int. J. Cardiol. 184 (2015) 198–207.)*

index), RV ejection fraction, RV fractional area change, and the tricuspid annular plane systolic excursion (TAPSE) [22–29]. Normal values for TAPSE in children have recently been published and should serve as a reference for children with PH [25]. The ratio of right ventricle to left ventricle size at end systole is a strong predictor of outcome (Fig. 30.3) [30]. An increasing right ventricle to left ventricle ratio systolic ratio is associated with an increasing hazard for a clinical event (hazard ratio, 2.49; 95% confidence interval, 1.92–3.24). Pulmonic valve insufficiency is frequently seen, and characteristics of the pulmonic regurgitant flow velocity or changes in the systolic flow velocity profile across the pulmonic valve also can be used to estimate noninvasively the pulmonary artery diastolic pressure and the mean pulmonary artery pressure [31]. The presence of a pericardial effusion is rare in children, but when present, suggests a poor prognosis [26,32]. As PH progresses and RV function worsens the systolic duration of the cardiac cycle lengthens leading to an increase in the systolic:diastolic (S:D) ratio. The S:D ratio is higher in PH patients than in controls (1.38 ± 0.61 vs. 0.72 ± 0.16, $P < .001$) and is associated with worse echocardiographic RV fractional area change, worse catheterization hemodynamics, and worse clinical outcomes independent of pulmonary resistance or pressures. As the right ventricle fails, the systolic duration increases and may ultimately impede left ventricular diastolic filling and cardiac output (Fig. 30.4) [29,33,34]. Tissue Doppler imaging (TDI) directly measures myocardial velocities and has been shown to be an accurate measure of RV and LV systolic and diastolic function. In recent pediatric studies, right ventricular TDI velocity was lower in children with PAH compared to healthy controls [35,36]. Moreover, tricuspid diastolic velocity (E′) had significant inverse correlations

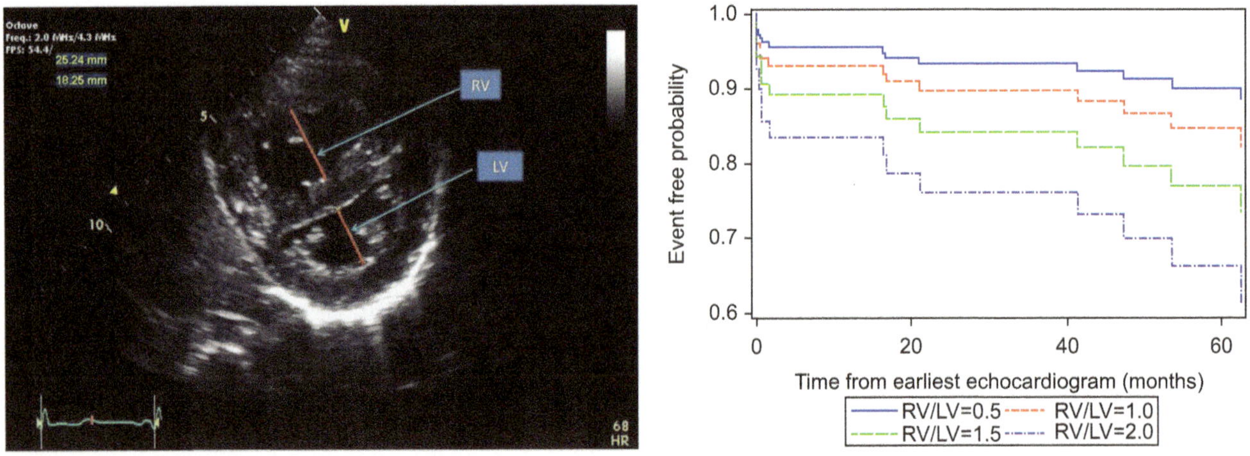

FIGURE 30.3 Parasternal short axis view of the right and left ventricles at the level of the papillary muscles. The right ventricle to left ventricle ratio (RV/LV) ratio is derived from RV diameter and LV diameter at end-systole. RV/LV end systole ratio is predictive of outcome. Estimated survival curves for four possible RV/LV ratios estimated from the Cox varying coefficients regression corresponding to a hazard ratio of 2.49 for RV/LV ratio. *(From Jone, et al., J. Am. Soc. Echocardiogr. 27 (2014) 172–178.)*

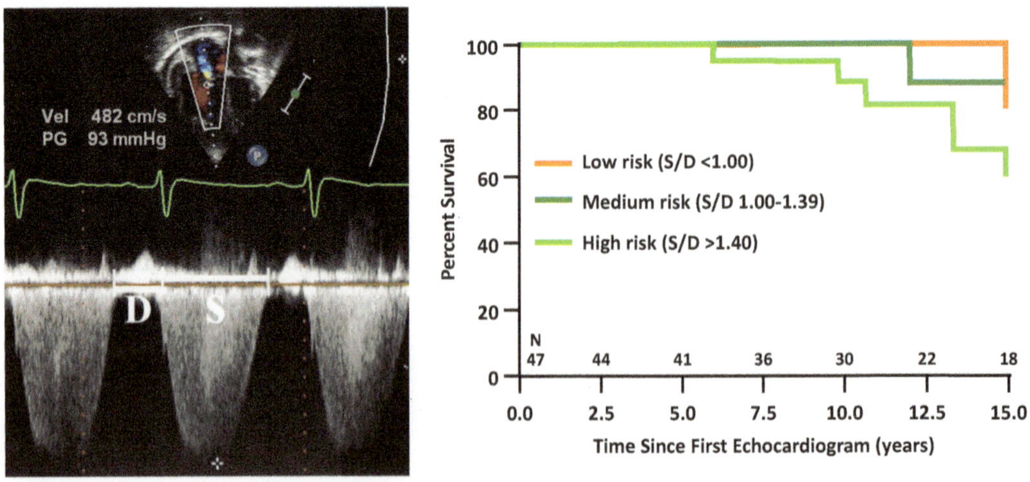

FIGURE 30.4 The systolic (S) to diastolic (D) time ratio from tricuspid regurgitation velocity can be measured as a measure of right ventricular function. An increase in the S/D ratio predicts worse outcome in children with PH. *(From J. Alkon, et al., Am. J. Cardiol. 106 (2010) 430–436.)*

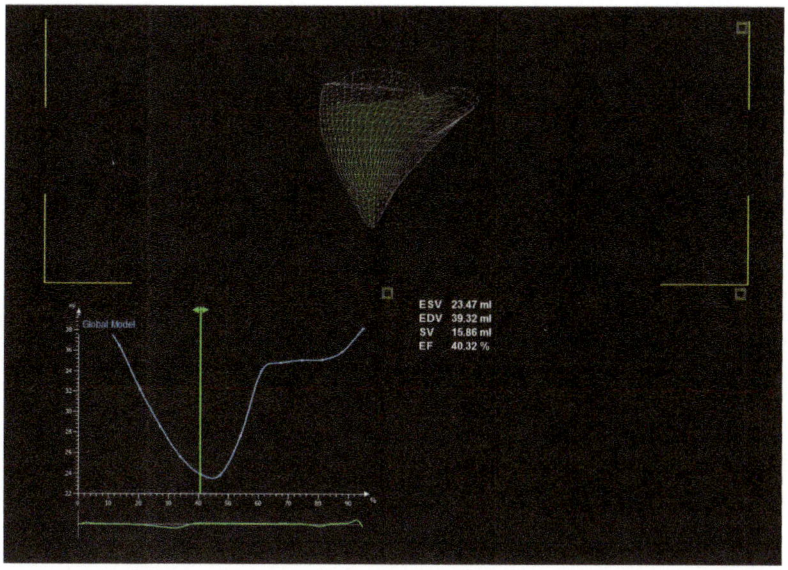

FIGURE 30.5 Real-time three-dimensional measurement of RV end systolic volume (ESV), end diastolic volume (EDV), stroke volume (SV), and ejection fraction (EF). *(Courtesy Dr. Pei-Ni Jone.)*

with right ventricular end-diastolic pressure and mean pulmonary arterial pressure, and cumulative event-free survival rate was significantly lower when tricuspid E′ velocity was ≤8 cm/s (log-rank test, $P<.001$, Fig. 30.10) [36]. The right ventricle contracts primarily in a longitudinal fashion, thus RV longitudinal strain measurement may play an important role in evaluation of RV function. RV longitudinal strain is a powerful tool to predict clinical outcome in adults with PH [37,38]. Finally, real time 3-dimensional echocardiography correlates well with cardiac MRI in children with congenital heart disease [39] and is being evaluated in children with PH (Fig. 30.5).

Cardiac MRI allows for more accurate determination of ventricular volume, mass, ejection fraction, and cardiac output. Further, stroke volume and gadolinium enhancement are important tools to evaluate right heart function. A recent study of 100 children with PH has shown that of the cardiac MRI parameters measured, right ventricular ejection fraction, and left ventricular stroke volume index were most strongly predictive of survival on univariate analysis (2.6- and 2.5-fold increase in mortality for every 1-SD decrease, respectively) [40]. Septal curvature measured by cardiac MRI correlates strongly with mean pulmonary artery pressure at baseline and during vasodilator testing [41]. Gadolinium enhancement at the hinge points of the tricuspid valve has been noted in adults and is likely a poor prognostic indicator; this has not been study in children. In an adult PH study right ventricular ejection fraction was a better predictor of survival than PVR (Fig. 30.6). Changes in right ventricular ejection fraction (HR: 0.929; $P=.014$) were associated with survival, but changes in PVR (HR: 1.000; $P=.820$) were not [42].

MANAGEMENT OF ACUTE RIGHT VENTRICULAR FAILURE

Although right ventricular failure is common in the intensive care unit, there have been no randomized control trials studying different management options. In a patient with acute elevations of pulmonary artery pressure and afterload, there is decreased in right ventricular contractility with right ventricular dilation in an effort to increase RV volume and improve cardiac output by the Frank–Starling mechanism. In patients with chronic PH, the right ventricle compensates with myocardial hypertrophy that reduces wall stress. Despite the hypertrophic mechanism the right ventricle can easily be overwhelmed and result in failure. Right ventricular hypertrophy is associated with an increase in myocardial demand leading to a supply demand mismatch. Thus, patients with chronic PAH who have an upper-respiratory infection, pneumonia, marked changes in preload, or medication noncompliance can rapidly develop right ventricular failure. As these compensatory mechanisms unravel, RV stroke volume continues to decrease leading to an under filled left ventricle with a drop in systemic blood pressure. This leads to a decrease in aortic and coronary perfusion and right ventricular ischemia. This circular abnormality mandates rapid changes in preload, ventricular function, and afterload (Fig. 30.1).

Management of right heart failure is complicated due to the complex interaction between the right ventricle and the left ventricle. The mainstays of treatment for acute RV failure include (1) RV afterload reduction; (2) improvement of RV contractility; (3) maintenance of systemic blood pressure to ensure coronary artery filling and to decrease IVS shift; and (4) maintain adequate but not excessive preload. Both hypovolemia and hypervolemia may impair RV function and perfusion. In many conditions, over aggressive volume administration may lead to worsening right heart failure, right ventricular dilation, and

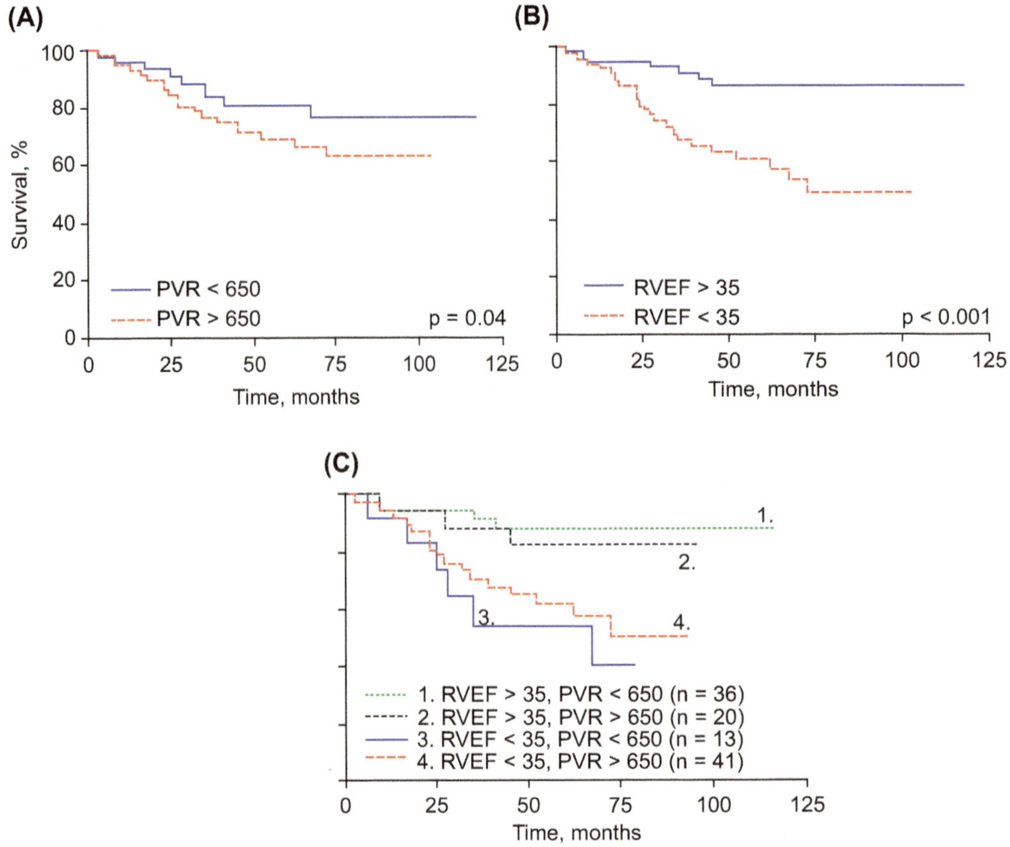

FIGURE 30.6 Survival rates of patients with pulmonary arterial hypertension (PAH) stratified according to pulmonary vascular resistance (PVR) and RVEF at baseline. (A) Patients with (PVR) < 650 dyne s cm^5 showed better survival rates than patients with PVR > 650 dyne s cm^5 (P = .04). (B) Patients with right ventricular ejection fraction (RVEF) > 35% showed better survival rates compared with patients with RVEF < 35% (P < .001). (C) Survival rates based on the coupling of PVR and RVEF. Note preserved RVEF even in the presence of high PVR is associated with improved survival. PAH, pulmonary arterial hypertension. *(From van de Veerdonk, et al., J. Am. Coll. Cardiol. 58 (24) (2011) 2511–2519.)*

impairment of left ventricular output. Adequate right ventricular volume is required, but a too aggressive strategy may impair output. In critical patients, central venous pressure monitoring may provide important clues as to right ventricular filling. The majority of patients with right heart failure will present with fluid overload and require diuretics. Although no optimal value of central venous pressure has been determined a reasonable target of central venous pressure is between 6 and 12 mmHg.

For most patients with acute right heart failure, inotropic medication is a mainstay of therapy. There is no perfect inotropic agent as most inotropes will have effects on the systemic circulation, which may impair right ventricular perfusion. For example, an agent that may lower PAP but also lead to systemic hypotension may decrease coronary profusion, worsen septal shift and thus right ventricular function. In fact, animal models of right heart dysfunction show an improvement in right ventricular output with aortic banding as right ventricular contractile function is partly dependent on left ventricular contractility, likely through shared myofibers between the two ventricles [43,44]. In severe RV failure, the use of high dose milrinone and dobutamine in isolation may lead to clinical worsening. Animal studies have shown improved contractility with a combination of epinephrine/milrinone and dopamine/milrinone compared to dobutamine alone [45]. Limitations of catecholamine agents include a potential increase in pulmonary vascular resistance and detrimental increase in heart rate. An ideal vasoactive agent will increase systemic resistance greater than pulmonary resistance and therefore maintain right coronary profusion. Some centers use vasopressin which increases systemic vascular resistance but may also lower pulmonary vascular resistance by the release of local nitric oxide [46,47].

The normal right ventricle, and even the hypertrophied right ventricle in the patient with PH, responds poorly to acute increases in right ventricular afterload. Therefore, a mainstay of therapy for right heart failure is reduction of right ventricular afterload. Inhaled nitric oxide is a selective pulmonary vasodilator that increases cyclic guanosine monophosphate. It has a short half-life due to inactivation of hemoglobin leading to a selective effect, make it an ideal initial therapy for many patients. Inhaled nitric oxide has been used in many different PH settings, including postoperative congenital heart

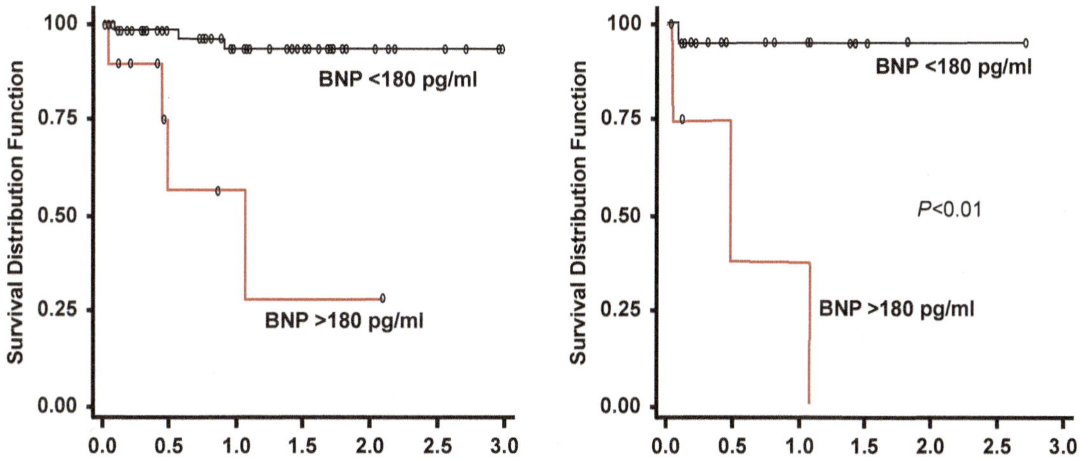

FIGURE 30.7 Kaplan–Meier survival curves for children with idiopathic pulmonary arterial hypertension (IPAH) and PAH associated with congenital heart disease. Survival curves are shown for all patients (left) and for the subgroup of IPAH patients (right) categorized with either brain natriuretic peptide (BNP) >180 or <180pg/mL. *(From A. Bernus, et al., Chest 135 (2009) 745–751.)*

Oral Therapy				Inhaled Therapy	Continuous Parenteral Therapy
ERAs	PDE5 Inhibitors	sGC Stimulator	Prostacyclin	Prostacyclins	
Ambrisentan	Sildenafil	Riociguat	Treprostinil	Iloprost	Epoprostenol (Flolan®)
Bosentan	Tadalafil		Selexipag	Treprostinil	RTS epoprostenol (Veletri®)
Macitentan					Treprostinil (SC or IV)

Note: No PAH-specific medication is FDA approved for use in pediatric populations. All PAH – specific medication use in pediatrics represents off-label use.

FIGURE 30.8 FDA approved pulmonary arterial hypertension-specific treatment options for adults failing acute vasoreactivity testing.

disease, heart transplantation, following left ventricular assist device implantation, and the postanesthetic period. Sildenafil may augment the nitric oxide response and may also facilitate weaning of nitric oxide to prevent rebound PH [48]. Further, PDE-5 inhibitors may also improve right ventricular performance [49].

MANAGEMENT OF CHRONIC RIGHT VENTRICULAR FAILURE

The goals of PH therapy are to improve survival, increase exercise tolerance, and reverse remodeling of the pulmonary vascular obstructive disease. WHO-functional class, N-terminal probrain natriuretic peptide, mean right atrial pressure, baseline PVRI, cardiac index, and acute vasodilator response have been shown consistently reported prognostic factors for outcome in pediatric PAH (Figs. 30.2 and 30.7) [50,51]. Most of these prognostic factors are directly related to right ventricular function. Conventional therapies typically used for heart failure in adults are also used for treatment of the patient with RV failure. Diuretic therapy should be initiated cautiously since patients with PAH are often preload dependent to maintain an optimal cardiac output. Digitalis may be beneficial in patients with overt right-sided cardiac dysfunction and clinical failure, but data are lacking [52].

Further understanding of the vascular biology of the pulmonary circulation has led to three different targeted therapies. These included prostacyclins, which (1) increase cyclic AMP, (2) the endothelin receptor antagonists, which block the endothelin receptors, and (3) the agents that lead to increase cyclic GMP, such as inhaled nitric oxide, or agents that block break down of cyclic GMP (PDE-5 inhibitors) or stimulate soluble guanylate cyclase (Fig. 30.8).

The Nice pediatric PH treatment algorithm was modeled from the 2009 consensus adult PH treatment algorithm and current pediatric experience [53]. The AHA/ATS guidelines modified and updated the Nice World Symposium proceedings [54]. Background therapy with diuretics, oxygen, anticoagulation, and digoxin should be considered on an individual basis. Following the complete evaluation for all causes of pulmonary hypertension, acute vasodilator testing at cardiac catheterization is recommended to help determine therapy.

In children with a positive AVT response, oral calcium channel blockers (CCB) may be initiated [55,56]. Therapy with amlodipine, nifedipine, or diltiazem have been used. Right heart failure is a contraindication to CCB therapy. Lower or higher risk criteria are used to determine initial therapy. Determinants of higher risk in children include clinical evidence of right ventricular failure, progression of symptoms, syncope, WHO functional class III or IV, significantly elevated or rising BNP levels, severe RV enlargement, or dysfunction and a pericardial effusion (Fig. 30.9). Additional hemodynamic parameters that predict higher risk include an elevated mean pulmonary artery pressure to systemic arterial pressure ratio greater than 0.75 [57], right atrial pressure greater than 10 mmHg, and the PVRI greater than 20 Wood units $\times$ m^2 (Fig. 30.9) [58]. Additional high-risk parameters include failure to thrive. In the child with a negative acute vasoreactivity response and lower risk, initiation of oral monotherapy is recommended. Treatment with an endothelin receptor antagonist (bosentan [58–66]; ambrisentan [67,68]; macitentan [69]) or PDE-5 inhibitor (sildenafil [70–77]; tadalafil [78,79]) is the treatment of choice. Little is known about the use of soluble guanylate cyclase stimulators (riociguat) [80], oral prostacyclin (treprostinil) [81,82], and selexipag [83] in children with PH.

Children who deteriorate on either an endothelin rector antagonist or PDE-5 inhibitor agents may benefit from consideration of early combination therapy (add-on or up front). If the child remains in a low-risk category, addition of inhaled prostacyclin (iloprost [84–88]; treprostinil [89,90]) to the background therapy may be beneficial [91]. In higher risk children, initiation of continuous epoprostenol [55,56,87,92–99], or treprostinil [92,94,95,99–101]. In the child deteriorating with high-risk features, early consideration of lung transplantation is important (Fig. 30.10).

PERCUTANEOUS AND SURGICAL INTERVENTIONS

In select patients who have been optimized from a medical standpoint, balloon atrial septostomy may be a viable option. The creation of an atrial shunt is based on early observational studies that suggested that patients with idiopathic PAH and a patent foramen ovale had an improved survival. The use of an atrial septostomy has been used in pediatric cardiology for

LOWER RISK	DETERMINANTS OF RISK	HIGHER RISK
No	Clinical evidence of RV failure	Yes
No	Progression of Symptoms	Yes
No	Syncope	Yes
	Growth	Failure to thrive
I,II	WHO Functional Class	III,IV
Minimally elevated	BNP / NTproBNP	Significantly elevated Rising level
	Echocardiography	Severe RV enlargement/dysfunction Pericardial Effusion
Systemic CI > 3.0 L/min/m^2 mPAP/mSAP < 0.75 Acute Vasoreactivity	Hemodynamics	Systemic CI < 2.5 L/min/m^2 mPAP/mSAP > 0.75 RAP > 10mmHg PVRI > 20 WU*m^2

FIGURE 30.9 Risk factors that should be considered when planning therapeutic management options in pulmonary hypertension. *CI*, cardiac index; *mPAp*, mean pulmonary artery pressure; *mSAp*, mean systemic aortic pressure; *NT-proBNP*, N-terminal-pro-brain natriuretic peptide; *PVRI*, indexed pulmonary vascular resistance; *RAP*, right atrial pressure; *RV*, right ventricle; *SBNP*, serum brain natriuretic peptide. *(From D. Ivy, et al., J. Am. Coll. Cardiol. 62 (2013) D117–D126.)*

over two decades. It is important to note that patient selection is crucial. Patients with evidence of right heart failure with high right atrial pressures may die following performance of an atrial septostomy due to marked hypoxemia. However, using a graded balloon dilation approach, a small fenestration may allow for decompression of the right ventricle and augmented left ventricular preload.

Over the last decade a Potts shunt has been reintroduced to treat a patient with ongoing right heart failure [102–105]. As opposed to a "diastolic pop off," the Potts shunt may allow a "systolic pop off" thus improving right ventricular function (Fig. 30.11). The Potts shunt was initially used for improving pulmonary blood flow in patients with severe tetralogy of Fallot in the 1950s but has been championed by the group in Paris as an important alternative. A further advantage of the Potts shunt is that it may maintain cerebral oxygenation at the expense of peripheral deoxygenation. In contrast, a significant right to left atrial level shunt will lead to hypoxemia of the brain and lower extremities.

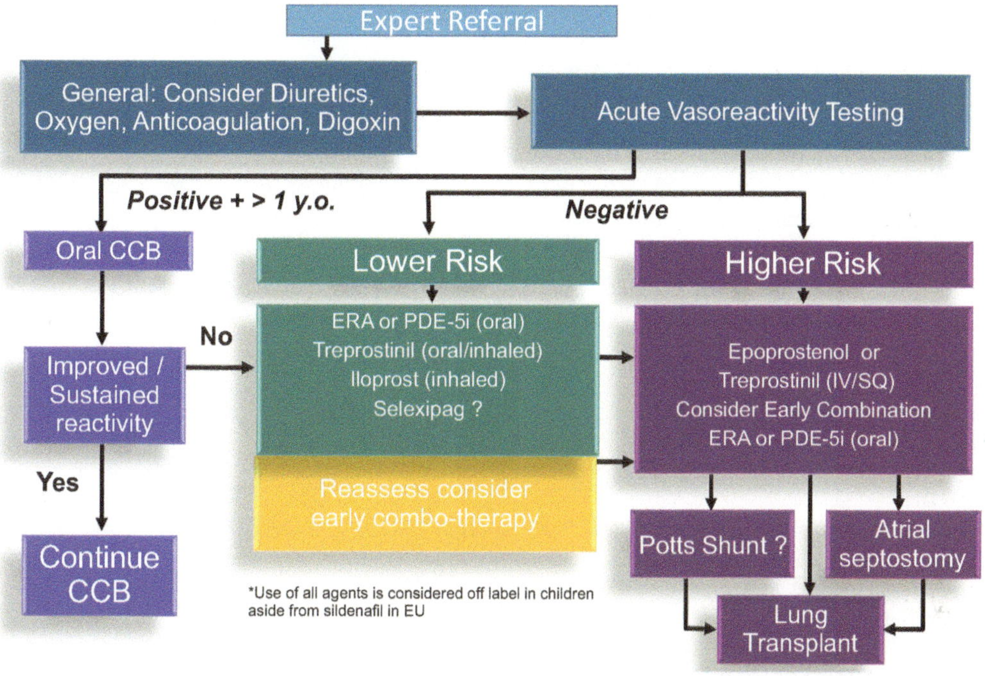

FIGURE 30.10 Treatment algorithm proposed in the management of pediatric patients with idiopathic or heritable pulmonary arterial hypertension. This may be translatable to other patients with pulmonary hypertension. *CCB*, calcium channel blocker; *ERA*, endothelin receptor antagonist; *PDE-5i*, phosphodiesterase 5 inhibitor. *(Adapted from D. Ivy, et al., J. Am. Coll. Cardiol. 62 (2013) D117–D126.)*

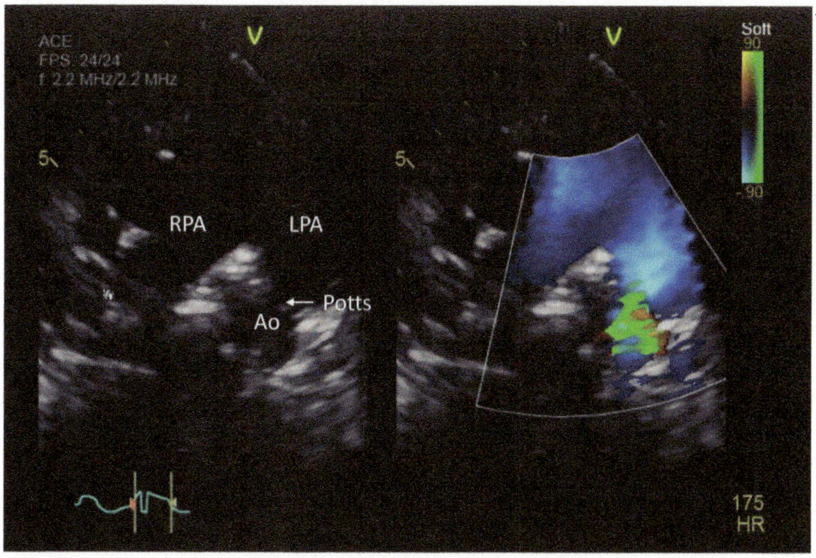

FIGURE 30.11 Echocardiogram with color compare of the Potts shunt in a patient with severe IPAH. *Ao*, aorta; *LPA*, left pulmonary artery; *RPA*, right pulmonary artery.

RIGHT VENTRICULAR ASSIST DEVICES

Failure of medical and other therapies in the patient with right heart failure may lead to the need of mechanical circulatory support. Many different devices and techniques have been performed. Many of these have been used as a bridge to lung transplantation. The classic use of mechanical support in patients with PAH is use of venoarterial extracorporeal membrane oxygenation (ECMO). VA ECMO can be implanted surgically or percutaneous and provide support the failing right ventricle by decompressing the right atrium as well as providing systemic output. Over the last decade the use of a Novalung or similar paracorporeal device has expanded. The Novalung is an external device that uses the patient's own heart function to decompress the pulmonary artery. Blood is removed from the pulmonary artery, sent through an oxygenating filter and is returned through the left atrium. This not only may decompress the right ventricle but also support left ventricular filling. This mode also provides CO_2 removal and limited improvement in oxygenation. Although, a limited number of cases of the NOVALUNG have been used, it may be particularly appealing in those patients waiting for lung transplantation for PH for a prolonged period of time [106,107].

CONCLUSION

The cause of death of many patients with PH is right ventricular dysfunction leading to right heart failure. Understanding of the pathophysiology of right heart failure in the patient with PH and the differences from left heart failure is crucial to determining management strategies. For most patients with PH, there is no cure but novel targeted PH therapies have improved survival. For patients failing conventional therapy, lung transplantation, and/or mechanical circulatory support as a bridge to lung transplantation may be necessary.

REFERENCES

[1] G. Simonneau, M.A. Gatzoulis, I. Adatia, D. Celermajer, C. Denton, A. Ghofrani, et al., Updated clinical classification of pulmonary hypertension, J. Am. Coll. Cardiol. 62 (25 Suppl.) (2013) D34–D41.

[2] D.D. Ivy, S.H. Abman, R.J. Barst, R.M. Berger, D. Bonnet, T.R. Fleming, et al., Pediatric pulmonary hypertension, J. Am. Coll. Cardiol. 62 (25 Suppl.) (2013) D117–D126.

[3] M. Rabinovitch, Pathobiology of pulmonary hypertension, Annu. Rev. Pathol. 2 (2007) 369–399.

[4] R. Naeije, Assessment of right ventricular function in pulmonary hypertension, Curr. Hypertens. Rep. 17 (5) (2015) 35.

[5] A. Vonk-Noordegraaf, F. Haddad, K.M. Chin, P.R. Forfia, S.M. Kawut, J. Lumens, et al., Right heart adaptation to pulmonary arterial hypertension: physiology and pathobiology, J. Am. Coll. Cardiol. 62 (25 Suppl.) (2013) D22–D33.

[6] J. Lumens, T. Arts, J.T. Marcus, A. Vonk-Noordegraaf, T. Delhaas, Early-diastolic left ventricular lengthening implies pulmonary hypertension-induced right ventricular decompensation, Cardiovasc. Res. 96 (2) (2012) 286–295.

[7] F. Sheehan, A. Redington, The right ventricle: anatomy, physiology and clinical imaging, Heart 94 (11) (2008) 1510–1515.

[8] N.F. Voelkel, R.A. Quaife, L.A. Leinwand, R.J. Barst, M.D. McGoon, D.R. Meldrum, et al., Right ventricular function and failure: report of a National Heart, Lung, and Blood Institute working group on cellular and molecular mechanisms of right heart failure, Circulation 114 (17) (2006) 1883–1891.

[9] Z. Su, W. Tan, R. Shandas, K.S. Hunter, Influence of distal resistance and proximal stiffness on hemodynamics and RV afterload in progression and treatments of pulmonary hypertension: a computational study with validation using animal models, Comput. Math. Methods Med. 2013 (2013):618326.

[10] N. Westerhof, J.W. Lankhaar, B.E. Westerhof, The arterial Windkessel, Med. Biol. Eng. Comput. 47 (2) (2009) 131–141.

[11] K.S. Hunter, P.F. Lee, C.J. Lanning, D.D. Ivy, K.S. Kirby, L.R. Claussen, et al., Pulmonary vascular input impedance is a combined measure of pulmonary vascular resistance and stiffness and predicts clinical outcomes better than pulmonary vascular resistance alone in pediatric patients with pulmonary hypertension, Am. Heart J. 155 (1) (2008) 166–174.

[12] K. Dyer, C. Lanning, B. Das, P.F. Lee, D.D. Ivy, L. Valdes-Cruz, et al., Noninvasive Doppler tissue measurement of pulmonary artery compliance in children with pulmonary hypertension, J. Am. Soc. Echocardiogr. 19 (4) (2006) 403–412.

[13] C.E. Weinberg, J.R. Hertzberg, D.D. Ivy, K.S. Kirby, K.C. Chan, L. Valdes-Cruz, et al., Extraction of pulmonary vascular compliance, pulmonary vascular resistance, and right ventricular work from single-pressure and Doppler flow measurements in children with pulmonary hypertension: a new method for evaluating reactivity: in vitro and clinical studies, Circulation 110 (17) (2004) 2609–2617.

[14] T. Thenappan, K.W. Prins, M.R. Pritzker, J. Scandurra, K. Volmers, E.K. Weir, The critical role of pulmonary arterial compliance in pulmonary hypertension, Ann. Am. Thorac. Soc. 13 (2) (2016) 276–284.

[15] J.M. Douwes, M.T. Roofthooft, B. Bartelds, M.D. Talsma, H.L. Hillege, R.M. Berger, Pulsatile haemodynamic parameters are predictors of survival in paediatric pulmonary arterial hypertension, Int. J. Cardiol. 168 (2) (2013) 1370–1377.

[16] I. Sajan, C. Manlhiot, J. Reyes, B.W. McCrindle, T. Humpl, M.K. Friedberg, Pulmonary arterial capacitance in children with idiopathic pulmonary arterial hypertension and pulmonary arterial hypertension associated with congenital heart disease: relation to pulmonary vascular resistance, exercise capacity, and survival, Am. Heart J. 162 (3) (2011) 562–568.

[17] M.K. Friedberg, J.A. Feinstein, D.N. Rosenthal, Noninvasive assessment of pulmonary arterial capacitance by echocardiography, J. Am. Soc. Echocardiogr. 20 (2) (2007) 186–190.

[18] S. Mahapatra, R.A. Nishimura, P. Sorajja, S. Cha, M.D. McGoon, Relationship of pulmonary arterial capacitance and mortality in idiopathic pulmonary arterial hypertension, J. Am. Coll. Cardiol. 47 (4) (2006) 799–803.

[19] S. Mahapatra, R.A. Nishimura, J.K. Oh, M.D. McGoon, The prognostic value of pulmonary vascular capacitance determined by Doppler echocardiography in patients with pulmonary arterial hypertension, J. Am. Soc. Echocardiogr. 19 (8) (2006) 1045–1050.

[20] L.L. Mertens, M.K. Friedberg, Imaging the right ventricle–current state of the art, Nat. Rev. Cardiol. 7 (10) (2010) 551–563.

[21] L.G. Rudski, W.W. Lai, J. Afilalo, L. Hua, M.D. Handschumacher, K. Chandrasekaran, et al., Guidelines for the echocardiographic assessment of the right heart in adults: a report from the American Society of Echocardiography endorsed by the European Association of Echocardiography, a registered branch of the European Society of Cardiology, and the Canadian Society of Echocardiography, J. Am. Soc. Echocardiogr. 23 (7) (2010) 685–713 quiz 86–88.

[22] P.R. Forfia, M.R. Fisher, S.C. Mathai, T. Housten-Harris, A.R. Hemnes, B.A. Borlaug, et al., Tricuspid annular displacement predicts survival in pulmonary hypertension, Am. J. Respir. Crit. Care Med. 174 (9) (2006) 1034–1041.

[23] N. Galie, A.L. Hinderliter, A. Torbicki, T. Fourme, G. Simonneau, T. Pulido, et al., Effects of the oral endothelin-receptor antagonist bosentan on echocardiographic and doppler measures in patients with pulmonary arterial hypertension, J. Am. Coll. Cardiol. 41 (8) (2003) 1380–1386.

[24] A.L. Hinderliter, W. PWt, R.J. Barst, S. Rich, L.J. Rubin, D.B. Badesch, et al., Effects of long-term infusion of prostacyclin (epoprostenol) on echocardiographic measures of right ventricular structure and function in primary pulmonary hypertension. Primary Pulmonary Hypertension Study Group, Circulation 95 (6) (1997) 1479–1486.

[25] M. Koestenberger, W. Ravekes, A.D. Everett, H.P. Stueger, B. Heinzl, A. Gamillscheg, et al., Right ventricular function in infants, children and adolescents: reference values of the tricuspid annular plane systolic excursion (TAPSE) in 640 healthy patients and calculation of z score values, J. Am. Soc. Echocardiogr. 22 (6) (2009) 715–719.

[26] R.J. Raymond, A.L. Hinderliter, P.W. Willis, D. Ralph, E.J. Caldwell, W. Williams, et al., Echocardiographic predictors of adverse outcomes in primary pulmonary hypertension, J. Am. Coll. Cardiol. 39 (7) (2002) 1214–1219.

[27] C. Tei, K.S. Dujardin, D.O. Hodge, K.R. Bailey, M.D. McGoon, A.J. Tajik, et al., Doppler echocardiographic index for assessment of global right ventricular function, J. Am. Soc. Echocardiogr. 9 (6) (1996) 838–847.

[28] K.L. Dyer, L.B. Pauliks, B. Das, R. Shandas, D. Ivy, E.M. Shaffer, et al., Use of myocardial performance index in pediatric patients with idiopathic pulmonary arterial hypertension, J. Am. Soc. Echocardiogr. 19 (1) (2006) 21–27.

[29] E. Kassem, T. Humpl, M.K. Friedberg, Prognostic significance of 2-dimensional, M-mode, and Doppler echo indices of right ventricular function in children with pulmonary arterial hypertension, Am. Heart J. 165 (6) (2013) 1024–1031.

[30] P.N. Jone, J. Hinzman, B.D. Wagner, D.D. Ivy, A. Younoszai, Right ventricular to left ventricular diameter ratio at end-systole in evaluating outcomes in children with pulmonary hypertension, J. Am. Soc. Echocardiogr. 27 (2) (2014) 172–178.

[31] T. Masuyama, K. Kodama, A. Kitabatake, H. Sato, S. Nanto, M. Inoue, Continuous-wave Doppler echocardiographic detection of pulmonary regurgitation and its application to noninvasive estimation of pulmonary artery pressure, Circulation 74 (3) (1986) 484–492.

[32] R.L. Benza, D.P. Miller, M. Gomberg-Maitland, R.P. Frantz, A.J. Foreman, C.S. Coffey, et al., Predicting survival in pulmonary arterial hypertension: insights from the registry to evaluate early and long-term pulmonary arterial hypertension disease management (REVEAL), Circulation 122 (2) (2010) 164–172.

[33] J. Alkon, T. Humpl, C. Manlhiot, B.W. McCrindle, J.T. Reyes, M.K. Friedberg, Usefulness of the right ventricular systolic to diastolic duration ratio to predict functional capacity and survival in children with pulmonary arterial hypertension, Am. J. Cardiol. 106 (3) (2010) 430–436.

[34] M.K. Friedberg, A.N. Redington, Right versus left ventricular failure: differences, similarities, and interactions, Circulation 129 (9) (2014) 1033–1044.

[35] A.E. Lammers, S.G. Haworth, G. Riley, K. Maslin, G.P. Diller, J. Marek, Value of tissue Doppler echocardiography in children with pulmonary hypertension, J. Am. Soc. Echocardiogr. 25 (5) (2012) 504–510.

[36] S. Takatsuki, T. Nakayama, P.N. Jone, B.D. Wagner, K. Naoi, D.D. Ivy, et al., Tissue Doppler imaging predicts adverse outcome in children with idiopathic pulmonary arterial hypertension, J. Pediatr. 161 (6) (2012) 1126–1131.

[37] K. Ozawa, N. Funabashi, H. Takaoka, N. Tanabe, N. Yanagawa, K. Tatsumi, et al., Utility of three-dimensional global longitudinal strain of the right ventricle using transthoracic echocardiography for right ventricular systolic function in pulmonary hypertension, Int. J. Cardiol. 174 (2) (2014) 426–430.

[38] N.M. Fine, L. Chen, P.M. Bastiansen, R.P. Frantz, P.A. Pellikka, J.K. Oh, et al., Outcome prediction by quantitative right ventricular function assessment in 575 subjects evaluated for pulmonary hypertension, Circ. Cardiovasc. Imaging 6 (5) (2013) 711–721.

[39] X. Lu, V. Nadvoretskiy, L. Bu, A. Stolpen, N. Ayres, R.H. Pignatelli, et al., Accuracy and reproducibility of real-time three-dimensional echocardiography for assessment of right ventricular volumes and ejection fraction in children, J. Am. Soc. Echocardiogr. 21 (1) (2008) 84–89.

[40] S. Moledina, B. Pandya, M. Bartsota, K.H. Mortensen, M. McMillan, S. Quyam, et al., Prognostic significance of cardiac magnetic resonance imaging in children with pulmonary hypertension, Circ. Cardiovasc. Imaging 6 (3) (2013) 407–414.

[41] B. Pandya, M.A. Quail, J.A. Steeden, A. McKee, F. Odille, A.M. Taylor, et al., Real-time magnetic resonance assessment of septal curvature accurately tracks acute hemodynamic changes in pediatric pulmonary hypertension, Circ. Cardiovasc. Imaging 7 (4) (2014) 706–713.

[42] M.C. van de Veerdonk, T. Kind, J.T. Marcus, G.J. Mauritz, M.W. Heymans, H.J. Bogaard, et al., Progressive right ventricular dysfunction in patients with pulmonary arterial hypertension responding to therapy, J. Am. Coll. Cardiol. 58 (24) (2011) 2511–2519.

[43] I. Belenkie, S.G. Horne, R. Dani, E.R. Smith, J.V. Tyberg, Effects of aortic constriction during experimental acute right ventricular pressure loading. Further insights into diastolic and systolic ventricular interaction, Circulation 92 (3) (1995) 546–554.

[44] C. Apitz, O. Honjo, T. Humpl, J. Li, R.S. Assad, M.Y. Cho, et al., Biventricular structural and functional responses to aortic constriction in a rabbit model of chronic right ventricular pressure overload, J. Thorac. Cardiovasc. Surg. 144 (6) (2012) 1494–1501.
[45] J.A. Hyldebrandt, C.A. Frederiksen, J. Heiberg, S. Rothmann, A.N. Redington, M.R. Schmidt, et al., Inotropic therapy for right ventricular failure in newborn piglets: effect on contractility, hemodynamics, and interventricular interaction, Pediatr. Crit. Care Med. 15 (7) (2014) e327–e333.
[46] J. Grinstein, M. Gomberg-Maitland, Management of pulmonary hypertension and right heart failure in the intensive care unit, Curr. Hypertens. Rep. 17 (5) (2015) 32.
[47] C.A. Kholdani, W.H. Fares, Management of right heart failure in the intensive care unit, Clin. Chest Med. 36 (3) (2015) 511–520.
[48] R.H. Steinhorn, J.P. Kinsella, C. Pierce, G. Butrous, M. Dilleen, M. Oakes, et al., Intravenous sildenafil in the treatment of neonates with persistent pulmonary hypertension, J. Pediatr. 155 (6) (2009) 841–847.e1.
[49] J. Nagendran, S.L. Archer, D. Soliman, V. Gurtu, R. Moudgil, A. Haromy, et al., Phosphodiesterase type 5 is highly expressed in the hypertrophied human right ventricle, and acute inhibition of phosphodiesterase type 5 improves contractility, Circulation 116 (3) (2007) 238–248.
[50] M.J. Ploegstra, W.M. Zijlstra, J.M. Douwes, H.L. Hillege, R.M. Berger, Prognostic factors in pediatric pulmonary arterial hypertension: a systematic review and meta-analysis, Int. J. Cardiol. 184 (2015) 198–207.
[51] A. Bernus, B.D. Wagner, F. Accurso, A. Doran, H. Kaess, D.D. Ivy, Brain natriuretic peptide levels in managing pediatric patients with pulmonary arterial hypertension, Chest 135 (3) (2009) 745–751.
[52] S. Rich, M. Seidlitz, E. Dodin, D. Osimani, D. Judd, D. Genthner, et al., The short-term effects of digoxin in patients with right ventricular dysfunction from pulmonary hypertension, Chest 114 (3) (1998) 787–792.
[53] V.V. McLaughlin, S.L. Archer, D.B. Badesch, R.J. Barst, H.W. Farber, J.R. Lindner, et al., ACCF/AHA 2009 expert consensus document on pulmonary hypertension a report of the American College of Cardiology Foundation Task Force on Expert Consensus Documents and the American Heart Association developed in collaboration with the American College of Chest Physicians, American Thoracic Society, Inc., and the Pulmonary Hypertension Association, J. Am. Coll. Cardiol. 53 (17) (2009) 1573–1619.
[54] S.H. Abman, G. Hansmann, S.L. Archer, D.D. Ivy, I. Adatia, W.K. Chung, et al., Pediatric pulmonary hypertension: guidelines from the American Heart Association and American Thoracic Society, Circulation 132 (21) (2015) 2037–2099.
[55] R.J. Barst, G. Maislin, A.P. Fishman, Vasodilator therapy for primary pulmonary hypertension in children, Circulation 99 (9) (1999) 1197–1208.
[56] D. Yung, A.C. Widlitz, E.B. Rosenzweig, D. Kerstein, G. Maislin, R.J. Barst, Outcomes in children with idiopathic pulmonary arterial hypertension, Circulation 110 (6) (2004) 660–665.
[57] J.M. Douwes, R.L. van Loon, E.S. Hoendermis, A. Vonk-Noordegraaf, M.T. Roofthooft, M.D. Talsma, et al., Acute pulmonary vasodilator response in paediatric and adult pulmonary arterial hypertension: occurrence and prognostic value when comparing three response criteria, Eur. Heart J. 32 (24) (2011) 3137–3146.
[58] D.D. Ivy, E.B. Rosenzweig, J.C. Lemarie, M. Brand, D. Rosenberg, R.J. Barst, Long-term outcomes in children with pulmonary arterial hypertension treated with bosentan in real-world clinical settings, Am. J. Cardiol. 106 (9) (2010) 1332–1338.
[59] R.J. Barst, D. Ivy, J. Dingemanse, A. Widlitz, K. Schmitt, A. Doran, et al., Pharmacokinetics, safety, and efficacy of bosentan in pediatric patients with pulmonary arterial hypertension, Clin. Pharmacol. Ther. 73 (4) (2003) 372–382.
[60] M. Beghetti, Bosentan in pediatric patients with pulmonary arterial hypertension, Curr. Vasc. Pharmacol. 7 (2) (2009) 225–233.
[61] M. Beghetti, S.G. Haworth, D. Bonnet, R.J. Barst, P. Acar, A. Fraisse, et al., Pharmacokinetic and clinical profile of a novel formulation of bosentan in children with pulmonary arterial hypertension: the FUTURE-1 study, Br. J. Clin. Pharmacol. 68 (6) (2009) 948–955.
[62] M. Beghetti, M.M. Hoeper, D.G. Kiely, J. Carlsen, B. Schwierin, E.S. Segal, et al., Safety experience with bosentan in 146 children 2–11 years old with pulmonary arterial hypertension: results from the European Postmarketing Surveillance program, Pediatr. Res. 64 (2) (2008) 200–204.
[63] N. Galie, M. Beghetti, M.A. Gatzoulis, J. Granton, R.M. Berger, A. Lauer, et al., Bosentan therapy in patients with Eisenmenger syndrome: a multicenter, double-blind, randomized, placebo-controlled study, Circulation 114 (1) (2006) 48–54.
[64] A.A. Hislop, S. Moledina, H. Foster, I. Schulze-Neick, S.G. Haworth, Long-term efficacy of bosentan in treatment of pulmonary arterial hypertension in children, Eur. Respir. J. 38 (1) (2011) 70–77.
[65] S. Maiya, A.A. Hislop, Y. Flynn, S.G. Haworth, Response to bosentan in children with pulmonary hypertension, Heart 92 (5) (2006) 664–670.
[66] E.B. Rosenzweig, D.D. Ivy, A. Widlitz, A. Doran, L.R. Claussen, D. Yung, et al., Effects of long-term bosentan in children with pulmonary arterial hypertension, J. Am. Coll. Cardiol. 46 (4) (2005) 697–704.
[67] S. Takatsuki, E.B. Rosenzweig, W. Zuckerman, D. Brady, M. Calderbank, D.D. Ivy, Clinical safety, pharmacokinetics, and efficacy of ambrisentan therapy in children with pulmonary arterial hypertension, Pediatr. Pulmonol. 48 (1) (2013) 27–34.
[68] W.A. Zuckerman, D. Leaderer, C.A. Rowan, J.D. Mituniewicz, E.B. Rosenzweig, Ambrisentan for pulmonary arterial hypertension due to congenital heart disease, Am. J. Cardiol. 107 (9) (2011) 1381–1385.
[69] T. Pulido, I. Adzerikho, R.N. Channick, M. Delcroix, N. Galie, H.A. Ghofrani, et al., Macitentan and morbidity and mortality in pulmonary arterial hypertension, N. Engl. J. Med. 369 (9) (2013) 809–818.
[70] S.H. Abman, J.P. Kinsella, E.B. Rosenzweig, U. Krishnan, T. Kulik, M. Mullen, et al., Implications of the U.S. Food and Drug Administration warning against the use of sildenafil for the treatment of pediatric pulmonary hypertension, Am. J. Respir. Crit. Care Med. 187 (6) (2013) 572–575.
[71] D. Abrams, I. Schulze-Neick, A.G. Magee, Sildenafil as a selective pulmonary vasodilator in childhood primary pulmonary hypertension, Heart 84 (2) (2000) E4.
[72] C. Apitz, J.T. Reyes, H. Holtby, T. Humpl, A.N. Redington, Pharmacokinetic and hemodynamic responses to oral sildenafil during invasive testing in children with pulmonary hypertension, J. Am. Coll. Cardiol. 55 (14) (2010) 1456–1462.

[73] R.J. Barst, D.D. Ivy, G. Gaitan, A. Szatmari, A. Rudzinski, A.E. Garcia, et al., A randomized, double-blind, placebo-controlled, dose-ranging study of oral sildenafil citrate in treatment-naive children with pulmonary arterial hypertension, Circulation 125 (2) (2012) 324–334.
[74] R.J. Barst, M. Beghetti, T. Pulido, G. Layton, I. Konourina, M. Zhang, et al., STARTS-2: long-term survival with oral Sildenafil monotherapy in treatment-naive pediatric pulmonary arterial hypertension, Circulation 129 (19) (2014) 1914–1923.
[75] T. Humpl, J.T. Reyes, S. Erickson, R. Armano, H. Holtby, I. Adatia, Sildenafil therapy for neonatal and childhood pulmonary hypertensive vascular disease, Cardiol. Young 21 (2) (2011) 187–193.
[76] T. Humpl, J.T. Reyes, H. Holtby, D. Stephens, I. Adatia, Beneficial effect of oral sildenafil therapy on childhood pulmonary arterial hypertension: twelve-month clinical trial of a single-drug, open-label, pilot study, Circulation 111 (24) (2005) 3274–3280.
[77] A.A. Karatza, A. Bush, A.G. Magee, Safety and efficacy of sildenafil therapy in children with pulmonary hypertension, Int. J. Cardiol. 100 (2) (2005) 267–273.
[78] E.B. Rosenzweig, Tadalafil for the treatment of pulmonary arterial hypertension, Expert Opin. Pharmacother. 11 (1) (2010) 127–132.
[79] S. Takatsuki, M. Calderbank, D.D. Ivy, Initial experience with tadalafil in pediatric pulmonary arterial hypertension, Pediatr. Cardiol. 33 (5) (2012) 683–688.
[80] H.A. Ghofrani, A.M. D'Armini, F. Grimminger, M.M. Hoeper, P. Jansa, N.H. Kim, et al., Riociguat for the treatment of chronic thromboembolic pulmonary hypertension, N. Engl. J. Med. 369 (4) (2013) 319–329.
[81] V.F. Tapson, Z.C. Jing, K.F. Xu, L. Pan, J. Feldman, D.G. Kiely, et al., Oral treprostinil for the treatment of pulmonary arterial hypertension in patients receiving background endothelin receptor antagonist and phosphodiesterase type 5 inhibitor therapy (the FREEDOM-C2 study): a randomized controlled trial, Chest 144 (3) (2013) 952–958.
[82] Z.C. Jing, K. Parikh, T. Pulido, C. Jerjes-Sanchez, R.J. White, R. Allen, et al., Efficacy and safety of oral treprostinil monotherapy for the treatment of pulmonary arterial hypertension: a randomized, controlled trial, Circulation 127 (5) (2013) 624–633.
[83] O. Sitbon, R. Channick, K.M. Chin, A. Frey, S. Gaine, N. Galie, et al., Selexipag for the treatment of pulmonary arterial hypertension, N. Engl. J. Med. 373 (26) (2015) 2522–2533.
[84] D.D. Ivy, Prostacyclin in the intensive care setting, Pediatr. Crit. Care Med. 11 (2 Suppl.) (2010) S41–S45.
[85] D.D. Ivy, A.K. Doran, K.J. Smith, G.B. Mallory Jr., M. Beghetti, R.J. Barst, et al., Short- and long-term effects of inhaled iloprost therapy in children with pulmonary arterial hypertension, J. Am. Coll. Cardiol. 51 (2) (2008) 161–169.
[86] A. Limsuwan, S. Wanitkul, A. Khosithset, S. Attanavanich, P. Samankatiwat, Aerosolized iloprost for postoperative pulmonary hypertensive crisis in children with congenital heart disease, Int. J. Cardiol. 129 (3) (October 13, 2008) 333–338.
[87] L. Melnick, R.J. Barst, C.A. Rowan, D. Kerstein, E.B. Rosenzweig, Effectiveness of transition from intravenous epoprostenol to oral/inhaled targeted pulmonary arterial hypertension therapy in pediatric idiopathic and familial pulmonary arterial hypertension, Am. J. Cardiol. 105 (10) (2010) 1485–1489.
[88] C. Tissot, M. Beghetti, Review of inhaled iloprost for the control of pulmonary artery hypertension in children, Vasc. Health Risk Manag. 5 (1) (2009) 325–331.
[89] U. Krishnan, D.D. Ivy, S. Takatsuki, J. Kerstein, M. Calderbank, E.B. Rosenzweig, Effectiveness and safety of inhaled treprostinil for the treatment of pulmonary arterial hypertension in children, Am. J. Cardiol. 110 (11) (2012) 1704–1709.
[90] S. Takatsuki, D.K. Parker, A.K. Doran, R.H. Friesen, D.D. Ivy, Acute pulmonary vasodilator testing with inhaled treprostinil in children with pulmonary arterial hypertension, Pediatr. Cardiol. 34 (4) (2013) 1006–1012.
[91] W.M. Zijlstra, J.M. Douwes, E.B. Rosenzweig, S. Schokker, U. Krishnan, M.T. Roofthooft, et al., Survival differences in pediatric pulmonary arterial hypertension: clues to a better understanding of outcome and optimal treatment strategies, J. Am. Coll. Cardiol. 63 (20) (2014) 2159–2169.
[92] A.K. Doran, D.D. Ivy, R.J. Barst, N. Hill, S. Murali, R.L. Benza, Guidelines for the prevention of central venous catheter-related blood stream infections with prostanoid therapy for pulmonary arterial hypertension, Int. J. Clin. Pract. Suppl. 160 (2008) 5–9.
[93] S.G. Haworth, A.A. Hislop, Treatment and survival in children with pulmonary arterial hypertension: the UK Pulmonary Hypertension Service for Children 2001–2006, Heart 95 (4) (2009) 312–317.
[94] D.D. Ivy, M. Calderbank, B.D. Wagner, S. Dolan, A.C. Nyquist, M. Wade, et al., Closed-hub systems with protected connections and the reduction of risk of catheter-related bloodstream infection in pediatric patients receiving intravenous prostanoid therapy for pulmonary hypertension, Infect. Control Hosp. Epidemiol. 30 (9) (2009) 823–829.
[95] D.D. Ivy, L. Claussen, A. Doran, Transition of stable pediatric patients with pulmonary arterial hypertension from intravenous epoprostenol to intravenous treprostinil, Am. J. Cardiol. 99 (5) (2007) 696–698.
[96] D.D. Ivy, A. Doran, L. Claussen, D. Bingaman, A. Yetman, Weaning and discontinuation of epoprostenol in children with idiopathic pulmonary arterial hypertension receiving concomitant bosentan, Am. J. Cardiol. 93 (7) (2004) 943–946.
[97] A.E. Lammers, A.A. Hislop, Y. Flynn, S.G. Haworth, Epoprostenol treatment in children with severe pulmonary hypertension, Heart 93 (6) (2007) 739–743.
[98] E.B. Rosenzweig, D. Kerstein, R.J. Barst, Long-term prostacyclin for pulmonary hypertension with associated congenital heart defects, Circulation 99 (14) (1999) 1858–1865.
[99] S.L. Siehr, D.D. Ivy, K. Miller-Reed, M. Ogawa, D.N. Rosenthal, J.A. Feinstein, Children with pulmonary arterial hypertension and prostanoid therapy: long-term hemodynamics, J. Heart Lung Transplant. 32 (5) (2013) 546–552.
[100] Bloodstream infections among patients treated with intravenous epoprostenol or intravenous treprostinil for pulmonary arterial hypertension–seven sites, United States, 2003–2006, MMWR Morb. Mortal. Wkly. Rep. 56 (8) (2007) 170–172.

[101] M. Levy, D.S. Celermajer, E. Bourges-Petit, M.J. Del Cerro, F. Bajolle, D. Bonnet, Add-on therapy with subcutaneous treprostinil for refractory pediatric pulmonary hypertension, J. Pediatr. 158 (4) (2011) 584–588.
[102] R.M. Grady, P. Eghtesady, Potts shunt and pediatric pulmonary hypertension: what we have learned, Ann. Thorac. Surg. 101 (4) (2015) 1539–1543.
[103] A.E. Baruteau, E. Belli, Y. Boudjemline, D. Laux, M. Levy, G. Simonneau, et al., Palliative Potts shunt for the treatment of children with drug-refractory pulmonary arterial hypertension: updated data from the first 24 patients, Eur. J. Cardiothorac. Surg. 47 (3) (2015) e105–e110.
[104] A.E. Baruteau, A. Serraf, M. Levy, J. Petit, D. Bonnet, X. Jais, et al., Potts shunt in children with idiopathic pulmonary arterial hypertension: long-term results, Ann. Thorac. Surg. 94 (3) (2012) 817–824.
[105] J. Blanc, P. Vouhe, D. Bonnet, Potts shunt in patients with pulmonary hypertension, N. Engl. J. Med. 350 (6) (2004) 623.
[106] D.M. Hoganson, A.Z. Gazit, U.S. Boston, S.C. Sweet, R.M. Grady, C.B. Huddleston, et al., Paracorporeal lung assist devices as a bridge to recovery or lung transplantation in neonates and young children, J. Thorac. Cardiovasc. Surg. 147 (1) (2014) 420–426.
[107] T.N. Machuca, M. de Perrot, Mechanical support for the failing right ventricle in patients with precapillary pulmonary hypertension, Circulation 132 (6) (2015) 526–536.

Chapter 31

Childhood Cardiorenal Syndrome

Ahmad Kaddourah[1,2], Stuart L. Goldstein[2]
[1]*Sidra Medical and Research Center, Doha, Qatar;* [2]*Cincinnati Children's Hospital Medical Center (CCHMC), Cincinnati, OH, United States*

INTRODUCTION

Organ cross talk is a biological concept that refers to different feedback pathways used by organs to communicate and incite physiologic or pathologic alterations in the function of other organs [1]. Cardiorenal syndrome (CRS) is one example of organ cross talk concept where acute or chronic reduced function of either the heart or kidney induces acute or chronic pathologic changes in the other organ [2]. Despite being described initially in the 1980s [3], the heart–kidney interaction was not formalized as a clinical entity until 2004 when the National Heart, Lung, and Blood Institute Working group introduced the CRS term [4]. The initial definition of CRS was as a state in which therapy to relieve heart failure symptoms was limited by worsening renal function. This primary definition of CRS raised many concerns about the accuracy of limiting the CRS definition to kidney dysfunction as a direct consequence of impaired renal blood flow in the setting of depressed left ventricular systolic function [5]. With the growing knowledge emphasizing the bidirectional cross talk between the failing heart and kidneys, the primary definition contradicted the pathophysiologic nature of CRS. Several groups have suggested that the CRS definition should be broadened to stress that each dysfunctional organ has the ability to initiate and perpetuate disease in the other organ through hemodynamic, neurohormonal, immunologic, and biochemical feedback pathways. In response to fill this gap, the Acute Dialysis Quality Initiative (ADQI) Group proposed that the term CRS be used to define different acute or chronic clinical conditions in which heart and kidney dysfunction overlap [6]. Accordingly, ADQI Working Group suggested classifying CRS into five types based on the primary involved organ and the chronicity of this involvement as shown in Table 31.1.

In this chapter, we will adopt the ADQI classification of CRS to review the current literature to highlight the significance of heart–kidney interactions in children and adolescents. Secondary CRS, or type-5 CRS, review is beyond the scope of this chapter.

CHILDHOOD TYPE-1 CARDIORENAL SYNDROME

Definition and Epidemiology

Type-1 CRS, or acute CRS, is defined as acute cardiac dysfunction leading to acute kidney injury (AKI). AKI has traditionally been used to describe an abrupt decline in renal function, however, a standardized definition for this condition did not exist until 2004 when the ADQI Group, recognizing the inconsistency of describing AKI in the literature, developed the first standardized multidimensional criteria, known as risk, injury, failure, loss and end-stage kidney disease (RIFLE), to define AKI [8]. A pediatric modified RIFLE criterion (pRIFLE) has been validated in children [9]. Subsequently, the Kidney Disease Improving Global Outcomes (KDIGO) working group harmonized pediatric and adult AKI definitions in 2012 [10]. The KDIGO AKI definition is illustrated Table 31.2.

In adults, the most common two examples of type-1 CRS are AKI following acute decompensated heart failure (ADHF) and coronary artery bypass grafting (CABG) procedures. Type-1 CRS occurs in about 25% of patients hospitalized for ADHF [11,12] and in 13% of patients undergoing CABG [13]. However, most of these patients have associated morbidities such as diabetes mellitus and systemic hypertension that might contribute to the AKI in the setting of the acute cardiac condition, leading to subsequent uncertainty that type-1 CRS is the only cause of AKI. For example, 60% of adult patients with ADHF and who meet AKI criteria have history of chronic kidney disease (CKD). Unlike adults, AKI following cardiac surgeries using cardiopulmonary bypass (CPB) and ADHF secondary to primary cardiomyopathies in infants and children represent a "purer" population than adults to study type-1 CRS since children lack such associated morbidities.

AKI is a common complication seen in neonates undergoing cardiopulmonary bypass (23%–52%) [14–16], and neonates receiving extracorporeal membrane oxygenation (ECMO) (71%) [17]. The reported need of renal replacement therapy (RRT) ranges between 2.1% and 17% following the bypass [18–22], with a mortality rate up to 40% in infants requiring RRT [19].

Heart Failure in the Child and Young Adult. http://dx.doi.org/10.1016/B978-0-12-802393-8.00031-4

TABLE 31.1 Classification of Cardiorenal Syndrome [7]

Class	Type	Description	Example
I	Acute cardiorenal syndrome	Abrupt worsening of cardiac function leads to acute kidney injury (AKI)	Hemodynamically mediated AKI secondary to acute heart failure or acute coronary syndrome
II	Chronic cardiorenal syndrome	Chronic abnormalities of cardiac function leads to chronic kidney disease (CKD)	CKD in patients with chronic heart failure
III	Acute renocardiac syndrome	Abrupt worsening of kidney function leads to acute cardiac dysfunction	Arrhythmias or acute pulmonary edema in patients with AKI
IV	Chronic renocardiac syndrome	CKD leads to chronic cardiac dysfunction	Cardiac hypertrophy and adverse cardiovascular events in patients with CKD
V	Secondary cardiorenal syndrome	Systemic disorders lead to both cardiac and renal dysfunction	Sepsis, leukemia, amyloidosis, etc.

Table modified from C. Ronco, P. McCullough, S.D. Anker, et al., Cardio-renal syndromes: report from the consensus conference of the acute dialysis quality initiative, Eur. Heart J. 31 (6) (March 2010) 703–711.

TABLE 31.2 Kidney Disease Improving Global Outcomes Staging System of Acute Kidney Injury

Stage	Serum Creatinine Criteria	Urine Output Criteria
1	1.5–1.9 times baseline within 7 days or ≥0.3 mg/dL (≥26.5 mmol/L) increase within 48 h	<0.5 mL/kg h for 6–12 h
2	2.0–2.9 times baseline	<0.5 mL/kg h for ≥12 h
3	3.0 times baseline or Increase in serum creatinine to ≥4.0 mg/dL (≥353.6 mmol/L) or Initiation of renal replacement therapy or, In patients <18 years, decrease in eGFR to <35 mL/min 1.73 m^2	Anuria for ≥12 h

Pathophysiology

Hemodynamic instability plays a major role in type-1 CRS. Acute decreased glomerular filtration rate (GFR) and the change of the nature of blood flow to the kidneys triggers an abrupt increase in intracellular oxygen demand, placing the metabolically active nephron units at risk for oxygen debt caused by global hypoperfusion and/or hypoxemia. During these periods, ATP stores are consumed rapidly, and energy availability becomes dependent on the local mitochondrial oxidative phosphorylation–mediated regeneration of ATP from adenosine diphosphate. Additionally, a second phase of ATP recovery occurs via neosynthesis and regeneration from purine precursors and AMP. Hence, recovery from an ischemic event is dependent on the length of the insult and the metabolic status of the patient before the insult [23].

Apart from hemodynamic pathophysiologic pathways, other nonhemodynamic mechanisms have been proposed as being involved in type-1 CRS, including systemic nervous system and renin–angiotensin–aldosterone system (RAAS) activation, chronic inflammatory status, impairment of reactive oxygen species/nitric oxide production, impaired macrophage activity, gut underperfusion and endotoxin release, and iatrogenic pharmacologic interactions [6].

TABLE 31.3 Diagnostic Utility of Different Acute Urinary Biomarkers to Predict Acute Kidney Injury Following Cardiopulmonary Bypass (CPB) in Children [24,27]

Biomarker	Area Under the Curve of AKI Prediction	Note
NGAL	0.90	Urinary concentration tested at 6h of CPB initiation
IL-18	0.82	
L-FABP	0.78	
[TIMP-2]·[IGFBP7]	0.85	Urinary concentration tested at 4h of CPB initiation

IGFBP7, insulin-like growth factor–binding protein; *IL-18*, interleukin 18; *KIM-1*, kidney injury molecule-1; *L-FABP*, liver-type fatty acid–binding protein; *NGAL*, neutrophil gelatinase-associated lipocalin; *TIMP-2*, tissue inhibitor of metalloproteinase-2.

Box 31.1 List of Biomarkers Evaluated for Early Detection of Acute Kidney Injury

- Alanine aminopeptidase
- Alpha-1 and beta-2 microglobulin (α1 and β2 microglobulin)
- Alpha and pi glutathione S-transferase (α-GST and π-GST)
- Alkaline phosphatase
- Clusterin
- Cystatin C
- Cysteine-rich protein
- Exosomal fetuin A
- γ-glutamyl transpeptidase
- Insulin-like growth factor–binding protein 7
- Interleukin 6
- Interleukin 18
- Kidney injury molecule-1
- Liver-type fatty acid–binding protein
- N-acetyl-β-D-glucosaminidase
- Na^+/H^+ exchanger isoform 3
- Netrin-1
- Neutrophil gelatinase-associated lipocalin
- Osteopontin
- Retinol-binding protein
- Tissue inhibitor of metalloproteinase-2

Diagnosis and Prediction

For decades, monitoring serum creatinine (SCr) concentration and urinary output has been the cornerstone of diagnosing AKI and initiating RRT in critically ill patients. Despite the standardization of AKI definition by ADQI and KDIGO working groups, early recognition of AKI has been limited by delayed elevation of SCr up to 24–48h following the insulting event to kidneys. Moreover, the absence of early AKI biomarkers has been a limiting factor to develop therapeutics interventions to treat or prevent AKI. Recognizing this gap, the last decade witnessed tremendous investigations to reveal kidney injury markers that can substitute for SCr. To date, numerous novel urinary biomarkers demonstrated excellent predictive characteristics of AKI before meeting RIFLE or KDIGO criteria. For example, urinary interleukin-18 (IL-18) and neutrophil gelatinase-associated lipocalin (NGAL) concentrations increased 2h after CPB surgery [24] and peaked 6h after cardiac surgery in patients with AKI 24–36h before SCr levels increased [25]. Moreover, a composite of two or more urinary injury markers showed a very good predictive value of AKI with area under the curve as good as 0.91 [24] with specificity up to 96% depending on the urinary concentration threshold and the injury biomarker used [26]. Table 31.3 shows the diagnostic utility of different biomarkers to predict AKI after CPB.

The increased awareness of the poor outcomes associated with AKI and the absence of availability of clinical biomarker to detect AKI early and accurately attracted medical industries to invest in developing such diagnostic tools. Some of these early biomarkers have been approved for clinical application such as kidney injury molecule-1 (KIM-1) and NGAL. Other markers such as insulin-like growth factor–binding protein 7 (IGFBP7) and tissue inhibitor of metalloproteinases 2 are available for commercial use in critically ill patients; however, their diagnostic utilities in type-1 CRS have not been extensively validated yet. Box 31.1 lists the markers used to predict AKI.

Prevention

It is conceivable that the speed and appropriateness of management might affect survival of critically ill patients with type-1 CRS. However, to date, there is no specific treatment or intervention that is proven to distinctly decrease the risk of AKI following CPB. Most procedures followed in practice to decrease the risk of AKI is limited to avoidance of risk factors known to be associated with post-CPB AKI such as avoiding preoperational use of nonsteroidal anti-inflammatory drugs, angiotensin-converting enzyme inhibitors (ACEi) ,and angiotensin receptor blockers (ARBs), avoiding preoperative and intraoperative hypotension and hypoxia, and maintaining good perfusion pressures. Several pharmacologic interventions have been attempted but showed different and sometimes conflicting results in preserving kidney function after CBP. Beneficial evidence accompanying administration of furosemide, dopamine, theophylline, mannitol, pentoxifylline, steroids, clonidine, diltiazem, atrial natriuretic peptide, and N-acetyl cysteine has been equivocal and none of these interventions provided convincing evidence to suggest applying them universally [28]. In a randomized prospective pediatric single-center trial, infusing fenoldopam at 1 μg/kg during CBP decreased urinary NGAL and cystatin C concentrations and was associated with less diuretics administration suggesting a renoprotective effect. The results of nonpharmacologic interventions came back with inconsistent results as well. One example of these approaches is the remote ischemic preconditioning prior to CBP surgery. The preconditioning hypothesis assumes that eliciting brief remote ischemia in upper or lower extremities may attenuate renal injury by releasing various molecules such as high-mobility group box damage associated protein that are filtered through the glomeruli and adhere to Toll-like receptors in the tubular cells, which result in intracellular signaling to induce natural defenses by arresting cell cycle [29,30]. The biggest three cohorts evaluating the outcomes of remote ischemic conditioning were published by Zarbock [31], Bein [32] and Hausenloy [33]. While the first trial showed that remote ischemic preconditioning significantly reduced the rate of AKI and use of RRT by more than 15% absolute reduction and the treated group showed lower urinary tubular injury biomarkers concentrations than the nontreated group, the latter data assessing different solitary and composite outcomes showed no improvement of clinical outcomes in patients who received remote ischemic preconditioning prior to the cardiac surgery. Single-center reports conducted in children showed conflicting results as well [34,35]. A comprehensive review regarding remote ischemic conditioning can be found elsewhere [36].

Role of Early Renal Replacement Therapy in Managing Type-1 Cardiorenal Syndrome

Until recently, approaching children with type-1 CRS following CPB was limited to careful observation and RRT initiation when significant volume overload developed. Recent evidence supports the beneficiary approach of starting RRT early in the course of AKI. Despite using different definitions of "early" RRT, studies concluded that starting RRT early after cardiac surgeries using CPB is associated with decreased in-hospital mortality, decreased hospital stay, shorter duration of RRT, and lower dialysis dependence [22,37–40].

At our institutions, patients undergoing CPB are screened and classified into high, moderate, and low-risk AKI groups to determine the need to prophylactically place a temporary PD catheter in the operating room (Table 31.4). We reported improved outcomes with this approach, showing earlier attainment of negative fluid balance, greater prevention of volume overload, and earlier discontinuation of mechanical ventilation [16,41].

TABLE 31.4 Cincinnati Children's Hospital Medical Center Protocol to Identify the Risk of Acute Kidney Injury (AKI) Following Cardiopulmonary Bypass (CPB) Surgeries

Risk Category	Patients' Criteria	Action
High-risk of AKI	1. Neonates ≤3 months undergoing any heart surgery using CPB. 2. Patients ≤6 months of age undergoing heart transplantation. 3. Patients ≤4 months of age undergoing Tetralogy of Fallot or double-outlet right ventricular repair.	**Plan** to prophylactically place a temporary peritoneal dialysis catheter in the operating room.
Moderate-risk of AKI	1. Patients >6 months of age undergoing heart transplantation. 2. Patients >4 months of age undergoing Tetralogy of Fallot or double-outlet right ventricular repair. 3. CPB time >120 min.	**Consider** placing peritoneal dialysis catheter prophylactically based on the patient's condition in the operating room and the surgeon assessment.
Low-risk of AKI	Patients do not meet the high- or the low-risk of AKI as above.	Peritoneal dialysis catheter placement is not indicated.

CHILDHOOD TYPE-2 CARDIORENAL SYNDROME

Definition and Epidemiology

Type-2 CRS, or chronic CRS, is defined as chronic heart failure leading to CKD. In adults, chronic cardiac abnormalities, such as myocarditis, ischemic heart disease with subsequent decreased systolic or diastolic function, hypertensive heart disease, and cardiomyopathies resulting in impaired kidney function are associated with adverse outcomes and prolonged hospitalizations [42,43]. The prevalence of type-2 CRS has been reported to be as high as 30% in adults with chronic heart failure [44]. That being said, a careful approach should be adopted when interpreting these data because a clear cut off between ADHF, with subsequent type-1 CRS, and chronic congestive heart failure, with subsequent type-2 CRS, is not evident. In children, studies evaluating epidemiology and risk-associated outcomes are sparse. We analyzed the data of the pediatric cardiomyopathy registry to determine the prevalence of decreased kidney function, defined as GFR < 90 mL/min 1.73 m^2, in children with dilated cardiomyopathy (DCM) [45]. We found that at least 25% of these patients had decreased kidney function at the time of cardiomyopathy diagnosis when compared to historical healthy controls. Interestingly, this rate was close to the reported range of 25%–30% prevalence of kidney dysfunction reported in adults with chronic heart failure [42,46]. However, in our report, we observed that children with DCM were more likely to have decreased kidney function at the time of DCM diagnosis up to 2 years after the diagnosis. After 2 years, the prevalence of type-2 CRS was similar in DCM patients and historical controls. We duplicated this finding in a cross-sectional study in a cohort of children with DCM patients without heart failure [47]. We found that hemodynamically stable DCM patients have normal eGFR, determined by SCr and cystatin C, and urinary protein. However, they have elevated urinary tubular injury markers concentrations when compared to a healthy cohort including subclinical tubular injury that cannot be detected using the conventional kidney function markers, i.e., SCr and urinary protein. Unfortunately, long-term prognostic data in children with type-2 CRS are not available.

Pathophysiology

The cardiorenal connection is an interactive network with positive and negative feedback loops in which multiple mechanisms have been suggested to contribute to CKD development in heart failure patients such as neurohormonal activation, kidney hypoperfusion, oxidative stress, inflammation, increased activity of the sympathetic nervous system, and venous congestion.

Heart failure experimental studies suggest that persistent decreased glomerular plasma flow in animals with heart failure is associated with histologic evidence of podocyte injury and segmental sclerosis in the glomeruli. Many of these changes were suggested as a result of dysregulation of sympathetic nervous system (SNS) nervous and RAAS [48]. This was supported by studies showing elevated venous renin concentration in patients with congestive heart failure [49]. Hence, reducing the activity of the renin–angiotensin system was one of the principles that clinical trials targeted to manage type-2 CRS. One of the most deleterious actions of RAAS upregulation in CRS is activation of NADPH-oxidase by angiotensin II, which results in formation of reactive oxygen species. This has been documented in the endothelial cells, vascular smooth muscle cells, renal tubular cells, and cardiomyocytes [48]. This context has been observed in the glomeruli of Dahl salt-sensitive rats with heart failure. NADPH-oxidase activity could be attenuated by ACE inhibition [50].

Diagnosis and Outcomes

The current diagnostic approach to recognize the presence and progression of type-2 CRS follows the same principals of CKD. Assessment of type-2 CRS has been limited to kidney function markers such as SCr and urinary albumin as these markers are well-recognized predictors of mortality, cardiovascular risk of morbidity and readmission rates in CKD patients. In patients with type-2 CRS, advanced CKD staging were associated with mortality in adults with heart failure independent of worsening heart failure and baseline kidney function [51].

In a pilot study in children with DCM, survival rates were similar in children with eGFR less or more than 90 mL/min 1.73 m^2 [45]. However, the study was not powered enough to preclude the significance of decreased eGFR on long term survival.

The role of cystatin C and the tubular injury biomarkers has been well presented in the literature and seems to carry future diagnostic utility in adults with type-2 CRS [11,42,52–56]. Unfortunately, pediatric data are limited in this field.

Management of Type-2 Cardiorenal Syndrome

Practice guidelines for management of heart failure in children were published in 2004 [57]. However, these guidelines were a product of adult-focused data as most of the available trials excluded pediatric patients. Unfortunately, pediatricians and pediatric cardiologists, in particular, have had comparatively minimal participation in the clinical practice guidelines realm [58]. As reflection on adult data, RAAS blockade using either ACEi and/or ARBs has been among the most prescribed agents in managing children with heart failure. Theoretically, ACEi or ARBs might delay kidney function deterioration due to eliminating RAAS dysregulation, which plays a significant role in type-2 CRS. Many trials have been conducted in adults to evaluate this hypothesis, but, at present, the evidence is inconclusive regarding the role of RAAS blockade in preventing progression of type-2 CRS [42]. The literature is limited in children as well. Aldosterone receptor inhibitor use was associated with decreased mortality in adults with heart failure despite worsening of kidney function [59], while another study suggested decrease in collagen synthesis suggesting a protective role against fibrosis [60]. Beta-blockers such as carvedilol, metoprolol, or bisoprolol are widely used in children with moderate and severe systolic dysfunction [61]. Current knowledge on the effect of these therapies on the progression on CKD in children is limited. The conclusion of the outcome of using beta-blockers in type-2 CRS is adult clinical trials is still controversial [62–64].

CHILDHOOD TYPE-3 CARDIORENAL SYNDROME

Definition and Epidemiology

Type-3 CRS, or acute renocardiac syndrome, occurs when acute or abrupt deterioration of kidney function, i.e., AKI, leads or contributes to the development of acute cardiac dysfunction or injury. The determination of the true epidemiology of type-3 CRS in children is difficult, mainly related to the AKI definition and epidemiology. First, standardized systemic definition of AKI in children had not been introduced till 2007 when the pRIFLE classification criteria have been published [9]. Second, AKI epidemiologic studies excluded the general pediatric population and looked at specific populations such as critically ill children or postsurgical cases. Hence, the current epidemiologic data on childhood type-3 CRS do not exist. Box 31.2 represents the most common causes and etiologies of childhood AKI.

Pathophysiology of Type-3 Cardiorenal Syndrome

AKI is a systemic inflammatory process with secondary impact on other organs including the cardiovascular system. Animal models show that AKI is associated with increased serum concentration of inflammatory markers such a TNF-α, IL-1, and IL-6 after induced ischemic AKI with subsequent depressant effects on the left ventricle represented by reduction of the ejection fraction and elevation of left ventricular end-diastolic and end-systolic volumes [6,42,65]. Infusion of TNF-α in animal models results in decreased coronary flow rate, negative inotropic effect [65] and increase oxygen consumption by the myocardial cells affecting contractility of these cells [66]. Moreover, increased expression of adhesion molecules such as ICAM-1 in the myocardium of rats with ischemia-induced AKI suggests the important role of the inflammation associated with AKI as a potent factor for developing type-3 CRS.

Box 31.2 Summary of Classification and Causes of Acute Kidney Injury (AKI) in Children

- Prerenal AKI (functional AKI)
  - Pathogenesis: Deceased perfusion to the kidney without intrinsic kidney injury
  - Causes: Dehydration, hemorrhage, shock, burns, arrhythmias, sepsis, and anaphylaxis.
- Intrinsic AKI (structural AKI)
  - Pathogenesis: pathologic process leads to pathologic changes in kidneys
  - Causes
    - Vascular disease: Thrombosis, hemolytic uremic syndrome, and vasculidities
    - Glomerular disease: Acute glomerulonephritis
    - Tubular and interstitial disease: Acute tubular necrosis secondary to prolonged prerenal AKI and Interstitial nephritis secondary to nephrotoxic agents such as aminoglycosides, amphotericin B, contrast agents, calcineurin inhibitors, and cisplatin
- Postrenal AKI
  - Pathogenesis: bilateral urinary tract obstruction or obstruction of the urinary tract of a solitary kidney
  - Causes: Renal calculi, clots, neurogenic bladder, and medications that cause urinary retention.

The hyperactivity of SNS and RAAS plays another role in the etiology as well. AKI is associated with higher angiotensin II release with subsequent vasoconstriction and myocardial cell apoptosis [67]. The AKI-associated release of catecholamines, such as norepinephrine, increases the oxygen demand of the cardiomyocytes and impairs the Ca^{+2} metabolism with potential inducing myocardial ischemia.

From clinical prospective, AKI is associated with volume overload, hypertension, metabolic acidosis, electrolytes abnormalities, progression to CKD, and uremia, all of which contribute negatively to the function of myocardium and the development of dysrhythmias [42].

Diagnosis and Management

Sensitive and specific biomarkers have been employed for early detection of cardiac dysfunction. Cardiac troponins, the traditional markers in general population, perform very well in renal patients [68]. Brain natriuretic peptide is a useful marker to diagnosis ADHF in patients with renal insufficiency and its high concentration is associated with progression of CKD. Other markers such as myeloperoxidase, TNF, IL-1, IL-6 have been employed for early detection of cardiac injury [6,42].

The management of type-3 CRS is targeted to early and appropriate management of AKI to prevent volume overload, treat electrolyte disturbances, and manage hypertension. Critically ill children might need RRT when AKI is severe. In such children, continuous, rather than intermittent, renal replacement modalities should be employed as children with type-3 CRS are sensitive to abrupt changes in fluid status.

CHILDHOOD TYPE-4 CARDIORENAL SYNDROME

Definition and Epidemiology

Among the five types of childhood CRS, type-4 probably is the most represented in literature in children. Type-4 CRS, or chronic renocardiac syndrome, is characterized by a condition of primary CKD contributing to different chronic cardiovascular morbidities. It is well established that CKD carries poor prognostic outcomes in children, for example, the mortality rate in children with kidney transplantation or on dialysis are 10 and 100 times higher than comparably aged healthy children, respectively [69,70]. Data from US Renal Data System listed cardiovascular disease as major cause of death in children between 0 and 19 years of age. Cardiovascular disease was the leading cause of death in children on hemodialysis and peritoneal dialysis and represented 32% and 28% of all death causes, respectively [70]. Moreover, cardiac cause was the second leading cause of mortality in kidney-transplanted children after infections. The reported causes of cardiac death were arrhythmias, congestive heart failure, cardiomyopathy, pericarditis, cerebrovascular disease, and acute myocardial infarction [70]. The data in children resemble those in adults where more than 50% of deaths in advanced CKD are attributed to cardiovascular disease and those with CKD carry a 10- to 20-fold increase in cardiac death compared to healthy controls [6,42,71,72].

Pathophysiology

Since type-4 CRS represents multiple cardiovascular manifestations, we will discuss the risk factors that potentiate CKD patients to develop type-4 CRS and then discuss the pathologic pathways that are associated with the development of cardiomyopathy and coronary atherosclerosis in CKD population.

Children with CKD have multiple risk factors known to cause cardiovascular disease. These risk factors include

- Hypertension: hypertension affects up to 54% of children with CKD [73,74] and despite using appropriate blood pressure lowering agents, blood pressure is controlled in only 52% [74].
- Obesity: 15% of children with CKD are obese [75].
- Dyslipidemia: 45% of children with CKD have dyslipidemia [76].
- Other risk factors such as hyperinsulinism, anemia, abnormal mineral metabolism, malnutrition, and inflammation that might contribute to cardiovascular disease development are common in children with CKD [70].

Children with CKD show evidence of myocardial alterations. Left ventricular hypertrophy (LVH) is the most observed abnormality, where up to 82% of children starting maintenance dialysis have evidence of a concentric or eccentric geometric LVH pattern [70]. Other studies demonstrate that children with CKD have evidence of diastolic dysfunction, depressed contractile reserve during exercise, and decreased reduction in myocardial blood flow [77]. At present, the mechanisms responsible for cardiac structure alterations in CKD patients are not well understood. The progression of CKD and progressive nephron loss leads to further salt and water retention and, hence, increase the preload of the myocardium. Moreover, the increased activity of RAAS and SNS leads to vasoconstriction and increases the myocardium afterload. In addition, the upregulated RAAS is associated with release of profibrotic factors such as TGF-β [78]. All of the above factors contribute to the myocardium modifications seen in CKD patients.

The atherosclerotic changes observed in adults with CKD start in childhood. In a study done on autopsies of deceased children with CKD, 28% of cadavers showed evidence of coronary artery calcifications [79]. In another study, 5 of 12 iliac artery samples obtained from 11 to 17 year old children on hemodialysis showed fibrous or fibroelastic intimal thickening, medial mucoid ground substance, and disruption of the internal elastic lamella and 2 of 12 showed evidence of calcifications. In adults with stage 3–5 CKD, 83% had evidence on coronary calcifications on CT scan [80]. There are many underlying causes of vascular calcification that initiate the process by transforming vascular smooth muscle cells to a chondrocyte or osteoblast-like cell, including hyperphosphatemia, uremia, hyperglycemia, and other metabolites. There is growing evidence that increased fibroblast growth factor 23 and decreased Klotho vascular factor play a crucial role in the development of vascular calcifications [81]. The role galectin-3, a member of the β-galactoside-binding lectin family, in the pathogenesis of type-4 CRS is still controversial [6]. Galectin-3 can bind to cardiac fibroblasts and increase collagen production in myocardium. In a recent study of more than 3500 adults with either renal or heart failure, galectin-3 concentrations increased with progressive renal impairment and independently associated with cardiovascular end points, infections, and all-cause death.

Outcome and Management

Despite the improvement of the mortality rates in pediatric end-stage renal disease (ESRD) in the last two decades, ESRD still carries a 30-fold higher risk of death compared to healthy children [82]. As mentioned previously, the majority of children with CKD carry at least one cardiovascular risk factor and half of them have at least two factors. This signifies the importance of eliminating the associated risk factors such as controlling hypertension, counseling for obesity, management of dyslipidemia, eliminating anemia, regulating RAAS and SNS upregulation, and addressing phosphorus, calcium, and parathyroid hormone levels. That being said, it should be noted here that most interventional therapeutic studies to decrease the risk factors associated with cardiac risk excluded CKD patients. Therefore, the recommendations of treating these risk factors in CKD patients are acquired from cohorts without renal disease. When the child develops ESRD, every effort should be done to conduct preemptive renal transplantation or to decrease the duration of RRT. Despite the fact they have shorter life span when compared to healthy children, children with kidney transplantation live 20–30 years more than those receiving maintenance dialysis [70]. In those who cannot achieve transplantation, aggressive management of hypertension, anemia, and volume overload cannot be overestimated. Unfortunately, standard thrice weekly hemodialysis even when achieving recommended clearance targets has not been shown to improve clinical outcomes [83]. The concept of intensified dialysis in high-risk patients has been supported by multiple studies in adults [84–86]. In one of these studies, six times weekly hemodialysis, as compared to three times weekly hemodialysis, was associated with favorable results with respect to the composite outcomes of death or change in left ventricular mass and death or change in a physical-health composite score [85]. Unlike adults, data in children are limited to single-center studies and case reports including the advantage of intensified hemodialysis protocols [87–89].

ABBREVIATIONS

ACEi Angiotensin-converting enzyme inhibitors
ADHF Acute decompensated heart failure
ADQI Acute Dialysis Quality Initiative
AKI Acute kidney injury
ARBs Angiotensin receptor blockers
AUC Area under the curve
CABG Coronary artery bypass grafting
CKD Chronic kidney disease
CPB Cardiopulmonary bypass
CRS Cardiorenal syndrome
DCM Dilated cardiomyopathy
ECMO Extracorporeal membrane oxygenation
FDA Food and Drug Administration
GFR Glomerular filtration rate
IGFBP7 Insulin-like growth factor–binding protein 7
IL-18 Interleukin-18
KDIGO Kidney Disease Improving Global Outcomes

LVH Left ventricular hypertrophy
NGAL Neutrophil gelatinase-associated lipocalin
RAAS Renin–angiotensin–aldosterone system
RRT Renal replacement therapy
SCr Serum creatinine
SNS Sympathetic nervous system
TIMP-2 Tissue inhibitor of metalloproteinases 2

REFERENCES

[1] F. Husain-Syed, P.A. McCullough, H.W. Birk, M. Renker, A. Brocca, W. Seeger, et al., Cardio-pulmonary-renal interactions: a multidisciplinary approach, J. Am. Coll. Cardiol. 65 (22) (2015) 2433–2448.

[2] T. Berl, W. Henrich, Kidney-heart interactions: epidemiology, pathogenesis, and treatment, Clin. J. Am. Soc. Nephrol. 1 (1) (2006) 8–18.

[3] R.J. Cody, S. Ljungman, A.B. Covit, S.H. Kubo, J.E. Sealey, K. Pondolfino, et al., Regulation of glomerular filtration rate in chronic congestive heart failure patients, Kidney Int. 34 (3) (1988) 361–367.

[4] J.S. Bock, S.S. Gottlieb, Cardiorenal syndrome: new perspectives, Circulation 121 (23) (2010) 2592–2600.

[5] C. Ronco, A.A. House, M. Haapio, Cardiorenal syndrome: refining the definition of a complex symbiosis gone wrong, Intensiv. Care Med. 34 (5) (2008) 957–962.

[6] C. Ronco, L. Di Lullo, Cardiorenal syndrome, Heart Fail. Clin. 10 (2) (2014) 251–280.

[7] C. Ronco, P. McCullough, S.D. Anker, I. Anand, N. Aspromonte, S.M. Bagshaw, et al., Cardio-renal syndromes: report from the consensus conference of the acute dialysis quality initiative, Eur. Heart J. 31 (6) (2010) 703–711.

[8] R. Bellomo, C. Ronco, J.A. Kellum, R.L. Mehta, P. Palevsky, Acute Dialysis Quality Initiative Workgroup, Acute renal failure – definition, outcome measures, animal models, fluid therapy and information technology needs: the Second International Consensus Conference of the Acute Dialysis Quality Initiative (ADQI) Group, Crit. Care 8 (4) (2004) R204–R212.

[9] A. Akcan-Arikan, M. Zappitelli, L.L. Loftis, K.K. Washburn, L.S. Jefferson, S.L. Goldstein, Modified RIFLE criteria in critically ill children with acute kidney injury, Kidney Int. 71 (10) (2007) 1028–1035.

[10] Kidney disease: improving global outcomes (KDIGO) acute kidney injury work group. KDIGO clinical practice guideline for acute kidney injury, Kidney Int. 2 (1) (March 2012).

[11] S.M. Bagshaw, D.N. Cruz, N. Aspromonte, L. Daliento, F. Ronco, G. Sheinfeld, et al., Epidemiology of cardio-renal syndromes: workgroup statements from the 7th ADQI Consensus Conference, Nephrol. Dial. Transplant. 25 (5) (2010) 1406–1416.

[12] K. Damman, G. Navis, A.A. Voors, F.W. Asselbergs, T.D. Smilde, J.G. Cleland, et al., Worsening renal function and prognosis in heart failure: systematic review and meta-analysis, J. Card. Fail. 13 (8) (2007) 599–608.

[13] L. Rydén, U. Sartipy, M. Evans, M.J. Holzmann, Acute kidney injury after coronary artery bypass grafting and long-term risk of end-stage renal disease, Circulation 130 (23) (2014) 2005–2011.

[14] C.D. Krawczeski, J.G. Woo, Y. Wang, M.R. Bennett, Q. Ma, P. Devarajan, Neutrophil gelatinase-associated lipocalin concentrations predict development of acute kidney injury in neonates and children after cardiopulmonary bypass, J. Pediatr. 158 (6) (2011) 1009.e1–1015.e1.

[15] J.J. Blinder, S.L. Goldstein, V.V. Lee, A. Baycroft, C.D. Fraser, D. Nelson, et al., Congenital heart surgery in infants: effects of acute kidney injury on outcomes, J. Thorac. Cardiovasc. Surg. 143 (2) (2012) 368–374.

[16] A. Kaddourah, S.L. Goldstein, Renal replacement therapy in neonates, Clin. Perinatol. 41 (3) (2014) 517–527.

[17] S.K. Gadepalli, D.T. Selewski, R.A. Drongowski, G.B. Mychaliska, Acute kidney injury in congenital diaphragmatic hernia requiring extracorporeal life support: an insidious problem, J. Pediatr. Surg. 46 (4) (2011) 630–635.

[18] K.R. Pedersen, J.V. Povlsen, S. Christensen, J. Pedersen, K. Hjortholm, S.H. Larsen, et al., Risk factors for acute renal failure requiring dialysis after surgery for congenital heart disease in children, Acta Anaesthesiol. Scand. 51 (10) (2007) 1344–1349.

[19] H. Boigner, W. Brannath, M. Hermon, E. Stoll, G. Burda, G. Trittenwein, et al., Predictors of mortality at initiation of peritoneal dialysis in children after cardiac surgery, Ann. Thorac. Surg. 77 (1) (2004) 61–65.

[20] K.L. Chan, P. Ip, C.S. Chiu, Y.F. Cheung, Peritoneal dialysis after surgery for congenital heart disease in infants and young children, Ann. Thorac. Surg. 76 (5) (2003) 1443–1449.

[21] A. Kuitunen, A. Vento, R. Suojaranta-Ylinen, V. Pettila, Acute renal failure after cardiac surgery: evaluation of the RIFLE classification, Ann. Thorac. Surg. 81 (2) (2006) 542–546.

[22] M. Bojan, S. Gioanni, P.R. Vouhe, D. Journois, P. Pouard, Early initiation of peritoneal dialysis in neonates and infants with acute kidney injury following cardiac surgery is associated with a significant decrease in mortality, Kidney Int. 82 (4) (2012) 474–481.

[23] N. Lameire, W. Van Biesen, R. Vanholder, Acute renal failure, Lancet 365 (9457) (2005) 417–430.

[24] C.D. Krawczeski, S.L. Goldstein, J.G. Woo, Y. Wang, N. Piyaphanee, Q. Ma, et al., Temporal relationship and predictive value of urinary acute kidney injury biomarkers after pediatric cardiopulmonary bypass, J. Am. Coll. Cardiol. 58 (22) (2011) 2301–2309.

[25] C.R. Parikh, P. Devarajan, M. Zappitelli, K. Sint, H. Thiessen-Philbrook, S. Li, et al., Postoperative biomarkers predict acute kidney injury and poor outcomes after pediatric cardiac surgery, J. Am. Soc. Nephrol. 22 (9) (2011) 1737–1747.

[26] R.K. Basu, H.R. Wong, C.D. Krawczeski, D.S. Wheeler, P.B. Manning, L.S. Chawla, et al., Combining functional and tubular damage biomarkers improves diagnostic precision for acute kidney injury after cardiac surgery, J. Am. Coll. Cardiol. 64 (25) (2014) 2753–2762.

[27] M. Meersch, C. Schmidt, H. Van Aken, J. Rossaint, D. Gorlich, D. Stege, et al., Validation of cell-cycle arrest biomarkers for acute kidney injury after pediatric cardiac surgery, PLoS One 9 (10) (2014) e110865.
[28] M.H. Rosner, M.D. Okusa, Acute kidney injury associated with cardiac surgery, Clin. J. Am. Soc. Nephrol. 1 (1) (2006) 19–32.
[29] R.K. Kharbanda, T.T. Nielsen, A.N. Redington, Translation of remote ischaemic preconditioning into clinical practice, Lancet 374 (9700) (2009) 1557–1565.
[30] N. Gassanov, A.M. Nia, E. Caglayan, F. Er, Remote ischemic preconditioning and renoprotection: from myth to a novel therapeutic option? J. Am. Soc. Nephrol. 25 (2) (2014) 216–224.
[31] A. Zarbock, C. Schmidt, H. Van Aken, C. Wempe, S. Martens, P.K. Zahn, et al., Effect of remote ischemic preconditioning on kidney injury among high-risk patients undergoing cardiac surgery: a randomized clinical trial, JAMA 313 (21) (2015) 2133–2141.
[32] P. Meybohm, B. Bein, O. Brosteanu, J. Cremer, M. Gruenewald, C. Stoppe, et al., A multicenter trial of remote ischemic preconditioning for heart surgery, N. Engl. J. Med. 373 (15) (2015) 1397–1407.
[33] D.J. Hausenloy, L. Candilio, R. Evans, C. Ariti, D.P. Jenkins, S. Kolvekar, et al., Remote ischemic preconditioning and outcomes of cardiac surgery, N. Engl. J. Med. 373 (15) (2015) 1408–1417.
[34] B.W. McCrindle, N.A. Clarizia, S. Khaikin, H.M. Holtby, C. Manlhiot, S.M. Schwartz, et al., Remote ischemic preconditioning in children undergoing cardiac surgery with cardiopulmonary bypass: a single-center double-blinded randomized trial, J. Am. Heart Assoc. 3 (4) (2014).
[35] M. Hepponstall, V. Ignjatovic, S. Binos, C. Attard, V. Karlaftis, Y. d'Udekem, et al., Remote ischemic preconditioning (RIPC) modifies the plasma proteome in children undergoing repair of tetralogy of fallot: a randomized controlled trial, PLoS One 10 (3) (2015) e0122778.
[36] G. Heusch, H.E. Bøtker, K. Przyklenk, A. Redington, D. Yellon, Remote ischemic conditioning, J. Am. Coll. Cardiol. 65 (2) (2015) 177–195.
[37] M.M. Elahi, M.Y. Lim, R.N. Joseph, R.R. Dhannapuneni, T.J. Spyt, Early hemofiltration improves survival in post-cardiotomy patients with acute renal failure, Eur. J. Cardiothorac. Surg. 26 (5) (2004) 1027–1031.
[38] S.M. Bagshaw, S. Uchino, R. Bellomo, H. Morimatsu, S. Morgera, M. Schetz, et al., Timing of renal replacement therapy and clinical outcomes in critically ill patients with severe acute kidney injury, J. Crit. Care 24 (1) (2009) 129–140.
[39] P. Bent, H.K. Tan, R. Bellomo, J. Buckmaster, L. Doolan, G. Hart, et al., Early and intensive continuous hemofiltration for severe renal failure after cardiac surgery, Ann. Thorac. Surg. 71 (3) (2001) 832–837.
[40] W.C. Sasser, R.J. Dabal, D.J. Askenazi, S. Borasino, A.B. Moellinger, J.K. Kirklin, J.A. Alten, Prophylactic peritoneal dialysis following cardiopulmonary bypass in children is associated with decreased inflammation and improved clinical outcomes, Congenit. Heart Dis. 9 (2) (March–April, 2014) 106–115. http://dx.doi.org/10.1111/chd.12072. Epub 2013 May 7. PubMed PMID: 23647999.
[41] D.M. Kwiatkowski, S. Menon, C.D. Krawczeski, S.L. Goldstein, D.L. Morales, A. Phillips, P.B. Manning, P. Eghtesady, Y. Wang, D.P. Nelson, D.S. Cooper, Improved outcomes with peritoneal dialysis catheter placement after cardiopulmonary bypass in infants, J. Thorac. Cardiovasc. Surg. 149 (1) (January 2015) 230–236. http://dx.doi.org/10.1016/j.jtcvs.2013.11.040. Epub 2013 Dec 31. PubMed PMID: 24503323.
[42] C. Ronco, M. Haapio, A.A. House, N. Anavekar, R. Bellomo, Cardiorenal syndrome, J. Am. Coll. Cardiol. 52 (19) (2008) 1527–1539.
[43] P. Jois, A. Mebazaa, Cardio-renal syndrome type 2: epidemiology, pathophysiology, and treatment, Semin. Nephrol. 32 (1) (2012) 26–30.
[44] H.L. Hillege, D. Nitsch, M.A. Pfeffer, K. Swedberg, J.J. McMurray, S. Yusuf, et al., Renal function as a predictor of outcome in a broad spectrum of patients with heart failure, Circulation 113 (5) (2006) 671–678.
[45] A. Kaddourah, S.L. Goldstein, S.E. Lipshultz, J.D. Wilkinson, L.A. Sleeper, M. Lu, S.D. Colan, J.A. Towbin, S.I. Aydin, J. Rossano, M.D. Everitt, J.G. Gossett, P. Rusconi, P.F. Kantor, R.K. Singh, J.L. Jefferies, Prevalence, predictors, and outcomes of cardiorenal syndrome in children with dilated cardiomyopathy: a report from the Pediatric Cardiomyopathy Registry, Pediatr. Nephrol. 30 (12) (December 2015) 2177–2188. http://dx.doi.org/10.1007/s00467-015-3165-8. Epub 2015 Jul 26. PubMed PMID: 26210985; PubMed Central PMCID: PMC4626312.
[46] J.J. Fadrowski, A.M. Neu, G.J. Schwartz, S.L. Furth, Pediatric GFR estimating equations applied to adolescents in the general population, Clin. J. Am. Soc. Nephrol. 6 (6) (2011) 1427–1435.
[47] A. Kaddourah, S.L. Goldstein, R. Basu, E.J. Nehus, T.C. Terrell, L. Brunner, M.R. Bennett, C. Haffner, J.L. Jefferies, Novel urinary tubular injury markers reveal an evidence of underlying kidney injury in children with reduced left ventricular systolic function: a pilot study, Pediatr. Nephrol. 31 (10) (October 2016) 1637–1645. http://dx.doi.org/10.1007/s00467-016-3360-2. Epub 2016 May 2. PubMed PMID: 27139898.
[48] L.G. Bongartz, M.J. Cramer, P.A. Doevendans, J.A. Joles, B. Braam, The severe cardiorenal syndrome: 'Guyton revisited', Eur. Heart J. 26 (1) (2005) 11–17.
[49] A.J. Merrill, J.L. Morrison, E.S. Branno, Concentration of renin in renal venous blood in patients with chronic heart failure, Am. J. Med. 1 (5) (1946) 468.
[50] A. Tojo, M.L. Onozato, N. Kobayashi, A. Goto, H. Matsuoka, T. Fujita, Angiotensin II and oxidative stress in Dahl Salt-sensitive rat with heart failure, Hypertension 40 (6) (2002) 834–839.
[51] N.A. Khan, I. Ma, C.R. Thompson, K. Humphries, D.N. Salem, M.J. Sarnak, et al., Kidney function and mortality among patients with left ventricular systolic dysfunction, J. Am. Soc. Nephrol. 17 (1) (2006) 244–253.
[52] W.H. Tang, F. Van Lente, K. Shrestha, R.W. Troughton, G.S. Francis, W. Tong, et al., Impact of myocardial function on cystatin C measurements in chronic systolic heart failure, J. Card. Fail. 14 (5) (2008) 394–399.
[53] K. Damman, S. Masson, H.L. Hillege, A.P. Maggioni, A.A. Voors, C. Opasich, et al., Clinical outcome of renal tubular damage in chronic heart failure, Eur. Heart J. 32 (21) (2011) 2705–2712.
[54] A. Yndestad, L. Landro, T. Ueland, C.P. Dahl, T.H. Flo, L.E. Vinge, et al., Increased systemic and myocardial expression of neutrophil gelatinase-associated lipocalin in clinical and experimental heart failure, Eur. Heart J. 30 (10) (2009) 1229–1236.
[55] C.G. Jungbauer, C. Birner, B. Jung, S. Buchner, M. Lubnow, C. von Bary, et al., Kidney injury molecule-1 and N-acetyl-beta-D-glucosaminidase in chronic heart failure: possible biomarkers of cardiorenal syndrome, Eur. J. Heart Fail. 13 (10) (2011) 1104–1110.

[56] C.G. Jungbauer, E. Uecer, S. Stadler, C. Birner, S. Buchner, L.S. Maier, A. Luchner, N-Acteyl-ß-D-glucosaminidase and kidney injury molecule-1: new predictors for long-term progression of chronic kidney disease in patients with heart failure, Nephrology (Carlton) 21 (6) (June 2016) 490–498. http://dx.doi.org/10.1111/nep.12632. PubMed PMID: 26422793.

[57] D. Rosenthal, M.R. Chrisant, E. Edens, L. Mahony, C. Canter, S. Colan, et al., International society for heart and lung transplantation: practice guidelines for management of heart failure in children, J. Heart Lung Transplant. 23 (12) (2004) 1313–1333.

[58] S.D. Colan, Review of the International Society for Heart and Lung Transplantation Practice guidelines for management of heart failure in children, Cardiol. Young 25 (Suppl. 2) (2015) 154–159.

[59] B. Pitt, F. Zannad, W.J. Remme, R. Cody, A. Castaigne, A. Perez, et al., The effect of spironolactone on morbidity and mortality in patients with severe heart failure. Randomized Aldactone Evaluation Study Investigators, N. Engl. J. Med. 341 (10) (1999) 709–717.

[60] J. Malyszko, H. Bachorzewska-Gajewska, B. Poniatowski, J.S. Malyszko, S. Dobrzycki, Urinary and serum biomarkers after cardiac catheterization in diabetic patients with stable angina and without severe chronic kidney disease, Ren. Fail. 31 (10) (2009) 910–919.

[61] P.F. Kantor, J. Lougheed, A. Dancea, M. McGillion, N. Barbosa, C. Chan, et al., Presentation, diagnosis, and medical management of heart failure in children: Canadian Cardiovascular Society guidelines, Can. J. Cardiol. 29 (12) (2013) 1535–1552.

[62] R.K. Wali, M. Iyengar, G.J. Beck, D.M. Chartyan, M. Chonchol, M.A. Lukas, et al., Efficacy and safety of carvedilol in treatment of heart failure with chronic kidney disease: a meta-analysis of randomized trials, Circ. Heart Fail. 4 (1) (2011) 18–26.

[63] D. Castagno, P.S. Jhund, J.J. McMurray, J.D. Lewsey, E. Erdmann, F. Zannad, et al., Improved survival with bisoprolol in patients with heart failure and renal impairment: an analysis of the cardiac insufficiency bisoprolol study II (CIBIS-II) trial, Eur. J. Heart Fail. 12 (6) (2010) 607–616.

[64] A. Cohen-Solal, D. Kotecha, D.J. van Veldhuisen, D. Babalis, M. Bohm, A.J. Coats, et al., Efficacy and safety of nebivolol in elderly heart failure patients with impaired renal function: insights from the SENIORS trial, Eur. J. Heart Fail. 11 (9) (2009) 872–880.

[65] N.J. Edmunds, H. Lal, B. Woodward, Effects of tumour necrosis factor-alpha on left ventricular function in the rat isolated perfused heart: possible mechanisms for a decline in cardiac function, Br. J. Pharmacol. 126 (1) (1999) 189–196.

[66] H. Miyano, T. Shishido, T. Kawada, H. Miyashita, T. Sato, M. Sugimachi, et al., Acute effect of tumor necrosis factor-alpha is minimal on mechanics but significant on energetics in blood-perfused canine left ventricles, Crit. Care Med. 27 (1) (1999) 168–176.

[67] J. Kajstura, E. Cigola, A. Malhotra, P. Li, W. Cheng, L.G. Meggs, et al., Angiotensin II induces apoptosis of adult ventricular myocytes in vitro, J. Mol. Cell. Cardiol 29 (3) (1997) 859–870.

[68] D.M. Needham, K.A. Shufelt, G. Tomlinson, J.W. Scholey, G.E. Newton, Troponin I and T levels in renal failure patients without acute coronary syndrome: a systematic review of the literature, Can. J. Cardiol. 20 (12) (2004) 1212–1218.

[69] T.J. Mathews, A.M. Minino, M.J. Osterman, D.M. Strobino, B. Guyer, Annual summary of vital statistics: 2008, Pediatrics 127 (1) (2011) 146–157.

[70] M.M. Mitsnefes, Cardiovascular disease in children with chronic kidney disease, J. Am. Soc. Nephrol. 23 (4) (2012) 578–585.

[71] C.A. Herzog, Dismal long-term survival of dialysis patients after acute myocardial infarction: can we alter the outcome? Nephrol. Dial. Transplant. 17 (1) (2002) 7–10.

[72] D.W. Johnson, A.M. Craven, N.M. Isbel, Modification of cardiovascular risk in hemodialysis patients: an evidence-based review, Hemodial. Int. 11 (1) (2007) 1–14.

[73] J.T. Flynn, M. Mitsnefes, C. Pierce, S.R. Cole, R.S. Parekh, S.L. Furth, et al., Blood pressure in children with chronic kidney disease: a report from the Chronic Kidney Disease in Children study, Hypertension 52 (4) (2008) 631–637.

[74] M. Mitsnefes, J. Flynn, S. Cohn, J. Samuels, T. Blydt-Hansen, J. Saland, et al., Masked hypertension associates with left ventricular hypertrophy in children with CKD, J. Am. Soc. Nephrol. 21 (1) (2010) 137–144.

[75] A.C. Wilson, M.F. Schneider, C. Cox, L.A. Greenbaum, J. Saland, C.T. White, et al., Prevalence and correlates of multiple cardiovascular risk factors in children with chronic kidney disease, Clin. J. Am. Soc. Nephrol. 6 (12) (2011) 2759–2765.

[76] J.M. Saland, C.B. Pierce, M.M. Mitsnefes, J.T. Flynn, J. Goebel, J.C. Kupferman, et al., Dyslipidemia in children with chronic kidney disease, Kidney Int. 78 (11) (2010) 1154–1163.

[77] D.K. Hothi, L. Rees, J. Marek, J. Burton, C.W. McIntyre, Pediatric myocardial stunning underscores the cardiac toxicity of conventional hemodialysis treatments, Clin. J. Am. Soc. Nephrol. 4 (4) (2009) 790–797.

[78] A.Y. Bagrov, J.I. Shapiro, Endogenous digitalis: pathophysiologic roles and therapeutic applications, Nat. Clin. Pract. Nephrol. 4 (7) (2008) 378–392.

[79] D.S. Milliner, A.R. Zinsmeister, E. Lieberman, B. Landing, Soft tissue calcification in pediatric patients with end-stage renal disease, Kidney Int. 38 (5) (1990) 931–936.

[80] J.S. Garland, R.M. Holden, P.A. Groome, M. Lam, R.L. Nolan, A.R. Morton, et al., Prevalence and associations of coronary artery calcification in patients with stages 3 to 5 CKD without cardiovascular disease, Am. J. Kidney Dis. 52 (5) (2008) 849–858.

[81] S. Paoli, M.M. Mitsnefes, Coronary artery calcification and cardiovascular disease in children with chronic kidney disease, Curr. Opin. Pediatr. 26 (2) (2014) 193–197.

[82] M.M. Mitsnefes, B.L. Laskin, M. Dahhou, X. Zhang, B.J. Foster, Mortality risk among children initially treated with dialysis for end-stage kidney disease, 1990–2010, JAMA 309 (18) (2013) 1921–1929.

[83] J.J. Fadrowski, D. Frankenfield, S. Amaral, T. Brady, G.H. Gorman, B. Warady, et al., Children on long-term dialysis in the United States: findings from the 2005 ESRD clinical performance measures project, Am. J. Kidney Dis. 50 (6) (2007) 958–966.

[84] R.S. Suri, G.E. Nesrallah, R. Mainra, A.X. Garg, R.M. Lindsay, T. Greene, et al., Daily hemodialysis: a systematic review, Clin. J. Am. Soc. Nephrol. 1 (1) (2006) 33–42.

[85] G.M. Chertow, N.W. Levin, G.J. Beck, T.A. Depner, P.W. Eggers, J.J. Gassman, et al., In-center hemodialysis six times per week versus three times per week, N. Engl. J. Med. 363 (24) (2010) 2287–2300.

[86] G.M. Chertow, N.W. Levin, G.J. Beck, J.T. Daugirdas, P.W. Eggers, A.S. Kliger, B. Larive, M.V. Rocco, T. Greene, Frequent Hemodialysis Network (FHN) Trials Group, Long-term effects of frequent in-center hemodialysis, J. Am. Soc. Nephrol. 27 (6) (June 2016) 1830–1836. http://dx.doi.org/10.1681/ASN.2015040426. Epub 2015 Oct 14. PubMed PMID: 26467779; PubMed Central PMCID: PMC4884113.

[87] E. Nehus, J. Goebel, M. Mitsnefes, A. Lorts, B. Laskin, Intensive hemodialysis for cardiomyopathy associated with end-stage renal disease, Pediatr. Nephrol. 26 (10) (2011) 1909–1912.

[88] M. Fischbach, C. Dheu, L. Seuge, S. Menouer, J. Terzic, In-center daily on-line hemodiafiltration: a 4-year experience in children, Clin. Nephrol. 69 (4) (2008) 279–284.

[89] M. Fischbach, J. Terzic, S. Menouer, C. Dheu, L. Seuge, A. Zalosczic, Daily on line haemodiafiltration promotes catch-up growth in children on chronic dialysis, Nephrol. Dial. Transplant. 25 (3) (2010) 867–873.

Chapter 32

Heart Failure in Pediatric Oncologic Disease

Neha Bansal[1], Jyothsna Akam-Venkata[1], Vivian I. Franco[1], Steven E. Lipshultz[1,2]
[1]Wayne State University School of Medicine and Children's Hospital of Michigan, Detroit, MI, United States; [2]Karmanos Cancer Institute, Detroit, MI, United States

INTRODUCTION

Epidemiology of Cardiotoxicity in Childhood Cancer Survivors

Between 2007 and 2011, the incidence of childhood cancer increased by 0.6% per year, making it the second most common cause of death in children 1–14 years old. Cancer accounts for one in every four deaths [1]. Fortunately, advances in cancer treatment have reduced childhood cancer mortality rates by 67%, from 6.3 per 100,000 in 1970 to 2.1 per 100,000 in 2011. The 5-year survival rate for all childhood cancers increased from 58% to 83% [1]. As of 2005, of the 328,652 survivors of childhood cancer in the United States, 24% have survived longer than 30 years since diagnosis [2].

These childhood cancer survivors are at risk for chronic health conditions, such as second malignancies, organ damage (cardiopulmonary, gonadal, etc.), impaired neurodevelopment, and poor cognitive function, all of which decrease quality of life [3]. Among survivors, the cumulative incidence of a chronic health conditions reached 73.4% (95% CI, 69%–78%) 30 years after cancer diagnosis, with a cumulative incidence of 42% (95% CI, 34%–51%) for severe, disabling, or life-threatening conditions or death from a chronic condition [4].

After the recurrence of primary and secondary malignancies, cardiovascular diseases are the most common cause of morbidity and mortality among cancer survivors [5]. The relative risk for heart failure (HF) and coronary artery disease (CAD) in cancer survivors is 15 and 10, respectively, compared to their healthy siblings [4]. Similarly, in cancer survivors, the hazard rate of pericardial diseases is 3–10 times as high, and that of valvar diseases is 5 times as high, as that of their sibling controls [6].

PATHOPHYSIOLOGY OF CARDIOVASCULAR TOXICITY

Anthracycline-Related Cardiovascular Toxicity

Chemotherapeutic medications interfere with neoplastic cell division and adversely affect normal cell division of highly mitotic cells. These medications have unpredictable effects on the cardiovascular system, which limits the regenerative capacity of the cardiovascular system. Cardiotoxic effects have been documented for several classes of cancer treatments, including anthracyclines (e.g., doxorubicin and epirubicin), alkylating agents (e.g., busulfan and cyclophosphamide), antimetabolites (including 5-fluorouracil and cytarabine), antimicrotubule agents (e.g., vinca alkaloids), targeted agents (e.g., lapatinib and trastuzumab), and radiation (Table 32.1) [7,8]. Newer antineoplastic compounds, such as tyrosine kinase inhibitors, are now being used to treat children. However, in adults these compounds can be cardiotoxic [9].

Anthracyclines enter cells by passive diffusion. Their concentrations can be much higher in the cytoplasmic compartment of cardiomyocytes because of the high concentrations of cardiolipin in these cells and the higher affinity of cardiolipin to anthracyclines [10,11]. Anthracyclines form complexes with intracellular iron and reduce the quinone moiety to subquinone, causing a cascade production of reactive oxygen species (ROS) [12–15]. These complexes also uncouple the electron transport chain, which also creates highly ROS and impairs ATP synthesis [11]. Oxidative stress produces nitric oxide and peroxynitrite by inducing the enzyme, nitric oxide synthase, which inactivates myofibrillar creatine kinase and other important cardiac enzymes [16,17]. Glutathione peroxidase, a cardiac antioxidant, is depleted in the presence of anthracyclines [18]. Thus, the already damaged mitochondria are unable to adjust to increased oxidative stress, which causes more damage and ultimately, cell death.

Heart Failure in the Child and Young Adult. http://dx.doi.org/10.1016/B978-0-12-802393-8.00032-6

Various other mechanisms of anthracycline-related cardiotoxicity have been hypothesized, including the induction of apoptosis, the production of vasoactive amines, the formation of toxic metabolites, the upregulation of nitric oxide synthase, and the inhibition of transcription and translation [19–21].

Cardiomyocytes exposed to anthracyclines show other changes, which may or may not depend on the oxidative pathway. These changes include depleted cardiac stem cells [22], impaired DNA synthesis [23], impaired cell signaling that triggers cell death [24], altered gene expression [25], inhibited calcium release from the sarcoplasmic reticulum [26], impaired formation of the protein titin in sarcomeres [27], and impaired mitochondrial creatine kinase activity and function [28]. These subcellular processes often continue for weeks after anthracycline exposure, thus explaining the mechanism of chronic cardiomyopathy [29].

Recently, topoisomerase-II β (Top2β) alterations, specifically the Top2β–doxorubicin–DNA ternary cleavage complex that induce DNA double-strand breaks, have been postulated to be another mechanism of doxorubicin-mediated cardiotoxicity [30–32]. A study in mice found that cardiomyocyte-specific deletion of Top2β was cardioprotective [30]. Another recent study found that peripheral blood leukocyte Top2β concentrations were higher in anthracycline-sensitive patients (with decreased left ventricular ejection fractions [LVEF] ≥10% from baseline and <50%, despite receiving a cumulative doxorubicin dose ≤250 mg/m^2) than in anthracycline-resistant patients (who received a cumulative doxorubicin dose ≥450 mg/m^2 with an LVEF ≥50%). These results indicate the potential for Top2β to be used as a surrogate marker for susceptibility to anthracycline-induced cardiotoxicity [33].

Radiotherapy-Related Cardiovascular Toxicity

The pathophysiology of cardiac damage from radiotherapy (RT) has been studied extensively. The hallmark of such damage is nonspecific, diffuse, interstitial fibrosis that can even include the conduction system [34–38]. Microscopically, the amount of type I collagenase increases disproportionately more than that of type III, including an overall increase in total collagen, which alters myocardial compliance, causing diastolic dysfunction [39]. Radiation also activates the inflammatory pathways that increase ROS production and oxidative damage [40,41]. This damage, in turn, leads to chronic

TABLE 32.1 Cardiotoxic Effects of Selected Cytotoxic Agents

Agents	Cardiotoxic Effect
Anthracyclines: Daunorubicin, doxorubicin, epirubicin, idarubicin, mitoxantrone	Arrhythmias, pericarditis, myocarditis, HF, LV dysfunction
Liposomal anthracyclines: Pegylated liposomal doxorubicin hydrochloride (DOXIL, CAELYX)	HF, LV dysfunction, arrhythmias
Antimetabolites: Capecitabine, carmustine, clofarabine, cytarabine, 5-fluorouracil, methotrexate	Ischemia, chest pain, MI, HF, arrhythmias, pericardial effusions, pericarditis, hemodynamic abnormalities
Antimicrotubules: Paclitaxel, vinca alkaloids	Hypotension or hypertension, ischemia, angina, MI, bradycardia, arrhythmias, conduction abnormalities, HF
Alkylating agents: Busulfan, chlormethine, cisplatin, cyclophosphamide, ifosfamide, mitomycin	Endomyocardial fibrosis, pericarditis, tamponade, ischemia, MI, hypertension, myocarditis, HF, arrhythmias
Small-molecule tyrosine kinase inhibitors: Dasatinib, gefitinib, imatinib mesylate, lapatinib, erlotinib, sorafenib, sunitinib	HF, edema, pericardial effusion, pericarditis, hypertension, arrhythmias, prolonged QT interval, ischemia, chest pain
Monoclonal antibodies: Alemtuzumab, bevacizumab, cetuximab, rituximab, trastuzumab	Hemodynamic abnormalities, LV dysfunction, HF, thromboembolism, angioedema, arrhythmias
Interleukins: Denileukin, IL-2	Hypotension, capillary leak syndrome, arrhythmias, coronary artery thrombosis, ischemia, LV dysfunction
Miscellaneous agents: All-trans-retinoic acid, arsenic trioxide, asparaginase, etoposide, IFN-α, lenalidomide, 6-mercaptopurine, pentostatin, teniposide, thalidomide	Electrocardiographic changes, QT prolongation, torsades de pointes, other arrhythmias, ischemia, angina, MI, HF, edema, hypotension, bradycardia, thromboembolism, and retinoid acid syndrome that includes fever, hypotension, respiratory distress, weight gain, peripheral edema, pleural–pericardial effusions

HF, heart failure; *IFN-α*, interferon alpha; *IL-2*, interleukin 2; *LV*, left ventricular; *MI*, myocardial infarction [128].

inflammation, which may increase the risk of clinically important plaque development and rupture [42]. Given the RT doses and techniques now used in children, extensive fibrotic thickening of the pericardium, including pericardial adhesions and excessive pericardial fluid, is now rare [43]. Irradiated valves, and left-sided valves more commonly, become fibrotic, with or without calcification [43–45]. The coronary ostia and proximal segments of the left anterior descending and the right coronary arteries are often affected after RT [43,44,46–48].

Differentiating between radiation-induced atherosclerotic plaque and typical nonradiation-related atherosclerotic CAD plaque remains controversial [43]. In the brain, an inflammation in the cerebral microvasculature causes endothelial perforation and increases platelet adherence and thrombus formation [49,50]. The loss of tight junctions leads to histopathological changes that also result in luminal narrowing, dilation, and tortuosity [49,51,52]. Neck irradiation increases the thickness of the intima and the media layer of the carotid wall, thus increasing the risk of stroke in the presence of preexisting atherosclerosis [53–55].

PROGRESSION OF CARDIOVASCULAR TOXICITY

Anthracycline cardiotoxicity can present any time after initial treatment, and early toxicity not a prerequisite for late toxicity [56,57]. Cardiotoxicity is classified as acute when the signs and symptoms appear within the first week of treatment, as early-onset chronic progressive toxicity when they appear between 1 week and 1 year after treatment begins, and late-onset toxicity when they appear 1 year after treatment (Table 32.2).

Acute toxicity manifests in less than 1% of the patients as arrhythmias, electrocardiographic abnormalities, and HF, or as a myocarditis–pericarditis syndrome [10,58–60]. The condition often resolves by stopping treatment, although fatal HF has been reported [10,60]. The effects of cardiotoxicity can be persistent and progressive and can even occur at lower cumulative anthracycline doses [61].

Early-onset cardiotoxicity presents between 1 week to 1 year and may present with left ventricular (LV) dysfunction, electrocardiographic changes, and potentially fatal HF [10,58,59,62–64].

In late-onset cardiotoxicity, the number of cardiomyocytes is often decreased, which results in LV dilation that progresses to a restrictive LV cardiomyopathy, LV wall thinning, and decreased LV contractility [61,65–67]. Echocardiographic findings include decreases in LV fractional shortening and decreased LV mass adjusted to body surface area, LV contractility, and LV end-diastolic posterior wall thickness adjusted to body surface area [10]. A 2005 study reported that dilated cardiomyopathy (DCM) progressed toward a restrictive-like pattern with extended follow-up (Fig. 32.1) [61]. Long-term follow-up found a decrease in LV dimension adjusted to body surface area with a subsequent increase in the LV thickness adjusted to body surface area that resulted in a normal LV thickness-to-dimension ratio, indicating ventricular remodeling. This shrinking myocardial cavity size that is too small for body surface area (a finding that we have characterized as the "Grinch Syndrome") is the chronic cardiomyopathy that may result in HF, heart transplantation, or death (Fig. 32.2) [68].

Radiation-induced cardiotoxicity may be insidious and can manifest almost a decade after exposure. Diastolic ventricular dysfunction is the most important clinical consequence. In adults with Hodgkin lymphoma, 14% have mild-to-moderate diastolic ventricular dysfunction [69]. Because many patients are asymptomatic, cardiovascular abnormalities

TABLE 32.2 Characteristics of the Different Types of Anthracycline Cardiotoxicity

Characteristic	Acute Cardiotoxicity	Early-Onset Progressive Cardiotoxicity	Late-Onset Progressive Cardiotoxicity
Onset	Within the first week of anthracycline treatment	<1 year after completing anthracycline treatment	≥1 year after completing anthracycline treatment
Risk factor dependence	Unknown	Yes	Yes
Clinical features in adults	Transient depression of myocardial contractility	Dilated cardiomyopathy	Dilated cardiomyopathy
Clinical features in children	Transient depression of myocardial contractility	Restrictive cardiomyopathy and/or dilated cardiomyopathy	Restrictive cardiomyopathy and/or dilated cardiomyopathy
Course	Usually reversible on discontinuation of anthracycline	Can be progressive	Can be progressive

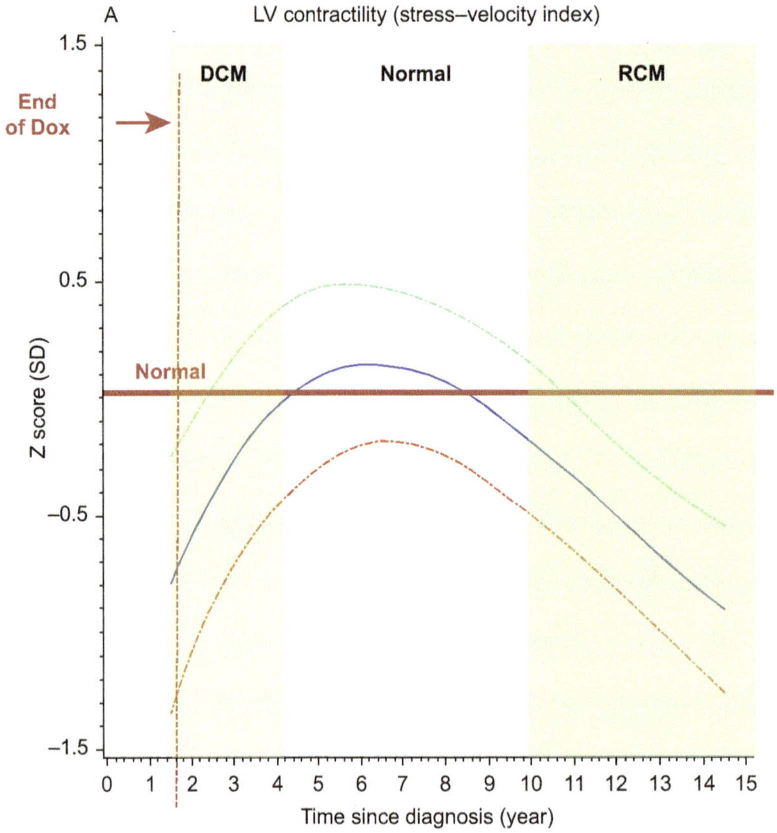

FIGURE 32.1 Cardiac measurements from 115 long-term survivors of acute lymphoblastic leukemia treated with doxorubicin, by years since diagnosis, showing how dilated cardiomyopathy evolves into restrictive cardiomyopathy about 10 years after treatment. *Solid line*, mean Z-score; *dashed lines*, 95% confidence band. *DCM*, dilated cardiomyopathy; *RCM*, restrictive cardiomyopathy; *LV*, left ventricular. *Published with permission from American Society of Clinical Oncology.*

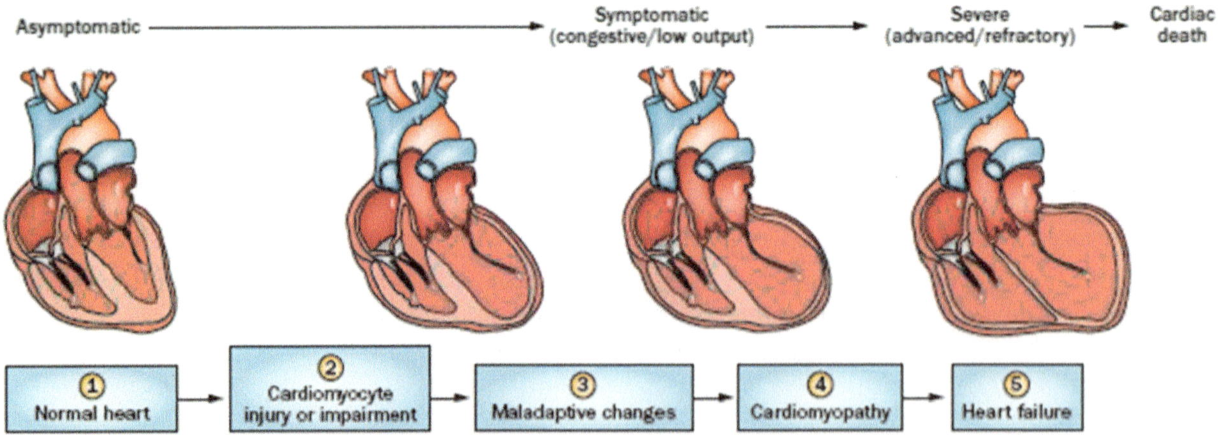

FIGURE 32.2 Stages in the development of pediatric ventricular dysfunction [128].

are unsuspected, although in our study, 37% of patients had LV end-diastolic systolic dysfunction [70]. We have found that low maximum oxygen consumption (VO_2 max) has been associated with a reduced quality of life assessment (P=.02) [71]. We also [70] noted that 47% of Hodgkin lymphoma survivors had valvar abnormalities, which could be progressive and likely increase the risk for endocarditis and HF [63]. Survivors with LV dysfunction tend to have poor cardiac event–free survival and a worse quality of life than those of survivors free of LV dysfunction [69,70,72]. Surveillance guidelines for these cardiovascular morbidities are currently lacking [73].

RISK FACTORS FOR ANTHRACYCLINE-INDUCED CARDIOTOXICITY

Cumulative Dose of Anthracycline

A higher cumulative dose of anthracycline is the strongest predictor of late cardiotoxicity [61,66]. Among 607 children treated with anthracyclines, the risk of cardiotoxicity was 11.8 times as high in those who received cumulative doses greater than 300 mg/m^2 than in those who received less than 300 mg/m^2 at a mean follow-up of 6.3 years [74]. In addition, a separate study reported that among 97 patients who received cumulative anthracycline doses of between 228 and 550 mg/m^2, 65% had a cardiac abnormality. In the same study, increased LV afterload and decreased LV contractility developed in all three patients who received greater than 500 mg/m^2. Of the 97 patients, 18 (17%) who received an anthracycline cumulative dose even as low as 45 mg/m^2 eventually experienced increased LV afterload secondary to decreases in LV wall thickness [66]. Thus, there is no safe dose of anthracycline that is free of cardiotoxicity, and this risk increases with higher cumulative doses and increased length of follow-up.

Genetic Factors

Hereditary factors and genetic variability may help explain the difference in the degree of cardiotoxicity among the cancer survivors. As described earlier, anthracyclines form complexes with iron that generate ROS, which in turn causes lipid peroxidation and DNA damage [75].

Hereditary hemochromatosis is a disorder of iron metabolism characterized by iron overload in the tissues. The most common mutation in this disorder is C282Y, and it is characterized by the replacement of cysteine with tyrosine at the 282nd position of the amino acid chain of the HFE protein. Heterozygous carriers of the C282Y mutation had higher concentrations of cardiac troponin T (cTnT), a marker of cardiac injury, than did noncarriers who received doxorubicin [76]. Patients with trisomy 21 may also have an increased risk of cardiotoxicity [59], perhaps because they are at risk for exposure to chemotherapeutic agents secondary to an increased incidence of both acute lymphoblastic leukemia (ALL) and acute myeloid leukemia (AML), and have a three- to fourfold increase in the generation of intracellular ROS [77].

A German non-Hodgkin lymphoma study reported that anthracycline-induced cardiotoxicity was associated with a polymorphism in the NAD(P)H oxidase subunit NCF4 gene. Mice deficient in NAD(P)H oxidase activity were resistant to the effects of chronic anthracycline exposure [78]. A study from the Children's Oncology Group found that a polymorphism in the gene coding for carbonyl reductase (CRB3), which converts anthracycline to cardiotoxic metabolites, was associated with an increased risk for cardiotoxicity at cumulative anthracycline doses of between 101 and 150 mg/m^2), although this risk was not found at high doses (>250 mg/m^2) [79].

In a recent study, DNA polymorphisms of metabolic and functional pathways of doxorubicin were thought to contribute to the risk stratification of anthracycline-mediated cardiotoxicity. Among the doxorubicin-treated childhood cancer survivors, the patients with the ABCC5 TT-1629 genotype, coding for an ATP-binding cassette transporter, had an 8%–12% decrease in their LV ejection fraction and LV shortening fraction. In the high-risk cancer patients, the NOS3 TT894 genotype of the endothelial nitric oxide synthase gene had a protective effect on the LV ejection fraction of childhood cancer patients treated with anthracyclines, even without using cardioprotective agents such as dexrazoxane [80].

Also associated with anthracycline-induced cardiotoxicity are several mutations in genes encoding the proteins involved in metabolizing anthracyclines, such as nucleoside transport (SLC28A3); anthracycline absorption, distribution, metabolism, and elimination (ATP-binding cassette transporters ABCB1, ABCB4, ABCC1); anthracycline hepatic uptake (SLC10A2); and anthracycline metabolite glucuronidation (UGT1A6) [81]. African–American ethnicity may also be associated with a higher risk for cardiotoxicity [59].

Endocrine Disorders

During cancer treatment, some patients may undergo neurosurgical procedures and cranial irradiation. These treatments may lead to growth hormone (GH) deficiency, which is a complication among childhood cancer survivors [82]. GH deficiency may also cause other endocrine disorders, such as dyslipidemia and metabolic syndrome. GH deficiency in childhood cancer survivors may result in inadequate LV mass and LV wall thickness. GH replacement therapy can increase LV wall thickness in cancer survivors exposed to anthracyclines. However, this effect was lost when GH was discontinued [83]. GH replacement therapy unfortunately did not abrogate the progressive LV dysfunction in these survivors [83].

Sex

Females have a higher risk of LV dysfunction than males exposed to equivalent doses of doxorubicin [65]. The reason for this association is not clear, although it may be related to why females benefit more from doxorubicin and remain in remission longer than do males [84,85]. These differences may be attributed to the fact that doxorubicin does not reach high concentrations in adipose tissue [86]. Because girls have more body fat than boys, but have still been dosed based on body surface area, they may have higher circulating concentrations of doxorubicin, along with higher nonadipose intracellular anthracycline concentrations shortly after administration.

Age

Survivors diagnosed before 4 years of age have a higher risk of late mortality [5,65,66], perhaps because they have a smaller LV mass and because doxorubicin accentuates the inhibition of myocardial growth. Also, infants and younger children have a higher percentage of body fat and may thus have higher circulating concentrations of the drug, as described above. Longer times since completing doxorubicin treatment are associated with decreased LV wall thickness and increased LV afterload [65], perhaps because of the higher cumulative doses of doxorubicin that were used several decades ago.

Lifestyle

High-risk behaviors, such as consuming cigarettes, alcohol, energy drinks, and illicit drugs, may increase the risk for late cardiotoxicity [87]. The incidence of smoking is not higher among cancer survivors than it is among their healthy siblings [88], and dietary habits and caloric intake are also similar [89]. However, male survivors have more body fat and dyslipidemia than do their healthy siblings [89,90]. Physical inactivity and hypothalamic-pituitary dysfunction that promotes obesity from cranial irradiation may cause this difference [90].

After a mean of 13.4 years since a childhood cancer diagnosis, the VO_2 max was lower in 72 survivors than in their 32 healthy siblings (males, 28.5 vs. 30.9 mL/kg/min; females, 19.81 vs. 23.4 mL/kg/min). Older age, more body fat, methotrexate exposure, and extremes of LV mass and function correlated with lower VO_2 max in survivors [91]. In a different study, at a median follow-up of 8.6 years, 355 survivors of childhood cancer had a lower health-related quality of life and poorer functional status than did the healthy children. In turn, lower quality of life and decreased functional status were associated with older age at diagnosis, lower socioeconomic status, LV size, and increased risk for death and transplant [92].

Comorbidities

Conventional risk factors for cardiovascular diseases, such as obesity, insulin resistance, type 2 diabetes mellitus, metabolic syndrome, dyslipidemia, hypertension, renal and pulmonary disorders, and so on, when present will continue to affect the survivors of childhood cancers and increase their risk for late cardiotoxicity. Survivors have a higher prevalence of hypertension and obesity and a greater rise in their BMI than their healthier siblings [93–95]. Survivors are also more likely to be insulin-resistant and to have dyslipidemia than their healthier siblings [96].

Concurrent Radiotherapy

The effect of concurrent RT with chemotherapy is not fully understood. Among 1909 patients treated with chemotherapy and radiation, there was no evidence that these treatments interacted in causing mortality (P=.40) [97]. Among 48 Hodgkin lymphoma survivors (of whom 4 also received anthracyclines), all but 1 had some form of cardiac abnormality, such as restrictive cardiomyopathy, valvar heart disease, and conduction abnormalities, at a mean of 14.3 years of follow-up. VO_2 max during exercise was decreased in 14 survivors [70]. A metaanalysis of 10 studies of circulatory diseases secondary to radiation exposure reported that the overall radiation-related mortality was about twice that of estimates based on cancer end points alone [98].

Concurrent Chemotherapy

The risk of anthracycline-induced cardiotoxicity increases with coadministration of other cardiotoxic chemotherapeutic agents, such as trastuzumab, cyclophosphamide, bleomycin, vincristine, and amsacrine [58,59]. One study reported that amsacrine-related cardiotoxicity depended on both the dose of anthracycline and the rate and dose of amsacrine. Cardiac abnormalities developed in none of the 6 patients who received greater than 400 mg/m^2 of anthracycline and less than

200 mg/m^2 of amsacrine, in 7 of 8 exposed to greater than 400 mg/m^2 of anthracycline and greater than 200 mg/m^2 of amsacrine, and in 9 of 11 patients who receive greater than 400 mg/m^2 and greater than 200 mg/m^2 of amsacrine [99].

MONITORING CARDIOTOXICITY

In 2007, the American Society of Clinical Oncology Survivorship Expert Panel identified the need for optimal screening strategies and evidence-based options for treating long-term cardiac and pulmonary toxicity secondary to chemotherapy or RT in both symptomatic and asymptomatic cancer survivors [100]. Currently, several such guidelines are available, such as those of the American Heart Association (AHA), which is nonspecific [101], and the Children's Oncology Group's risk-based guidelines for long-term cardiac morbidity [102]. The optimal timing and frequency of cardiovascular monitoring in cancer survivors remains controversial because the evidence is limited and the existing guidelines are inconsistent.

Cardiac troponins are biomarkers specific for myocardial damage. Increased concentrations indicate irreversible cardiomyocyte cell death [103,104]. Two serum cardiac biomarkers, cTnT, and N-terminal prohormone of brain natriuretic peptide (NT-proBNP), are validated surrogate end points for late cardiotoxicity in long-term cancer survivors [105]. Among 134 children, reduced LV end-diastolic posterior wall thickness and LV mass and increased LV remodeling 4 years later were significantly associated with serum cTnT concentrations elevated during the first 90 days of anthracycline treatment [105]. Also, NT-proBNP concentrations elevated during the first 90 days of treatment correlated with abnormal LV thickness-to-dimension ratios 4 years after therapy (Fig. 32.3). These markers can be used to tailor anticancer therapy. Furthermore, monitoring NT-proBNP concentrations during therapy might predict which children are at higher risk of cardiotoxicity, allowing treatment to be modified before cardiomyocyte damage is irreversible [106].

Patients should be monitored annually with a thorough history and physical examination with careful screening for signs of cardiac dysfunction. However, these traditional methods often detect changes only after they become irreversible. Electrocardiography is universally available and inexpensive, but it lacks specificity and sensitivity [107,108]. Echocardiography can measure variables such as LV systolic function using M-mode LV fractional shortening measurements [109,110]. However, these measurements are load dependent and variable, providing rates of subclinical cardiotoxicity of from 0% to 57% [111]. Angle-independent, speckle-tracking echocardiography has been validated in both adults [112] and children [113] and shows great promise in detecting subclinical cardiac dysfunction, although the results vary with image quality [114,115].

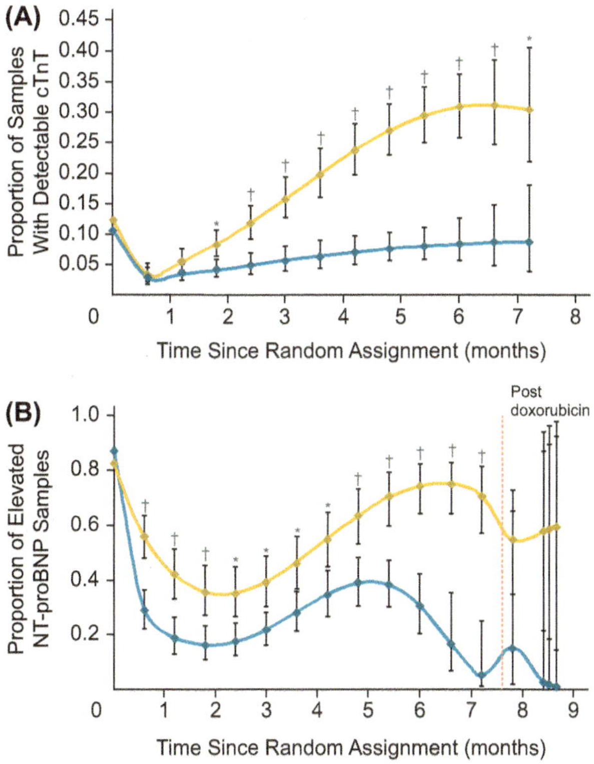

FIGURE 32.3 (A) Model-based estimated probability of having an elevated cardiac troponin T (cTnT) concentration over time in patients treated with doxorubicin, with or without dexrazoxane. The doxorubicin–dexrazoxane group is indicated by the *blue line*, and the doxorubicin group by the *gold line*. Vertical bars are 95% confidence intervals. Increased cTnT concentration is defined as a value greater than 0.01 ng/mL. *P versus dexrazoxane group, ≤.05; †P versus dexrazoxane group, ≤.001. An overall test for dexrazoxane effect during treatment was significant (P<.001). (B) Model-based estimated probability of having an elevated N-terminal probrain natriuretic peptide (NT-proBNP) concentration over time in patients treated with doxorubicin, with or without dexrazoxane. The doxorubicin–dexrazoxane group is indicated by the *blue line*, and the doxorubicin group by the *gold line*. Vertical bars are 95% confidence intervals. Increased NT-proBNP concentration is defined as a value 150 pg/mL or greater for children less than 1 year old and 100 pg/mL or greater for children 1 year older or older. *P versus dexrazoxane group, ≤.05; †P versus dexrazoxane group, ≤.001. An overall test for a dexrazoxane effect was significant (P<.001) during treatment but not after treatment (P=.24). *Published with permission from American Society of Clinical Oncology.*

Characterizing ultrasonic tissue by integrated backscatter is a noninvasive method. In this technique, the magnitude of backscatter decreases in both ischemic and nonischemic myocardial diseases, making it highly sensitive but nonspecific for detecting subclinical changes [116–118]. However, results vary with the angle and motion of the heart, and further research is required to determine the usefulness of this modality.

Cardiac magnetic resonance imaging, although time-consuming and often requiring sedation in younger children, has been evaluated in some small studies. It has shown great promise in detecting perfusion abnormalities and subendocardial damage undetected by any other method. It does not use ionizing radiation and provides high-resolution pictures with numerous windows [119–121].

PREVENTING CARDIOTOXICITY

The cardiotoxic effects of cancer therapy cause substantial morbidity and mortality. Therefore, preventing cardiac damage without reducing the efficacy of chemotherapy is a major consideration in managing cardiotoxicity.

Anthracycline-Induced Cardiotoxicity

Anthracycline Dosing

As discussed earlier, higher cumulative anthracycline dose is the largest risk factor for cardiotoxicity. Before this fact was recognized in 1970s, cumulative doses greater than 400 mg/m^2 were used in all children with ALL [66]. Since then, the maximum cumulative doses have been decreased to 45–60 mg/m^2 for patients with standard-risk ALL and to 300–360 mg/m^2 for those with high-risk ALL and this has decreased the risk for late cardiotoxicity [122]. Two decades later, a study of 189 patients found less cardiotoxicity in those receiving less than 300 mg/m^2 than in those who received more than 300 mg/m^2 [123]. This study led to decreasing the cumulative dose to 300 mg/m^2 for patients with high-risk ALL [124]. Late cardiotoxicity has occurred in patients receiving as low as 45 mg/m^2 of doxorubicin [66]; hence, there is no safe dose of anthracyclines and decreasing the dose may reduce its efficacy.

Anthracycline Derivatives

There is not clear evidence that the use of anthracycline analogues in children results in less cardiotoxicity in survivors do to issues of dose equivalency. Although many studies have suggested there is less cardiotoxicity, other studies have shown that higher cumulative doses must be given to achieve comparable oncologic efficacy. Therefore, studies noted below do not provide evidence that there is any cardioprotection if the goal is to maintain oncologic efficacy. Epirubicin, a 4′-doxorubicin epimer, is less cardiotoxic than doxorubicin and is safe at even double the maximum cumulative dose of doxorubicin, which allows higher doses and more treatment cycles [125]. In adults with breast cancer, idarubicin, a synthetic derivative of daunorubicin, has been reported to be less cardiotoxic than doxorubicin (in 0 of 37 vs. 6 of 19 patients, respectively) [126]. Mitoxantrone, a synthetic anthraquinone with antitumor, antiinfective properties, causes less-severe cardiac damage than doxorubicin in adults [127]. However, the safety and balance of efficacy and toxicities of epirubicin, idarubicin, and mitoxantrone treatment in children requires more study [128].

Continuous Versus Bolus Infusion

Studies in adults have shown that continuous infusion of anthracyclines may prevent cardiac damage by decreasing peak anthracycline concentrations [129]. However, in a randomized trial of children with high-risk ALL after a median follow-up of 8 years, continuous infusion of doxorubicin was not cardioprotective and provided no long-term benefit over bolus infusions [130].

Liposomal Anthracycline

When encapsulated within a liposome, doxorubicin has a higher affinity for malignant cells with neovascularization and has a lesser volume of distribution [131]. The cardiac syncytium is comprised of tight junctions and does not allow this form of the drug to reach the cardiomyocytes. The only current FDA-approved liposomal doxorubicin is Doxil, which decreases the risk of cardiotoxicity without decreasing the efficacy of treatment in adults with cancer, but pediatric studies are limited [132].

Dexrazoxane

Dexrazoxane, an ethylene diamine tetraacetic acid, such as bisdioxopiperazine, becomes hydrolyzed within the cardiomyocyte to form a potent chelator of heavy metals, especially iron. Hence, it acts by chelating intracellular iron and decreasing free radical formation [133]. It provides long-term cardioprotection without decreasing the efficacy of doxorubicin in patients with high-risk ALL [134]. Its cardioprotective effect is seen more in girls than in boys in one study but affects both sexes equally in others [134].

One of the mechanisms of doxorubicin-related cardiotoxicity is mitochondrial inhibition. Studies of anthracycline exposure in the mitochondria have shown disruption of the oxidative phosphorlylation enzymes, particularly the nicotinamide adenine dinucleotide dehydrogenase and cytochrome c oxidase activity, in addition to mitochondrial DNA (mtDNA) changes such as mutations, deletions, and reduced copy numbers per cardiomyocyte [135–138].

mtDNA and its function were assessed in peripheral blood mononuclear cells of survivors of ALL who were treated with doxorubicin, with or without dexrazoxane. As a compensatory response to impaired mitochondrial function, mtDNA copy numbers within each cell were increased in patients who received doxorubicin alone. Patients receiving both doxorubicin and dexrazoxane had a lower number of mtDNA copy numbers/cell, indicating that dexrazoxane preserves mitochondrial structure and function during doxorubicin treatment. Even at a median follow-up of 7.8 years after treatment, the median number of mtDNA copies per cell were higher in patients who received doxorubicin alone (1106.3 vs. 310.5, $P=.001$) [139].

Dexrazoxane is approved by the FDA for use in women with stage 4 breast cancer who have received a cumulative doxorubicin dose of 300 mg/m^2. Its use can be considered in patients with any malignancy in which more than 300 mg/m^2 of doxorubicin is used [140]. The FDA designated dexrazoxane as an orphan drug for preventing anthracycline-related cardiotoxicity in children less than 16 years of age [141]. Even though dexrazoxane is approved for use when anthracycline cumulative doses exceed 300 mg/m^2 we have found that it is most effective when used with the initial dose of anthracycline and before each subsequent anthracycline dose.

Asselin et al. assessed the cardiac effects of 537 patients with T-cell ALL and lymphoblastic non-Hodgkin's lymphoma randomly assigned into two groups that received doxorubicin alone and the group that received both doxorubicin and dexrazoxane. LV fractional shortening, LV thickness, and LV thickness-to-dimension ratio was lower in patients treated with doxorubicin alone than they were in patients receiving both dexrazoxane and doxorubicin. This cardioprotection was observed even at cumulative doxorubicin doses of 360 mg/m^2, and the efficacy of chemotherapy was similar in both groups. The 5-year event-free survival was not different between the two groups (76.7% for the dexrazoxane group vs. 76% for the doxorubicin only group) [142].

Dexrazoxane decreases the incidence and severity of both acute and late anthracycline-induced cardiotoxicity in children with solid tumors [143]. Dexrazoxane reduced subclinical cardiotoxicity in 5 randomized-controlled trials and both subclinical and clinical cardiotoxicity in 12 nonrandomized-controlled trials. The risk for secondary malignant neoplasms was marginally higher in patients who received dexrazoxane and doxorubicin than in those who received doxorubicin alone (2.7% vs. 1.1%) [144]. Dexrazoxane is well-tolerated, and its only major adverse effect is dose-dependent but reversible myelosuppression [145]. Tebbi et al. reported that dexrazoxane might increase the risk of secondary malignant neoplasms in children with Hodgkin lymphoma at a median follow-up of 4 years, although this result has not since been reported [146]. Citing the Tebbi study, the European Medicines Agency in 2011 reported that dexrazoxane increased the risk of second malignancies in children with diseases such as AML and myelodysplastic syndrome [147]. Chow et al. examined the long-term mortality (median follow-up of 12.6 years) of patients with T-cell ALL/lymphoma and low, intermediate, and high-risk Hodgkin lymphoma from the results of the three randomized clinical trials (Children's Oncology Group trials P9404, P9425, and P9426), including those reported on by Tebbi but now with longer follow-up. Among 1008 patients with T-cell ALL/lymphoma or Hodgkin lymphoma, 507 received dexrazoxane with doxorubicin. Overall mortality rates were similar in both groups (12.8% in dexrazoxane-treated patients vs. 12.2% in doxorubicin-treated patients). Similarly, mortality rates from AML/myelodysplastic syndrome did not differ (7 of 12 in dexrazoxane-treated patients vs. 5 of 12 who did not receive dexrazoxane) [148]. In children and adolescents with metastatic osteosarcoma treated with doxorubicin, dexrazoxane was not only cardioprotective but also did not reduce the efficacy of chemotherapy, allowed intensification of chemotherapy, and did not increase the risk for secondary malignancies [149]. Several studies published between 2011 and 2014, including a Cochrane review, have confirmed the efficacy of dexrazoxane in preventing cardiotoxicity in childhood cancer survivors without decreasing the antitumor efficacy of chemotherapy and without increased risk for second malignancies [150].

The Dana-Farber Cancer Institute's Childhood Acute Lymphoblastic Leukemia Consortium has incorporated dexrazoxane into all its clinical protocols involving anthracyclines since 2000 with no adverse effects. The Children's Oncology Group also includes dexrazoxane in protocols that use 150 mg/m^2 of doxorubicin or more or any dose of anthracycline with planned RT that may affect the heart [150]. The AHA and the American Academy of Pediatrics have endorsed the use of dexrazoxane for cardioprotection in patients receiving dexrazoxane [122].

Amifostine

Amifostine can decrease damage to cardiomyocytes by its cytoprotective and antioxidant properties. It acts by decreasing lipid peroxidation, stabilizing DNA, increasing glutathione, and reducing free radicals by forming disulfide bonds [151].

It is cardioprotective in rats [152]. It did not affect the efficacy of chemotherapy in 28 children with osteosarcoma, and the number of amifostine-treated patients with subclinical HF was lower than that in the placebo group (0 of 28 vs. 2 of 28) [153].

Angiotensin Converting Enzyme Inhibitors and Beta-Adrenergic Antagonists

Angiotensin converting enzyme inhibitors (ACEI), such as enalapril, can prevent or partially reverse LV remodeling, decrease LV chamber stiffness, decrease LV mass, prevent LV dilatation, and therefore decrease the afterload in adults with severe LV systolic dysfunction [154]. However, a long-term follow-up study of doxorubicin-treated childhood cancer survivors with asymptomatic LV dysfunction found that enalapril improved LV structure and function for only 6–10 years [155]. However, in the same study anthracycline-treated childhood cancer survivors presenting with HF had a transient improvement in LV function when treated with enalapril but all had failed medical management within 5 years of starting enalapril and received a heart transplant or died a cardiac death.

In adults with increased troponin I concentrations after receiving high-dose chemotherapy, LV end-systolic and end-diastolic volumes were lower in those treated with ACEI than in controls [156]. In the ACEI after anthracyclines study, childhood cancer survivors who had been treated with anthracyclines were randomly assigned to receive an ACEI or placebo. Enalapril reduced LV end-systolic wall stress by reducing blood pressure but did not influence exercise performance [157].

Beta-adrenergic antagonists can decrease mortality and morbidity rates in adults with HF [158,159]. The proposed mechanism of action is the attenuation of adrenergically mediated LV remodeling and LV dysfunction [160]. Metoprolol increased mean LV fractional shortening by 23% and mean LV ejection fraction by 41% in children with HF from various causes, including anthracycline-induced cardiomyopathy [161]. More randomized trials are needed to validate the use of beta-adrenergic antagonists in preventing cardiotoxicity in cancer survivors.

Radiation-Induced Cardiotoxicity

The mechanism of radiation-induced cardiotoxicity has been described [122]; however, the extent of cardiovascular damage is variable and depends on several factors, such as radiation dosage, the RT technique, the duration and time since exposure, age, concomitant chemotherapy, and other conventional risk factors for cardiovascular diseases.

Dosage and Volume of Radiation

The standard radiation dosing for treating Hodgkin lymphoma has been decreased from 35–45 Gy to 15–25 Gy [122]. Cardiac protection by adding a subcarinal block has reduced the risk of nonischemic cardiac causes of deaths from 5.3 to 1.4 [162,163]. Also, the volume of radiation has been decreased from regional RT to involved-field RT and further to involved-node RT. The mean heart dose from involved-node RT has decreased by 50% from that in involved-field RT [164].

Intensity-Modulated Radiotherapy

Intensity-modulated RT is similar to 3-dimensional conformational RT except that it may provide better target coverage and less exposure to normal tissue when treating soft-tissue tumors, such as nasopharyngeal carcinoma [165]. It may be beneficial for treating mediastinal tumors, as well as for decreasing radiation exposure to cardiac tissue and thus preventing RT-induced cardiac damage.

MANAGING CARDIAC MORBIDITY IN CANCER SURVIVORS

Managing late cardiotoxicity requires considering several factors, including the underlying mechanism of cardiotoxicity, stage of HF, and comorbidities. The main goals of therapy are to prevent or reverse LV remodeling and to relieve symptoms using medical therapy or surgery in cases refractory to medical therapy.

Chemotherapy-Induced Morbidity

Guidelines for diagnosing and managing HF in adults were developed by American College of Cardiology/AHA in 2005 and updated in 2009 [166]. They are based on the classification of slowly progressive cardiac changes into four stages of HF from patients at risk for ventricular dysfunction (stage A) to intractable HF refractory to medical therapy (stage D). This classification is applicable to all children and to childhood cancer survivors [167].

Stage A: Patients at Risk for Ventricular Dysfunction

In stage A, patients have risk factors for heart disease in the absence of symptomatic or structural heart disease. Patients exposed to chemotherapeutic agents, with or without other risk factors, such as metabolic syndrome, hypertension, dyslipidemia, CAD, and so on, are in this category. The main aim of intervention in this stage is primary prevention to delay disease onset. The main steps for preventing heart disease are lifestyle changes or behavior modification, such as dietary changes, increased physical activity to prevent metabolic syndrome, and not using tobacco, alcohol, or illicit drugs.

Stage B: Patients With Structural Heart Disease Without Symptoms of Heart Failure

Patients in stage B have structural heart disease without symptoms of HF. Because HF develops slowly and is irreversible, patients are in stage B for a long period, allowing for interventions to delay disease progression. Beta-blockers and ACEI can delay or partially reverse LV remodeling in adult cancer survivors [166]. In 135 long-term survivors of pediatric cancers, ACEI did not alter exercise performance but did reduce LV end-systolic wall stress [157]. Evidence is insufficient to suggest that enalapril or beta-adrenergic antagonist treatment will improve long-term outcomes in childhood survivors. However, lifestyle changes discussed in stage A are also important in preventing disease progression in stage B.

Stage C: Patients With Ventricular Dysfunction With Symptomatic Heart Failure

Patients in stage C have ventricular dysfunction with symptomatic HF. Reducing LV preload with diuretic therapy is recommended for symptom relief [122]. Lipshultz et al. followed 18 doxorubicin-treated children for 10 years after they started enalapril. Enalapril provided only transient improvement in LV structure and function: after 6 years, all 6 symptomatic patients and 3 of 12 asymptomatic patients had either died or required a heart transplant, indicating the rapid deterioration of cardiac function [155]. Carvedilol therapy did not substantially improve clinical outcomes in children with HF [168].

Stage D: Decompensated Heart Failure Refractory to Medical Treatment

Patients in Stage D have decompensated HF that is refractory to medical management. Heart transplantation is indicated in such cases [169]. Intermediate cardiac support with extracorporeal membranous oxygenation or with a continuous or pulsatile LV assist device can be used as a bridge to heart transplantation [170,171], which in one study of 2375 patients was successful in 86% [172]. The 10-year survival rate after cardiac transplant in children with DCM is 72% [173]. However, mechanical support can have adverse events, such as infection, bleeding, thrombosis, and neurological complications. Hence, the benefits of mechanical support should outweigh the risk of these adverse events.

The Conundrum of Angiotensin Converting Enzyme Inhibitor Use in Anthracycline-Treated Survivors

- Enalapril-induced improvement in LV structure and function was transient. Enalapril did not prevent, but merely delayed, progression, for a 6–10 year benefit for patients with asymptomatic LV dysfunction before returning to baseline. For enalapril-treated HF patients on this study there was only a 2- to 6-year benefit. All HF patients progressed to cardiac transplantation or cardiac death within 2–6 years [155].
- Enalapril did not prevent progressive LV wall thinning, the primary defect that results in increased LV afterload and decreased LV fractional shortening. Limiting hypertrophic growth in a developing child may have detrimental consequences over a lifespan related to the long-term exacerbation of inadequate hypertrophy related to doxorubicin and then to enalapril [155].
- Enalapril did not address the primary defect of an inappropriately thin LV wall. Enalapril reduced LV afterload by a short-term lowering of diastolic blood pressure and LV dilation [155].
- The "AAA (ACEI After Anthracycline) Randomized, Double-blind, Placebo-controlled Trial of Enalapril" of 146 childhood cancer survivors showed the only significant finding: A fall in end-systolic stress in the first year of therapy based on a fall in blood pressure due to ACEI (P=.036) [157].
- It becomes important to understand the differences between anthracycline cardiomyopathy (ACM) and DCM. ACM differs from ischemic, postinfectious, and idiopathic DCM. In both the AAA study and our study there was a notable absence of ventricular remodeling in response to the fall in wall stress. In most DCM patients ACEIs induce reverse ventricular remodeling with a reduction in ventricular volume and an improved mass-to-volume ratio, which further reduces wall stress and improves cardiac function. In both studies despite a marked fall in wall stress ventricular size and thickness did not change. In contrast to other forms of DCM, the natural history of ACM is characterized by minimal,

nonprogressive dilation. The natural history of ACM and the response to ACEI therapy is unlike that of DCM but is more characteristic of a restrictive cardiomyopathy, a disease class that does not benefit from ACEI therapy. Further, many AAA study participants also received cardiac irradiation, a therapy also associated with the development of a late restrictive cardiomyopathy [157].

- The available data do not address whether the risk of ACEI therapy in patients with ACM exceeds those in other forms of DCM [174].
- The wisdom of recommending ACEI use based on the applicability of trials conducted in other patient groups should be questioned [174].
- The clinical pattern of a dominantly restrictive cardiomyopathy predicts a reduced likelihood of benefit [174].
- Data are also inadequate to address the risk associated with ACEI therapy of asymptomatic LV dysfunction in this population [155].
- Any adverse effects of long-term therapy clearly increase the risks for these patients, purely on the basis of markedly longer exposure [174].
- Further these patients may be at increased risk for potential adverse events [155].
- Therefore, these findings argue against the routine use of ACEI therapy in patients with asymptomatic LV dysfunction secondary to ACM.

Theoretical Enalapril Concerns in This Population

- An excess rate of gastrointestinal cancers relative to placebo has been observed in several large trials of nononcology adult patients receiving pronged ACEI therapy. This may be more of a concern to younger cancer survivors already at increased risk for relapsed primary or secondary malignancies [175].
- Survivors are at increased global risk for premature atherosclerotic heart disease, a risk that may also be affected by ACEI therapy [55].
- The unknown effects of chronic neurohormonal suppression or other side effects of long-term enalapril therapy in this population are a concern. Dizziness, hypotension, and fatigue were common problems for enalapril-treated AAA participants [157].
- The considerable cost of an unproven potentially life-long therapy in a young patient population with large past-medical expenses and lifetime insurance limits [174].
- Daily potentially life-long ACEI use for asymptomatic patients raises compliance issues. The effects do not appear to last forever raising other concerns [174].
- The unknown understanding of other potentially adverse drug interactions with this therapy for this population [155].
- For females of childbearing age, ACEI use may cause fetal kidney abnormalities if taken during pregnancy [176].
- The potential for healthy, asymptomatic survivors to feel or be treated differently from their peers for taking chronic medications, may increase the likelihood of these children feeling like "cardiac cripples" [174].

Conclusions About the Efficacy of Angiotensin Converting Enzyme Inhibitor Therapy in Anthracycline-Treated, Long-Term Survivors of Childhood Cancer

- This remains an unanswered, but important question [174].
- No study has shown any beneficial effects of ACEI in childhood survivors on improving quality of life, long-term benefit, or reducing progression to HF or death [174].
- The potential adverse effects of this therapy in patients with ACM argue against using this therapy, especially without convincing evidence of efficacy [174].

Radiation-Induced Morbidity

Abdominal RT or whole-body irradiation increases the risk of insulin resistance, metabolic syndrome, type 2 diabetes mellitus, and obesity. Cranial irradiation increases the risk for the GH deficiency, in addition to these conditions. Radiation therapy is also associated with increased risk for restrictive cardiomyopathy and valvar heart diseases.

Dietary modification and increased physical activity with parental involvement is associated with better outcomes in metabolic syndrome. Given its beneficial effect on metabolism and coronary vascular disease risk factors, GH replacement increases overall quality of life. Longer studies have not revealed an increased risk for diabetes mellitus from GH replacement, which was a concern raised by short-term studies. GH therapy may increase the risk for secondary malignancies, but the evidence is not strong [122]. Radiation therapy-induced restrictive cardiomyopathy is treated in the same way as is idiopathic restrictive cardiomyopathy, with fluid management, diuretics, and surgery if medical therapy is unsuccessful.

CONCLUSION

With advancements in cancer treatment, the cardiovascular-related health burden among survivors has become more important. The chemotherapeutic agents and their mechanism of cardiotoxicity are not well understood. Symptoms of cardiac damage may manifest years to decades after treatment. Injury to cardiomyocytes is progressive and irreversible; hence, identifying early signs of cardiac insult is critical in these patients. Standardized guidelines for optimal cardiac monitoring of these patients are still needed. The main goals in protecting the cardiac health of chemotherapy recipients should be to prevent or reduce the risk for treatment-related cardiotoxicity by using cardioprotectants, such as dexrazoxane, identifying evidence-based serial cardiac monitoring, identifying high-risk groups for closer follow-up, and incorporating lifestyle changes to prevent comorbidities.

REFERENCES

[1] Society AC, Cancer Facts & Figures 2015, American Cancer Society, Atlanta, 2015.
[2] A.B. Mariotto, J.H. Rowland, K.R. Yabroff, S. Scoppa, M. Hachey, L. Ries, et al., Long-term survivors of childhood cancers in the United States, Cancer Epidemiol. Biomark. Prev. 18 (4) (2009) 1033–1040.
[3] K.C. Oeffinger, M.M. Hudson, Long-term complications following childhood and adolescent cancer: foundations for providing risk-based health care for survivors, CA Cancer J. Clin. 54 (4) (2004) 208–236.
[4] K.C. Oeffinger, A.C. Mertens, C.A. Sklar, T. Kawashima, M.M. Hudson, A.T. Meadows, et al., Chronic health conditions in adult survivors of childhood cancer, N. Engl. J. Med. 355 (15) (2006) 1572–1582.
[5] A.C. Mertens, Q. Liu, J.P. Neglia, K. Wasilewski, W. Leisenring, G.T. Armstrong, et al., Cause-specific late mortality among 5-year survivors of childhood cancer: the childhood cancer survivor study, J. Natl. Cancer Inst. 100 (19) (2008) 1368–1379.
[6] D.A. Mulrooney, M.W. Yeazel, T. Kawashima, A.C. Mertens, P. Mitby, M. Stovall, et al., Cardiac outcomes in a cohort of adult survivors of childhood and adolescent cancer: retrospective analysis of the childhood cancer survivor study cohort, BMJ 339 (2009) b4606.
[7] J.M. Fulbright, Review of cardiotoxicity in pediatric cancer patients: during and after therapy, Cardiol. Res. Pract. 2011 (2011) 942090.
[8] V.C. Simbre, S.A. Duffy, G.H. Dadlani, T.L. Miller, S.E. Lipshultz, Cardiotoxicity of cancer chemotherapy: implications for children, Paediatr. Drugs 7 (3) (2005) 187–202.
[9] R. Kerkela, L. Grazette, R. Yacobi, C. Iliescu, R. Patten, C. Beahm, et al., Cardiotoxicity of the cancer therapeutic agent imatinib mesylate, Nat. Med. 12 (8) (2006) 908–916.
[10] S.E. Lipshultz, J.A. Alvarez, R.E. Scully, Anthracycline associated cardiotoxicity in survivors of childhood cancer, Heart 94 (4) (2008) 525–533.
[11] T. Simunek, M. Sterba, O. Popelova, M. Adamcova, R. Hrdina, V. Gersl, Anthracycline-induced cardiotoxicity: overview of studies examining the roles of oxidative stress and free cellular iron, Pharmacol. Rep. 61 (1) (2009) 154–171.
[12] N. Ashley, J. Poulton, Mitochondrial DNA is a direct target of anti-cancer anthracycline drugs, Biochem. Biophys. Res. Commun. 378 (3) (2009) 450–455.
[13] D. Lebrecht, B. Setzer, U.P. Ketelsen, J. Haberstroh, U.A. Walker, Time-dependent and tissue-specific accumulation of mtDNA and respiratory chain defects in chronic doxorubicin cardiomyopathy, Circulation 108 (19) (2003) 2423–2429.
[14] K.L. Thompson, B.A. Rosenzweig, J. Zhang, A.D. Knapton, R. Honchel, S.E. Lipshultz, et al., Early alterations in heart gene expression profiles associated with doxorubicin cardiotoxicity in rats, Cancer Chemother. Pharmacol. 66 (2) (2010) 303–314.
[15] K.B. Wallace, Doxorubicin-induced cardiac mitochondrionopathy, Pharmacol. Toxicol. 93 (3) (2003) 105–115.
[16] S. Fogli, P. Nieri, M.C. Breschi, The role of nitric oxide in anthracycline toxicity and prospects for pharmacologic prevention of cardiac damage, FASEB J. 18 (6) (2004) 664–675.
[17] M.J. Mihm, J.A. Bauer, Peroxynitrite-induced inhibition and nitration of cardiac myofibrillar creatine kinase, Biochimie 84 (10) (2002) 1013–1019.
[18] J.H. Doroshow, G.Y. Locker, C.E. Myers, Enzymatic defenses of the mouse heart against reactive oxygen metabolites: alterations produced by doxorubicin, J. Clin. Invest. 65 (1) (1980) 128–135.
[19] B. Chen, X. Peng, L. Pentassuglia, C.C. Lim, D.B. Sawyer, Molecular and cellular mechanisms of anthracycline cardiotoxicity, Cardiovasc. Toxicol. 7 (2) (2007) 114–121.
[20] H. Ito, S.C. Miller, M.E. Billingham, H. Akimoto, S.V. Torti, R. Wade, et al., Doxorubicin selectively inhibits muscle gene expression in cardiac muscle cells in vivo and in vitro, Proc. Natl. Acad. Sci. U.S.A. 87 (11) (1990) 4275–4279.
[21] X. Peng, B. Chen, C.C. Lim, D.B. Sawyer, The cardiotoxicology of anthracycline chemotherapeutics: translating molecular mechanism into preventative medicine, Mol. Interv. 5 (3) (2005) 163–171.
[22] A. De Angelis, E. Piegari, D. Cappetta, L. Marino, A. Filippelli, L. Berrino, et al., Anthracycline cardiomyopathy is mediated by depletion of the cardiac stem cell pool and is rescued by restoration of progenitor cell function, Circulation 121 (2) (2010) 276–292.
[23] B. Kalyanaraman, J. Joseph, S. Kalivendi, S. Wang, E. Konorev, S. Kotamraju, Doxorubicin-induced apoptosis: implications in cardiotoxicity, Mol. Cell Biochem. 234–235 (1–2) (2002) 119–124.

[24] R. Jurcut, H. Wildiers, J. Ganame, J. D'Hooge, R. Paridaens, J.U. Voigt, Detection and monitoring of cardiotoxicity-what does modern cardiology offer? Support Care Cancer 16 (5) (2008) 437–445.

[25] P. Rusconi, O. Gomez-Marin, M. Rossique-Gonzalez, E. Redha, J.R. Marin, M. Lon-Young, et al., Carvedilol in children with cardiomyopathy: 3-year experience at a single institution, J. Heart Lung Transplant. 23 (7) (2004) 832–838.

[26] S. Lowis, I. Lewis, A. Elsworth, C. Weston, F. Doz, G. Vassal, et al., A phase I study of intravenous liposomal daunorubicin (DaunoXome) in paediatric patients with relapsed or resistant solid tumours, Br. J. Cancer 95 (5) (2006) 571–580.

[27] D. Lebrecht, A. Kokkori, U.P. Ketelsen, B. Setzer, U.A. Walker, Tissue-specific mtDNA lesions and radical-associated mitochondrial dysfunction in human hearts exposed to doxorubicin, J. Pathol. 207 (4) (2005) 436–444.

[28] M. Ryberg, D. Nielsen, G. Cortese, G. Nielsen, T. Skovsgaard, P.K. Andersen, New insight into epirubicin cardiac toxicity: competing risks analysis of 1097 breast cancer patients, J. Natl. Cancer Inst. 100 (15) (2008) 1058–1067.

[29] M. Tokarska-Schlattner, M. Zaugg, C. Zuppinger, T. Wallimann, U. Schlattner, New insights into doxorubicin-induced cardiotoxicity: the critical role of cellular energetics, J. Mol. Cell Cardiol. 41 (3) (2006) 389–405.

[30] S. Zhang, X. Liu, T. Bawa-Khalfe, L.S. Lu, Y.L. Lyu, L.F. Liu, et al., Identification of the molecular basis of doxorubicin-induced cardiotoxicity, Nat. Med. 18 (11) (2012) 1639–1642.

[31] S. Khiati, I. Dalla Rosa, C. Sourbier, X. Ma, V.A. Rao, L.M. Neckers, et al., Mitochondrial topoisomerase I (top1mt) is a novel limiting factor of doxorubicin cardiotoxicity, Clin. Cancer Res. 20 (18) (2014) 4873–4881.

[32] Y.L. Lyu, J.E. Kerrigan, C.P. Lin, A.M. Azarova, Y.C. Tsai, Y. Ban, et al., Topoisomerase IIbeta mediated DNA double-strand breaks: implications in doxorubicin cardiotoxicity and prevention by dexrazoxane, Cancer Res. 67 (18) (2007) 8839–8846.

[33] P. Vejpongsa, E.T. Yeh, Prevention of anthracycline-induced cardiotoxicity: challenges and opportunities, J. Am. Coll. Cardiol. 64 (9) (2014) 938–945.

[34] F. Orzan, A. Brusca, F. Gaita, C. Giustetto, M.C. Figliomeni, L. Libero, Associated cardiac lesions in patients with radiation-induced complete heart block, Int. J. Cardiol. 39 (2) (1993) 151–156.

[35] S.I. Cohen, S. Bharati, J. Glass, M. Lev, Radiotherapy as a cause of complete atrioventricular block in Hodgkin's disease. An electrophysiological-pathological correlation, Arch. Intern. Med. 141 (5) (1981) 676–679.

[36] L. La Vecchia, Physiologic dual chamber pacing in radiation-induced atrioventricular block, Chest 110 (2) (1996) 580–581.

[37] M.J. Adams, P.H. Hardenbergh, L.S. Constine, S.E. Lipshultz, Radiation-associated cardiovascular disease, Crit. Rev. Oncol. Hematol. 45 (1) (2003) 55–75.

[38] L.F. Fajardo, J.R. Stewart, K.E. Cohn, Morphology of radiation-induced heart disease, Arch. Pathol. 86 (5) (1968) 512–519.

[39] M. Chello, P. Mastroroberto, R. Romano, S. Zofrea, I. Bevacqua, A.R. Marchese, Changes in the proportion of types I and III collagen in the left ventricular wall of patients with post-irradiative pericarditis, Cardiovasc. Surg. 4 (2) (1996) 222–226.

[40] S. Schultz-Hector, K.R. Trott, Radiation-induced cardiovascular diseases: is the epidemiologic evidence compatible with the radiobiologic data? Int. J. Radiat. Oncol. Biol. Phys. 67 (1) (2007) 10–18.

[41] M.E. Robbins, W. Zhao, Chronic oxidative stress and radiation-induced late normal tissue injury: a review, Int. J. Radiat. Biol. 80 (4) (2004) 251–259.

[42] M.P. Little, E.J. Tawn, I. Tzoulaki, R. Wakeford, G. Hildebrandt, F. Paris, et al., A systematic review of epidemiological associations between low and moderate doses of ionizing radiation and late cardiovascular effects, and their possible mechanisms, Radiat. Res. 169 (1) (2008) 99–109.

[43] F.C. Brosius 3rd, B.F. Waller, W.C. Roberts, Radiation heart disease. Analysis of 16 young (aged 15 to 33 years) necropsy patients who received over 3,500 rads to the heart, Am. J. Med. 70 (3) (1981) 519–530.

[44] J.P. Veinot, W.D. Edwards, Pathology of radiation-induced heart disease: a surgical and autopsy study of 27 cases, Hum. Pathol. 27 (8) (1996) 766–773.

[45] R.G. Carlson, W.R. Mayfield, S. Normann, J.A. Alexander, Radiation-associated valvular disease, Chest 99 (3) (1991) 538–545.

[46] P.T. McEniery, K. Dorosti, W.A. Schiavone, T.J. Pedrick, W.C. Sheldon, Clinical and angiographic features of coronary artery disease after chest irradiation, Am. J. Cardiol. 60 (13) (1987) 1020–1024.

[47] V. King, L.S. Constine, D. Clark, R.G. Schwartz, A.G. Muhs, M. Henzler, et al., Symptomatic coronary artery disease after mantle irradiation for Hodgkin's disease, Int. J. Radiat. Oncol. Biol. Phys. 36 (4) (1996) 881–889.

[48] L.S. Annest, R.P. Anderson, W. Li, M.D. Hafermann, Coronary artery disease following mediastinal radiation therapy, J. Thorac. Cardiovasc. Surg. 85 (2) (1983) 257–263.

[49] H. Yuan, M.W. Gaber, K. Boyd, C.M. Wilson, M.F. Kiani, T.E. Merchant, Effects of fractionated radiation on the brain vasculature in a murine model: blood-brain barrier permeability, astrocyte proliferation, and ultrastructural changes, Int. J. Radiat. Oncol. Biol. Phys. 66 (3) (2006) 860–866.

[50] M. Verheij, L.G. Dewit, M.N. Boomgaard, H.J. Brinkman, J.A. van Mourik, Ionizing radiation enhances platelet adhesion to the extracellular matrix of human endothelial cells by an increase in the release of von Willebrand factor, Radiat. Res. 137 (2) (1994) 202–207.

[51] L.F. Fajardo, The pathology of ionizing radiation as defined by morphologic patterns, Acta Oncol. 44 (1) (2005) 13–22.

[52] Y.Q. Li, P. Chen, A. Haimovitz-Friedman, R.M. Reilly, C.S. Wong, Endothelial apoptosis initiates acute blood-brain barrier disruption after ionizing radiation, Cancer Res. 63 (18) (2003) 5950–5956.

[53] K. Muzaffar, S.L. Collins, N. Labropoulos, W.H. Baker, A prospective study of the effects of irradiation on the carotid artery, Laryngoscope 110 (11) (2000) 1811–1814.

[54] D.H. O'Leary, J.F. Polak, R.A. Kronmal, T.A. Manolio, G.L. Burke, S.K. Wolfson Jr., Carotid-artery intima and media thickness as a risk factor for myocardial infarction and stroke in older adults. Cardiovascular health study collaborative research group, N. Engl. J. Med. 340 (1) (1999) 14–22.

[55] G.L. Smith, B.D. Smith, T.A. Buchholz, S.H. Giordano, A.S. Garden, W.A. Woodward, et al., Cerebrovascular disease risk in older head and neck cancer patients after radiotherapy, J. Clin. Oncol. 26 (31) (2008) 5119–5125.
[56] A.M. Goorin, A.R. Chauvenet, A.R. Perez-Atayde, J. Cruz, R. McKone, S.E. Lipshultz, Initial congestive heart failure, six to ten years after doxorubicin chemotherapy for childhood cancer, J. Pediatr. 116 (1) (1990) 144–147.
[57] B.H. Trachtenberg, D.C. Landy, V.I. Franco, J.M. Henkel, E.J. Pearson, T.L. Miller, et al., Anthracycline-associated cardiotoxicity in survivors of childhood cancer, Pediatr. Cardiol. 32 (3) (2011) 342–353.
[58] A. Giantris, L. Abdurrahman, A. Hinkle, B. Asselin, S.E. Lipshultz, Anthracycline-induced cardiotoxicity in children and young adults, Crit. Rev. Oncol. Hematol. 27 (1) (1998) 53–68.
[59] J.P. Krischer, S. Epstein, D.D. Cuthbertson, A.M. Goorin, M.L. Epstein, S.E. Lipshultz, Clinical cardiotoxicity following anthracycline treatment for childhood cancer: the pediatric oncology group experience, J. Clin. Oncol. 15 (4) (1997) 1544–1552.
[60] M.R. Bristow, J.W. Mason, M.E. Billingham, J.R. Daniels, Doxorubicin cardiomyopathy: evaluation by phonocardiography, endomyocardial biopsy, and cardiac catheterization, Ann. Intern. Med. 88 (2) (1978) 168–175.
[61] S.E. Lipshultz, S.R. Lipsitz, S.E. Sallan, V.M. Dalton, S.M. Mone, R.D. Gelber, et al., Chronic progressive cardiac dysfunction years after doxorubicin therapy for childhood acute lymphoblastic leukemia, J. Clin. Oncol. 23 (12) (2005) 2629–2636.
[62] E. Barry, J.A. Alvarez, R.E. Scully, T.L. Miller, S.E. Lipshultz, Anthracycline-induced cardiotoxicity: course, pathophysiology, prevention and management, Expert Opin. Pharmacother. 8 (8) (2007) 1039–1058.
[63] M.J. Adams, S.E. Lipshultz, Pathophysiology of anthracycline- and radiation-associated cardiomyopathies: implications for screening and prevention, Pediatr. Blood Cancer 44 (7) (2005) 600–606.
[64] M.A. Grenier, S.E. Lipshultz, Epidemiology of anthracycline cardiotoxicity in children and adults, Semin. Oncol. 25 (4 Suppl. 10) (1998) 72–85.
[65] S.E. Lipshultz, S.R. Lipsitz, S.M. Mone, A.M. Goorin, S.E. Sallan, S.P. Sanders, et al., Female sex and drug dose as risk factors for late cardiotoxic effects of doxorubicin therapy for childhood cancer, N. Engl. J. Med. 332 (26) (1995) 1738–1743.
[66] S.E. Lipshultz, S.D. Colan, R.D. Gelber, A.R. Perez-Atayde, S.E. Sallan, S.P. Sanders, Late cardiac effects of doxorubicin therapy for acute lymphoblastic leukemia in childhood, N. Engl. J. Med. 324 (12) (1991) 808–815.
[67] D.H. Kim, A.B. Landry 3rd, Y.S. Lee, A.M. Katz, Doxorubicin-induced calcium release from cardiac sarcoplasmic reticulum vesicles, J. Mol. Cell Cardiol. 21 (5) (1989) 433–436.
[68] S.E. Lipshultz, R.E. Scully, K.E. Stevenson, V.I. Franco, D.S. Neuberg, S.D. Colan, et al., Hearts too small for body size after doxorubicin for childhood leukemia: Grinch Syndrome, J. Clin. Oncol. 32 (2014) 10021 Abstr.
[69] P.A. Heidenreich, S.L. Hancock, R.H. Vagelos, B.K. Lee, I. Schnittger, Diastolic dysfunction after mediastinal irradiation, Am. Heart J. 150 (5) (2005) 977–982.
[70] M.J. Adams, S.R. Lipsitz, S.D. Colan, N.J. Tarbell, S.T. Treves, L. Diller, et al., Cardiovascular status in long-term survivors of Hodgkin's disease treated with chest radiotherapy, J. Clin. Oncol. 22 (15) (2004) 3139–3148.
[71] M.J. Adams, A.K. Ng, P. Mauch, S.R. Lipsitz, P. Winters, S.E. Lipshultz, Peak oxygen consumption in Hodgkin's lymphoma survivors treated with mediastinal radiotherapy as a predictor of quality of life 5 years later, Prog. Pediatr. Cardiol. 39 (2, Part A) (2015) 93–98.
[72] P.A. Heidenreich, I. Schnittger, H.W. Strauss, R.H. Vagelos, B.K. Lee, C.S. Mariscal, et al., Screening for coronary artery disease after mediastinal irradiation for Hodgkin's disease, J. Clin. Oncol. 25 (1) (2007) 43–49.
[73] Y. Xie, W.J. Collins, M.W. Audeh, S.L. Shiao, R.A. Gottlieb, M.T. Goodman, et al., Breast cancer survivorship and cardiovascular disease: emerging approaches in cardio-oncology, Curr. Treat. Options Cardiovasc. Med. 17 (12) (2015) 60.
[74] L.C. Kremer, E.C. van Dalen, M. Offringa, J. Ottenkamp, P.A. Voute, Anthracycline-induced clinical heart failure in a cohort of 607 children: long-term follow-up study, J. Clin. Oncol. 19 (1) (2001) 191–196.
[75] G. Link, R. Tirosh, A. Pinson, C. Hershko, Role of iron in the potentiation of anthracycline cardiotoxicity: identification of heart cell mitochondria as a major site of iron-anthracycline interaction, J. Lab. Clin. Med. 127 (3) (1996) 272–278.
[76] S.E. Lipshultz, S.R. Lipsitz, J.L. Kutok, T.L. Miller, S.D. Colan, D.S. Neuberg, et al., Impact of hemochromatosis gene mutations on cardiac status in doxorubicin-treated survivors of childhood high-risk leukemia, Cancer 119 (19) (2013) 3555–3562.
[77] J. Busciglio, B.A. Yankner, Apoptosis and increased generation of reactive oxygen species in Down's syndrome neurons in vitro, Nature 378 (6559) (1995) 776–779.
[78] L. Wojnowski, B. Kulle, M. Schirmer, G. Schluter, A. Schmidt, A. Rosenberger, et al., NAD(P)H oxidase and multidrug resistance protein genetic polymorphisms are associated with doxorubicin-induced cardiotoxicity, Circulation 112 (24) (2005) 3754–3762.
[79] J.G. Blanco, C.L. Sun, W. Landier, L. Chen, D. Esparza-Duran, W. Leisenring, et al., Anthracycline-related cardiomyopathy after childhood cancer: role of polymorphisms in carbonyl reductase genes–a report from the children's oncology group, J. Clin. Oncol. 30 (13) (2012) 1415–1421.
[80] M. Krajinovic, J. Elbared, S. Drouin, L. Bertout, A. Rezgui, M. Ansari, et al., Polymorphisms of ABCC5 and NOS3 genes influence doxorubicin cardiotoxicity in survivors of childhood acute lymphoblastic leukemia, Pharmacogenomics J. 16 (6) (November 2016) 530–535.
[81] H. Visscher, C.J. Ross, S.R. Rassekh, A. Barhdadi, M.P. Dube, H. Al-Saloos, et al., Pharmacogenomic prediction of anthracycline-induced cardiotoxicity in children, J. Clin. Oncol. 30 (13) (2012) 1422–1428.
[82] S.E. Oberfield, C.A. Sklar, Endocrine sequelae in survivors of childhood cancer, Adolesc. Med. 13 (1) (2002) 161–169 viii.
[83] S.E. Lipshultz, S.A. Vlach, S.R. Lipsitz, S.E. Sallan, M.L. Schwartz, S.D. Colan, Cardiac changes associated with growth hormone therapy among children treated with anthracyclines, Pediatrics 115 (6) (2005) 1613–1622.
[84] C.C. Gotay, P.H. Phillips, B.D. Cheson, Male-female differences in the impact of cancer therapy, Oncology (Williston Park) 7 (2) (1993) 67–74 discussion, 7.

[85] H.O. Adami, R. Bergstrom, L. Holmberg, L. Klareskog, I. Persson, J. Ponten, The effect of female sex hormones on cancer survival. A register-based study in patients younger than 20 years at diagnosis, JAMA 263 (16) (1990) 2189–2193.
[86] E. Piazza, N. Natale, A. Trabattoni, C. Mariscotti, L. Mosca, A. Libretti, et al., Plasma and tissue distribution of adriamycin in patients with pelvic cancer, Tumori 67 (6) (1981) 533–537.
[87] S.E. Lipshultz, M.J. Adams, Cardiotoxicity after childhood cancer: beginning with the end in mind, J. Clin. Oncol. 28 (8) (2010) 1276–1281.
[88] L.S. Kahalley, L.A. Robinson, V.L. Tyc, M.M. Hudson, W. Leisenring, K. Stratton, et al., Risk factors for smoking among adolescent survivors of childhood cancer: a report from the childhood cancer survivor study, Pediatr. Blood Cancer 58 (3) (2012) 428–434.
[89] D.C. Landy, S.R. Lipsitz, J.M. Kurtz, A.S. Hinkle, L.S. Constine, M.J. Adams, et al., Dietary quality, caloric intake, and adiposity of childhood cancer survivors and their siblings: an analysis from the cardiac risk factors in childhood cancer survivors study, Nutr. Cancer 65 (4) (2013) 547–555.
[90] T.L. Miller, S.R. Lipsitz, G. Lopez-Mitnik, A.S. Hinkle, L.S. Constine, M.J. Adams, et al., Characteristics and determinants of adiposity in pediatric cancer survivors, Cancer Epidemiol. Biomark. Prev. 19 (8) (2010) 2013–2022.
[91] A.M. Miller, G. Lopez-Mitnik, G. Somarriba, S.R. Lipsitz, A.S. Hinkle, L.S. Constine, et al., Exercise capacity in long-term survivors of pediatric cancer: an analysis from the cardiac risk factors in childhood cancer survivors study, Pediatr. Blood Cancer 60 (4) (2013) 663–668.
[92] L.A. Sleeper, J.A. Towbin, S.D. Colan, D. Hsu, E.J. Orav, M.S. Lemler, et al., Health-related quality of life and functional status are associated with cardiac status and clinical outcome in children with cardiomyopathy, J. Pediatr. 170 (2016) 173–180 e4.
[93] L.R. Meacham, E.J. Chow, K.K. Ness, K.Y. Kamdar, Y. Chen, Y. Yasui, et al., Cardiovascular risk factors in adult survivors of pediatric cancer–a report from the childhood cancer survivor study, Cancer Epidemiol. Biomark. Prev. 19 (1) (2010) 170–181.
[94] K.C. Oeffinger, A.C. Mertens, C.A. Sklar, Y. Yasui, T. Fears, M. Stovall, et al., Obesity in adult survivors of childhood acute lymphoblastic leukemia: a report from the childhood cancer survivor study, J. Clin. Oncol. 21 (7) (2003) 1359–1365.
[95] E.G. Garmey, Q. Liu, C.A. Sklar, L.R. Meacham, A.C. Mertens, M.A. Stovall, et al., Longitudinal changes in obesity and body mass index among adult survivors of childhood acute lymphoblastic leukemia: a report from the childhood cancer survivor study, J. Clin. Oncol. 26 (28) (2008) 4639–4645.
[96] J. Steinberger, A.R. Sinaiko, A.S. Kelly, W.M. Leisenring, L.M. Steffen, P. Goodman, et al., Cardiovascular risk and insulin resistance in childhood cancer survivors, J. Pediatr. 160 (3) (2012) 494–499.
[97] M. Tukenova, C. Guibout, O. Oberlin, F. Doyon, A. Mousannif, N. Haddy, et al., Role of cancer treatment in long-term overall and cardiovascular mortality after childhood cancer, J. Clin. Oncol. 28 (8) (2010) 1308–1315.
[98] M.P. Little, T.V. Azizova, D. Bazyka, S.D. Bouffler, E. Cardis, S. Chekin, et al., Systematic review and meta-analysis of circulatory disease from exposure to low-level ionizing radiation and estimates of potential population mortality risks, Environ. Health Perspect. 120 (11) (2012) 1503–1511.
[99] L.J. Steinherz, P.G. Steinherz, D. Mangiacasale, C. Tan, D.R. Miller, Cardiac abnormalities after AMSA administration, Cancer Treat. Rep. 66 (3) (1982) 483–488.
[100] J.R. Carver, C.L. Shapiro, A. Ng, L. Jacobs, C. Schwartz, K.S. Virgo, et al., American Society of Clinical Oncology clinical evidence review on the ongoing care of adult cancer survivors: cardiac and pulmonary late effects, J. Clin. Oncol. 25 (25) (2007) 3991–4008.
[101] S.A. Hunt, W.T. Abraham, M.H. Chin, A.M. Feldman, G.S. Francis, T.G. Ganiats, et al., ACC/AHA 2005 guideline update for the diagnosis and management of chronic heart failure in the adult: a report of the American College of Cardiology/American Heart Association task force on practice guidelines (writing committee to update the 2001 guidelines for the evaluation and management of heart failure): developed in collaboration with the American College of Chest Physicians and the International Society for Heart and Lung Transplantation: endorsed by the Heart Rhythm Society, Circulation 112 (12) (2005) e154–235.
[102] W. Landier, S. Bhatia, D.A. Eshelman, K.J. Forte, T. Sweeney, A.L. Hester, et al., Development of risk-based guidelines for pediatric cancer survivors: the children's oncology group long-term follow-up guidelines from the children's oncology group late effects committee and nursing discipline, J. Clin. Oncol. 22 (24) (2004) 4979–4990.
[103] S.E. Lipshultz, N. Rifai, S.E. Sallan, S.R. Lipsitz, V. Dalton, D.B. Sacks, et al., Predictive value of cardiac troponin T in pediatric patients at risk for myocardial injury, Circulation 96 (8) (1997) 2641–2648.
[104] D. Cardinale, M.T. Sandri, A. Colombo, N. Colombo, M. Boeri, G. Lamantia, et al., Prognostic value of troponin I in cardiac risk stratification of cancer patients undergoing high-dose chemotherapy, Circulation 109 (22) (2004) 2749–2754.
[105] S.E. Lipshultz, T.L. Miller, R.E. Scully, S.R. Lipsitz, N. Rifai, L.B. Silverman, et al., Changes in cardiac biomarkers during doxorubicin treatment of pediatric patients with high-risk acute lymphoblastic leukemia: associations with long-term echocardiographic outcomes, J. Clin. Oncol. 30 (10) (2012) 1042–1049.
[106] S.E. Lipshultz, V.I. Franco, T.L. Miller, S.D. Colan, S.E. Sallan, Cardiovascular disease in adult survivors of childhood cancer, Annu. Rev. Med. 66 (2015) 161–176.
[107] H. Nakamae, K. Tsumura, M. Akahori, Y. Terada, T. Yamane, T. Hayashi, et al., QT dispersion correlates with systolic rather than diastolic parameters in patients receiving anthracycline treatment, Intern. Med. 43 (5) (2004) 379–387.
[108] R. Altena, P.J. Perik, D.J. van Veldhuisen, E.G. de Vries, J.A. Gietema, Cardiovascular toxicity caused by cancer treatment: strategies for early detection, Lancet Oncol. 10 (4) (2009) 391–399.
[109] L.J. Steinherz, T. Graham, R. Hurwitz, H.M. Sondheimer, R.G. Schwartz, E.M. Shaffer, et al., Guidelines for cardiac monitoring of children during and after anthracycline therapy: report of the cardiology committee of the childrens cancer study group, Pediatrics 89 (5 Pt 1) (1992) 942–949.
[110] M.D. Cheitlin, W.F. Armstrong, G.P. Aurigemma, G.A. Beller, F.Z. Bierman, J.L. Davis, et al., ACC/AHA/ASE 2003 guideline update for the clinical application of echocardiography: summary article. A report of the American College of Cardiology/American Heart Association task force on practice guidelines (ACC/AHA/ASE committee to update the 1997 guidelines for the clinical application of echocardiography), J. Am. Soc. Echocardiogr. 16 (10) (2003) 1091–1110.

[111] L.C. Kremer, H.J. van der Pal, M. Offringa, E.C. van Dalen, P.A. Voute, Frequency and risk factors of subclinical cardiotoxicity after anthracycline therapy in children: a systematic review, Ann. Oncol. 13 (6) (2002) 819–829.
[112] B.H. Amundsen, T. Helle-Valle, T. Edvardsen, H. Torp, J. Crosby, E. Lyseggen, et al., Noninvasive myocardial strain measurement by speckle tracking echocardiography: validation against sonomicrometry and tagged magnetic resonance imaging, J. Am. Coll. Cardiol. 47 (4) (2006) 789–793.
[113] G.K. Singh, B. Cupps, M. Pasque, P.K. Woodard, M.R. Holland, A. Ludomirsky, Accuracy and reproducibility of strain by speckle tracking in pediatric subjects with normal heart and single ventricular physiology: a two-dimensional speckle-tracking echocardiography and magnetic resonance imaging correlative study, J. Am. Soc. Echocardiogr. 23 (11) (2010) 1143–1152.
[114] J. Ganame, P. Claus, A. Uyttebroeck, M. Renard, J. D'Hooge, B. Bijnens, et al., Myocardial dysfunction late after low-dose anthracycline treatment in asymptomatic pediatric patients, J. Am. Soc. Echocardiogr. 20 (12) (2007) 1351–1358.
[115] S. Kaul, J.G. Miller, P.A. Grayburn, S. Hashimoto, M. Hibberd, M.R. Holland, et al., A suggested roadmap for cardiovascular ultrasound research for the future, J. Am. Soc. Echocardiogr. 24 (4) (2011) 455–464.
[116] P. Colonna, R. Montisci, L. Galiuto, L. Meloni, S. Iliceto, Effects of acute myocardial ischemia on intramyocardial contraction heterogeneity: a study performed with ultrasound integrated backscatter during transesophageal atrial pacing, Circulation 100 (17) (1999) 1770–1776.
[117] Z. Vered, G.A. Mohr, B. Barzilai, C.J. Gessler Jr., S.A. Wickline, K.A. Wear, et al., Ultrasound integrated backscatter tissue characterization of remote myocardial infarction in human subjects, J. Am. Coll. Cardiol. 13 (1) (1989) 84–91.
[118] J.E. Perez, J.B. McGill, J.V. Santiago, K.B. Schechtman, A.D. Waggoner, J.G. Miller, et al., Abnormal myocardial acoustic properties in diabetic patients and their correlation with the severity of disease, J. Am. Coll. Cardiol. 19 (6) (1992) 1154–1162.
[119] K. Oberholzer, R.P. Kunz, M. Dittrich, M. Thelen, Anthracycline-induced cardiotoxicity: cardiac MRI after treatment for childhood cancer, Rofo 176 (9) (2004) 1245–1250.
[120] E.Z. Basar, F. Corapcioglu, K. Babaoglu, Y. Anik, G. Gorur Daglioz, R. Dedeoglu, Are cardiac magnetic resonance imaging and radionuclide ventriculography good options against echocardiography for evaluation of anthracycline induced chronic cardiotoxicity in childhood cancer survivors? Pediatr. Hematol. Oncol. 31 (3) (2014) 237–252.
[121] M.A. Lunning, S. Kutty, E.T. Rome, L. Li, A. Padiyath, F. Loberiza, et al., Cardiac magnetic resonance imaging for the assessment of the myocardium after doxorubicin-based chemotherapy, Am. J. Clin. Oncol. 38 (4) (2015) 377–381.
[122] S.E. Lipshultz, M.J. Adams, S.D. Colan, L.S. Constine, E.H. Herman, D.T. Hsu, et al., Long-term cardiovascular toxicity in children, adolescents, and young adults who receive cancer therapy: pathophysiology, course, monitoring, management, prevention, and research directions: a scientific statement from the American Heart Association, Circulation 128 (17) (2013) 1927–1995.
[123] K. Nysom, K. Holm, S.R. Lipsitz, S.M. Mone, S.D. Colan, E.J. Orav, et al., Relationship between cumulative anthracycline dose and late cardiotoxicity in childhood acute lymphoblastic leukemia, J. Clin. Oncol. 16 (2) (1998) 545–550.
[124] S.E. Lipshultz, N. Rifai, V.M. Dalton, D.E. Levy, L.B. Silverman, S.R. Lipsitz, et al., The effect of dexrazoxane on myocardial injury in doxorubicin-treated children with acute lymphoblastic leukemia, N. Engl. J. Med. 351 (2) (2004) 145–153.
[125] G.L. Plosker, D. Faulds, Epirubicin. A review of its pharmacodynamic and pharmacokinetic properties, and therapeutic use in cancer chemotherapy, Drugs 45 (5) (1993) 788–856.
[126] A. Martoni, E. Piana, M. Guaraldi, G. Cilenti, A. Farris, F. Saccani, et al., Comparative phase II study of idarubicin versus doxorubicin in advanced breast cancer, Oncology 47 (5) (1990) 427–432.
[127] T.D. Shenkenberg, D.D. Von Hoff, Mitoxantrone: a new anticancer drug with significant clinical activity, Ann. Intern. Med. 105 (1) (1986) 67–81.
[128] S.E. Lipshultz, T.R. Cochran, V.I. Franco, T.L. Miller, Treatment-related cardiotoxicity in survivors of childhood cancer, Nat. Rev. Clin. Oncol. 10 (12) (2013) 697–710.
[129] S.S. Legha, R.S. Benjamin, B. Mackay, M. Ewer, S. Wallace, M. Valdivieso, et al., Reduction of doxorubicin cardiotoxicity by prolonged continuous intravenous infusion, Ann. Intern. Med. 96 (2) (1982) 133–139.
[130] S.E. Lipshultz, T.L. Miller, S.R. Lipsitz, D.S. Neuberg, S.E. Dahlberg, S.D. Colan, et al., Continuous versus bolus infusion of doxorubicin in children with ALL: long-term cardiac outcomes, Pediatrics 130 (6) (2012) 1003–1011.
[131] A. Gabizon, F. Martin, Polyethylene glycol-coated (pegylated) liposomal doxorubicin. Rationale for use in solid tumours, Drugs 54 (Suppl. 4) (1997) 15–21.
[132] M.E. O'Brien, N. Wigler, M. Inbar, R. Rosso, E. Grischke, A. Santoro, et al., Reduced cardiotoxicity and comparable efficacy in a phase III trial of pegylated liposomal doxorubicin HCl (CAELYX/Doxil) versus conventional doxorubicin for first-line treatment of metastatic breast cancer, Ann. Oncol. 15 (3) (2004) 440–449.
[133] G. Minotti, S. Recalcati, P. Menna, E. Salvatorelli, G. Corna, G. Cairo, Doxorubicin cardiotoxicity and the control of iron metabolism: quinone-dependent and independent mechanisms, Methods Enzymol. 378 (2004) 340–361.
[134] S.E. Lipshultz, R.E. Scully, S.R. Lipsitz, S.E. Sallan, L.B. Silverman, T.L. Miller, et al., Assessment of dexrazoxane as a cardioprotectant in doxorubicin-treated children with high-risk acute lymphoblastic leukaemia: long-term follow-up of a prospective, randomised, multicentre trial, Lancet Oncol. 11 (10) (2010) 950–961.
[135] D. Lebrecht, J. Kirschner, A. Geist, J. Haberstroh, U.A. Walker, Respiratory chain deficiency precedes the disrupted calcium homeostasis in chronic doxorubicin cardiomyopathy, Cardiovasc. Pathol. 19 (5) (2010) e167–e174.
[136] K. Chandran, D. Aggarwal, R.Q. Migrino, J. Joseph, D. McAllister, E.A. Konorev, et al., Doxorubicin inactivates myocardial cytochrome c oxidase in rats: cardioprotection by Mito-Q, Biophys. J. 96 (4) (2009) 1388–1398.
[137] D. Lebrecht, A. Geist, U.P. Ketelsen, J. Haberstroh, B. Setzer, U.A. Walker, Dexrazoxane prevents doxorubicin-induced long-term cardiotoxicity and protects myocardial mitochondria from genetic and functional lesions in rats, Br. J. Pharmacol. 151 (6) (2007) 771–778.

[138] D. Lebrecht, U.A. Walker, Role of mtDNA lesions in anthracycline cardiotoxicity, Cardiovasc. Toxicol. 7 (2) (2007) 108–113.
[139] S.E. Lipshultz, L.M. Anderson, T.L. Miller, M. Gerschenson, K.E. Stevenson, D.S. Neuberg, et al., Impaired mitochondrial function is abrogated by dexrazoxane in doxorubicin-treated childhood acute lymphoblastic leukemia survivors, Cancer 122 (6) (2016) 946–953.
[140] L.M. Schuchter, M.L. Hensley, N.J. Meropol, E.P. Winer, Update of recommendations for the use of chemotherapy and radiotherapy protectants: clinical practice guidelines of the American Society of Clinical Oncology, J. Clin. Oncol. 20 (2002) 2895–2903.
[141] J.K. Hewitt, J.L. Silberg, M. Rutter, E. Simonoff, J.M. Meyer, H. Maes, et al., Genetics and developmental psychopathology: 1. Phenotypic assessment in the Virginia twin study of adolescent behavioral development, J. Child Psychol. Psychiatr. 38 (8) (1997) 943–963.
[142] B. Asselin, M. Devidas, T. Zhou, B.M. Camitta, S.E. Lipshultz, Cardioprotection and safety of dexrazoxane in patients treated for newly diagnosed T-cell acute lymphoblastic leukemia or advanced-stage lymphoblastic non-Hodgkin lymphoma: a report of the children's cncology group randomized trial 940, J. Clin. Oncol. 34 (8) (March 10, 2016) 854–862.
[143] H.S. Choi, E.S. Park, H.J. Kang, H.Y. Shin, C.I. Noh, Y.S. Yun, et al., Dexrazoxane for preventing anthracycline cardiotoxicity in children with solid tumors, J. Korean Med. Sci. 25 (9) (2010) 1336–1342.
[144] F. Shaikh, L.L. Dupuis, S. Alexander, A. Gupta, L. Mertens, P.C. Nathan, Cardioprotection and second malignant neoplasms associated with dexrazoxane in children receiving anthracycline chemotherapy: a systematic review and meta-analysis, J. Natl. Cancer Inst. 108 (4) (2016).
[145] R.S. Cvetkovic, L.J. Scott, Dexrazoxane: a review of its use for cardioprotection during anthracycline chemotherapy, Drugs 65 (7) (2005) 1005–1024.
[146] C.K. Tebbi, W.B. London, D. Friedman, D. Villaluna, P.A. De Alarcon, L.S. Constine, et al., Dexrazoxane-associated risk for acute myeloid leukemia/myelodysplastic syndrome and other secondary malignancies in pediatric Hodgkin's disease, J. Clin. Oncol. 25 (5) (2007) 493–500.
[147] Assessment Report Dexrazoxane-Containing Medicinal Products Medicines Agency European, 2011. Available from: www.ema.europa.eu.
[148] E.J. Chow, B.L. Asselin, C.L. Schwartz, D.R. Doody, W.M. Leisenring, S. Aggarwal, et al., Late mortality after dexrazoxane treatment: a report from the children's oncology group, J. Clin. Oncol. 33 (24) (2015) 2639–2645.
[149] C.L. Schwartz, L.H. Wexler, M.D. Krailo, L.A. Teot, M. Devidas, L.J. Steinherz, et al., Intensified chemotherapy with dexrazoxane cardioprotection in newly diagnosed nonmetastatic osteosarcoma: a report from the children's oncology group, Pediatr. Blood Cancer 63 (1) (2016) 54–61.
[150] S.E. Lipshultz, V.I. Franco, S.E. Sallan, P.C. Adamson, R.K. Steiner, S.M. Swain, et al., Dexrazoxane for reducing anthracycline-related cardiotoxicity in children with cancer: an update of the evidence, Prog. Pediatr. Cardiol. 36 (1–2) (2014) 39–49.
[151] D.J. Grdina, Y. Kataoka, J.S. Murley, Amifostine: mechanisms of action underlying cytoprotection and chemoprevention, Drug Metabol. Drug Interact. 16 (4) (2000) 237–279.
[152] P. Nazeyrollas, C. Frances, A. Prevost, B. Costa, M. Lorenzato, J.P. Kantelip, et al., Efficiency of amifostine as a protection against doxorubicin toxicity in rats during a 12-day treatment, Anticancer Res. 23 (1a) (2003) 405–409.
[153] S. Gallegos-Castorena, A. Martinez-Avalos, A. Mohar-Betancourt, G. Guerrero-Avendano, M. Zapata-Tarres, A. Medina-Sanson, Toxicity prevention with amifostine in pediatric osteosarcoma patients treated with cisplatin and doxorubicin, Pediatr. Hematol. Oncol. 24 (6) (2007) 403–408.
[154] H. Pouleur, M.F. Rousseau, C. van Eyll, L. Stoleru, W. Hayashida, J.A. Udelson, et al., Effects of long-term enalapril therapy on left ventricular diastolic properties in patients with depressed ejection fraction. SOLVD Investigators, Circulation 88 (2) (1993) 481–491.
[155] S.E. Lipshultz, S.R. Lipsitz, S.E. Sallan, V.C. Simbre 2nd, S.L. Shaikh, S.M. Mone, et al., Long-term enalapril therapy for left ventricular dysfunction in doxorubicin-treated survivors of childhood cancer, J. Clin. Oncol. 20 (23) (2002) 4517–4522.
[156] D. Cardinale, A. Colombo, M.T. Sandri, G. Lamantia, N. Colombo, M. Civelli, et al., Prevention of high-dose chemotherapy-induced cardiotoxicity in high-risk patients by angiotensin-converting enzyme inhibition, Circulation 114 (23) (2006) 2474–2481.
[157] J.H. Silber, A. Cnaan, B.J. Clark, S.M. Paridon, A.J. Chin, J. Rychik, et al., Enalapril to prevent cardiac function decline in long-term survivors of pediatric cancer exposed to anthracyclines, J. Clin. Oncol. 22 (2004) 820–828.
[158] P.A. Heidenreich, T.T. Lee, B.M. Massie, Effect of beta-blockade on mortality in patients with heart failure: a meta-analysis of randomized clinical trials, J. Am. Coll. Cardiol. 30 (1) (1997) 27–34.
[159] P. Lechat, M. Packer, S. Chalon, M. Cucherat, T. Arab, J.P. Boissel, Clinical effects of beta-adrenergic blockade in chronic heart failure: a meta-analysis of double-blind, placebo-controlled, randomized trials, Circulation 98 (12) (1998) 1184–1191.
[160] M.R. Bristow, Mechanism of action of beta-blocking agents in heart failure, Am. J. Cardiol. 80 (11A) (1997) 26L–40L.
[161] R.E. Shaddy, L.Y. Tani, S.S. Gidding, E. Pahl, G.S. Orsmond, E.M. Gilbert, et al., Beta-blocker treatment of dilated cardiomyopathy with congestive heart failure in children: a multi-institutional experience, J. Heart Lung Transplant. 18 (3) (1999) 269–274.
[162] S.L. Hancock, M.A. Tucker, R.T. Hoppe, Factors affecting late mortality from heart disease after treatment of Hodgkin's disease, JAMA 270 (16) (1993) 1949–1955.
[163] R.J. Carmel, H.S. Kaplan, Mantle irradiation in Hodgkin's disease. An analysis of technique, tumor eradication, and complications, Cancer 37 (6) (1976) 2813–2825.
[164] D.C. Weber, N. Peguret, G. Dipasquale, L. Cozzi, Involved-node and involved-field volumetric modulated arc vs. fixed beam intensity-modulated radiotherapy for female patients with early-stage supra-diaphragmatic Hodgkin lymphoma: a comparative planning study, Int. J. Radiat. Oncol. Biol. Phys. 75 (5) (2009) 1578–1586.
[165] B. Zhang, Z. Mo, W. Du, Y. Wang, L. Liu, Y. Wei, Intensity-modulated radiation therapy versus 2D-RT or 3D-CRT for the treatment of nasopharyngeal carcinoma: a systematic review and meta-analysis, Oral Oncol. 51 (11) (2015) 1041–1046.
[166] S.A. Hunt, W.T. Abraham, M.H. Chin, A.M. Feldman, G.S. Francis, T.G. Ganiats, et al., 2009 focused update incorporated into the ACC/AHA 2005 guidelines for the diagnosis and management of heart failure in adults: a report of the American College of Cardiology Foundation/American Heart Association task force on practice guidelines: developed in collaboration with the International Society for heart and lung transplantation, Circulation 119 (14) (2009) e391–479.

[167] D. Rosenthal, M.R. Chrisant, E. Edens, L. Mahony, C. Canter, S. Colan, et al., International society for heart and lung transplantation: practice guidelines for management of heart failure in children, J. Heart Lung Transplant. 23 (12) (2004) 1313–1333.

[168] R.E. Shaddy, M.M. Boucek, D.T. Hsu, R.J. Boucek, C.E. Canter, L. Mahony, et al., Carvedilol for children and adolescents with heart failure: a randomized controlled trial, JAMA 298 (10) (2007) 1171–1179.

[169] A.I. Dipchand, D.C. Naftel, B. Feingold, R. Spicer, D. Yung, B. Kaufman, et al., Outcomes of children with cardiomyopathy listed for transplant: a multi-institutional study, J. Heart Lung Transplant. 28 (12) (2009) 1312–1321.

[170] E.S. Pincott, M. Burch, Mechanical bridging to orthotopic heart transplantation in children, Future Cardiol. 8 (5) (2012) 753–763.

[171] G. Brancaccio, S. Filippelli, G. Michielon, R. Iacobelli, S. Alfieri, F. Gandolfo, et al., Ventricular assist devices as a bridge to heart transplantation or as destination therapy in pediatric patients, Transplant. Proc. 44 (7) (2012) 2007–2012.

[172] E.D. Blume, D.C. Naftel, H.J. Bastardi, B.W. Duncan, J.K. Kirklin, S.A. Webber, Outcomes of children bridged to heart transplantation with ventricular assist devices: a multi-institutional study, Circulation 113 (19) (2006) 2313–2319.

[173] R. Kirk, D. Naftel, T.M. Hoffman, C. Almond, G. Boyle, R.L. Caldwell, et al., Outcome of pediatric patients with dilated cardiomyopathy listed for transplant: a multi-institutional study, J. Heart Lung Transplant. 28 (12) (2009) 1322–1328.

[174] S.E. Lipshultz, S.D. Colan, Cardiovascular trials in long-term survivors of childhood cancer, J. Clin. Oncol. 22 (5) (2004) 769–773.

[175] S. Bangalore, S. Kumar, S.E. Kjeldsen, H. Makani, E. Gressman, J. Wetterslev, et al., Antihypertensive drugs and risk of cancer: network meta-analyses and trial sequential analyses of 324,168 participants from randomised trials, Lancet Oncol. 12 (1) (January 2011) 65–82.

[176] R.A. Martin, K.L. Jones, A. Mendoza, M. Barr Jr., K. Benirschke, Effect of ACE inhibition on the fetal kidney: decreased renal blood flow, Teratology 46 (4) (October 1992) 317–321.

Chapter 33

The Failing Myocardium in Sepsis

Mahsun Yuerek[1], Scott L. Weiss[1,2], Maryam Y. Naim[1,2]

[1]*Children's Hospital of Philadelphia, Philadelphia, PA, United States;* [2]*The University of Pennsylvania Perelman School of Medicine, Philadelphia, PA, United States*

EPIDEMIOLOGY

The sepsis syndrome is a life-threatening immunoinflammatory response to infection that often requires intensive care management. Current consensus guidelines define sepsis along a spectrum of illness severity beginning with a systemic inflammatory response to an invasive infection that can progress (sometimes rapidly) to cardiovascular dysfunction (septic shock) or multiple organ dysfunction syndrome (severe sepsis) [1]. Worldwide, sepsis remains one of the most common causes of pediatric deaths, as it can occur secondary to pneumonia, diarrhea, malaria, influenza (and other viral infections), and other invasive bacterial diseases [2]. Recent evidence suggests that the overall prevalence of pediatric severe sepsis is increasing in large part driven by a rising number of cases of infantile sepsis [3–6]. An expanding vulnerable population with chronic comorbid conditions [7,8], increasing rates of multidrug resistant organisms and healthcare-acquired infections [9], and a surge in sepsis surveillance [10,11] may be contributing as well.

In the United States (US), there was an estimated 75,000 pediatric hospitalizations involving severe sepsis, up to 42,000 in 1995, and corresponding to an increase in prevalence from 0.56 to 0.89 cases per 1000 pediatric-aged persons [4]. While the mortality rate for pediatric sepsis has declined dramatically in the US since the mid-1900s, latest reports of the overall case fatality for pediatric severe sepsis range from 4% to 9% [3,4,12]. However, for critically ill children with severe sepsis who require treatment in a pediatric intensive care unit (PICU), hospital morality rates are much higher [5,6,13–15]. The recent SPROUT point prevalence study involving 128 PICUs across 26 countries reported 25% all-cause hospital mortality and a 17% rate of new moderate functional disability in survivors [16]. It has been estimated that over one-third of children who die in a tertiary care PICU in the US have severe sepsis [6,17].

Involvement of the heart in the pathophysiology of the cardiovascular dysfunction in septic shock has been considered since the 1980s and develops in nearly 50% of patients with septic shock [18,19]. Ceneviva and colleagues examined the hemodynamic profile of 50 consecutive children with fluid refractory septic shock with pulmonary artery catheter data and found that 58% of children had low cardiac index indicating myocardial dysfunction, 20% had high cardiac index and low systemic vascular resistance indicating vascular dysfunction, and 22% had both low cardiac index and low systemic vascular resistance indicating both myocardial and vascular dysfunction [20].

PATHOPHYSIOLOGY

Septic shock is characterized by inadequate oxygen delivery and utilization, leading to anaerobic metabolism and lactic acid production. The cardiovascular consequences of septic shock include myocardial dysfunction, abnormal vascular tone, increased capillary permeability, decreased oxygen delivery, and altered oxygen metabolism. The majority of existing knowledge of the pathophysiology of myocardial dysfunction in sepsis is based on research done in adult patients with septic shock and in vitro studies. Pediatric studies are limited.

In the 1960s, before objective bedside cardiac output assessment was routinely available, septic shock was divided into two categories: "warm" shock, characterized by bounding pulses, hypotension, and peripheral vasodilation, and "cold" shock, which was described by cold skin and peripheral vasoconstriction [21,22]. Hemodynamic data were available in a few adult patients showing high cardiac output state in patients with "warm" shock, where as patients in "cold" shock had low cardiac output. "Warm" shock was regarded as the initial physiologic response to infection. Patients with sepsis would either recover from "warm" shock or develop heart failure and progress to hypodynamic shock and death [23]. Some animal studies supported this theory [24,25], although others opposed this theory, showing that low cardiac output was a rare finding in septic shock [26]. Wilson et al. measured the hemodynamic profile in 53 adult patients treated for septic shock

Heart Failure in the Child and Young Adult. http://dx.doi.org/10.1016/B978-0-12-802393-8.00033-8

in the "shock unit" of the Detroit Receiving Hospital, describing septic shock as a state of high cardiac output and low systemic vascular resistance [26]. Despite these results Wilson's theory of cardiovascular dysfunction in septic shock was not accepted. Routine use of pulmonary artery catheter for determination of cardiac output and pulmonary artery wedge pressure, in the following years, led to deeper understanding of the hemodynamic profile in patients with septic shock [27,28]. Subsequent studies confirmed the initial findings of Wilson et al. supporting that patients in "cold" shock experience a transition into the hyperdynamic phase after volume resuscitation for qualitative hypovolemia [29–32].

The concept of sepsis-induced cardiac dysfunction emerged from a research group lead by Parker and Parrillo in 1984 [19]. Using radionucleotide ventriculography and thermodilution for cardiac output determination in adult patients with septic shock, they demonstrated a high cardiac output state and low systemic vascular resistance. 13 of 20 patients survived. Remarkably, survivors had a reduced ejection fraction with increased end-systolic and end-diastolic volumes compared to nonsurvivors, who had no reduction in their ejection fraction and unchanged ventricular volumes. The ventricular dysfunction in the group of survivors recovered after 7–10 days of illness [19]. Further clinical and experimental studies confirmed the concept of reversible ventricular dilation and dysfunction in septic shock [33–37]. Based on the results of Parker et al., the idea of left ventricular (LV) dilation having protective effects in septic patients emerged, however, subsequent studies did not confirm these "compensatory effects" to be beneficial [18,38–41]. On the contrary, Parrillo et al. showed in another study published in 1990 a significantly increased mortality rate of 70%–90% in adult patients with cardiovascular dysfunction compared with 20% in adult septic patients without cardiovascular dysfunction [42]. Further research confirmed that biventricular systolic function is decreased in the early phase in adult humans regardless of the type of bacteria [33].

Historically, it was thought that the heart of patients in septic shock is the last organ to fail. This concept was opposed by Suffredini et al. in a study done in 1987 [43]. The investigators administered *Escherichia coli* endotoxin to healthy volunteer adults to analyze the cardiovascular effects by this mediator of septic shock, providing insight into the early hemodynamic changes in humans in response to endotoxemia. The ejection fraction decreased and fluid administration resulted in increased end-diastolic volume index and pulmonary capillary wedge pressure, which was not observed in healthy adult patients not exposed to endotoxin [43]. Unlike adults, children with fluid refractory septic shock more frequently demonstrate decreased cardiac output and increased LV afterload [20].

During the past 2 decades, research has been focused in investigating the underlying causes of cardiac dysfunction. A variety of pathophysiological mechanisms have been proposed.

Myocardial Ischemia, Coronary Blood Flow, and Myocardial Cell Changes During Septic Shock

Decreased coronary blood flow causing myocardial ischemia was proposed as underlying cause for cardiac dysfunction in septic patients until the late 1980s. Direct measurement of coronary blood flow and metabolites ruled this hypothesis out [44]. Dhainaut et al. studied the coronary hemodynamics and myocardial metabolism in 40 septic adult patients and 13 control patients [45]. Surprisingly, coronary arteries were found to be dilated and coronary blood flow was normal and increased in patients with septic shock. Myocardial oxygen extraction was diminished, lactate uptake was elevated, uptake of free fatty acids, glucose, and ketone bodies was decreased suggesting abnormal myocardial cell metabolism [45].

Structural myocardial changes have also been suggested as contributing factors for sepsis-related myocardial dysfunction. Rossi et al. histologically investigated the myocardium of eight patients with septic shock caused by infection and compared those with 11 specimens from patients who deceased from either noninfectious disease processes causing systemic inflammatory response syndrome or accidental nonthoracic trauma [46]. The myocardium of patients with septic shock showed greater interstitial cellular infiltration and increased intracardiomyocyte lipid accumulation likely influencing the contractile function of the myocardium [46].

Immunohistochemical analysis of myocardial cells in nonsurvivors of septic shock showed disruption of myofilaments, potentially caused by metalloproteinase activity [46]. Matrix metalloproteinases can degrade the contractile apparatus and the cytoskeleton [47,48]. Degradation of the contractile apparatus is associated with a decrease in the sensitivity of myofilaments to calcium ions [49,50].

Several studies in pediatric patients and adult patients with septic shock have described elevation of the biomarker troponin I, which has been shown to correlate with the severity of cardiac dysfunction [51,52]. Based on current research the elevated troponin I levels are mainly caused by abnormal myocardial cell integrity with increased leakage of the biomarker [53]. Necrosis was not detected in heart specimens of patients who died from septic shock [54]. However, microcirculatory abnormalities may be the cause of myocardial ischemia [55,56].

As mentioned above, necrosis has not been observed as the underlying mechanism of myocardial cell death leading to cardiac function in septic patients [54], however, apoptosis is thought to be the involved in myocardial cell depletion during septic shock [57]. Caspases, which are effectors of apoptosis, are activated by tumor necrosis factor alpha (TNFα) and release of cytochrome C from mitochondrial cells. Endotoxin-induced cardiac dysfunction has been associated with activation of caspases [58,59]. Inhibition of caspase-3, a protease found in myocardial cells undergoing apoptosis, prevents development of cardiac dysfunction and apoptosis [58,59]. Similarly, administration of cyclosporine A prevents apoptosis in myocardial cells by blocking release of cytochrome C from the inner mitochondrial membrane through mitochondrial permeability transition pores [60]. Overexpression of bcl-2, an antiapoptotic factor, has been reported to be protective against endotoxin-induced myocardial dysfunction, by altering the diameter of mitochondrial permeability transition pores [61].

Circulating Myocardial Depressant Factors

More than 40 years ago circulating myocardial depressant factors were proposed to be present in septic patients causing myocardial dysfunction [62], but it was not until the late 1980s that serum factors were identified to play a role. Parrillo et al. exposed myocardial cells in vitro to serum of patients with septic shock during the acute and recovery phases and assessed the contractile function of the myocardial cells [63]. When exposed to serum from the acute phase, there was a decrease in the extent and velocity of myocardial cell contraction. Such changes of myocardial cell function were not observed, when cells were exposed to serum obtained during the recovery phase. Further research identified these serum factors as proteins and polypeptides including TNFα, interleukin-1 (IL-1), IL-6, and lipopolysaccharide (LPS) [63–66].

Toll-like receptors (TLRs) are transmembrane glycoproteins that have an important role in the innate immune response. TLRs recognize specific molecular patterns of pathogens and activate nuclear factor kappa B (NF-κB), a transcription factor that regulates the expression of inflammatory cytokine genes. Among the TLRs studied, TLR4 has been found to be involved most in sepsis induced myocardial dysfunction. TLR4 deficient mice were found to be protected against myocardial contractile abnormalities in a sepsis model [67].

LPS effects on myocardial function are mainly caused by an increased production of cytokines (IL-1, TNFα) through stimulation of the CD14 and TLR4 receptors by LPS-binding protein complex. Removal of TNFα and IL-1 by immunoabsorption resulted in loss of depressant activity in the rodent myocardial cells [67a]. Early studies showed improved LV function in patients with septic shock who received anti-TNFα antibodies [68], however, subsequent studies failed to show any benefit in survival [69–71]. Similarly, targeting IL-1 in septic patients with monoclonal antibodies did not show any statistical survival benefit [72]. This discrepancy between animal and human studies may be related to the early treatment of animals under controlled experimental settings as opposed to septic patients who have likely already developed some degree of organ dysfunction prior to receiving antiinflammatory therapies. This also indicates that circulating myocardial depressant factors are not solely the cause for myocardial dysfunction in septic patients.

Endothelin-1 is a potent vasoconstrictor peptide originating from endothelial cells. Many different cell types and disease processes stimulate the overexpression of endothelin-1, which leads to vascular dysfunction by activating proinflammatory cascades (increased production of TNFα, IL-1, and IL-6), mitogenic and proliferative effects, stimulation of free radical formation, and platelet activation [73]. In an experimental study of endotoxemic shock, tezosentan, an endothelin receptor antagonist, improved cardiac index, stroke volume index, and LV stroke work index [74].

Prostanoids are other circulating factors associated with sepsis induced myocardial dysfunction. Prostacyclin and thromboxane levels are elevated in humans with sepsis [75]. Increased mortality has been associated with elevated levels of these prostanoids. Elevation of prostanoids is coupled with increased activity of cyclooxygenase enzyme 2, the expression of which is induced by LPS and other cytokines [76]. The exact pathophysiological mechanism has yet to be fully elucidated, and is hypothesized to be related to altered coronary autoregulation, activation of leukocytes, and impaired function of the endothelium.

Nitric Oxide

Nitric oxide (NO) is known to have multifaceted effects in health and disease states. The role of NO and its metabolites during septic shock has undergone extensive investigation. In healthy individuals, low-dose NO improved LV function [77]. Inhibition of endogenous NO release by infusion of an NO synthase (NOS) inhibitor led to decreased LV contractility [77]. NO in higher doses can cause myocardial dysfunction by alteration of the myocardial energy generating processes [78]. Sepsis can lead to increased expression of inducible NOS, which contributes to myocardial dysfunction by increased NO production and generation of cytotoxic peroxynitrite [79–82]. Although cardiac function in NOS deficient mice is preserved after endotoxin challenge [83], infusion of the NOS inhibitor N^G-nitro-L-arginine-methyl-ester does not restore cardiac function back to normal after endotoxin challenge in animals sufficient in NOS, which indicates that NO has also indirect effects in the pathophysiology of myocardial dysfunction during sepsis [84,85]. However, in a study by Hwang et al. nonselective inhibition of NOS restored cardiac output after endotoxin challenge in septic rats [86]. Similarly, infusion of the nonselective NOS inhibitor methylene blue in septic patients improves mean arterial pressure, stroke volume and LV stroke work [87]. Other studies have investigated peroxynitrite, a metabolite generated from the reaction between NO and superoxide radicals. Peroxynitrites have a cardio-depressant effect by causing calcium flux abnormalities, depressing mitochondrial respiration, and by denaturating proteins [82,88,89]. The role of peroxynitrite in septic cardiomyopathy was proven by the use of peroxynitrite neutralizers, which improved cardiac dysfunction in a sepsis animal model. In a recent study, it was proposed that mitochondrial NOS have a significant role in septic cardiomyopathy by NO overproduction and alteration of mitochondrial transition pore opening, leading to mitochondrial cell swelling and further sequelae [90].

Altered β–Adrenergic Signaling in Sepsis and Autonomic Dysfunction

Most studies have shown that the β-adrenergic pathway is altered in septic patients. Elevated levels of catecholamines in septic patients have been documented [91–93]. It is well known that prolonged β-adrenergic stimulation of myocardial cell is associated intracellular calcium elevation leading to myocardial cell damage [94]. In an experimental septic rat model it was found that the density of β-adrenergic receptors was decreased [95,96]. Similarly, in another experimental study it was shown that exposing cultured neonatal cardiomyocytes to the serum of septic patients treated with norepinephrine for 48 h lead to a decreased density of β-adrenergic receptors [97]. In yet another investigation it was shown myocardial cells of rats had increased β-adrenergic stimulation of calcium current after 12 h, however, a decrease was noted after 36 h [98]. The changes in the β-adrenergic receptor pathway are most likely time dependent [99].

In addition to the changes in the receptor density, changes in the G-protein activity have been described. Matsuda et al. reported a decrease in the stimulatory G-proteins in endotoxemic rabbits [100]. On the contrary, inhibitory G-proteins were found to be increased in nonsurvivors of septic shock and septic animals [101,102]. The above changes led to decreased levels of cyclic adenosine monophosphate levels.

Another feature of critical illness is narrow heart rate variability, which is associated with severity of illness and mortality [103,104]. The narrowed heart rate variability is a sign of autonomic dysfunction, which implies an imbalance between the vagal tone and sympathetic tone [105,106]. It appears that both sympathetic and parasympathetic autonomic systems are affected in sepsis unlike patients with primary cardiac disease, in whom sympathetic tone typically dominates over the vagal tone [104]. In a study of healthy volunteers, administration of endotoxin caused reversible narrowed heart rate variability [107]. A clear correlation between septic cardiomyopathy and autonomic dysfunction has yet to be found.

Calcium and Sodium Homeostasis

Calcium uptake and myofilament sensitivity to calcium in the myocardial cells are altered during sepsis [108]. Endotoxin and cytokines reduce the density and activity of L-type Ca-channels, leading to a decreased intracellular calcium levels [109]. The availability of intracellular calcium declines further by decreased activity of the ryanodine receptor [110]. Various models have confirmed the decreased sensitivity of myofilaments to calcium [49,50]. The exact mechanisms are not well delineated, however, phosphorylation of troponin I may be involved [84], leading to a decreased activation of troponin I by calcium [111].

Recently, Koester et al. studied the cardiac excitability in a rat model of sepsis [112]. They reported impaired depolarization by altered sodium current, resulting in decreased ventricular contractility. It was proposed that the altered sodium current caused a decrease in peak depolarization. This resulted in reduced opening of calcium channels, and decreased levels of intracellular calcium available for electromechanical coupling, ultimately leading to decreased contractility.

Mitochondrial Dysfunction

Mitochondrial dysfunction has been considered to be key mechanism of multiorgan dysfunction in sepsis [113]. Recent studies have shown that mitochondrial dysfunction occurs during pediatric septic shock, however, further studies are needed to delineate the significance on disease process and outcome [114,115]. Structurally abnormal mitochondria were found in cardiac specimens of humans with septic shock [116]. Cardiac mitochondrial dysfunction was also evident in most well-established animal models for septic shock [117]. The degree of mitochondrial dysfunction correlated with the degree of myocardial dysfunction. Decrease in oxidative phosphorylation decreased mitochondrial membrane potential and decreased ATP production are some characteristics of mitochondrial dysfunction during sepsis [118].

The production of NO by the mitochondrial NOS and decreased neutralization of NO lead to increased production of peroxynitrite, which is a very powerful oxidant [119,120]. Peroxynitrite causes impairment in the function of the oxidative phosphorylation and decreased ATP production [120].

Mitochondrial calcium homeostasis is important for regulating the mitochondrial permeability transition pore opening [118]. Hassoun et al. showed calcium uptake by the mitochondria is increased in an LPS induced endotoxemia model in rats [121]. Calcium overload is a trigger for mitochondrial permeability transition pore opening, which leads to loss of the mitochondrial membrane potential, decrease of oxidative phosphorylation, mitochondrial swelling, rupture of the outer membrane, and ultimately activation of apoptosis pathway [118].

The role of mitochondrial uncoupling by alteration of uncoupling proteins has yet to be determined. Overall, mitochondrial uncoupling leads to a decreased hydrogen ion gradient across the mitochondrial membrane leading to decreased ATP production [122,123]. Studies have been controversial regarding the role of mitochondrial uncoupling protein's in septic cardiomyopathy [118].

There are studies that have shown recovery of myocardial function when the mitochondrial pathophysiological mechanism was targeted by experimental drug therapy [118]. This implies the role of myocardial energetics rather than cardiac inflammation as underlying caused for cardiac dysfunction.

Heat Shock Proteins

Heat shock proteins (HSP) are known to protect cells in reaction to stress, a mechanism described as thermotolerance [124]. Previously, HSPs were thought to function as chaperones during folding and intracellular transport of peptides [125], however, other research showed that HSPs may have also immune modulating effects, similar to cytokines [126]. Studies have shown that HSPs may have protective effects on cardiomyocytes from damage by oxidative stress and endotoxins [124]. The most studied HSPs are HSP70, categorized by their weight (i.e., 70 kD). The family of the HSP70 includes the inducible HSP70 (also known as HSP72), HSC70 (heat shock cognate protein 70, also known as HSP73), and GRP75 (found in mitochondria). Extracellular HSP70 has been mainly studied in association with sepsis. Elevated serum levels of HSP70 have been associated with clinical outcome [127]. Animal studies have shown that pretreatment with exogenous HSP70 can improve septic shock and decrease mortality [128,129].

GRP75 has a potential role in protection of mitochondrial cell from proteolytic damage. Downregulation of GRP75 during sepsis has been associated with decreased production of respiratory chain enzymes and their function [130].

In vitro studies have shown that HSP70 induction inhibits TNFα production from macrophages [131]. Another study showed that preconditioning of macrophages with HSP70 led to decreased LPS-induced production of NO, which as mentioned previously is known to have detrimental effects on myocardial function during sepsis [129]. A recent study by Hsu et al. showed that preconditioning mice with HSC70 attenuates the TNFα response to endotoxins, decreased function of NF-κB, and induces tolerance of cardiac cells to endotoxins [132].

DIAGNOSIS

Echocardiography is the primary modality for diagnosis of myocardial dysfunction in sepsis and is easily available at the bedside. Early echocardiography studies quantifying LV performance with M-mode imaging and wall stress found a reversible impairment in ventricular contractility [133]. In sepsis, methods to quantitate systolic function with ejection fraction and shortening fraction have limitations as changes to the preload and afterload of the myocardium occur commonly. Newer methods measure myocardial strain and have been shown to more accurately detect myocardial dysfunction. Recent work by Basu et al. in children with septic shock showed that speckle tackle imaging to assess myocardial strain showed impairments in myocardial function that were not seen by standard echocardiographic measurements of shortening and ejection fraction [134]. Diastolic dysfunction can be assessed by measurement of mitral valve inflow velocities by blood flow Doppler analysis and mitral valve annular velocities by tissue Doppler analysis [135].

Pulmonary artery catheters allow measurement of the hemodynamic profile of children with sepsis and can identify myocardial and vascular dysfunction by measurement of cardiac index and systemic vascular resistance [20]. However, pulmonary artery catheters give inaccurate information in the presence of an intracardiac shunt and their use in general has decreased in pediatrics and adults since large adult studies questioned the risk to benefit ratio of pulmonary artery catheters [136]. Central venous catheters allow measurement of right sided pressures (which reflects right ventricular diastolic pressure in the absence of tricuspid pathology) and measurement of superior vena cava oximetry, which is an accurate estimation of mixed venous saturation in the absence of an intracardiac shunt. Superior vena cava oximetry in the presence of an arterial line also allows measurement of arterial-venous oxygen difference that can be impaired in patients with septic shock.

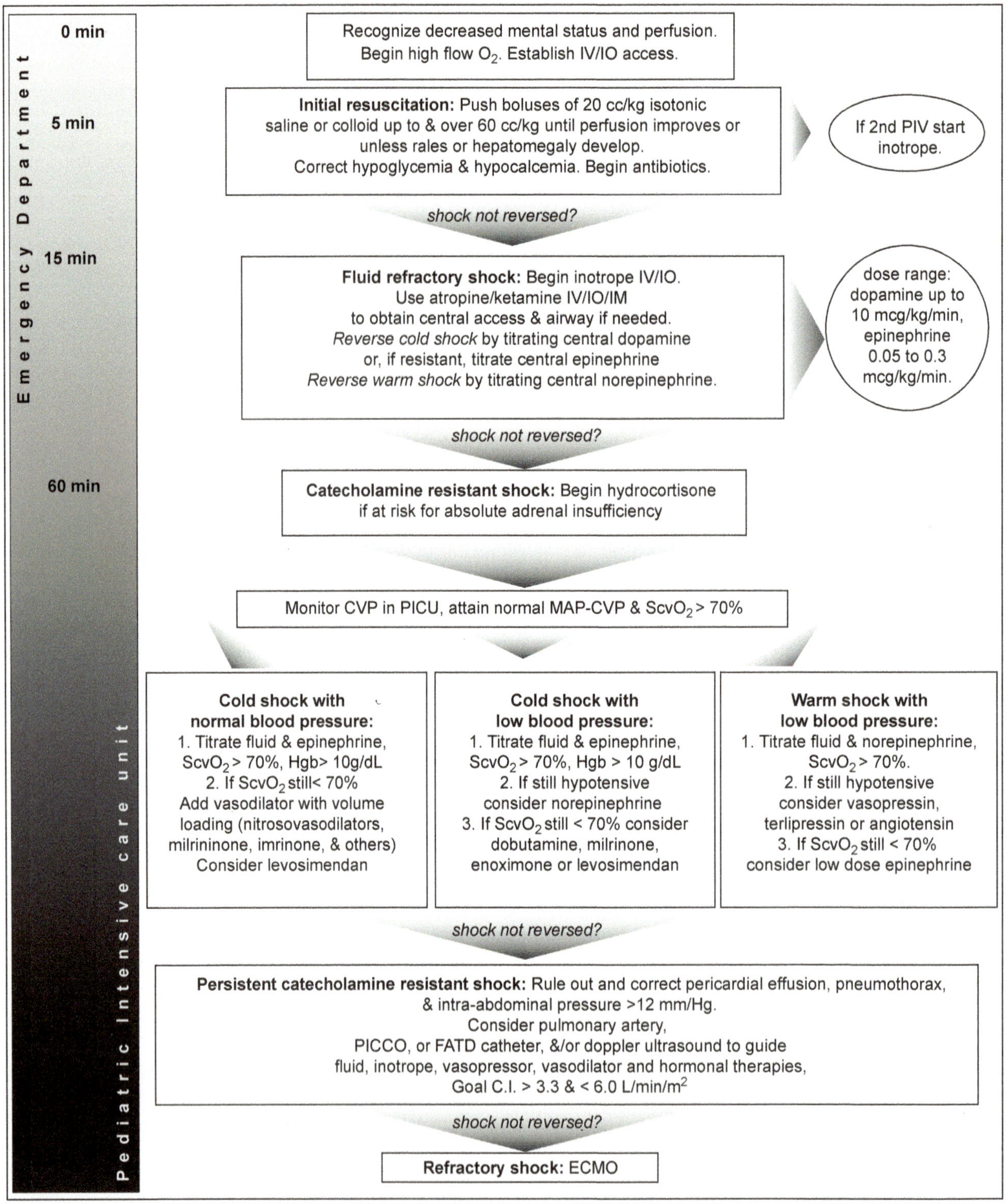

FIGURE 33.1 Algorithm for time sensitive, goal-directed stepwise hemodynamic support of infant and children in septic shock. *CVP*, central venous pressure; *ECMO*, extracorporeal membrane oxygenation; *FATD*, femoral artery thermodilution; *IM*, intramuscular; *IO*, intraosseous; *IV*, intravenous; *MAP*, mean arterial pressure; *PICCO*, pulse contour cardiac output; *PICU*, pediatric intensive care unit; *PIV*, peripheral intravenous line. *(From J. Brierley, et al., Clinical practice parameters for hemodynamic support of pediatric and neonatal septic shock: 2007 update from the American College of Critical Care Medicine. Crit. Care Med. 37 (2) (2009) 666–688.)*

In sepsis, children without myocardial dysfunction have a decreased arterial-venous oxygen difference, where as those with myocardial dysfunction have an increased arterial-venous oxygen difference.

Brain-type naturetic peptide is a hormone that is released from the myocardium in response to cardiac wall stretch. Brain-type naturetic peptide elevation has been observed in sepsis and sepsis induced cardiomyopathy [137] and has been correlated with severity of illness and myocardial dysfunction [138].

As mentioned previously troponin I is a very sensitive and specific biomarker of myocardial injury and levels are elevated in patients with sepsis. Fenton et al. observed elevated troponin I levels in just over half of children with septic shock. Troponin I levels correlated with myocardial dysfunction by echocardiogram and increased severity of illness [52]. Similarly, Lodha et al. found that 88% of children with septic shock had elevated troponin levels and demonstrated a correlation with troponin I levels and the risk of mortality using the pediatric index of mortality score 2 [139].

MANAGEMENT

The management strategy myocardial dysfunction in sepsis is the same as the treatment of sepsis without myocardial dysfunction, with initial fluid resuscitation and timely administration of antibiotic therapy for the suspected source of infection. Delays in antibiotic therapy have been associated with mortality and prolonged organ dysfunction in pediatric sepsis [140]. There are guidelines for hemodynamic support of pediatric and neonatal septic shock [141]. See Fig. 33.1.

Fluid Resuscitation

Initial aggressive volume resuscitation has been shown to improve survival in children presenting in septic shock [142] and has remained a mainstay of a goal-directed approach to the management of sepsis. Either isotonic crystalloids or colloids can be the initial fluid of choice [143]. However, care should be taken as fluid resuscitation can have complications especially in a child with impaired myocardial function and high left atrial pressures, pulmonary edema, and respiratory failure can occur necessitating intubation and mechanical ventilation. A recent study from a critical care resource limited setting in sub-Saharan Africa in children with severe febrile illness, with impaired consciousness, respiratory distress, or both, and impaired perfusion found that fluid resuscitation with bolus fluids was associated with decreased survival compared to the use of maintenance fluids [144]. In this population the lack of additional critical care therapies to aid respiratory failure and circulatory failure such as mechanical ventilation and inotropic support were likely an important cause of mortality.

Inotropic Support

The majority of children with septic shock have a state of low cardiac output state with variable systemic vascular resistance [20]. In children with sepsis with low cardiac output and elevated systemic vascular resistance who are normotensive dobutamine have been the initial inotrope of choice and have been shown to have an effective hemodynamic profile with increasing cardiac index and decreasing systemic vascular resistance in children with cardiogenic and septic shock [145]. In comparison the phosophodiesterase inhibitor milrinone has inotropic and vasodilatory effects similar to dobutamine but has a longer half-life and cannot be easily titrated off with hypotension. In children with sepsis with low cardiac output and elevated systemic vascular resistance with hypotension epinephrine and historically dopamine have been the initial inotropes of choice. In a recent clinical trial in infants and children with septic shock refractory to fluid administration, children who received epinephrine had a more rapid resolution of shock and less organ failure–free days compared to those who received dopamine; however, no difference in mortality was observed between the two groups [146]. In children with low cardiac output with low systemic vascular resistance, it is reasonable to initiate norepinephrine an initial agent; however, epinephrine is usually needed to augment cardiac output [147].

Hydrocortisone

In children with purpura fulminans, recent steroid treatment, and known adrenal insufficiency, hydrocortisone should be administered early with fluid resuscitation and in children with catecholamine resistant shock. Routine use of steroids in pediatric sepsis without these indications is not recommended.

Mechanical Circulatory Support

Mechanical circulatory support with venoarterial (VA) and venovenous (VV), extracorporeal membrane oxygenation (ECMO) has been used for refractory pediatric septic shock with recent survival rates reported at 68% from the Extracorporeal Life Support Organization Registry in 4332 children [148], with higher survival for VV (79%) compared to VA (64%) ECMO. A single center study where children with refractory septic shock were cannulated with central VA–ECMO cannulation showed a 74% survival to hospital discharge suggesting that higher flow rates achieved with central cannulation in this study compared to peripheral cannulaiton in previous reports were associated with improved outcome.

Prognosis

Encouragingly, adult and pediatric studies have shown that myocardial dysfunction is reversible in 3–7 days after initiation of treatment for sepsis [19,150,151]. However, although there have been significant advances in pediatric sepsis, a recent global point prevalence study showed that hospital mortality of children with severe sepsis was 25% and did not differ by age or between developed and resource limited countries [16]. These data indicate that further investigation is needed to improve outcomes of patients with severe sepsis.

REFERENCES

[1] B. Goldstein, B. Giroir, A. Randolph, International pediatric sepsis consensus conference: definitions for sepsis and organ dysfunction in pediatrics, Pediatr. Crit. Care Med. 6 (1) (2005) 2–8.

[2] L. Liu, et al., Global, regional, and national causes of child mortality in 2000–13, with projections to inform post-2015 priorities: an updated systematic analysis, Lancet 385 (9966) (2015) 430–440.

[3] F. Balamuth, et al., Pediatric severe sepsis in U.S. children's hospitals, Pediatr. Crit. Care Med. 15 (9) (2014) 798–805.

[4] M.E. Hartman, et al., Trends in the epidemiology of pediatric severe sepsis, Pediatr. Crit. Care Med. 14 (7) (2013) 686–693.

[5] J.C. Jaramillo-Bustamante, et al., Epidemiology of sepsis in pediatric intensive care units: first Colombian Multicenter Study, Pediatr. Crit. Care Med. 13 (5) (2012) 501–508.

[6] A. Ruth, et al., Pediatric severe sepsis: current trends and outcomes from the pediatric health information systems database, Pediatr. Crit. Care Med. 15 (9) (2014) 828–838.

[7] S.W. Wen, et al., Epidemiology of preterm birth and neonatal outcome, Semin. Fetal Neonatal Med. 9 (6) (2004) 429–435.

[8] J.C. Magee, et al., Pediatric transplantation in the United States, 1997-2006, Am. J. Transplant. 8 (4 Pt 2) (2008) 935–945.

[9] C. Gudiol, et al., Changing aetiology, clinical features, antimicrobial resistance, and outcomes of bloodstream infection in neutropenic cancer patients, Clin. Microbiol. Infect. 19 (5) (May 2013) 474–479.

[10] A.T. Cruz, et al., Implementation of goal-directed therapy for children with suspected sepsis in the emergency department, Pediatrics 127 (3) (2011) e758–e766.

[11] G.Y. Larsen, N. Mecham, R. Greenberg, An emergency department septic shock protocol and care guideline for children initiated at triage, Pediatrics 127 (6) (2011) e1585–e1592.

[12] F.O. Odetola, A. Gebremariam, G.L. Freed, Patient and hospital correlates of clinical outcomes and resource utilization in severe pediatric sepsis, Pediatrics 119 (3) (2007) 487–494.

[13] S. Nadel, et al., Drotrecogin alfa (activated) in children with severe sepsis: a multicentre phase III randomised controlled trial, Lancet 369 (9564) (2007) 836–843.

[14] F. Proulx, et al., Epidemiology of sepsis and multiple organ dysfunction syndrome in children, Chest 109 (4) (1996) 1033–1037.

[15] S.L. Weiss, et al., Defining pediatric sepsis by different criteria: discrepancies in populations and implications for clinical practice, Pediatr. Crit. Care Med. 13 (4) (2012) e219–e226.

[16] S.L. Weiss, et al., Global epidemiology of pediatric severe sepsis: the sepsis prevalence, outcomes, and therapies study, Am. J. Respir. Crit. Care Med. 191 (10) (2015) 1147–1157.

[17] J.P. Burns, et al., Epidemiology of death in the PICU at five U.S. teaching hospitals*, Crit. Care Med. 42 (9) (2014) 2101–2108.

[18] J. Charpentier, et al., Brain natriuretic peptide: a marker of myocardial dysfunction and prognosis during severe sepsis, Crit. Care Med. 32 (3) (2004) 660–665.

[19] M.M. Parker, et al., Profound but reversible myocardial depression in patients with septic shock, Ann. Intern. Med. 100 (4) (1984) 483–490.

[20] G. Ceneviva, et al., Hemodynamic support in fluid-refractory pediatric septic shock, Pediatrics 102 (2) (1998) e19.

[21] L.D. MacLean, et al., Patterns of septic shock in man–a detailed study of 56 patients, Ann. Surg. 166 (4) (1967) 543–562.

[22] B.A. Waisbren, Bacteremia due to gram-negative bacilli other than the *Salmonella*; a clinical and therapeutic study, AMA Arch. Intern. Med. 88 (4) (1951) 467–488.

[23] G.H. Clowes Jr., M. Vucinic, M.G. Weidner, Circulatory and metabolic alterations associated with survival or death in peritonitis: clinical analysis of 25 cases, Ann. Surg. 163 (6) (1966) 866–885.

[24] J. Postel, P.R. Schloerb, Cardiac depression in bacteremia, Ann. Surg. 186 (1) (1977) 74–82.

[25] L.D. Maclean, et al., Studies on the circulatory changes in the dog produced by endotoxin from gram-negative microorganisms, J. Clin. Investig. 35 (11) (1956) 1191–1198.
[26] L.W. Wilson, D. Powers, L.A. Soloff, The hemodynamic effects of infusions of long chain saturated fatty acids into dogs, Am. J. Med. Sci. 249 (1965) 75–78.
[27] R.D. Weisel, et al., Myocardial depression during sepsis, Am. J. Surg. 133 (4) (1977) 512–521.
[28] E.C. Rackow, et al., Hemodynamic response to fluid repletion in patients with septic shock: evidence for early depression of cardiac performance, Circ. Shock 22 (1) (1987) 11–22.
[29] E.J. Winslow, et al., Hemodynamic studies and results of therapy in 50 patients with bacteremic shock, Am. J. Med. 54 (4) (1973) 421–432.
[30] M.M. Krausz, et al., Cardiopulmonary effects of volume loading in patients in septic shock, Ann. Surg. 185 (4) (1977) 429–434.
[31] M.M. Parker, et al., Serial cardiovascular variables in survivors and nonsurvivors of human septic shock: heart rate as an early predictor of prognosis, Crit. Care Med. 15 (10) (1987) 923–929.
[32] A.J. Ahmed, et al., Hemodynamic responses to gram-positive versus gram-negative sepsis in critically ill patients with and without circulatory shock, Crit. Care Med. 19 (12) (1991) 1520–1525.
[33] C. Natanson, et al., Role of endotoxemia in cardiovascular dysfunction and mortality. *Escherichia coli* and *Staphylococcus aureus* challenges in a canine model of human septic shock, J. Clin. Investig. 83 (1) (1989) 243–251.
[34] C. Natanson, et al., Cardiovascular performance with *E. coli* challenges in a canine model of human sepsis, Am. J. Physiol. 254 (3 Pt 2) (1988) H558–H569.
[35] C. Natanson, et al., Endotoxin and tumor necrosis factor challenges in dogs simulate the cardiovascular profile of human septic shock, J. Exp. Med. 169 (3) (1989) 823–832.
[36] C. Natanson, et al., Gram-negative bacteremia produces both severe systolic and diastolic cardiac dysfunction in a canine model that simulates human septic shock, J. Clin. Investig. 78 (1) (1986) 259–270.
[37] A.G. Ellrodt, et al., Left ventricular performance in septic shock: reversible segmental and global abnormalities, Am. Heart J. 110 (2) (1985) 402–409.
[38] F. Jardin, et al., Persistent preload defect in severe sepsis despite fluid loading: a longitudinal echocardiographic study in patients with septic shock, Chest 116 (5) (1999) 1354–1359.
[39] A. Vieillard Baron, et al., Early preload adaptation in septic shock? A transesophageal echocardiographic study, Anesthesiology 94 (3) (2001) 400–406.
[40] A. Vieillard-Baron, et al., Actual incidence of global left ventricular hypokinesia in adult septic shock, Crit. Care Med. 36 (6) (2008) 1701–1706.
[41] J.L. Vincent, et al., Myocardial depression characterizes the fatal course of septic shock, Surgery 111 (6) (1992) 660–667.
[42] J.E. Parrillo, et al., Septic shock in humans. Advances in the understanding of pathogenesis, cardiovascular dysfunction, and therapy, Ann. Intern. Med. 113 (3) (1990) 227–242.
[43] A.F. Suffredini, et al., The cardiovascular response of normal humans to the administration of endotoxin, N. Engl. J. Med. 321 (5) (1989) 280–287.
[44] R.E. Cunnion, et al., The coronary circulation in human septic shock, Circulation 73 (4) (1986) 637–644.
[45] J.F. Dhainaut, et al., Coronary hemodynamics and myocardial metabolism of lactate, free fatty acids, glucose, and ketones in patients with septic shock, Circulation 75 (3) (1987) 533–541.
[46] M.A. Rossi, et al., Myocardial structural changes in long-term human severe sepsis/septic shock may be responsible for cardiac dysfunction, Shock 27 (1) (2007) 10–18.
[47] C.Q. Gao, et al., Matrix metalloproteinase-2 mediates cytokine-induced myocardial contractile dysfunction, Cardiovasc. Res. 57 (2) (2003) 426–433.
[48] W. Wang, et al., Intracellular action of matrix metalloproteinase-2 accounts for acute myocardial ischemia and reperfusion injury, Circulation 106 (12) (2002) 1543–1549.
[49] K. Takeuchi, et al., Increased myocardial calcium cycling and reduced myofilament calcium sensitivity in early endotoxemia, Surgery 126 (2) (1999) 231–238.
[50] L.L. Wu, C. Tang, M.S. Liu, Altered phosphorylation and calcium sensitivity of cardiac myofibrillar proteins during sepsis, Am. J. Physiol. Regul. Integr. Comp. Physiol. 281 (2) (2001) R408–R416.
[51] P. Ammann, et al., Troponin as a risk factor for mortality in critically ill patients without acute coronary syndromes, J. Am. Coll. Cardiol. 41 (11) (2003) 2004–2009.
[52] K.E. Fenton, et al., Increases in serum levels of troponin I are associated with cardiac dysfunction and disease severity in pediatric patients with septic shock, Pediatr. Crit. Care Med. 5 (6) (2004) 533–538.
[53] A.H. Wu, Increased troponin in patients with sepsis and septic shock: myocardial necrosis or reversible myocardial depression? Intensive Care Med. 27 (6) (2001) 959–961.
[54] S. Lanone, et al., Muscular contractile failure in septic patients: role of the inducible nitric oxide synthase pathway, Am. J. Respir. Crit. Care Med. 162 (6) (2000) 2308–2315.
[55] M.J. Herbertson, et al., Myocardial oxygen extraction ratio is decreased during endotoxemia in pigs, J. Appl. Physiol. (1985) 79 (2) (1995) 479–486.
[56] R.J. Powell, et al., Oxygen free radicals: effect on red cell deformability in sepsis, Crit. Care Med. 19 (5) (1991) 732–735.
[57] U. Buerke, et al., Apoptosis contributes to septic cardiomyopathy and is improved by simvastatin therapy, Shock 29 (4) (2008) 497–503.
[58] H. Fauvel, et al., Differential effects of caspase inhibitors on endotoxin-induced myocardial dysfunction and heart apoptosis, Am. J. Physiol. Heart Circ. Physiol. 280 (4) (2001) H1608–H1614.

[59] R. Neviere, et al., Caspase inhibition prevents cardiac dysfunction and heart apoptosis in a rat model of sepsis, Am. J. Respir. Crit. Care Med. 163 (1) (2001) 218–225.
[60] H. Fauvel, et al., Protective effects of cyclosporin A from endotoxin-induced myocardial dysfunction and apoptosis in rats, Am. J. Respir. Crit. Care Med. 165 (4) (2002) 449–455.
[61] S. Lancel, et al., Expression of apoptosis regulatory factors during myocardial dysfunction in endotoxemic rats, Crit. Care Med. 33 (3) (2005) 492–496.
[62] S.L. Wangensteen, et al., Relationship between splanchnic blood flow and a myocardial depressant factor in endotoxin shock, Surgery 69 (3) (1971) 410–418.
[63] J.E. Parrillo, et al., A circulating myocardial depressant substance in humans with septic shock. Septic shock patients with a reduced ejection fraction have a circulating factor that depresses in vitro myocardial cell performance, J. Clin. Investig. 76 (4) (1985) 1539–1553.
[64] J.W. Horton, et al., Nitric oxide modulation of TNF-alpha-induced cardiac contractile dysfunction is concentration dependent, Am. J. Physiol. Heart Circ. Physiol. 278 (6) (2000) H1955–H1965.
[65] S.E. Francis, et al., Interleukin-1 in myocardium and coronary arteries of patients with dilated cardiomyopathy, J. Mol. Cell. Cardiol. 30 (2) (1998) 215–223.
[66] N. Pathan, et al., Role of interleukin 6 in myocardial dysfunction of meningococcal septic shock, Lancet 363 (9404) (2004) 203–209.
[67] G. Baumgarten, et al., Toll-like receptor 4, nitric oxide, and myocardial depression in endotoxemia, Shock 25 (1) (2006) 43–49.
[67a] A. Kumar, V. Thota, L. Dee, J. Olson, E. Uretz, J.E. Parrillo, Tumor necrosis factor alpha and interleukin 1beta are responsible for in vitro myocardial cell depression induced by human septic shock serum, J. Exp. Med. 183 (3) (March 1, 1996) 949–958.
[68] J.L. Vincent, et al., Administration of anti-TNF antibody improves left ventricular function in septic shock patients. Results of a pilot study, Chest 101 (3) (1992) 810–815.
[69] C.J. Fisher Jr., et al., Treatment of septic shock with the tumor necrosis factor receptor: Fc fusion protein. The Soluble TNF Receptor Sepsis Study Group, N. Engl. J. Med. 334 (26) (1996) 1697–1702.
[70] E. Abraham, et al., Double-blind randomised controlled trial of monoclonal antibody to human tumour necrosis factor in treatment of septic shock. NORASEPT II Study Group, Lancet 351 (9107) (1998) 929–933.
[71] E. Abraham, et al., p55 Tumor necrosis factor receptor fusion protein in the treatment of patients with severe sepsis and septic shock. A randomized controlled multicenter trial. Ro 45-2081 Study Group, JAMA 277 (19) (1997) 1531–1538.
[72] S.M. Opal, et al., Confirmatory interleukin-1 receptor antagonist trial in severe sepsis: a phase III, randomized, double-blind, placebo-controlled, multicenter trial. The Interleukin-1 Receptor Antagonist Sepsis Investigator Group, Crit. Care Med. 25 (7) (1997) 1115–1124.
[73] L.L. Yang, et al., Conditional cardiac overexpression of endothelin-1 induces inflammation and dilated cardiomyopathy in mice, Circulation 109 (2) (2004) 255–261.
[74] D. Konrad, et al., Differentiated and dose-related cardiovascular effects of a dual endothelin receptor antagonist in endotoxin shock, Crit. Care Med. 32 (5) (2004) 1192–1199.
[75] H.D. Reines, et al., Plasma thromboxane concentrations are raised in patients dying with septic shock, Lancet 2 (8291) (1982) 174–175.
[76] S.F. Liu, et al., Differential regulation of cyclo-oxygenase-1 and cyclo-oxygenase-2 gene expression by lipopolysaccharide treatment in vivo in the rat, Clin. Sci. (Lond) 90 (4) (1996) 301–306.
[77] T. Rassaf, et al., Positive effects of nitric oxide on left ventricular function in humans, Eur. Heart J. 27 (14) (2006) 1699–1705.
[78] M. Kelm, et al., Nitric oxide induced contractile dysfunction is related to a reduction in myocardial energy generation, Cardiovasc. Res. 36 (2) (1997) 185–194.
[79] J.C. Preiser, et al., Time course of inducible nitric oxide synthase activity following endotoxin administration in dogs, Nitric Oxide 5 (2) (2001) 208–211.
[80] F.H. Khadour, et al., Enhanced NO and superoxide generation in dysfunctional hearts from endotoxemic rats, Am. J. Physiol. Heart Circ. Physiol. 283 (3) (2002) H1108–H1115.
[81] P. Pacher, J.S. Beckman, L. Liaudet, Nitric oxide and peroxynitrite in health and disease, Physiol. Rev. 87 (1) (2007) 315–424.
[82] H. Ishida, et al., Peroxynitrite-induced cardiac myocyte injury, Free Radic. Biol. Med. 20 (3) (1996) 343–350.
[83] R. Ullrich, et al., Congenital deficiency of nitric oxide synthase 2 protects against endotoxin-induced myocardial dysfunction in mice, Circulation 102 (12) (2000) 1440–1446.
[84] B. Tavernier, et al., Cardiac contractile impairment associated with increased phosphorylation of troponin I in endotoxemic rats, FASEB J. 15 (2) (2001) 294–296.
[85] U.K. Decking, et al., Endotoxin-induced contractile dysfunction in guinea pig hearts is not mediated by nitric oxide, Am. J. Physiol. 268 (6 Pt 2) (1995) H2460–H2465.
[86] T.L. Hwang, C.C. Yeh, Hemodynamic and hepatic microcirculational changes in endotoxemic rats treated with different NOS inhibitors, Hepatogastroenterology 50 (49) (2003) 188–191.
[87] M.Y. Kirov, et al., Infusion of methylene blue in human septic shock: a pilot, randomized, controlled study, Crit. Care Med. 29 (10) (2001) 1860–1867.
[88] Y.W. Xie, P.M. Kaminski, M.S. Wolin, Inhibition of rat cardiac muscle contraction and mitochondrial respiration by endogenous peroxynitrite formation during posthypoxic reoxygenation, Circ. Res. 82 (8) (1998) 891–897.
[89] S. Lancel, et al., Peroxynitrite decomposition catalysts prevent myocardial dysfunction and inflammation in endotoxemic rats, J. Am. Coll. Cardiol. 43 (12) (2004) 2348–2358.
[90] C. Xu, et al., Mitochondrial nitric oxide synthase participates in septic shock myocardial depression by nitric oxide overproduction and mitochondrial permeability transition pore opening, Shock 37 (1) (2012) 110–115.

[91] D. Annane, et al., Inappropriate sympathetic activation at onset of septic shock: a spectral analysis approach, Am. J. Respir. Crit. Care Med. 160 (2) (1999) 458–465.
[92] J.K. Bocking, et al., Plasma catecholamine levels and pulmonary dysfunction in sepsis, Surg. Gynecol. Obstet. 148 (5) (1979) 715–719.
[93] G. Bernardin, et al., Beta-adrenergic receptor-dependent and -independent stimulation of adenylate cyclase is impaired during severe sepsis in humans, Intensive Care Med. 24 (12) (1998) 1315–1322.
[94] L.H. Opie, Heart Physiology: From Cell to Circulation, fourth ed., Lippincott Williams & Wilkins, Philadelphia, 2004. xix, 648 p., 8 p. of plates.
[95] C. Tang, M.S. Liu, Initial externalization followed by internalization of beta-adrenergic receptors in rat heart during sepsis, Am. J. Physiol. 270 (1 Pt 2) (1996) R254–R263.
[96] R.E. Shepherd, C.H. Lang, K.H. McDonough, Myocardial adrenergic responsiveness after lethal and nonlethal doses of endotoxin, Am. J. Physiol. 252 (2 Pt 2) (1987) H410–H416.
[97] C. Reithmann, et al., Desensitization of rat cardiomyocyte adenylyl cyclase stimulation by plasma of noradrenaline-treated patients with septic shock, Circ. Shock 41 (1) (1993) 48–59.
[98] N. Abi-Gerges, et al., Sequential changes in autonomic regulation of cardiac myocytes after in vivo endotoxin injection in rat, Am. J. Respir. Crit. Care Med. 160 (4) (1999) 1196–1204.
[99] C. Rabuel, A. Mebazaa, Septic shock: a heart story since the 1960s, Intensive Care Med. 32 (6) (2006) 799–807.
[100] N. Matsuda, et al., Impairment of cardiac beta-adrenoceptor cellular signaling by decreased expression of G(s alpha) in septic rabbits, Anesthesiology 93 (6) (2000) 1465–1473.
[101] L.L. Wu, et al., G protein and adenylate cyclase complex-mediated signal transduction in the rat heart during sepsis, Shock 19 (6) (2003) 533–537.
[102] M. Bohm, et al., Increase of myocardial inhibitory G-proteins in catecholamine-refractory septic shock or in septic multiorgan failure, Am. J. Med. 98 (2) (1995) 183–186.
[103] R.J. Winchell, D.B. Hoyt, Spectral analysis of heart rate variability in the ICU: a measure of autonomic function, J. Surg. Res. 63 (1) (1996) 11–16.
[104] H. Schmidt, et al., Autonomic dysfunction predicts mortality in patients with multiple organ dysfunction syndrome of different age groups, Crit. Care Med. 33 (9) (2005) 1994–2002.
[105] P.K. Stein, R.E. Kleiger, Insights from the study of heart rate variability, Annu. Rev. Med. 50 (1999) 249–261.
[106] H.B. Schmidt, K. Werdan, U. Muller-Werdan, Autonomic dysfunction in the ICU patient, Curr. Opin. Crit. Care 7 (5) (2001) 314–322.
[107] H.J. Silverman, et al., Impaired beta-adrenergic receptor stimulation of cyclic adenosine monophosphate in human septic shock: association with myocardial hyporesponsiveness to catecholamines, Crit. Care Med. 21 (1) (1993) 31–39.
[108] B. Tavernier, et al., Myofilament calcium sensitivity is decreased in skinned cardiac fibres of endotoxin-treated rabbits, Cardiovasc. Res. 38 (2) (1998) 472–479.
[109] W.Y. Lew, et al., Endotoxin-induced cardiac depression is associated with decreased cardiac dihydropyridine receptors in rabbits, J. Mol. Cell. Cardiol. 28 (6) (1996) 1367–1371.
[110] L.W. Dong, et al., Impairment of the ryanodine-sensitive calcium release channels in the cardiac sarcoplasmic reticulum and its underlying mechanism during the hypodynamic phase of sepsis, Shock 16 (1) (2001) 33–39.
[111] J. Layland, et al., Protection against endotoxemia-induced contractile dysfunction in mice with cardiac-specific expression of slow skeletal troponin I, FASEB J. 19 (9) (2005) 1137–1139.
[112] A. Koesters, K.L. Engisch, M.M. Rich, Decreased cardiac excitability secondary to reduction of sodium current may be a significant contributor to reduced contractility in a rat model of sepsis, Crit. Care 18 (2) (2014) R54.
[113] M.C. Exline, E.D. Crouser, Mitochondrial mechanisms of sepsis-induced organ failure, Front. Biosci. 13 (2008) 5030–5041.
[114] S.L. Weiss, et al., Differential expression of the nuclear-encoded mitochondrial transcriptome in pediatric septic shock, Crit. Care 18 (6) (2014) 623.
[115] S.L. Weiss, et al., Mitochondrial dysfunction in peripheral blood mononuclear cells in pediatric septic shock, Pediatr. Crit. Care Med. 16 (1) (2015) e4–e12.
[116] O. Takasu, et al., Mechanisms of cardiac and renal dysfunction in patients dying of sepsis, Am. J. Respir. Crit. Care Med. 187 (5) (2013) 509–517.
[117] L. Smeding, et al., Structural changes of the heart during severe sepsis or septic shock, Shock 37 (5) (2012) 449–456.
[118] M.C. Cimolai, et al., Mitochondrial mechanisms in septic cardiomyopathy, Int. J. Mol. Sci. 16 (8) (2015) 17763–17778.
[119] A. Boveris, S. Alvarez, A. Navarro, The role of mitochondrial nitric oxide synthase in inflammation and septic shock, Free Radic. Biol. Med. 33 (9) (2002) 1186–1193.
[120] G. Escames, et al., Attenuation of cardiac mitochondrial dysfunction by melatonin in septic mice, FEBS J. 274 (8) (2007) 2135–2147.
[121] S.M. Hassoun, et al., Prevention of endotoxin-induced sarcoplasmic reticulum calcium leak improves mitochondrial and myocardial dysfunction, Crit. Care Med. 36 (9) (2008) 2590–2596.
[122] S. Krauss, C.Y. Zhang, B.B. Lowell, The mitochondrial uncoupling-protein homologues, Nat. Rev. Mol. Cell Biol. 6 (3) (2005) 248–261.
[123] M.D. Brand, T.C. Esteves, Physiological functions of the mitochondrial uncoupling proteins UCP2 and UCP3, Cell Metab. 2 (2) (2005) 85–93.
[124] K.C. Kregel, Heat shock proteins: modifying factors in physiological stress responses and acquired thermotolerance, J. Appl. Physiol. (1985) 92 (5) (2002) 2177–2186.
[125] P. Srivastava, Roles of heat-shock proteins in innate and adaptive immunity, Nat. Rev. Immunol. 2 (3) (2002) 185–194.
[126] A. Asea, et al., HSP70 stimulates cytokine production through a CD14-dependant pathway, demonstrating its dual role as a chaperone and cytokine, Nat. Med. 6 (4) (2000) 435–442.
[127] D.P. Gelain, et al., Serum heat shock protein 70 levels, oxidant status, and mortality in sepsis, Shock 35 (5) (2011) 466–470.
[128] G.A. Kustanova, et al., Exogenous heat shock protein 70 mediates sepsis manifestations and decreases the mortality rate in rats, Cell Stress Chaperones 11 (3) (2006) 276–286.

[129] E. Rozhkova, et al., Exogenous mammalian extracellular HSP70 reduces endotoxin manifestations at the cellular and organism levels, Ann. N.Y Acad. Sci. 1197 (2010) 94–107.

[130] H.W. Chen, et al., Heat shock pretreatment prevents cardiac mitochondrial dysfunction during sepsis, Shock 20 (3) (2003) 274–279.

[131] X. Meng, A.H. Harken, The interaction between Hsp70 and TNF-alpha expression: a novel mechanism for protection of the myocardium against post-injury depression, Shock 17 (5) (2002) 345–353.

[132] J.H. Hsu, et al., Exogenous heat shock cognate protein 70 pretreatment attenuates cardiac and hepatic dysfunction with associated anti-inflammatory responses in experimental septic shock, Shock 42 (6) (2014) 540–547.

[133] T.F. Feltes, et al., Quantitated left ventricular systolic mechanics in children with septic shock utilizing noninvasive wall-stress analysis, Crit. Care Med. 22 (10) (1994) 1647–1658.

[134] S. Basu, et al., Two-dimensional speckle tracking imaging detects impaired myocardial performance in children with septic shock, not recognized by conventional echocardiography, Pediatr. Crit. Care Med. 13 (3) (2012) 259–264.

[135] S. Raj, et al., Myocardial dysfunction in pediatric septic shock, J. Pediatr. 164 (1) (2014) 72–77 e2.

[136] A.P. Wheeler, et al., Pulmonary-artery versus central venous catheter to guide treatment of acute lung injury, N. Engl. J. Med. 354 (21) (2006) 2213–2224.

[137] J. Papanikolaou, et al., New insights into the mechanisms involved in B-type natriuretic peptide elevation and its prognostic value in septic patients, Crit. Care 18 (3) (2014) R94.

[138] M. Domico, et al., Elevation of brain natriuretic peptide levels in children with septic shock, Pediatr. Crit. Care Med. 9 (5) (2008) 478–483.

[139] R. Lodha, et al., Myocardial cell injury is common in children with septic shock, Acta Paediatr. 98 (3) (2009) 478–481.

[140] S.L. Weiss, et al., Delayed antimicrobial therapy increases mortality and organ dysfunction duration in pediatric sepsis. Crit. Care Med. 42 (11) (2014) 2409–2417.

[141] J. Brierley, et al., Clinical practice parameters for hemodynamic support of pediatric and neonatal septic shock: 2007 update from the American College of Critical Care Medicine, Crit. Care Med. 37 (2) (2009) 666–688.

[142] J.A. Carcillo, A.L. Davis, A. Zaritsky, Role of early fluid resuscitation in pediatric septic shock, JAMA 266 (9) (1991) 1242–1245.

[143] M. Upadhyay, et al., Randomized evaluation of fluid resuscitation with crystalloid (saline) and colloid (polymer from degraded gelatin in saline) in pediatric septic shock, Indian Pediatr. 42 (3) (2005) 223–231.

[144] K. Maitland, et al., Mortality after fluid bolus in African children with severe infection, N. Eng. J. Med. 364 (26) (2011) 2483–2495.

[145] R.M. Perkin, et al., Dobutamine: a hemodynamic evaluation in children with shock, J. Pediatr. 100 (6) (1982) 977–983.

[146] K.N. Ramaswamy, et al., Double-blind randomized clinical trial comparing dopamine and epinephrine in pediatric fluid-refractory hypotensive septic shock, Pediatr. Crit. Care Med. 17 (11) (2016) e502–e512.

[147] A. Deep, et al., Evolution of haemodynamics and outcome of fluid-refractory septic shock in children, Intensive Care Med. 39 (9) (2013) 1602–1609.

[148] S.C. Skinner, et al., Improved survival in venovenous vs venoarterial extracorporeal membrane oxygenation for pediatric noncardiac sepsis patients: a study of the Extracorporeal Life Support Organization registry, J. Pediatr. Surg. 47 (1) (2012) 63–67.

[149] F. Carmona, et al., Inflammation, myocardial dysfunction, and mortality in children with septic shock: an observational study, Pediatr. Cardiol. 35 (3) (2014) 463–470.

[150] H. Knoester, et al., Cardiac function in pediatric septic shock survivors, Arch. Pediatr. Adolesc. Med. 162 (12) (2008) 1164–1168.

Chapter 34

Outpatient Management of Pediatric HF

Paul F. Kantor[1], Kristen George[2], Judith Wilson[2], Jennifer L. Conway[1]
[1]University of Alberta, Edmonton, AB, Canada; [2]The Hospital for Sick Children and the University of Toronto, Toronto, ON, Canada

INTRODUCTION

The outpatient subspecialty Pediatric Heart Failure (HF) Clinic is a recent development in ambulatory pediatric cardiology care. It has developed directly as a result of the recognition that HF medicine is an area of special expertise and training. A range of patients with established HF as well as those considered at risk (HF stage A) are commonly encountered in the outpatient setting (Table 34.1), and therefore a coherent approach to their management is required. It follows logically that there are substantial differences between patients at different levels of HF severity, and that the management objectives will vary. A simplified framework of the objectives of outpatient care for such patients is listed in Table 34.1.

The priorities of care for patients with HF can be summarized as:

- Improved quality of life, with minimized symptoms of HF.
- Maintained compliance with guideline directed therapy.
- Anticipation and avoidance of risks related to HF.
- Timely recognition of the need for advanced care.

The unstated objective is in fact to avoid or minimize any admission related to HF. The reasons for this are manifold, both related to the expansive costs [1], chronicity, and impact on quality of life when children are hospitalized with chronic illness. Registry data from the 1990 to 2005 era suggest that only 54% of children with dilated cardiomyopathy survive the first 5 years after diagnosis without a heart transplant. In the adult experience with HF, hospitalization itself is a robust predictor of later mortality either from worsening HF or sudden death. Hence the importance of avoiding hospitalization and maintaining children with HF in a stable fashion by detailed and attentive outpatient care whenever possible.

THE VALUE OF THE HEART FAILURE CLINIC

Families and children experience significant anxiety associated with illness and hospitalization [2]. Feelings of isolation, loneliness, fears of abandonment, and fears related to finances are prominent. Following children in a specialized pediatric HF outpatient setting is more cost-effective and can improve anxiety associated with hospitalization [3]. Consultation with the HF team while the child is in hospital initiates a relationship and plan of care with the family that can continue in the outpatient setting. Coordinating the care of children with HF in an outpatient setting is multifaceted and requires a holistic team approach. To provide the complex specialized care required, dedicated HF clinics play a fundamental role [4–11]. Experience in adult HF care has demonstrated that noncompliance with the medical plan and subsequent readmission for worsening HF arises frequently from faulty discharge planning and suboptimal outpatient follow-up planning [7]. However, with a dedicated HF clinic, patient-referrals can be streamlined, and an improved care-system results [12]. Once embedded in an outpatient HF clinic, identifying patients at risk of worsening HF requires regular and consistent assessment to detect changes in symptoms. Patients who are in New York Heart Association (NYHA) functional class I will require less frequent follow up than those in NYHA class II–III, while those in NYHA class IV will require more frequent follow up.

Optimization of medical and nonmedical therapy as well as a supportive environment for the child and family, are necessary to deliver comprehensive care and prevent hospital readmission. Despite well-established guidelines for HF management with angiotensin-converting enzyme inhibitor (ACEi) and beta-blocker (BB) therapy [13–16], these medications are commonly underprescribed or given at subtherapeutic doses [4]. Within the structure of a multidisciplinary pediatric HF clinic, evidence-based standards of care can be tailored to create pediatric clinical practice protocols. This allows for less variation in the approach to management, and the elimination of nonevidence-based practices. Pediatric HF clinics also offer a dedicated setting to monitor the uptitration of vasoactive medications to achieve optimal therapeutic dosage. Clinical

Heart Failure in the Child and Young Adult. http://dx.doi.org/10.1016/B978-0-12-802393-8.00034-X

TABLE 34.1 Descriptive Overview of the Patient Specific Objectives of Care in a Pediatric Heart Failure (HF) Clinic

AHA/ACC HF Staging	Patient Description	Diseases Commonly Encountered	Key Outpatient Clinic Activity	Objective of Outpatient Care
A	At risk for HF, without structural disease or symptoms of HF	Family history: • Hypertrophic Cardiomyopathy • ARVC Suspected: • Skeletal myopathy • Metabolic disorders	Screening with: • Echocardiography • MRI • Biochemical panel • Genetic Counseling/testing	• Early and accurate diagnosis. • Effective patient and family reassurance.
B	Structural heart disease without prior or current symptoms of HF.	• Hypertrophic cardiomyopathy. • Familial dilated cardiomyopathy • Postanthracycline exposure • LV noncompaction	• Exclude any treatable causes of LV dysfunction. • Investigations to stratify risk profile: (MRI, holter, exercise testing) • Biomarker assay. • Initiate medical therapy to prevent progression (ACEi, BB). • Optimize nutrition. • Look for/manage other risk factors.	• Prevent the occurrence of symptoms. • Minimize disease progression and secondary consequences of disease.
C	Structural heart disease with prior or current symptoms of HF.	• Congenital heart disease with LV dysfunction • Fontan with circulatory failure • Restrictive cardiomyopathy • Dilated cardiomyopathy • Postacute myocarditis.	• Optimize medical therapy, consider adding other drugs • Treat electromechanical dyssynchrony, • Treat nutritional deficit, anemia, and other modifiable risk factors.	• Reduce symptoms, and improve quality of life.
D	Refractory HF requiring advanced therapy	• Any of the above	• Optimize medical therapy. • Outpatient inotropic therapy • CPAP • VAD	• Consider inpatient admission to stabilize. • Review patient/family wishes. • Consider transplant, VAD. • Involve palliative care team.

ACEi, angiotensin-converting enzyme inhibitor; *ARVC*, arrhythmogenic right ventricular cardiomyopathy; *BB*, beta-blocker; *CPAP*, continuous positive airway pressure; *LV*, left ventricular; *MRI*, magnetic resonance imaging; *VAD*, ventricular assist device.

visits can provide a multidisciplinary venue to address other aspects of care such as activity, nutritional, and psychosocial needs of the child and family.

Goals of Care

Goals of care should be patient-specific. They can nevertheless change, as disease progresses, to suit patient and family wishes. While the ultimate goal of care is improvement in cardiac function this is not always achievable in the setting of advanced disease. For all patients, defining the baseline status, and establishing medical, nutritional, and physical activity plans on that basis, can set the stage for attaining success. Patients with end-stage HF who do not improve despite optimal medical therapy are then more readily identified, and either listed for cardiac transplantation or directed to advanced therapy or palliative care. Individualized plans of care can help to guide patient management with the objective of reducing readmission rates, improving quality of life, and decreasing morbidity and mortality [4]. The goals of care may change over time as cardiac function either improves (stability with decreased diuretic needs, delisting, ventricular assist device (VAD) removal) or the child deteriorates (inotropes, VAD, listed for transplant, and palliative care). Multidisciplinary collaboration in care planning must primarily take into account the wishes of the child and family [5].

THE MULTIDISCIPLINARY APPROACH

Regular outpatient follow-up for patients with symptomatic HF allows for interaction with multiple team members. Key providers of outpatient care include physicians and nurses with specialty HF management training, who together with ensuring education of patients and caregivers regarding diagnosis, signs of increasing HF symptoms, can ensure adherence to medication and dietary advice. McAlister [10,11] describes a dynamic interchange between medical, behavioral, and psychosocial elements, which is better managed by a multidisciplinary approach. Furthermore, in a systematic review, multidisciplinary care was found to reduce HF-related hospitalizations and mortality [10,11]. The availability of healthcare professionals and the capacity to provide this frequent follow up have been identified as key contributors to establishing and maintaining successful HF programs [4,5,7]. Table 34.2 outlines possible HF clinic team members and their roles in providing care to patients and their caregivers.

Cardiologists with experience in managing HF are primarily responsible for determining the level of care required and ensuring comprehensive testing and directing treatment plans [17]. Cardiologist-led multidisciplinary HF programs frequently have nurse-specialists providing a vital role in day-to-day management of patient care. Much of the literature regarding successful outpatient management of HF patients has emphasized the importance of specially trained nurses in providing education and access to medical care [4,5,7,8,10–12,18]. Nurse-practitioners (NP) have been identified as one group of specialists who can care for patients throughout the continuum of care in both the inpatient and outpatient settings. NPs combine nursing and medical models of care and function both independently and collaboratively within a multidisciplinary team [18].

During inpatient stays the pharmacist provides medication teaching and schedules to the patient and family, which may be adjusted in the outpatient setting as needed by the cardiologist or NP. Written instructions and education regarding the name, indications, dose, timing, and side effects of medications assist with promoting adherence and improving clinical stability [5,7,8,11,15–17].

It is important to draw on the expertise of pediatric dieticians, and occupational, physical, and child life therapists, who add to the physical well-being of the child by providing nutritional, developmental, and activity advice together with psychological support. Many children with HF have poor growth; dieticians evaluate the child and provide recommendations to optimize caloric intake while balancing the challenges imposed by fluid restrictions [17]. If the child is unable to gain weight or is intolerant of oral feeds, placement of a nasogastric or gastrostomy tube is often necessary. Placement of a feeding tube can be distressing for the child and family, and ongoing support is needed to explain the rationale and benefits of this approach.

Occupational therapists may be able to assist with improving oral feeding and should be consulted to assess developmental status in infants as well as provide direction to parents with regard to gaining development milestones in a child with a chronic disease. Children with significant HF may have limited physical capabilities, so physiotherapists can assess endurance and physical ability and provide exercise programs to maintain or improve physical capacity. For the child who has limited capacity or is too young to participate in a cardiopulmonary exercise test, a 6-min walk test can be performed on consecutive occasions to assess changes in activity tolerance.

Child life therapists, or psychologists can play a role in assessing the child's developmental stage and assisting with coping strategies in relation to managing illness. If the child is experiencing anxiety, depression, or is thought to have an underlying psychiatric disorder, referral for assessment and treatment by a psychiatrist may occasionally be necessary.

The financial burden and disruption to the family's social system adds to the stress on caregivers. Social workers are tasked with assessing the family's needs and navigating the systems that can offer financial and caregiver support. Consultation with other specialists either because of primary disease or for management of comorbidities occurs on an as-needed basis. Finally, early involvement of the palliative care team is essential in determining goals of treatment in advance of a critical event. Collaborating with community caregivers is necessary to ensure that a consistent plan of care is conveyed to the patient and family [5].

Counseling Effectively: Educational Materials, Support Services, Engaging With Other Specialties

Counseling the child and family regarding their underlying cardiac condition and uncertain prognosis; signs and symptoms of worsening HF, medications, dietary, and fluid restrictions; and activity plans is complex and time-intensive. Nevertheless, it is essential to provide education and information at a level that is understandable for the child and family and in appropriate quantity, so that it can be absorbed. Even when well understood, it is important to reiterate the message and to

TABLE 34.2 The Multidisciplinary Team and Key Roles That are Needed in a Pediatric Heart Failure Clinic

Professional	Key Roles
HF MD	• Overall responsibility for medical care plan • Chooses comprehensive assessment investigations • Establishes treatment plan • Requests external consultations • Communicates overall plan with family
RN/NP	• Primary care coordinator and patient/family liaison • Provides written and verbal information to family regarding: Signs and symptoms of HF Fluid restriction and weight monitoring Medication adjustment and uptitration Whom to contact with concerns. • Clinical assessment and laboratory result review–response
Dietician	• Nutritional assessment and written recommendations • Optimization of caloric intake (fortifying feeds) • Review of food records/daily intake and growth • Recommendations regarding enteral (NG, G tube, GJ tube) or parenteral nutrition
Social worker	• Assessment of psychosocial, cultural, and financial needs • Support/assist access to social benefits/resources • Letters of support for employer/school regulators
Pharmacist	• Update immunization and allergy information • Medication teaching (names, purpose, dose, frequency, and side effects) • Provides a medication schedule; coordinates timing to optimize compliance • Support for insurance/paying agency drug approval
OT/PT	• Initial activity and developmental assessment, • Serial rehabilitation/evaluation of activity tolerance • Assessment of progress of developmental milestones • Feeding and swallowing assessments
Child life	• Consideration of child's developmental stage • Procedural support, coping strategies
Psychologist or Psychiatrist	• Developmental assessment, coping strategies for school, anxiety, and depression • Support with psychiatric/behavioral disorder management
Palliative care specialist	• Support for uncertain prognosis (e.g., deterioration while awaiting transplant), • Development of an advance directive care-plan • Community-based palliative care.
Electrophysiologist	• Guides antiarrhythmic drug therapy • Advises regarding device indications. • EP studies in cases of tachycardiomyopathy
VAD specialist	• Outpatient VAD management including anticoagulation, infectious markers, pump function evaluation/ alarm response.
Respiratory therapist	• Home oxygen and CPAP care and management
Community caregivers (GP/pediatrician/RN)	• Collaboration and care coordination/support for fragile patients with complex needs. • Respite care, in-home nursing evaluation/assistance.
Genetic counselor	• Counseling regarding genetic testing for suspected genetic disorders in index case • Counseling regarding genetic testing and cardiac screening in first degree relatives • Counseling regarding future pregnancies and inheritance patterns
Clinic coordinator	• Coordinating clinic visits and tests, coordinating visits with other specialists. • Maintaining statistics regarding clinic activity • Coordinating care transition to adult care. • Family screening

CPAP, continuous positive airway pressure; *EP*, electrophysiologic; *G*, gastrostomy; *GJ*, gastrojejunal; *GP*, general practitioner; *HF*, heart failure; *MD*, medical doctor; *NG*, nasogastric; *NP*, nurse practitioner; *OT*, occupational therapist; *PT*, physical therapist; *RN*, registered nurse; *VAD*, ventricular assist device.

provide written reference material to support verbal instruction. If there is a language barrier, use of interpreter services and language-specific written information is crucial to ensure both the caregiver and the healthcare professional have a mutual understanding of goals of care and treatment plans.

Optimal communication with patients and caregivers involves a coordinated multidisciplinary approach across the continuum of care [9]. Engaging all team members to provide education also provides an added support network for the child and family. Child life therapists, for example, are invaluable in offering age appropriate methods of teaching the child about their illness. While many patients and caregivers will use the internet as a resource for discovering medical information, the health care team can provide direction with regard to reputable websites and assist with appraising the information obtained from these sources [19].

Comorbidities require collaboration with other specialists who are involved in the child's care and can ensure optimal medical management of underlying disorders to help support overall cardiac function. Specific expertise in clinical genetics, metabolic diseases, neuromuscular diseases, and palliative care may be necessary. A close relationship with cardiac transplantation service expertise becomes beneficial if end-stage disease is believed to be likely.

Outside of the multidisciplinary HF team it is also important to liaise with the community services that support the child and family at home. The family doctor, pediatrician, community nurse, and palliative care team are part of a wider team who are integral members of the patient's health care team. Communication with these community-based partners is essential to ensuring a cohesive plan of care, since poor communication can easily result in contradictory plans of care, medication errors, and other mishaps [4].

Finally, the social and financial stressors associated with having a child with HF may take a toll on the child and family. Writing letters to employers to support work absences and assistance with accessing financial and respite services can ease some of the burden. Continued integration from an educational and psychological perspective may be offered by collaborating with the child's school with regard to how to support the child, activity restrictions, or the need for home schooling.

COMMON MANAGEMENT ISSUES

Outpatient Medication Uptitration

Pharmacotherapy remains the lynchpin of symptom-free maintenance for most patients with HF. Recent guidelines for both adults and pediatric patients have continued to endorse the concept of multidrug management. The specific drugs and their mechanisms are dealt with in detail elsewhere in this book. We will address practical aspects of sequence, uptitration, and common pitfalls of medical therapy. Fig. 34.1 is provided as a conceptual guide to stepwise therapy in HF patients. In reality, these steps are often blurred, and overlap significantly.

Diuretic Therapy

Typically patients with HF stage C require maintenance therapy with diuretics. A single agent loop diuretic at a dose of 1 mg/kg given 12 hourly would be considered low-level therapy, and usually does not result in significant electrolyte derangement, or kidney function impairment in normotensive patients. In this setting, patients with ROSS/NYHA symptoms class I–II may be able to be weaned off therapy altogether. Serial assays of B-type natriuretic peptide (BNP) or N-terminal proBNP (NT-proBNP) can provide reassurance that the patient is progressing adequately, and in the setting of stable and normal levels of BNP or NT-proBNP, it is often possible to sustain good functional capacity and euvolemia in the absence of diuretics. As a rule of thumb, such patients will not have significant right ventricular (RV) dysfunction or mitral regurgitation, and will have an LV ejection fraction of >25%. Regardless, it is desirable to minimize diuretic exposure to the level required for active symptom relief alone.

If patients remain symptomatic on a loop diuretic given at optimal and frequent (q6h) doses, additional diuretics may be required. Patients unresponsive to furosemide may indeed respond to ethacrynic acid, despite a similar mechanism of action. If this is unsuccessful, addition of a thiazide agent to the loop diuretic regimen is almost always effective. One choice is metolazone a quinazoline derivative with a prolonged half-life, but conventional shorter-acting thiazides are also effective. The risks associated with this approach are of excessive intravascular volume depletion, hyponatremia, hypokalemia and hypomagnesemia.

Angiotensin-Converting Enzyme Inhibitors

As of 2017, ACEi retain a class I indication, level of evidence A, for outpatient management of HF, as a result of several randomized clinical trials conducted in the 1980s and early 1990s in adult HF. The evidence in children is more empirical.

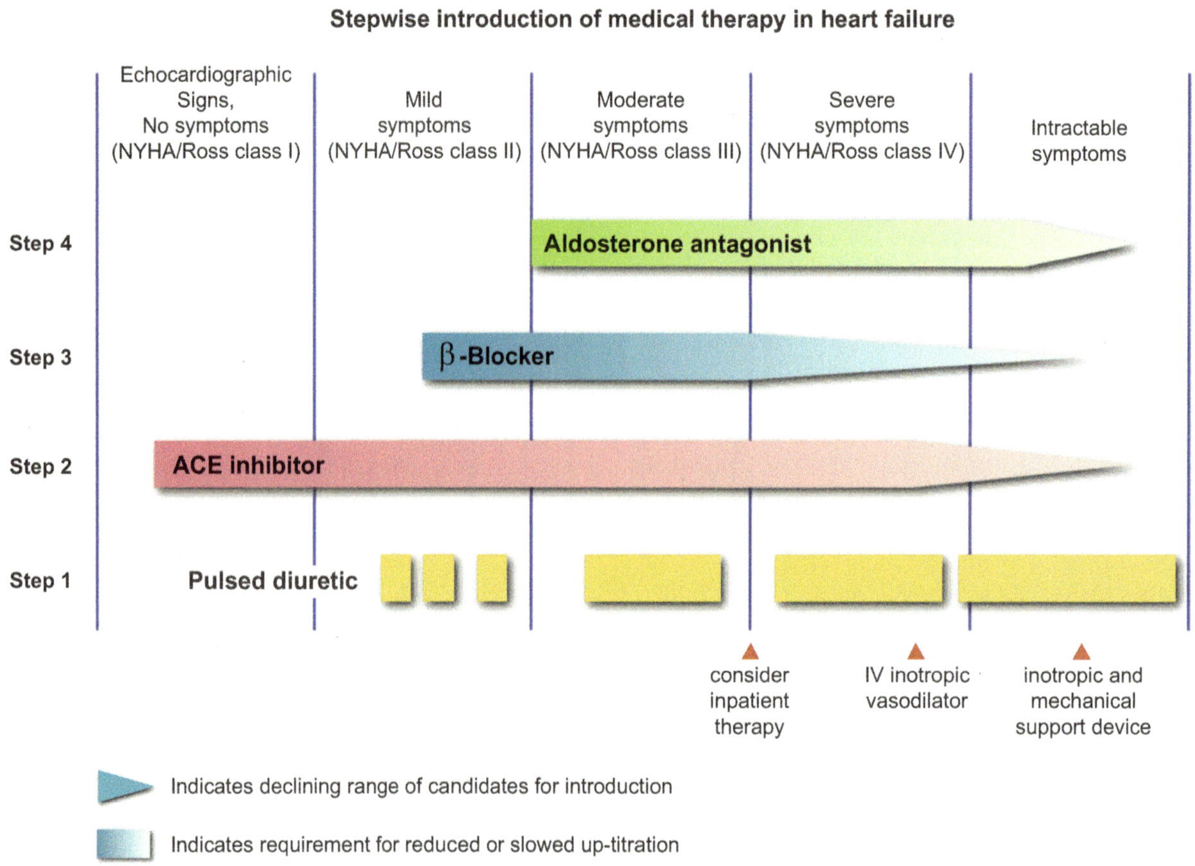

FIGURE 34.1 The introduction of oral maintenance therapy for children in chronic heart failure (HF). This approach is based on patient symptoms. Lighter shading for each drug indicates when the possibility of a lower target dose, or slower increment than usual is needed, due to advanced HF with severely compromised systolic function. Narrowing of the bars indicates the possibility that fewer patients will tolerate the introduction of that agent at that given symptomatic stage. Note the preferred use of pulsed diuretic therapy, which becomes more frequent as symptoms advance. *Red arrows* indicate the point at which admission to hospital and additional support therapies may be required. *NYHA*, New York Heart Association. *From P.F. Kantor, J. Lougheed, A. Dancea, M. McGillion, N. Barbosa, C. Chan, et al., Presentation, diagnosis, and medical management of heart failure in children: Canadian Cardiovascular Society guidelines, Can. J. Cardiol. 29 (2013) 1535–1552.*

The optimal choice of ACEi remains somewhat debatable. In young infants, captopril is often chosen because of its shorter half-life, although enalapril is a suitable alternative for anyone over 6 months of age. Although there is biologic evidence of enhanced efficacy for tissue-specific ACEi (ramipril, perindopril), there is no clinical trial evidence that these agents are actually superior in HF. Thus most patients with decreased left ventricular (LV) systolic function (typically an ejection fraction of <50%) and some evidence of symptoms, past or present, having a biventricular circulation are likely to benefit from ACEi therapy. There are certain challenges which arise in specific circumstances:

- Outpatients on inotropic infusions: The aim for patients in this group is not necessarily to achieve a full therapeutic dose of an ACEi, as this will commonly result in symptomatic hypotension and provoke renal dysfunction. Some recommend to gradually uptitrate to a dose of around 40%–50% of therapeutic target range, or until an increment in serum creatinine over >50% of baseline is encountered. In the author's experience, the introduction of ACEi is well tolerated in most patients while still on a milrinone infusion.
- Impaired renal function: This is one of the most commonly encountered adverse effects of ACEi in patients with reduced cardiac index. A rapid uptitration is therefore not a universal requirement, especially in patients with significant RV dysfunction or with recent cardiogenic shock. Following a test dose, incremental increases can be performed periodically (e.g., every 48 h) with a periodic (e.g., weekly) follow-up assessment. The patient's electrolyte, urea, and creatinine levels must be checked, and uptitration should be held, if a significant creatinine increment (e.g., of >100% over baseline) occurs, or in the setting of hyperkalemia. If the patient is hypotensive, with elevated potassium levels, the dosage should be reduced to a preceding lower dose.
- Single ventricle physiology: To date, there has been little or no evidence that ACEi actually helps single ventricle patients at any stage of their course. The Single Ventricle Reconstruction Trial demonstrated no increment in somatic

growth, improvement in ejection fraction or HF symptoms in patients randomized to receive enalapril up to 14 months of age, when compared to placebo [20]. While cross-sectional registry data suggest that approximately 57% of patients with Fontan physiology are treated with ACEi [21], there is no evidence from either adolescent [22] or adult cohorts with the Fontan circulation, that improved systolic function or improved clinical outcomes will result from this treatment choice.

Mineralocorticoid Receptor Antagonists

To completely block the effects of increased serum renin, angiotensin, and aldosterone, the mineralocorticoid receptor must also be targeted. The typical choice for this purpose is spironolactone. This drug has been used empirically in children with overcirculation symptoms since the 1970s [23], although to this day no prospective randomized-controlled trial data support its efficacy in children with cardiac disease. Therefore, current practice is extrapolated from the adult experience [24]. In general, a mineralocorticoid antagonist (MRA) is indicated in patients with persistent, moderate, or severe dysfunction who have stable tolerance of ACEi. Careful monitoring of serum potassium levels, and for gynecomastia in males is essential. Eplerenone is a second-generation MRA with more specific receptor-blockade, and a lower risk of gynecomastia, however, the cost at this time is substantially higher.

Beta-Blocker Therapy

Beta-blockers retain a class I indication in HF with reduced ejection fraction, of at least moderate severity. Despite the lack of positive supportive evidence from the Pediatric Carvedilol Study [25] (which was conducted in a heterogeneous study population, conservatively dosed, for a limited time frame, and with a debatable end point), these drugs remain widely used in pediatric HF. The recommended choices are carvedilol, metoprolol, and bisoprolol, often selected based on the half-life (least to greatest as listed). In adults, a BB is indicated in any patient with an EF of <40% after establishing adequate dosing of ACEi. This is independent of symptom status. Uptitration can typically be achieved in weekly or two-weekly increments by doubling the preliminary tolerated dose. Tolerance is usually assessed by the blood pressure response, with hypotension, or symptoms of hypotension being an indication to scale-back therapy. A cardioselective BB is usually well tolerated with few side effects. Occasionally, a short stay admission is required to introduce a BB in a patient with tenuous hemodynamics and concerns due to lack of community follow-up.

ADVANCED HEART FAILURE MANAGEMENT IN OUTPATIENTS

Outpatient Ventricular Assist Device Management Priorities

VAD therapy has had a significant impact on the survival for children with end-stage HF awaiting transplant [26]. While most of these patients have been supported as inpatients with an extracorporeal pulsatile pump, there has been an increasing trend of implanting intracorporeal continuous flow devices in children. These devices, such as the Thoratec Heartmate II and Heartware HVAD provide an opportunity for discharge from hospital and subsequently outpatient management.

Outpatient management, as with other complex pediatric patients, benefits from a dedicated and cohesive multidisciplinary team to assist families in the transition to the outpatient setting. The goals of outpatient therapy are to prevent and manage complications, to optimize pump function, and to address barriers that may impede the family and patient from achieving an acceptable quality of life. The components of the VAD team will vary depending on the resources available. Regardless of the composition of the team, expert advice should readily available at all times, for the families and patients, as well as other healthcare providers.

The outpatient literature in pediatric VAD usage is limited to a few small case series. Schweiger et al. [27] have reported on 12 patients implanted with the HVAD at nine different centers who were discharged home. This series demonstrated that a majority of children required readmission to hospital with an average of 2.5 admissions per patient. Driveline infections, anticoagulation issues, and VAD alarms comprised the top three reasons for readmission. In addition, patients were admitted for epistaxis, infectious symptoms, technical issues, acute renal failure, and hemolysis. A smaller single-center study showed similar trend in readmission, and reason for readmission, with pump thrombosis also reported [28]. While these small studies point to ongoing morbidity in this patient population, larger-scale studies are truly required to have a better understanding of the outpatient course in children, especially those with longer duration of support.

As highlighted above, recognition of abnormal trends and prevention of complications are essential components of outpatient management. Education of the patient and family starts well before discharge, by reviewing common presenting symptoms of complications, acceptable pump function, and the importance of anticoagulation management. Written materials can supplement teaching and be a guide for the families when they are at home. Having a preset plan for readmission and how to deal with complications will prevent delays in treatment especially for families who live far from the VAD center.

This component of advanced HF therapy is still developing in pediatrics, with most of the knowledge generated from adult experiences and a small number of pediatric patients. As we move forward in this field collaboration between centers is essential to understand how to optimize the outpatient experience and maximize the quality of life in this unique patient population.

Outpatient Parenteral Inotropic Therapy

Patients listed for heart transplantation may face prolonged wait times, due to a shortage of donor hearts. Pediatric VAD therapy addresses this problem in part, and prolonged inotropic administration in an outpatient setting is an alternate option, sometimes allowing children with advanced HF to be discharged home. Outpatient intravenous inotropic therapies in adults have previously been demonstrated as an effective bridge to transplantation [29–31], with milrinone, a phosphodiesterase-III inhibitor, substituting well for catecholamines [32]. To date, there are three pediatric studies examining the use of home inotropic therapy, with milrinone being the most commonly prescribed [3,33,34]. Birnbaum et al. [34] examined the results of 106 pediatric and young adult patients discharged home on inotropic therapy (91% on milrinone). The age of patients supported ranged from 0.2 to 26 years with the average being 10.1 years. One-third of the patients were less than 5 years of age. The majority (85%) were bridged to heart transplant, with 19 of these being rehospitalized for HF, remaining inpatients until transplantation. A small percentage (6%) of children died, half of them from progressive HF. Overall, more than half of these patients required readmission with 94% of the hospitalizations explained by worsening HF, infections or central line malfunction. This study highlights the relative safety and effectiveness of home inotropic therapy in the outpatient pediatric setting.

A home inotropic program requires a collaborative effort between the HF team, home-care services, and the family. The extent of outpatient support will depend on the comfort level of the home-care team as well as the services they provide. At a minimum, assistance with pump issues and central line–dressing care should be expected. The family must be willing to take on the responsibility of caring for the pump and central line, learning how to change the medication and troubleshooting issues that arise. Access to the HF team should be readily available to support the home-care team and family should issues arise.

As clinical HF is a significant cause of readmission frequent assessment and evaluation for worsening congestive HF is essential. Some programs opt to start standard oral HF medications while a patient is on milrinone as part of an inotropic weaning strategy [34].

Outpatient Continuous Positive Airway Pressure

Continuous Positive airway pressure (CPAP) therapy may be an additional tool for HF management in pediatrics, but has not yet been systematically investigated in children with HF due to reduced ejection fraction. Respiratory symptoms are commonly seen in pediatric HF and the interaction between the cardiac and respiratory systems can alter cardiac output [35]. HF has been associated with sleep-disordered breathing, including primary central sleep apnea in adults and to a lesser degree in children [36,37]. Positive pressure ventilation has the potential to improve cardiac output in those with left heart dysfunction by altering LV afterload [35]. Positive pressure can also assist in recruiting alveoli and decreasing pulmonary edema resulting in improvement in oxygen delivery. However, randomized trials of CPAP in adult patients with HF have to date not demonstrated a reduction in mortality.

If indicated, CPAP therapy for HF management should be initiated during an inpatient stay with assessment of tolerance prior to discharge. Where this initiation occurs will depend on the patient's clinical status, institutional policy, and comfort level with CPAP. Therapy can be started on a general cardiology ward in stable patients, or in the intensive care setting if used as a rescue effort. CPAP may be used during sleep or continuously depending on patient tolerance and developmental requirements. Enteral tube feeds can be continued during CPAP, although venting of the tube may be necessary to avoid abdominal distention. Close collaboration with the respirology team and respiratory therapist can help in assessment of sleep-disordered breathing (which may or may not coexist with HF), and acquiring necessary equipment for home usage.

Parents are trained to use the CPAP machine and a schedule for CPAP is determined prior to discharge. Outpatient management of CPAP consists of troubleshooting issues that may arise with the machine and developing a weaning plan in clinically stable patients. Tracking hours of usage and patient symptoms can help determine the frequency and speed of weaning.

Advanced Directives and End of Life Care

Assessment of the family and child's understanding of their diagnosis and prognosis is crucial, and usually only achieved over several encounters. Since cardiomyopathy and therefore pediatric HF are frequently not "curable" conditions, discussion must also focus on the possibility of end of life care. The objectives of this dialogue are to establish a preparedness plan for families, and to permit an early and ongoing discussion of what measures are to be taken if symptoms are worsening. This is the crux of a so-called "advanced directive" as to the intensity of care desired by the patient. It is best to involve children in this discussion, but the age and level of involvement will vary according to the child and the family preference. Focusing on what the team will undertake to do in a given situation as opposed to what the team will not do is important [38]. Since children have an active imagination (and often imagine the worst), exclusion of the child from the care plan is not optimal.

The content and structure of the discussion involving the possibility of death, or an advanced directive being developed, has been dealt with in detail by Xafis et al. using a linguistic rubric [39]. The approach proposed is to (1) establish the quantity of information and complexity desired by families; (2) convey the factual information, and then the possible outcomes and implications of these facts, adapted to the specific circumstances, acknowledging the unknown elements; (3) employ honesty and compassion and avoid generic statements, which may convey false hope to families and children, using joint consultations with other experts where necessary; (4) using straightforward terminology, assess and question how the information is being received both at a cognitive and at an emotional level.

The goals of end of life care are to provide care for all aspects of the child's needs, while supporting their family [40]. The palliative care team is an integrated member of HF team and should be involved in the care of children with cardiomyopathy and HF at some level. At a minimum, the palliative care team should be consulted when a family inquires, for patients dependent on inotropes or more advance therapy, being assessed for heart transplantation, and those deemed not to be a transplant candidate.

TRANSITION MANAGEMENT

Planning transitioning from pediatric to adult care can begin when the child is as young as age 10. Some centers may have a formal transition program which the child and family can access to assist in the transition process. Individualized planning is calibrated to the child and family in question, and occurs in phases. Caregivers should be informed and included in the plan as the entire family adjusts to changes in care. Early stages of transition aim to empower the child by educating and reviewing their diagnosis, medications, tests, and treatment options. This may be an ideal time to introduce the role of the Adolescent Medicine service, if available. As the child gets older they should be expected to know the name and dose of their medications and demonstrate responsibility for taking their medication. In the final phase of transition the adolescent should take on primary responsibility for their medications including ordering refills.

REFERENCES

[1] C.A. Wittlieb-Weber, K.Y. Lin, T.E. Zaoutis, M.J. O'Connor, K. Gerald, S.M. Paridon, et al., Pediatric versus adult cardiomyopathy and heart failure-related hospitalizations: a value-based analysis, J. Card. Fail. 21 (2015) 76–82.

[2] F. Muscara, M.C. McCarthy, C. Woolf, S.J. Hearps, K. Burke, V.A. Anderson, Early psychological reactions in parents of children with a life threatening illness within a pediatric hospital setting, Eur. Psychiatry 30 (2015) 555–561.

[3] A.M. Berg, L. Snell, W.T. Mahle, Home inotropic therapy in children, J. Heart Lung Transplant. 26 (2007) 453–457.

[4] P.J. Hauptman, M.W. Rich, P.A. Heidenreich, J. Chin, N. Cummings, M.E. Dunlap, et al., The heart failure clinic: a consensus statement of the Heart Failure Society of America, J. Card. Fail. 14 (2008) 801–815.

[5] A Systematic Approach to Chronic Heart Failure Care: A Consensus Statement, 2013. https://heartfoundation.org.au/images/uploads/publications/HF_CHF_consensus_web_FINAL_SP.pdf.

[6] N.M. Albert, G.C. Fonarow, C.W. Yancy, A.B. Curtis, W.G. Stough, M. Gheorghiade, et al., Influence of dedicated heart failure clinics on delivery of recommended therapies in outpatient cardiology practices: findings from the registry to improve the use of evidence-based heart failure therapies in the outpatient setting (IMPROVE HF), Am. Heart J. 159 (2010) 238–244.

[7] K.L. Grady, K. Dracup, G. Kennedy, D.K. Moser, M. Piano, L.W. Stevenson, et al., Team management of patients with heart failure: a statement for healthcare professionals from the Cardiovascular Nursing Council of the American Heart Association, Circulation 102 (2000) 2443–2456.

[8] C.O. Phillips, R.M. Singa, H.R. Rubin, T. Jaarsma, Complexity of program and clinical outcomes of heart failure disease management incorporating specialist nurse-led heart failure clinics. A meta-regression analysis, Eur. J. Heart Fail. 7 (2005) 333–341.

[9] M. Glogowska, R. Simmonds, S. McLachlan, H. Cramer, T. Sanders, R. Johnson, et al., Managing patients with heart failure: a qualitative study of multidisciplinary teams with specialist heart failure nurses, Ann. Fam. Med. 13 (2015) 466–471.

[10] F.A. McAlister, F.M. Lawson, K.K. Teo, P.W. Armstrong, A systematic review of randomized trials of disease management programs in heart failure, Am. J. Med. 110 (2001) 378–384.

[11] F.A. McAlister, S. Stewart, S. Ferrua, J.J. McMurray, Multidisciplinary strategies for the management of heart failure patients at high risk for admission: a systematic review of randomized trials, J. Am. Coll. Cardiol. 44 (2004) 810–819.

[12] N.M. Albert, Managing a heart failure clinic, in: P.M. McCarthy, J.B. Young (Eds.), Heart Failure: A Combined Medical and Surgical Approach, Blackwell Publishing, Malden, Massachusetts, USA, 2007. http://dx.doi.org/10.1002/9780470994795. (Chapter 6).

[13] S.A. Hunt, W.T. Abraham, M.H. Chin, A.M. Feldman, G.S. Francis, T.G. Ganiats, et al., ACC/AHA 2005 guideline update for the diagnosis and management of chronic heart failure in the adult: a report of the American College of cardiology/American heart association Task Force on practice guidelines (writing committee to update the 2001 guidelines for the evaluation and management of heart failure): developed in collaboration with the American College of chest physicians and the International Society for Heart and Lung Transplantation: endorsed by the Heart Rhythm Society, Circulation 112 (2005) e154–235.
[14] Heart Failure Society of America, HFSA 2006 comprehensive heart failure practice guideline, J. Card. Fail. 12 (2006) e1–2.
[15] D. Moyer-Knox, T.M. Mueller, K. Vuckovic, L. Mischke, R.E. Williams, Remote titration of carvedilol for heart failure patients by advanced practice nurses, J. Card. Fail. 10 (2004) 219–224.
[16] M. Ansari, M.G. Shlipak, P.A. Heidenreich, D. Van Ostaeyen, E.C. Pohl, W.S. Browner, et al., Improving guideline adherence: a randomized trial evaluating strategies to increase beta-blocker use in heart failure, Circulation 107 (2003) 2799–2804.
[17] T. Jaarsma, Inter-professional team approach to patients with heart failure, Heart 91 (2005) 832–838.
[18] K.D.H.J. Rasmusson, J.C. Vesty, S.B. Brush, J.S. Sampson, K. Van Wagenen, A.G. Kfoury, L.C. Hofmann, D.G. Renlund, Managing the heart failure epidemic: the evolving role of nurse specialists, Top. Adv. Pract. Nurs. 5 (4) (2005).
[19] J.A. Diaz, R.A. Griffith, J.J. Ng, S.E. Reinert, P.D. Friedmann, A.W. Moulton, Patients' use of the internet for medical information, J. Gen. Intern. Med. 17 (2002) 180–185.
[20] D.T. Hsu, V. Zak, L. Mahony, L.A. Sleeper, A.M. Atz, J.C. Levine, et al., Enalapril in infants with single ventricle: results of a multicenter randomized trial, Circulation 122 (2010) 333–340.
[21] P.A. Anderson, R.E. Breitbart, B.W. McCrindle, L.A. Sleeper, A.M. Atz, D.T. Hsu, et al., The Fontan patient: inconsistencies in medication therapy across seven pediatric heart network centers, Pediatr. Cardiol. 31 (2010) 1219–1228.
[22] A.A. Kouatli, J.A. Garcia, T.M. Zellers, E.M. Weinstein, L. Mahony, Enalapril does not enhance exercise capacity in patients after Fontan procedure, Circulation 96 (1997) 1507–1512.
[23] S.M. Hobbins, R.S. Fowler, R.D. Rowe, A.G. Korey, Spironolactone therapy in infants with congestive heart failure secondary to congenital heart disease, Arch. Dis. Child. 56 (1981) 934–938.
[24] B. Pitt, F. Zannad, W.J. Remme, R. Cody, A. Castaigne, A. Perez, et al., The effect of spironolactone on morbidity and mortality in patients with severe heart failure. Randomized Aldactone Evaluation Study Investigators, N. Engl. J. Med. 341 (1999) 709–717.
[25] R.E. Shaddy, M.M. Boucek, D.T. Hsu, R.J. Boucek, C.E. Canter, L. Mahony, et al., Carvedilol for children and adolescents with heart failure: a randomized controlled trial, JAMA 298 (2007) 1171–1179.
[26] C.S. Almond, D.L. Morales, E.H. Blackstone, M.W. Turrentine, M. Imamura, M.P. Massicotte, et al., Berlin Heart EXCOR pediatric ventricular assist device for bridge to heart transplantation in US children, Circulation 127 (2013) 1702–1711.
[27] M. Schweiger, C. Vanderpluym, A. Jeewa, C.E. Canter, P. Jansz, P.E. Parrino, et al., Outpatient management of intra-corporeal left ventricular assist device system in children: a multi-center experience, Am. J. Transplant. 15 (2015) 453–460.
[28] J. Sparks, D. Epstein, S. Baltagi, M.E. Mehegan, K.E. Simpson, C.E. Canter, et al., Continuous flow device support in children using the HeartWare HVAD: 1000 days of lessons learned from a single center experience, ASAIO J. 61 (2015) 569–573.
[29] K.J. Harjai, M.R. Mehra, H.O. Ventura, Y.M. Lapeyre, J.P. Murgo, D.D. Stapleton, et al., Home inotropic therapy in advanced heart failure: cost analysis and clinical outcomes, Chest 112 (1997) 1298–1303.
[30] S. Upadya, F.A. Lee, C. Saldarriaga, S. Verma, A. Sedrakyan, K. Nystrom, et al., Home continuous positive inotropic infusion as a bridge to cardiac transplantation in patients with end-stage heart failure, J. Heart Lung Transplant. 23 (2004) 466–472.
[31] S.C. Brozena, C. Twomey, L.R. Goldberg, S.S. Desai, B. Drachman, A. Kao, et al., A prospective study of continuous intravenous milrinone therapy for status IB patients awaiting heart transplant at home, J. Heart Lung Transplant. 23 (2004) 1082–1086.
[32] P. Siostrzonek, M. Koreny, G. Delle-Karth, M. Haumer, J. Koller-Strametz, G. Heinz, Milrinone therapy in catecholamine-dependent critically ill patients with heart failure, Acta Anaesthesiol. Scand. 44 (2000) 403–409.
[33] J.F. Price, J.A. Towbin, W.J. Dreyer, B.S. Moffett, N.J. Kertesz, S.K. Clunie, et al., Outpatient continuous parenteral inotropic therapy as bridge to transplantation in children with advanced heart failure, J. Card. Fail. 12 (2006) 139–143.
[34] B.F. Birnbaum, K.E. Simpson, T.A. Boschert, J. Zheng, M.J. Wallendorf, K. Schechtman, et al., Intravenous home inotropic use is safe in pediatric patients awaiting transplantation, Circ. Heart Fail. 8 (2015) 64–70.
[35] L. Shekerdemian, D. Bohn, Cardiovascular effects of mechanical ventilation, Arch. Dis. Child. 80 (1999) 475–480.
[36] S. Al-Saleh, P.F. Kantor, N.K. Chadha, Y. Tirado, A.L. James, I. Narang, Sleep-disordered breathing in children with cardiomyopathy, Ann. Am. Thorac. Soc. 11 (2014) 770–776.
[37] S.L. den Boer, K.F. Joosten, S. van den Berg, A.P. Backx, R.B. Tanke, G.J. du Marchie Sarvaas, et al., Prospective evaluation of sleep apnea as manifestation of heart failure in children, Pediatr. Cardiol. 37 (2) (February 2016) 248–254.
[38] K.S.R. Widger, K. Oberle, B. Davies, Exploring the supportive care model as a framework for pediatric palliative care, J. Hosp. Palliat. Nurs. 11 (2009) 209–216.
[39] V. Xafis, A. Watkins, D. Wilkinson, Death talk: basic linguistic rules and communication in perinatal and paediatric end-of-life discussions, Patient Educ. Couns. 99 (4) (April 2016) 555–561.
[40] M. McSherry, K. Kehoe, J.M. Carroll, T.I. Kang, M.T. Rourke, Psychosocial and spiritual needs of children living with a life-limiting illness, Pediatr. Clin. N. Am. 54 (2007) 609–629 ix-x.
[41] P.F. Kantor, J. Lougheed, A. Dancea, M. McGillion, N. Barbosa, C. Chan, et al., Presentation, diagnosis, and medical management of heart failure in children: Canadian Cardiovascular Society guidelines, Can. J. Cardiol. 29 (2013) 1535–1552.

Chapter 35

Quality of Life and Psychosocial Care in Pediatric Heart Failure

Ivan Wilmot[1], Bradley S. Marino[2]
[1]Cincinnati Children's Hospital Medical Center, Cincinnati Children's Hospital Medical Center, Cincinnati, OH, United States; [2]Ann & Robert Lurie Children's Hospital of Chicago, Northwestern University Feinberg School of Medicine, Chicago, IL, United States

INTRODUCTION

Advances in both medical and surgical management of children living with cardiovascular disease have resulted in improved survival in this population. However, children living with cardiovascular disease are often required to abide by physical activity restrictions, medications, and chronic long-term follow-up, which can impair health-related quality of life (HRQOL). Additionally, advanced therapies including implantable cardioverter–defibrillators (ICDs), cardiac resynchronization therapy (CRT), and increasingly utilized mechanical circulatory support (MCS) in this population can further affect HRQOL. Additionally, heart failure (HF) is increasingly appreciated as a syndrome affecting many organ systems including the brain, mental health, and HRQOL. HRQOL is appreciated as an important long-term outcome measure in the management of adults living with HF and is increasingly appreciated as such in the pediatric HF population [1].

EPIDEMIOLOGY

HF in the pediatric population is an increasing concern. HF can be seen in children with congenital heart disease (CHD), cardiomyopathy, and those with acquired heart disease. HF is estimated to affect nearly 35,000 children in the United States of America and results in >15,000 pediatric HF-related admissions per year [2,3]. Increasing survival of children with CHD has led to an expanding population of adults living with congenital heart disease [4]. However, in those children with CHD who develop HF the mortality is significantly elevated. In a study evaluating the KID inpatient hospital database children living with CHD or cardiomyopathies who present with HF were found to have a greater than 20-fold increase in risk of hospital mortality compared to those without HF [5]. Additionally, advances in the diagnosis of cardiac muscle disease have led to a significant increase in the number of children followed in cardiomyopathy-specific clinics. Identification of those affected with cardiomyopathy and at risk of developing cardiac muscle disease has improved as the hereditary nature of such cardiomyopathies is appreciated. Published surveillance guidelines for first-degree relatives of those affected with cardiomyopathy have contributed to this growing population [6,7]. The International Society for Heart and Lung Transplantation Guidelines for the Management of Pediatric Heart Failure published in 2014 recommends such surveillance and monitoring of psychosocial performance. Psychosocial concerns in the growing population of children with HF can significantly affect HRQOL.

PSYCHOSOCIAL

Recognition of the cognitive, psychosocial, and psychological effects of HF in children is essential. Children with HF are at risk of cognitive and psychosocial delays in development. Increasing utilization of MCS can not only introduce risk in the form of ischemic brain injury or hemorrhage but also benefit in the form of improved mobility, social interactions, and cognitive stimulation. Psychological effects such as depression and impaired functioning are well reported comorbidities of HF. Depression in adults with HF has been studied extensively and has been associated with elevated risk of arrhythmia, hospitalization, death, and poor HRQOL [8–10]. For adults with HF and a ventricular assist device (VAD) there are reports of increased rates of depression, impaired social interaction, disorders involving body perception, self-image, and self [11]. In regard to VAD use in children with HF, anxiety and/or depression is noted to be more common in this population [12]. Interestingly, parents of children with HF managed on a VAD are reported to have similar increased anxiety and depression also [12]. Advanced therapies such as ICDs in children with HF have been associated with increased anxiety, depression,

Heart Failure in the Child and Young Adult. http://dx.doi.org/10.1016/B978-0-12-802393-8.00035-1

and diminished HRQOL [13–15]. Additionally, increased anxiety and depression has been noted in children with ICDs who received an inappropriate or recent shock [16]. Directed therapies addressing the cognitive, psychosocial, and psychological effects of HF in these children can improve outcomes including HRQOL.

DEFINITION OF HEALTH-RELATED QUALITY OF LIFE

HRQOL refers to the impact of a specific illness, injury, medical treatment, or health service policy on quality of life (QOL). QOL describes a child's ability to function in situational contexts (family, school, peer) and derive personal satisfaction from doing so. QOL can further be divided into physical health or physical functioning, psychologic functioning, and social functioning. As such the study of HRQOL is a critical component for the evaluation of long-term outcomes of chronic conditions and how they can affect physical, psychologic, and social functioning [17–19].

ASSESSMENT OF HEALTH-RELATED QUALITY OF LIFE

Assessment of HRQOL in the pediatric HF population can be challenging when dealing with a variety of etiologies causing HF, a developmental spectrum in patients, and a variety of therapies with a spectrum of outcomes. In addition, HF severity may impact HRQOL, and developmental changes in children have made adoption of a universal system for grading HF severity in children difficult. Use of the modified American Heart Association (AHA) staging for pediatric HF is promoted in the 2014 International Society for Heart and Lung Transplant Guidelines for the Management of Pediatric Heart Failure [20,21]. Increasing use of this modified AHA HF staging system has allowed for assessment of HRQOL in the pediatric population with varying stages of HF [22,23]. The modified AHA staging for pediatric HF includes individuals at risk (Stage A), those with identified structural heart disease (Stage B), individuals with structural heart disease and cardiovascular symptoms (Stage C), and those with heart disease and refractory symptoms requiring advanced therapies (Stage D) such as inotropes, CRT, ICD, and MCS [20]. The modified AHA staging is a major advance in assessing HF severity in children. This staging system provides the ability to assess HF severity using a single system across all age groups and includes at-risk children (Stage A) who may develop future HF. Additionally, the AHA staging of HF allows for assessment of how changes in HF severity may influence HRQOL.

PEDIATRIC QUALITY OF LIFE INVENTORY

The Pediatric Quality of Life Inventory (PedsQL) is a questionnaire assessment tool used to evaluate HRQOL in children. The PedsQL is reliable and valid in children who are healthy, ethnically diverse, or diagnosed with acute and chronic disease [24–29]. The generic PedsQL 4.0 has been used in a variety of pediatric populations creating a large normative database of HRQOL in ethnically diverse children and children with chronic diseases. It is composed of 23 items that gauge function in the following four areas: physical (eight items), emotional (five items), social (five items), and school (five items). Patients report their function using a 5-point Likert scale ranging from 0 to 4. These responses are reverse scored and linearly transformed to a 0 to 100 scale, with a higher score indicating a higher QOL.

The Psychosocial Health Summary score is a computed mean of the emotional, social, and school functioning subscales of the PedsQL. The physical functioning scale is the same as the Physical Summary score. In addition, the computed mean of the Emotional, Social, School functioning, and Physical scales are used to generate a Total Summary score. PedsQL scales are composed of parallel child self-report and parent–proxy report formats.

The PedsQL 3.0 Cardiac Module is a reliable and valid, disease-specific module that includes items specific to heart disease [29]. It includes the following five scales; symptoms (seven items), perceived physical appearance (three items), treatment anxiety (four items), cognitive problems (five items), and communication (three items). The module uses the same format as the PedsQL.

HEALTH-RELATED QUALITY OF LIFE IN HEART FAILURE

Advancements in pediatric HF management have resulted in improved survival and a focus on long-term outcomes including HRQOL. HF severity has been noted to have significant effects on HRQOL. HRQOL in adult HF patients is noted to decrease with increasing severity of AHA HF stage [30]. Increasing reports of a similar decrease in HRQOL with increasing HF severity in children exists [1]. In a study evaluating HRQOL in children with HF authors noted QOL scores to be significantly lower in children living with HF when compared to healthy children, and progressively lower with advancing HF stage [1]. Children with HF had PedsQL scores similar to those with seen in children with chronic illness (e.g., end-stage renal disease requiring dialysis) [1]. Interestingly, parental perceptions appeared to underestimate the impairment in HRQOL in this study [1]. Children with Stage C HF reported HRQOL scores similar to children with moderate and severe CHD including surgically palliated single ventricle lesions (Fig. 35.1). Additional studies evaluating HRQOL in children with HF have identified children with only a family history of cardiomyopathy (Stage A) who are at risk of developing cardiomyopathy had reduced QOL scores [23]. This study too identified parent–proxy reports underestimating the impairment in HRQOL in their children with HF [23]. These studies emphasize the importance of including both parent–proxy and child self-report when assessing HRQOL in children, as perceptions between children and their parents often vary.

It must be noted that individuals with HF who remain asymptomatic are also noted to have significant impairment in HRQOL. In the CHARM study young patients with HF had significantly impaired HRQOL relative to the older population, yet few clinical or radiological signs of HF were present [31]. Friess and colleagues report similarly impaired HRQOL in children with a family history of cardiomyopathy (Stage A) when compared to healthy children [23]. As previously discussed, this impairment is often underappreciated by parents. Although children with HF may lack external signs or symptoms of a chronic condition, they too have significantly impaired HRQOL.

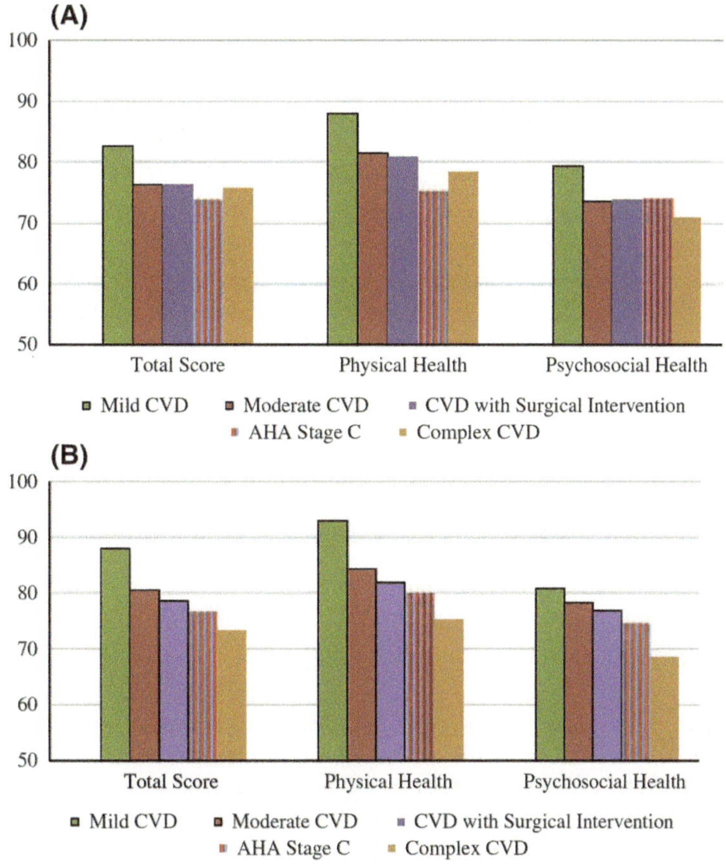

FIGURE 35.1 PedsQL scores by self-report and parent–proxy for children with AHA Stage C HF compared with children with cardiovascular disease. (A) Mean PedsQL scores by self-report for children with AHA Stage C HF compared with children with cardiovascular disease (CVD). CVD includes the following: (1) Mild including disease requiring no therapy or effectively treated nonoperatively (catheter therapy), (2) Moderate including those requiring no therapy or surgically corrected (curative), (3) CVD requiring surgical correction (≥1 procedure) with significant residua or need for additional surgery, and (4) Complex or severe CVD including uncorrectable or palliated, includes single ventricle; two sample t-tests were performed between patient groups using a Bonferroni correction for four comparisons with a statistically significant P value $< .0125$. Health-related quality of life (HRQOL) scores for Stage C patients are significantly lower than those with mild CVD for total ($P = .011$) and physical health summary scales ($P = .001$). Stage C patients reported no significant differences in all HRQOL measures compared with children with moderate CVD, surgically treated CVD, and severe CVD. (B) Mean PedsQL scores by parent–proxy for children with AHA Stage C HF compared with children with CVD. HRQOL scores for Stage C patients are significantly lower than all HRQOL measures of those with mild CVD ($P < .0125$). Stage C parents reported no significant differences in all HRQOL measures compared with children with moderate CVD, surgically treated CVD, and severe CVD. *AHA*, American Heart Association; *HF*, herat failure; *PedsQL*, pediatric quality of life inventory. *(Adapted from Wilmot and colleagues publication on HRQOL in children with heart failure as perceived by children and parents [1].)*

TABLE 35.1 Risk Factors Associated With Diminished Health-Related Quality of Life in Children With Heart Failure [1,13,23,29,33–35]

Risk Factor
1. Older age at diagnosis of cardiomyopathy
2. Need for cardiovascular medication
3. Physical activity restriction
4. Implantable cardioverter–defibrillator implant
5. Severity of American Heart Association Heart Failure Stage
6. Severity of cardiovascular disease
7. Severity of congenital heart disease

Additional factors that have been associated with decreased HRQOL in children with HF include need for cardiovascular medications and/or ICD/Pacemaker implantation, severity of cardiovascular disease, severity of CHD, and exercise restriction (Table 35.1) [23,29,32–34]. A recent evaluation of the Pediatric Cardiomyopathy Registry identified risk factors associated with decreased HRQOL and functional status including older age at diagnosis, lower socioeconomic status, and increased left ventricular size [35]. Interestingly, diminished HRQOL and functional status were associated with an increased risk of death and need for transplant in this population [35].

CONCLUSION

HRQOL is significantly impaired in children living with HF. Parental perceptions appear to underestimate the HRQOL impairments in this population, especially in individuals without symptoms. Use of HRQOL as a screening tool in all children with HF is recommended and can assist in identifying at-risk individuals who may benefit from a multidisciplinary approach including psychosocial intervention, school interventions, and targeted genetic testing and counseling.

FUTURE DIRECTIONS

Additional studies evaluating HRQOL in the expanding population of children with HF is needed. Given the heterogeneity of cardiovascular disease in children, and the expanding population of children and young adults living with CHD, there are likely some unique yet unidentified risk factors that contribute to diminished HRQOL in each of these populations. Expanding awareness of the importance of HRQOL in assessing children with HF will contribute to the understanding of this as a long-term outcome metric in the care of these children.

REFERENCES

[1] I. Wilmot, C.E. Cephus, A. Cassedy, I. Kudel, B.S. Marino, J.L. Jefferies, Health-related quality of life in children with heart failure as perceived by children and parents, Cardiol. Young 26 (2016) 885–893.

[2] D.T. Hsu, G.D. Pearson, Heart failure in children: part I: history, etiology, and pathophysiology, Circ. Heart Fail. 2 (2009) 63–70.

[3] J.W. Rossano, Cost of heart failure admission in children in the United States, J. Card. Fail. 16 (2010) S86.

[4] K.K. Stout, C.S. Broberg, W.M. Book, et al., Chronic heart failure in congenital heart disease: a scientific statement from the American heart association, Circulation 133 (2016) 770–801.

[5] J.W. Rossano, J.J. Kim, J.A. Decker, et al., Prevalence, morbidity, and mortality of heart failure-related hospitalizations in children in the United States: a population-based study, J. Card. Fail. 18 (2012) 459–470.

[6] E.L. Burkett, R.E. Hershberger, Clinical and genetic issues in familial dilated cardiomyopathy, J. Am. Coll. Cardiol. 45 (2005) 969–981.

[7] R.E. Hershberger, J. Lindenfeld, L. Mestroni, et al., Genetic evaluation of cardiomyopathy–a heart failure society of America practice guideline, J. Card. Fail. 15 (2009) 83–97.

[8] N. Holzapfel, C. Zugck, T. Muller-Tasch, et al., Routine screening for depression and quality of life in outpatients with congestive heart failure, Psychosomatics 48 (2007) 112–116.

[9] T. Rutledge, V.A. Reis, S.E. Linke, B.H. Greenberg, P.J. Mills, Depression in heart failure a meta-analytic review of prevalence, intervention effects, and associations with clinical outcomes, J. Am. Coll. Cardiol. 48 (2006) 1527–1537.

[10] A. Sherwood, J.A. Blumenthal, A.L. Hinderliter, et al., Worsening depressive symptoms are associated with adverse clinical outcomes in patients with heart failure, J. Am. Coll. Cardiol. 57 (2011) 418–423.

[11] A. Baba, G. Hirata, F. Yokoyama, et al., Psychiatric problems of heart transplant candidates with left ventricular assist devices, J. Artif. Organs 9 (2006) 203–208.

[12] B. Ozbaran, S. Kose, T. Yagdi, et al., Psychiatric evaluation of children and adolescents with left ventricular assist devices, Psychosom. Med. 74 (2012) 554–558.

[13] R.J. Czosek, W.J. Bonney, A. Cassedy, et al., Impact of cardiac devices on the quality of life in pediatric patients, Circ. Arrhythmia Electrophysiol. 5 (2012) 1064–1072.

[14] H.M. Koopman, C.M. Vrijmoet-Wiersma, J.N. Langius, et al., Psychological functioning and disease-related quality of life in pediatric patients with an implantable cardioverter defibrillator, Pediatr. Cardiol. 33 (2012) 569–575.

[15] S.F. Sears, A.G. Hazelton, J. St Amant, et al., Quality of life in pediatric patients with implantable cardioverter defibrillators, Am. J. Cardiol. 107 (2011) 1023–1027.

[16] A. Eicken, C. Kolb, S. Lange, et al., Implantable cardioverter defibrillator (ICD) in children, Int. J. Cardiol. 107 (2006) 30–35.

[17] J.E. Ware Jr., Methodology in behavioral and psychosocial cancer research. Conceptualizing disease impact and treatment outcomes, Cancer 53 (1984) 2316–2326.

[18] N.K. Aaronson, Quality of life: what is it? How should it be measured? Oncology 2 (1988) 69–76 64.

[19] D. Drotar, Measuring child health: scientific questions, challenges, and recommendations, Ambul. Pediatr. 4 (2004) 353–357.

[20] C.W. Yancy, M. Jessup, B. Bozkurt, et al., 2013 ACCF/AHA guideline for the management of heart failure: a report of the American College of Cardiology Foundation/American heart association task force on practice guidelines, J. Am. Coll. Cardiol. 62 (2013) e147–239.

[21] R. Kirk, A.I. Dipchand, D.N. Rosenthal, et al., The international society of heart and lung transplantation guidelines for the management of pediatric heart failure: executive summary, J. Heart Lung Transplant. 33 (2014) 888–909.

[22] I. Wilmot, C.E. Cephus, A. Cassedy, I. Kudel, B.S. Marino, J.L. Jefferies, Health-related quality of life in children with heart failure as perceived by children and parents, Cardiol. Young (2015) 1–9.

[23] M.R. Friess, B.S. Marino, A. Cassedy, I. Wilmot, J.L. Jefferies, A. Lorts, Health-related quality of life assessment in children followed in a cardiomyopathy clinic, Pediatr. Cardiol. 36 (2015) 516–523.

[24] J.W. Varni, T.M. Burwinkle, M. Seid, D. Skarr, The PedsQL 4.0 as a pediatric population health measure: feasibility, reliability, and validity, Ambul. Pediatr. 3 (2003) 329–341.

[25] J.W. Varni, M. Seid, P.S. Kurtin, PedsQL 4.0: reliability and validity of the pediatric quality of life inventory version 4.0 generic core scales in healthy and patient populations, Med. Care 39 (2001) 800–812.

[26] J.W. Varni, C.A. Limbers, T.M. Burwinkle, Impaired health-related quality of life in children and adolescents with chronic conditions: a comparative analysis of 10 disease clusters and 33 disease categories/severities utilizing the PedsQL 4.0 generic core scales, Health Qual. Life Outcomes 5 (2007) 43.

[27] J.W. Varni, T.M. Burwinkle, M.A. Rapoff, J.L. Kamps, N. Olson, The PedsQL in pediatric asthma: reliability and validity of the pediatric quality of life inventory generic core scales and asthma module, J. Behav. Med. 27 (2004) 297–318.

[28] S.L. Goldstein, N. Graham, T. Burwinkle, B. Warady, R. Farrah, J.W. Varni, Health-related quality of life in pediatric patients with ESRD, Pediatr. Nephrol. 21 (2006) 846–850.

[29] K. Uzark, The pediatric quality of life inventory in children with heart disease, Prog. Pediatr. Cardiol. 18 (2003) 141–148.

[30] A. Azevedo, P. Bettencourt, M. Alvelos, et al., Health-related quality of life and stages of heart failure, Int. J. Cardiol. 129 (2008) 238–244.

[31] C.M. Wong, N.M. Hawkins, P.S. Jhund, et al., Clinical characteristics and outcomes of young and very young adults with heart failure the CHARM programme (candesartan in heart failure assessment of reduction in mortality and morbidity), J. Am. Coll. Cardiol. 62 (2013) 1845–1854.

[32] I. Lesman-Leegte, T. Jaarsma, J.C. Coyne, H.L. Hillege, D.J. Van Veldhuisen, R. Sanderman, Quality of life and depressive symptoms in the elderly: a comparison between patients with heart failure and age- and gender-matched community controls, J. Card. Fail. 15 (2009) 17–23.

[33] B.S. Marino, R.S. Tomlinson, G. Wernovsky, et al., Validation of the pediatric cardiac quality of life inventory, Pediatrics 126 (2010) 498–508.

[34] R.L. Knowles, T. Day, A. Wade, et al., Patient-reported quality of life outcomes for children with serious congenital heart defects, Arch. Dis. Child. 99 (2014) 413–419.

[35] L.A. Sleeper, J.A. Towbin, S.D. Colan, et al., Health-related quality of life and functional status are associated with cardiac status and clinical outcome in children with cardiomyopathy, J. Pediatr. 170 (2016) 173–180 e1–4.

Chapter 36

Quality Metrics and Quality Improvement in Pediatric Heart Failure

Steven J. Kindel[1], Samuel Hanke[2], Jeffrey B. Anderson[2]
[1]*Children's Hospital of Wisconsin, Milwaukee, WI, United States;* [2]*Cincinnati Children's Hospital Medical Center, Cincinnati, OH, United States*

DEFINITIONS OF QUALITY IMPROVEMENT

In the 2000 report, Crossing the Quality Chasm, the Institute of Medicine broadly outlined the changes needed to reinvent the delivery of health care in the United States [1]. This report highlighted the limitations of traditional scientific discovery methods to translate knowledge into consistent, high-quality medical care. Since the release of this report, the health care industry has seen an increased application of quality improvement methods developed by Dr. Walter Shewhart and implemented with great success by W. Edwards Deming in the manufacturing industries. This systems-based approach is predicated on the concept of learning from sequential changes and establishing objective measures to assess if those changes result in improvement [2].

The definition and measurement of quality improvement differs from measurement in traditional research methods. While research measurement focuses on discovering new knowledge by eliminating all bias, performing one large test and using statistical tests to determine superiority, quality improvement measurement accepts a consistent bias, performs sequential tests and uses statistical process control to determine improvement in the system [3]. An understanding of these differences and the differences in accountability metrics are critical in the appropriate application of quality improvement metrics.

Many of the quality metrics discussed in this chapter have been developed with the purpose of evaluating the performance of providers or medical groups. While these are important measures to evaluate and compare provider/medical group performance, the focus of these measures is not always on improvement of the system being measured. This distinction between performance and quality improvement measurement is of increased importance as the United States health system transitions from a fee-for-service system to value directed payment models as directed in the Medicare Access and CHIP Reauthorization Act of 2015 (MACRA) [4]. Having said that, quality metrics, based ideally on good evidence, provide a starting point to identify variation in practice and a target for quality improvement efforts that would be expected to improve clinical outcomes.

PERFORMANCE MEASURES FOR HEART FAILURE POPULATIONS

Adult heart failure has been discussed as an epidemic since the 2000s and more recently confirmed as such in scientific study that represents one of the largest health-care expenditures in the United States [5]. Due to the prevalence, morbidity, mortality, and expense associated to heart failure admissions and the overall burden to societal health, heart failure was one of the early targets of medical quality initiatives in the United States. In 1995 the Joint Commission (JCH) announced its ORYX, initiative which was its first attempt at measuring hospital quality on a national scale [6,7]. In 1999 the American Heart Association (AHA) and American College of Cardiology (ACC) convened a special meeting to determine quality goals for metrics in care of heart failure patients [8]. Starting in 2002 JCH required accredited hospitals to collect and report performance metrics for at least half of four areas of focus (including heart failure). In 2005 the ACC/AHA went one step further and released performance guidelines for the care of adults with heart failure [9]. In 2009 the ACC/AHA released new clinical practice guidelines that were closely followed by revised performance metrics recommendations in 2011, which will be discussed below. These performance and quality metrics have become increasingly aligned with the ACC/AHA Heart Failure Management Guidelines over time and will be discussed as they relate to the individual metrics.

Pediatric heart failure, while recognized as an important clinical condition, has prevalence estimates considerably lower than those in adult populations [10]. While research has explored the frequency of etiologies, admissions, expenses, and

Heart Failure in the Child and Young Adult. http://dx.doi.org/10.1016/B978-0-12-802393-8.00036-3

clinical outcomes, little data exist to guide therapies [11–15]. Despite increasing study in the field and production of two recent guideline statements for the care of children with heart failure, very little data have been developed to guide quality metric development in the field. A recent pediatric heart failure guideline has been produced under the umbrella of the International Society of Heart and Lung Transplantation (ISHLT) and relevant guidelines will be discussed in relation to available adult quality and performance metrics. Because of the lack of specific pediatric quality metrics the following discussion will revolve around the available quality performance metrics in adult congestive heart failure (CHF), with focus on metrics that could potentially be applied in the pediatric realm.

Adult Heart Failure Performance Metrics

Cardiac Imaging

The 2011 combined AHA/ACC performance measures define metrics appropriate for both the inpatient and outpatient settings [9]. With respect to outpatient management of patients with CHF, formal imaging-based measurement of systolic function is recommended. Specifically ejection fraction (EF) should be acquired at diagnosis or with new onset symptoms. This metric is in line with the most recent ACC/AHA guidelines on the care of heart failure that recommend echocardiographic assessment of anatomy and function for all new heart failure admissions or outpatient diagnoses [16]. Metrics regarding follow-up echocardiography regimens are not formally addressed as a performance metric as data regarding the benefit of routine imaging has not been established and routine (nonsymptom based) follow-up is not recommended in the most recent guidelines. The rationale for this recommendation is that cardiac imaging including assessment of EF in patients with newly symptomatic heart failure provides important clinical information to guide targeted therapy and management.

This metric may be applicable for children with heart failure and systolic dysfunction and the most recent pediatric heart failure guidelines recommend assessment of left ventricular (LV) dimensions and function in patients with newly discovered or symptomatic heart failure (Class I; level of evidence B) as well as monitoring of LV remodeling in the chronic setting (Class I; level of evidence B) [17]. However, quality studies on the value and necessary timing of interval studies in pediatrics have not been presented. Further the heterogeneity of pediatric heart failure phenotypes limits to some extent the ability to use transthoracic echocardiography alone in the assessment of cardiac function. In particular the imaging of children with systemic right ventricles or single ventricle anatomy has not proven to be easily acquired by standard transthoracic echocardiographic measures [18–20]. While ensuring initial echocardiographic assessment is a reasonable quality metric to institute at a local level, there is a lack of evidence to support this as a performance metric at this time in pediatric heart failure management.

It is worth noting that there are disease-specific practice statements that have produced recommendations for echocardiographic screening and assessment outside of the general pediatric heart failure guidelines. For instance, patients with Duchene's muscular dystrophy (DMD) or other heritable neuromuscular disease are currently recommended to have cardiac assessment annually starting at age 10 or at the onset of cardiac symptoms [21]. Similarly asymptomatic carriers of a known cardiomyopathy causing genetic variant are recommended to have annual screening based on phenotype starting in childhood and continuing into late adolescence or early adulthood [22]. In addition, various chemotherapy regimens are associated to their individual screening protocols, and many well-known dysmorphic syndromes (e.g., Noonan's Syndrome and other RAS-opathies) and metabolic syndromes (e.g., Dannon Syndrome or mitochondrial disease) are associated to cardiomyopathies with recommendations for screening. At this stage development of performance measures based on success meeting these standards would be premature; however, local sites can utilize these various guidelines to help drive their individual quality-monitoring programs and data development.

Clinical Status Assessment and Management Plan

To ensure assessment and documentation of clinical findings associated with heart failure progression and facilitate improved patient monitoring, it is recommended that all patients have a clinical status assessment of the fluid volume status by clinical means. Additionally, associated symptoms and the degree of activity/limitation should be performed and documented. Documentation is recommended to include a New York Heart Association symptom score and AHA/ACC heart failure stage. This measure is to be applied in both the inpatient and outpatient setting at each visit. This performance measure is once again tied tightly to the most recent ACC/AHA Heart Failure Management Guidelines where assessment of volume status, vital signs, weight, and estimates of fluid overload are a Class I, level of evidence (LOE) B recommendation [16].

In addition to a clinical assessment, the 2011 AHA/ACC Performance Measures included a new quality metric to include development and documentation of a heart failure action plan and follow-up interval changes in symptoms. The action plan serves as a defined therapeutic intervention strategy with goals of improving derangements in fluid status and patient symptoms. The goal of this new metric is to utilize ongoing assessments of congestive symptoms and activity level as a means of titrating medication management. Due to the various clinical assessment approaches and diverse measurement options, this symptom-specific measurement is designed to allow for institutional level quality assessment but is not recommended for inclusion in pay-for-performance, physician or hospital system ranking.

Ultimately decreasing symptoms is the primary goal of heart failure management, particularly in the outpatient setting, and is associated to decreased hospitalizations, mortality, and health care utilization [23]. The pediatric application of regular assessment of symptoms and documentation of these findings seems a reasonable measure and are supported by the ISHLT Pediatric Heart Failure Guidelines, which indicate an assessment of the degree of congestion and adequacy of perfusion as a Class I, LOE C recommendation [17]. It is worth noting that pediatric heart failure symptoms remain more protean and are less commonly associated to pure congestive physiology, and assessment of activity levels can be very challenging especially in younger children and infants [24,25]. Further assessments of growth and development likely need to be included in any symptom assessment; however, these measures have not specifically been endorsed by pediatric guidelines at this time.

Specific Therapeutics

Beta-blocker initiation is a quality metric for the most recent AHA/ACC Performance Measures in patients with systolic dysfunction and EF <40% in both the inpatient and outpatient setting. The rationale for this quality metric comes from the vast body of evidence that initiation of beta-blocker therapy in this group of patients provides improved survival. This has been reflected in the 2009 and 2013 ACC/AHA Heart Failure Management Guidelines. Further, evidence is now adequate to indicate that all beta-blockers are not equal in their survival improvement for adults with heart failure. The current quality measures specifically look to measure the appropriate use of beta-blockers with known survival benefits: bisoprolol, carvedilol, or sustained-release metoprolol. Similarly the use of angiotensin converting enzyme inhibitors (ACE-i) are well-established therapy for systolic heart failure with EF <40% and should be initiated in addition to beta-blockade in these patients. As some patients have been converted to Angiotensin Receptor Blockers (ARBs) for various forms of ACE-i intolerance and class IIB evidence exists for similar benefit between these two drug classes in heart failure populations the ACC/AHA Performance Metrics included a quality measure for the use of either medication in systolic heart failure.

The data on the use of beta-blockade, ACE-i, and ARB therapeutics in pediatric heart failure are quite limited with only a single, negative, randomized control trial of beta-blockers in children [26]. While the current practice at many pediatric heart failure centers is to use these medications in similar fashion to adult populations this is not a data-driven management strategy [27]. Despite mixed data in children and based largely on adult studies the most recent pediatric heart failure guidelines recommend ACE-i for patients with symptomatic LV dysfunction (Class I; LOE B) and beta-blockers for patients with symptomatic heart failure and low EF(Class II LOE B) [17]. In pediatrics the data taken as a whole are inadequate to propose initiation of any specific medication as a performance or global quality metric in children with new onset heart failure. Again specific situations do exist where stronger recommendations have been made such as the initiation of ACE-i in children with DMD with asymptomatic decrement in ejection fraction or with onset of heart failure symptoms [17].

While the level of evidence remains relatively low in general, the initiation of medication to treat symptoms and the monitoring for side effects seems reasonable for programs seeking to provide best care for these patients. Further, monitoring and documentation of these interventions, particularly for children with systolic dysfunction with an EF <40% would be reasonable center specific metrics to monitor in attempting to provide uniform care to this population. Ultimately the ability to strongly recommend the monitoring of particular medications would require large randomized control trials that showed clear survival benefit, which is unlikely to occur in this population. The small numbers of patients, compared to the adult population of heart failure, give rise to the opportunity to use multicenter learning networks or registries to answer these types of questions within the field of pediatric heart failure. This concept will be discussed later in the chapter.

Counseling on Implantable Cardioversion-Defibrilator Device Implantation

In adult guidelines implantable cardioversion-defibrilator device (ICD) placement is recommended (Class IA) for patients greater than 40-days post–myocardial infarction (MI) with reduced EF <35% and class 2–3 symptoms while on guideline directed medical therapy (GDMT) and who are expected to live >1 year. In addition those patients with class 1 symptoms and EF <30% who are >40 days post-MI on GDMT and expected to live 1 year are recommended to receive ICD implantation as a class IB recommendation. In light of this the most recent performance measures have instituted a measure of counseling regarding the placement of ICD in patients with heart failure. As these recommendations are grounded in a solid evidence base of improved survival the writing committee considered ICD placement as a quality metric; however, the overall complexity of patient selection led them to focus solely on counseling.

In the pediatric setting, a similar guideline would not seem appropriate at this juncture. The data to drive the placement of ICDs in children with various forms of cardiomyopathy and heart failure are sparse, and there are data that sudden death events are significantly less frequent in this population (likely in part due to disease heterogeneity and etiologies) [28]. Further, the complications of lead fracture, device malfunction, placement complications, and inappropriate shock rates all make the determination to place an ICD in pediatric patients much more complex in pediatric patients. Such decisions likely should be made in a multidisciplinary setting and with significant education and involvement of the family, caregivers, and patient (when age appropriate).

Postdischarge Appointment for Inpatients With Heart Failure

The final quality metric recommended in the 2011 ACC/AHA Performance Metrics was the provision of out-patient follow up appointment for in-patients with heart failure prior to discharge. This is a new quality metric that was designed to address the important transition from inpatient to outpatient care to prevent early readmission and morbidities associated with poor follow-up.

In pediatric heart failure patients the need for family and patient education prior to discharge is equally if not more important. Assurance of discharge instructions with a scheduled follow-up visit would be a reasonable local quality metric that would seem attainable and likely high yield for practitioners caring for these high-risk patients. Taken further, additional discharge education goals including specific education on new medications with potential side effects and a clear symptom drive action plan including signs and symptoms for which to contact the care team could be assessed. One model that could be utilized to develop a quality approach to improved discharge education and transition would be various interstage monitoring programs that exist at many pediatric heart centers [29]. The interstage period following primary surgical intervention for children with single ventricle anatomy has been a particular area of collaborative and site-specific success in quality assessment and improvement science [30].

At the current stage, no specific quality metrics exist for the management of heart failure in children. One barrier to the development of such metrics is the lack of large randomized trials showing intervention superiority. Since pediatric heart failure represents a much smaller population than adults, defining and refining internal quality metrics within heart failure programs is a recommended initial step toward site-specific improvement. Specific metrics that would seem easily applicable would be those of routine imaging, routine clinical assessment of symptoms, documentation, and monitoring of interventions, and provision of education and in-depth discharge instructions including a specific follow-up appointment for patients at discharge from the hospital or clinic. Further additional pediatric metrics may include monitoring of growth and development as well as involvement of multidisciplinary teams in the evaluation and follow-up of these complex children.

STRATEGIES FOR IMPROVING OUTCOMES

Addressing clinical processes and outcomes can be carried out at the local practice level and can be accelerated in involvement with clinical networks and registries. Regardless of whether work is done on a local level or with the cooperation of a clinical network, a framework for quality improvement should be used. While there are several potential frameworks to follow, we recommend use of the Model for Improvement as a foundation for this work. The Model for Improvement is a simple, yet powerful tool that teams can use to accelerate improvement [2]. The Model for Improvement uses a planned experimentation framework to make changes to a system to improve processes and outcomes. This framework (Fig. 36.1) begins with the definition of what is trying to be improved, followed by defining measures of change and finally outlining what interventions will result in an improvement. The application of these interventions is performed through sequential Plan-Do-Study-Act cycles. This method of improvement is rooted in the ability to accurately define quality.

Practical Approach to Quality Improvement at the Local Level

Improvement efforts at the local level require identification of appropriate clinical metrics, creation of systems to allow tracking of these metrics, and application of improvement principles while monitoring for metric changes. This effort typically involves a team of individuals, ideally including clinical experts (physicians, nurses, and other ancillary health care providers), information specialists for data collection and analytics, quality improvement coaching, and importantly

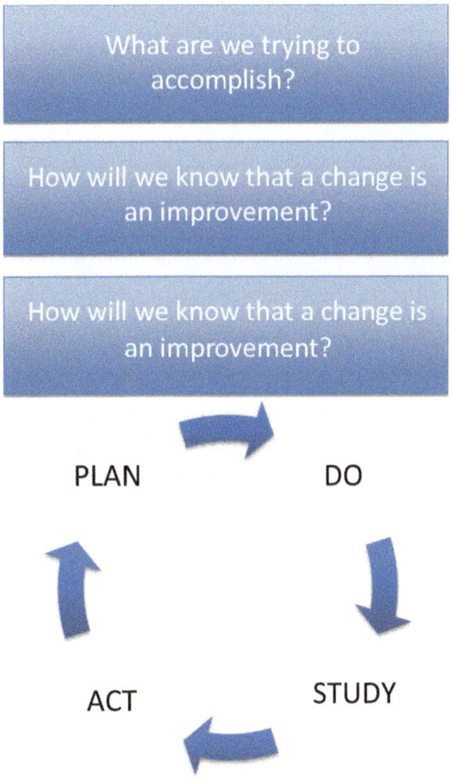

FIGURE 36.1 Model for Improvement.

patients and/or families. Each of these groups brings specific expertise but also brings an important viewpoint to the improvement process.

Once a team has been established the work can commence in determining the most important outcomes that should be addressed and the key processes involved with moving those outcomes. A Key Driver Diagram (Fig. 36.2) is a useful tool to begin thinking about what the team wants to accomplish and what changes are needed to see improvement. Targets for improvement may be found in national or specialty society benchmarking metrics, hospital metrics, or metrics that are important to the team. These metrics may include adhering to appropriate practices in the patient population (e.g., yearly influenza immunization), outcome metrics (e.g., readmission to the hospital), or cost metrics. The next step in the process of improving outcomes is to create clear definitions of the metrics and design tools to collect the current local performance of these metrics. This step ideally will involve cooperation from the local information technology team, as proper integration with the electronic medical record will allow for efficiency in data entry. Visualization of metric performance in a way that allows meaningful interpretation is also beneficial. The use of statistical process control charts or similar techniques allows the most accurate tracking of metrics and will allow early identification of improvement to the system and tracking of long-term sustained improvement.

Role of Clinical Networks and Registries

As a supplement to work done by local teams, clinical networks and registries are useful vehicles to aid in understanding variation in clinical care, and to test changes in clinical practice that can standardize care and improve clinical outcomes. This is especially true when dealing with rare diseases, such as pediatric heart failure where large randomized control trials are unlikely to be feasible. Registries and networks provide the infrastructure to gather information on patients from multiple treatment locations and groups and to understand differences in care processes and clinical outcomes. Regional and national networks and databases have been established to better understand care of several diseases including pediatric cancer, neonatal management, and cystic fibrosis [31–34]. Working within a registry has proved important in reducing variation and improving care for patients with chronic illness [31]. In pediatric cardiology and cardiac surgery, registries (e.g., Pediatric Heart Network, Society for Thoracic Surgery Registry, Mid-Atlantic Group of Interventional Cardiology Registry, Pediatric Cardiology Care Consortium, Pediatric Electrophysiology Society Ablation Registry,

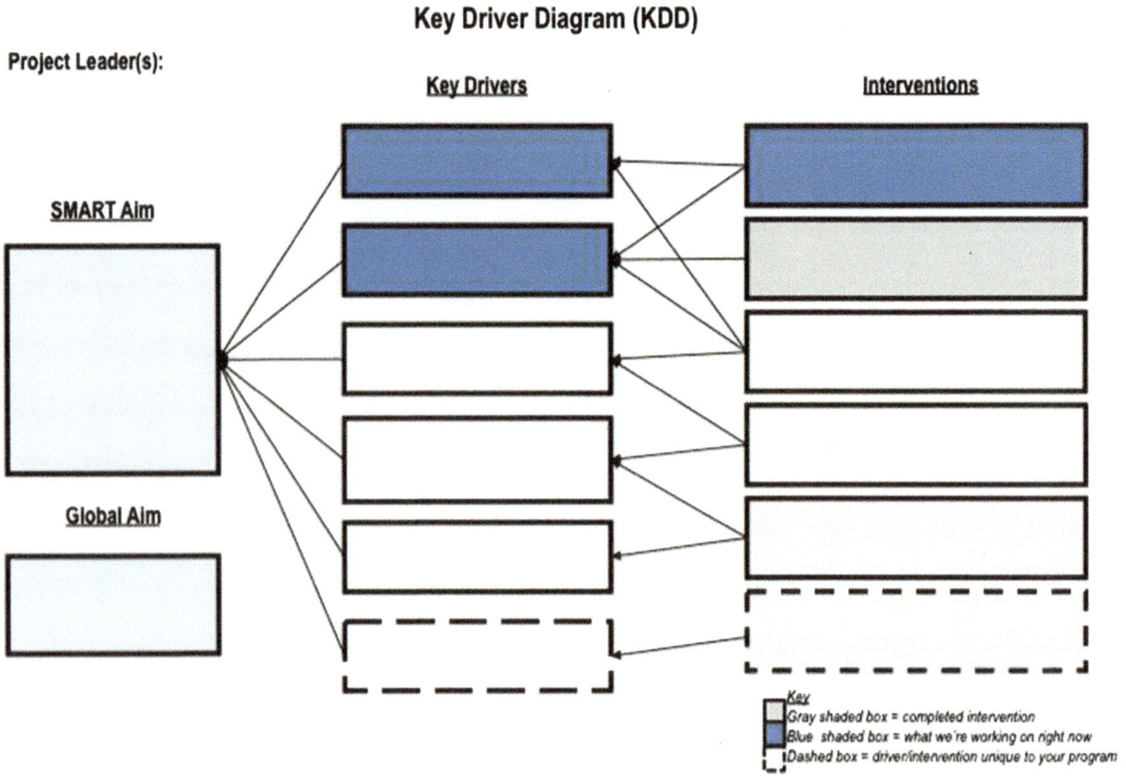

FIGURE 36.2 Key Driver Diagram for planning quality improvement work.

IMPACT Registry) have generated comparative data between centers and identified clinical outcomes that are related to variation in care [35–38].

A learning network not only collects and compares information through the use of the registry but also uses a multisite clinical network for both research and improvement. Successful learning network models include the Northern New England Cardiovascular Disease Study Group, Vermont Oxford Network, and the Children's Oncology Group [32,33,39]. These types of networks can offer epidemiologic, statistical, and translational advantages, which allow for creation of "laboratories" for conducting comparative effectiveness and translational research [40–42]. Learning networks allow for coordinated testing through planned experimentation, which also can lead to more rapid discovery. Learning networks allow not only for data collection but also for structured implementation of changes in practice through quality improvement science methodology. Improvement activities in the pediatric subspecialties, including pediatric cardiology, have been catalyzed in part by the adoption of Maintenance of Certification (MOC) requirements for involvement in quality improvement by the American Board of Pediatrics [43]. MOC emphasizes ongoing assessment and documentation of performance, and participation in quality improvement activities, as a requirement for ongoing certification.

Pediatric registries focused on the management of children with heart failure or in need of heart transplantation have been developing over the last two decades with many recently formed groups. The Pediatric Heart Transplant Study Foundation is a voluntary registry of patients less than 18 years of age listed for heart transplant that now includes more than 50 centers in North America and Europe. While this study has focused primarily on heart transplantation outcomes and research collaboration with more than 65 publications produced to date, they also provide member institutions with quality data regarding listings, wait-list times, wait-list mortality, and transplant outcomes. More recently PEDIMACS the pediatric arm of the Interagency Registry for Mechanically Assisted Circulatory Support has developed as a voluntary database of children supported via mechanical circulatory support. PEDIMACS provides annual data on MCS usage in children as well as allowing for database research to better understand outcomes in these children. The MEDAMACS database sponsored through the NHLBI will provide similar data regarding medical management of patients with heart failure with plans to include pediatric patients as the database evolves.

CONCLUSION

Improvement in clinical outcomes in any field begins with understanding and defining important metrics. The field of adult heart failure has spent years defining important clinical process metrics, some of which have application in pediatric heart failure patients. Pediatric heart failure specialists continue to learn about and understand disease processes that affect pediatric patients and identify the most important clinical outcomes and process metrics in this diverse population. At the same time, improvement science can be used to move outcomes by increasing compliance with adult heart failure quality metrics that apply to the pediatric population. This can be done at the level of a local practice, or more powerfully, through collaborative efforts within a learning network. Either approach would benefit from the framework offered by the Model for Improvement.

REFERENCES

[1] America IoMCoQoHCi, Crossing the Quality Chasm: A New Health System for the 21st Century, National Academy Press, 2001.

[2] G.J. Langley, R. Moen, K.M. Nolan, T.W. Nolan, C.L. Norman, L.P. Provost, The Improvement Guide: A Practical Approach to Enhancing Organizational Performance, John Wiley & Sons, 2009.

[3] L.P. Provost, S. Murray, The Health Care Data Guide: Learning from Data for Improvement, John Wiley & Sons, 2011.

[4] Medicare Access and CHIP Reauthorization Act of 2015, H.R.2 114th Congress, 2015.

[5] P.A. McCullough, E.F. Philbin, J.A. Spertus, et al., Confirmation of a heart failure epidemic: findings from the resource utilization among congestive heart failure (REACH) study, J. Am. Coll. Cardiol. 39 (1) (January 2, 2002) 60–69.

[6] K.J. Lee, J.M. Loeb, D. Nadzam, L. Hanold, Special report: an overview of the Joint Commission's ORYX initiative and proposed statistical methods, Health Serv. Outcomes Res. Methodol. 1 (1) (2000) 63–73.

[7] B.I. Braun, R.G. Koss, J.M. Loeb, Integrating performance measure data into the Joint Commission accreditation process, Eval. Health Prof. 22 (3) (September 1999) 283–297.

[8] H.M. Krumholz, D.W. Baker, C.M. Ashton, et al., Evaluating quality of care for patients with heart failure, Circulation 101 (12) (March 28, 2000) E122–E140.

[9] R.O. Bonow, S. Bennett, D.E. Casey Jr., et al., ACC/AHA clinical performance measures for adults with chronic heart failure: a report of the American College of Cardiology/American Heart Association Task Force on performance measures (writing committee to develop heart failure clinical performance measures): endorsed by the Heart Failure Society of America, Circulation 112 (12) (September 20, 2005) 1853–1887.

[10] J.W. Rossano, J.J. Kim, J.A. Decker, et al., Prevalence, morbidity, and mortality of heart failure-related hospitalizations in children in the United States: a population-based study, J. Card. Fail. 18 (6) (June 2012) 459–470.

[11] S.P. Law, J.J. Kim, J.A. Decker, et al., Hospital charges for pediatric heart transplant hospitalizations in the United States from 1997 to 2006, J. Heart Lung Transplant. 31 (5) (May 2012) 485–491.

[12] S.D. Colan, S.E. Lipshultz, A.M. Lowe, et al., Epidemiology and cause-specific outcome of hypertrophic cardiomyopathy in children: findings from the Pediatric Cardiomyopathy Registry, Circulation 115 (6) (February 13, 2007) 773–781.

[13] J.A. Towbin, A.M. Lowe, S.D. Colan, et al., Incidence, causes, and outcomes of dilated cardiomyopathy in children, JAMA 296 (15) (October 18, 2006) 1867–1876.

[14] P.M. Alexander, P.E. Daubeney, A.W. Nugent, et al., Long-term outcomes of dilated cardiomyopathy diagnosed during childhood: results from a national population-based study of childhood cardiomyopathy, Circulation 128 (18) (October 29, 2013) 2039–2046.

[15] R.E. Andrews, M.J. Fenton, D.A. Ridout, M. Burch, British Congenital Cardiac Association, New-onset heart failure due to heart muscle disease in childhood: a prospective study in the United Kingdom and Ireland, Circulation 117 (1) (January 1, 2008) 79–84.

[16] C.W. Yancy, M. Jessup, B. Bozkurt, et al., 2013 ACCF/AHA guideline for the management of heart failure: a report of the American College of Cardiology Foundation/American Heart Association Task Force on Practice Guidelines, J. Am. Coll. Cardiol. 62 (16) (October 15, 2013) e147–239.

[17] R. Kirk, A.I. Dipchand, D.N. Rosenthal, et al., The International Society for Heart and Lung Transplantation Guidelines for the management of pediatric heart failure: executive summary. [Corrected], J. Heart Lung Transplant. 33 (9) (September 2014) 888–909.

[18] M.D. Puchalski, R.V. Williams, B. Askovich, L.L. Minich, C. Mart, L.Y. Tani, Assessment of right ventricular size and function: echo versus magnetic resonance imaging, Congenit. Heart Dis. 2 (1) (January–February 2007) 27–31.

[19] R. Margossian, M.L. Schwartz, A. Prakash, et al., Comparison of echocardiographic and cardiac magnetic resonance imaging measurements of functional single ventricular volumes, mass, and ejection fraction (from the Pediatric Heart Network Fontan Cross-Sectional Study), Am. J. Cardiol. 104 (3) (August 1, 2009) 419–428.

[20] B.D. Soriano, M. Hoch, A. Ithuralde, et al., Matrix-array 3-dimensional echocardiographic assessment of volumes, mass, and ejection fraction in young pediatric patients with a functional single ventricle: a comparison study with cardiac magnetic resonance, Circulation 117 (14) (April 8, 2008) 1842–1848.

[21] L.H. Cripe, B.J. Barber, R.L. Spicer, et al., Outpatient continuous inotrope infusion as an adjunct to heart failure therapy in Duchenne muscular dystrophy, Neuromuscul. Disord. 16 (11) (November 2006) 745–748.

[22] R.E. Hershberger, J. Cowan, A. Morales, J.D. Siegfried, Progress with genetic cardiomyopathies: screening, counseling, and testing in dilated, hypertrophic, and arrhythmogenic right ventricular dysplasia/cardiomyopathy, Circ. Heart Fail. 2 (3) (May 2009) 253–261.

[23] G.C. Fonarow, L.W. Stevenson, J.A. Walden, et al., Impact of a comprehensive heart failure management program on hospital readmission and functional status of patients with advanced heart failure, J. Am. Coll. Cardiol. 30 (3) (September 1997) 725–732.

[24] S.M. Macicek, C.G. Macias, J.L. Jefferies, J.J. Kim, J.F. Price, Acute heart failure syndromes in the pediatric emergency department, Pediatrics 124 (5) (November 2009) e898–904.

[25] D.T. Hsu, G.D. Pearson, Heart failure in children: part II: diagnosis, treatment, and future directions, Circ. Heart Fail. 2 (5) (September 2009) 490–498.

[26] R.E. Shaddy, M.M. Boucek, D.T. Hsu, et al., Carvedilol for children and adolescents with heart failure: a randomized controlled trial, JAMA 298 (10) (September 12, 2007) 1171–1179.

[27] P.F. Kantor, J.R. Abraham, A.I. Dipchand, L.N. Benson, A.N. Redington, The impact of changing medical therapy on transplantation-free survival in pediatric dilated cardiomyopathy, J. Am. Coll. Cardiol. 55 (13) (March 30, 2010) 1377–1384.

[28] E. Pahl, L.A. Sleeper, C.E. Canter, et al., Incidence of and risk factors for sudden cardiac death in children with dilated cardiomyopathy: a report from the Pediatric Cardiomyopathy Registry, J. Am. Coll. Cardiol. 59 (6) (February 7, 2012) 607–615.

[29] N.A. Rudd, M.A. Frommelt, J.S. Tweddell, et al., Improving interstage survival after Norwood operation: outcomes from 10 years of home monitoring, J. Thorac. Cardiovasc. Surg. 148 (4) (October 2014) 1540–1547.

[30] J.B. Anderson, R.H. Beekman 3rd, J.D. Kugler, et al., Improvement in interstage survival in a national pediatric cardiology learning network, Circ. Cardiovasc. Qual. Outcomes 8 (4) (July 2015) 428–436.

[31] T. Bodenheimer, Interventions to improve chronic illness care: evaluating their effectiveness, Dis. Manag. 6 (2003) 63–71.

[32] National Cancer Policy Board, Childhood Cancer Survivorship: Improving Care and Quality of Life, National Academies Press, Washington, DC, 2003.

[33] C. Pui, W. Evans, Acute lymphoblastic leukemia, N. Engl. J. Med. 339 (1998) 605–615.

[34] J. Hobar, J. Rogowskiu, P. Plsek, et al., Collaborative quality improvement for neonatal intensive care. NIC/Q Project Investigators of the Vermont Oxford Network, Pediatrics 107 (2001) 14–22.

[35] D.T. Hsu, V. Zak, L. Mahony, et al., Enalapril in infants with single ventricle: results of a multicenter randomized trial, Circulation 122 (4) (July 27, 2010) 333–340.

[36] J.R. Kaltman, D.B. Andropoulos, P.A. Checchia, et al., Report of the pediatric heart network and national heart, lung, and blood institute working group on the perioperative management of congenital heart disease, Circulation 121 (25) (June 29, 2010) 2766–2772.

[37] R.G. Ohye, L.A. Sleeper, L. Mahony, et al., Comparison of shunt types in the Norwood procedure for single-ventricle lesions, N. Engl. J. Med. 362 (21) (May 27, 2010) 1980–1992.

[38] G.R. Martin, R.H. Beekman, F.F. Ing, et al., The IMPACT registry: improving pediatric and adult congenital treatments, Semin. Thorac. Cardiovasc. Surg. Pediatr. Card Surg. Annu. 13 (1) (2010) 20–25.

[39] J. Simone, J. Lyons, Superior Cancer Survival in Children Compared to Adults: A Superior System of Cancer Care? Institute of Medicine, Washington, DC, 2003.

[40] P. Conway, C. Clancy, Charting a path from comparative effectiveness funding to improved patient-centered health care, JAMA 303 (2010) 985–986.

[41] P. Margolis, L. Provost, P. Schoettker, M. Britto, Quality improvement, clinical research and quality improvement research: opportunities for integration, Pediatr. Clin. N. Am. 56 (4) (2009) 831–841.

[42] L. Simpson L. Peterson, C.M. Lannon, S. Murphy, C. GoodmanZ. Ren, A, Zajicek. Special challenges in comparative effectiveness research on children's and adolescents' health, Health Affairs 29 (10) (October 2010) 1849–1856.

[43] American Board of Pediatrics, Maintenance of Certification (MOC) – Pediatrics, June 15, 2008. https://http://www.abp.org/ABPWebSite/.

Chapter 37

Nursing Aspects of Heart Failure

Christine Benhase[1], Theresa J. Faulkner[2], Karen Hendricks[3], Juli Sublett[4,5]

[1]*Xavier University, Cincinnati, OH, United States;* [2]*UC Health University Cincinnati Medical Center (UCMS), Cincinnati, OH, United States;* [3]*Nursing Informatics at Chamberlain College of Nursing, Chicago, IL, United States;* [4]*Miami University, Oxford, OH, United States;* [5]*The University of Cincinnati College of Nursing, Cincinnati, OH, United States*

INTRODUCTION

Nursing care of pediatric and young adult HF patients is challenging due to many different etiologies and presentations. Additionally, pediatric HF nurses must care for and educate not only the patient but also the caregivers to ensure successful outcomes. The main objective is to achieve and maintain patient clinical stability in and out of the hospital setting. Nurses must understand and support different types of medical management to improve patient quality of life, reduce hospitalizations, and increase survival rates [1,2]. This chapter focuses on the HF nurse's collaborative role in contributing to optimal clinical outcomes in this patient population.

INCIDENCE AND EPIDEMIOLOGY

While the vast majority of HF patients in the United States are adults, children are also affected. Kanter, Lamour, and Pierce reported that 12,000–35,000 children in the United States have HF due to either congenital heart disease or cardiomyopathy [3]. Towbin et al. reported an annual incidence of dilated cardiomyopathy to be 1.13 out of 100,000 infants and children [4]. It is also estimated that 15%–25% of children with congenital heart disease develop HF [5]. While the typical adult risk factors, such as dyslipidemia, smoking, diabetes mellitus, a sedentary lifestyle and obesity may influence the development of HF in children, and they are less common. Pediatric HF can be attributed to various causes including genetic triggers, myocardial toxins, neuromuscular disorders, metabolic disorders, or structural heart defects (Table 37.1) [4,6].

NURSING THEORETICAL FRAMEWORKS

HF nurses may use a variety of theoretical frameworks to individualize care plans for patients of different ages and diagnoses. By utilizing relevant evidence-based theories in their education, nurses assist in patient comprehension and retention. For a list of potential frameworks, please refer to Table 37.2 [7].

For this chapter, the authors chose to focus the nursing care of this patient population on Dorothea Orem's Theory of Self-Care. This theory is based on individuals purposefully performing self-care actions to regulate their own physiological

TABLE 37.1 Common Causes of Heart Failure and Differences in Pediatrics Versus Adults

Pediatric	Adult
Genetic mutations or syndromes	Myocardial Infarction
Myocardial toxins (such as chemotherapy)	Dyslipidemia
Neuromuscular disorders	Smoking
Metabolic disorders	Obesity/sedentary lifestyle
Infective agents	Diabetes
Structural heart defects	Hypertension

Heart Failure in the Child and Young Adult. http://dx.doi.org/10.1016/B978-0-12-802393-8.00037-5

TABLE 37.2 Nursing Theories Applicable to Pediatric Heart Failure [8]

Potential Frameworks to Guide Pediatric Heart Failure Care
The situation-specific theory of heart failure self-care
Theory of planned behavior
Stages of change
Health belief model

TABLE 37.3 Differences in Heart Failure Symptomology in Pediatrics Versus Adults

Pediatrics	Adults
Retractions or grunting	Shortness of breath or tachypnea
Dyspnea or tachypnea	Cough/congestion
Feeding difficulties	Decreased appetite
Diaphoresis, particularly when feeding	Edema
Failure to thrive	Weight gain
Activity intolerance or fatigue	Activity intolerance or fatigue
Tachycardia	Tachycardia

functioning. Patients or their caregivers must be successful in learning self-care techniques to effectively manage HF. It is the nurse's responsibility to not only meet the pediatric patient's self-care demands as an inpatient but also to teach the patient and family how to meet these needs at home [8]. In Orem's theory, health deviations, such as HF exacerbation, increase the demand for self-care. By learning to recognize signs of deterioration, effectively communicating with the patient's health-care team, and following prescribed treatment regimens, families and caregivers of pediatric HF patients can learn self-management skills [8].

NURSING ASSESSMENT

HF is defined as an inability of the heart to pump an adequate amount of blood to the systemic circulation to meet metabolic demands [9]. One of the primary causes of HF in pediatrics is cardiomyopathy, which refers to a set of heart muscle diseases that impair the ability of cardiac muscles to contract [9]. Nurses must recognize that HF symptomatology in pediatrics differs, and can be unique across pediatric age ranges and diagnoses. Infants may exhibit feeding difficulties, dyspnea, retractions, tachypnea, grunting, tachycardia, fatigue, or diaphoresis [5]. Children experiencing HF may manifest decreased activity, failure to thrive, anorexia, or more classic adult-like symptoms such as cough, shortness of breath, or peripheral edema [5]. Palpitations, presyncope or syncope can be attributed to associated rhythm disturbances and warrant further assessment. By constantly assessing symptoms, particularly during telephone triage, nurses can recognize changes in clinical status, allowing for quicker interventions. Treatment of HF has both short- and long-term objectives. The short-term goal is to achieve hemodynamic stability and relieve symptoms. The long-term goal is to improve quality of life and prolong survival by reversing disease progression (Table 37.3) [6].

NURSING DIAGNOSES

Many **nursing diagnoses** can be identified for pediatric and adult patients in HF. It is imperative that nurses identify pertinent diagnoses so that appropriate interventions can be applied. Activity intolerance, excess fluid volume, and decreased cardiac output are perhaps the most commonly recognized North American Nursing Diagnosis Association and American Association of Heart Failure Nurses (AAHFN) diagnoses in this disease process [10]. Pediatric HF nurses should also identify educational and psychosocial diagnoses applicable to this patient population such as

TABLE 37.4 Heart Failure Symptoms and Related Nursing Diagnoses [6]

Symptom	Nursing Diagnoses
Tachycardia	Arrhythmia; anxiety; impaired psychomotor activity; vasogenic shock; cardiogenic shock; decreased cardiac output; increased cardiac output; knowledge deficit regarding arrhythmia; chest discomfort; cardiac rate changes; abnormal heart rhythm; nausea; dizziness.
Dyspnea	Conflicting attitude in relation to physical activity; adherence to the physical activity regime; respiratory acidosis; impaired self-performance activity; knowledge about physical activity; functional dyspnea; dyspnea at rest; impaired deglutition; knowledge deficit regarding physical activity; lack of capacity to manage the physical activity regime; fatigue; altered respiratory rate; intolerance to activity; altered respiratory pattern; impaired physical activity pattern; altered respiratory rhythm; impaired respiratory system; impaired sleep; impaired gas exchange, impaired ventilation.
Edema	Metabolic acidosis due to electrolyte alteration; ascites; metabolic acidosis due to fluid alteration; metabolic acidosis due to fluid and electrolyte alteration; adherence to fluid volume; imbalance of fluids and electrolytes; exhaustion from the treatment; knowledge deficit regarding fluid volume; impaired skin integrity; impaired movement in bed; dry skin; altered cardiac tissue perfusion; decreased blood pressure; increased blood pressure; impaired urinary system process, impaired peripheral vascular process; water retention, fluid volume deficit; unsatisfactory response to fluid therapy.
Congestion	Impaired ability to dress self; impaired ability to perform hygiene; impaired ability to groom self; impaired ability to bathe self; impaired ability to transfer self; impaired airway clearance; knowledge deficit regarding the response to medication; lack of response to the treatment; hypoxia due to congestion, lack of adherence to the therapeutic regimen; unsatisfactory response to medication; productive cough; dry cough; excessive fluid volume.

knowledge deficit, readiness for enhanced learning, ineffective self-health management, caregiver role strain, anxiety, grieving, interrupted family processes, impaired attachment, and noncompliance. Please refer to Table 37.4 for a list of nursing diagnoses related to prominent HF symptoms [6]. Nurses play a key role in helping families adjust to new diagnoses and their implications on the family's lifestyle. Children and adolescents should always be encouraged to share their feelings and ask their own questions during these discussions. By partnering with the family, nurses can provide needed educational and psychosocial support. Potential nursing interventions based on nursing diagnoses are described in Table 37.5 [6].

NURSING INTERVENTIONS

Whether the cause of HF in pediatrics is due to congenital heart disease, genetically inherited cardiomyopathy, or acquired cardiomyopathy, standardization of care is always a goal to improve patient outcomes [11]. Much of the data that exist regarding HF were studied among the adult population but can be extrapolated for the pediatric population. Nursing care and interventions among the pediatric HF population are highly specialized in the inpatient and outpatient setting. As outlined previously, nursing diagnoses, and subsequent interventions are focused on symptom recognition and management, education, and assisting to meet patient self-care needs.

As with adult HF, the inpatient setting may be the first introduction to the diagnosis of heart disease with subsequent HF and management in the pediatric patient. The bedside nurse has to consider many social aspects affecting the care of the patient in addition to providing safe and effective medical care. The role of the nurse is to be a liaison between the family and the health-care team. Nurses must consider complex social situations, family anxiety, and difficulty coping as inherent to a new diagnosis of a chronic illness [11]. In the hospitalized pediatric patient, nursing interventions begin with admission and should always be anticipatory of discharge with a goal of preventing readmissions [8].

One of the most important interventions is medication reconciliation, which should be done at admission, any time there is a transfer of care, and at transition to home. Medication reconciliation involves reviewing and updating the patient's medication list to ensure the most accurate and current information is available. In 2012, a systematic review [12] of 26 controlled studies pertaining to hospital processes of medication reconciliation highlighted important interventions related to medication reconciliation that correlated with reduction in medication discrepancies, potential adverse drug events, adverse drug events, and health-care utilization (i.e., rate of readmission). The following list outlines the medication reconciliation process:

- An accurate preadmission medication list (this may be performed by pharmacy or nursing).
- An accurate list of medications being taken by the patient at the time of transfer and discharge.
- Patient/caregiver counseling with documentation of patient/caregiver understanding of what each medication is used for and when to take it.

TABLE 37.5 Nursing Diagnoses and Related Interventions [6]

Nursing Diagnoses	Associated Nursing Interventions
Arrhythmia	Analyze cardiovascular function and imminent risk of arrhythmia after patient exertion and reduce exertion.
	Institute basic life support maneuvers.
	Observe frequency and regularity of the pulse if altered.
	Verify signs of lethal arrhythmias (ventricular fibrillation, ventricular tachycardia) such as decreased level of consciousness.
Cardiogenic shock	Note variations in blood pressure (orthostatic hypotension).
	Be familiar with the presence of the third heart sound.
	Observe signs of oliguria.
	Prepare circulatory containment measures (preparation of cardiotonic drugs).
	Report episodes of rapid and thin pulse and altered peripheral perfusion, and initiate fluid resuscitation and basic support maneuvers.
Increased cardiac output	Control fluid volume gains.
	Monitor changes in cardiac rate after physical exertion.
	Appropriately position the patient in the bed.
	Reduce physical exertion.
Functional dyspnea	Be familiar with the clinical conditions of the degree of congestive heart failure and its aggravations.
	Determine the hemodynamic status and compare with previous respiratory rate values.
	Examine pulmonary conditions.
	Observe the pulse oximetry values if <90%.
Fatigue	Monitor serum electrolyte levels (Ht, Hb, Na).
	Assist in social contact.
	Develop an individualized management plan for physical and social rehabilitation.
	Plan rest/activity periods.
Impaired gas exchange	Assist in arterial puncture for diagnostic examinations.
	Evaluate respiratory ventilation/perfusion.
	Maintain elevation of the bed at 90 degrees.
	Maintain airway permeability.
	Monitor level of consciousness, arterial pressure, pulse, temperature, and breathing pattern.

- Patient/caregiver demonstration of knowledge of medication changes during hospitalization and the reasons for the changes.
- Prescriptions sent to appropriate pharmacy at the time of discharge.
- Written documentation in patient chart, follow-up letter to next provider and, paper copy given to patient at discharge (see Chart 37.1) [12].

The systematic review [12] outlined heavy pharmacist involvement in the medication reconciliation process and nursing focusing on discharge counseling. Readiness for discharge is something that should be reviewed continuously throughout the admission and education should be tailored to the patient/caregiver education level, age of the patient, learning style preferences, language barriers, and psychosocial stressors [8]. The following criteria should be met prior to discharge (Table 37.6).

The discharge nurse may spend a substantial amount of time completing one-on-one education to assist the transition to home. In previous studies, the HF nurse educator spent approximately 60 min completing discharge teaching with patients.

Clinic/Nurse Contact Information: Updated: Date

Medication	Directions	AM	PM
Carvedilol (Coreg) [25mg tablet]	Take 1 tablet (25mg) twice daily	X	X
Chlorothiazide (Diuril) [500mg tablet]	Take 1 tablet (500mg) every morning	X	
Furosemide (Lasix) [20mg tablet]	Take 1 tablet (20mg) every morning AS NEEDED	X	
Multi-vitamin	Take 1 tablet every morning	X	
Ranitidine (Zantac) [150mg tablet]	Take 1 tablet (150mg) twice daily	X	X
Sacubitril-Valsartan (Entresto) [49-51mg tablet]	Take 1 tablet (49-51mg) twice daily	X	X
Warfarin (Coumadin) [5mg tablet]	Take 1 tablet (5mg) every evening		X

CHART 37.1 Example of heart failure medication chart.

TABLE 37.6 Discharge Criteria

Adequate control of presenting symptoms
Near euvolemic volume status
Off intravenous therapies (inotropic support and diuretic therapy) for 24 h
Initiation and stable on oral therapies for 24 h (ACE inhibitor, beta blocker, diuretic therapy, or documentation of intolerance)
Documentation of current left ventricular ejection fraction
Ambulatory (if an appropriate age)
Discharge education completed with patient/family
Initial follow-up visit scheduled (7–10 days after initial inpatient admission but may be 1–3 months in a chronic pediatric heart failure patient)
Supplies and home nursing care established, if indicated, prior to discharge (scale in older children/adults)
24-h care has been completed by the caregiver [11]

This intervention has shown to reduce HF readmission rates by as much as 50% in a 6-month period [13]. Pediatric HF is unique in that it does not have the same signs and symptoms of the typical adult HF, so teaching points will be different. Adult guidelines suggest the teach-back method [8]. In pediatrics, this includes the patient or caregiver completing a self-care trial where they manage medications and symptoms independently for 24 h while still admitted in the hospital. During this time period, known as 24-h care, nursing staff is available for assistance, but the goal is that the family recognizes the patient's care needs. Lerret [14] reported that meaningful interactions and confidence building are vital concepts related to parental discharge readiness. Prior to going home, the patient or caregiver should be able to verbalize the following (Table 37.7).

Discharge education is not a stand-alone intervention but rather prepares the patient and family for interventions in outpatient setting and home care coordination [13]. The outpatient HF nurse seeks to teach self-management skills as well as coordinate care among the complex health-care system. These interventions usually begin with a postdischarge phone call to ascertain clinical status and ensure follow-up appointments are appropriate. The initial follow-up phone call (within the first 72 h after discharge) is perhaps not only the simplest form of telemonitoring but also the most important since it allows the nurse to assess symptoms as well as the family's understanding of needed care [11]. Further telemonitoring can include parents/patient reporting health data such as vital signs, oral intake, and weight. This information can be communicated via phone, email, or text. The nurse triages the patient information and notifies the appropriate member of the multidisciplinary team of any concerns.

Additionally, telemonitoring can include information from implantable devices such as loop recorders, implantable cardio defibrillators, and resynchronization devices. This can provide real-time monitoring of heart rhythms and correlate them with reported symptoms [11]. The AAHFN wrote a position statement in 2014 regarding appropriate nursing care

TABLE 37.7 Patient/Caregiver Discharge Criteria

Accurate discharge medication regimen and reason for taking it
Vital signs and Weight monitoring (monitoring for appropriate growth in younger children and fluid retention in older children)
Daily physical activity level and activity restrictions (i.e., are there sports restrictions)
Nutritional plan: sodium restrictions in older children, appropriate caloric intake in younger children
Follow-up appointments
Recognition of worsening symptoms
Instructions to follow if symptoms worsen

TABLE 37.8 Outpatient Interventions

Multidisciplinary team evidence–based approach in disease management using nurses, advanced practice nurses, physicians, pharmacists, dieticians, social workers, child life specialists, medical assistants, and cardiac rehab specialists.
Multimodal teaching multisensory input (visual, auditory, skill practice) enhances retention of information
Multisensory input covers more preferred learning styles: use of lecture, group discussion, CD, TV, workbooks may be used
Telemonitoring interventions: this covers a wide range of intervention including, postdischarge telephone calls, home devices with transmission of data to central monitoring site
Enhancing patient engagement: use of decision aids for shared decision making, targeting education toward skill mastery and empowerment, focus on individualized care with attention to comorbidities
Cognitive-based interventions: cognitive strategies may help memory and spatial problems
Motivational interviewing: based on cognitive dissonance to move patients to a higher level of change to facilitate learning and behavior change
Including families and caregivers in education: educating families and caregivers along with patients improves adherence with dietary sodium restriction [8]

and interventions in the adult population. The following table from their paper is an excellent comprehensive summary of interventions in an outpatient program and can be applied to the pediatric population (Table 37.8).

Enhancing self-care is an important aspect in transitioning to outpatient monitoring. The outpatient nurse may initially be heavily involved but ideally the patient or caregiver will eventually take over their own management. Caregivers that do not become engaged in the patient's care pose higher risk for exacerbations [15]. Interventions on behalf of the nurse to promote this should not only provide information to the patient but also have a theoretical background to guide the content, such as Dorothea Orem's theory. Basing care on a theoretical approach will provide the rationale behind interventions and outcomes [16]. A specific aspect in the pediatric population is consideration of the age and developmental level of the child. Interventional and educational tools should be adjusted for patient cooperation and understanding. Initial interventions are focused on the caregiver, but as the child ages he or she should be involved decisions to promote future adherence [11].

The Cardiomyopathy and Advanced Heart Failure clinic at Cincinnati Children's Hospital Medical Center sees approximately 900 patients annually. To provide robust, comprehensive care to such a large population, care coordination measures are utilized. To stratify patients based on risk, two RN Care Managers and two social workers meet weekly to tier patients based on medical and psychosocial complexity. The highest risk patients are assigned an RN Care Manager, social worker, or both. Assigned team members are then responsible for patient communication and follow-up, allowing for consistency in care delivery. Since patient assignments are visible in the Electronic Medical Record, the assigned care team members also receive alerts when patients are admitted, seen in the emergency room, or complete ordered testing. These alerts assist the health-care team members in preventing duplicate testing, following up on results and maintaining up-to-date care plans. The care team assignments also enhance communication across subspecialties, as health-care team members in other divisions can identify the appropriate cardiology contact for questions regarding interdisciplinary management.

NURSING EDUCATION

Working with HF patients across all socioeconomic classes, categories of age, and phases of the HF trajectory, nurses are in a key position to prevent complications, recognize early signs and symptoms of worsening HF, and tailor education and treatment strategies to ensure high-quality care [17]. Deficiencies in nurse training have been recognized related to HF. Nursing's ability to influence patient outcomes must take into account the nurses ability to understand, identify, and teach the types of HF, testing, interventions, and outcome measures. By regularly contacting patients and their caregivers, nurses can identify early clinical deterioration and facilitate optimization of medical management. Nurses who have received specialized training in HF management are better able to recognize and overcome deficiencies in care. Consistent assessment and incorporation of therapies such as exercise, dietary assessment, and immunization education are some examples where nursing coordination can have an effective impact. Another area nursing can be influential is medication education. Many hospital admissions are related to medication nonadherence. Patients often do not adhere to their medication regimen for a number of reasons, including

- Lack of knowledge related to what each medication is used for
- Not understanding the importance of right medication at the right time and what to do if a dose is missed
- Inability to obtain or financially afford their medication

The AAHFN recommends a formal orientation, education, and certification of the nursing staff that are involved in HF care. Understanding important factors for HF management for the nurse to assess and teach effectively should be evidence-based, HF guideline-directed content. HF nursing orientation education curriculum should address these topics:

- Definition
- Etiologies
- Types of HF
- HF reduced ejection fraction (EF)
- HF preserved EF
- Diagnosis
- Testing
- Treatments
- Medications, interventions, surgeries
- Device therapies
- Managing comorbid conditions
- Self-care Programs that enhance nurses' knowledge of HF self-care through a sound educational curriculum
- Diet, lifestyle, activity, weight tracking, symptom recognition/management, alcohol recommendations, smoking cessation, influenza/pneumococcal vaccinations
- Preventing readmissions
- Disease progression
- Coping with HF
- Advanced directives
- End-stage therapies, heart transplant, and mechanical circulatory support
- Palliative care and end-of-life preferences [8].

The AAHFN also states that effective HF patient education is a complex endeavor that must meet the unique needs of the individual and the family. Patient engagement and activation with self-care needs to be fostered. No single approach will work for all patients, and many factors need to be considered while providing personalized education. Recommendations for special considerations by the nurse and HF team, when educating patients with HF, are listed in Table 37.9 [8].

In many instances, nursing staff executes HF patient education without formalized documentation that addresses a measurable patient learning assessment, educational process, or patient comprehension, in an effort to complete documentation of discharge instructions. Such education has been performed using wide-ranging methods with uncertain effectiveness. Meaningful education needs to go beyond basic education. Utilization of a variety of learning tools that can reinforce information should include verbal discussions, written handouts, and evidence-based websites. These tools can reinforce information as well as help patients gain knowledge, skills, and mastery of the content provided. Data suggest that outcomes improve when we educate patients with the intent for them to become active participants in their own care. Patient activation and engagement are key features of patient-centered care, which is supported through individualized education. Patients or parents who are not engaged in care have higher readmission rates [8]. Transitional care by providers should be the highest consideration [8].

TABLE 37.9 Factors to Consider While Educating Hear Failure Patients

Special Considerations	Specific Actions to Consider
Limited cognition population	Reminders
	Repetition
	Engage family/caregiver
	Follow-up calls
Comorbidities	Consider how comorbid conditions impact self-care
	Consider referral to multispecialty clinic that uses mental health professionals
	Refer to mental health professional to treat illness and enhance adherence
	Support groups
Low health literacy	Assess learning preference and literacy level
	Multimedia approach
	Use teach-back method
	Teach to goal
	Repetition
	Literacy appropriate tools
	Education tools in native language
Cognitive dysfunction	Assess for cognitive dysfunction (speech therapy for neurocognitive evaluation)
	Consider cognitive, behavioral interventions
	Repetition
Lack of social support	Support groups
	Group visits
	Family support
Caregiver burden	Support groups
	Group visits
	Educational plan for caregivers
Socioeconomic challenges	Social work and/or financial counselor consultation
	Pharmacy assistance programs
	Transportation assistance
Racial, cultural, gender, and religious preferences	Assess for patient's preferences
	Offer options when considering treatment decisions
	Include culturally relevant content

Outpatient clinic and home visit interventions should focus on medications, symptom management, diet, activity, sleep, medical follow-up, and the emotional status of patients and caregivers. A variety of strategies that reinforce teaching include teach-back, written instructions and medication schedules. Home care visits and telephone follow-up allow nurses to timely address questions or concerns from patients or caregivers. By monitoring the patient's progress and communicating effectively with collaborating physicians, nurses can facilitate therapy adjustments and needed referrals. Discharge summaries need to be reviewed with patients and caregivers, with special emphasis on medication adjustments. Written summaries that include care plans, goals, and care team contact information should be provided to all patients, caregivers, and comanaging providers.

Outcome measures need to be collected and evaluated, including hospital readmission rates related to any cause, recurrence or exacerbation of the index hospitalization diagnosis related groupers, comorbid conditions, or new health problems. The primary intervention efficacy test should be defined on the basis of time to first readmission for any reason. Secondary outcomes are cumulative days of rehospitalization, mean readmission length of stay, number of unscheduled acute care visits after discharge, estimated cost of postindex hospitalization health services, functional status, depression, and patient satisfaction [8].

HF is a complicated disease process that can affect multiple aspects of a patient's life. One of the most demanding components of HF management for the HF nurse and patient is compliance and adherence. Newly diagnosed patients are often overwhelmed with a diagnosis of HF. The lifelong changes that must occur to continue quality of life and control progression of this chronic disease process related to symptoms can be confusing. Patients and their families are often educated on diet, exercise, medications, self-care management, smoking cessation, the need for consistent follow-up appointments, and recognition of acute exacerbation of HF symptoms. Health-care providers often do not realize that patients and their families face many barriers to successful management. Barriers that must be investigated before a patient is discharged are

- Educational level of patients and family members
- Financial burden
- Physical limitations
- Denial of disease
- Access to care/transportation
- Polypharmacy
- Lack of support
- Insufficient education by medical staff
- Depression
- Diet restrictions
- Inability to recognize HF symptoms

PATIENT/FAMILY EMPOWERMENT AND SELF-MANAGEMENT

Given the complexity of the disease state, many patients struggle with required lifestyle modifications. Defining an individualized HF plan of care that assesses, identifies, and addresses barriers is important for successful patient empowerment, self-care, and adherence. One recognized nursing barrier to successful disease education is the lack of time to teach patients and their caregivers. The HF core measurement goal to decrease hospital length of stay further complicates disease management [13].

Financial barriers are often the most difficult to manage as most patients are not given opportunity to discuss their finances prior to discharge. Given current changes and uncertainty in health-care coverage, medical providers are changing the ways they practice. Many providers are more cognizant that families experience tremendous financial strains regarding deductibles, copays, and cost of medications. Educating and having a financial plan of care for the patients and caregivers that discusses outpatient follow-up care may include cardiac MRIs, catheterizations, laboratory testing, echocardiograms, EKGs, and supportive measures of nutritional education and cardiac rehabilitation. In addition, most insurance companies now require prior authorizations on testing and medications, creating delays in treatment as well as increased stress on families.

The physical limitations caused by congestive HF lead to a multitude of barriers on patients and their families. Decreased energy levels create an environment wherein the patient and family must budget extra time to get to appointments and adjust activities of daily living. Depression is a significant concern to be discussed with HF patients. HF is a life changing event that ebbs and flows with time. Approximately one in five patients with HF meets criteria for major depressive disorder, and a greater percentage reports depressive symptoms [18]. Without continual evaluation and treatment, patients with depression and HF continue to exhibit poor outcomes. It has been shown that depression has been linked to decreased adherence to medication regimens, daily weights, and recognition of acute exacerbations of HF [19]. In addition, many patients with end-stage HF exhibit anxiety due to breathlessness while sleeping. Depression screenings, support groups, and patient education should be introduced early in the disease process to reduce the emotional strain of HF.

Transportation can be another barrier that inhibits access to care. Many institutions do not provide transportation due to limited financial resources. In addition, in rural areas, patients may not have access to health-care facilities and may have to travel long distances. This patient population is at a significant risk for poor outcomes and my benefit from telemedicine technologies. Clear, concise, and open communication must be established and maintained between all medical providers, including the primary care provider, to provide consistent communication to the family [20].

Patients with HF face many dietary challenges. Infants and young children often require increased calories to account for the increased metabolic demands of HF. Older children and adults require education on sodium and fluid restrictions [21]. Dieticians are essential members of the HF multidisciplinary team who are responsible for closely monitoring growth and ensuring adequate nutrition. While restaurants are mandated to provide dietary information, it usually is not readily displayed. In addition, purchasing healthy foods can be expensive for families. HF dietary control is a lifelong commitment with education specifically addressing nutritional labels and sodium intake [22].

Patients and caregivers often experience denial when faced with the diagnosis of HF. HF symptoms may be intermittent, which can support the reaction of denial and nonadherence behavior. Additionally, children are resilient and tend to remain largely asymptomatic until end stages of the disease. Young adults may struggle to adhere to recommendations regarding diet, exercise, and smoking. The social issues facing young adults are further complicated by HF management. Parents of small children may want their children to participate in activities to avoid their children from being excluded from school activities. In addition, patients who identify themselves as athletes struggle with limitations placed on them due to HF. Medical providers should emphasize patient capabilities rather than limitations.

Perhaps one of the most complex aspects of medical management involving HF is polypharmacy related to other comorbidities. Many patients will, at some point, experience other chronic disease processes such as diabetes, obstructive lung disease, gastrointestinal disorders (due to decreased blood flow), cachexia, thyroid and kidney dysfunction, and pain. With each new diagnosis, new medical subspecialists are often added. Each provider's unique treatments can include medications that may interfere with HF medications or exacerbate symptoms.

Patients or their caregivers' inability to recognize HF exacerbations are perhaps the most crucial of barriers to breach. Failure to identify symptoms such as increased dyspnea, increased fatigue, inability to lay flat, anorexia, nausea or edema, etc., can lead to disease exacerbations or hospital admissions. Each successive readmission leads to decreased quality of life, poor patient outcomes, and higher health-care costs.

PALLIATIVE CARE

As previously mentioned, HF is a progressive disease that eventually leads to pump failure. Due to the progressive nature of HF, medical providers must be proactive in initiating discussions involving palliative and hospice care. Many health-care providers use palliative care and hospice interchangeably, but they are distinct phases of care. Oftentimes, medical providers are more focused on curative measures with little dialogue on end-of-life options.

Palliative care, defined by Centers for Medicare and Medicaid Services (CMS), is the treatment for the relief of pain and other uncomfortable symptoms through the appropriate coordination of all aspects of care needed to maximize personal comfort and relieve distress [19]. Palliative care should be initiated at diagnosis to maintain quality of life. The goal of palliative care is to allow patients and their families to effectively manage symptoms and minimize acute HF exacerbations. Please refer to Chart 37.2 for a model of HF phases of care.

End-stage HF, as defined by American College of Cardiology and the American Heart Association (stage D), occurs when symptoms exist at rest despite optimal medical management [19]. Hospice care is an arm of palliative care that is introduced when a patient reaches Stage D and refractory symptoms require special interventions, such as transplantation or ventricular assistive devices, are contraindicated. Please refer to Chart 37.3 for HF staging and interventions. Hospice providers support patients and their family members by providing comfort care instead of curative care within the home or hospice facility. CMS defines hospice care as the ability to allow the terminally ill patient to remain at home as long as

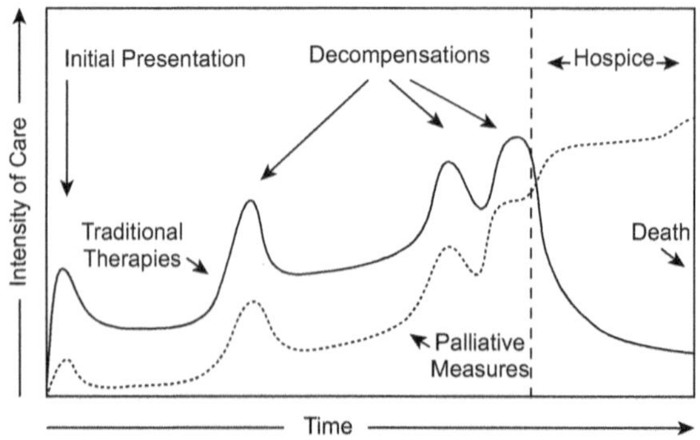

CHART 37.2 Phases of care.

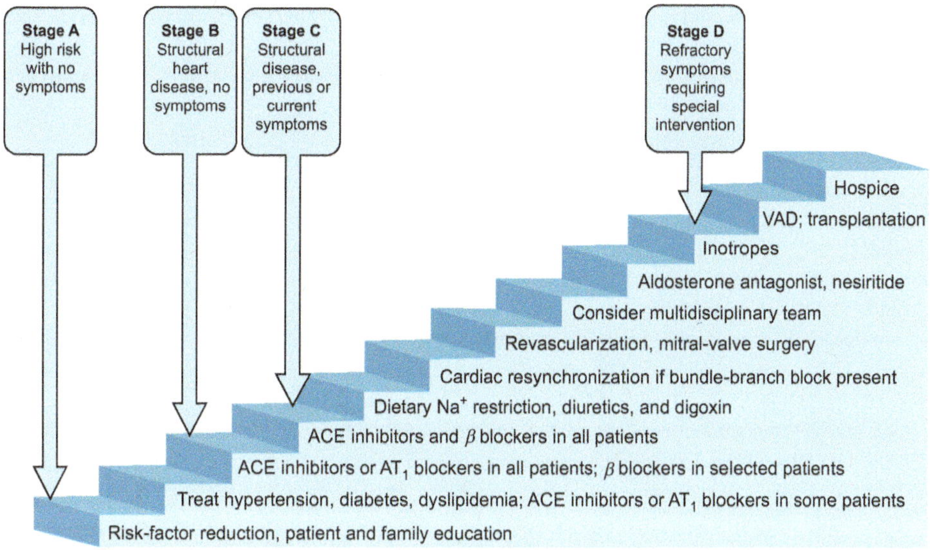

CHART 37.3 Heart failure staging and interventions [25]. *ACE*, Ang-converting enzyme; AT_1, type 1 Ang receptor; *VAD*, ventricular assist device.

possible by providing support to the patient and family and keeping the patient as comfortable as possible while maintaining his or her dignity and quality of life [19]. The goal of hospice care is not to prolong life but to allow patients and their families to feel comfortable and emotionally supported throughout the dying process.

The heightened risk of sudden cardiac death and decreased life expectancy by HF should be recognized, and patients should be educated on the progressive nature of the disease. Evidence is needed to direct care at the end of life, including use of HF medications, and to define management of multiple sources of distress for HF patients and their families [23].

The American Heart Association's "Get with the Guidelines" program reported that less than 10% of eligible HF patients use hospice care [19]. Referrals to hospice care should be made when patients have recurrent hospitalizations, worsening functional status, or need for continuous intravenous inotropic therapy despite attempts to optimize overall management [19]. Initiating palliative care discussions early in disease progression helps reduce emotional distress when making end-of-life decisions.

According to Bakitas et al., referrals to palliative care are often late in the trajectory of illness, preventing patients from receiving full benefit [24]. A multidisciplinary team approach assists patients and their families throughout the chronic disease process. Palliative care teams collaborate with the health-care team and patients to achieve patient and family goals, values, and preferences, communicating prognostic information, and articulating potential options for, and outcomes, of treatment [25].

Nursing has the ability to impact pediatric and young adult HF management through barrier assessment, education, and care coordination. Certified HF nurses have demonstrated expertise in providing effective care and education to this patient population. As influential members of multidisciplinary care teams, nurses have the responsibility to incorporate evidence-based practices that will lead to optimal outcomes.

REFERENCES

[1] International Standards Organization (ISO), ISO 18104:2003 Health Informatic-Integration of a Reference Terminology Model for Nursing, Geneva, 2003.

[2] International Council of Nurses (ICN), Guidelines for ICNP Catalogue Development, Geneva, 2008.

[3] K. Kanter, J. Lamour, F.B. Pearce, Epidemiology, natural history and prognosis of heart failure, in: R. Kirk, A.I. Dipchand, D.N. Rosenthal (Eds.), ISHLT Guidelines for the Management of Pediatric Heart Failure, 2014, pp. 5–17. Birmingham.

[4] J.A. Towbin, A.M. Lowe, S.D. Colan, L.A. Sleeper, E.J. Orav, S. Clunie, J. Messere, G.F. Cox, P.L. Lurie, D. Hsu, C. Canter, J.D. Wilkinson, S.E. Lipshultz, Incidence, causes and outcomes of dilated cardiomyopathy in children, JAMA 296 (2006) 1867–1875.

[5] E. Madriago, M. Silberbach, Heart failure in infants and children, Pediatr. Rev. 31 (2010) 4–12.

[6] A.A. Araujo, M.M.L. Nobrega, T.R. Garcia, Nursing diagnoses and interventions for patients with congestive heart failure using the ICNP, Rev. Esc. Enferm. USP 47 (2013) 385–392.

[7] N.T. Artinian, M. Magnan, M. Sloan, M.P. Lange, Issues Cardiovasc. Nurs. 31 (2002) 161–172.

[8] K. Rasmusson, M. Flattery, L.S. Baas, American association of heart failure nurses position paper on educating patients with heart failure, Heart Lung 44 (2015) 173–177.

[9] S.K. Clunie, Nursing and psychosocial aspects of heart failure, in: A.C. Chang, J.T. Towbin (Eds.), Heart Failure in Children and Young Adults, 2006, pp. 438–450.

[10] V. Souza, S.S. Zeitoun, C.T. Lopes, A.P.D. Oliveria, J.L. Lopes, A.L.B.L. Barros, Content validation of the operational definitions of the nursing diagnoses of activity intolerance, excess fluid volume and decreased cardiac output in patients with heart failure, Int. J. Nurs. Knowl. 25 (2013) 85–89.

[11] L. Bannister, E.D. Blume, A. Dubin, D.M. McMullan, A. Petropoulos, C. White-Williams, Health care delivery, in: R. Kirk, A.I. Dipchand, D.N. Rosenthal (Eds.), ISHLT Guidelines for the Management of Pediatric Heart Failure, 2014, pp. 259–271. Birmingham.

[12] S.K. Mueller, K.C. Sponsler, S. Kripalani, J.L. Schnipper, Hospital-based medication reconciliation practices: a systemic review, Arch. Intern. Med. 172 (2012) 1057–1069.

[13] R. Regalbuto, M.S. Maurer, D. Chapel, J. Mendez, J.A. Shaffer, Joint commission requirements for discharge instructions for patients with heart failure: is understanding important for preventing readmissions? J. Card. Fail. 20 (2014) 641–647.

[14] S.M. Lerret, Discharge readiness: an integrative review focusing on discharge following pediatric hospitalization, J. Spec. Pediatr. Nurs. 14 (2009) 245–255.

[15] D. Bjork, J. Rinker, MHealth and pediatric chronic conditions, Benefits Mag. (2014) 34–36.

[16] S. Boisvert, A. Proulx-Bellhumenaur, N. Goncalves, M. Dore, J. Francoeur, M.C. Gallani, An integrative literature review on nursing interventions aimed at increasing self-care among heart failure patients, Rev. Lat. Am. Enferm. 23 (2015) 753–768.

[17] Committee on the Robert Wood Johnson Foundation Initiative on the Future of Nursing at the Institute of Medicine, The Future of Nursing: Leading Change, Advancing Health, first ed., The National Academies Press, Washington, DC, 2011.

[18] L. LeMond, L. Allen, Palliative care and hospice in advanced heart failure, PCD 54 (2011) 168–178.

[19] D. Whellan, S. Goodlin, M. Dickinson, P. Heidenrich, C. Jaenicke, W. Stough, M. Rich, End-of-life care in patients with heart failure, JCF 20 (2014) 121–134.

[20] R. Simmonds, M. Glogowska, S. McLachlan, H. Cramer, T. Sanders, R. Johnson, U. Kadam, D. Lasserson, S. Purdy, Unplanned admissions and the organizational management of heart failure: a multicenter ethnographic, qualitative study, BMJ 5 (2015) 1–12.

[21] D.N. Rosenthal, M. Everett, Co-morbidities, in: R. Kirk, A.I. Dipchand, D.N. Rosenthal (Eds.), ISHLT Guidelines for the Management of Pediatric Heart Failure, 2014, pp. 5–17. Birmingham.

[22] R. Oosterom-Calo, A.J. van Ballegooijen, C.B. Terwee, S.J. te Velde, I.A. Brouwe, T. Jaarsma, J. Brug, Determinants of heart failure self-care: a systematic literature review, HFR 17 (2012) 367–385, http://dx.doi.org/10.1007/s10741-001-9292-9.

[23] S.J. Goodlin, Palliative Care in Congestive Heart Failure Patient-Centered Education and Research, Salt Lake City, Utah Received 5 October 2008, Revised 6 February 2009, Accepted 9 February 2009, Available online 22 July 2009, 2009.

[24] M. Bakitas, M. Macmarti, K. Trzepkowski, A. Robert, L. Jackson, J. Brown, J. Dionne-Odom, A. Kono, Palliative care consultations for heart failure patients: how many, when, and why? JCF 19 (3) (2013) 193–201.

[25] https://medicine1journal.wordpress.com/category/chronic-heart-failure-pathophysiology.http://www.uptodate.com/contents/hospital-discharge-and-readmission#H10.

Section III

Medical Treatment for Pediatric Heart Failure

Chapter 38

Diuretics and Invasive Fluid Management Strategies

Jack F. Price
Texas Children's Hospital, Houston, TX, United States

INTRODUCTION

Congestion is one of the most common clinical features of heart failure. Fluid overload may occur in patients with acute or chronic heart failure and can lead to symptoms independent of cardiac output. Among children, signs and symptoms of congestion frequently include hepatomegaly, abdominal pain, gallop heart rhythm, poor appetite, tachypnea, and wheezing. Peripheral edema, hyponatremia, and jugular venous distention occur in more advanced stages of heart failure. Symptomatic relief may be obtained with diuresis as cardiac filling pressures are lowered and extravascular fluid is mobilized from the lungs and peripheral tissues. Cardiac performance may also improve with diuresis as left ventricular end-diastolic pressure is reduced and mitral regurgitation is decreased [1].

Diuretics are the most commonly prescribed medications for the treatment of symptomatic heart failure. The overwhelming majority of adults and children who are hospitalized with acute heart failure are treated with intravenous loop diuretics [2,3]. Although diuretics may improve symptoms of congestion, they can also cause side effects such as electrolyte disturbances, dehydration, and neurohormonal activation. Excessive diuresis is sometimes associated with worsening renal function that frequently improves with discontinuation or decreased dosing of diuretics.

The purpose of this chapter is to provide an overview of the rationale for diuretic use in heart failure, the types, sites of action, and side effects of the most commonly prescribed diuretics and adjunct therapies that may be applied in diuretic-resistant cases. Doses and pharmacokinetics of diuretics are listed in Tables 38.1 and 38.2 [4–12].

DIURETIC CLASSES AND SITES OF ACTION

Loop Diuretics

The loop diuretics (furosemide, bumetanide, torsemide, ethacrynic acid) are sodium–potassium–chloride ($Na^+/K^+/2Cl^-$) cotransporter inhibitors. They are secreted into the proximal tubule lumen then transported to the thick ascending loop (see Fig. 38.1) [13]. They act by inhibiting the $Na^+/K^+/2Cl^-$ transporter of the luminal surface in the ascending limb of the loop of Henle, decreasing reabsorption of sodium, potassium, chloride, and water (see Fig. 38.2) [4]. Sodium reabsorption is reduced by approximately 25%, resulting in natriuresis. Decreased sodium reabsorption causes increased sodium delivery and an increase in sodium reabsorption in the distal and collecting tubules. The increased sodium delivery leads to increased potassium secretion [4]. The loop agents are quite potent at mobilizing fluid, relative to other diuretics, and are therefore called "high ceiling" diuretics.

Furosemide

Furosemide is considered a mainstay of treatment in fluid-overloaded heart failure patients. It is the most commonly prescribed diuretic in children [3,14]. About 60%–80% of orally administered furosemide is absorbed in healthy individuals. Bioavailability is not affected in congestive heart failure but time to peak serum drug concentration is delayed [15,16]. Furosemide is metabolized by hepatic and renal mechanisms. The half-life is prolonged in term and preterm newborns [14,17]. Mirochnick and colleagues evaluated the pharmacokinetics of furosemide in 10 preterm infants [18]. A starting dose of 1 mg/kg was increased to 1–2 mg/kg every 12 or 24 h, depending on clinical response. Oral bioavailability of furosemide was ~84% and protein binding was almost 95%. Clearance was prolonged in preterm infants, with half-life values

Heart Failure in the Child and Young Adult. http://dx.doi.org/10.1016/B978-0-12-802393-8.00038-7

TABLE 38.1 The Pharmacokinetics (PK) and Pharmacodynamics (PD) of Diuretics in Children, Where Pediatric Data are not Available; Data From Adults are Included [5–12]

Drug Class/Drug	PK From	Elimination	$t_{1/2}$ (h)	Excretion	PD From	Route	Onset of Effect	Duration of Effect (h)
Carbonic Anhydrase Inhibitors								
Acetazolamide	Adults	Renal	≈4	Renal	Adults	Oral	<1 h	8–12
					Adults	IV	<5 min	4–5
Osmotic Diuretics								
Mannitol	Adults	Renal	2–4	Renal	Children	IV	30–60 min	2–4
Loop diuretics								
Furosemide	Preterm Term Infants/children	Hepatic/renal Hepatic/renal Hepatic/renal	≈12–24 ≈4–8 ≈1–2	Renal/biliary Renal/biliary Renal/biliary	Infants/children Infants/children	Oral IV	30–60 min 15–30 min	4–6 2–3
Bumetanide	Preterm Term Infants/children	Hepatic/renal Hepatic/renal Hepatic/renal	≈6 ≈2 ≈1–2	Renal/biliary Renal/biliary Renal	Infants/children Infants/children	Oral IV	60 min 20–30 min	4–6 3–4
Thiazide Diuretics								
Hydrochlorothiazide	Adults	Renal	6–15	Renal	Adults	Oral	1–4 h	10–12
Chlorothiazide	Preterm	Renal	≈5	Renal	Adults	Oral	<1 h	6–12
Metolazone	Adults	Renal/hepatic	5–6	Renal	Adults	Oral	<1 h	12–24
Potassium-Sparing Diuretics								
Spironolactone	Adults	Hepatic	1.5	Renal/biliary	Adults	Oral	48–72 h	72
Amiloride	Adults	Hepatic	2–9	Renal	Adults	Oral	2–6 h	10–24
Triamterene	Adults	Hepatic	≈4	Renal	Adults	Oral	2–6 h	7–9

IV, intravenous; $t_{1/2}$, elimination half-life.
Table is From M.K. van der Vorst, et al., Diuretics in pediatrics: current knowledge and future practice. Pediatr. Drugs 8 (2006) 245–264.

TABLE 38.2 Recommended Dosages for Diuretics and Dosage Adjustment for Renal Failure in Children

Type of Diuretic	Age Group Data From	Pediatric Dosage	Interval (h)	Route
Carbonic Anhydrase Inhibitors				
Acetazolamide	Adults	5–12.5 mg/kg 24 h	24	Oral/IV
Osmotic Diuretics				
Mannitol	Adults	0.25–1 g/kg dose	6	IV
Loop Diuretics				
Furosemide (frusemide)	Neonates	1 mg/kg dose	12–24	Oral/IV
	Infant/child	1–4 mg/kg 24 h	6–12	Oral
		1–2 mg/kg dose	6–12	IV
Bumetanide	Neonates	0.01–0.05 mg/kg dose	24–48	Oral/IV
	Infant/child	0.015–0.1 mg/kg dose	6–24	Oral/IV
Thiazide Diuretics				
Hydrochlorothiazide	<6 mo	2–3.3 mg/kg 24 h	12	Oral
	>6 mo	2 mg/kg 24 h	12	Oral
Chlorothiazide	<6 mo	20–40 mg/kg 24 h	12	Oral
	>6 mo	20 mg/kg 24 h	12	Oral
Metolazone	Adults	0.2–0.4 mg/kg 24 h	12–24	Oral
Potassium-Sparing Diuretics				
Amiloride	Adults	0.625 mg/kg 24 h	12–24	Oral
Triamterene	Adults	1–4 mg/kg 24 h	12	Oral
Spironolactone	Preterm <32 week	1 mg/kg 24 h	24	Oral
	Term	1–2 mg/kg 24 h	12	Oral
	Infant/child	1–3 mg/kg 24 h	6–12	Oral

IV, intravenous.
Table is From M.K. van der Vorst, et al., Diuretics in pediatrics: current knowledge and future practice, Pediatr. Drugs 8 (2006) 245–264.

ranging from 1.8 to 67.3 h. Renal clearance improved with increasing age. By 36 weeks, the mean half-life had decreased to 4 h, similar to that of term neonates [18,19]. In children and adults, onset of action after intravenous administration is typically within 5 min with peak effect generally occurring within 1–2 h and duration of action is usually 2–6 h [5,19,20]. The majority of furosemide is excreted in the urine as unchanged drug, and the remainder undergoes glucuronidation in the kidneys and liver [13,21]. The active metabolites are eliminated by renal and nonrenal mechanisms [4,18,22]. Because furosemide displaces bilirubin from its albumin binding sites, premature newborns who are treated with furosemide may be at increased risk of hyperbilirubinemia. Recommended dosages are listed in Table 38.2.

Bumetanide

Approximately 50% of bumetanide is metabolized by the kidney and liver, while the remainder is eliminated into the urine as unchanged drug [4,5,23]. Therefore, its half-life is prolonged in patients with hepatic insufficiency [13,21]. Renal clearance of bumetanide increases during the first 6 months of age as tubular organic acid secretion matures [7,8,15]. Recommended dosages are listed in Table 38.2. Doses as high as 0.1 mg/kg appear to be well-tolerated in volume overloaded newborns and infants [8].

Torsemide

The bioavailability of oral torsemide is approximately 80% and the half-life is about 3.5 h. Like furosemide and bumetanide, it is eliminated by hepatic and renal mechanisms. Several studies have shown that torsemide may be more effective than

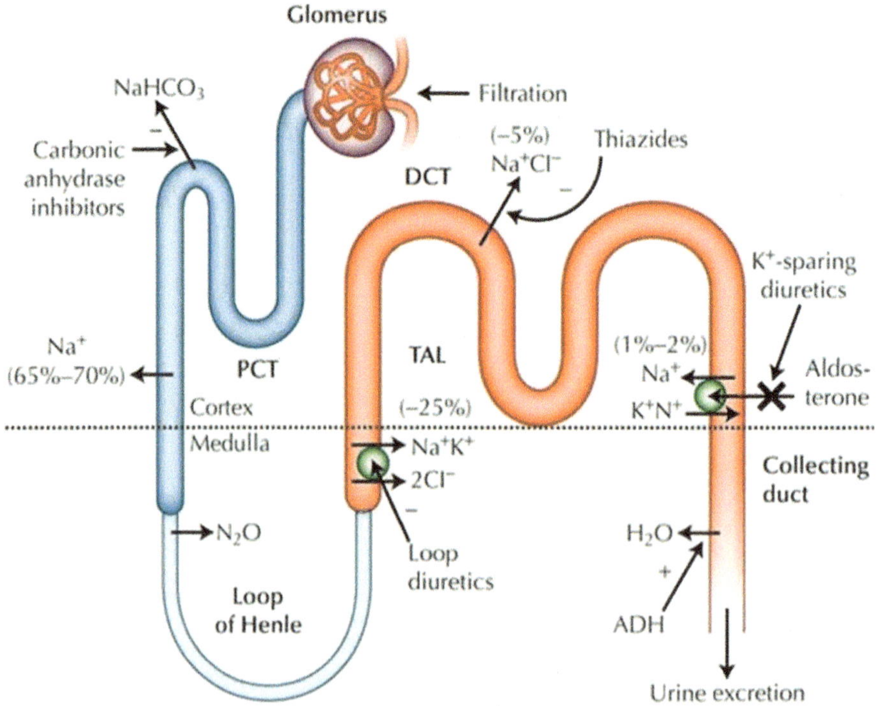

FIGURE 38.1 Diuretic site of action in the renal tubule. The amount of sodium absorbed at each site is in parentheses. Free water is reabsorbed proportionately to the amount of sodium reabsorption and the osmotic gradient across the membrane. Most sodium reabsorption occurs in the proximal tubule. As sodium reabsorption is inhibited (as with diuretics), free water is excreted and diuresis ensues. *ADH*, antidiuretic hormone; *DCT*, distal convoluting tubule; *PCT*, proximal convoluting tubule; *TAL*, thick ascending limb. *From J. Goebel, A.B. Van Bakel, Rational use of diuretics in acute decompensated heart failure, Curr. Heart Fail. Rep. 5 (2008) 153–162.*

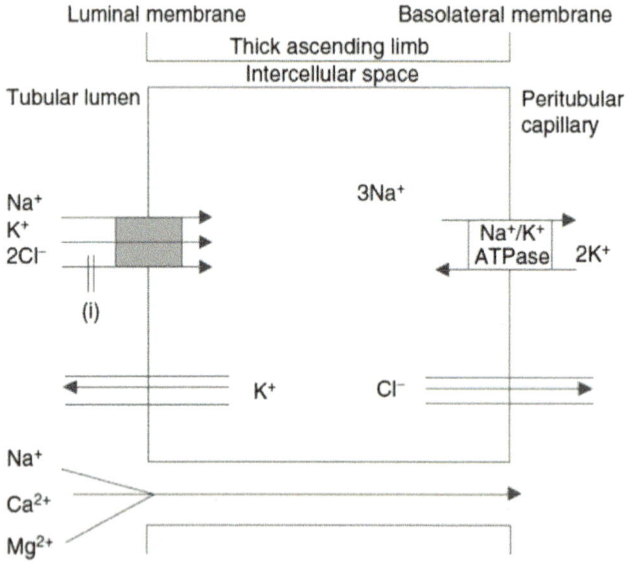

FIGURE 38.2 Passive sodium transport into the tubular cell, via the sodium–potassium–chloride ($Na^+/K^+/2Cl^-$) membrane carrier, and active sodium transport out of the cell via the Na^+/K^+-adenosine triphosphatase (ATPase) pump, and reabsorption of the cations Na^+, Ca^{2+}, and Mg^{2+}. (i) Loop diuretics block chloride uptake in the $Na^+/K^+/2Cl^-$ membrane carrier, leading to decreased sodium reabsorption. *From M.K. Von der Vorst, et al., Diuretics in pediatrics: current knowledge and future practice. Pediatr. Drugs 8 (2006) 245–264.*

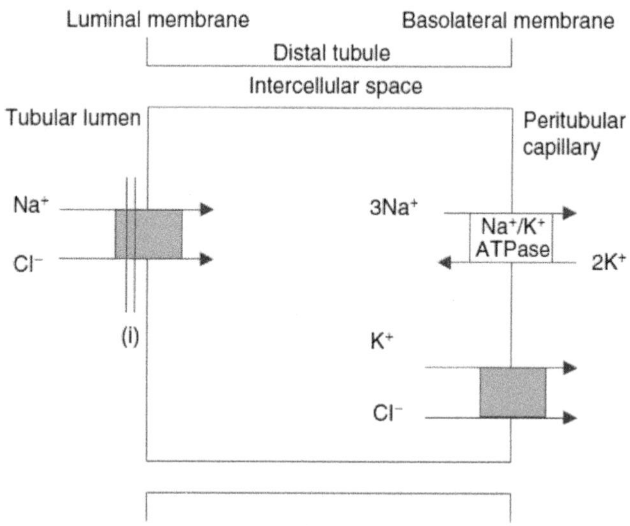

FIGURE 38.3 Diagram demonstrates the passive sodium transport into the tubular cell via the Na^+/Cl^- membrane carrier and the active sodium transport out of the cell via the Na^+/K^+ adenosine triphosphatase (ATPase) pump; (i) thiazide diuretics block the passive sodium transport into the cell. *From M.K. Von der Vorst, J.E. Kist, A.J. van der Heijden, J. Burggraaf, Diuretics in pediatrics: current knowledge and future practice, Pediatr. Drugs 8 (2006) 245–264.*

furosemide in treating volume overloaded heart failure patients [24–26] Murray et al. found that compared with furosemide-treated patients, torsemide-treated patients were less likely to need readmission for heart failure (32% vs. 19 17%, $P<.01$) or for all cardiovascular causes [24]. Patients treated with torsemide had significantly fewer hospital days for heart failure (106 vs. 296 days, $P=.02$) and had greater improvements in dyspnea and fatigue scores from baseline.

Ethacrynic Acid

The onset of action is rapid, usually 5 min within administration of an intravenous dose. Maximum response occurs within 15–30 min and persists for approximately hours [27]. Ethacrynic acid is often diuretic of choice when treating patients who have true sulfa allergies.

Thiazide Diuretics

Thiazides (hydrochlorothiazide, chlorothiazide, and metolazone) are less potent than loop diuretics. Their role should be viewed as an adjunct to further augment urine output in patients already treated with a loop diuretic. They act as inhibitors of the sodium–chloride (Na^+/Cl^-) cotransporter in the distal convoluted tubule, inhibiting reabsorption of sodium and chloride and increasing their urinary excretion (Fig. 38.3). Oral absorption is variable, with a peak effect of chlorothiazide when given intravenously occurring in ~30 min [13]. The duration of effect is about 6–12 h for hydrochlorothiazide and chlorothiazide. Metolazone oral absorption is also unpredictable and its duration of action is longer, generally reported to be 12–24 h. Metolazone is not structurally a thiazide but it has thiazide-like activity in the distal tubule [13]. It has a long half-life (2 days) and may be synergistic with the other thiazides [28].

Carbonic Anhydrase Inhibitor

The carbonic anhydrase inhibitors (acetazolamide) are relatively weak diuretics and are used mainly for the treatment of glaucoma. This class of diuretics acts by decreasing sodium and bicarbonate reabsorption in the proximal tubule. When carbonic anhydrase in the tubular cell is blocked, water reabsorption is deceased and a concomitant loss of bicarbonate in the urine results in a metabolic acidosis within 2–4 days of therapy [4]. This effect may be desirable and useful in heart failure patients who develop a hypochloremic metabolic alkalosis while being treated with loop diuretics. In a study of 74 adult patients with severe congestive heart failure and hypochloremic metabolic alkalosis while treated with furosemide, a combination of acetazolamide and spironolactone was administered for hypochloremic metabolic alkalosis [29]. Most of the patients experienced significant weight loss, even when furosemide dosing was held briefly, as well as correction of the metabolic abnormality.

Aldosterone Antagonist

The aldosterone antagonists (spironolactone, eplerenone) act on the collecting duct of the nephron, competing with aldosterone for the mineralocorticoid receptor and preventing aldosterone-induced potassium excretion and sodium resorption [13]. Spironolactone is more frequently prescribed than eplerenone in the pediatric heart failure population. It is a weak diuretic and is typically administered for its potassium-sparing and antifibrotic effects in heart failure patients. The Randomized Aldactone Evaluation Study (RALES) was designed to determine the mortality benefit of low-dose spironolactone among adult heart failure patients [30]. A 30% reduction in all-cause mortality was demonstrated in patients receiving spironolactone compared to those receiving placebo. Subsequently, the benefits of spironolactone in the RALES study were reproduced with eplerenone in the EMPHASIS-HF trial [31]. Spironolactone is only available as an oral preparation. Its pharmacokinetics is not well understood in infants and children. Serum potassium and creatinine concentrations should be monitored regularly when administering to children with heart failure.

Mannitol

Mannitol is an osmotic diuretic that is filtered freely in the glomerulus. Unlike other diuretics, tubular reabsorption does not occur. Water and potassium are shifted from the intracellular space to the extracellular fluid causing volume expansion, hyperkalemia, and hyponatremia. Pulmonary edema and worsening heart failure may occur, especially in patients with preexisting renal insufficiency. Because of this, mannitol and other osmotic diuretics are not recommended for the treatment of volume overloaded heart failure [28].

ADVERSE EFFECTS OF DIURETICS

All diuretics are associated with adverse effects such as dizziness, lightheadedness, nausea, cramping, blurred vision, weakness, paresthesia, acid–base disturbances, and electrolyte abnormalities.

Electrolyte Abnormalities

Potassium

Hypokalemia is the most common diuretic-associated electrolyte disturbance and diuretic therapy is the most common cause of hypokalemia [32]. In the ascending loop, diuretics have a direct kaliuretic effect. Furosemide activates the renin–angiotensin system and thus aldosterone-mediated potassium secretion in the collecting duct. In the distal tubule, sodium delivery is enhanced leading to potassium secretion [13]. Hypokalemia in heart failure is associated with an increased incidence of dysrhythmias and death [33,34]. Leier and colleagues recommend keeping serum potassium levels ≥4.5 mEq/L [35]. Hyperkalemia may also occur with administration of aldosterone antagonists such as spironolactone. Potassium concentrations should be monitored in heart failure patients who are treated with spironolactone, especially if angiotensin-converting enzyme inhibitors or digoxin are used concurrently as hyperkalemia may cause life-threatening arrhythmias.

Calcium

Loop diuretics may lead to hypocalcemia by enhancing the renal excretion of calcium. The inhibition of sodium reabsorption in the loop of Henle causes reduced reabsorption of calcium. Additionally, chronic loop diuretic use may cause volume contraction and alkalosis thereby increasing the concentration of serum proteins and protein-bound calcium leading to decreased free-calcium levels [36–38]. Hypocalcemia may also occur as a result of loop diuretic-induced hypomagnesemia [39]. High urinary excretion rates of calcium increases the risk of nephrolithiasis and nephrocalcinosis [40,41], especially in preterm infants. Nephrocalcinosis resolves in about 50 percent of premature infants, 5–6 months after furosemide has been discontinued [42]. Hydrochlorothiazide and spironolactone have also been linked to hypercalciuria in infants [43].

Magnesium

Serum magnesium concentration may be decreased in patients receiving potassium-wasting diuretic therapy, although the prevalence is low [44]. Among a group of hospitalized elderly patients, only those who were taking a thiazide diuretic were found to have reduced serum concentrations of diuretics [45]. An analysis of 199 adult patients with congestive heart failure who were receiving diuretics showed that serum magnesium concentration was <1.6 mEq/L in 19% of the cohort [46]. Hypomagnesemic patients had more frequent episodes of premature ventricular contractions and ventricular tachycardia compared to patients with normal magnesium levels. They also had worse survival rates at 1 and 2 years. The need for and benefit of magnesium replacement in patients receiving chronic diuretic therapy is uncertain.

Sodium

Hyponatremia is a common comorbidity in heart failure patients and portends a poor prognosis in patients hospitalized with decompensated heart failure [47,48]. In volume overloaded patients, it is thought that vasopressin acts on V2 receptors in the kidney to promote free-water retention, leading to dilutional hyponatremia. Some patients develop diuretic-induced hyponatremia while being treated for heart failure. This occurs more commonly in those receiving thiazides than in those receiving loop diuretics. The exact mechanisms are not fully understood but are likely related to increased water intake, reduced free-water clearance, and renal Na^+ and/or K^+ loss [49]. Mild to moderate hyponatremia may be reversed by instituting a fluid restriction, eliminating hypotonic fluids, and discontinuing thiazide diuretics. Vasopressin antagonists such as tolvaptan can be considered in hospitalized patients who are hyponatremic with hypervolemia (this is discussed in more detail later in the chapter). Patients who are symptomatic with severe hyponatremia should be considered for treatment with hypertonic saline.

Ototoxicity

Transient and permanent hearing loss and tinnitus have been described in patients treated with both oral and intravenous loop diuretics. Hearing impairment appears to occur more frequently with the use of ethacrynic acid and furosemide than with bumetanide. It is also more likely to occur when other ototoxic medications (e.g., aminoglycosides) are used simultaneously. The $Na^+/K^+/2Cl^-$ cotransporter is expressed in mammalian cochlea and thought to play an important role in ototoxicity. The mechanism of hearing loss may be due to electrolyte disturbances in the endolymph, edema of the stria vascularis in the cochlea, and alterations of the endocochlear potential [50,51].

Dehydration and Worsening Renal Function

Worsening renal function occurs commonly in adults and children with heart failure during treatment with diuretics. Aggressive diuresis can lead to dehydration and hypovolemia, even in fluid-overloaded heart failure patients. Fortunately, worsening renal function in this situation is often transient and resolves or improves once the diuretic is discontinued or the dose is decreased. Transient worsening renal function is associated with lower risk of mortality compared to persistent worsening renal function in adults with acute heart failure syndromes [52].

Although the mechanisms are not fully understood, diminished cardiac function coupled with renal dysfunction, or the cardiorenal syndrome, has been observed in both the acute and chronic care settings. The use of intravenous diuretics such as furosemide can activate the renin–angiotensin–aldosterone system leading to systemic vasoconstriction and fluid retention [53]. Intravenous furosemide can augment urine output but it does so at the expense of glomerular filtration rate after administration of a single dose of furosemide in adults with heart failure [54]. The renal insufficiency that occurs during the treatment of decompensated heart failure, however, cannot be attributed to diuretic therapy alone. Low blood pressure, elevated central venous pressure, and the use of potentially nephrotoxic medications also contribute to the cardiorenal syndrome in patients with heart failure.

Several studies have demonstrated the prognostic importance of increasing serum creatinine concentrations for predicting morbidity and mortality in adult patients with heart failure [54–58]. Among patients hospitalized for acute decompensated heart failure, worsening renal function is associated with longer length of stay, higher in-hospital costs, and an increased risk of in-hospital mortality [59]. Even a modest increase in serum creatinine (i.e., >0.3 mg/dL) can predict mortality in patients hospitalized for heart failure [60]. The largest study examining combined heart failure and renal dysfunction in children described the prevalence of renal insufficiency in 73 consecutive patient hospitalizations with a primary diagnosis of acute decompensated heart failure [61]. All patients were treated with intravenous furosemide. Worsening renal function was defined as an increase in serum creatinine of ≥0.3 mg/dL at any time during hospitalization. Renal failure at the time of admission was uncommon in this cohort but serum creatinine subsequently increased in 82% and worsening renal function occurred during 48% of hospitalizations. In this cohort of children, worsening renal function was found to be an independent predictor of death or the need for mechanical circulatory assistance during hospitalization and was associated with a longer observed length of stay.

RATIONAL USE OF DIURETICS IN PEDIATRIC HEART FAILURE

The principal goal of diuretic therapy in patients suffering from heart failure is to alleviate symptoms and ultimately eliminate or reduce clinical evidence of fluid retention. This is a Class I recommendation from the American Heart Association and the American College of Cardiology in fluid-overloaded patients with heart failure and reduced ejection fraction [62]. Furosemide has become the first-line diuretic of choice in adults and children in this condition. If patients require hospitalization for fluid overload, they should initially be treated with loop diuretics, preferably intravenously [63]. Data from the Acute Decompensated Heart Failure Registry showed that approximately 90% of adults hospitalized with acute heart failure were treated with intravenous loop diuretics [2]. In a study of children hospitalized with acute decompensated heart failure, diuretics were prescribed in 90.1% of patients [3]. Furosemide was the most commonly prescribed diuretic during pediatric hospitalization, administered intravenously in 72% of patients and enterally in 71%. Intravenous furosemide was administered for a median of 4 days before patients were transitioned to oral therapy.

Evidence of congestion is frequently present in children with advanced heart failure. In a study of 141 children hospitalized with heart failure, manifest signs or symptoms of volume overload included dyspnea or increased work of breathing (63%), gallop rhythm (55%), hepatomegaly (45%), and rales (20%) [47]. Chest radiography demonstrated pulmonary vascular congestion in 54% and pleural effusions in 26%. Nearly 86% of children who present to the emergency department with acute heart failure have at least one respiratory-related sign or symptom of congestion [64]. More than half of children with end-stage heart failure who undergo cardiac catheterization are found to have elevated filling pressures, with a pulmonary capillary wedge pressure of >18 mmHg or a right atrial pressure >8 mmHg [65]. Thus, the use of a diuretic as first-line therapy in pediatric decompensated heart failure is a rational choice. Furthermore, diuretics may also improve cardiac performance. Lowered ventricular filling pressures may lessen subendomyocardial ischemia, decrease myocardial wall stress, and reduce mitral regurgitation leading to improved cardiac output [1].

Inpatient therapy should be commenced in the emergency center without delay as early treatment with intravenous heart failure therapies may be associated with better outcomes [66–68]. Delays in diuretic administration at hospital presentation have been reported in both adults and children with heart failure [64,69]. In a cohort of 60 children who presented to the hospital with heart failure exacerbation and clinical evidence of fluid retention, the median time to first administration of a diuretic was 5.8 h when given in the emergency department [64]. This time from "door-to-diuretic" has recently become a focus of quality improvement [70].

During inpatient treatment with diuretics, patients should be monitored closely for ongoing response to therapy and side effects. Documentation of fluid balance and daily weights is recommended and may helpful to determine adequacy of decongestion therapy [62]. However, these measures can be difficult to obtain with accuracy and discrepancy between fluid balance and weight loss, which is common in hospitalized patients [71]. Daily or frequent measurement of electrolytes and serum creatinine are recommended in the early treatment with intravenous diuretics or when used in combination with digitalis or angiotensin-converting enzyme inhibitors.

Inadequate diuresis during hospitalization is not uncommon [72]. Data from the ADHERE Registry show that approximately 42% of adult patients are discharged with persistent symptoms of fluid overload, one-third lose fewer than 5 pounds, while hospitalized and 16% actually gain weight during hospitalization [73]. One potential contributor to the inability to adequately decongest the fluid-overloaded patient is the coadministration of intravenous fluids and diuretics. In a review of over 130,000 adult hospitalizations for heart failure management, 11% of patients were treated with intravenous fluids and loop diuretics during the first 2 days of admission [74]. The use of intravenous fluids was associated with worse outcomes, including higher rates of subsequent critical care admission, mechanical ventilation, renal replacement therapy, and hospital death, when compared to patients who were not treated with fluids.

Once the symptoms of congestion are ameliorated, the route of administration can be transitioned from intravenous to enteral. Most patients who are discharged home following a heart failure hospitalization should be maintained on diuretics through the first follow-up visit. Inadequate diuresis during hospitalization or shortly after discharge, along with many cofactors, may contribute to rehospitalization. Among adults discharged following inpatient treatment for heart failure, nearly 20% were readmitted within 30 days [75]. The readmission rate is lower in children, with only 13% requiring rehospitalization for heart failure–related illness within 30 days of hospital discharge [76].

DIURETIC RESISTANCE

In some situations, the recommended use of diuretics does not achieve the intended results and heart failure patients remain congested. A failure to adequately decongest despite escalating doses of diuretics has been termed "diuretic resistance." There are several physiologic and pharmacologic causes of diuretic resistance.

An important concept in understanding diuretic resistance is the development of diminished natriuresis (or the "breaking phenomenon") that occurs with chronic administration of diuretics. Several physiologic and pharmacologic mechanisms lead to decreased urinary sodium excretion, shifting the dose–response curve downward and to the right in patients with heart failure (Fig. 38.4) [77]. During treatment with diuretics, decreased extracellular fluid volume leads to increased solute and fluid reabsorption in the proximal tubule [78]. Reduced interstitial pressure caused by volume contraction further enhances proximal solute and fluid reabsorption. Stimulation of renin and renal efferent sympathetic nerves also contributes to increased sodium reabsorption and reduced sodium excretion due to decreased renal blood flow. Chronic administration of diuretics to rats leads to hypertrophy and hyperplasia of the epithelial cells of the distal convoluted tubule, causing increased sodium reabsorption in this segment of the nephron [79–81] (Fig. 38.5).

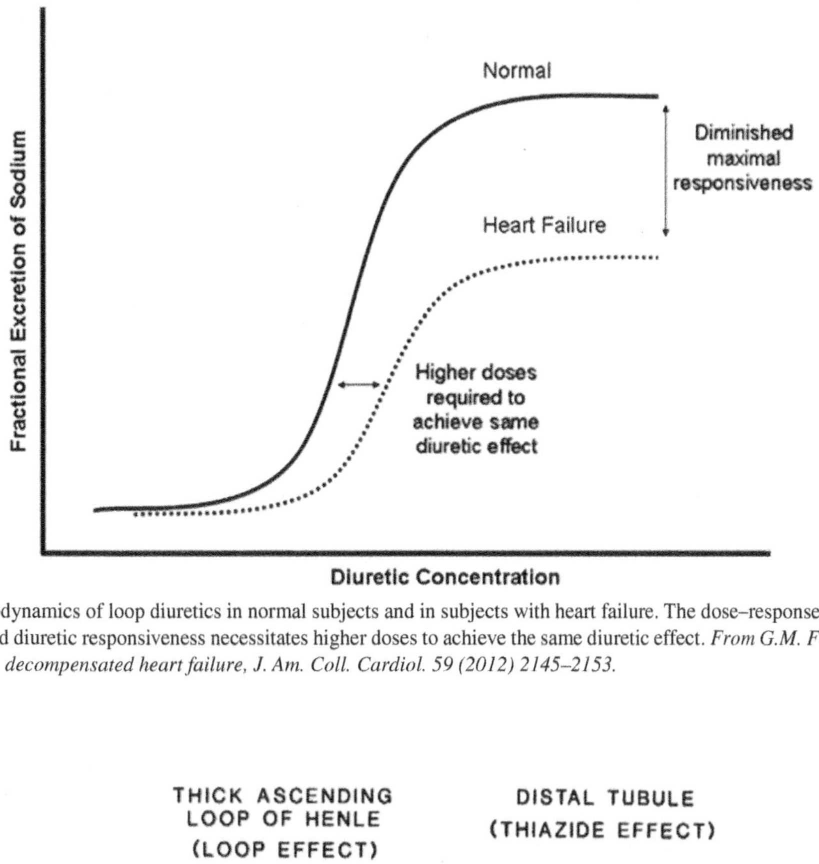

FIGURE 38.4 Pharmacodynamics of loop diuretics in normal subjects and in subjects with heart failure. The dose–response curve is shifted downward and to the right. Diminished diuretic responsiveness necessitates higher doses to achieve the same diuretic effect. *From G.M. Felker, R.J. Mentz, Diuretics and ultrafiltration in acute decompensated heart failure, J. Am. Coll. Cardiol. 59 (2012) 2145–2153.*

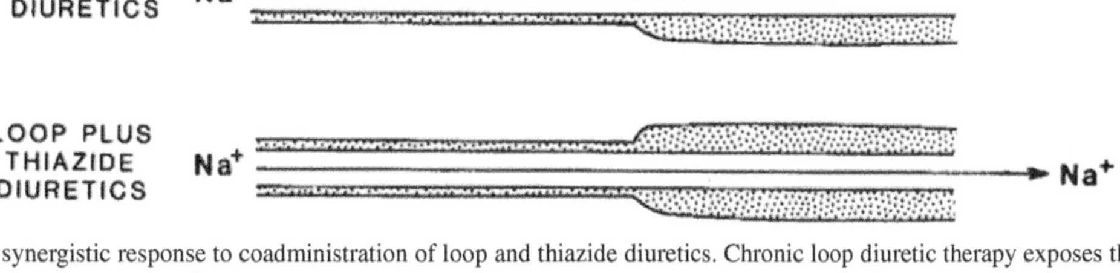

FIGURE 38.5 The synergistic response to coadministration of loop and thiazide diuretics. Chronic loop diuretic therapy exposes the distal nephron to excess sodium causing cellular hypertrophy. Blocking the thickened nephrons leads to improved natriuresis due to the synergism of loop and thiazide diuretics. *From D.C. Brater, Update in diuretic therapy: Clinical pharmacology. Semin. Nephrol. 31 (2011) 483–494.*

The treatment of diuretic resistance requires that heart failure therapies be optimized and nephrotoxic therapies be minimized or eliminated. Invasive monitoring of central venous pressure may be helpful in some situations. Hemodynamic perturbations such as systemic hypotension and cardiac arrhythmias must be corrected. The use of sympathomimetic agents in patients who are normotensive may compromise renal perfusion and their use should be limited. Nonsteroidal antiinflammatory agents should also be discontinued due to their potential nephrotoxic effects and small risk for fluid retention. In patients with low cardiac output and a wide-QRS rhythm, cardiac resynchronization therapy should be considered to optimize atrioventricular conduction. Implantation of a short-term or long-term ventricular assist device may significantly improve cardiac output and lower central venous pressures, allowing for improved renal perfusion.

In some situations, ineffective dosing may lead to perceived diuretic resistance. In heart failure patients with renal insufficiency the response to diuretics is decreased compared to patients with preserved renal function [82]. Simply using higher doses of diuretics may be sufficient to improve urine output. In the Diuretic Optimization Strategies Evaluation (DOSE) trial, adults with acute decompensated heart failure who were treated with intravenous high-dose diuretics (2.5 times their total daily oral dose of furosemide) had greater relief from symptoms of dyspnea, change in weight, and change in fluid balance at 72 h than those who received low-dose furosemide [83]. When administering intravenous diuretics, it is important to remember that the use of diuretics has been reported to activate the renin–angiotensin–aldosterone system [53,84]. An upregulated neurohormonal system is associated with progression of heart failure. However, a recent study by Mentz et al. found that high-dose diuretic was not associated with activation of the renin–angiotensin–aldosterone system compared to low-dose diuretic [85]. In that study, neurohormonal activation was measured at a specific time point (72 or 96 h after diuretic dose) as opposed to the earlier studies that measured biomarkers within hours of therapy and that may explain the discrepancy in findings.

Administering a different type of diuretic in combination with loop diuretics may also augment urine output [86–90]. The chronic use of a loop diuretic leads to increased delivery of sodium to the distal tubule causing hypertrophy of the nephron and increased reabsorption. The addition of a thiazide diuretic will block sodium at the distal tubule and enhance diuresis in a synergistic fashion (See Fig. 38.5). This strategy of sequential nephron blockade was utilized in a study of 20 adult patients with severe congestive heart failure and diuretic resistance while receiving high-dose furosemide. The addition of hydrochlorothiazide resulted in improved urine output and decreased creatinine clearance [86]. Hypokalemia was an important side effect of this strategy and occurred in the majority of the patients. Kiyingi et al. reported on the combination of oral metolazone with a loop diuretic in adults with New York Heart AssociationClass IV congestive heart failure who failed to adequately respond to the loop diuretic alone [91]. 12 of 17 patients responded with a brisk diuresis and weight loss. Metolazone therapy was associated with transient hypokalemia in 7 patients and renal insufficiency in 1. Most patients were subsequently discharged with improved symptoms despite their initial inadequate response to the loop diuretics.

In children who remain symptomatic with evidence of fluid overload and despite adequate diuretic dosing, decongestion may be enhanced by administering a continuous infusion of loop diuretic rather than bolus injections. Luciani et al. demonstrated that among critically ill neonates and infants who have undergone cardiac surgery, a continuously infused loop diuretic afforded lower total diuretic dosing with comparable urine output to bolus dosing and lesser fluctuations in urine output and need for fluid replacement [92]. A metaanalysis performed by Salvador et al. showed that urine output was greater in adult heart failure patients receiving continuous infusions of diuretic compared to patients receiving intermittent dosing. Continuous infusions were also associated with fewer adverse effects (tinnitus and hearing loss), shortened hospital stay and lower all-cause mortality than in patients receiving bolus injections [93]. However, results from the DOSE trial suggest that continuous infusions have no added benefit to adult patients hospitalized with decompensated heart failure [83]. In that study, bolus furosemide was compared to continuous infusion. There was no difference in the two types of therapies with regard to patients' assessment of symptoms, serum creatinine, change in weight, or net fluid balance.

The nonosmotic release of vasopressin in advanced heart failure leads to increased water reabsorption and hyponatremia in some patients. Vasopressin antagonists that block the V2 receptors of the kidney have been shown to enhance free-water excretion, correct hyponatremia and improve symptoms [94–96]. In a small series of pediatric patients with heart failure, tolvaptan was associated with increased urine output at 24 h [97]. More recently, however, two well-designed studies in adults with acute heart failure study showed that the addition of tolvaptan to standard therapy did not result in significant improvement in dyspnea despite greater fluid loss and weight loss [98,99]. The role of vasopressin antagonists in acute heart failure and diuretic resistance is not clear at this time.

Recent studies have described the concomitant use of small-volume hypertonic saline and a loop diuretic for the treatment of diuretic resistance in patients with advanced heart failure [100–103]. The administration of hypertonic saline with intravenous diuretic was associated with increased diuresis, reduced hospital readmissions, reduced hospital length of stay, improved neurohormonal biomarker concentrations, and reduced mortality. It is thought that hypertonic saline causes a shift of fluid from the extravascular space into the intravascular space thereby affecting the baroreceptor signals and reducing systemic vascular resistance. This decrease in afterload results in improved cardiac output and end-organ perfusion, including the kidneys. There is little evidence for the use of hypertonic saline in children with heart failure and diuretic resistance.

The addition of spironolactone to standard therapy may promote increased urine output in patients with refractory congestive heart failure. Van Vliet et al. described a small cohort of adults with advanced heart failure and diuretic resistance who remained fluid overloaded despite treatment with high-dose loop diuretic and an angiotensin-converting enzyme inhibitor [104]. After 1 week of combination therapy with 100 mg spironolactone per day, marked natriuresis and diuresis were observed in most of the patients. The effectiveness of this combination was thought to be due to enhanced antagonism of the renin–angiotensin–aldosterone system. When high doses of spironolactone such as this are used it is important to closely monitor serum potassium levels and hydration status.

ULTRAFILTRATION

Ultrafiltration is sometimes utilized in decompensated heart failure as an alternative therapy to diuretics for restoring fluid balance. It is a tool for rapid and stabilized fluid removal with volume extraction rates as high as 500 mL/h in adults. Venovenous ultrafiltration can be performed with either peripheral, midline, or central access. Two venous lines are necessary and a minimum blood flow rate of 10 mL/min is necessary. Anticoagulation with heparin is generally recommended. The ultrafiltrate circuit is portable and consists of blood and ultrafiltrate pumps, filter, pressure sensors, and collection bag (See Fig. 38.6) [77].

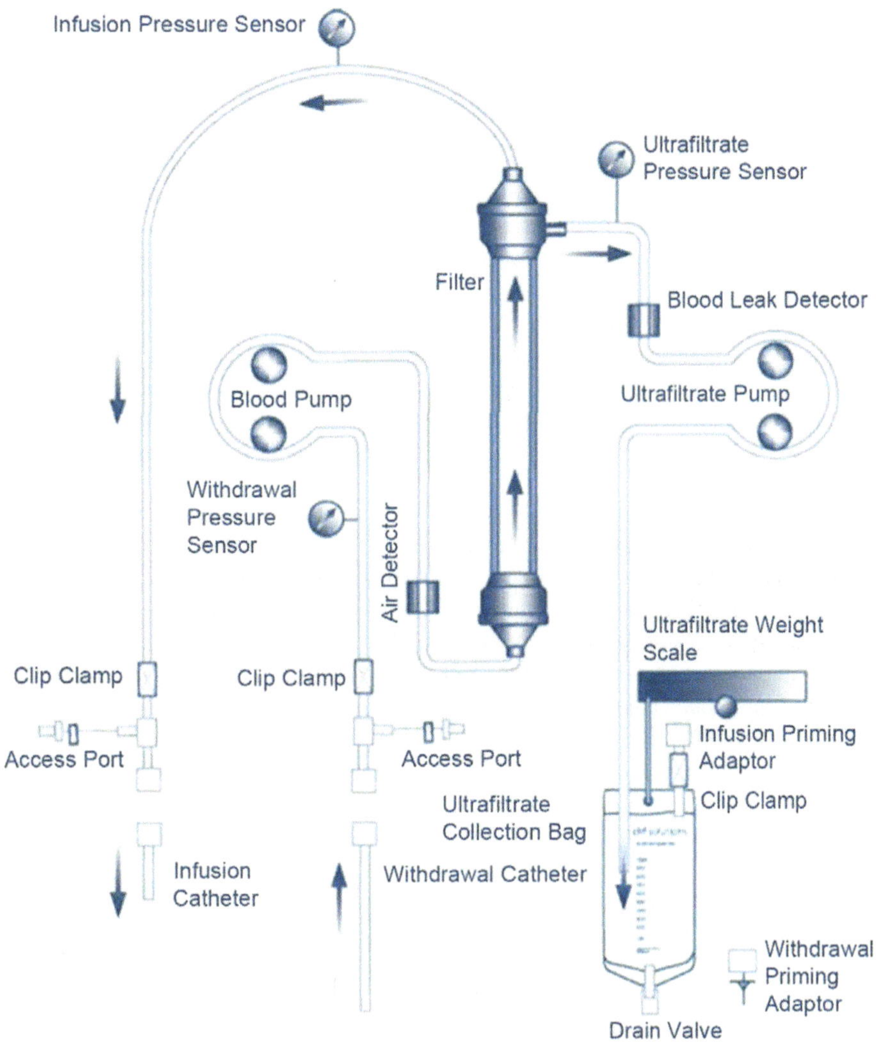

FIGURE 38.6 Ultrafiltration system for fluid overload in acute decompensated heart failure. *From G.M. Felker, R.J. Mentz, Diuretics and ultrafiltration in acute decompensated heart failure, J. Am. Coll. Cardiol. 59 (2012) 2145–2153.*

For several years, clinical trials have attempted to determine the safety and efficacy of ultrafiltration in fluid-overloaded states [105–108]. Some potential advantages of ultrafiltration over conventional therapy with diuretics include minimal or no neurohormonal activation, fewer electrolyte disturbances, greater sodium clearance, rapid symptomatic relief, and improved fluid removal in diuretic resistance. Early studies in small cohorts reported favorable findings. In a study of 22 adults with congestive heart failure, measurements of plasma renin activity as well as aldosterone, and norepinephrine concentrations decreased significantly after 48 h of treatment and a 20% decreased in plasma volume [105]. In a similarly small study of adults with refractory congestive heart failure, cardiac hemodynamics (right atrial pressure, pulmonary artery pressure, wedge pressure) improved during the procedure and cardiac output increased by the end of treatment with no instability in blood pressure or intravascular volume status [106]. Because the ultrafiltrate is isotonic, more sodium can be extracted at a similar volume loss than what is achieved with diuretics, and natriuresis/diuresis may be enhanced with improved hemodynamics [106,109].

These small early studies had no follow up or findings beyond the immediate effects of the procedure. Larger clinical trials have given more insight into the efficacy and role of ultrafiltration in decompensated heart failure. The RAPID-CHF (Relief for Acutely Fluid-Overloaded Patients with Decompensated Congestive Heart Failure) trial randomized patients who were hospitalized with decompensated heart failure and fluid overload to an 8 h session of ultrafiltration or to standard care [108]. After 24 h of treatment, patients who received ultrafiltration had greater fluid removal than subjects who received standard care but there was no significant difference in weight loss between the two groups. Dyspnea and heart failure symptoms were improved in the ultrafiltration group compared to the standard care group. Costanzo et al. examined the use of ultrafiltration in heart failure patients with renal insufficiency and diuretic resistance [110] and found similar favorable results. After fluid removal with ultrafiltration, subjects experienced significant weight loss, improved measures of quality of life, and decreased B-type natriuretic peptide concentrations.

The UNLOAD (Ultrafiltration vs. Intravenous Diuretics for Patients Hospitalized for Acute Decompensated Congestive Heart Failure) trial randomized 200 adult heart failure subjects to treatment with either ultrafiltration or intravenous loop diuretic with primary end-points of weight loss and dyspnea assessment at 48 h after randomization [111]. At 48 h, weight loss was greater in the ultrafiltration group compared to the diuretic group but no difference in dyspnea scores between the two groups. At 90 days, rehospitalization rates and length of stay were lower in the ultrafiltration group.

In the smaller but more recent CARRESS-HF (Cardiorenal Rescue Study in Acute Decompensated Heart Failure) trial, investigators sought to determine the efficacy and safety of ultrafiltration in decompensated heart failure complicated by persistent congestion and worsening renal function [112]. One hundred and eighty-eight subjects were randomized to either ultrafiltration or stepped medical therapy. The primary end point was the bivariate change in serum creatinine and weight at 96 h after randomization. Serum creatinine increased in the ultrafiltration group compared to the medical therapy group and there was no difference in weights at 96 h. Additionally, the ultrafiltration group experienced a higher incidence of adverse events than the medical group. Enrollment ended early as there was no evidence of benefit and the adverse event rate was unacceptably high. The study's design has been criticized since subjects in the ultrafiltration group were not allowed to receive vasoactive agents and the rate of ultrafiltration could not be adjusted although the medical group was allowed to have their pharmacologic therapy adjusted.

The most recent trial to study the efficacy of ultrafiltration in heart failure is the AVOID-HF (Study of Heart Failure Hospitalizations after Aquapheresis Therapy Compared with Intravenous Diuretic Treatment) trial [113]. In this multicenter study, patients were randomized to receive either adjustable ultrafiltration or diuretics. The primary outcome was time to first heart failure event after hospital discharge. The study was terminated prematurely due to slow enrollment and failed to show that ultrafiltration prolonged the time to first heart failure event.

The role of ultrafiltration in the treatment of heart failure remains uncertain at this time. Societal guidelines for the use of ultrafiltration in acute decompensated heart failure are vague. The need for central venous access, cost, provider inexperience, and lack of clear understanding of safety and efficacy in special groups makes the use of ultrafiltration somewhat problematic. Currently, there is no clear role for ultrafiltration in the treatment of children with heart failure and fluid overload.

REFERENCES

[1] A. Ramierez, W.H. Abelmann, Hemodynamic effects of diuresis by ethacrynic acid, Arch. Intern. Med. 121 (1968) 320–326.

[2] C.L. Emerman, T.D. Marco, M.R. Costanzo, W.F. Peacock, For the ASAC. Impact of intravenous diuretics on the outcomes of patients hospitalized with acute decompensated heart failure: insights from the ADHERE(R) Registry, J. Card. Fail. 10 (2004) S116–S117.

[3] B.S. Moffett, J.F. Price, National prescribing trends for heart failure medications in children, Congenit. Heart Dis. 10 (2015) 78–85.

[4] M.K. Von der Vorst, J.E. Kist, A.J. van der Heijden, J. Burggraaf, Diuretics in pediatrics: Current knowledge and future practice, Pediatr. Drugs 8 (2006) 245–264.

[5] S.K. Eades, M.L. Christensen, The clinical pharmacology of loop diuretics in the pediatric patient, Pediatr. Nephrol. 12 (1998) 603–616.
[6] J.E. Sullivan, M.K. Witte, T.S. Yamashita, C.M. Myers, J.L. Blumer, Analysis of the variability in the pharmacokinetics and pharmacodynamics of bumetanide in critically ill infants, Clin. Pharmacol. Ther. 60 (1996) 414–423.
[7] J.E. Sullivan, M.K. Witte, T.S. Yamashita, C.M. Myers, J.L. Blumer, Pharmacokinetics of bumetanide in critically ill infants, Clin. Pharmacol. Ther. 60 (1996) 405–413.
[8] J.E. Sullivan, M.K. Witte, T.S. Yamashita, C.M. Myers, J.L. Blumer, Dose-ranging evaluation of bumetanide pharmacodynamics in critically ill infants, Clin. Pharmacol. Ther. 60 (1996) 424–434.
[9] J.D. Marshall, T.G. Wells, L. Letzig, G.L. Kearns, Pharmacokinetics and pharmacodynamics of bumetanide in critically ill pediatric patients, J. Clin. Pharmacol. 38 (1998) 994–1002.
[10] A.M. Lopez, M.W. Modi, J.A. Adams, Pharmacokinetics of bumetanide in the newborn infant, Pediatr. Res. 27 (1990) 62A.
[11] S. Shankaran, N. Ilagan, K.C. Liang, Bumetanide pharmacokinetics in preterm neonates, Pediatr. Res. 25 (1989) 72A.
[12] R. Nau, Osmotherapy for elevated intracranial pressure: a critical reappraisal, Clin. Pharmacokinet. 38 (2000) 23–40.
[13] J. Goebel, A.B. Van Bakel, Rational use of diuretics in acute decompensated heart failure, Curr. Heart Fail. Rep. 5 (2008) 132–162.
[14] J.V. Aranda, J. Perez, D.S. Sitar, J. Collinage, A. Portuguez-Malavasi, B. Duffy, C. Dupont, Pharmacokinetic disposition and protein binding of furosemide in newborn infants, J. Pediatr. 93 (1978) 507–511.
[15] L. Lowrie, Diuretic therapy of heart failure in infants and children, Prog. Pediatr. Cardiol. 12 (2000) 45–55.
[16] D.C. Brater, Pharmacokinetics of loop diuretics in congestive heart failure, Br. Heart J. 72 (1994) S40–S43.
[17] S. Tuck, P. Morselli, M. Broquaire, P. Vert, Plasma and urinary kinetics of furosemide in newborn infants, J. Pediatr. 103 (1983) 481–485.
[18] M.H. Mirochnick, J.J. Miceli, P.A. Kramer, D.J. Chapron, J.R. Raye, Furosemide pharmacokinetics in very low birth weight infants, J. Pediatr. 112 (4) (1988) 653–657.
[19] M.L. Buck, Furosemide: a review of its use in infants and children, Pediatr. Pharm. 15 (8) (2009).
[20] J. Prandota, Clinical pharmacology of furosemide in children: a supplement, Am. J. Ther. 8 (2001) 275–289.
[21] D.C. Brater, Diuretic pharmacokinetics and pharmacodynamics, in: C.J. van Boxtel, N.H.G. Holford, M. Danhof (Eds.), The in Vivo Study of Drug Action: Principles and Applications of Kinetic-dynamic Modeling, Elsevier Science, Amsterdam, 1992, pp. 253–275.
[22] R.K. Verbeeck, J.F. Gerkens, G.R. Wilkinson, R.A. Branch, Disposition of furosemide in functionally hepatectomized dogs, J. Pharmacol. Exp. Ther. 216 (3) (1981) 479–483.
[23] L.A. Marcantonio, W.H. Auld, G.G. Skellern, C.A. Howes, W.R. Murdoch, R. Purohit, The pharmacokinetics and pharmacodynamics of bumetanide in normal subjects, J. Pharmacokinet. Biopharm. 10 (1982) 393–409.
[24] M.D. Murray, M.M. Deer, J.A. Ferguson, P.R. Dexter, S.J. Bennett, S.M. Perkins, F.E. Smith, K.A. Lane, L.D. Adams, W.M. Tierney, D.C. Brater, Open-label randomized trial of torsemide compared with furosemide therapy for patients with heart failure, Am. J. Med. 111 (2001) 513–520.
[25] J. Cosin, J. Diez, Toric Investigators, Torasemide in chronic heart failure: results of the TORIC study, Eur. J. Heart Fail. 4 (2002) 507–513.
[26] K. Mueller, G. Gamba, F. Jaquet, B. Hess, Torasemide vs. furosemide in primary care patients with chronic heart failure NYHA II to IV–efficacy and quality of life, Eur. J. Heart Fail. 5 (2003) 793–801.
[27] J. Molnar, J.C. Somber, The clinical pharmacology of ethacrynic acid, Am. J. Ther. 16 (2009) 86–92.
[28] H.A. Dickerson, A.C. Chang, Diuretics, in: Chang, Towbin (Eds.), Heart Failure in Children and Young Adults, Elsevier, Philadelphia, 2006.
[29] M.I. Khan, Treatment of refractory congestive heart failure and normokalemic hypochloremic alkalosis with acetazolamide and spironolactone, Can. Med. Assoc. J. 123 (1980) 883–887.
[30] B. Pitt, F. Zannad, W.J. Remme, R. Cody, A. Castaigne, A. Perez, J. Palensky, J. Wittes, The effect of spironolactone on morbidity and mortality in patients with severe heart failure. Randomized Aldactone Evaluation Study Investigators, N. Engl. J. Med. 341 (1999) 709–717.
[31] F. Zannad, J.J. McMurray, H. Krum, D.J. van Veldhuisen, K. Swedberg, H. Shi, J. Vincent, S.J. Pocock, B. Pitt, EMPHASIS-HF Study Group, Eplerenone in patients with systolic heart failure and mild symptoms, N. Engl. J. Med. 364 (2011) 11–21.
[32] J.P. Knochel, Diuretic-induced hypokalemia, Am. J. Med. 77 (1984) 18–27.
[33] J.G.F. Cleland, H.J. Dargie, Arrhythmias, catecholamines and electrolytes, Am. J. Cardiol. 62 (1988) 55A–59A.
[34] H.J. Dargie, J.G.F. Cleland, V.J. Leckie, C.G. Inglis, B.W. East, I. Ford, Relation of arrhythmias and electrolyte abnormalities to survival in patients with severe chronic heart failure, Circulation 75 (1987) 98–107.
[35] C.V. Leier, L. Dei Cas, M. Metro, Clinical relevance and management of the major electrolyte abnormalities in congestive heart failure: hyponatremia, hypokalemia, and hypomagnesemia, Am. Heart J. 128 (1994) 564–574.
[36] G. Liamis, H.J. Milionis, M. Ellisaf, A review of drug-induced hypocalcemia, J. Bone Miner. Metab. 27 (2009) 635–642.
[37] B.D. Rose, Diuretics, Kidney Int. 39 (1991) 336–352.
[38] M. Haas, The Na–K–Cl cotransporters, Am. J. Physiol. 267 (1994) C869–C885.
[39] H.J. Milionis, G.E. Alexandrides, E.N. Liberopoulos, E.T. Bairaktari, J. Goudevenos, M.S. Elisaf, Hypomagnesemia and concurrent acid–base and electrolyte abnormalities in patients with congestive heart failure, Eur. J. Heart Fail. 4 (2002) 167–173.
[40] H.N. Noe, J.F. Bryant, S. Roy III, F.B. Stapleton, Urolithiasis in pre-term neonates associated with furosemide therapy, J. Urol. 132 (1984) 93–94.
[41] K.G. Hufnagle, S.N. Khan, D. Penn, A. Cacciarelli, P. Williams, Renal calcifications: a complication of long-term furosemide therapy in preterm infants, Pediatrics 70 (1982) 360–363.
[42] J.C. Pope, L.A. Trusler, A.M. Klein, W.F. Walsh, A. Yared, J.W. Brock, The natural history of nephrocalcinosis in premature infants treated with loop diuretics, J. Urol. 156 (1996) 709–712.

[43] S.A. Atkinson, J.K. Shah, C. McGee, B.T. Steele, Mineral excretion in premature infants receiving various diuretic therapies, J. Pediatr. 113 (1988) 540–545.
[44] K. Kroenke, D.R. Wood, J.F. Hanley, The value of serum magnesium determination in hypertensive patients receiving diuretics, Arch. Intern. Med. 147 (9) (1987) 1553–1556.
[45] B.J. Martin, K. Milligan, Diuretic-associated hypomagnesemia in the elderly, Arch. Intern. Med. 147 (1987) 1768–1771.
[46] S.S. Gottlieb, L. Baruch, M.L. Kukin, J.L. Bernstein, M.L. Fisher, M. Packer, Prognostic importance of the serum magnesium concentrations in patients with congestive heart failure, J. Am. Coll. Cardiol. 16 (1990) 827–831.
[47] J.F. Price, P.F. Kantor, R.E. Shaddy, J.W. Rossano, J.F. Goldberg, J. Hagan, T.J. Humlicek, A.G. Cabrera, A. Jeewa, S.W. Denfield, W.J. Dreyer, A. Akcan-Arikan, Incidence, severity, and association with adverse outcome of hyponatremia in children hospitalized with heart failure, Am. J. Cardiol. 118 (2016) 1006–1010.
[48] M. Sonnenblick, Y. Friedlander, A.J. Rosin, Diuretic-induced severe hyponatremia. Review and analysis of 129 reported patients, Chest 103 (1993) 601.
[49] K.S. Hwang, G.H. Kim, Thiazide-Induced Hyponatremia, vol. 8, Electrolyte Blood Press, 2010, pp. 51–57.
[50] K. Ikeda, T. Oshima, H. Hidaka, T. Takasak, Molecular and clinical implications of loop diuretic ototoxicity, Hear. Res. 107 (1997) 1–8.
[51] L.P. Rybak, Furosemide ototoxicity: clinical and experimental aspects, Laryngoscope (Suppl. 38) (1985) 1–14.
[52] D. Aronson, A.J. Burger, The relationship between transient and persistent worsening renal function and mortality in patients with acute decompensated heart failure, J. Card. Fail. 16 (2010) 541–547.
[53] J. Bayliss, M. Norell, Canepa-Anelson, G. Sutton, P. Poole-Wilson, Untreated heart failure: clinical and neuroendocrine effects of introducing diuretics, Br. Heart J. 57 (1987) 17–22.
[54] S.S. Gottlieb, W. Abraham, J. Butler, D.E. Forman, E. Loh, B.M. Massie, C.M. O'connor, M.W. Rich, L.W. Stevenson, J. Young, H.M. Krumholz, The prognostic importance of different definitions of worsening renal function in congestive heart failure, J. Card. Fail. 8 (2002) 136–141.
[55] M.S. Weinfeld, G.M. Chertow, L.W. Stevenson, Aggravated renal dysfunction during intensive therapy for advanced heart failure, Am. Heart J. 138 (1999) 285–290.
[56] H.L. Hillege, A.R. Girbes, P.J. de Kam, F. Boomsma, D. de Zeeuw, A. Charlesworth, J.R. Hampton, D.J. van Veldhuisen, Renal function, neurohormonal activation, and survival in patients with chronic heart failure, Circulation 102 (2000) 203–210.
[57] N.G. Mahon, E.H. Blackstone, G.S. Francis, R.C. Starling 3rd, J.B. Young, M.S. Lauer, The prognostic value of estimated creatinine clearance alongside functional capacity ambulatory patients with chronic congestive heart failure, J. Am. Coll. Cardiol. 40 (2002) 1106–1113.
[58] D.E. Forman, J. Butler, Y. Wang, W.T. Abraham, C.M. O'Connor, S.S. Gottlieb, E. Loh, B.M. Massie, M.W. Rich, L.W. Stevenson, J.B. Young, H.M. Krumholz, Incidence, predictors at admission, and impact of worsening renal function among patients hospitalized with heart failure, J. Am. Coll. Cardiol. 43 (2004) 61–67.
[59] H.M. Krumholz, Y.T. Chen, V. Vaccarino, Y. Wang, M.J. Radford, W.D. Bradford, R.I. Horwitz, Correlates and impact on outcomes of worsening renal function in patients ≥65 years of age with heart failure, Am. J. Cardiol. 85 (2000) 1110–1113.
[60] G.L. Smith, V. Vaccarino, M. Kosiborod, J.H. Lichtman, S. Cheng, S.G. Watnick, H. Krumholz, Worsening renal function: what is a clinically meaningful change in creatinine during hospitalization with heart failure? J. Card. Fail. 9 (2003) 13–25.
[61] J.F. Price, A.R. Mott, H.A. Dickerson, J.L. Jefferies, D.P. Nelson, A.C. Chang, E. O'Brian Smith, J.A. Towbin, W.J. Dreyer, S.W. Denfield, S.L. Goldstein, Worsening renal function in children hospitalized with decompensated heart failure: evidence for a pediatric cardiorenal syndrome? Pediatr. Crit. Care Med. 9 (2008) 279–284.
[62] C.W. Yancy, M. Jessup, B. Bozkurt, J. Butler, D.E. Casey, M.H. Drazner, G.C. Fonarow, S.A. Geraci, T. Horwich, J.L. Januzzi, M.R. Johnson, E.K. Kasper, W.C. Levy, F.A. Masoudi, P.E. McBride, J.J. McMurray, J.E. Mitchell, P.N. Peterson, B. Riegel, F. Sam, L.W. Stevenson, W.H. Tang, E.J. Tsai, B.L. Wilkoff, 2013 ACCF/AHA guideline for the management of heart failure: a report of the American College of Cardiology Foundation/American Heart Association Task Force on Practice Guidelines, Circulation 128 (2013) e240–e327.
[63] M. Jessup, W.T. Abraham, D.E. Casey, A.M. Feldman, G.S. Francis, T.G. Ganiats, M.A. Konstam, D.M. Mancini, P.S. Rahko, M.A. Silver, L.W. Stevenson, C.W. Yancy, 2009 focused update: ACCFAHA guidelines for the diagnosis and management of heart failure in adults: A report of the American College of Cardiology Foundation/American Heart Association Task Force on Practice Guidelines developed in collaboration with the International Society for Heart and Lung Transplantation, J. Am. Coll. Cardiol. 53 (2009) 1343–1382.
[64] S.M. Macicek, C.G. Macias, J.L. Jefferies, J.J. Kim, J.F. Price, Acute heart failure syndromes in the pediatric emergency department, Pediatrics 124 (2009) e898–904.
[65] S. Chen, R.J. Gajarski, A. Lin, L.J. May, D.N. Rosenthal, M.D. Everitt, D.M. McElhinney, A.Y. Shin, S.A. Hollander, E. Pruitt, C.S. Almond, Hemodynamic profiles in children with end-stage heart failure: an analysis of data from the Pediatric Heart Transplant Study Group, J. Heart Lung Transplant. 34 (2015) S35.
[66] W.F. Peacock, G.C. Fonarow, C.L. Emerman, R.M. Mills, J. Wynne, ADHERE Scientific Advisory Committee and Investigators, Adhere Study Group, Impact of early initiation of intravenous therapy for acute decompensated heart failure on outcomes in ADHERE, Cardiology 107 (2007) 44–51.
[67] W.F. Peacock, C. Emerman, M.R. Costanzo, D.B. Diercks, M. Lopatin, G.C. Fonarow, Early vasoactive drugs improve heart failure outcomes, Congest. Heart Fail. 15 (2009) 256–264.
[68] A.S. Maisel, W.F. Peacock, N. McMullin, R. Jessie, G.C. Fonarow, J. Wynne, R.M. Mills, Timing of immunoreactive B-type natriuretic peptide levels and treatment delay in acute decompensated heart failure: an ADHERE (Acute Decompensated Heart Failure National Registry) analysis, J. Am. Coll. Cardiol. 52 (2008) 534–540.
[69] A.H. Rosenstein, J.B. Hanel, C. Martin, Timing is everything: impact of emergency department care on hospital length of stay, J. Clin. Outcomes Manage. 7 (2000) 31–36.

[70] V. Singh, S. Luthra, V. Singhal, N. Divakaran, A. Magno, M. Krishnamurthy, R. Kouides, Door-to-di uretic time: a promising strategy for improving delivery of care to patients hospitalized with decompensated heart failure, a community-based single center experience, J. Am. Coll. Cardiol. 65 (2015) A866.

[71] J.M. Testani, M.A. Birsco, R.D. Kocio, D. Jacoby, L. Bellumkonda, C.R. Parikh, S.T. Coca, W.H. Tang, Substantial discrepancy between fluid and weight loss during acute decompensated heart failure treatment: important lessons for research and clinical care, Am. J. Med. 128 (2015) 776–783.

[72] K.F. Adams Jr., G.C. Fonarow, C.L. Emerman, T.H. LeJemtel, M.R. Costanzo, W.T. Abraham, R.L. Berkowitz, M. Galvao, D.P. Horton, ADHERE Scientific Advisory Committee and Investigators, Characteristics and outcomes of patients hospitalized for heart failure in the United States: rationale, design, and preliminary observations from the first 100,000 cases in the Acute Decompensated Failure National Registry (ADHERE), Am. Heart J. 149 (2005) 209–216.

[73] M. Gheorghiade, G. Filippatos, Reassessing treatment of acute heart failure syndromes: the ADHERE registry, Eur. Heart J. 7 (Suppl. B) (2005) B131–B139.

[74] B. Bikdeli, K.M. Strait, K. Dharmarajan, S.X. Li, P. Mody, C. Partovian, S.G. Coca, et al., Intravenous fluids in acute decompensated heart failure, J. Am. Coll. Cardiol. 3 (2015) 127–133.

[75] S.F. Jencks, M.V. Williams, E.A. Coleman, Rehospitalizations among patients in the medicare fee-for-service program, N. Engl. J. Med. 364 (2011) 1582.

[76] B.S. Moffet, T.J. Humlicek, J.W. Rossano, J.F. Price, A.G. Cabrera, Readmissions for heart failure in children, J. Pediatr. 177 (2016) 153–158.

[77] G.M. Felker, R.J. Mentz, Diuretics and ultrafiltration in acute decompensated heart failure, J. Am. Coll. Cardiol. 59 (2012) 2145–2153.

[78] D.H. Ellison, Diuretic therapy and resistance in congestive heart failure, Cardiology 96 (2001) 132–143.

[79] B. Kaissling, B.A. Stanton, Adaptation of distal tubule and collecting duct to increased sodium delivery. I. Ultrastructure, Am. J. Physiol. 255 (1988) F1256–F1268.

[80] D.H. Ellison, H. Velázquez, F.S. Wright, Adaptation of the distal convoluted tubule of the rat: structural and functional effects of dietary salt intake and chronic diuretic infusion, J. Clin. Investig. 83 (1989) 113–126.

[81] D.H. Ellison, Diuretic resistance: physiology and therapeutics, Semin. Nephrol. 19 (1999) 581–597.

[82] D.C. Brater, Update in diuretic therapy: clinical pharmacology, Semin. Nephrol. 31 (2011) 483–494.

[83] G.M. Felker, K.L. Lee, D.A. Bull, M.M. Redfield, L.W. Stevenson, S.R. Goldsmith, M.M. LeWinter, A. Deswal, J.L. Rouleau, E.O. Ofili, K.J. Anstrom, A.F. Hernandez, S.E. McNulty, E.J. Velazquez, A.G. Kfoury, H.H. Chen, M.M. Givertz, M.J. Semigran, B.A. Bart, A.M. Mascette, E. Bruanwald, C.M. O'Connor, Diuretic strategies in patients with acute decompensated heart failure, N. Engl. J. Med. 364 (2011) 797–805.

[84] G.S. Francis, R.M. Siegel, S.R. Goldsmith, M.T. Olivari, T.B. Levine, J.N. Cohn, Acute vasoconstrictor response to intravenous furosemide in patients with chronic congestive heart failure. Activation of the neurohumoral axis, Ann. Intern. Med. 103 (1985) 1–6.

[85] R.J. Mentz, S.R. Stevens, A.D. DeVore, A. Lala, J.M. Vader, O.F. AbouEzzeddine, P. Khazanie, M.M. Redfield, L.W. Stevenson, C.M. O'Connor, S.R. Goldsmith, B.A. Bart, K.J. Anstrom, A.F. Hernandez, E. Braunwald, G.M. Felker, Decongestion strategies and renin-angiotensin-aldosterone system activation in acute heart failure, J. Am. Coll. Cardiol. 3 (2015) 97–107.

[86] T.P.J. Dormans, P.G.G. Gerlag, Combination of high-dose furosemide and hydrochlorothiazide in the treatment of refractory congestive heart failure, Eur. Heart J. 17 (1996) 1867–1874.

[87] D. Fliser, M. Schroter, M. Neubeck, E. Ritz, Coadministration of thiazides increases the efficacy of loop diuretics even in patients with advanced renal failure, Kidney Int. 46 (1994) 482–488.

[88] K.S. Channer, K.A. McLean, P. Lawson-Matthew, M. Richardson, Combination of diuretic treatment in severe heart failure: a randomized controlled trial, Br. Heart J. 71 (1994) 146–150.

[89] J.C. Jentzer, T.A. DeWald, A.F. Hernandez, Combination of loop diuretics with thiazide-type diuretics in heart failure, J. Am. Coll. Cardiol. 56 (2010) 1527–1534.

[90] T.P. Dormans, P.G. Gerla, F.G. Russel, P. Smits, Combination diuretic therapy in severe congestive heart failure, Drugs 55 (1998) 165–172.

[91] A. Kiyingi, M.J. Field, C.C. Pawsey, J. Yiannikas, J.R. Lawrence, W.J. Arter, Metolazone in treatment of severe refractory congestive cardiac failure, Lancet 335 (1990) 29–31.

[92] G.B. Luciani, S. Nichani, A.C. Chang, W.J. Wells, C.J. Newth, V.A. Starnes, Continuous versus intermittent furosemide infusion in critically ill infants after open heart operations, Ann. Thorac. Surg. 64 (1997) 1133–1139.

[93] D.R. Salvador, N.R. Rey, G.C. Ramos, F.E. Punzalan, Continuous infusion versus bolus injection of loop diuretics in congestive heart failure, Cochrane Database Syst. Rev. (3) (2005) CD003178.

[94] J.E. Udelson, C. Orlandi, J. Ouyang, H. Krasa, C.A. Zimmer, G. Frivold, W.H. Haught, S. Meymandi, C. Macarie, D. Raef, P. Wedge, M.A. Konstam, M. Gheorghiade, Acute hemodynamic effects of tolvaptan, a vasopressin V2 receptor blocker, in patients with symptomatic heart failure and systolic dysfunction: an international, multicenter, randomized, placebo-controlled trial, J. Am. Coll. Cardiol. 52 (2008) 1540–1545.

[95] M. Gheorghiade, M.A. Konstam, J.C. Burnett, L. Grinfield, A.P. Maggioni, K. Swedberg, J.E. Udelson, F. Zannad, T. Cook, J. Ouyang, C. Zimmer, C. Orlandi, Efficacy of Vasopressin Antagonism in Heart Failure Outcome Study with Topvaptan (EVEREST) Investigators, J. Am. Med. Assoc. 297 (2007) 1332–1343.

[96] M.A. Konstam, M. Gheorghiade, J.C. Burnett, L. Grinfeld, A.P. Maggioni, K. Swedberg, J.E. Udelson, F. Zannad, T. Cook, J. Ouyang, C. Zimmer, C. Orlandi, Efficacy of Vasopressin Antagonism in heart Failure Outcome Study With Tolvaptan (EVEREST) Investigators, Efficacy of oral tolvaptan in patients hospitalized for worsening heart failure: the EVEREST Outcome Trial, J. Am. Med. Assoc. 297 (2007) 1319–1331.

[97] R.B. Regen, A. Gonzalez, K. Zawodniak, D. Leonard, R. Quigley, A.P. Barnes, J.D. Koch, Tolvaptan increases serum sodium in pediatric patients with heart failure, Pediatr. Cardiol. 34 (2013) 1463–1468.

[98] G.M. Felker, R.J. Mentz, R.T. Cole, K.F. Adams, G.F. Egnaczyk, M. Fiuzat, C.B. Patel, M. Echols, M.G. Khouri, J.M. Tauras, D. Gupta, P. Monds, R. Roberts, C.M. O'Connor, Efficacy and safety of tolvaptan in patients hospitalized with acute heart failure, J. Am. Coll. Cardiol. 69 (2017) 1399–1406.

[99] M.A. Konstam, M. Kiernan, A. Chandler, R. Dhingra, F.V. Mody, H.E. Eisen, W.H. Haught, Short-term effects of tolvaptan in patients with acute heart failure and volume overload, J. Am. Coll. Cardiol. 69 (2017) 1409–1419.

[100] S. Paterna, P. Di Pasquale, G. Parrinello, E. Fornaciari, F. Di Guadio, S. Fasullo, M. Giammanco, F.M. Sarullo, G. Licata, Changes in brain natriuretic peptide levels and bioelectrical impedance measurements after treatment with high-dose furosemide and hypertonic saline solution versus high-dose furosemide alone in refractory congestive heart failure: a double-blind study, J. Am. Coll. Cardiol. 45 (2005) 1997–2003.

[101] G. Parrinello, S. Paterna, P. Di Pasquale, D. Torres, M. Mezzero, M. Cardillo, S. Fasullo, G. La Rocca, G. Licata, Changes in estimating echocardiography pulmonary capillary wedge pressure after hypersaline plus furosemide versus furosemide alone in decompensated heart failure, J. Card. Fail. 17 (2011) 331–339.

[102] A. Tuttolomondo, A. Pinto, G. Parrinello, G. Licata, Intravenous high-dose furosemide and hypertonic saline solutions for refractory heart failure and ascites, Semin. Nephrol. 31 (2011) 513–522.

[103] S. Gandhi, W. Mosleh, R.B.H. Myers, Hypertonic saline with furosemide for the treatment of acute congestive heart failure: a systematic review and meta-analysis, Int. J. Cardiol. 173 (2014) 139–145.

[104] A.A. Van Vliet, A.M. Donker, J.P. Nauta, F.W. Verheugt, Spironolactone in congestive heart failure refractory to high-dose loop diuretic and low-dose angiotensin-converting enzyme inhibitor, Am. J. Cardiol. 71 (1993) 21A–28A.

[105] M.D. Guazzi, P. Agostoni, B. Perego, G. Lauri, A. Salvioni, F. Giraldi, M. Matturri, M. Guazzi, G. Marenzi, Apparent paradox of neurohumoral axis inhibition after body fluid volume depletion in patients with chronic congestive heart failure and water retention, Br. Heart J. 72 (1994) 534–539.

[106] G. Marenzi, G. Lauri, M. Grazi, E. Assanelli, J. Campodonico, P. Agostoni, Circulatory response to fluid overload removal by extracorporeal ultrafiltration in refractory congestive heart failure, J. Am. Coll. Cardiol. 38 (2001) 963–968.

[107] P. Agostoni, G. Marenzi, G. Lauri, G. Perego, M. Schianni, P. Sganzerla, M.D. Guazzi, Sustained improvement in functional capacity after removal of body fluid with isolated ultrafiltration in chronic cardiac insufficiency: failure of furosemide to provide the same result, Am. J. Med. 96 (1994) 191–199.

[108] B.A. Bart, A. Boyle, A.J. Bank, et al., Ultrafiltration versus usual care for hospitalized patients with heart failure: the relief for acutely fluid-overloaded patients with decompensated congestive heart failure (RAPID-CHF) trial, J. Am. Coll. Cardiol. 46 (2005) 2043–2046.

[109] S.S. Ali, C.C. Olinger, P.A. Sobotka, S. Bernard, T.G. Dahle, M.C. Bunte, et al., Enhanced sodium extraction with ultrafiltration compared to intravenous diuretics, J. Card. Fail. 12 (2006) S114.

[110] M.R. Costanzo, M. Saltzberg, J. O'Sullivan, P. Sobotka, Early ultrafiltrations in patients with decompensated heart failure and diuretic resistance, J. Am. Coll. Cardiol. 46 (2005) 2047–2051.

[111] M.R. Costanzo, M.E. Guglin, M.T. Saltzberg, M.L. Jessup, B.A. Bart, J.R. Teerlink, B.E. Jaski, J.C. Fang, E.D. Feller, G.J. Haas, A.S. Anderson, M.P. Schollmeyer, P.A. Sobotka, UNLOAD Trial Investigators, Ultrafiltration versus intravenous diuretics for patients hospitalized for acute decompensated heart failure, J. Am. Coll. Cardiol. 49 (2007) 675–683.

[112] B.A Bart, S.R. Goldsmith, K.L. Lee, M.M. Givertz, C.M. O'Connor, D.A. Bull, M.M. Redfield, A. Deswal, J.L. Rouleau, M.M. LeWinter, E.O. Ofili, L.W. Stevenson, M.J. Semigran, G.M. Felker, H.H. Chen, A.F. Hernandez, McN.S.E. AnstromKJ, E.J. Velazquez, J.C. Ibarra, A.M. Mascette, E. Braunwald, Heart Failure Clinical Research Network, Ultrafiltration in decompensated heart failure with cardiorenal syndrome, N. Engl. J. Med. 367 (2012) 2296–2304.

[113] M.R. Costanzo, D. Negoianu, B.E. Jaski, B.A. Bart, J.T. Heywood, I.S. Anand, J.M. Smelser, A.M. Kaneshige, D.B. Chomsky, E.D. Adler, G.J. Haas, J.A. Watts, J.L. Nabut, M.P. Schollmeyer, G.C. Fonarow, Aquapheresis versus intravenous diuretics and hospitalizations for heart failure, JACC Heart Fail. 4 (2016) 95–105.

Chapter 39

The Use of Inotropic Agents in Acute Decompensated Heart Failure

Alejandro A. Floh, Emily Jean-St.-Michel, Steven M. Schwartz
The Hospital for Sick Children and the University of Toronto, Toronto, ON, Canada

INTRODUCTION

The use of inotropic agents to increase myocardial contractility can be desirable in the treatment of children with decompensated heart failure. However, despite numerous studies showing an immediate improvement in cardiac output and baseline hemodynamics, these effects wane over time and have failed to demonstrate a longer-term reduction in clinical complications in adults. This chapter will review the physiologic underpinnings by which inotropic medications exert their effects and explore under which settings they should be used and avoided.

MECHANISMS OF ACTION

Inotropic medications, often referred simply as inotropes, include several classes of drugs that increase the strength of myocardial contraction, resulting in a higher stroke volume and cardiac output. Although widely used, a single classification system has never been universally adopted. One practical approach is to categorize inotropes according to their physiologic mechanism of action [1]. Feldman proposed grouping inotropes into four groups that improve function by means of (1) increasing 3′-5′cyclic adenosine monophosphate (cAMP) concentrations, (2) interacting with receptors on the sarcoplasmic reticulum, (3) increasing calcium sensitivity, or (4) through a combination of mechanisms. This approach can be particularly useful as it helps account for all known physiologic effects of these drugs, both cardiac-specific and systemic.

Increase in cardiac performance is most commonly mediated through activation of the cAMP second messenger system. In the cardiac myocyte, generation of cAMP activates Protein Kinase A leading to a biochemical cascade that releases calcium from the sarcoplasmic reticulum into the cytosol [2]. The higher concentration of calcium promotes binding to Troponin-C, increases actin–myosin bridging, and augments strength of myocardial contraction. cAMP is then degraded back to 5′-adenosine monophosphate by the phosphodiesterase (PDE) enzyme.

Sympathomimetics, the most widely used inotropic class whose members include Epinephrine, Dopamine, and Dobutamine, exert their effects through activation of adrenergic system and increase of cAMP. The binding of these exogenous catecholamines to myocardial membrane β-adrenergic receptors triggers the cAMP pathway through induction of a stimulatory G_s-protein. The resulting configuration change in G_s results in activation of adenylate cyclase and the production of cAMP. Stimulation of β_1-receptors also induces a dose-dependent heart rate response. The nonselective binding of these drugs to systemic endothelial α and β receptors can also result in variable amounts of vasoconstriction or vasodilation.

PDE inhibitors, such as milrinone and amrinone, also mediate their inotropic effects through increased cAMP. This drug class binds to PDE 3 in a competitive fashion, preventing cAMP binding and degradation. PDE 3 inhibitors also contribute to systemic and pulmonary vasodilation through inhibition of PDE 3 in vascular smooth muscle. The increase in cAMP in the vasculature leads to higher myosin light chain kinase activity and smooth muscle relaxation.

CLINICAL EVIDENCE FOR USE OF INOTROPIC SUPPORT

Dobutamine is one of the earliest inotropes studied for the treatment of heart failure in adult patients. Dobutamine is a synthetic catecholamine and was initially considered to be a highly selective inotrope that improved contractility but, unlike other sympathomimetics, resulted in minimal increase in heart rate and vasoconstriction. In the earliest studies,

Heart Failure in the Child and Young Adult. http://dx.doi.org/10.1016/B978-0-12-802393-8.00039-9

dobutamine infusions demonstrated a favorable physiologic response that included an immediate increase in cardiac output with associated reduction in afterload of both systemic and pulmonary circulations [3]. Similar hemodynamic effects were subsequently observed in adults with heart failure and resulted in a rapid improvement in their hemodynamic profile, echocardiographic and invasive metrics of cardiac performance and were associated with symptomatic relief [4,5]. Nevertheless, the symptomatic improvements were limited due to emergence of tachyphylaxis if the infusions were extended beyond a few days; intermittent dosing was required to provide longer-term symptom relief. It was ultimately shown that despite its initial promise, subjective reductions in symptoms, and reduction in NYHA (New York Heart Association) class, intermittent dobutamine infusions did not prove to provide sustained hemodynamic benefit nor improvement in mortality rate compared to patients receiving conventional therapy [6,7].

The use of PDE 3 inhibitors for decompensated heart failure was also studied extensively due to their positive inotropic effects and reduction of systemic afterload, without an associated increase in myocardial oxygen demand [8]. However, similar to β-agonists, treatment with several drug formulations, including amrinone, imazodan, and milrinone, consistently failed to demonstrate improvement in clinical symptoms or reduction mortality [9–11]. Moreover, patients on chronic PDE 3 inhibitor therapy had higher rates of complications. The PROMISE trial was a randomized, placebo control study that examined the effects of oral milrinone on all-cause mortality in patients with severe heart failure [12]. Milrinone was not associated with any symptomatic or functional change but was associated with an increase in all-cause mortality of 28% leading to early termination of the trial. The majority of the deaths were attributed to a primary cardiovascular etiology, disproportionately affecting the highest risk patients (53% increase in NYHA IV patients). Common side effects included line infections, headache, diarrhea, hypotension, syncope, and palpitations. Similarly, milrinone also failed to show a clinical benefit when administered for 48–72 h at an initial dose of 0.5 mcg kg/min [8]. Milrinone infusion did not shorten the duration of initial hospitalization nor did it reduce the rate of readmission. Subjects receiving milrinone were more likely to experience adverse events including hypotension, atrial fibrillation, and ventricular arrhythmias.

Several mechanisms have been postulated to explain the poor long-term efficacy and complication burden of catecholamines and PDE 3 inhibitors. Sympathomimetics increase cardiac output at the expense of increased myocardial work and oxygen consumption [13]. It is possible that early administration may favor cardiac output while over time the equilibrium tips toward a state of negative energy balance predisposing to progressive failure, especially in adult heart failure patients, many of whom have ischemic heart disease as an underlying cause of their myocardial dysfunction. Sympathomimetics also act synergistically with the endogenous catecholamines and an intrinsically upregulated neuroendocrine axis. Increased morbidity may arise from maladaptive cardiac remodeling and cellular apoptosis that result from sustained cAMP–induced increases in intracellular calcium [14]. Increased sequestration of calcium within the sarcoplasmic reticulum system may be proarrhythmic through spontaneous calcium release. Chronic exposure to catecholamines causes downregulation of adrenergic receptors leading to tachyphylaxis.

Despite the poor long-term clinical outcomes and recognized hazards associated with these inotropes, milrinone and dobutamine continue to have a role in the stabilization of hospitalized patients in acute decompensated heart failure. Along with diuretics, they are considered as first-line agents in patients who present with evidence of low cardiac output syndrome and organ dysfunction. In smaller studies, milrinone has proven an effective component in the treatment strategy for hospitalized patients who failed to wean off inotropic support and were being bridged to transplant [15,16]. In one retrospective, single-center study of patients who did not tolerate discontinuation of milrinone support, over 75% were successfully supported for a mean of 60 days until reaching transplantation with the remainder undergoing insertion of a ventricular assist device at an average 93 days. Unlike earlier studies, 93% of all subjects had an automated implantable cardioverter–defibrillator that delivered shocks in 13% of patients, possibly mitigating some of the morbidity associated with longer-term milrinone infusions and reducing the risk of sudden death. In a separate study, the use of milrinone did not reduce or mitigate the risk for receiving mechanical circulatory support (MCS) with an intraaortic balloon pump or ventricular assist device. In the current era in which use of devices for MCS and treatment of life-threatening arrhythmias are much more common than they were in the era that these drugs were originally studied, the implication is that they can be seen as a bridge to device implantation and/or transplantation, but should probably not be seen as long-term therapy on their own other than as palliative treatment. This approach is supported by the recommendations regarding inotropic support from the 2013 American College of Cardiology Foundation/American Heart Association guidelines on heart failure management (see insert) [17]. Similarly, the International Society of Heart and Lung Transplantation recommend inotropic support as Class IIa for "symptomatic relief in the palliative setting." These authors suggest that "intermittent of chronic inotropic therapy other than as a bridge to transplant is not recommended" and label this as a Class III recommendation (potentially harmful) [18].

Inotropic Support: Recommendations.

Adapted from 2013 ACCF/AHA Guideline for the Management of Heart Failure: A Report of the American College of Cardiology Foundation/American Heart Association Task Force on Practice Guidelines.

Class I

1. Until definitive therapy (e.g., coronary revascularization, MCS, heart transplantation) or resolution of the acute precipitating problem, patients with cardiogenic shock should receive temporary intravenous inotropic support to maintain systemic perfusion and preserve end-organ performance. (*Level of Evidence: C*)

Class IIa

1. Continuous intravenous inotropic support is reasonable as "bridge therapy" in patients with stage D heart failure refractory to guideline-directed medical therapy and device therapy who are eligible for and awaiting MCS or cardiac transplantation. (*Level of Evidence: B*)

Class IIb

1. Short-term, continuous intravenous inotropic support may be reasonable in those hospitalized patients presenting with documented severe systolic dysfunction who present with low blood pressure and significantly depressed cardiac output to maintain systemic perfusion and preserve end-organ performance. (*Level of Evidence: B*)
2. Long-term, continuous intravenous inotropic support may be considered as palliative therapy for symptom control in select patients with stage D heart failure despite optimal guideline-directed medical therapy and device therapy who are not eligible for either MCS or cardiac transplantation. (*Level of Evidence: B*)

Class III: Harm

1. Long-term use of either continuous or intermittent, intravenous parenteral positive inotropic agents, in the absence of specific indications or for reasons other than palliative care, is potentially harmful in the patient with heart failure. (*Level of Evidence: B*)
2. Use of parenteral inotropic agents in hospitalized patients without documented severe systolic dysfunction, low blood pressure, or impaired perfusion and evidence of significantly depressed cardiac output, with or without congestion, is potentially harmful. (*Level of Evidence: B*)

Levosimendan is a drug whose properties of increased inotropy, lusitropy, and systemic and pulmonary vasodilation positioned it potentially as an ideal drug in the treatment of heart failure. By binding to Troponin-C in a calcium-dependent fashion, Levosimendan induces a conformational change in tropomyosin and increases actin–myosin cross-bridging [19–21]. Vasodilation occurs due to ATP-sensitive potassium channel activation and smooth muscle. As a calcium sensitizer, levosimendan does not increase intracellular calcium, thereby increasing contractility while potentially avoiding some of the negative side effects of other inotropes. Levosimendan is degraded to the active metabolites OR-1855 and OR-1896, which allows a 24-h infusion to have a duration of action of up to 1 week [22].

A series of early clinical studies showed promise. In the 2002 LIDO trial, a study of hospitalized adult patients requiring inotropic support, subjects were randomized to receive levosimendan or continuous dobutamine infusion [23]. Levosimendan was associated with greater hemodynamic benefit in that a larger proportion of subjects receiving Levosimendan showed improved cardiac output (28% vs. 15%) and reduced pulmonary artery capillary wedge pressure at 24h. Levosimendan was also associated with improved markers of end-organ function, the levosimendan group tended to be less symptomatic. Interestingly, the hemodynamic differences were most marked in patients treated with β–blockade in whom the effects of dobutamine were diminished. The benefits of Levosimendan were reinforced in the RUSSLAN trial, a multicenter, international trial of adults with ischemic cardiomyopathy [24]. Compared to placebo, levosimendan infusion was not associated with symptom relief but conferred a survival advantage without a significant increase in complications.

Despite early optimism, these types of positive results were not replicated in the North American–based SURVIVE trial. This was a multicenter, international study of 1327 patients admitted to hospital with acute decompensated heart failure randomized to levosimendan or dobutamine therapy and powered to detect differences in survival. Kaplan–Meier survival curves converged and no difference in 31 or 180-day (primary outcome) survival was observed [20]. An equal number of subjects in each arm required a second dose of dobutamine or levosimendan to be administered. Levosimendan was associated with more tachycardia and lower blood pressure within the first week of drug administration, but fewer episodes of arrhythmia and hypokalemia. The similar survival across treatment arms was possibly attributed to a lower mortality rate of dobutamine-treated patients compared to previous studies. Most recently, the REVIVE trial in 2013 [25] compared levosimendan infusion to placebo. Levosimendan was associated with a larger proportion of patients reporting symptom relief and fewer subjectively worsening, and these benefits were associated with a significant drop in plasma B-type natriuretic peptide (BNP) early in management course, which normalized by 1-month follow-up. However, patients on levosimendan had an increased risk of side effects, including a 14% higher incidence of hypotension, 8% higher incidence of ventricular dysrhythmias, and a 6% increase in atrial fibrillation. Most concerning was a trend to higher risk of all-cause mortality in patients treated with levosimendan. This was reinforced by a recent metaanalysis in which levosimendan was found to be superior to dobutamine but did not show a survival advantage to placebo [26]. Levosimendan has not been approved for use in either the United States or Canada.

Although previous efforts failed to identify medications and regimens to modify the natural-history of end-stage heart failure, a persistent poor prognosis and increasing number of at-risk patients have driven investigators to explore other synthetic inotropes. Istaroxime was identified as possible alternative agent given that its effects are produced through a separate biochemical pathway. Istaroxime is a synthetic drug that enhances calcium-handling activity by combining the inhibition of a sodium–potassium antiport and stimulation of SERCA2a, a membrane-bound enzyme that moves calcium from the cytosol back into the sarcoplasmic reticulum. The aggregate effect improves myocardial contraction by increasing sequestered calcium in the endoplasmic reticulum available for myocardial contraction and enhances ventricular relaxation by lowering concentrations during diastole [27]. In the single randomized clinical trial HORIZON-HF, istaroxime was found to improve systolic blood pressure and lower pulmonary vascular resistance. It had no significant impact on ventricular relaxation as evaluated by echocardiography but decreased left ventricular volume. The effect of istaroxime on clinical outcomes has yet to be evaluated.

PEDIATRIC CONSIDERATIONS

The overwhelming volume of research on the use of inotropic agents in heart failure has been conducted in adult cohorts, a much larger at-risk population. Comparative studies evaluating the chronic use of inotropes in pediatrics are lacking. The evidence for inotropic support for children is therefore limited and based predominantly on observational studies with surrogate clinical end points [28,29].

With relative paucity of pediatric-specific data it is tempting, and even necessary to extrapolate the findings of adult studies into children, but this should be done with an abundance of caution and a recognition of the significant differences between adult and pediatric heart failure patients. Most importantly, the most common causes of cardiomyopathy and heart failure in adults are different than they are in pediatrics and response to therapy may therefore also differ. Most adult heart failure is attributed to hypertension, ischemic heart disease, and diabetes [30]. All of these entities are either rare in children or when present are unlikely to cause heart failure in the pediatric age range. Children have a higher representation of familial and idiopathic cardiomyopathy as well as heart failure in the setting of congenital heart disease. These differences can potentially have significant impact. For example, agents that increase myocardial oxygen demand may have very different costs in a patient with coronary insufficiency compared to one who can increase myocardial oxygen supply if overall cardiac output increases. In a secondary posthoc analysis of the OPTIME-CHF study, patients with nonischemic cardiomyopathy responded differently to milrinone therapy [11]. Whereas milrinone had no clinical impact on those with heart failure from ischemic origin, patients with nonischemic cardiomyopathy tended to decrease duration of hospitalization, inhospital mortality, and composite end point of death and hospitalization. That said, it is also important to recognize that molecular processes in heart failure tend to follow common pathways despite different causes of heart failure. Dismissing the adverse long-term effects of inotropic agents, many of which seem to occur at a molecular level, as being germane only to adult patients seems unwise as well.

Despite the deficiency of pediatric-specific studies, the use of milrinone has become standard of care in the emergent treatment and acute stabilization of children with decompensated heart failure. The addition of sympathomimetic support is confined to presence of hypotension, low cardiac output, or evolving end-organ dysfunction. Once stabilized, efforts are then made to wean off inotropic support and transition patients to chronic antifailure therapy. For those unable to wean from inotropes, long-term therapy as a bridge to transplant or as destination therapy has been shown to be a safe and viable alternative [31,32]. In a retrospective review of seven patients, chronic home-based parenteral inotropic support was shown to reduce number of emergency department visits and hospital admissions [32]. One patient with a failing Fontan physiology and preexisting ventricular arrhythmia died. The group was treated with a consistent inotropic strategy that included dopamine, milrinone, or a combination of the two. For those in shock there is recent evidence that epinephrine is preferable to dopamine in pediatric septic shock [33] although there have been no similar studies in pediatric cardiac patients. Of note, one small study in postoperative Norwood patients suggested that dopamine was of little benefit in terms of cardiac output but did increase oxygen consumption [34].

A major focus of emerging research surrounds the pediatric use of levosimendan. Most of the studies have looked at the postoperative management of children with congenital heart disease and myocardial dysfunction or low cardiac output who are poorly responsive to usual inotropic support. From these selective studies, levosimendan was shown to be safe, have a similar pharmacokinetic profile as seen in adults [35], and effectively reduce postoperative low cardiac output syndrome [36]. In the first study in pediatric heart failure, there was an observed increase in left ventricular ejection fraction and reduction in dobutamine infusion with a single dose of levosimendan [37]. Nearly three quarters of the children (11/15) survived to hospital discharge and 46% were alive at time of publication. Ventricular tachycardia occurred in one patient, which was successfully terminated. Similar outcomes were seen with levosimendan use for chemotherapy-induced heart dysfunction [38]. In this small case series, levosimendan was associated with discontinuation of inotropic support and mechanical ventilation and transition to standard heart failure therapy. Finally, in the most recent retrospective review, levosimendan was used to help bridge children with heart failure to ventricular assist device and transplantation [39]. In a study that included six patients (median age 2 years) with diagnoses of idiopathic dilated cardiomyopathy (4), maternal lupus-induced cardiomyopathy (1) and Epstein–Barr virus myocarditis (1), a 24-h infusion of levosimendan was followed by a drop in BNP by day 2. This decrease, however, was short-lived, and BNP returned to baseline by day 8. Furthermore, left ventricular ejection fraction did not statistically increase but that may have reflected small sample size. All patients received multiple doses (range 5–32), and this strategy was associated with a delay for patients to reach institutional criteria for MCS. Ultimately, five patients were successfully bridged to transplantation.

CONCLUSION

Inotropic support has an important role in the treatment of pediatric decompensated heart failure. Regardless of mechanism of action, inotropes have been shown to acutely improve cardiac performance and facilitate transition to chronic heart failure management, but they have not shown consistent clinical benefit and may pose potential harm when administered long term without clear end points such as MCS or transplantation. Although children differ from adults, use of inotropes in pediatrics is generally guided by adult studies as little evidence exists to support different indications for long-term use in children. Further investigation is required to determine if children with different etiologies to heart failure respond similarly to inotropic agents, have different risk profiles, or if there are important pharmacogenomic determinants of response to these commonly used drugs. Ongoing study into novel agents required.

REFERENCES

[1] A.M. Feldman, Classification of positive inotropic agents, J. Am. Coll. Cardiol. 22 (4) (1993) 1223–1227.

[2] M. Zaccolo, cAMP signal transduction in the heart: understanding spatial control for the development of novel therapeutic strategies, Br. J. Pharmacol. 158 (1) (2009) 50–60.

[3] N. Akhtar, E. Mikulic, J.N. Cohn, et al., Hemodynamic effect of dobutamine in patients with severe heart failure, Am. J. Cardiol. 36 (2) (1975) 202–205.

[4] M.M. Applefeld, K.A. Newman, W.R. Grove, et al., Intermittent, continuous outpatient dobutamine infusion in the management of congestive heart failure, Am. J. Cardiol. 51 (3) (1983) 455–458.

[5] C.V. Leier, J. Webel, C.A. Bush, The cardiovascular effects of the continuous infusion of dobutamine in patients with severe cardiac failure, Circulation 56 (3) (1977) 468–472.

[6] M.J. Krell, E.M. Kline, E.R. Bates, et al., Intermittent, ambulatory dobutamine infusions in patients with severe congestive heart failure, Am. Heart J. 112 (4) (1986) 787–791.

[7] F. Oliva, R. Latini, A. Politi, et al., Intermittent 6-month low-dose dobutamine infusion in severe heart failure: DICE multicenter trial, Am. Heart J. 138 (2 Pt 1) (1999) 247–253.

[8] M.S. Cuffe, R.M. Califf, K.F. Adams Jr., et al., Short-term intravenous milrinone for acute exacerbation of chronic heart failure: a randomized controlled trial, JAMA 287 (12) (2002) 1541–1547.

[9] A.D. Goldberg, J. Nicklas, S. Goldstein, Effectiveness of imazodan for treatment of chronic congestive heart failure. The Imazodan Research Group, Am. J. Cardiol. 68 (6) (1991) 631–636.

[10] B. Massie, M. Bourassa, R. DiBianco, et al., Long-term oral administration of amrinone for congestive heart failure: lack of efficacy in a multicenter controlled trial, Circulation 71 (5) (1985) 963–971.

[11] G.M. Felker, R.L. Benza, A.B. Chandler, et al., Heart failure etiology and response to milrinone in decompensated heart failure: results from the OPTIME-CHF study, J. Am. Coll. Cardiol. 41 (6) (2003) 997–1003.

[12] M. Packer, J.R. Carver, R.J. Rodeheffer, et al., Effect of oral milrinone on mortality in severe chronic heart failure. The PROMISE Study Research Group, N. Engl. J. Med. 325 (21) (1991) 1468–1475.

[13] D.J. Penny, T. Sano, J.J. Smolich, Increased systemic oxygen consumption offsets improved oxygen delivery during dobutamine infusion in newborn lambs, Intensive Care Med. 27 (9) (2001) 1518–1525.

[14] J.I. Goldhaber, M.A. Hamilton, Role of inotropic agents in the treatment of heart failure, Circulation 121 (14) (2010) 1655–1660.

[15] C. Assad-Kottner, D. Chen, J. Jahanyar, et al., The use of continuous milrinone therapy as bridge to transplant is safe in patients with short waiting times, J. Card. Fail. 14 (10) (2008) 839–843.

[16] M.R. Mehra, H.O. Ventura, C. Kapoor, et al., Safety and clinical utility of long-term intravenous milrinone in advanced heart failure, Am. J. Cardiol. 80 (1) (1997) 61–64.

[17] 2013 ACCF/AHA guideline for the management of heart failure: a report of the American College of Cardiology Foundation/American heart association task force on practice guidelines, Circulation 128 (2013) e240–e327.

[18] L. Bannister, R. Caruthers, B. Feingold, et al., Pharmacological treatment of chronic heart failure with reduced EF (systolic heart failure), in: in: R. Kirk, A.I. Dipchand, D.N. Rosenthal (Eds.), ISHLT Guidelines for the Management of Pediatric Heart Failure. ISHLT Monograph Series, vol. 8, UAB Printing, 2014, pp. 119–141. J.K. Kirklin, series editor.

[19] S. Archan, W. Toller, Levosimendan: current status and future prospects, Curr. Opin. Anaesthesiol. 21 (1) (2008) 78–84.

[20] A. Mebazaa, M.S. Nieminen, M. Packer, et al., Levosimendan vs dobutamine for patients with acute decompensated heart failure: the SURVIVE randomized trial, JAMA 297 (17) (2007) 1883–1891.

[21] T.M. Hoffman, Newer inotropes in pediatric heart failure, J. Cardiovasc. Pharmacol. 58 (2) (2011) 121–125.

[22] M. Kivikko, S. Antila, J. Eha, L. Lehtonen, P.J. Pentikäinen, Pharmacokinetics of levosimendan and its metabolites during and after a 24-hour continuous infusion in patients with severe heart failure, Int. J. Clin. Pharmacol. Ther. 40 (10) (October 2002) 465–471.

[23] F. Follath, J.G. Cleland, H. Just, et al., Efficacy and safety of intravenous levosimendan compared with dobutamine in severe low-output heart failure (the LIDO study): a randomised double-blind trial, Lancet 360 (9328) (2002) 196–202.

[24] V.S. Moiseyev, P. Poder, N. Andrejevs, et al., Safety and efficacy of a novel calcium sensitizer, levosimendan, in patients with left ventricular failure due to an acute myocardial infarction. A randomized, placebo-controlled, double-blind study (RUSSLAN), Eur. Heart J. 23 (18) (2002) 1422–1432.

[25] M. Packer, W. Colucci, L. Fisher, et al., Effect of levosimendan on the short-term clinical course of patients with acutely decompensated heart failure, JACC Heart Fail. 1 (2) (2013) 103–111.

[26] A. Delaney, C. Bradford, J. McCaffrey, et al., Levosimendan for the treatment of acute severe heart failure: a meta-analysis of randomised controlled trials, Int. J. Cardiol. 138 (3) (2010) 281–289.

[27] S.J. Shah, J.E. Blair, G.S. Filippatos, et al., Effects of istaroxime on diastolic stiffness in acute heart failure syndromes: results from the hemodynamic, echocardiographic, and neurohormonal effects of istaroxime, a novel intravenous inotropic and lusitropic agent: a randomized controlled trial in patients hospitalized with heart failure (HORIZON-HF) trial, Am. Heart J. 157 (6) (2009) 1035–1041.

[28] C. Vilaboa Pedrosa, C. Martinez Roca, P. Yanez Gomez, et al., Experience with levosimendan in 32 paediatric patients, Pediatr. Cardiol. 36 (5) (2015) 1038–1041.

[29] P.K. Suominen, Single-center experience with levosimendan in children undergoing cardiac surgery and in children with decompensated heart failure, BMC Anesthesiol. 11 (2011) 18.

[30] V.L. Roger, Epidemiology of heart failure, Circ. Res. 113 (2013) 646–659.

[31] A.M. Berg, L. Snell, W.T. Mahle, Home inotropic therapy in children, J. Heart Lung Transplant. 26 (5) (2007) 453–457.

[32] J.F. Price, J.A. Towbin, W.J. Dreyer, et al., Outpatient continuous parenteral inotropic therapy as bridge to transplantation in children with advanced heart failure, J. Card. Fail. 12 (2) (2006) 139–143.

[33] A.M.C. Ventura, H.H. Shieh, A. Bousso, et al., Double-blind prospective randomized controlled trial of dopamine versus epinephrine as first-line vasoactive drugs in pediatric septic shock, Crit. Care Med. 43 (2015) 2292–2302.

[34] J. Li, H. Zhang, H. Holtby, et al., Adverse effects of dopamine on systemic hemodynamic status and oxygen transport in neonates after the Norwood procedure, J. Am. Coll. Cardiol. 48 (2006) 1859–1864.

[35] M. Turanlahti, T. Boldt, T. Palkama, et al., Pharmacokinetics of levosimendan in pediatric patients evaluated for cardiac surgery, Pediatr. Crit. Care Med. 5 (5) (2004) 457–462.

[36] J.R. Egan, A.J. Clarke, S. Williams, et al., Levosimendan for low cardiac output: a pediatric experience, J. Intensive Care Med. 21 (3) (2006) 183–187.

[37] P. Namachivayam, D.S. Crossland, W.W. Butt, et al., Early experience with levosimendan in children with ventricular dysfunction, Pediatr. Crit. Care Med. 7 (5) (2006) 445–448.

[38] A. Tosoni, A.I. Dipchand, H. Mohseni-Bod, The use of levosimendan in children with cancer with severe acute cardiac dysfunction: case series and a review of the literature, Cardiol. Young 24 (3) (2014) 524–527.

[39] P.E. Seguela, P. Mauriat, J.B. Mouton, et al., Single-centred experience with levosimendan in paediatric decompensated dilated cardiomyopathy, Arch. Cardiovasc. Dis. 108 (6–7) (2015) 347–355.

Chapter 40

Phosphodiesterase Inhibitors

Timothy M. Hoffman
University of North Carolina, Chapel Hill, NC, United States

INTRODUCTION

In pediatric medicine, the use of phosphodiesterase inhibitors has evolved despite the paucity of research evaluating efficacy and the inherent flaw of attempting to extrapolate adult data to the pediatric population. Phosphodiesterase 3 (PDE3) inhibitors, namely milrinone, have been used in the management of acute and chronic heart failure with the majority of studies evaluating infants and children in the postoperative setting. However, phosphodiesterase 5 (PDE5) inhibitors, namely sildenafil, have been used in patients with pulmonary hypertension as well as in those with single ventricle physiology for poor hemodynamics attributable to elevated pulmonary artery pressures status post cavopulmonary palliation. The mechanism of action is the inhibition of cyclic nucleotide phosphodiesterase activity thus leading to an increase in intracellular cyclic adenosine monophosphate (cAMP) and cyclic guanosine monophosphate (cGMP) [1]. PDE3 inhibitors yield increased intracellular cAMP in cardiac and vascular smooth muscle, whereas PDE5 inhibitors raise cGMP in vascular smooth muscle with a propensity for pulmonary versus the systemic vasculature [1].

PHOSPHODIESTERASE 5 INHIBITION AND HEART FAILURE

There are animal model data and theoretical benefits of PDE5 inhibitors in heart failure including blunting of cardiac hypertrophy, afterload reduction for the right ventricle due to pulmonary vasodilation, a lesser afterload reduction for the left ventricle due to systemic vasodilation, and a preconditioning-like cardioprotective effect against ischemia and reperfusion injury [1,2]. In adult and pediatric heart failure practice, there is a role for PDE5 inhibitors in those with heart failure and secondary pulmonary hypertension. Additionally, adult studies are ongoing as to the role of sildenafil in those patients with heart failure with preserved ejection fraction. However, despite recent publications regarding pediatric heart failure guidelines, no recommendations exist that address the use of PDE5 inhibitors for pediatric heart failure management although it is alluded that there may be a role in those with heart failure and secondary pulmonary hypertension similar to the practice in adult care [3,4]. Despite the lack of formal recommendations, there are several compelling studies that suggest PDE5 inhibitors are beneficial in those with single ventricle physiology. One such study was a double-blind, placebo-controlled, crossover trial conducted in children and young adults after the Fontan operation where patients were randomized to placebo or sildenafil for 6 weeks [5]. After that period of time, the subjects crossed over and all patients had an exercise physiology study at the start and end of each phase. In short, sildenafil was associated with improved ventilatory efficiency during exercise and in some subgroups, a suggestion of improved oxygen consumption at the anaerobic threshold [5]. Another study evaluated sildenafil in the postoperative period after extracardiac Fontan completion as compared to a similar group that did not receive vasodilators in the same institution [6]. Those receiving sildenafil had less pleural effusion chest tube output, a lower mean pulmonary artery pressure, lower inotropic score, and less ventilator time [6]. Finally, catheterization data have been evaluated in children status postbidirectional Glenn procedure after a single dose of sildenafil, which was deemed well tolerated [7]. Patients had improvement in saturations and pulmonary blood flow in those with pulmonary vascular resistances above 2 Wood units. However, there was no change in myocardial performance or cardiac index [7]. With the evolving management strategies for those with single ventricle physiology either postoperatively or long term to augment functional capacity, quality of life, and outcomes, it is paramount to continue to investigate the role of PDE5 inhibitors in this patient population.

PHOSPHODIESTERASE 3 INHIBITION

PDE3 inhibition leads to an increase in cAMP concentration in the myocardium as well in vascular smooth muscle [8]. The main effect in heart failure is felt to be inotropic but certainly there is a vasodilatory component based on relaxation of smooth muscle and dilation of the vascular bed [8]. Inotropic support in pediatrics has centered on agents that act via

Heart Failure in the Child and Young Adult. http://dx.doi.org/10.1016/B978-0-12-802393-8.00040-5

alterations of intracellular myocardial cAMP, which include catecholamines and PDE3 inhibitors. Catecholamines act via stimulation of adrenergic receptors, which in turn yields increased cAMP production, whereas PDE3 inhibitors bind to the esteratic site of the enzyme in a competitive fashion with cAMP, which begets increased concentration and accumulation of cAMP in the myocyte [9]. Catecholamines are limited by several factors, including downregulation of adrenergic receptors in those with heart failure, increased myocardial oxygen consumption, and excessive chronotropy at higher dosing strategies [9]. PDE3 inhibitors not only have intropic and vasodilatory effects but also enhance lusitropy while not increasing myocardial oxygen consumption [9].

The cellular mechanism for PDE3 inhibition to invoke the inotropic, lusitropic, and vasodilating properties via relaxation of vascular smooth muscle is independent of adrenergic receptors. Intracellular cAMP and calcium increase, as does the sensitivity of the actin–myosin complex to calcium, thus leading to enhanced myocardial contractility [10]. Additionally, intracellular cAMP begets an increase in protein kinase A activity [11]. Protein kinase A leads to an opening of L-type calcium channels of the cell membrane, which allows for entry of calcium into the myocardium [11]. This phenomenon stimulates calcium release in the sarcoplasmic reticulum but also promotes phosphorylation of phospholamban [11]. Phospholamban is thus activated that accelerates removal of calcium from the cytosol by the sarcoplasmic reticulum, which in turn shortens the contraction time. This phenomenon allows for more relaxation time of the myocardium in each cardiac cycle, which accounts for enhanced lusitropy [10]. Finally, PDE3 inhibition increases levels of cGMP in the vascular smooth muscle lending to a dilation of the coronary, pulmonary, and systemic vascular beds [10].

Historically, the first PDE3 inhibitor to be introduced was amrinone in 1972 [12]. Its use was limited by a concerning side effect profile, and as with many other inotropic agents in adult patients with heart failure, the use of the drug was associated with increased mortality [12]. A metaanalysis of PDE3 inhibitors in adult heart failure noted an approximate 3% increase in cardiac mortality and a similar increase in sudden cardiac death [13]. The proarrhythmic effect of PDE3 inhibition in adults is well documented but the underlying mechanism is unclear [8]. There is speculation whether this is due to an increase in intracellular calcium cycling or cAMP-mediated pathologic modeling associated with apoptosis [8]. Since amrinone had considerable limitations and a prolonged half-life, a series of additional phosphodiesterase inhibitors were discovered each with unique properties, namely milrinone, enoximone, vesnarinone, pentoxifylline, and cilostazol [12]. Since milrinone is arguably the most commonly used and studied PDE3 inhibitor in adults and pediatrics, the remainder of the chapter will focus on milrinone.

In the adult heart failure world, if a patient were on optimal enteral heart failure therapy and still decompensated, the addition of PDE3 inhibition might be considered especially for those patients on beta-blockade. Since PDE3 inhibitors act independently of the beta-adrenergic receptors, their use becomes theoretically palatable knowing that beta-adrenergic receptors downregulate with time in chronic heart failure. Additionally, catecholamine dosing strategies would have to be potentially altered to obtain the desired effect especially in light of those patients on chronic beta-blockade. At higher doses of catecholamines, potential undesirable alpha adrenergic effects might occur thus raising systemic vascular resistance in a setting where that physiology is counterproductive. All of these theoretical pharmacodynamic properties of PDE3 inhibitors lead to the development of enteral and intravenous milrinone. However, the PROMISE trial (Prospective Randomized Milrinone Survival Evaluation) randomized adult subjects with New York Heart Association Class III–IV classification with heart failure with reduced ejection fraction of less than 35% (HFrEF) to enteral milrinone versus placebo [14]. This trial was stopped early by the data safety monitoring board for a 28% increase in mortality in those receiving what in retrospect was considered a high dose of enteral milrinone [14]. Some criticisms of the study after subsequent research on PDE3 inhibitors include that the subjects were provided doses of study drug that were construed empirically without previous pharmacokinetic data, subjects on beta-blockers were excluded thus eliminating a potentially protective medication, and finally that the study group had severe heart failure [12]. Subsequent studies of oral enoximone at low doses and in combination with usual heart failure care including beta-blockers showed improvement in ejection fraction [15]. Despite a few studies on low-dose enteral PDE3 inhibitors in combination with usual heart failure pharmacologic interventions, research and development on enteral milrinone as a viable strategy has ceased.

No ideal inotrope has been discovered that would garner all of the following properties: (1) improves systolic and diastolic cardiac function, (2) decreases systemic and pulmonary vasoconstriction, (3) has a favorable effect on myocardial oxygen dynamics, (4) has little to no adverse effects, and (5) improves quality of life and survival [9,15]. In adult heart failure care, all-cause mortality is increased when a patient with decompensated heart failure receives intravenous inotropic support [16]. This phenomenon is not felt to be noted in pediatrics and adverse effects of milrinone, for example, are infrequent in children. In 1995, a study of 10 neonates with postoperative low cardiac output were provided milrinone and the hemodynamic impact included a decrease in both right and left atrial pressures, a decrease in the mean systemic arterial and pulmonary arterial pressures after loading but not during steady-state infusion, and an increase in cardiac index [17]. There was also an increase in heart rate during the loading stage but an eventual slight decrease during infusion. All of these hemodynamic effects were noted without a change in myocardial oxygen consumption [17]. Several years after this study, the first pharmacokinetic studies were performed in children [18,19]. In essence, the studies did not find congruent results and utilized different compartment models. Nonetheless, similar favorable hemodynamic effects were noted, yet 58% of patients did experience thrombocytopenia postoperatively and the risk of such raised in concert with an increase in the length of infusion [18]. In contrast to amrinone, milrinone did not bind to cardiopulmonary circuits [18]. In summary, however, an increased elimination clearance was noted with older age children. It was also felt to be intuitive that larger pediatric patients would be able to clear milrinone per unit time more effectively as this elimination is felt to be associated with body mass [18]. Milrinone is known to be renally excreted as the main form of metabolism with 70% bound to plasma proteins [19]. Populations at risk for decreased glomerular filtration rates such as preterm infants, neonates, heart failure patients with renal compromise, and in those status post congenital heart surgery with the use of cardiopulmonary bypass are at times in need of an appropriate dose adjustment. These aforementioned studies all included a bolus followed by an infusion for a period of time.

With the knowledge of low cardiac output occurring in approximately 25% of patients postoperatively and in light of these aforementioned studies, a large multicenter randomized trial of prophylactic milrinone versus placebo was designed and carried out by 31 centers in North America, namely the PRIMACORP trial (Prophylactic Intravenous use of Milrinone After Cardiac OpeRation in Pediatrics) [20]. It was felt to be safest to follow a similar practice of providing a bolus after the surgery in the intensive care unit followed by an infusion even though this was not common practice at the time. Most centers had already started providing a bolus in the operating room followed by an infusion prior to arriving in the post-operative setting. However, for ultimate safety of the trial and assuring appropriate observation of the pharmacodynamic impact of study drug albeit in a blinded fashion, the design assured an observed bolus over 1 h in the intensive care setting followed by an infusion for 35 h. The design was a double-blind, placebo-controlled trial with three parallel groups (low-dose milirinone 25 μg/kg bolus followed by 25 μg/kg/min infusion; high-dose milirinone 75 μg/kg bolus followed by 75 μg/kg/min infusion, and placebo). A clinical endpoint for low cardiac output syndrome (LCOS) was designed and a composite endpoint of death or the development of LCOS was evaluated for up to a month after initiation of study drug. The clinical endpoint of LCOS became a criticism of the trial, albeit a necessary aspect, as direct measurement of hemodynamic impact such as cardiac output in patients ranging from neonates to 6 years of age was neither practical nor feasible. Despite this limitation, the endpoint was only reached if there was clinical evidence as per defined criteria and there were additional alterations in care to treat the LCOS either via additional pharmacological or mechanical support within the first 36 h after initiation of study drug. Among 238 treated patients, high-dose milrinone was found to significantly reduce the risk of development of LCOS as compared to placebo [20]. There was a trend toward decreasing LCOS in those on low dose as well with 25.9% experiencing LCOS in the placebo group, whereas 17.5% and 11.7% were noted to have LCOS in the low and high-dose milrinone groups, respectively [20]. In those subjects receiving high-dose milrinone, there was a relative risk reduction of 55% in the 238 treated patients and in 64% of 227 patients without major protocol violations (Fig. 40.1) [20]. Safety analyses performed showed no significant difference in the rate of thrombocytopenia or arrhythmias in those receiving milrinone regardless of dosing strategy as compared to placebo. This trial was also accompanied by a population pharmacokinetic study, although this analysis was unique in that for study safety reasons, the bolus was provided over 1 h [21]. Nonetheless, it was noted that both the volume of distribution and clearance increased with increasing body weight with both parameters being directly proportional to weight. Most importantly, in this trial and pharmacokinetic model,

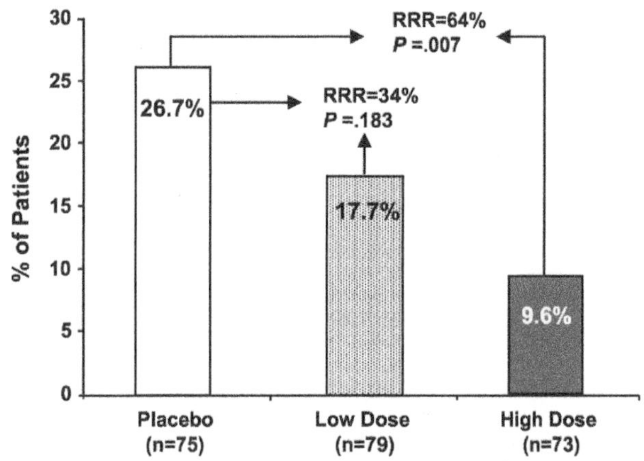

FIGURE 40.1 PRIMACORP study relative risk reduction (RRR) of low cardiac output syndrome composite endpoint.

clearance increases linearly with patient age, which could reflect a delayed maturation of drug clearance processes [21]. For example, the clearance in neonates was less than 25% of that in children indicating that in a neonate, a constant rate infusion will take longer to approach steady-state, but the steady-state concentration will be higher in neonates as compared to older children. The key understanding is that constant rate infusions will eventually result in higher blood concentrations in younger patients, however, the longer half-life in younger patients means that it will take longer to approach steady-state [21]. With a longer duration of administration, dose reductions in neonates especially theoretically could be accomplished without lowering the plasma concentrations below therapeutic [21].

The PRIMACORP trial was helpful in several regards to understanding the efficacy and safety of prophylactic milrinone in the postoperative setting, although the dosing strategies were not congruent with general practice of 0.5 mcg/kg/min. Secondly, by this time, most centers were providing a bolus in the operating suite prior to modified ultrafiltration. Another criticism of the trial was that the most at risk patients, namely those with single ventricle physiology, were excluded from enrollment. Subsequently, a single center pharmacokinetic milrinone study was performed in patients with hypoplastic left heart syndrome undergoing Stage I palliation [22]. The study was a blinded, randomized design where neonates received either 100 or 250 µg/kg into the cardiopulmonary bypass circuit at the initiation of rewarming. A modified ultrafiltration concentrating effect was noted in all patients and the initial loading dose of 100 µg/kg resulted in therapeutic plasma concentrations [22]. Modified ultrafiltration yielded an increase in plasma milrinone concentrations by approximately 35% (Fig. 40.2) [22]. Similar to what was noted in the PRIMACORP pharmacokinetic study, the expected decrease postoperatively of glomerular filtration rate resulted in impaired clearance albeit transient. To that end, the study elicited a speculative conclusion that in the setting of impaired renal function, an infusion dose of 0.2 µg/kg/min may be adequate and sustain steady-state therapeutic concentration in these high-risk neonates [22].

The PRIMACORP trial begets interest in other populations such as premature infants and patients with cardiomyopathy with acute and chronic heart failure. One such study in premature infants encompassed a known entity of decreased systemic blood flow that occurs in 35% of those infants 30 weeks gestation and in 61% of infants 27 weeks gestational age [23]. The study involved open label milrinone in a dose-escalation fashion in patients at risk for this hemodynamic phenomenon. None of the subjects received a bolus and the dosing was either 0.25 µg/kg/min for 24 h, 0.5 µg/kg/min for 24 h, or 0.75 µg/kg/min for 3 h followed by an infusion of 0.2 µg/kg/min for 18 h [9,23]. The measured outcome datum was the maintenance of superior vena cava flow via echocardiography at 0.45 mL/kg/min, which correlated with a good cardiac output. All patients receiving the milrinone dosing strategy of 0.75 µg/kg/min for 3 h followed by 0.2 µg/kg/min for 18 h maintained the desired superior vena cava flow and thus was deemed the "optimal dosing strategy" [23]. There was a subpar response with the other two dosing arms of the pilot study. Ultimately, there were no adverse effects noted and the elimination half-life of milrinone in this premature population was 10 h [23].

This study was followed by a double-blind, randomized trial using the "optimal dosing strategy" versus placebo in subjects less than 30 weeks gestation using the same endpoint, maintenance of superior vena caval flow above the aforementioned threshold [24]. Ninety infants were randomized and no difference was noted between those receiving milrinone versus placebo. Secondary hemodynamic effects also showed no difference in incidence of hypotension, need for additional inotropic support, time to initiating inotropic support, or mean dose of inotropes [24]. The only difference noted was that those in the milrinone arm experienced an increased incidence of sinus tachycardia. Since milrinone was not efficacious, it

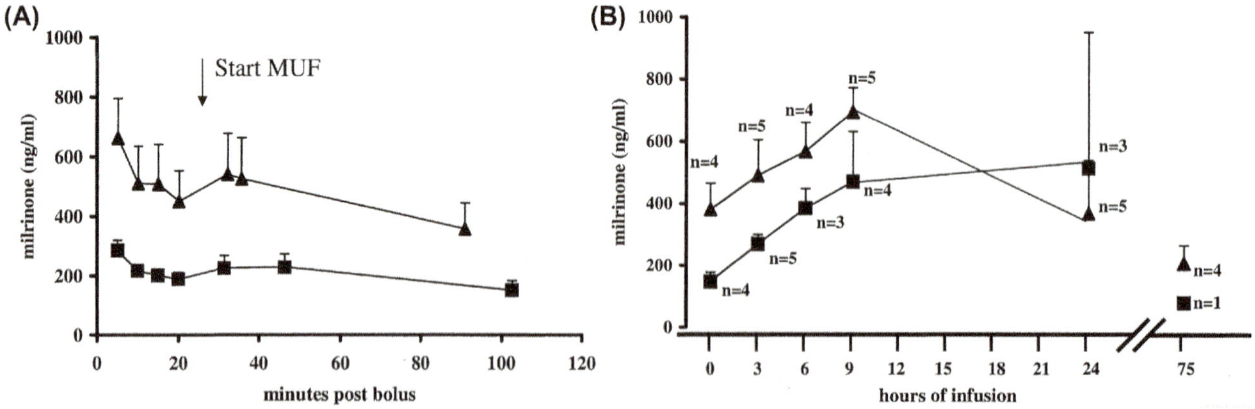

FIGURE 40.2 (A) Plasma concentrations during intraoperative period, including modified ultrafiltration (MUF). Squares represent the 100 µg/kg bolus group; triangles represent the 250 µg/kg bolus group. (B) Plasma concentration during postoperative period. Squares represent the 100 µg/kg bolus group; triangles represent the 250 µg/kg bolus group. Subject included in this figure received a continuous infusion of 0.5 µg · kg^{-1} · min^{-1}.

was speculated that milrinone has a decreased effectiveness in the immature myocardium similar to a phenomenon noted in animal studies. Secondly, there was concern on behalf of the authors that the intervention with milrinone may have been at the wrong timing to see an effect and in turn may have led to the wrong therapeutic target [24]. Milrinone use in premature infants has not become standard practice in most settings. Although, theoretical use of milrinone in certain clinical situations, such as postductal ligation in premature infants, has been discussed. A case report exists outlining the postoperative course of a low birth weight infant born at 26 weeks gestation who underwent patent ductus arteriosus ligation and received milrinone due to hemodynamic instability [25]. Preterm infants are prone to hemodynamic instability and alterations in left ventricular performance after ductal ligation based on the acute change in loading conditions in association with an increase in systemic vascular resistance [25]. Milrinone affords a decrease in systemic vascular resistance, positive inotropy, and enhanced lusitropy all of which would be beneficial effects for this clinical situation. The patient in the case report experienced an increase in blood pressure after ligation but evidence of diastolic dysfunction and low cardiac output via echocardiography. Once milrinone was initiated with a bolus of 50 μg/kg followed by an infusion of 0.3 μg/kg/min for 18 h, repeat echocardiography showed an improvement in diastolic and cardiac output parameters, which also correlated with an improvement clinically [25]. Therefore, speculation exists as to whether milrinone has a role in other populations including the premature infant although again, concern exists that PDE3 inhibitors are felt to be less effective in the immature myocardium.

The extrapolation of the PRIMACORP trial among other published experiences has elicited the conclusion that pediatric patients do not experience the same side effect frequency or mortality rates on PDE3 inhibitors as compared to adults. A very eloquent study was performed on both adults and prepubertal children whose explanted heart tissue was utilized for quantification of cAMP, phosphodiesterase activity, and phospholamban phosphorylation at the time of transplant [26]. The experience of the researchers with 53 pediatric patients bridged to transplant as an outpatient on home milrinone infusions without any incidence of sudden death prompted the investigation of differences in children and adults with end-stage heart failure. It was expected that the clinical differences are likely due to age-related variations in cellular adaptation and signaling thus yielding less adverse events and side effects in children who receive PDE3 inhibitors. In short, elevated cAMP levels and higher phospholamban phosphorylation in children likely contribute to the sustained hemodynamic benefit of milrinone in pediatrics [26]. Additionally, the higher phosphodiesterase activity noted in adults while on milrinone may beget lower myocardial cAMP and phopholamban phosphorylation therefore limiting the potential benefit of PDE3 inhibition [26]. This study helps fuel the argument that children likely not only have age-related differences in metabolic and cellular mechanisms that may allow for perpetuated benefit of milrinone therapy, but it is obvious that the underlying disease pathophysiology (i.e., nonischemic heart failure) is grossly different than that in the adult population. It is then reasonable to speculate that inotropic support with PDE inhibitors will not beget the same adverse effect profile or detriment to overall survival that is noted in the adult population. In contrast, however, to children with dilated cardiomyopathy, milrinone has been less studied in those with specifically a single right ventricle physiology. Milrinone is often used in this population for failed Fontan physiology despite the cause as a bridge to transplant or recovery [27]. However, researchers have now found that the molecular adaptation associated in patients with single right ventricular physiology is different than the aforementioned response in children with dilated cardiomyopathy. In other words, the single right ventricle molecular response is similar to that of a nonfailing right ventricle [27]. To that end, chronic PDE3 inhibition may theoretically not be efficacious due to the different adaptation mechanisms in those with single right ventricles. This paradigm emphasizes that extrapolation of data to all populations is fraught with limitations. Clearly, the efficacy and safety of PDE inhibition will vary based on a myriad of variables including age, underlying anatomic substrate, pathophysiology of heart failure, and metabolic differences. In essence, much has yet to be learned about common assumed practices in pediatric heart failure especially the use and potential overuse of PDE inhibition.

CONCLUSION

Over two decades of experience and research with PDE inhibition in pediatric heart failure lead to more questions than answers. The role of PDE5 inhibition in those with congenital heart disease and elevated pulmonary artery pressures is still theoretical yet the studies published to date are compelling. PDE3 inhibition in pediatrics, namely milrinone, has been used in LCOS and various conditions that beget heart failure. The molecular response to milrinone is different depending on the underlying anatomic substrate. Not only does this have an effect on efficacy but this phenomenon also influences safety. In general, most pediatric studies have described a far better safety profile of milrinone as compared to what has been noted in adults. Arrhythmia, thrombocytopenia, and mortality are seemingly less common in pediatrics as compared to that noted in adult heart failure care. In summary, via clinical studies, translational projects, and ongoing basic science research, the journey to optimal use of these medications is facilitated.

REFERENCES

[1] M. Movsesian, J. Stehlik, F. Vandeput, M.R. Bristow, Phosphodiesterase inhibition in heart failure, Heart Fail. Rev. 14 (4) (December 2009) 255–263.
[2] P. Kumar, G.S. Fracis, W.H. Tang, Phosphodiesterase 5 inhibition in heart failure: mechanisms and clinical implications, Nat. Rev. Cardiol. 6 (5) (May 2009) 349–355.
[3] P.F. Kantor, J. Lougheed, A. Dancea, et al., Presentation, diagnosis, and medical management of heart failure in children: Canadian cardiovascular society guidelines, Can. J. Caridol. 29 (12) (December 2013) 1535–1552.
[4] R. Kirk, A.I. Dipchand, D.N. Rosenthal, et al., The international society of heart and lung transplantation guidelines for the management of pediatric heart failure: executive summary, J. Heart Lung Transplant. 33 (9) (September 2014) 888–909.
[5] D.J. Goldberg, B. French, M.G. McBride, et al., Impact of oral sildenafil on exercise performance in children and young adults after the Fontan operation: a randomized, double-blind, placebo-controlled, crossover trial, Circulation 123 (11) (March 22, 2011) 1185–1193.
[6] R. Giordano, G. Palma, V. Poli, et al., First experience with sildenafil after Fontan operation: short-term outcomes, J. Cardiovasc. Med. 16 (8) (August 2015) 552–555.
[7] K.D. Hill, R.D. Tunks, P.C. Barker, et al., Sildenafil exposure and hemodynamic effect after stage II single-ventricle surgery, Pediatr. Crit. Care Med. 14 (6) (July 2013) 593–600.
[8] M.A. Movsesian, R.C. Kukreja, Phosphodiesterase inhibition in heart failure, Handb. Exp. Pharmacol. 204 (2011) 237–249.
[9] T.M. Hoffman, New inotropes in pediatric heart failure, J. Cardiovasc. Pharmacol. 58 (2) (August 2011) 121–125.
[10] B. Duggal, U. Pratap, Z. Slavik, J. Kaplanova, D. Macrae, Milrinone and low cardiac output following cardiac surgery in infants: is there a direct myocardial effect? Pediatr. Cardiol. 26 (5) (September–October 2005) 642–645.
[11] R. Feneck, Phosphodiesterase inhibitors and the cardiovascular system. Continuing education in anaesthesia, Crit. Care Pain 7 (6) (November 2007) 203–207.
[12] A.M. Feldman, D.M. McNamara, Reevaluating the role of phosphodiesterase inhibitors in the treatment of cardiovascular disease, Clin. Cardiol. 25 (6) (June 2002) 256–262.
[13] E. Amsallem, C. Kasparian, G. Haddour, J.P. Boissel, P. Nony, Phosphodiesterase III inhibitors for heart failure, Cochrane Database Syst. Rev. (1) (January 25, 2005) CD002230.
[14] M. Packer, J.R. Carver, R.J. Rodeheffer, et al., Effect of oral milrinone on mortality in severe chronic heart failure. The PROMISE Study Research Group, N. Engl. J. Med. 325 (1991) 1468–1475.
[15] S.F. Shakar, W.T. Abraham, E.M. Gilbert, et al., Combined oral positive inotropic and beta-blocker therapy for treatment of refractory class IV heart failure, J. Am. Coll. Cardiol. 31 (1998) 1336–1340.
[16] U. Elkayam, G. Tasissa, C. Binanay, et al., Use and impact of inotropes and vasodilator therapy in hospitalized patients with severe heart failure, Am. Heart J. 153 (2007) 98–104.
[17] A.C. Chang, A.M. Atz, G. Wernovsky, R.P. Burke, D.L. Wessel, Milrinone: systemic and pulmonary hemodynamic effects in neonates after cardiac surgery, Crit. Care Med. 23 (11) (November 1995) 1907–1914.
[18] C. Ramamoorthy, G.D. Anderson, G.D. Williams, A.M. Lynn, Pharmacokinetics and side effects of milrinone in infants and children after open heart surgery, Anesth. Analg. 86 (2) (February 1998) 283–289.
[19] R.M. Stroshane, R.F. Koss, C.E. Biddlecome, et al., Oral and intravenous pharmacokinetics of milrinone in human volunteers, J. Pharm. Sci. (1984) 731438–731441.
[20] T.M. Hoffman, G. Wernovsky, A.M. Atz, et al., Efficacy and safety of milrinone in preventing low cardiac output syndrome in infants and children after corrective surgery for congenital heart disease, Circulation 107 (7) (February 25, 2003) 996–1002.
[21] J.M. Bailey, T.M. Hoffman, D.L. Wessel, et al., A population pharmacokinetic analysis of milrinone in pediatric patients after cardiac surgery, J. Pharmacokinet. Pharmacodyn. 31 (1) (February 2004) 43–59.
[22] A.F. Zuppa, S.C. Nicholson, P.C. Adamson, et al., Population pharmacokinetics of milrinone in neonates with hypoplastic left heart syndrome undergoing stage I reconstruction, Anesth. Analg. 102 (4) (April 2006) 1062–1069.
[23] M. Paradisis, N. Evans, M. Kluckow, D. Osborn, A.J. McLachlan, Pilot study of milrinone for low systemic blood flow in very preterm infants, J. Pediatr. 148 (3) (March 2006) 306–313.
[24] M. Paradisis, N. Evans, M. Kluckow, D. Osborn, Randomized trial of milrinone versus placebo for prevention of low systemic blood flow in very preterm infants, J. Pediatr. 154 (2) (February 2009) 189–195.
[25] A. Sehgal, J.V. Francis, A.I. Lewis, Use of milrinone in the management of haemodynamic instability following duct ligation, Eur. J. Pediatr. 170 (1) (January 2011) 115–119.
[26] S.J. Nakano, S.D. Miyamoto, M. Movsesian, P. Nelson, B.L. Stauffer, C.C. Sucharov, Age-related differences in phosphodiesterase activity and effects of chronic phosphodiesterase inhibition in idiopathic dilated cardiomyopathy, Circ. Heart Fail. 8 (1) (January 2015) 57–63.
[27] S.J. Nakano, P. Nelson, C.C. Sucharov, S.D. Miyamoto, Myocardial response to milrinone in single right ventricular heart disease, J. Pediatr. (16) (May 12, 2016) 30057–30059 pii: S0022-3476.

Chapter 41

Use of Vasodilators in Heart Failure

Michael Burch, Jacob Simmonds, Timothy Thiruchelvam
Great Ormond Street Hospital, London, Great Britain

Chapter 41.1

Section 1. Oral Therapies in the Treatment of Heart Failure in the Young

Oral vasodilator therapy remains the cornerstone of treatment for heart failure in the young, but the evidence base is limited. The vast majority of clinical trials (as well as many physiological and pathological studies) in heart failure have taken place in adult populations; the pediatric cardiologist is therefore forced to base much of their knowledge on extrapolation on these. It is important, however, to bear in mind the axiom "children are not small adults," and many oral vasodilator drugs of proven benefit in adults have shown unconvincing use in children [1–6]. The reasons for these discrepancies remain opaque [7], but certainly some studies have been underpowered [3]. What is certain is that the dearth of large-scale, multicenter, high-quality trials in pediatric cardiology is a frustration commonly found in major guidelines on the subject [8,9].

Previously, with limited understanding of the pathophysiology of heart failure, therapies were aimed at improving myocardial function directly. Although this must still be the approach in the acute setting, there is evidence that this strategy worsens both long-term morbidity and mortality [10–12]. As knowledge has increased, greater importance has been placed on preventing the deleterious effects of long-term compensatory mechanisms, not only to improve cardiac function in the acute setting but also to prolong the long-term viability of the myocardium. This has led to treatment according to the "neuroendocrine" model of heart failure. In this model, heart failure is initially compensated for by increases in sympathetic drive, angiotensin, and endothelins, but this results in adverse changes in myocardial structure, function, and electrical stability, and a progressive cycle of worsening clinical heart failure develops. Interrupting this cycle with neuroendocrine antagonists may result in a transient deterioration but may modify the unfavorable natural history of chronic heart failure.

ANGIOTENSIN CONVERTING ENZYME INHIBITORS

Angiotensin converting enzyme (ACE) inhibitors were one of the great leaps forward in drug therapies for cardiovascular diseases. In the mid-1950s ACE was identified as the enzyme responsible for the conversion of angiotensin I to the vasoconstrictor substance, angiotensin II. By opposing the constricting action of angiotensin II the potential for reversing the neurohormonal effects of heart failure was conceived. In London in the 1960s the Nobel laureate, John Vane, demonstrated ACE activity was inhibited by peptides from the Brazilian viper's venom. Vane's work led to the US pharmaceutical company, ER Squibb and Sons researching ACE inhibitors, and eventually in the mid 1970s the first effective oral ACE inhibitor, captopril was discovered. It was released in the 1980s but the initial doses advised were far higher than currently used and hypotension was common. Another ACE inhibitor, enalapril, was developed by Merck a few years later. For both drugs there was concern from clinicians that hypotension would limit their use in heart failure because of the exaggerated activation of the renin–angiotensin system caused by the dehydration from diuretics. In 1987 the Cooperative North Scandinavian Enalapril Survival Study was published, which showed a huge reduction in mortality at 1 year in patients with severe heart failure who were treated with enalapril using a permissive approach to dose reduction for hypotension. Many other studies

Heart Failure in the Child and Young Adult. http://dx.doi.org/10.1016/B978-0-12-802393-8.00041-7

showed the benefits of ACE inhibitors in heart failure including SAVE and SOLVD, the latter showing a benefit in asymptomatic patients. ATLAS demonstrated that better results were obtained with higher doses of Lisinopril, a longer acting drug. The paradigm of a test dose of ACE inhibitor and then gradually increasing up to higher doses as tolerated became accepted.

As mentioned, the evidence base for heart failure drugs is limited in the young, and there are no large randomized studies for ACE inhibitors that show the mortality benefit seen in older adults. However, there are studies showing echocardiographic improvement [13,14], and others showing the beneficial effect of ACE inhibitors in Duchenne Muscular Dystrophy patients, with delay in onset and progression of cardiomyopathy [15–17].

In contrast, there is no evidence of mortality benefit of ACE inhibitors in congenital heart disease, and only limited evidence of improvement in "soft" markers such as exercise tolerance and echocardiography. Interestingly, this extends across the range of single ventricle patients and two ventricle patients, including those with systemic right ventricles such as congenitally corrected transposition or intraatrial baffle for transposition [5,18], and those with failing subpulmonic right ventricles (ramipril had little effect in patients with Tetralogy of Fallot) [19]. ACE inhibitors will increase cyanosis in Glenn shunts [20] and offer no benefit in the medium term [2]. Even after the Fontan there is no evidence for benefit in exercise ability [21].

ACE inhibitors can produce angioedema and must be used cautiously in hypotensive patients or those with renal insufficiency or elevated serum potassium. ACE inhibitors also inhibit kininase and this will therefore increase levels of bradykinin, elevated bradykinin can cause a dry cough, although it can also help heart failure by increasing vasodilation. Children tend to tolerate cough well, and cessation of ACE inhibitors in such circumstances appears less common than in adults. Renal function and serum potassium need to be monitored carefully with ACE inhibition in children and particularly in neonates.

In young children the use of ACE inhibitors is rather different to adult practice. In Europe captopril is commonly used and in North America enalapril, rather than longer acting ACE inhibitors. This reflects the years of experience with these older drugs. Enalapril is a prodrug and is converted to the active component enalaprilat, but the ability to convert it varies in the very young and can conversely lead to higher doses being needed. Captopril has a rapid onset and hypotension is common with test doses. It is often given 3 times a day in infants. There are different formulations of these medications, and a current EU grant sponsors a trial to develop a mini tablet of enalapril, which can offer accurate small doses in young children and infants and will investigate the pharmacokinetics (LENA: Labeling of Enalapril from Neonates up to Adolescents). Longer acting, once a day ACE inhibitors are commonly used in older children and adolescents such as lisinopril, ramipril, and perindopril.

There are specific ACE gene polymorphisms, which result in a range of ACE levels in humans. As yet there is limited evidence of varying genetic influences on the response to ACE inhibitors in childhood, but it does seem relevant in adults [22].

The current advice from the American Heart Association [23] (Yancy 2016: Pharmacological Treatment for Stage C HF With Reduced Ejection Fraction: Recommendations) states: angiotensin system inhibition with angiotensin-converting enzyme inhibitor or angiotensin receptor blocker (ARB) or angiotensin receptor–neprilysin inhibitor (ARNI): Recommendations: a level of evidence A and strength or recommendation 1.

In the pediatric heart failure guidelines from ISHLT 2014 [8], the use of ACE inhibitors for symptomatic left ventricular dysfunction is given a strength of recommendation 1 and level of evidence B. Similarly it was stated that ACE inhibitors should be considered for Duchenne muscular dystrophy although the optimal age of starting is unclear. It was, however, recommended that ACE inhibitors are not routinely used in patients with a single ventricle but could be considered in specific cases.

Angiotensin Receptor Blockers

The recognition that angiotensin II production continues in the presence of ACE inhibition via alternative pathways led to the development of ARBs. Dual blockade of the renin–angiotensin system seems logical and may have seemingly beneficial effects on certain surrogate end points. In metaanalysis and systematic review dual therapy failed to reduce mortality and was associated with an excessive risk of adverse events such as hyperkalemia, hypotension, and renal failure compared with monotherapy [24]. It is rarely used in pediatrics.

Unlike ACE inhibitors, ARBs do not inhibit kininase and therefore are associated with a much lower incidence of cough and angioedema. In pediatrics, the main use of ARBs is in patients who are intolerant of ACE inhibitors because of cough.

As with ACE inhibitors they must be used carefully in those with hypotension, renal insufficiency, or elevated serum potassium. The clinical benefit of ARBs is similar to ACE inhibitors in chronic heart failure [25,26]; and again higher doses appear to give better outcomes [27].

As with ACE inhibitors, results for the use of ARBs in congenital heart disease have been disappointing. For example, a study by Dore et al. demonstrated no improvement in exercise capacity or reduction NT-proBNP levels in patients with systemic right ventricles treated with losartan [4]. The authors noted that there was minimal baseline activation of the renin–angiotensin system, which they speculated may explain this lack of benefit and imply an alternative pathophysiological mechanism for the progressive ventricular dysfunction and impaired exercise capacity observed in such patients.

Combination for Hydralazine and Isosorbide Dinitrate

The V-Heft Trial showed a benefit of hydralazine and isosorbide dinitrate in adult heart failure [28] and V-Heft II compared the combination to enalapril [29]. Although the second study showed superiority of enalapril in all races, there was a beneficial effect of the combination therapy in African Americans but not in the white population. There was a greater history of hypertension in African Americans although hypertensive patients were excluded. A-Heft examined whether fixed dose of the combination was beneficial when given in addition to standard treatment and showed a mortality benefit of hydralazine and isosorbide dinitrate [30]. This suggests that the renin–angiotensin–aldosterone (RAAS) system may be less important than nitric oxide pathways in African Americans with heart failure. It seems likely that hypertension has a greater role in the etiology of heart failure in this group. It is very difficult to extrapolate these results to children, and, the current ISHLT guidelines do not advise the use of hydralazine and isosorbide dinitrate in pediatric heart failure (strength class III level of evidence C) [8].

CARVEDILOL (A VASODILATING β-BLOCKER)

The paradigm that β-blockers worsen heart failure was questioned by Waagstein in 1975 [31], and over the following years small studies confirmed that β-blockers were tolerated in most stable chronic heart and associated with clinical improvement. Post hoc analysis of secondary prevention trials after myocardial infarction demonstrated β-blockade had the greatest effect in patients with left ventricular dysfunction. As with ACE inhibitors and ARBs, it is the neurohormonal model of heart failure that is the rationale behind the use of β-blockers in heart failure. The aim is to prevent and reverse adrenergically mediated intrinsic myocardial dysfunction and remodeling, one of the initially compensatory but ultimately deleterious factors in the progression of heart failure.

This model provides a rationale for the use of β-blockers in combination with ACE inhibitors. The Metoprolol in Dilated Cardiomyopathy Trial [32] and the Cardiac Insufficiency Bisoprolol Study-I (CIBIS-I) [33] demonstrated hemodynamic improvements and reduced hospitalization rates for acute heart failure but were underpowered to detect an effect on survival. Larger multicenter trials in adults have shown their benefit in mortality in heart failure. The first of these was the US Carvedilol trial in 1996 [34]. Carvedilol is not only a nonselective β1-, β2-blocker but also is an alpha antagonist with antioxidant properties. The alpha antagonist effect means that it is a vasodilating beta-blocker. CIBIS II [35] and MERIT-HF [36] showed mortality benefit with selective beta-blockers. The Effect of Carvedilol on Survival in Severe Chronic Heart Failure study [37] showed that the previously reported benefits of carvedilol with regard to morbidity and mortality in patients with mild-to-moderate heart failure were also apparent in the patients with severe heart failure who were evaluated in this trial. The additional properties of carvedilol such as alpha-adrenergic blockade, antioxidant activity, and antiendothelin effect promote vasodilatation, and it is quite possibly this mechanism that enables carvedilol to be used successfully in severe heart failure unlike other beta-blockers.

Disappointingly, the pediatric carvedilol study showed no benefit of carvedilol versus placebo on clinical outcomes in children with symptomatic systemic ventricular systolic dysfunction and heart failure [3]. The authors of the study have implicated a higher than expected placebo response rate, and a possible interaction between systemic ventricular anatomy and primary outcome as possible reasons for the disappointing result. In contrast, however, in a small study on nine pediatric patients with dilated cardiomyopathy, carvedilol was found to significantly reduce neurohormonal activity (reduced renin–angiotensin system activation, reduced norepinephrine, aldosterone, and dopamine) and improve left ventricular ejection fraction, with significant reductions in ventricular diameters [38]. The differences in the conclusions from these two articles highlighting the difficulties inherent in pediatric heart failure research.

ANGIOTENSIN RECEPTOR–NEPRILYSIN INHIBITOR

ARNIs are a combination drug of an ARB with an inhibitor of neprilysin. The latter is an enzyme that breaks down vasoactive peptides, including natriuretic peptides, bradykinin, adrenomedullin. Omapatrilat, a neprilysin inhibitor combined with an ACE inhibitor (not an ARB) and an aminopeptidase P inhibitor, was associated with a threefold increased risk of angioedema compared with enalapril and development of this drug has ceased. A history of angioedema is a contraindication to ARNI therapy, despite the lower risk with an ARB compared to ACE inhibitor.

In the PARADIGM-HF (a RCT of over 8000 patients) study, the drug LCZ696 was superior to enalapril in reducing the risks of death and of hospitalization for heart failure with reduced ejection fraction [39]. The drug is now approved and marketed as Entresto. As with ACE inhibitors and ARBs, the use of ARNI is associated with the risk of hypotension and renal insufficiency. There is also a risk of angioedema but this may be less than with ACE inhibitors. This drug may replace ACE inhibitors as part of the neurohormonal treatment for heart failure and is now represented in the latest heart failure guidelines [23]. At present it is not approved in pediatrics, although pediatric trials are likely in the near future. Pharmacokinetic data and clinical experience with hypotension and concomitant drugs will guide clinicians on the optimal titration and tolerability of ARNI.

REFERENCES

[1] P.F. Kantor, J.R. Abraham, A.I. Dipchand, L.N. Benson, A.N. Redington, The impact of changing medical therapy on transplantation-free survival in pediatric dilated cardiomyopathy, J. Am. Coll. Cardiol. 55 (13) (March 30, 2010) 1377–1384.

[2] D.T. Hsu, V. Zak, L. Mahony, L.A. Sleeper, A.M. Atz, J.C. Levine, P.C. Barker, C. Ravishankar, B.W. McCrindle, R.V. Williams, K. Altmann, N.S. Ghanayem, R. Margossian, W.K. Chung, W.L. Border, G.D. Pearson, M.P. Stylianou, S. Mital, Enalapril in infants with single ventricle: results of a multicenter randomized trial, Circulation 122 (4) (July 27, 2010) 333–340.

[3] R.E. Shaddy, M.M. Boucek, D.T. Hsu, R.J. Boucek, C.E. Canter, L. Mahony, R.D. Ross, E. Pahl, E.D. Blume, D.A. Dodd, D.N. Rosenthal, J. Burr, B. LaSalle, R. Holubkov, M.A. Lukas, L.Y. Tani, Carvedilol for children and adolescents with heart failure: a randomized controlled trial, JAMA 298 (10) (September 12, 2007) 1171–1179.

[4] A. Dore, C. Houde, K.L. Chan, A. Ducharme, P. Khairy, M. Juneau, F. Marcotte, L.A. Mercier, Angiotensin receptor blockade and exercise capacity in adults with systemic right ventricles: a multicenter, randomized, placebo-controlled clinical trial, Circulation 112 (16) (October 18, 2005) 2411–2416.

[5] S.J. Hechter, P.M. Fredriksen, P. Liu, G. Veldtman, N. Merchant, M. Freeman, J. Therrien, L. Benson, S. Siu, G. Webb, Angiotensin-converting enzyme inhibitors in adults after the Mustard procedure, Am. J. Cardiol. 87 (5) (March 1, 2001) 660–663 A11.

[6] T. van der Bom, M.M. Winter, B.J. Bouma, M. Groenink, H.W. Vliegen, P.G. Pieper, A.P. van Dijk, G.T. Sieswerda, J.W. Roos-Hesselink, A.H. Zwinderman, B.J. Mulder, Effect of valsartan on systemic right ventricular function: a double-blind, randomized, placebo-controlled pilot trial, Circulation 127 (3) (January 22, 2013) 322–330.

[7] J.W. Rossano, R.E. Shaddy, Update on pharmacological heart failure therapies in children: do adult medications work in children and if not, why not? Circulation 129 (5) (February 4, 2014) 607–612.

[8] R. Kirk, A.I. Dipchand, D.N. Rosenthal, L. Addonizio, M. Burch, M. Chrisant, A. Dubin, M. Everitt, R. Gajarski, L. Mertens, S. Miyamoto, D. Morales, E. Pahl, R. Shaddy, J. Towbin, R. Weintraub, The International Society of Heart and Lung Transplantation Guidelines for the management of pediatric heart failure: executive summary, J. Heart Lung Transplant. 33 (9) (September 2014) 888–909.

[9] P.F. Kantor, J. Lougheed, A. Dancea, M. McGillion, N. Barbosa, C. Chan, R. Dillenburg, J. Atallah, H. Buchholz, C. Chant-Gambacort, J. Conway, L. Gardin, K. George, S. Greenway, D.G. Human, A. Jeewa, J.F. Price, R.D. Ross, S.L. Roche, L. Ryerson, R. Soni, J. Wilson, K. Wong, Presentation, diagnosis, and medical management of heart failure in children: Canadian Cardiovascular Society guidelines, Can. J. Cardiol. 29 (12) (December 2013) 1535–1552.

[10] J.F. Price, A.R. Mott, H.A. Dickerson, J.L. Jefferies, D.P. Nelson, A.C. Chang, S.E. O'Brian, J.A. Towbin, W.J. Dreyer, S.W. Denfield, S.L. Goldstein, Worsening renal function in children hospitalized with decompensated heart failure: evidence for a pediatric cardiorenal syndrome? Pediatr. Crit. Care Med. 9 (3) (May 2008) 279–284.

[11] W.T. Abraham, K.F. Adams, G.C. Fonarow, M.R. Costanzo, R.L. Berkowitz, T.H. LeJemtel, M.L. Cheng, J. Wynne, In-hospital mortality in patients with acute decompensated heart failure requiring intravenous vasoactive medications: an analysis from the Acute Decompensated Heart Failure National Registry (ADHERE), J. Am. Coll. Cardiol. 46 (1) (July 5, 2005) 57–64.

[12] M. Packer, J.R. Carver, R.J. Rodeheffer, R.J. Ivanhoe, R. DiBianco, S.M. Zeldis, G.H. Hendrix, W.J. Bommer, U. Elkayam, M.L. Kukin, Effect of oral milrinone on mortality in severe chronic heart failure. The PROMISE Study Research Group, N. Engl. J. Med. 325 (21) (November 21, 1991) 1468–1475.

[13] H. Stern, J. Weil, T. Genz, W. Vogt, K. Buhlmeyer, Captopril in children with dilated cardiomyopathy: acute and long-term effects in a prospective study of hemodynamic and hormonal effects, Pediatr. Cardiol. 11 (1) (January 1990) 22–28.

[14] M. Eronen, E. Pesonen, E.I. Wallgren, I. Tikkanen, F. Fyhrquist, S. Andersson, Enalapril in children with congestive heart failure, Acta Paediatr. Scand. 80 (5) (May 1991) 555–558.

[15] D. Duboc, C. Meune, G. Lerebours, J.Y. Devaux, G. Vaksmann, H.M. Becane, Effect of perindopril on the onset and progression of left ventricular dysfunction in Duchenne muscular dystrophy, J. Am. Coll. Cardiol. 45 (6) (March 15, 2005) 855–857.

[16] D. Duboc, C. Meune, B. Pierre, K. Wahbi, B. Eymard, A. Toutain, C. Berard, G. Vaksmann, S. Weber, H.M. Becane, Perindopril preventive treatment on mortality in Duchenne muscular dystrophy: 10 years' follow-up, Am. Heart J. 154 (3) (September 2007) 596–602.

[17] J.L. Jefferies, B.W. Eidem, J.W. Belmont, W.J. Craigen, S.M. Ware, S.D. Fernbach, S.R. Neish, E.O. Smith, J.A. Towbin, Genetic predictors and remodeling of dilated cardiomyopathy in muscular dystrophy, Circulation 112 (18) (November 1, 2005) 2799–2804.

[18] B. Robinson, C.T. Heise, J.W. Moore, J. Anella, M. Sokoloski, E. Eshaghpour, Afterload reduction therapy in patients following intraatrial baffle operation for transposition of the great arteries, Pediatr. Cardiol. 23 (6) (November 2002) 618–623.

[19] S.V. Babu-Narayan, A. Uebing, P.A. Davlouros, M. Kemp, S. Davidson, K. Dimopoulos, S. Bayne, D.J. Pennell, D.G. Gibson, M. Flather, P.J. Kilner, W. Li, M.A. Gatzoulis, Randomised trial of ramipril in repaired tetralogy of Fallot and pulmonary regurgitation: the APPROPRIATE study (ACE-inhibitors for Potential PRevention of the deleterious effects of Pulmonary Regurgitation in Adults with repaired TEtralogy of Fallot, Int. J. Cardiol. 154 (3) (February 9, 2012) 299–305.

[20] K.J. Lee, S.J. Yoo, H. Holtby, B. Grant, D. Mroczek, D. Wong, L. Grosse-Wortmann, L.N. Benson, R.R. Chaturvedi, Acute effects of the ACE inhibitor enalaprilat on the pulmonary, cerebral and systemic blood flow and resistance after the bidirectional cavopulmonary connection, Heart 97 (16) (August 2011) 1343–1348.

[21] A.A. Kouatli, J.A. Garcia, T.M. Zellers, E.M. Weinstein, L. Mahony, Enalapril does not enhance exercise capacity in patients after Fontan procedure, Circulation 96 (5) (September 2, 1997) 1507–1512.

[22] B. Andersson, C. Sylven, The DD genotype of the angiotensin-converting enzyme gene is associated with increased mortality in idiopathic heart failure, J. Am. Coll. Cardiol. 28 (1) (July 1996) 162–167.

[23] C.W. Yancy, M. Jessup, B. Bozkurt, J. Butler, D.E. Casey Jr., M.M. Colvin, M.H. Drazner, G. Filippatos, G.C. Fonarow, M.M. Givertz, S.M. Hollenberg, J. Lindenfeld, F.A. Masoudi, P.E. McBride, P.N. Peterson, L.W. Stevenson, C. Westlake, 2016 ACC/AHA/HFSA focused update on new pharmacological therapy for heart failure: an update of the 2013 ACCF/AHA guideline for the management of heart failure: a report of the American College of Cardiology/American Heart Association Task Force on clinical practice guidelines and the heart failure society of America, J. Am. Coll. Cardiol. (May 17, 2016).

[24] H. Makani, S. Bangalore, K.A. Desouza, A. Shah, F.H. Messerli, Efficacy and safety of dual blockade of the renin-angiotensin system: meta-analysis of randomised trials, BMJ 346 (2013) f360.

[25] J.N. Cohn, G. Tognoni, A randomized trial of the angiotensin-receptor blocker valsartan in chronic heart failure, N. Engl. J. Med. 345 (23) (December 6, 2001) 1667–1675.

[26] M.A. Pfeffer, J.J. McMurray, E.J. Velazquez, J.L. Rouleau, L. Kober, A.P. Maggioni, S.D. Solomon, K. Swedberg, F. Van de Werf, H. White, J.D. Leimberger, M. Henis, S. Edwards, S. Zelenkofske, M.A. Sellers, R.M. Califf, Valsartan, captopril, or both in myocardial infarction complicated by heart failure, left ventricular dysfunction, or both, N. Engl. J. Med. 349 (20) (November 13, 2003) 1893–1906.

[27] M.A. Konstam, J.D. Neaton, K. Dickstein, H. Drexler, M. Komajda, F.A. Martinez, G.A. Riegger, W. Malbecq, R.D. Smith, S. Guptha, P.A. Poole-Wilson, Effects of high-dose versus low-dose losartan on clinical outcomes in patients with heart failure (HEAAL study): a randomised, double-blind trial, Lancet 374 (9704) (November 28, 2009) 1840–1848.

[28] J.N. Cohn, D.G. Archibald, S. Ziesche, J.A. Franciosa, W.E. Harston, F.E. Tristani, W.B. Dunkman, W. Jacobs, G.S. Francis, K.H. Flohr, Effect of vasodilator therapy on mortality in chronic congestive heart failure. Results of a Veterans Administration Cooperative Study, N. Engl. J. Med. 314 (24) (June 12, 1986) 1547–1552.

[29] J.N. Cohn, G. Johnson, S. Ziesche, F. Cobb, G. Francis, F. Tristani, R. Smith, W.B. Dunkman, H. Loeb, M. Wong, A comparison of enalapril with hydralazine-isosorbide dinitrate in the treatment of chronic congestive heart failure, N. Engl. J. Med. 325 (5) (August 1, 1991) 303–310.

[30] A.L. Taylor, S. Ziesche, C. Yancy, P. Carson, R. D'Agostino Jr., K. Ferdinand, M. Taylor, K. Adams, M. Sabolinski, M. Worcel, J.N. Cohn, Combination of isosorbide dinitrate and hydralazine in blacks with heart failure, N. Engl. J. Med. 351 (20) (November 11, 2004) 2049–2057.

[31] F. Waagstein, A. Hjalmarson, E. Varnauskas, I. Wallentin, Effect of chronic beta-adrenergic receptor blockade in congestive cardiomyopathy, Br. Heart J. 37 (10) (October 1975) 1022–1036.

[32] F. Waagstein, M.R. Bristow, K. Swedberg, F. Camerini, M.B. Fowler, M.A. Silver, E.M. Gilbert, M.R. Johnson, F.G. Goss, A. Hjalmarson, Beneficial effects of metoprolol in idiopathic dilated cardiomyopathy. Metoprolol in Dilated Cardiomyopathy (MDC) Trial Study Group, Lancet 342 (8885) (December 11, 1993) 1441–1446.

[33] A randomized trial of beta-blockade in heart failure. The cardiac insufficiency bisoprolol study (CIBIS). CIBIS investigators and committees, Circulation 90 (4) (October 1994) 1765–1773.

[34] M. Packer, M.R. Bristow, J.N. Cohn, W.S. Colucci, M.B. Fowler, E.M. Gilbert, N.H. Shusterman, The effect of carvedilol on morbidity and mortality in patients with chronic heart failure. U.S. Carvedilol Heart Failure Study Group, N. Engl. J. Med. 334 (21) (May 23, 1996) 1349–1355.

[35] The cardiac insufficiency bisoprolol study II (CIBIS-II): a randomised trial, Lancet 353 (9146) (January 2, 1999) 9–13.

[36] Effect of metoprolol CR/XL in chronic heart failure: metoprolol CR/XL randomised intervention trial in congestive heart failure (MERIT-HF), Lancet 353 (9169) (June 12, 1999) 2001–2007.

[37] M. Packer, A.J. Coats, M.B. Fowler, H.A. Katus, H. Krum, P. Mohacsi, J.L. Rouleau, M. Tendera, A. Castaigne, E.B. Roecker, M.K. Schultz, D.L. DeMets, Effect of carvedilol on survival in severe chronic heart failure, N. Engl. J. Med. 344 (22) (May 31, 2001) 1651–1658.

[38] A. Giardini, R. Formigari, G. Bronzetti, D. Prandstraller, A. Donti, M. Bonvicini, F.M. Picchio, Modulation of neurohormonal activity after treatment of children in heart failure with carvedilol, Cardiol. Young 13 (4) (August 2003) 333–336.

[39] J.J. McMurray, M. Packer, A.S. Desai, J. Gong, M.P. Lefkowitz, A.R. Rizkala, J.L. Rouleau, V.C. Shi, S.D. Solomon, K. Swedberg, M.R. Zile, Angiotensin-neprilysin inhibition versus enalapril in heart failure, N. Engl. J. Med. 371 (11) (September 11, 2014) 993–1004.

Chapter 41.2

Section 2. Intravenous Vasodilator Therapies in the Treatment of Heart Failure in the Young

INTRODUCTION AND PHYSIOLOGICAL CONCEPTS

Section 1 has discussed the clinical trials in adult heart failure that have demonstrated therapeutic benefit with oral therapies in chronic heart failure, sadly there has not been similar advances in the treatment of "acute heart failure" (AHF) [1–3]. Clinical practice guidelines recognize heart failure to be a complex clinical diagnosis and "AHF" [4,5] but in hospitalized patients, the left ventricular ejection fraction (EF) is an important discriminator when classifying patients with heart failure by demographics, comorbid condition, prognosis, and response to therapies [6]. Yet in both children and adults, heart failure may be associated with a wide spectrum of abnormalities in ventricular function, this may range or even progress from patients with normal size left ventricle (LV) and preserved EF to those with severe dilatation and/or markedly reduced EF. Abnormalities of both systolic and diastolic dysfunctions often coexist.

In children additional complexity is encountered when AHF is encountered in association with structural heart disease and can be exacerbated by catheter or surgical therapies designed to palliate or cure the underlying lesion. Might using systemic vasodilators to treat dilated cardiomyopathy with moderate mitral regurgitation yield a similar reduction in arterial elastance and improved cardiac performance compared to an infant with a functional single ventricle, diastolic dysfunction that ejects into an aortic arch that has been reconstructed by the Norwood technique?

Despite systolic blood pressure being an understandable therapeutic target, it is not equivalent to "cardiac afterload" and systemic vascular resistance (SVR) forms only a component of this dynamic afterload [7]. At rest and exercise the cardiovascular system is designed to enable ample blood flow at sufficient pressure to nourish all organs without large disturbances in blood pressure. This "ventriculo–arterial interaction," its adaptations with age, gender, rest or exercise, and also its maladaptations in disease states including hypertension and heart failure are now better understood [8,9]. In an isolated canine heart Sagawa described how "elastance" of the LV may serve as a load independent index of left ventricular contractility (end-systolic stiffness) [10]. Sunagawa et al. used a three element Windkessel model in the isolated canine heart to characterize arterial load as a composite of (1) characteristic impedance or proximal resistance to pulsatile flow in the ascending aorta, (2) distal arteriolar resistance (mean SVR), and (3) total arterial compliance alongside their relative contributions during systole and diastole [11]. However, this model does not account for the effects of reflected waves, which interfere with flow but augment pressure; with increased vascular stiffness this augmentation may adversely affect late ventricular systolic load and diastolic relaxation. It is important to recognize cardiac performance and myocardial energetics are optimal when the ratio of ventricular stiffness (Es) to arterial elastance (Ea) are approximately equal and absolute values are low [8,12]. The hydraulic efficiency of the LV (and myocardial oxygen consumption) is best conserved when the mechanical energy of the LV is transferred to kinetic energy of blood within the arterial tree.

The drugs discussed in this chapter act predominantly as "systemic vasodilators" that can be used to optimize left "ventricular–arterial coupling" reduce LV wall tension and myocardial oxygen consumption by reducing Ea enabling more efficient maintenance of cardiac output and oxygen delivery when heart rate, rhythm and preload are optimal. The properties of these agents will be highlighted and a brief description of how the vasodilator has been used in various patient groups (or subgroups) associated with acute decompensation or an intervention.

MILRINONE

Milrinone is a bipyridine derivative commonly classified as an "inodilator" whose mechanism of action is through the inhibition of phosphodiesterase type III (PDE3). It is this intracellular mechanism that evades the receptor-mediated downregulation experienced with exposure to endogenous or exogenous catecholamines. Moreover, the desired cardiovascular effects of PDE3 inhibitors may be obtained in the presence of beta-blockade [13,14]. The result of PDE3 inhibition in the cardiac myocyte is the accumulation of cyclic adenosine monophosphate, which activates protein kinases that increase calcium flux. Inotropic and lusitropic effects are consequent to the increased activation of contractile proteins, augmenting myocardial contractility but reducing the contractile time as a proportion of the cardiac cycle. In contrast, the effect on coronary, pulmonary, and peripheral vascular smooth muscle cells is afforded by an increase cGMP levels [15,16].

When administered intravenously, onset of action is within 5–10 min, the drug is 70% protein bound and the effective plasma concentration is 100–300 ng/mL for all age-groups [17]. The volume of distribution of milrinone is between 0.32 and 0.45 L/kg being greater in neonates than adults [18], the majority of the drug is actively eliminated by tubular secretion in the urine with 12% metabolized in the liver. The clearance of milrinone in neonates is less than in older children where the elimination half-life is approximately 2.5 h. In those patients experiencing renal dysfunction or requiring continuous venovenous hemofiltration the clearance of milrinone can be delayed [19].

An early report in 11 adults with congestive heart failure describes a comparable increase in cardiac index and reduction in coronary artery resistance between milrinone and dobutamine, while increased myocardial oxygen extraction was observed with dobutamine as opposed to milrinone where left ventricular end-diastolic pressure and atrial pressures were reduced to a greater extent. This is in keeping with its more potent vasodilator properties [20]. However, nearly 30 years later and in light of observational data from the ADHERE registry of over 65,000 episodes of acute decompensated heart failure whereby patients receiving milrinone or dobutamine exhibited greater in-hospital mortality than those receiving nesiritide or nitroglycerine (GTN), the use of milrinone in adult heart failure has waned [21,22]. It is still widely used in pediatric heart failure and is probably the most commonly used vasoactive medication [23]. In a recent was and long-term infusion has been shown to be safe in pediatric patients awaiting transplantation [24].

The hemodynamic profile is similar in children; with increased cardiac index, reduced cardiac filling pressures, SVR and PVR without an increase in myocardial oxygen consumption when milrinone was administered to 10 neonates following cardiac surgery with low cardiac output (cardiac index $<3.0\,L/min/m^2$) [25]. Subsequently Hoffman et al. conducted a prospective randomized placebo controlled trial to investigate the safety and efficacy of milrinone in the prevention of low cardiac output state. The study enrolled 242 children under 6 years of age undergoing biventricular surgery and observed a 64% relative risk reduction of low cardiac output syndrome (LCOS) at 36 h using high-dose milrinone (0.75 mcg/kg load followed by 0.75 mcg/kg/min for 35 h) compared to the parallel treatment arms of placebo or low-dose milrinone (0.25 mcg/kg bolus followed by 0.25 mcg/kg/min infusion for 35 h). In what was the largest randomized control trial in the pediatric cardiac surgical population at the time, safety data suggested there was no increased risk of arrhythmia, hypotension, or thrombocytopenia.

Zuppa et al. undertook a blinded randomized pharmacokinetic study of milrinone in a different population, 16 neonates undergoing stage 1 reconstruction for hypoplastic left heart syndrome. Following an initial administration of 100 or 250 mcg/kg of milrinone at the start of rewarming on cardiopulmonary bypass a continuous infusion was titrated to clinical need. The authors noted clearance of milrinone to be impaired, with an infusion of 0.5 mcg/kg/min resulting in drug accumulation and concluding that an infusion rate of 0.2 mcg/kg/min be considered in this population [26]. Low-dose infusions are probably most appropriate in neonates with renal insufficiency where the adverse effects of milrinone accumulation such as hypotension may become apparent.

Other adverse effects have been reported where milrinone use at admission to the intensive care unit was found to be risk factor for tachyarrhythmia requiring an intervention in a single center prospective study of 603 pediatric patients. This association was independent of age less than 1 month, cardiopulmonary bypass use and duration, surgical complexity, or the use of dopamine or epinephrine [27]. The authors acknowledge the use of milrinone at their institution to be the rule, the dose of milrinone and thresholds for treatment of tachyarrhythmia may have varied and some arrhythmias occurred after the cessation of milrinone.

The widespread adoption of milrinone in clinical practice as a prophylactic treatment for children undergoing cardiac surgery is not only born out in a survey of European practice but also highlights the adoption of varying dose regimes and modes of administration [28,29]. Similar practice variations are also evident in therapeutic studies of milrinone in the pediatric population.

A Cochrane systematic review by Burkhadt et al. of studies using prophylactic milrinone to prevent LCOS and mortality in children undergoing surgery for congenital heart disease identified five randomized control trials in which the use of milrinone, in isolation or combination with other vasoactive agents, was compared to placebo or other inotropic combinations. These trials included children up to the age of 12 years undergoing palliative or corrective surgery, primary outcome measures included 30-day mortality and LCOS as defined by the authors. Secondary outcomes included duration of mechanical ventilation, duration ICU stay, hospital stay, and the need for mechanical circulatory support or transplantation. Safety outcomes included the incidence of adverse events such as arrhythmia, tachycardia, hypotension, and thrombocytopenia. The PRIMACOR study of Hoffman et al. compared milrinone with placebo, while another compared milrinone with dobutamine [30] and the remaining studies compared milrinone with the calcium channel sensitizer levosimendan [31–33]. This review concluded that there was insufficient evidence of a prophylactic effect when milrinone is used to prevent mortality or LCOS and no significant differences were found in secondary or safety outcomes. This conclusion was supported by firstly the small number of small trials, no single treatment arm contained more than

80 patients. Secondly, the lack of evidence of a mortality benefit and thirdly the emphasis given to the short-term benefit of milrinone in the immediate postoperative period where the definition of LCOS is not standardized and the reporting of safety outcomes is inconsistent.

Although milrinone is clearly used as the perioperative drug of choice for children undergoing cardiac surgery further studies have seemingly not better defined or strengthen the evidence for its use in this population. However, it is with these reported early benefits following pediatric cardiac surgery that more novel drugs are often compared.

LEVOSIMENDAN

Levosimendan, an inodilator, was identified 20 years ago in the search for molecules that increase the sensitivity of contractile apparatus to calcium, increasing the force of contraction without increasing oxygen consumption. Levosimendan is capable if increasing calcium binding to cardiac troponin C, the myofibrillar receptor protein that activates actin–myosin interaction, resulting in inotropy. Calcium-dependent binding to troponin C is weaker when intracellular calcium levels are low during diastole; inotropy is achieved without impairment of ventricular relaxation or increased oxygen demand. Vasodilation is achieved by opening of sarcolemmal adenosine triphosphate sensitive potassium channels in smooth muscle cells [34,35]. Levosimendan is also capable of inhibiting PDE3 although not at therapeutic doses.

Levosimendan is administered intravenously, it is 98% protein bound and is entirely metabolized by the liver and not affected by renal or moderate liver impairment. Whereas the elimination half-life of levosimendan is 1–2 h the most active metabolite is OR-1896, which exhibits similar cardiovascular effects is 75–80 h. Although the hemodynamic effects of this metabolite may persist for 7–9 days, it is less clear to what extent the more pleiotropic cardioprotective, antiinflammatory, and antiapoptotic effects associated with levosimendan are also present with OR-1896 [36,37]. A similar pharmacokinetic profile was seen in 13 children with congenital heart disease where a 12 mcg/kg bolus of levosimendan over 10 min followed by an infusion of 0.2 mcg/kg/min for 24 h [38]. The hemodynamic effects of levosimendan are not attenuated by the use of beta-adrenergic blockade and neither tolerance has been reported [39,40].

In clinical practice levosimendan has demonstrated the ability to increase stroke volume and cardiac output, while reducing pulmonary vascular resistance, pulmonary capillary wedge, SVR, and natriuretic peptide levels, which may reduce symptoms of heart failure. Two early phase III randomized controlled trials suggests a mortality benefit in adults with decompensated heart failure treated with levosimendan [41,42]. This benefit was not demonstrated in two subsequent large studies that highlighted hypotension as being more frequent with levosimendan than placebo with an increased incidence of tachyarrhythmia compared to placebo or dobutamine [43,44]. A recent large metaanalysis looked at randomized controlled studies of the impact of levosimendan on mortality and hospitalization in the adult medical and surgical population. This incorporated 45 trials including 5480 patients and concluded levosimendan might reduce mortality in the cardiology and cardiac surgical setting with data from 17 studies suggesting that levosimendan was associated with a reduced length of stay [45]. Although widely available in Europe levosimendan has not received Food and Drug Administration approval and although further large-scale trials of levosimendan in adult heart failure seem unlikely, interest in the adult surgical population remains.

In an infant model of cardiopulmonary bypass Stocker et al. report both milrinone and levosimendan to illicit similar improvements in afterload and ventricular–vascular coupling but with levosimendan having greater effects on contractility [46]. Multiple case series and four randomized control trials have been reported suggesting that levosimendan is well tolerated whether used for children with heart failure or those undergoing cardiac surgery with only transient hypotension and tachycardia reported when the infusion commences. In a double-blind study with milrinone 36 patients under 5 years of age demonstrated levosimendan to have similar hemodynamics in the early postoperative phase [32]. A randomized control trial of 40 infants of mixed surgical complexity but excluding single ventricle palliation levosimendan was found to be safe with a nonsignificant trend toward increased cardiac output overtime as assessed by transoesophageal Doppler, with no significant differences in other hemodynamic end points [31]. A further 63 neonates undergoing higher complexity surgery (RACHS 3 and 4) demonstrated improved metabolic parameters and significantly lower inotrope scores with levosimendan compared to conventional therapy [47]. In another phase 1 study of 20 neonates receiving either milrinone or levosimendan following cardiac surgery, in addition to providing pharmacokinetic data on milrinone, levosimendan, and its metabolites OR 1855 and OR-1896, monitoring of physiological variables revealed the milrinone (n = 9)-treated neonates to have lower pH, higher blood sugar, lactate, and inotrope score in the early postoperative phase [33]. Although levosimendan does not appear inferior to standard therapy in the pediatric studies to date, meaningful end points including better appreciation of the side effect profile of levosimendan, evidence of mortality or morbidity benefit and cost-effectiveness are required before levosimendan can be confidently adopted in the pediatric population.

NITRODILATORS

Two types of nitrodilators are in clinical use, those that are spontaneous donors of nitric oxide (NO) such as sodium nitroprusside and the organic nitrates that require an enzymatic process to release NO such as GTN and the oral preparations isosorbide dinitrate and isosorbide mononitrate.

Nitric oxide mediates vasodilation predominantly by three mechanisms. (1) Activating soluble guanylate cyclase to increase intracellular cGMP and reduce intracellular calcium to enable smooth muscle relaxation. (2) Activating K^+ channels that induce smooth muscle cell hyperpolarization and relaxation. (3) Increased stimulation of cGMP-dependent kinases that activate myosin light chain phosphatase inducing relaxation and dilatation.

Discovered in 1849, the therapeutic applications of nitroprusside in adults with heart disease were described over 120 years later [48–50]. Nitroprusside has a rapid onset of action and elimination half-life of less than 5 min. Nitroprusside can be administered via a peripheral line but is light sensitive. This pharmacokinetic profile is desirable in the acute setting permitting the titration of nitroprusside up to 6 mcg/kg/min in neonates and 10 mcg/kg/min in children [51]. Nitroglycerin has a similar pharmacokinetic profile with a rapid onset of action and elimination half-life of 1–3 min. Nitroglycerin, like other organic nitrates but unlike nitroprusside, exhibits attenuation of beneficial hemodynamic properties through early tolerance (pseudotolerance) and true tolerance. Pseudotolerance is caused by counterregulatory neurohormonal responses, such as increased noradrenaline and plasma renin activity but true tolerance results from impaired responsiveness to stimuli for the release of endothelial-derived NO. Tolerance may be overcome by the concomitant use of angiotensin converting enzyme inhibitors and confer additional benefit in patients with AHF requiring organic nitrate therapy [52].

Nitroprusside can improve aortic blood flow in heart failure patients with little effect on heart rate and minimal reduction in aortic pressure. This is achieved by altering the pulsatile flow and steady flow components of the vascular load both increasing aortic compliance and systemic arteriolar vasodilatation [53,54]. A similar reduction in afterload associated with increasing arterial elastance has also been reported with the use of nitroglycerin [55]. Nitroprusside is more commonly considered a "balanced" veno-, arteriolar, and pulmonary vasodilator that has successfully been used in the treatment of adults with advanced low-output cardiac failure [49,56], whereas intravenous nitroglycerin predominantly dilates venous capacitance vessels to rapidly reduce atrial pressures and alleviate pulmonary congestion [57]. However, the use of nitroprusside in patients with acute myocardial ischemia has been tempered by concerns regarding coronary steal in these patients and nitroglycerin may be the preferred vasodilator in this setting because of its coronary vasodilatory effects. International AHF guidelines have not sought to distinguish which nitrodilator to use but the European Society of Cardiology guidelines advocate the use of nitrates when patients with AHF have a systolic blood pressure over 100 mmHg. The American College of Cardiology/American Heart Association advocate nitrate use in the absence of systemic hypotension [4,5].

In the first reported use of nitroprusside in the pediatric surgical population Kirklin et al. titrated nitroprusside with blood volume expansion in 16 infants aged less than 18 months old following intracardiac surgery. The infusion was commenced within 3 h of surgery and titrated to achieve a normal blood pressure requiring doses of between 2.5 and 12 mcg/kg/min. An increase in cardiac index of 17% without an increase in heart rate with an associated fall in atrial filling pressures and pulmonary artery pressure was observed that was incompletely reversed on cessation of nitroprusside. This favorable observation was in keeping with observations in adults and suggested this strategy of targeted afterload reduction might reduce myocardial oxygen consumption particularly when compared to a catecholamine-based approach. In contrast, nitroglycerin was not effective in reducing blood pressure and increasing cardiac index when compared with nitroprusside in a prospective randomized trial carried out in 14 children and adolescents [58].

The postoperative hypertension seen after coarctation of the aorta repair may require dual therapy with an intravenous beta-blocker (esmolol) and nitroprusside [59]. In children with mitral regurgitation-induced heart failure nitroprusside may reduce pulmonary capillary wedge and increase stroke volume and cardiac output [60]. Although vasodilator therapy is generally contraindicated in severe aortic stenosis, nitroprusside has been shown to be effective in critically ill patients with aortic stenosis where peripheral vasoconstriction is contributing to afterload [61,62].

The main adverse effect of nitrate therapy is hypotension particularly when cardiac filling pressures are lower than anticipated. An important complication of nitroprusside therapy is cyanide toxicity that may manifest with confusion, convulsions and hyperreflexia and lactic acidosis. Toxicity is more likely with high dose or prolonged infusions particularly if renal impairment is present. Suspected toxicity or thiocyanate levels above 2 mcg/mL should be treated by thiosulfate infusion or hemodialysis.

ALPHA-ADRENERGIC RECEPTOR BLOCKERS

The nonselective alpha-adrenergic receptor blockers phenoxybenzamine and phentolamine have been best studied in children following the first stage in single ventricle palliation.

Both are nonselective competitive inhibitors of alpha 1 and alpha 2 receptors in the systemic vasculature [63]. Phenoxybenzamine combines irreversibly with alpha adrenoreceptors, which accounts for its long elimination half-life of 19h, whereas phentolamine binds reversibly with a short onset of action and comparatively short half-life of 19min allowing the possibility of dose titration.

In an observational study of 60 infants undergoing cardiac repair on cardiopulmonary bypass, half the population received a 1mg/kg bolus of phenoxybenzamine and the remaining infants received an infusion of 2–5mcg/kg/min of nitroprusside [64]. Those treated with phenoxybenzamine reportedly had greater flow on cardiopulmonary bypass with improvements in perfusion sustained on the intensive care unit evidenced by a significant reduction in left atrial pressure, base deficit, and core-to-peripheral temperature gradient.

Following stage I palliation of single ventricle anatomy, milrinone appears to have been the most commonly used vasoactive agent with only 8 of 14 centers involved in the single ventricle reconstruction trial used alpha-blockers to a varied extent [65,66].

Over the last two decades, mathematical modeling [67,68], invasive hemodynamic assessments [69,70], and single center case series [71–74] have shifted early strategic efforts from controlling the pulmonary vascular resistance to manipulating the SVR to improve oxygen delivery and meet metabolic demands. In the absence of residual lesions (e.g., residual arch obstruction), this strategy may yield early hemodynamic benefits regardless of whether a systemic to pulmonary artery shunt, right ventricle to pulmonary artery, or hybrid palliation are used [68,69].

In a prospective observational study, when phenoxybenzamine in addition to standard treatment (n=7) was compared to standard treatment alone (n=8), the use of phenoxybenzamine was associated with a greater systemic venous oxygenation and improved pulmonary to systemic flow ratios in the early postoperative period following the Norwood procedure [74]. Further observations from this expanded cohort suggest improved systemic venous oxygenation and arteriovenous content difference are more readily achieved with the use of phenoxybenzamine but when therapeutic targets are not attained there is an increased risk of organ failure, extracorporeal membrane oxygenation and death [72,73]. Other groups have reported similar findings following the implementation of a postoperative strategy that included alpha-blockade observing the use of phenoxybenzamine as independently associated with a reduced risk of early circulatory collapse following the Norwood operation [71].

Maintaining adequate perfusion pressure with long acting alpha-blockade may prove difficult to titrate, particularly with the concomitant use of other drugs with vasodilator properties or presence of sepsis. In these situations, noradrenaline, and vasopressin have been used to overcome the effects of phenoxybenzamine [75]. Coupled with the limited supply of phenoxybenzamine and perhaps the apparent lack of benefit of the use ACE inhibitors in the ongoing treatment of children following stage 1 palliation there has been restricted adoption of alpha-blockade. However, the principle of sustained afterload reduction early following interventional or surgical stage 1 palliation remains an attractive physiological goal.

NESIRITIDE

In patients with heart failure, circulating human B-type natriuretic peptide has diagnostic and prognostic value. The properties of its recombinant form "Nesiritide" have understandably generated therapeutic interest in adult and pediatric populations.

Venous, arterial, and coronary vasodilations are achieved by increasing cGMP levels without reflex tachycardia or discernible inotropic effect. The reduction in preload and afterload is accompanied by enhanced natriuresis and suppression the RAAS [76]. Nesiritide has an elimination half-life of 8min.

In seven adult subjects with congestive heart failure an infusion of atrial natriuretic factor at 0.01mcg/kg/min result in a significant decrease in pulmonary capillary wedge and SVR and an increase in cardiac index at 60min [77]. These benefits were replicated using nesiritide in a randomized placebo controlled trial (n=103) using three dosing regimens for 24h with no significant effect on heart rate observed [78]. These hemodynamic improvements were encouraging and could be prospectively associated with improved dyspnea relief, which was sustained at 7days, with no suggestion of tolerance [79].

These and other positive reports led to a randomized double-blind Vasodilatation in the Management of Acute Congestive Heart Failure trial studying 489 adults with acute decompensated heart failure and dyspnea, 246 of whom received pulmonary artery catheterization. Nesiritide (n=143), nitroglycerin (n=143), or placebo was added to standard therapy for 3h followed by nesiritide (n=278) or nitroglycerin (n=216) to standard medication for 24h [80]. Nesiritide was found to significantly decrease pulmonary capillary wedge compared to placebo at 3h and nitroglycerin at 24h but relief of dyspnea was improved when compared with placebo. However, no differences in 30-day hospital readmission or 6-month mortality were observed.

Subsequent metaanalysis of the use of nesiritide in acute decompensated heart failure raised the possibility of adverse effects on survival and renal function prompting a large multicenter randomized double-blind placebo controlled trial of nesiritide in addition to standard of care [81]. The study included 7141 patients from 398 centers worldwide and was conducted in just over 3 years. This well powered study found treatment with nesiritide in combination with other therapies neither to be associated with a significant change in death rate, dyspnea, or hospital readmission at 30 days nor worsening renal function although there was an increased risk of hypotension. Interest in the use of nesiritide for heart failure has waned but it is important to recognize that following cardiac surgery on cardiopulmonary bypass, a phase II placebo controlled trial of nesiritide in adults with LV dysfunction, patients who received nesiritide were reported to have improved renal function, a shorter length of stay and reduced mortality at 6 months.

Two small case series have suggested nesiritide could be used in children with heart failure to achieve symptomatic improvements and effective diuresis without evidence of harm [82,83]. Mahle et al. retrospectively reviewed the open-label use of nesiritide in children (n = 30) with heart failure receiving inotropic and diuretic therapy [84]. The population included 19 children had congenital heart disease (of which five were single ventricle defects), DCM (n = 7), and postheart transplantation (n = 5). In the 16 children who had undergone heart surgery during the same admission, the median time from surgery to initiation of nesiritide was 4.5 days, the duration of therapy between 1 and 24 days. Survival to hospital discharge for the cohort was reported as 80% in this population of sick children nesiritide could be administered safely, possible side effects were noted in two subjects (arrhythmia and hypotension). The administration of nesiritide was associated with an improvement in fluid balance at 24 h with a nonsignificant trend toward a lower right atrial pressure and without adversely affecting serum creatinine or blood urea nitrogen.

Further safety and efficacy data were reported from 63 subjects under 21 years of age with acquired or congenital heart disease in whom a clinical diagnosis of decompensated heart failure (without evidence of hypotension) requiring admission to the intensive care unit was made. The study not only included 140 infusions of nesiritide but also included a prospective subgroup analysis of neurohormonal markers of heart failure in 20 patients. All patients received loop diuretics and where possible nesiritide was the first parenteral vasoactive to be administered. Two infusions were discontinued because of hypotension although overall no significant difference in blood pressure was seen. A significant decrease in heart with increased urine output at days 1 and 3 were noted. Renal parameters were not adversely affected and a nonsignificant decrease in neurohormonal markers at 72 h was reported.

More invasive hemodynamic data were obtained Behera et al. The group randomized 20 patients less than 21 years old, with a diagnosis of dilated cardiomyopathy and Swan-Ganz catheters in situ, to receive nesiritide (n = 9) or placebo (n = 11). The authors were able to demonstrate significant reductions in pulmonary capillary wedge, pulmonary pressure and systolic blood pressure following an infusion of 24 h duration [85].

Data from pediatric surgical cohorts have also been sought, particularly as decreased activity of the natriuretic system may occur in children following cardiopulmonary bypass [86,87]. A cohort of 20 patients (mean age 8 years) who underwent surgery received nesiritide administered as a bolus prior to weaning from bypass and continued as an infusion up to 24 h [88]. Three children were excluded from analysis because of sepsis (n = 2) and junctional ectopic tachycardia (n = 1), hospital survival was 100%. A nonsignificant drop of mean blood pressure by 7% was noted following loading with nesiritide that did not require intervention. In 15 of the patients, nesiritide was the only postoperative vasoactive medication, 2 patients receiving milrinone in addition to nesiritide. The authors acknowledge the small numbers, older cohort, and lack of control group and recommended further prospective comparative studies in the perioperative pediatric patients.

In one such study, primary Fontan patients, a group in whom perioperative trials are uncommon, were selected for a single center randomized double-blind placebo controlled trial comparing parallel arms of placebo, milrinone, or nesiritide infusions administered on cardiopulmonary bypass [89]. The primary outcome measure was the number of days alive out of hospital within 30 days of surgery, with secondary outcome measures including cardiovascular, renal, resource use, and neurohormonal variables. Baseline characteristics of the 106 patients randomized, including echocardiographic and cardiac catheterization parameters, were similar. The authors concluded neither milrinone nor nesiritide could be recommended for routine use in children undergoing primary Fontan repair when no significant differences were found in the stated primary or secondary outcome measures. Furthermore, milrinone was discontinued in one quarter of the patients who received it because hypotension and an increased rate of accelerated junctional rhythm were reported. This study, whilst questioning the routine use of milrinone does not preclude the possibility that vasodilators may provide benefit to a subpopulation of children undergoing primary Fontan repair associated with severe ventricular dysfunction or systemic atrioventricular valve regurgitation. The study also raises the possibility of quiescent harm caused by the use of therapy in the absence of pediatric data in specific patient groups.

SERELAXIN

Relaxin (H2) is a naturally occurring peptide hormone that accounts for many of the cardiovascular adaptations achieved in pregnancy. These include increased arterial compliance with systemic and renovascular dilatation, diuresis and natriuresis [90]. Its effects are conveyed by stimulation of endogenous NO production, vascular endothelial growth factor, and inhibition of endogenous vasoconstrictors such as angiotensin II and endothelin [91–93].

Serelaxin is a recombinant protein developed to take advantage of these changed that allow the physiological stress of pregnancy to be tolerated. The RELAXin acute heart failure (RELAX-AHF) study randomized 1,161 adults with AHF and systolic blood pressure >125 mmHg, to either serelaxin (n=581) or placebo (n=580) in addition to the standard of care AHF treatment [94]. The 48-h IV infusion resulted in an improvement in dyspnea at 24 h that was not sustained at 5 days, the primary end point. Neither was a reduction in hospital readmission rate or death at 60 days seen. However, at the prespecified end point of mortality at 180 days a significant reduction in both all-cause and cardiovascular mortality was reported.

Subsequent subgroup analysis reported significant interactions between some patient subgroups and the effects of serelaxin on 180 days cardiovascular and all-cause mortality, but it was felt these should be interpreted cautiously due to the number of comparisons and the low incidence of deaths in the subgroups at lower risk [95]. In addition to a larger (n=6375) multicentre phase III mortality trial in adults (RELAX-AHF II), a pediatric multicentre, dose escalation, safety, and pharmacokinetic study of serelaxin in children hospitalized with AHF is currently underway.

REFERENCES

[1] P.S. Pang, M. Komajda, M. Gheorghiade, The current and future management of acute heart failure syndromes, Eur. Heart J. 31 (7) (2010) 784–793.

[2] W.F. Peacock, et al., National Heart, Lung, and Blood Institute working group on emergency department management of acute heart failure: research challenges and opportunities, J. Am. Coll. Cardiol. 56 (5) (2010) 343–351.

[3] N.L. Weintraub, et al., Acute heart failure syndromes: emergency department presentation, treatment, and disposition: current approaches and future aims: a scientific statement from the American Heart Association, Circulation 122 (19) (2010) 1975–1996.

[4] J.J. McMurray, et al., ESC guidelines for the diagnosis and treatment of acute and chronic heart failure 2012: the task force for the diagnosis and treatment of acute and chronic heart failure 2012 of the European society of cardiology. Developed in collaboration with the heart failure association (HFA) of the ESC, Eur. J. Heart Fail. 14 (8) (2012) 803–869.

[5] C.W. Yancy, et al., 2013 ACCF/AHA guideline for the management of heart failure: a report of the American College of Cardiology Foundation/American Heart Association Task Force on practice guidelines, J. Am. Coll. Cardiol. 62 (16) (2013) e147–239.

[6] G.C. Fonarow, et al., Characteristics, treatments, and outcomes of patients with preserved systolic function hospitalized for heart failure: a report from the OPTIMIZE-HF Registry, J. Am. Coll. Cardiol. 50 (8) (2007) 768–777.

[7] D.A. Kass, R.P. Kelly, Ventriculo-arterial coupling: concepts, assumptions, and applications, Ann. Biomed. Eng. 20 (1) (1992) 41–62.

[8] B.A. Borlaug, D.A. Kass, Ventricular-vascular interaction in heart failure, Heart Fail. Clin. 4 (1) (2008) 23–36.

[9] P.D. Chantler, E.G. Lakatta, S.S. Najjar, Arterial-ventricular coupling: mechanistic insights into cardiovascular performance at rest and during exercise, J. Appl. Physiol. (1985) 105 (4) (2008) 1342–1351.

[10] K. Sagawa, et al., End-systolic pressure/volume ratio: a new index of ventricular contractility, Am. J. Cardiol. 40 (5) (1977) 748–753.

[11] K. Sunagawa, et al., Left ventricular interaction with arterial load studied in isolated canine ventricle, Am. J. Physiol. 245 (5 Pt 1) (1983) H773–H780.

[12] M.R. Starling, Left ventricular-arterial coupling relations in the normal human heart, Am. Heart J. 125 (6) (1993) 1659–1666.

[13] S.F. Shakar, et al., Combined oral positive inotropic and beta-blocker therapy for treatment of refractory class IV heart failure, J. Am. Coll. Cardiol. 31 (6) (1998) 1336–1340.

[14] B.D. Lowes, et al., Inotropes in the beta-blocker era, Clin. Cardiol. 23 (3 Suppl.) (2000) III11–I16.

[15] A.A. Alousi, D.C. Johnson, Pharmacology of the bipyridines: amrinone and milrinone, Circulation 73 (3 Pt 2) (1986) III10–24.

[16] D. el Allaf, V. D'Orio, J. Carlier, The new inotropic phosphodiesterase inhibitors, Arch. Int. Physiol. Biochim. 92 (4) (1984) S69–S79.

[17] J.M. Bailey, et al., The pharmacokinetics of milrinone in pediatric patients after cardiac surgery, Anesthesiology 90 (4) (1999) 1012–1018.

[18] C. Ramamoorthy, et al., Pharmacokinetics and side effects of milrinone in infants and children after open heart surgery, Anesth. Analg. 86 (2) (1998) 283–289.

[19] T. Taniguchi, et al., Pharmacokinetics of milrinone in patients with congestive heart failure during continuous venovenous hemofiltration, Intensive Care Med. 26 (8) (2000) 1089–1093.

[20] R. Grose, et al., Systemic and coronary effects of intravenous milrinone and dobutamine in congestive heart failure, J. Am. Coll. Cardiol. 7 (5) (1986) 1107–1113.

[21] W.T. Abraham, et al., In-hospital mortality in patients with acute decompensated heart failure requiring intravenous vasoactive medications: an analysis from the Acute Decompensated Heart Failure National Registry (ADHERE), J. Am. Coll. Cardiol. 46 (1) (2005) 57–64.

[22] L.A. Allen, et al., Hospital variation in intravenous inotrope use for patients hospitalized with heart failure: insights from Get with the Guidelines, Circ. Heart Fail. 7 (2) (2014) 251–260.

[23] B.S. Moffett, et al., Readmissions for heart failure in children, J. Pediatr. (2016).

[24] B.F. Birnbaum, et al., Intravenous home inotropic use is safe in pediatric patients awaiting transplantation, Circ. Heart Fail. 8 (1) (2015) 64–70.

[25] A.C. Chang, et al., Milrinone: systemic and pulmonary hemodynamic effects in neonates after cardiac surgery, Crit. Care Med. 23 (11) (1995) 1907–1914.

[26] A.F. Zuppa, et al., Population pharmacokinetics of milrinone in neonates with hypoplastic left heart syndrome undergoing stage I reconstruction, Anesth. Analg. 102 (4) (2006) 1062–1069.

[27] A.H. Smith, et al., Relation of milrinone after surgery for congenital heart disease to significant postoperative tachyarrhythmias, Am. J. Cardiol. 108 (11) (2011) 1620–1624.

[28] W. Vogt, S. Laer, Treatment for paediatric low cardiac output syndrome: results from the European EuLoCOS-Paed survey, Arch. Dis. Child. 96 (12) (2011) 1180–1186.

[29] W. Vogt, S. Laer, Prevention for pediatric low cardiac output syndrome: results from the European survey EuLoCOS-Paed, Paediatr. Anaesth. 21 (12) (2011) 1176–1184.

[30] A. Cavigelli-Brunner, et al., Therapy of low cardiac output syndrome after cardiac surgery in infants and children: a double blind randomized study comparing Dobutamine and Milrinone, Cardiol. Young 23 (Suppl. S1) (2013) S34.

[31] E. Lechner, et al., Levosimendan versus milrinone in neonates and infants after corrective open-heart surgery: a pilot study, Pediatr. Crit. Care Med. 13 (5) (2012) 542–548.

[32] M. Momeni, et al., Levosimendan in congenital cardiac surgery: a randomized, double-blind clinical trial, J. Cardiothorac. Vasc. Anesth. 25 (3) (2011) 419–424.

[33] A. Pellicer, et al., Phase 1 study of two inodilators in neonates undergoing cardiovascular surgery, Pediatr. Res. 73 (1) (2013) 95–103.

[34] H. Haikala, et al., Cardiac troponin C as a target protein for a novel calcium sensitizing drug, levosimendan, J. Mol. Cell Cardiol. 27 (9) (1995) 1859–1866.

[35] H. Yokoshiki, et al., Levosimendan, a novel Ca^{2+} sensitizer, activates the glibenclamide-sensitive K^+ channel in rat arterial myocytes, Eur. J. Pharmacol. 333 (2–3) (1997) 249–259.

[36] D. Farmakis, et al., Levosimendan beyond inotropy and acute heart failure: evidence of pleiotropic effects on the heart and other organs: an expert panel position paper, Int. J. Cardiol. 222 (2016) 303–312.

[37] A. Pathak, et al., Pharmacology of levosimendan: inotropic, vasodilatory and cardioprotective effects, J. Clin. Pharm. Ther. 38 (5) (2013) 341–349.

[38] M. Turanlahti, et al., Pharmacokinetics of levosimendan in pediatric patients evaluated for cardiac surgery, Pediatr. Crit. Care Med. 5 (5) (2004) 457–462.

[39] M. Kivikko, L. Lehtonen, W.S. Colucci, Sustained hemodynamic effects of intravenous levosimendan, Circulation 107 (1) (2003) 81–86.

[40] A. Mebazaa, et al., Levosimendan vs. dobutamine: outcomes for acute heart failure patients on beta-blockers in SURVIVE, Eur. J. Heart Fail. 11 (3) (2009) 304–311.

[41] F. Follath, et al., Efficacy and safety of intravenous levosimendan compared with dobutamine in severe low-output heart failure (the LIDO study): a randomised double-blind trial, Lancet 360 (9328) (2002) 196–202.

[42] V.S. Moiseyev, et al., Safety and efficacy of a novel calcium sensitizer, levosimendan, in patients with left ventricular failure due to an acute myocardial infarction. A randomized, placebo-controlled, double-blind study (RUSSLAN), Eur. Heart J. 23 (18) (2002) 1422–1432.

[43] A. Mebazaa, et al., Levosimendan vs dobutamine for patients with acute decompensated heart failure: the SURVIVE randomized trial, JAMA 297 (17) (2007) 1883–1891.

[44] M. Packer, et al., Effect of levosimendan on the short-term clinical course of patients with acutely decompensated heart failure, JACC Heart Fail. 1 (2) (2013) 103–111.

[45] G. Landoni, et al., Effects of levosimendan on mortality and hospitalization. A meta-analysis of randomized controlled studies, Crit. Care Med. 40 (2) (2012) 634–646.

[46] C.F. Stocker, et al., Mechanisms of a reduced cardiac output and the effects of milrinone and levosimendan in a model of infant cardiopulmonary bypass, Crit. Care Med. 35 (1) (2007) 252–259.

[47] Z. Ricci, et al., Levosimendan infusion in newborns after corrective surgery for congenital heart disease: randomized controlled trial, Intensive Care Med. 38 (7) (2012) 1198–1204.

[48] N.H. Guiha, et al., Treatment of refractory heart failure with infusion of nitroprusside, N. Engl. J. Med. 291 (12) (1974) 587–592.

[49] R.F. Palmer, K.C. Lasseter, Drug therapy. Sodium nitroprusside, N. Engl. J. Med. 292 (6) (1975) 294–297.

[50] J.H. Tinker, J.D. Michenfelder, Sodium nitroprusside: pharmacology, toxicology and therapeutics, Anesthesiology 45 (3) (1976) 340–354.

[51] W.E. Benitz, et al., Use of sodium nitroprusside in neonates: efficacy and safety, J. Pediatr. 106 (1) (1985) 102–110.

[52] D. Gupta, et al., Nitrate therapy for heart failure: benefits and strategies to overcome tolerance, JACC Heart Fail. 1 (3) (2013) 183–191.

[53] J.P. Merillon, et al., Aortic input impedance in heart failure: comparison with normal subjects and its changes during vasodilator therapy, Eur. Heart J. 5 (6) (1984) 447–455.

[54] C.J. Pepine, et al., Aortic input impedance during nitroprusside infusion. A reconsideration of afterload reduction and beneficial action, J. Clin. Investig. 64 (2) (1979) 643–654.

[55] H.L. Haber, et al., Bolus intravenous nitroglycerin predominantly reduces afterload in patients with excessive arterial elastance, J. Am. Coll. Cardiol. 22 (1) (1993) 251–257.

[56] W. Mullens, et al., Sodium nitroprusside for advanced low-output heart failure, J. Am. Coll. Cardiol. 52 (3) (2008) 200–207.

[57] U. Elkayam, et al., Comparison of effects on left ventricular filling pressure of intravenous nesiritide and high-dose nitroglycerin in patients with decompensated heart failure, Am. J. Cardiol. 93 (2) (2004) 237–240.

[58] M. Yaster, et al., A comparison of nitroglycerin and nitroprusside for inducing hypotension in children: a double-blind study, Anesthesiology 65 (2) (1986) 175–179.
[59] S. Tabbutt, et al., Perioperative course in 118 infants and children undergoing coarctation repair via a thoracotomy: a prospective, multicenter experience, J. Thorac. Cardiovasc. Surg. 136 (5) (2008) 1229–1236.
[60] R.H. Beekman, et al., Vasodilator therapy in children: acute and chronic effects in children with left ventricular dysfunction or mitral regurgitation, Pediatrics 73 (1) (1984) 43–51.
[61] H. Ikram, et al., Hemodynamic effects of nitroprusside on valvular aortic stenosis, Am. J. Cardiol. 69 (4) (1992) 361–366.
[62] U.N. Khot, et al., Nitroprusside in critically ill patients with left ventricular dysfunction and aortic stenosis, N. Engl. J. Med. 348 (18) (2003) 1756–1763.
[63] C.A. Hamilton, J.L. Reid, D.J. Sumner, Acute effects of phenoxybenzamine on alpha-adrenoceptor responses in vivo and in vitro: relation of in vivo pressor responses to the number of specific adrenoceptor binding sites, J. Cardiovasc. Pharmacol. 5 (5) (1983) 868–873.
[64] P. Motta, et al., Comparison of phenoxybenzamine to sodium nitroprusside in infants undergoing surgery, J. Cardiothorac. Vasc. Anesth. 19 (1) (2005) 54–59.
[65] S.K. Pasquali, et al., Variation in perioperative care across centers for infants undergoing the Norwood procedure, J. Thorac. Cardiovasc. Surg. 144 (4) (2012) 915–921.
[66] G. Wernovsky, et al., Hypoplastic left heart syndrome: consensus and controversies in 2007, Cardiol. Young 17 (Suppl. 2) (2007) 75–86.
[67] O. Barnea, et al., Estimation of oxygen delivery in newborns with a univentricular circulation, Circulation 98 (14) (1998) 1407–1413.
[68] E.L. Bove, et al., Use of mathematic modeling to compare and predict hemodynamic effects of the modified Blalock-Taussig and right ventricle-pulmonary artery shunts for hypoplastic left heart syndrome, J. Thorac. Cardiovasc. Surg. 136 (2) (2008) 312–320 e2.
[69] J. Li, et al., Comparison of the profiles of postoperative systemic hemodynamics and oxygen transport in neonates after the hybrid or the Norwood procedure: a pilot study, Circulation 116 (11 Suppl.) (2007) I179–I187.
[70] J. Li, et al., Profiles of hemodynamics and oxygen transport derived by using continuous measured oxygen consumption after the Norwood procedure, J. Thorac. Cardiovasc. Surg. 133 (2) (2007) 441–448.
[71] N.C. De Oliveira, et al., Prevention of early sudden circulatory collapse after the Norwood operation, Circulation 110 (11 Suppl. 1) (2004) II133–II138.
[72] G.M. Hoffman, et al., Alteration of the critical arteriovenous oxygen saturation relationship by sustained afterload reduction after the Norwood procedure, J. Thorac. Cardiovasc. Surg. 127 (3) (2004) 738–745.
[73] J.S. Tweddell, et al., Mixed venous oxygen saturation monitoring after stage 1 palliation for hypoplastic left heart syndrome, Ann. Thorac. Surg. 84 (4) (2007) 1301–1310 discussion 1310-1.
[74] J.S. Tweddell, et al., Phenoxybenzamine improves systemic oxygen delivery after the Norwood procedure, Ann. Thorac. Surg. 67 (1) (1999) 161–167 discussion 167-8.
[75] S.B. O'Blenes, et al., Vasopressin reversal of phenoxybenzamine-induced hypotension after the Norwood procedure, J. Thorac. Cardiovasc. Surg. 123 (5) (2002) 1012–1013.
[76] S.J. Holmes, et al., Renal, endocrine, and hemodynamic effects of human brain natriuretic peptide in normal man, J. Clin. Endocrinol. Metab. 76 (1) (1993) 91–96.
[77] R.J. Cody, et al., Atrial natriuretic factor in normal subjects and heart failure patients. Plasma levels and renal, hormonal, and hemodynamic responses to peptide infusion, J. Clin. Investig. 78 (5) (1986) 1362–1374.
[78] R.M. Mills, et al., Sustained hemodynamic effects of an infusion of nesiritide (human b-type natriuretic peptide) in heart failure: a randomized, double-blind, placebo-controlled clinical trial. Natrecor Study Group, J. Am. Coll. Cardiol. 34 (1) (1999) 155–162.
[79] W.S. Colucci, et al., Intravenous nesiritide, a natriuretic peptide, in the treatment of decompensated congestive heart failure. Nesiritide Study Group, N. Engl. J. Med. 343 (4) (2000) 246–253.
[80] Publication Committee for the VMAC Investigators, Intravenous nesiritide vs nitroglycerin for treatment of decompensated congestive heart failure: a randomized controlled trial, JAMA 287 (12) (2002) 1531–1540.
[81] C.M. O'Connor, et al., Effect of nesiritide in patients with acute decompensated heart failure, N. Engl. J. Med. 365 (1) (2011) 32–43.
[82] B. Feingold, Y.M. Law, Nesiritide use in pediatric patients with congestive heart failure, J. Heart Lung Transplant. 23 (12) (2004) 1455–1459.
[83] J.L. Jefferies, et al., A prospective evaluation of nesiritide in the treatment of pediatric heart failure, Pediatr. Cardiol. 27 (4) (2006) 402–407.
[84] W.T. Mahle, et al., Nesiritide in infants and children with congestive heart failure, Pediatr. Crit. Care Med. 6 (5) (2005) 543–546.
[85] S.K. Behera, et al., Nesiritide improves hemodynamics in children with dilated cardiomyopathy: a pilot study, Pediatr. Cardiol. 30 (1) (2009) 26–34.
[86] J.M. Costello, et al., Effect of cardiopulmonary bypass and surgical intervention on the natriuretic hormone system in children, J. Thorac. Cardiovasc. Surg. 130 (3) (2005) 822–829.
[87] M.C. Seghaye, et al., Endogenous nitric oxide production and atrial natriuretic peptide biological activity in infants undergoing cardiac operations, Crit. Care Med. 25 (6) (1997) 1063–1070.
[88] J.M. Simsic, et al., Perioperative effects and safety of nesiritide following cardiac surgery in children, J. Intensive Care Med. 21 (1) (2006) 22–26.
[89] J.M. Costello, et al., Impact of empiric nesiritide or milrinone infusion on early postoperative recovery after Fontan surgery: a randomized, double-blind, placebo-controlled trial, Circ. Heart Fail. 7 (4) (2014) 596–604.
[90] K.P. Conrad, Maternal vasodilation in pregnancy: the emerging role of relaxin, Am. J. Physiol. Regul. Integr. Comp. Physiol. 301 (2) (2011) R267–R275.

[91] D. Bani, et al., Relaxin activates the L-arginine-nitric oxide pathway in vascular smooth muscle cells in culture, Hypertension 31 (6) (1998) 1240–1247.
[92] T. Dschietzig, et al., Relaxin, a pregnancy hormone, is a functional endothelin-1 antagonist: attenuation of endothelin-1-mediated vasoconstriction by stimulation of endothelin type-B receptor expression via ERK-1/2 and nuclear factor-kappaB, Circ. Res. 92 (1) (2003) 32–40.
[93] X.J. Du, et al., Cardiovascular effects of relaxin: from basic science to clinical therapy, Nat. Rev. Cardiol. 7 (1) (2010) 48–58.
[94] J.R. Teerlink, et al., Serelaxin, recombinant human relaxin-2, for treatment of acute heart failure (RELAX-AHF): a randomised, placebo-controlled trial, Lancet 381 (9860) (2013) 29–39.
[95] M. Metra, et al., Effects of serelaxin in subgroups of patients with acute heart failure: results from RELAX-AHF, Eur. Heart J. 34 (40) (2013) 3128–3136.

Chapter 42

Beta-Adrenergic Receptor Blockade

David J. Goldberg[1], Robert E. Shaddy[2]

[1]The Perelman School of Medicine at the University of Pennsylvania, Philadelphia, PA, United States; [2]Children's Hospital Los Angeles and the Keck School of Medicine of the University of Southern California

He was a bold man that first ate an oyster.
Jonathan Swift

Up until the seminal publication by Waagstein in 1975 in which he described the beneficial effects of beta-adrenergic receptor (beta) blockers in a small group of adults with heart failure, beta blockers had been considered contraindicated in the management of heart failure [1]. This and other publications soon to follow generated a large amount of interest in the potential benefit of beta blockers in heart failure. There were suggestions that beta blockers could be beneficial, but these early studies were underpowered to demonstrate definite benefit [2,3]. Thus it was not until 20 years after Waagstein's initial report that beta blockers were conclusively proven to improve symptoms, left ventricular function, and survival in adults with heart failure with reduced ejection fraction (HFrEF). This was based on five major prospective, randomized trials in adults (Table 42.1). Two large trials, the US Carvedilol Study and the Multidose Oral Carvedilol in Heart Failure Assessment (MOCHA) trial, did not show a benefit in the primary end point (submaximal exercise) but showed a significant survival benefit [4,5]. Subsequent large trials in adults with HFrEF showed similar benefit from other beta blockers (bisoprolol) [3] and with the beta blocker carvedilol in patients with severe chronic heart failure [6]. There may be differences in therapeutic outcomes between beta blockers. In one large multicenter trial, carvedilol was shown to be superior to metoprolol in adult with HFrEF [7]. Not all beta blockers have shown benefit in heart failure in adults; the most notable example of this is the lack of benefit seen from bucindolol in the BEST trial [8]. There are many theories as to why bucindolol failed to show benefit in contrast to other beta blockers, but one hypothesis is that there is a single nucleotide polymorphism in the beta-1 adrenergic receptor that determines responsiveness to bucindolol [9]. Thus, based on the multiple prospective, randomized trials in adults with heart failure with reduced ejection fraction (HFrEF), beta-blockers (specifically bisoprolol, carvedilol, and metoprolol) are currently recommended as a Class I recommendation Level of Evidence A treatment in adults with Stage C HFrEF [9a]. There is every reason to think that adolescents with dilated cardiomyopathy or with congenital heart disease and a systemic left ventricle would benefit from beta-blocker therapy similar to adults. It is much less clear in very young children or children with systemic ventricles that are not of a left ventricular (LV) morphology.

There are many proposed mechanisms for the beneficial effects of beta blockers in patients with HFrEF, including reduced intracellular calcium, slower heart rate, improved diastolic function, upregulation of beta receptors, coronary vasodilation, and antioxidant effects [10]. The recent discovery that slowing of the heart rate alone in HFrEF with ivabradine results in improved symptoms, survival and left ventricular function makes the slowing of the heart rate appear to be more important than initially thought [11].

Once metoprolol and carvedilol were approved for use in adults, many small studies were published assessing the value of beta blockers in children with heart failure. Most of the studies focused on pediatric patients with systemic systolic ventricular dysfunction (HFrEF). However, some studies showed benefit in patients with pulmonary overcirculation due to large left-to-right shunts [12,13]. In those children with HFrEF, many small retrospective and prospective studies suggested improvement in echocardiographic parameters of ventricular function and symptoms [14–19]. These trials mainly included children with dilated cardiomyopathy and used echocardiographic parameters as endpoints. A few trials used clinical outcomes and were able to demonstrate a suggestion of benefit in those patients with dilated cardiomyopathy. However, the prospective, randomized, double-blind trial of carvedilol in children with symptomatic heart failure due to systemic ventricular systolic dysfunction failed to show benefit as measured by a composite clinical end point [20]. Using a prespecified analysis, there appeared to be a relationship between ventricular morphology and response to carvedilol, in that those children with a left ventricular morphology had a significantly better response to carvedilol that those with right or single ventricular morphology. In those children with a systemic left ventricle, there were significant improvements in

Heart Failure in the Child and Young Adult. http://dx.doi.org/10.1016/B978-0-12-802393-8.00042-9

TABLE 42.1 Seminal Randomized Trials of Beta-Blockers in Adults

Trial	β Blocker	Patients	End Point	Mortality Benefit
MOCHA 1996	Carvedilol	345 NYHA 1–3	Submaximal exercise	Dose-dependent survival
US Coreg 1996	Carvedilol	1094 NYHA 1–3	Submaximal exercise	67%
MERIT-HF 1997	Metoprolol	3991 NYHA 1–3	All-cause mortality	35%
CIBIS-II 1999	Bisoprolol	2647 NYHA 1–3	All-cause mortality	29%
COPERNICUS 2001	Carvedilol	2289 severe HF	All-cause mortality	35%

CIBIS, cardiac insufficiency bisoprolol study; *COPERNICUS*, carvedilol prospective randomized cumulative survival; *HF*, heart failure; *MERIT-HF*, metoprolol controlled-release randomised intervention trial in heart failure; *MOCHA*, multicenter oral carvedilol heart failure assessment; *NYHA*, New York heart association.

echocardiographic parameters of left ventricular performance, compared to placebo. The reasons for this lack of benefit of carvedilol in this population are unclear but may be related to the heterogeneity of the population (children with systemic ventricles of left ventricular and right ventricular morphology), possible underdosing of carvedilol [21], and possibly that children do not receive the same benefit from carvedilol as adults. Soon after the pediatric carvedilol trial was published, Albers and colleagues published a pharmacokinetic study of carvedilol in children [21a]. This study demonstrated that the pharmacokinetics of carvedilol was significantly different than in adults, particularly in the very young. In infants and toddlers, the dose of carvedilol required to achieve therapeutic levels were much higher than in adolescents or adults. The half-life was also shorter, suggesting that some very young children may benefit from dosing every 8 h, rather than every 12 h in adolescents and adults. Other factors that can influence the inability to demonstrate a beneficial response may be challenges in study design in pediatric heart failure, the different response of children to medications compared with adults, the fact that children with heart failure have different diseases than adults, and the possibility that the pediatric myocardium has a different substrate than the adult myocardium in cardiomyopathies [22,23].

While many questions remain regarding the use of beta blockers in children with heart failure but structurally normal hearts, even less is known regarding their use in children with functional single ventricle physiology. The use of beta blockers in this anatomy is further complicated by the morphologic difference between single left ventricles and single right ventricles. It's possible that the two ventricles may respond differently to beta blockers, particularly when in the heart failure state.

In one recent study that sought to examine myocellular changes in the myocardium of those with hypoplastic left heart syndrome, it was noted that while beta-adrenergic receptor density was decreased in the systemic right ventricle, it was decreased differently than what was noted in children with left ventricular failure due to cardiomyopathy. Rather than equal downregulation of both beta-1 and beta-2 receptors, those with failing single right ventricles demonstrated downregulation of beta-1 receptors with preservation of beta-2 expression [24]. This difference in receptor expression may mediate a different response to beta blockers via altered downstream signaling. These findings lend support to the notion of differential response based on morphology.

Aside from the pediatric carvedilol trial, the only other report of beta blocker use in those with single ventricle physiology is a single case report and subsequent retrospective review of carvedilol use in a series from Japan [25,26]. While the retrospective nature of the study and the heterogeneity of the included subjects make the conclusions of this paper difficult to interpret, the authors do report an improvement in ejection fraction, measured by echocardiography, in those with single right ventricles. Interestingly, this was not accompanied by an improvement in serum B-type natriuretic peptide levels. In those with single left ventricle, the findings were just the opposite: an improvement in serum B-type natriuretic peptide levels, but no improvement in ventricular function.

Given the dearth of data and varied findings of the utility of beta blockers in those with single ventricle physiology, it is not surprising that there is no consensus on their utility. In a position paper of the Working Group of Grown-Up Congenital Heart Disease and the Heart Failure Association of the European Society of Cardiology there was reference to the findings from the group from Japan and a mention of the possible utility of carvedilol in those with single ventricle physiology although there was no strong recommendation regarding their use [27]. In a paper from the Pediatric Heart Network evaluating medication use in their Fontan cross-sectional cohort, only 19 of the 546 enrolled subjects were treated with a beta blocker of any kind suggesting that the idea of carvedilol as a treatment for those with single ventricle physiology is the exception rather than the rule [28].

In a Cochrane review of beta-blockers for congestive heart failure in children in 2009, the authors reviewed three studies with 203 participants. They concluded that "there are not enough data to recommend or discourage the use of beta-blockers in children with congestive heart failure" [29]. A more recent systematic review and metaanalysis of carvedilol in the treatment of children with systemic ventricular systolic dysfunction reviewed eight prospective/observational trials that examined carvedilol and standard treatment efficacy in children with systemic systolic ventricular dysfunction. Their analysis showed that carvedilol could prevent one death or heart transplantation by treating 14 children with systemic ventricular systolic dysfunction [30]. Ultimately, the challenge presented by the small number of children with heart failure makes it very difficult to discern whether beta blockers have a significant role to play in management. Given the variation in the types of heart failure encountered in the pediatric community and the further complication of treating both failing left and failing right ventricles, it is very difficult to know with certainty whether beta blockers should be used routinely as part of the treatment strategy. While there is likely sufficient evidence to support the use of beta blockers in those with a failing left ventricle, the use of beta blockers in those with failing single right ventricles is not strongly supported. The most recent recommendations from the International Society of Heart and Lung Transplantation for the management of pediatric heart failure are a Class IIa recommendation: Following adult heart failure guidelines, systolic dysfunction, particularly if the systemic ventricle has a LV morphology. Therapy should start at a small dose and slowly up-titrate. Level of Evidence B [31]. Even in those in whom beta blockers may provide a benefit, more work is needed to understand the myocellular mechanisms of heart failure in pediatrics and thus whether carvedilol or a differently selective beta blocker would be the most appropriate medication to choose.

REFERENCES

[1] F. Waagstein, A. Hjalmarson, E. Varnauskas, I. Wallentin, Effect of chronic beta-adrenergic receptor blockade in congestive cardiomyopathy, Br. Heart J. 37 (1975) 1022–1036.

[2] F. Waagstein, M.R. Bristow, K. Swedberg, F. Camerini, M.B. Fowler, M.A. Silver, E.M. Gilbert, M.R. Johnson, F.G. Goss, A. Hjalmarson, Metoprolol in dilated cardiomyopathy (MDC) trial study group, Beneficial effects of metoprolol in idiopathic dilated cardiomyopathy, Lancet 342 (1993) 1441–1446.

[3] CIBIS investigators and committees, A randomized trial of beta-blockade in heart failure. The cardiac insufficiency bisoprolol study (CIBIS), Circulation 90 (1994) 1765–1773.

[4] M. Packer, M.R. Bristow, J.N. Cohn, W.S. Colucci, M.B. Fowler, E.M. Gilbert, N.H. Shusterman, U.S. carvedilol heart failure study group, [See comments], The effect of carvedilol on morbidity and mortality in patients with chronic heart failure, N. Engl. J. Med. 334 (1996) 1349–1355.

[5] M.R. Bristow, E.M. Gilbert, W.T. Abraham, K.F. Adams, M.B. Fowler, R.E. Hershberger, S.H. Kubo, K.A. Narahara, H. Ingersoll, S. Krueger, S. Young, N. Shusterman, MOCHA investigators, Carvedilol produces dose-related improvements in left ventricular function and survival in subjects with chronic heart failure, Circulation 94 (1996) 2807–2816.

[6] M. Packer, A.J.S. Coats, M.B. Fowler, H.A. Katus, H. Krum, P. Mohacsi, J.L. Rouleau, M. Tendera, A. Castaigne, E.B. Roecker, M.K. Schultz, C. Staiger, E.L. Curtin, D.L. DeMets, The carvedilol prospective randomized cumulative survival study group, Effect of carvedilol on survival in severe chronic heart failure, N. Engl. J. Med. 344 (2001) 1651–1658.

[7] P.A. Poole-Wilson, K. Swedberg, J.G. Cleland, A. Di Lenarda, P. Hanrath, M. Komajda, J. Lubsen, B. Lutiger, M. Metra, W.J. Remme, C. Torp-Pedersen, A. Scherhag, A. Skene, Comparison of carvedilol and metoprolol on clinical outcomes in patients with chronic heart failure in the carvedilol or metoprolol European trial (COMET): randomised controlled trial, Lancet 362 (2003) 7–13.

[8] A trial of the beta-blocker bucindolol in patients with advanced chronic heart failure, N. Engl. J. Med. 344 (2001) 1659–1667.

[9] S.B. Liggett, J. Mialet-Perez, S. Thaneemit-Chen, S.A. Weber, S.M. Greene, D. Hodne, B. Nelson, J. Morrison, M.J. Domanski, L.E. Wagoner, W.T. Abraham, J.L. Anderson, J.F. Carlquist, H.J. Krause-Steinrauf, L.C. Lazzeroni, J.D. Port, P.W. Lavori, M.R. Bristow, A polymorphism within a conserved beta(1)-adrenergic receptor motif alters cardiac function and beta-blocker response in human heart failure, Proc. Natl. Acad. Sci. U.S.A. 103 (2006) 11288–11293.

[9a] C.W. Yancy, M. Jessup, B. Bozkurt, J. Butler, D.E. Casey Jr., M.M. Colvin, M.H. Drazner, G.S. Filippatos, G.C. Fonarow, M.M. Givertz, S.M. Hollenberg, J. Lindenfeld, F.A. Masoudi, P.E. McBride, P.N. Peterson, L.W. Stevenson, C. Westlake, 2017 ACC/AHA/HFSA Focused Update of the 2013 ACCF/AHA Guideline for the Management of Heart Failure, J. Am. Coll. Cardiol (2017). http://dx.doi.org/10.1016/j.jacc.2017.04.025.

[10] M.R. Bristow, Mechanism of action of beta-blocking agents in heart failure, Am. J. Cardiol. 80 (1997) 26L–40L.

[11] K. Swedberg, M. Komajda, M. Bohm, J.S. Borer, I. Ford, A. Dubost-Brama, G. Lerebours, L. Tavazzi, S. Investigators, Ivabradine and outcomes in chronic heart failure (SHIFT): a randomised placebo-controlled study, Lancet 376 (2010) 875–885.

[12] R. Buchhorn, D. Bartmus, W. Siekmeyer, M. Hulpke-Wette, R. Schulz, J. Bursch, Beta-blocker therapy of severe congestive heart failure in infants with left to right shunts, Am. J. Cardiol. 81 (1998) 1366–1368.

[13] R. Buchhorn, M. Hulpke-Wette, R. Hilgers, D. Bartmus, A. Wessel, J. Bursch, Propranolol treatment of congestive heart failure in infants with congenital heart disease: the CHF-PRO-INFANT trial. Congestive heart failure in infants treated with propanol, Int. J. Cardiol. 79 (2001) 167–173.

[14] L.A. Bruns, M.K. Chrisant, J.M. Lamour, R.E. Shaddy, E. Pahl, E.D. Blume, S. Hallowell, L.J. Addonizio, C.E. Canter, Carvedilol as therapy in pediatric heart failure: an initial multicenter experience, J. Pediatr. 138 (2001) 505–511.

[15] P. Rusconi, O. Gomez-Marin, M. Rossique-Gonzalez, E. Redha, J.R. Marin, M. Lon-Young, G.S. Wolff, Carvedilol in children with cardiomyopathy: 3-year experience at a single institution, J. Heart Lung Transplant. 23 (2004) 832–838.

[16] R.E. Shaddy, Beta-blocker therapy in young children with congestive heart failure under consideration for heart transplantation, Am. Heart J. 136 (1998) 19–21.

[17] R.E. Shaddy, Beta-adrenergic receptor blockers as therapy in pediatric chronic heart failure, Minerva Pediatr. 53 (2001) 297–304.

[18] E. Azeka, J.A. Franchini Ramires, C. Valler, E. Alcides Bocchi, Delisting of infants and children from the heart transplantation waiting list after carvedilol treatment, J. Am. Coll. Cardiol. 40 (2002) 2034–2038.

[19] E.D. Blume, C.E. Canter, R. Spicer, K. Gauvreau, S. Colan, K.J. Jenkins, Prospective single-arm protocol of carvedilol in children with ventricular dysfunction, Pediatr. Cardiol. 27 (2006) 336–342.

[20] R.E. Shaddy, M.M. Boucek, D.T. Hsu, R.J. Boucek, C.E. Canter, L. Mahony, R.D. Ross, E. Pahl, E.D. Blume, D.A. Dodd, D.N. Rosenthal, J. Burr, B. LaSalle, R. Holubkov, M.A. Lukas, L.Y. Tani, Pediatric carvedilol study group, Carvedilol for children and adolescents with heart failure: a randomized controlled trial, JAMA 298 (2007) 1171–1179.

[21] S. Albers, B. Meibohm, T.S. Mir, S. Laer, Population pharmacokinetics and dose simulation of carvedilol in paediatric patients with congestive heart failure, Br. J. Clin. Pharmacol. 65 (2008) 511–522.

[21a] S. Albers, B. Meihbohm, T. Mir, S. Laer, Br. J. Clin, Pharmacol 65 (4) (2008) 511–522.

[22] J.W. Rossano, R.E. Shaddy, Update on pharmacological heart failure therapies in children: do adult medications work in children and if not, why not? Circulation 129 (2014) 607–612.

[23] S.D. Miyamoto, B.L. Stauffer, S. Nakano, R. Sobus, K. Nunley, P. Nelson, C.C. Sucharov, Beta-adrenergic adaptation in paediatric idiopathic dilated cardiomyopathy, Eur. Heart J. 35 (2014) 33–41.

[24] S.D. Miyamoto, B.L. Stauffer, J. Polk, A. Medway, M. Friedrich, K. Haubold, V. Peterson, K. Nunley, P. Nelson, R. Sobus, K.R. Stenmark, C.C. Sucharov, Gene expression and beta-adrenergic signaling are altered in hypoplastic left heart syndrome, J. Heart Lung Transplant. 33 (2014) 785–793.

[25] N. Ishibashi, I.S. Park, Y. Takahashi, M. Nishiyama, Y. Murakami, K. Mori, S. Mimori, M. Ando, Y. Takahashi, T. Nakanishi, Effectiveness of carvedilol for congestive heart failure that developed long after modified Fontan operation, Pediatr. Cardiol. 27 (2006) 473–475.

[26] N. Ishibashi, I.S. Park, T. Waragai, T. Yoshikawa, Y. Murakami, K. Mori, S. Mimori, M. Ando, Y. Takahashi, S. Doi, S. Mizutani, T. Nakanishi, Effect of carvedilol on heart failure in patients with a functionally univentricular heart, Circ. J. 75 (2011) 1394–1399.

[27] W. Budts, J. Roos-Hesselink, T. Radle-Hurst, A. Eicken, T.A. McDonagh, E. Lambrinou, M.G. Crespo-Leiro, F. Walker, A.A. Frogoudaki, Treatment of heart failure in adult congenital heart disease: a position paper of the working group of grown-up congenital heart disease and the heart failure association of the European society of cardiology, Eur. Heart J. 37 (2016) 1419–1427.

[28] P.A. Anderson, R.E. Breitbart, B.W. McCrindle, L.A. Sleeper, A.M. Atz, D.T. Hsu, M. Lu, R. Margossian, R.V. Williams, The Fontan patient: inconsistencies in medication therapy across seven pediatric heart network centers, Pediatr. Cardiol. 31 (2010) 1219–1228.

[29] A.K. Frobel, M. Hulpke-Wette, K.G. Schmidt, S. Läer, Beta-blockers for congestive heart failure in children, Cochrane Database of Syst. Rev (1) (2009). http://dx.doi.org/10.1002/14651858.CD007037.pub2. article no. CD007037.

[30] S. Prijic, R. Bucchorn, J. Kosutic, V. Vukomanovic, A. Prijic, B. Bjelokavic, M. Zdravkovic, Beta-blockers (Carvedilol) in children with systemic ventricle systolic dysfunction—systematic review and meta-analysis, Rev. Recent Clin. Trials (9) (2014) 68–75.

[31] R. Kirk, A.I. Dipchamd, D.N. Rosenthal, et al., The International Society for Heart and Lung Transplantation Guidelines for the management of pediatric heart failure: Executive summary, J. Heart Lung Transplant 33 (9) (September 2014) 888–909.

Chapter 43

Recognition and Treatment of Low Cardiac Output States in Pediatric Cardiac Intensive Care

Jonathan W. Byrnes, David P. Nelson
The Heart Institute at Cincinnati Children's Hospital, Cincinnati, OH, United States

HISTORY AND SIGNIFICANCE

The transient decline in cardiac output in neonates, infants, and young children following cardiac surgery is well documented. The initial description is credited to Parr where in observation of 139 children less than 48 months, mortality was high (27%) in this group, which was associated with the interaction of cardiac output and venous oximetry [5]. Death was rare if venous partial pressure of oxygen was no lower than 35 mm of mercury or cardiac index was no lower than 2.5 L/min/m^2. Blood pressure was realized to be unrelated to either cardiac output or venous oximetry. In fact, systemic vascular resistance was remarkably high (mean of 30 Woods units indexed), resulting in the speculation that vasodilators should be applied early in children with low cardiac index after cardiac surgery. Wernovsky et al. reported an average drop in cardiac index of 24% in neonates undergoing arterial switch operation, with a cardiac index nadir of <2 L/min/m^2 after surgery in nearly 1 in 4 of the patients [6]. Wall-stress analysis in a subgroup of these patients 1–2 weeks after surgery demonstrated normal myocardial function, indicating the postoperative myocardial dysfunction was transient [7]. The PRIMACORP study similarly observed low cardiac output syndrome (LCOS) in 27% of the patients in the control group and 10% of patients in the high-dose milrinone group [8].

Since morbidity and mortality associated with LCOS remains significant, rapid recognition and treatment of LCOS is paramount to improving outcomes in the cardiac intensive care unit (ICU). Patients with LCOS have higher rates of cardiac arrest, necrotizing enterocolitis, infection, neurologic events, renal dysfunction, resource utilization, longer hospital length of stay and possibly even long-term cognitive sequelae [9–11]. In addition, patients with a marginal cardiac reserve may be unable to recover from LCOS and thus progress to cardiogenic shock, requiring escalating care and possibly mechanical support. The predictability of LCOS in postoperative patients should enable the clinician to quickly recognize and treat low output states in these patients.

CLINICAL SIGNS OF LOW CARDIAC OUTPUT SYNDROME

The clinical findings of low cardiac output are the result of systemic and/or pulmonary venous congestion, with inadequate systemic blood flow to maintain end-organ perfusion. Respiratory compromise from pulmonary venous congestion is often an early sign of heart failure in children, but this can be difficult to detect in a mechanically ventilated postoperative patient. Systemic venous congestion manifests as hepatomegaly, peripheral edema, pleural effusions, and ascites. Typical signs of inadequate systemic blood flow, or cardiogenic shock, are tachycardia, delayed capillary refill, oliguria, and metabolic acidosis. Clinical assessment of systemic perfusion is an important indicator of LCOS. Assessment of capillary refill time and core extremity–temperature gradient may be helpful, although neither has been carefully validated independently, although structured clinical exams that incorporate assessment of multiple physical exam findings shows the ability to more accurately predict low cardiac output [12]. Hypotension may result from the low cardiac output state following cardiac surgery; however, systemic blood pressure is not a reliable marker of systemic perfusion in children who have rapid regulation of vascular tone. Hypotension thus tends to be a late manifestation of cardiogenic shock and is usually not seen until cardiac arrest is imminent. Persistent LCOS results in unrelenting metabolic acidosis and ultimately multiorgan failure, including acute renal failure, gastrointestinal complications, and central nervous system compromise. Patients with palliated single ventricle physiology are much more likely to have multisystem organ dysfunction from low cardiac output.

Heart Failure in the Child and Young Adult. http://dx.doi.org/10.1016/B978-0-12-802393-8.00043-0

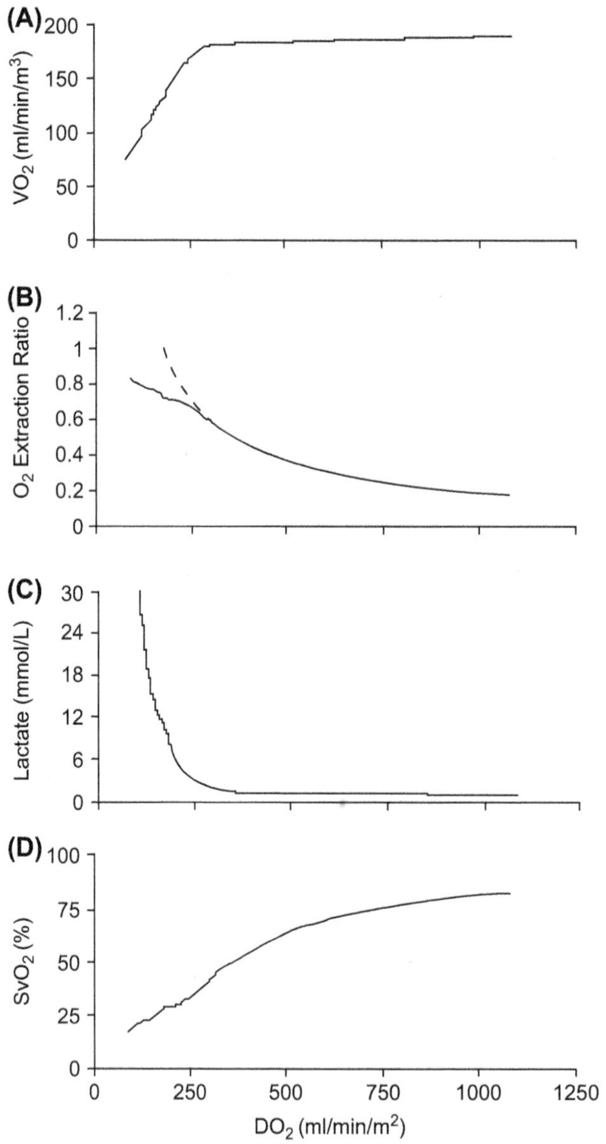

FIGURE 43.1 Changes in systemic oxygen consumption (VO_2), the oxygen extraction ratio, serum lactate, and mixed-venous oxygen saturation (SvO_2) as systemic oxygen delivery (DO_2) falls. VO_2 remains constant until a critical point (A), which is accomplished by an increase in oxygen extraction by tissues (B). To maintain oxygen consumption, the extraction ratio must approach unity (*dashed curve*, B). When oxygen delivery is insufficient to meet metabolic demands, mixed-venous saturation falls (D) and serum lactate rises (C).

Fig. 43.1 illustrates the physiologic response as systemic oxygen delivery falls. Panel A shows a biphasic response in oxygen consumption as oxygen delivery declines. Assuming oxygen demands are constant, oxygen consumption remains relatively unchanged by a compensatory increase in oxygen extraction (represented by the solid line in panel B) until a critical oxygen delivery value is reached, at which point oxygen consumption falls as oxygen delivery falls further. If oxygen consumption were to remain constant below the critical oxygen delivery, the oxygen extraction ratio would have to exceed a fixed, critical oxygen extraction ratio (dashed line, Panel B). As oxygen consumption falls, tissue ischemia results and serum lactate levels accumulate rapidly (panel C). Mixed-venous saturation reflects the ratio of oxygen supply to demand; as the oxygen delivery decreases, mixed-venous saturation falls (panel D).

Respiratory insufficiency after congenital heart surgery can manifest as changes in pulmonary vascular resistance, compliance, or as defects in lung gas exchange. Cardiopulmonary bypass (CPB) results in acute lung injury through complement and inflammatory mediators [13,14] and may cause changes in pulmonary vascular reactivity. Pulmonary edema, pleural effusions, and ascites decrease pulmonary compliance and interfere with pulmonary mechanics, thereby impairing gas exchange.

Acute renal insufficiency manifested by oliguria is a sensitive sign of LCOS, especially in infants who cannot maintain adequate renal blood flow in cardiogenic shock. Acute renal insufficiency leading to acute renal failure is a well-known complication after neonatal open heart surgeries and has been shown to occur more frequently in patients with complex operations requiring long bypass times [15,16]. It has been associated with a high risk of mortality and prolonged stay in the ICU [15]. The incidence of renal failure requiring renal replacement therapy after cardiac surgery ranges from 2.4% to 8%, but transient acute kidney injury with reduced creatinine clearance is common [6,17]. Perioperative ischemia, hypotension, and acidosis increase the risk of developing renal failure [18]. Fortunately, most of these patients will regain normal renal function prior to hospital discharge [16,19,20]. Nonetheless, supportive therapy with inotropes, fluids, and intravenous diuretics is ineffective in up to 9% of children undergoing CPB and renal replacement therapy is required [18]. Hemofiltration and peritoneal dialysis are the two mechanisms for renal replacement therapy in pediatrics. Peritoneal dialysis has been shown to be well tolerated and effective in pediatric patients [16,17,19], and may be preferential over hemodialysis, which requires systemic anticoagulation and may be difficult in patients with intravenous access difficulties [21]. Description of how to define CPB associated renal insufficiency through a combination of clinical and biomarker parameters has led to multiple scoring systems where the pediatric-modified Risk, Injury, Failure and Loss, and End-Stage is the most sensitive and the Acute Kidney Injury Network is the most specific with the Kidney Disease: Improving Global Outcomes having a combination of sensitivity and specificity; however, no matter the score utilized all are associated with mortality [22].

Limited perfusion to the gastrointestinal organs is common in patients with low cardiac output. This is likely to contribute to feeding difficulties, which is quite common, especially in neonates after congenital heart surgery. The inflammatory response from CPB leads to bowel edema and abnormal intestinal permeability [23]. The splanchnic circulation may also be compromised by high-dose inotropes and will worsen the degree of feeding difficulties. These patients are thus vulnerable to poor nutrition and often require parenteral nutrition. However, since bacteremia or sepsis may result from poor intestinal mucosal integrity, the early institution of trophic enteral feeding is thought to be beneficial [24]. Poor perfusion may also lead to hepatic insufficiency and coagulation abnormalities. LCOS may also result in gastric bleeding, mesenteric ischemia, and necrotizing enterocolitis, which are all associated with a high incidence of mortality [25,26].

Neurologic abnormalities are also relatively common after congenital heart surgery. In children requiring hypothermic circulatory arrest or continuous low-flow bypass for vital organ support during cardiac repair, up to 20% experienced some form of neurologic dysfunction shortly after surgery [10]. Patients who are placed on CPB commonly have abnormal electroencephalogram recordings, seizure activity, and long-term motor and cognitive delays [10,27–34]. Although these neurologic outcomes are thought to be related to CPB [35], postoperative low cardiac output may contribute to cerebral hypoperfusion and hypoxia to further exacerbate neurologic injury and impact developmental outcomes.

CAUSES OF LOW CARDIAC OUTPUT AFTER CONGENITAL HEART SURGERY

The etiology of LCOS after congenital heart surgery is multifactorial. Although LCOS is often associated with ventricular dysfunction, one must always investigate other potential causes of LCOS. Contractile dysfunction is not always the primary cause of LCOS; i.e., LCOS is not always ameliorated just by increasing inotropic support! Altered ventricular loading and residual cardiac lesions can also cause or exacerbate LCOS.

Changes in ventricular loading are integral to myocardial performance after congenital heart surgery. Ventricular preload is often inadequate, due to blood loss, perioperative fluid shifts, positive pressure ventilation, altered diastolic compliance, and/or physiologic changes resulting from the surgical procedure (e.g., Fontan or shunted single ventricle physiology) [36]. Cardiac tamponade, which limits preload by reducing diastolic compliance, should also always be considered in patients showing signs of LCOS. Increases in intrathoracic pressure resulting from tamponade, pneumothorax or positive pressure ventilation limit venous return and impede ventricular filling. It is vital to recognize myocardial tamponade can result from either global diffuse intrathoracic fluid accumulation or a localized collection of blood clot or fluid that limits venous return to a single chamber of the heart (usually right of left atrium).

Ventricular afterload is often increased after CPB, resulting from bypass-mediated vascular injury and altered vascular reactivity. Both systemic and pulmonary endothelial dysfunction have been observed following CPB (with or without circulatory arrest), presumably resulting from ischemia-reperfusion injury to the vascular endothelium [37–40]. The "classic" pulmonary hypertensive crisis results from an acute rise in right ventricular (RV) afterload, which shifts the interventricular septum toward the systemic ventricle, decreasing preload of that ventricle and thereby diminishing stroke volume and cardiac output. Early signs of a pulmonary hypertensive crisis include: acute systemic hypotension, diminished perfusion, and a rapid fall in lung compliance. Arterial oxygen saturation decreases only when right-to-left intracardiac shunting is present.

Residual anatomic defects such as outflow obstruction or valvar insufficiency reduce the effective stroke volume, increase myocardial work and oxygen demands, and lower cardiac output. Similarly, persistence of a left-to-right shunt will yield excessive pulmonary blood flow and diminish systemic blood flow. Careful evaluation for residual cardiac abnormalities is imperative in any patient with low cardiac output, especially when patients do not follow their expected postoperative course.

Arrhythmias are relatively common after congenital heart surgery [41,42]. Low cardiac output is typically exacerbated by arrhythmias, which often impair ventricular filling, especially if atrioventricular synchrony is disrupted. There is correlation between LCOS and most rhythm disturbances, especially junctional ectopic tachycardia (JET) and atrial automatic tachycardia. Since an arrhythmia may not be persistent, telemetry is imperative to allow retrospective review for rhythm disturbances.

Endocrine abnormalities in the immediate postoperative period further exacerbate LCOS. Altered or deficient levels of hormones impair the body's stress response to surgery. In particular, adrenal and thyroid dysfunctions as well as vasopressin deficiency are potentially treatable causes of catecholamine-resistant LCOS that is especially common after CPB [43]. Replacement therapy should be considered in patients with refractory LCOS; however, there have not been convincing studies regarding cortisol cutoffs to guide treatment of relative adrenal insufficiency as a cause of LCOS [44,45].

Hyperglycemia is often seen following cardiopulmonary bypass. The mechanisms attributed to hyperglycemia include stress response to surgery, perioperative steroids, dextrose containing fluids, and possibly intraoperative oxygenation strategies [46,47]. In the past perioperative morbidity and mortality was attributed to hyperglycemia, so some investigators advocated for strict glucose control [48]. More recently Agus demonstrated in a randomized-controlled trial in children less than 36 months who underwent surgery with CPB that tight glycemic control did not modify infection rate, mortality, length of stay, or measures of organ failure, as compared with standard care [49]. Although intraoperative hyperglycemia was not associated with worse neurologic outcome in the Boston Circulatory Arrest Trial, hypoglycemia may be associated with an increased risk for seizure activity in the early postoperative period [49,50]. Although tight glycemic control has been demonstrated to not be advantageous, it is unclear if and at what threshold glycemic control after cardiac surgery is advantageous.

Molecular Mechanisms of Bypass-Mediated Myocardial Injury

Despite advances in perfusion technology, patients undergoing CPB uniformly develop biochemical inflammation and approximately 40% develop a systemic inflammatory response resulting in tissue injury with transient myocardial and vascular dysfunction, which contributes to postoperative morbidity and mortality [1–4,6,51,52]. The mechanism for bypass-mediated tissue injury is multifactorial. Circulatory support with CPB involves obligate periods of myocardial and pulmonary ischemia with subsequent reperfusion, resulting in reperfusion injury from oxygen-derived free radicals. Hypothermic circulatory arrest is still utilized during congenital heart surgery, resulting in global ischemia/reperfusion. These periods of ischemia/reperfusion, combined with activation of blood components by the extracorporeal circuit, initiate tissue and vascular injury throughout the body [6,18,53,54]. The CPB-mediated inflammatory response involves cytokine and endotoxin release [54–57]; initiation of the complement, coagulation, and fibrinolytic cascades [51,58]; and leukocyte-endothelial interactions [59]. This process ultimately leads to the development of edema, tissue injury, and organ damage, most notably in the heart and lungs [2]. Mechanisms of contractile dysfunction after cardiac surgery remain elusive, but evidence suggests cardiomyocytes are injured by oxygen-derived free radicals and intracellular calcium overload during early reperfusion [53,60,61]. Other potential causes of myocardial dysfunction after congenital heart surgery include cytokine-mediated myocardial depression [62,63], cardiomyocyte apoptosis [64], alterations in adrenergic receptor signaling [65,66], and decreases in calcium responsiveness of the sarcomeric contractile apparatus due to troponin degradation [67–71].

Various interventions have been implemented to decrease the inflammatory response following CPB. Conventional and modified ultrafiltration have been shown to improve fluid balance and increase cardiac output in patients after bypass [72,73], which may be a result of the removal of inflammatory cytokines or other proinflammatory agents which may participate in the inflammatory cascade or which may have direct effects on cardiomyocytes. Peritoneal dialysis has also been shown to remove inflammatory mediators [74], but its effect on cardiac performance has not been assessed. Heparin-coated and miniaturized bypass circuits may blunt leukocyte activation and decrease cytokine production by reducing the contact of blood with artificial circuit surfaces [58,75–77]. Although these modalities have been shown to reduce levels of circulating cytokines and inflammatory mediators, correlation with clinical outcomes has not been established [78].

Efforts to attenuate the inflammatory response to CPB include administration of agents directed against cytokines, adhesion molecules [37,38,54,79,80], or activated complement [81]. Most of these agents have only been tested in animal models. Although the data are somewhat inconsistent, perioperative glucocorticoid treatment may reduce postoperative inflammation by altering levels of inflammatory mediators and cytokines, which has been associated with improved oxygen delivery in the postoperative period [82–85].

DIAGNOSIS OF LOW CARDIAC OUTPUT SYNDROME

LCOS is a predictable postoperative phenomenon; therefore, prompt recognition and aggressive management should be emphasized in the care of these patients to reduce morbidity and mortality. Optimal postoperative management includes continuous monitoring of pulse oximetry, end-tidal CO_2, atrial and arterial waveforms, and multiple electrocardiographic leads [86,87]. Since direct measure of myocardial performance and/or cardiac output is not feasible for routine clinical monitoring in children, cardiac output and systemic perfusion are usually assessed indirectly by monitoring vital signs, peripheral perfusion, urine output, and acid–base status. The length of time spent in the ICU and the amount and duration of ventilatory and inotropic support correlate with cardiac output and systemic oxygen delivery [15,88]. Furthermore, some data suggest ICU acuity scores may accurately predict mortality in pediatric cardiac surgery patients [89].

In addition to external monitoring, various serum markers reflect the adequacy of cardiac output in the perioperative patient. Studies have demonstrated persistent elevation of serum lactate suggests inadequate systemic perfusion [90–92]. Lactate is produced as cells transition to an anaerobic metabolic pathway to produce ATP. As cardiac output falls following cardiopulmonary bypass, systemic oxygen delivery decreases and serum lactate levels rise as tissues and end-organs depend on catabolic pathways for energy production (Fig. 43.1C) [93–97]. Elevated lactate levels correlate with an increased postoperative morbidity and mortality [93–97]. A progressive rise in serum lactate predicts impending cardiovascular collapse better than following hemodynamic parameters, such as blood pressure or physical exam findings [96]. Unfortunately, monitoring serum lactate is not a sensitive test. Lactate does not start to rise until oxygen delivery is below the critical threshold, where oxygen consumption becomes dependent on oxygen delivery [98]. In addition, elevated serum lactate does not reflect the current circulatory state, but reflects prior periods of diminished tissue perfusion.

Cardiac output is most accurately predicted by systemic venous saturation. Both mixed-venous oxygen saturation (SvO_2) and the arterial-venous oxygen saturation difference ($AVDO_2$) are valid predictors of cardiac output [99,100]. In patients with intracardiac shunts, superior vena cava (SVC) saturation is the best estimate of SvO_2 [101], and many investigators have advocated continuous or intermittent monitoring of SVC saturation in perioperative patients [102–105]. Low SvO_2 and elevated $AVDO_2$ indicate low systemic blood flow and inadequate systemic oxygen delivery. An $AVDO_2$ greater than 40 suggests impairment in cardiac output and inadequate tissue delivery of oxygen [106]. SVC saturation monitoring is particularly useful after Norwood palliation, since systemic output in these patients depends on both myocardial performance and the balance of systemic and pulmonary blood flow. In these patients, anaerobic metabolism and metabolic acidosis are more common when the absolute SvO_2 falls below 30% [107]. The relationship between oxygen delivery and oxygen demand can be calculated as the oxygen extraction ratio [$O_2ER=(SaO_2-SvO_2)/SaO_2$)]. Excessive oxygen extraction reflects a limited supply of oxygen to the tissues, thus increasing the risk for tissue anaerobic metabolism, lactic acid production, and end-organ injury. As depicted in Fig. 43.1B, an oxygen extraction ratio value over 0.4 reflects inadequate oxygen delivery and increased mortality [102].

Twittenwein et al. analyzed postoperative hemodynamic and laboratory data from 218 pediatric patients to establish entry criteria for postoperative cardiac extracorporeal membrane oxygenation (ECMO) after pediatric open heart surgery [106]. Multiple regression analysis revealed SvO_2 and serum lactate as independent predictors of death, so combined assessment of serum lactate and SvO_2 may improve accuracy of LCOS determination [106].

Cerebral saturation monitoring using near-infrared spectroscopy (NIRS) has been studied as a noninvasive surrogate for mixed-venous saturation [108]. Biologic materials have good transparency to light in the near-infrared spectrum. Oxyhemoglobin and deoxyhemoglobin absorb light at different wavelengths, which can be quantified as an absolute tissue oxygen index (TOI) [109]. This index is a measure of local tissue oxygenation. Although several studies report good correlation between cerebral NIRS and SvO_2 in critically ill neonates and children [108], other studies have observed differences between SvO_2 and cerebral oxygen saturation (ScO_2) measured by NIRS [108,110–112]. Although ScO_2 and SvO_2 do not always correlate, changes in ScO_2 seem to reflect changes in cardiac output, which can be used as a clinical marker for cardiac output. Trends in TOI may thus help predict trends in cardiac output, but serum saturation data, although more invasive, is a more accurate surrogate for cardiac output/oxygen delivery.

Brain natriuretic peptide (BNP) levels have been shown to reflect decompensated heart failure with limited tissue perfusion. Higher levels also correlate with excessive pulmonary blood flow and elevated pulmonary to systemic flow ratios (Qp:Qs) in infants and children with congenital heart disease [113]. Recent studies suggest elevated perioperative serum BNP correlates with ventricular dysfunction and length of stay in the ICU [114–117]. One study demonstrated the maximal BNP level occurred within 12h after cardiopulmonary bypass, when cardiac output is typically at its postsurgical nadir [114]. Limited data suggest serial BNP levels may predict which patients are at greater risk for developing LCOS postoperatively.

Cardiac output and myocardial performance have been measured directly in postoperative pediatric patients after congenital heart surgery [4]. Measurement of cardiac output by the thermodilution method can be accomplished in the ICU, but results may be unreliable in patients with low output, atrioventricular valvar regurgitation, or intracardiac shunts. It should be recognized thermodilution measurements are misleading if tissue oxygen demand is not considered; thermodilution measurements fail to detect interactions between oxygen delivery and tissue oxygen extraction [118,119]. For example, "normal" cardiac output may be inadequate in times of increased oxygen demand, while "reduced" cardiac output might be sufficient during times of lower oxygen demand. Measurement of mixed-venous saturation or oxygen extraction better reflects the relationship between oxygen supply and demand to identify patients at risk for LCOS [102]. An excellent alternative to thermodilution cardiac output assessment is the Fick method, especially in patients with intracardiac shunts or low cardiac output [118,120]. Since the Fick method requires accurate measurement of systemic oxygen consumption, the presence of an endotracheal tube leak can seriously confound Fick cardiac output analysis.

Other methods of cardiac output assessment used in pediatric cardiac surgery patients include thoracic impedance measurements and detachable aortic Doppler ultrasound flow probes [121]. More recently semiinvasive measures of cardiac output such as pressure-recording analytical method have been adopted, but validation studies are lacking in perioperative pediatric cardiac patients [122,123]. Most recently electrical cardiometry was validated in pediatric patients intraoperatively [124]. Considering all of these modalities, it should be recognized that only Fick cardiac output measurements reflect the interaction between oxygen delivery and tissue oxygen extraction [118].

Accurate measurement of myocardial performance in the postoperative pediatric cardiac surgical patient is extremely difficult. Poor echocardiographic windows, hemodynamic instability, and variable inotropic support have confounded noninvasive analyses of myocardial function in children. Conductance catheters have been used to assess load-independent measures of both left ventricular (LV) and RV function in the early postoperative period after cardiac surgery, although this is primarily a research tool [4,125]. Recent studies using microconductance catheters to record ventricular pressure–volume loops postoperatively demonstrated depressed systolic function in patients undergoing uncomplicated corrective cardiac surgical procedures even with short bypass and aortic cross-clamp times [4].

When myocardial dysfunction contributes to LCOS in the perioperative period, transthoracic or transesophageal echocardiography can provide some insight into myocardial function. Transthoracic echocardiography is often limited due to surgical dressings and various drains and intravascular lines. Echocardiography has been used to detect restrictive RV physiology (RV diastolic dysfunction) after corrective repair for tetralogy of Fallot, by determining the presence of antegrade flow into the pulmonary artery during ventricular diastole [60]. Although diastolic dysfunction likely plays an important role in LCOS, accurate assessment in this patient population remains elusive.

TREATMENT OF LOW CARDIAC OUTPUT SYNDROME

Management of postoperative LCOS includes: reduction of tissue oxygen demands; optimization of preload and afterload; prompt diagnosis of residual cardiac lesions; prevention of hypoxia, anemia, and acidosis; and administration of pharmacologic agents to improve myocardial contractile function and to regulate vascular tone [126]. In addition, in low cardiac output associated with right heart failure, some children may benefit from an atrial "pop-off" shunt to unload the failing right ventricle (e.g., residual atrial septal defect in a neonatal tetralogy of Fallot repair).

Minimize Oxygen Requirements

The combination of increased systemic oxygen consumption and reduction in cardiac output adversely alters systemic oxygen balance after cardiopulmonary bypass. One study of children aged 2 months to 15 years demonstrated a significant increase in oxygen consumption following CPB [119]. Since peak oxygen consumption correlates with increases in central temperature, fever in the setting of LCOS should be treated aggressively with antipyretic medication or surface cooling. A cooling blanket may be useful, but shivering should be avoided since it may increase oxygen consumption. Total oxygen consumption can be decreased by sedation, paralysis, and/or mild hypothermia that reduces metabolic rate [127]. Case reports of moderate hypothermia for patients with refractory LCOS suggest this as a potential therapy for LCOS [128,129].

Ensure Adequate Preload

Inadequate preload can result from various factors, including bleeding, hypovolemia, ultrafiltration during cardiopulmonary bypass, peripheral vasodilation from rewarming, or excessive afterload reduction in the postoperative period [36]. Cardiac tamponade, which impairs preload by altering atrial and/or ventricular diastolic compliance, should also always be considered in patients showing signs of LCOS. Increased mediastinal pressure, with fluid or extrapleural air, can lead to myocardial compression with a resultant low cardiac output and should be treated promptly. Myocardial swelling can limit myocardial filling and may necessitate sternal reopening. Delayed sternal closure has been successfully used to treat persistent low cardiac output with hemodynamic instability in postoperative pediatric and adult patients, without a significant increase in morbidity or mortality [130–135].

Although true ventricular preload is the end-diastolic ventricular volume, preload assessment can be estimated from right or left atrial pressure. Continual reassessment of optimal preload is essential, as ventricular compliance and subsequent preload needs are often dynamic in the perioperative period. The top panel of Fig. 43.2 graphically demonstrates how preload determination is predominantly a "trial and error" process. When atrial pressure is low, fluid administration augments end-diastolic volume (EDV) and increases stroke volume. With successive fluid administration, however, increases in stroke volume become limited due to the nonlinear nature of ventricular diastolic compliance. Preload augmentation is also limited by elevations in ventricular end-diastolic pressure (EDP), which results in clinically significant systemic and/or pulmonary venous congestion and potential impairment of myocardial perfusion. Interpretation of hemodynamic pressure monitoring data must always be made with an understanding of the patient's underlying physiology. A poorly compliant ventricle, such as with RV dysfunction after tetralogy of Fallot repair will be associated with elevated RV EDP and correspondingly higher right atrial pressure than a normal heart, which may necessitate higher filling pressures to generate an adequate cardiac output. Patients with diastolic dysfunction may require more extensive postoperative volume administration to maintain preload and cardiac output. These patients may also benefit from lusitropic therapy and/or a relatively lower heart rate to improve diastolic ventricular filling. Fig. 43.2, panel B illustrates how a change in ventricular diastolic compliance affects atrial pressure. Enhanced lusitropy should result in a greater stroke volume for a comparable atrial pressure.

Prompt Recognition of Arrhythmias

Prompt recognition of arrhythmias is imperative in the perioperative period. A baseline postoperative surface electrocardiogram should always be obtained for comparison with preoperative and subsequent postoperative tracings. Continuous electrocardiographic monitoring during the postoperative period is also essential. Sinus bradycardia, bundle branch block, and atrioventricular block can occur after many cardiac surgical procedures; thus, temporary atrial and ventricular pacing wires are often placed to facilitate pacing, if necessary. Overdrive pacing, and electrical or pharmacologic cardioversion may be necessary for the treatment of reentrant tachyarrhythmias [41]. Hoffman et al. reviewed the incidence of arrhythmias in postoperative cardiac surgical patients and observed that the most common rhythm disturbances were nonsustained ventricular and supraventricular tachycardia, with incidences of 22% and 12%, respectively. The incidence of sustained ventricular, junctional, and supraventricular arrhythmias were 6%, 5%, and 4%, respectively [41]. Loss of atrioventricular synchrony (the atrial "kick") decreases preload, resulting in increased venous congestion and reduced cardiac output, so maintenance of atrioventricular synchrony is imperative in postoperative patients (via dual-chamber pacing, if necessary).

JET is a common dysrhythmia that usually occurs within the first 48–72 h following surgery, especially after procedures involving ventricular septal defect closure [41]. It is generally poorly tolerated, especially in patients with already unstable hemodynamics. Early recognition of JET and other arrhythmias may be aided by careful surveillance of atrial pressure waveforms. Loss of the distinct "a" and "v" waves, indicating loss of atrioventricular synchrony, is often the first indication of a dysrhythmia and/or atrioventricular dyssynchrony. There is some controversy about the role of hypomagnesemia as a trigger for JET. One study suggested reduction in the incidence of JET with administration of intravenous magnesium in the early postoperative period [136]. The primary treatment of JET is directed toward the reestablishment of atrioventricular synchrony. Atrial or atrioventricular sequential pacing is the initial therapy of choice. Since adrenergic agents may exacerbate or increase the JET rate, the infusion doses should be limited when possible. If the junctional rate is too fast to allow pacing, pharmacological therapy should be implemented to provide rate control and allow atrial or dual-chamber pacing. While intravenous amiodarone is generally considered the drug of choice [137], induction of hypothermia and procainamide administration has also been shown to be effective [57]. Finally, since the risk of JET is greater in the presence of low output, the diagnosis of JET should prompt a search for other causes of LCOS, including residual cardiac lesions.

Prompt Diagnosis of Residual Cardiac Lesions

Residual cardiac lesions in the postoperative patient can cause or exacerbate LCOS and result in increased morbidity and mortality. Pressure and oximetry data from indwelling intracardiac catheters and transesophageal or surface echocardiography should be used to identify residual structural lesions in patients with LCOS following CPB. Catheterization should be promptly considered if LCOS persists and the etiology remains elusive. Careful evaluation for residual cardiac abnormalities is indicated, especially when patients do not follow their expected postoperative course after congenital heart surgery.

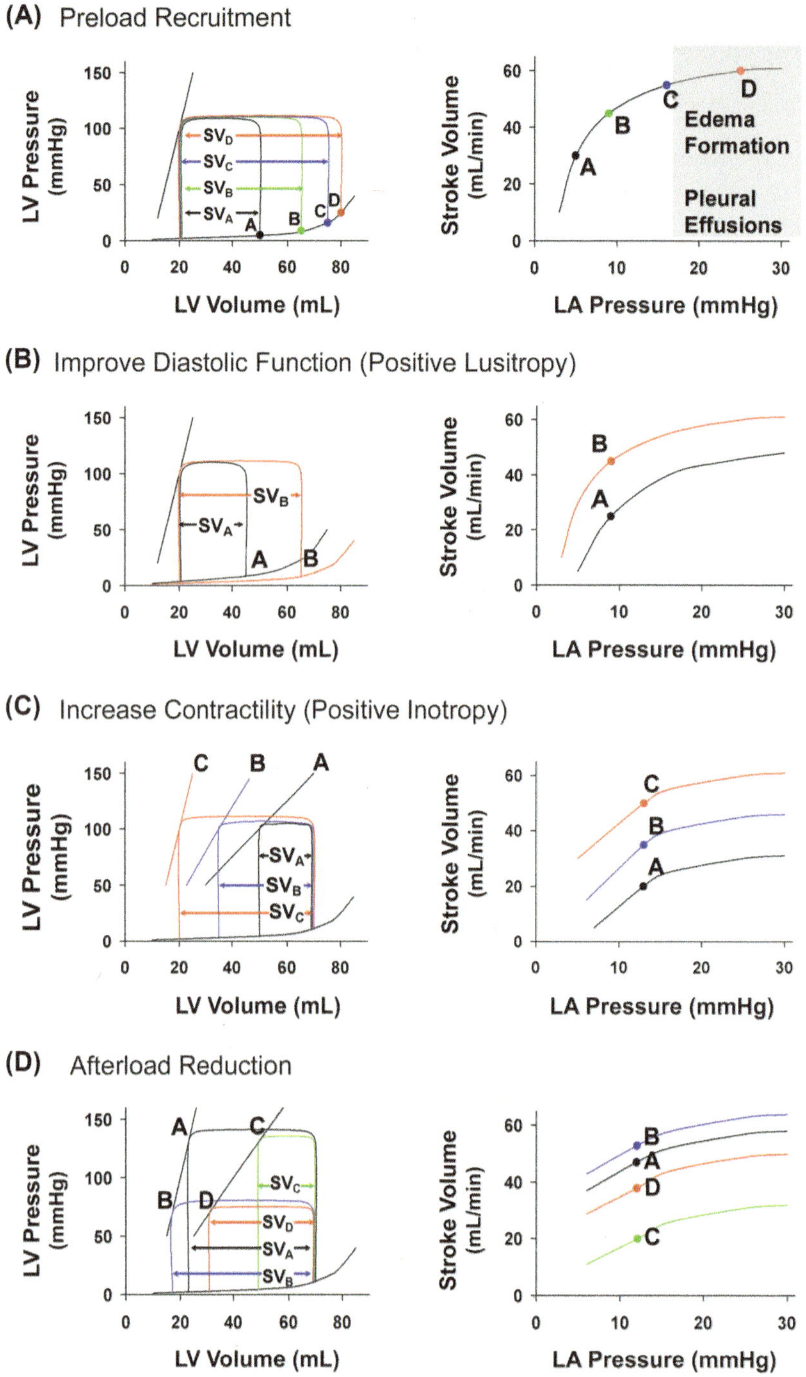

FIGURE 43.2 Paired changes in the pressure–volume and Starling relationship with isolated manipulations in preload (A), diastolic compliance (B), contractility, and (C) afterload (D). The ventricular end-diastolic volume (EDV) and stroke volume at point A (SV_A) for each pair of graphs represents the initial baseline hemodynamic condition.

(A) The top panel demonstrates the effect of preload recruitment on the pressure–volume and Starling relationships. Fluid volume administration augments end-diastolic volume from point A to point B, with the resultant increase in stroke volume from SV_A to SV_B. Since diastolic compliance is nonlinear, increases in stroke volume are progressively less with further fluid administration (SV_C and SV_D). EDVs A, B, C, and D represent the ventricular diastolic compliance. Preload augmentation is limited by elevations in left ventricular (LV) end-diastolic pressure (EDP), which result in impaired myocardial perfusion and elevations in atrial pressure, with resultant transcapillary leak and edema formation.

(B) Panel B demonstrates beneficial effects of positive lusitropy on the pressure–volume and Starling relationships. Enhanced ventricular compliance corresponds to an increased EDV for the same EDP, thereby augmenting stroke volume without increasing atrial pressure. *Enhanced lusitropy results in a greater stroke volume for a comparable atrial pressure.*

(C) Panel C demonstrates beneficial effects of positive inotropy on the pressure–volume and Starling relationships. Increases in contractility are shown as enhancement of the end-systolic pressure–volume relationship (ESPVR), demonstrated by increases in the slopes of lines A through line C on the left-hand graph. At constant preload, increased contractility enhances ejection during isovolumetric contraction, decreasing the end-systolic volume and increasing stroke volume (from SV_A to SV_B and to SV_C). *Enhanced contractility results in a greater stroke volume for a comparable preload.*

(D) The bottom panel demonstrates beneficial effects of afterload reduction on the pressure–volume and Starling relationships. From baseline conditions A or C, afterload reduction allows the heart to eject to a lower systolic pressure and volume (points B and D), enhancing ejection and augmenting stroke volume (SV_A to SV_B and SV_C to SV_D). At normal contractility (slope AB), the ventricle responds to altered afterload with only small changes in stroke volume (SV_A to SV_B). On the other hand, neonatal and failing hearts are more sensitive to alterations in afterload. Benefits of afterload reduction are more pronounced in neonatal hearts and in the setting of poor contractility. With reduced contractility (as shown by the reduced slope of ESPVR CD), the increase in stroke volume is greater for a comparable change in afterload. *Afterload reduction results in a greater stroke volume for a comparable preload.*

Treatment of Depressed Myocardial Contractility

Since low cardiac output after pediatric heart surgery is often associated with some level of contractile dysfunction, inotropic support in the early postoperative period is usually necessary. Panel C of Fig. 43.2 demonstrates the beneficial effects of positive inotropy on the pressure–volume and Starling relationships. At constant preload, increased contractility should enhance ejection during isovolumetric contraction to increase stroke volume. Since inotropic agents have unwanted side effects, it is important to assess efficacy of these agents following initiation or dosage adjustment. Fig. 43.2 illustrates the potential utility of Starling curves to assess efficacy of most hemodynamic interventions. The Starling relationship specifies the therapeutic goal of all inotropic agents—*enhanced contractility should result in a greater stroke volume for a comparable preload.* Unfortunately, measurement of stroke volume is not routine in postoperative patients, so an alternative to the true Starling relationship is illustrated in Fig. 43.3. Since stroke volume is not easily monitored, indirect measures of cardiac output (such as venous oxygen saturation) or measures of end-organ perfusion (such as urine output) may be plotted against atrial pressure to attain a "modified" Starling relationship. Points A–C of Fig. 43.3 illustrate how preload recruitment is used to increase venous saturation or urine output. Since preload recruitment is limited, however, inotropic agents are typically necessary to augment venous saturation and urine output by shifting the Starling relationship leftward (point D). Using the modified Starling relationship, *the therapeutic goal of enhanced contractility is improvement in systemic blood flow for a comparable preload* (reflected as improved venous saturation and enhanced organ perfusion).

Inotropic agents and vasodilators are routinely used in pediatric cardiac surgical patients to help reestablish adequate myocardial function during and after surgery. Table 43.1 lists the agents most commonly used in pediatric cardiac intensive care for LCOS. Support is often initiated with a low-dose infusion of an adrenergic agent. The infusion rate is then titrated to achieve the desired perfusion and systemic blood pressure. Higher doses of adrenergic agents are typically avoided because of the increasing vasoconstrictor and chronotropic effects at higher doses. Dobutamine generally produces less tachycardia than dopamine and decreases systemic afterload because of its affinity to β receptors. These effects may be desirable, especially when treating patients with dilated cardiomyopathies or volume-loaded ventricles with excessive pulmonary blood flow. Epinephrine is a more potent inotrope than dopamine or dobutamine because of its greater myocardial α_1- and β_1-adrenergic effects and is preferred for treatment of severe ventricular dysfunction. High-dose epinephrine (>0.1 μg/kg/min) frequently results in tachycardia and systemic vasoconstriction. Epinephrine is often used in combination with intravenous vasodilators such as milrinone, sodium nitroprusside, or phenoxybenzamine to treat ventricular dysfunction and decrease

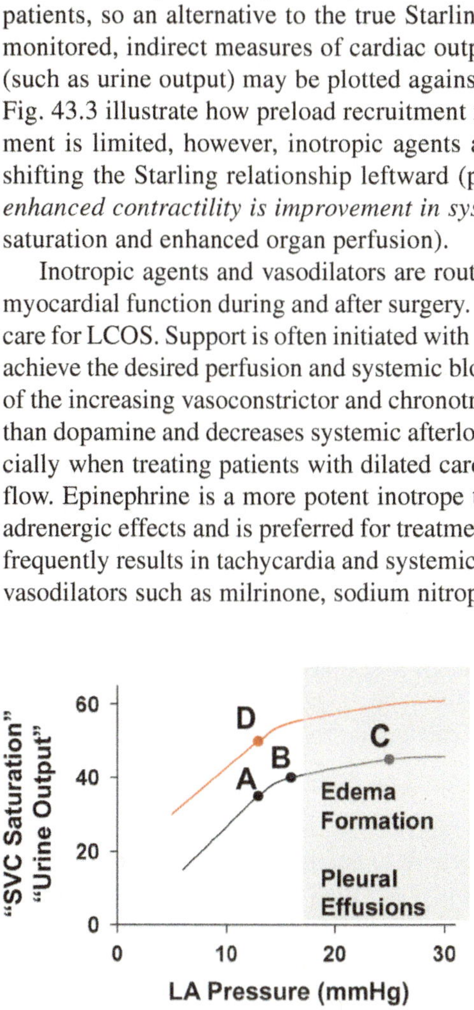

FIGURE 43.3 **Modified Starling relationship.** Since stroke volume is not easily monitored, indirect measures of cardiac output (such as venous saturation) or measures of end-organ perfusion (such as urine output) may be plotted against atrial pressure to attain a "modified" Starling relationship. Fluid administration augments preload and leads to improvement in superior vena cava (SVC) saturation and end-organ perfusion (point A to point B). Preload augmentation is limited, however; so progressive fluid administration will increase atrial pressure and ultimately lead to edema formation (point C). Alternate ways to improve SVC saturation or urine output may include increased inotropic support, afterload reduction, or improved lusitropy, which all shift the Starling relationship leftward (point D). *The therapeutic goal of enhanced lusitropy, increased contractility, or afterload reduction is higher venous saturation and enhanced organ perfusion for a comparable preload.*

TABLE 43.1 Common Inotropic Agents for Treatment of Low Cardiac Output Syndrome

Inotropic Agent	Loading Dose	Typical Dose Range
Dobutamine	None	3–20 μg/kg/min
Epinephrine	None	0.02–0.2 μg/kg/min
Norepinephrine	None	0.02–0.2 μg/kg/min
Milrinone	50–100 μg/kg	0.25–1 μg/kg/min
Calcium chloride	None	5–20 mg/kg/h

systemic afterload (or at least attenuate the α_1-effects of epinephrine). The use of high-dose catecholamines for inotropic support has disadvantages, as they can increase afterload substantially, promote tachycardia and arrhythmias, increase myocardial oxygen consumption, and depress the myocardial adrenergic response by downregulating β-adrenergic receptors. Furthermore, prolonged use of high-dose catecholamines may further amplify cardiomyocyte injury, thus aggravating diastolic and systolic ventricular dysfunction [138].

The perioperative use of the phosphodiesterase (PDE) inhibitor, milrinone has increased considerably over the past few years. Milrinone improves cardiac output by enhancing both systolic and diastolic function, while reducing systemic and pulmonary vascular resistance. It is less arrhythmogenic than other inotropic agents. Its mechanism of action is to inhibit breakdown of cyclic adenosine monophosphate (cAMP) by the PDE III isozyme [139], resulting in enhanced calcium transport into the cell and improved myocyte contractility. In addition, reuptake of calcium is a cAMP-dependent process, so these agents may enhance diastolic relaxation of the myocardium by increasing the rate of calcium reuptake after systole. PDE inhibitors increase cardiac muscle contractility and vascular muscle relaxation without increasing myocardial oxygen consumption or ventricular afterload [140]. Milrinone is usually the preferred PDE inhibitor, because of its shorter half-life and lower incidence of thrombocytopenia [8,141–144].

The ability to achieve a rapid hemodynamic response on initiation of milrinone is extremely important after separation from CPB, when uncompensated LCOS can quickly result in the deterioration of hemodynamic status and subsequent secondary organ dysfunction. For patients at high risk for LCOS, some centers prefer to load with milrinone during CPB to avoid potential hypotension associated with loading. The clinical utility of PDE inhibitors in the pediatric population is similar to that of milrinone in adult heart failure patients [145–147]. The PRIMACORP study demonstrated milrinone administration in children early after congenital heart surgery reduces the incidence of LCOS [8]. Since renal dysfunction results in delayed clearance of milrinone, patients with renal insufficiency are at risk for toxicity due to excessive drug levels [143,148]. Continuous infusion rates should thus be adjusted based on creatinine clearance to avoid excessive and prolonged vasodilation, especially in neonates.

Calcium supplementation and calcium sensitizing agents also warrant discussion. Cardiac contraction and relaxation are mediated by cyclic fluctuations in cytoplasmic calcium concentration. In the adult heart, calcium released from the sarcoplasmic reticulum accounts for the majority of the calcium that binds to troponin C. In the neonate, the sarcoplasmic reticular system is relatively sparse and undifferentiated, so the neonatal myocardium is more dependent on extracellular calcium stores for contractile function [67]. Maintenance of adequate extracellular calcium is essential for normal myocardial contractile function in all patients, but especially in neonates. Hypocalcemia occurs frequently in the postoperative period and may be pronounced in patients with a 22q11 deletion syndrome or transient hypoparathyroidism. Transfusion of citrate-treated blood, which chelates calcium, and administration of loop diuretics may exacerbate hypocalcemia. Ionized calcium, the physiologically active form of calcium, should be monitored frequently perioperatively and normal or supernormal levels maintained with supplementation. Many centers routinely use calcium infusions in neonates after CPB to augment and stabilize extracellular ionized calcium, especially in patients with a 22q11 deletion.

Calcium sensitizing agents are a relatively new class of drugs that have been used mostly in adults for the treatment of heart failure and low cardiac output states. These drugs act directly on the contractile protein system and are believed to increase cardiac contractility by sensitizing cardiac myofibrils to calcium without increasing intracellular calcium. They may also increase cAMP through PDE inhibition, enhancing contractility and decreasing afterload. These effects occur without increasing myocardial oxygen consumption or impairing diastolic function. Levosimendan, one of the first calcium sensitizers, has been shown to be beneficial in adult patients in acute severe heart failure [149,150]. Pediatric clinical trials have demonstrated improvements in hemodynamics, myocardial oxygen demand, cardiac injury biomarkers, and reduction of inotropic requirement without adverse effects, although no reduction in morbidity and mortality has been recognized [151–155].

TABLE 43.2 Agents Used for Treatment of Catecholamine-Resistant Low Cardiac Output Syndrome

Agent	Typical Dose Range
Arginine vasopressin	0.2–3 m-U/kg/min infusion
Hydrocortisone	50 mg/m^2/day (dosed every 6 h)
Liothyronine (triostat)	0.05–0.2 µg/kg/h infusion

Postoperative patients may develop a prolonged low cardiac output state that is refractory to escalating inotropic support. In these patients, hormone replacement therapy may improve cardiac output. Table 43.2 lists several agents used in the treatment of catecholamine-resistant low cardiac output. Although it is unclear the exact mechanism that these agents play in development of persistent LCOS, they may prevent the need for mechanical support. Indeed, if these medications do not improve cardiac output, mechanical support should be initiated to maintain end-organ perfusion as a bridge to recovery.

Thyroid dysfunction has been shown to occur following CPB with decreased levels of free triiodothyronine (T_3), total T_3, and thyroxine (T_4) [156,157]. These deficiencies can persist for several days and may play a role in postoperative myocardial depression [157]. Thyroid replacement therapy has been shown to raise serum T_3 levels and improve cardiac performance [158,159]. A randomized, double-blind, placebo-controlled trial demonstrated infants undergoing aortic arch surgery had higher systolic blood pressures and improved urine output in the early postoperative period with continuous T_3 infusions [160]. Therefore, postoperative thyroid replacement therapy may be beneficial, especially in patients at highest risk for low cardiac output, such as younger patients with more complex congenital heart disease requiring longer CPB times [161].

Arginine vasopressin has been advocated in the treatment of and possibly in the prophylaxis from refractory hypotension in postsurgical pediatric patients [162–164]. Vasopressin deficiency has been well described in adult patients who undergo cardiac surgery and develop vasodilatory shock after CPB that is refractory to inotropic therapy. Vasopressin administration improved cardiac output and reduced the need for postoperative inotropic support [165–167]. Rosenzwieg et al. observed improvement in blood pressure and perfusion following vasopressin infusion in young children with LCOS following CPB [162]. Vasopressin has also been shown to be effective for refractory hypotension in patients on mechanical circulatory support [165,168].

Data suggest relative adrenal dysfunction contributes to morbidity and mortality in critically ill adult and pediatric patients; and glucocorticoid administration improves hemodynamics and reduces the need for inotropic support for these patients with refractory LCOS [169,170]. In a retrospective study of postoperative neonates receiving escalating doses of epinephrine, inotrope requirements decreased significantly within 24h of corticosteroid treatment [170]. Some patients demonstrated low random cortisol levels with a normal adrenocorticotrophic hormone (ACTH) stimulation test, suggesting adrenal insufficiency. These data suggest stress–dose hydrocortisone (50 $mg/m^2/day$) may help reduce inotropic requirements in pediatric patients with LCOS refractory to conventional therapy. The physiologic basis for the reduction in inotropic support after both vasopressin and corticosteroid therapy remains obscure, but they may share a similar mechanism, since vasopressin serves as a potent stimulus for ACTH [171].

Afterload Reduction for Systemic Ventricular Failure

Elevated afterload is particularly detrimental to the neonatal heart, especially when compounded by postoperative myocardial dysfunction. Afterload reduction is thus often beneficial in postoperative patients showing signs of LCOS. Furthermore, if high-dose catecholamines cannot be avoided, vasodilator therapy should be considered to counter catecholamine vasoconstrictor effects. The lower panel of Fig. 43.2 demonstrates the beneficial effects of afterload reduction on pressure–volume and Starling relationships. This panel also demonstrates an important principle: benefits of afterload reduction are particularly pronounced in neonatal hearts and patients with poor contractility. With neonatal hearts or impaired contractility, afterload reduction is particularly useful to augment stroke volume and overall cardiac output. As with inotropic agents, it is important to assess efficacy of these agents following initiation or dosage adjustment since vasodilator agents also have unwanted side effects. As shown in Fig. 43.2, *the therapeutic goal of afterload reduction should be a greater stroke volume for a comparable preload.* As noted previously, however, since measurement of stroke volume is not routine in postoperative patients, the modified Starling relationship can be used to assess efficacy of most hemodynamic interventions, including afterload reduction. As shown in Fig. 43.3, *the therapeutic goal of afterload reduction is improvement in systemic blood flow for a comparable preload.*

Phenoxybenzamine is a potent adrenergic blocking agent in selected patients after cardiac surgery [104]. Since phenoxybenzamine is a potent vasodilator with a very long half-life (>24h), its use may be complicated by severe hypotension. Although clinically useful in skilled hands, phenoxybenzamine use has been largely abandoned due to lack of availability. For this reason, fast-acting vasodilators are the typical agents (e.g., sodium nitroprusside or nicardipine) for afterload reduction and vasodilator therapy in patients with congenital heart disease. Although nitroprusside or nicardipine are less effective vasodilators than phenoxybenzamine, the therapeutic effects are easier to titrate due to the shorter half-life and rapid onset of action. Systemic vasodilation is also beneficial in patients with excessive pulmonary blood flow after Norwood palliation [103]. In such patients, the dual effects of vasodilation include: (1) afterload reduction for improvement of myocardial performance and (2) reduction of systemic vascular resistance to balance pulmonary and systemic blood flow.

PDE inhibitors are also commonly used for afterload reduction in pediatric patients with congenital heart disease. These agents are particularly useful in the postoperative pediatric cardiac surgical patient because enhanced inotropic and lusitropic effects are combined with systemic and pulmonary vasodilation. In patients who require high-dose adrenergic agents, it is especially important to use one or more vasodilator agents concurrently.

Mechanical Support

When LCOS persists despite adequate medical therapy, mechanical circulatory support should be considered [172]. In pediatric patients, mechanical support is provided by ECMO or ventricular assist devices. The choice may depend on the patient's weight and/or presence of pulmonary dysfunction. ECMO can be used in patients with life-threatening pulmonary disease or postcardiotomy ventricular failure, whereas a ventricular assist device can be used in infants with adequate pulmonary function. With both techniques, patients are sedated and sometimes paralyzed and receive minimal inotropic support. However, over the last decade increased liberation from ICU-related therapies (mechanical ventilation, sedation, paralysis) and even discharge has been realized with pediatric durable devices [173,174]. If feasible from a pulmonary perspective, it is preferable to convert to ventricular assist device support from ECMO if greater than 14 days of support will be required as morbidity, mortality, and posttransplant outcomes are worsened with mid-term and long-term ECMO support [175–177]. Early intervention and aggressive management are key to the overall outcome with mechanical circulatory support.

MANAGEMENT OF PULMONARY HYPERTENSION

Elevation in pulmonary vascular resistance (PVR) may lead to LCOS by increasing the afterload of the right ventricle. Children with many forms of congenital heart disease, particularly those with elevated pulmonary pressure or blood flow before surgery, may have elevated PVR after congenital heart surgery. Furthermore, bypass-mediated inflammation may result in increased pulmonary vascular reactivity, due to pulmonary vascular endothelial injury [40]. This endothelial injury is mediated by thromboxane production, decreased production of endogenous nitric oxide synthase, and pulmonary microemboli. A reduction in exhaled nitric oxide, endogenously produced by the pulmonary vascular endothelium, may be a marker of endothelial injury [178,179]. Furthermore, endothelin-1 in the pulmonary vascular endothelium is increased after CPB and deep hypothermic circulatory arrest [66]. Increases in PVR will increase RV afterload aggravating RV dysfunction and potentiating low cardiac output. In patients with elevated pulmonary artery pressures, careful assessment for anatomic causes of pulmonary hypertension is indicated, such as pulmonary venous obstruction or residual shunts.

Prevention should be the first line therapy for postoperative pulmonary hypertension. Infants and children at risk for postoperative pulmonary hypertension should be identified preoperatively. For these patients, strategies to minimize stimuli known to increase PVR should be initiated, such as avoidance of hypoxia, hypercarbia, acidosis, agitation, pain, and tracheal suction/stimulation. Therapy may include deep sedation/analgesia with a continuous opioid infusion alone or in combination with a benzodiazepine. Neuromuscular blockade may be indicated to obtain precise control of ventilation. Elevated PVR can be managed by increasing arterial pH through the induction of alkalosis. Since hyperventilation may increase mean airway pressure and compromise venous return, administration of sodium bicarbonate may be the preferred way to induce alkalosis. Induction of metabolic alkalosis with bicarbonate administration in postoperative neonates has been shown to reduce PVR and pulmonary arterial pressure, with a corresponding increase in cardiac index [180]. As discussed below, ventilation strategies should aim to avoid atelectasis and maintain end-expiratory lung volume at functional residual capacity (FRC), while minimizing intrathoracic pressure. This usually entails utilizing an appropriate tidal volume and inspiratory time, and judicious use of positive end-expiratory pressure (PEEP). Ventilation strategies should aim to avoid higher mean airway pressures.

Another way to lower pulmonary arterial pressure and PVR is with the use of pulmonary vasodilators. In addition to its systemic vasodilation effects, milrinone is an effective pulmonary vasodilator. Isoproterenol is also an effective pulmonary vasodilator, although its side effect profile (tachycardia, increased myocardial O_2 uptake) may limit use [181]. The use of other nonspecific vasodilators, such as sildenafil, may be limited by deleterious systemic effects, including systemic hypotension and aggravation of existing defects in pulmonary gas exchange. Inhaled nitric oxide (iNO), however, acts selectively on the pulmonary vasculature. Studies have demonstrated that iNO is an effective way to reduce pulmonary vascular resistance [182], with fewer pulmonary hypertensive crises in the postoperative neonates [183]. PDE inhibitors, both type III (milrinone) and type V (such as sildenafil), have been shown to enhance pulmonary vasodilatory effects of iNO and reduce rebound pulmonary hypertension after discontinuation of nitric oxide therapy [184]. The endothelin-receptor antagonist, bosentan, also acts to dilate the pulmonary vasculature [185]. Limited data with L-arginine and substance P suggest a benefit of these agents in restoring pulmonary endothelial function [186].

MANAGEMENT OF RIGHT VENTRICULAR FAILURE

Right heart failure is common after congenital heart surgery and often contributes to LCOS. Factors contributing to postoperative RV dysfunction include: difficulties with right heart myocardial protection; a right ventriculotomy and CPB-mediated myocardial injury resulting in diastolic dysfunction. Patients undergoing right heart procedures, including tetralogy of Fallot repair and Fontan procedures, often demonstrate restrictive physiology (diastolic RV dysfunction), characterized by antegrade diastolic pulmonary arterial flow coinciding with atrial systole [187,188].

Children with acute RV restrictive physiology have a decreased cardiac index because the stiff right ventricle has impaired diastolic filling [60]. These patients typically have a slower postoperative recovery and a prolonged stay in the ICU. Impairment in LV filling may occur as the hypertensive RV impinges on the LV. Due to altered ventricular compliance, patients with RV failure are particularly sensitive to alterations in venous return caused by intrathoracic pressure changes. These patients therefore benefit from ventilation strategies that minimize intrathoracic pressure [187–190]. In addition, these patients may benefit from manipulation of PVR to minimize RV afterload. PDE inhibitors are particularly beneficial in these patients, due to the combined lusitropic and pulmonary vasodilatory effects.

In patients with RV dysfunction, preserving a right-to-left shunt at the atrial level is beneficial. In patients undergoing the modified Fontan procedure, fenestration of the Fontan pathway is associated with reduced pleural effusion and significantly shorter hospital stays [191]. In patients who undergo tetralogy of Fallot repair, a right-to-left atrial shunt can be similarly facilitated by maintaining patency of the foramen ovale or by creating a small fenestration in the atrial septum.

VENTILATION STRATEGIES AFTER CARDIAC SURGERY

Cardiopulmonary Interactions

The cardiorespiratory system functions as a unit, and as a result, ventilation can have a profound effect on hemodynamics. These effects may particularly pronounced in infants following cardiac surgery. An understanding of the complex interactions between the cardiovascular and respiratory systems is thus crucial to the management of these patients. Alterations in intrathoracic pressure and lung volume affect dynamic and loading conditions of the right ventricle and left ventricle differently, often having opposing effects. Thus, the right ventricle and left ventricle are traditionally considered separately in discussions of cardiopulmonary interactions. These effects highlight the central role of cardiopulmonary interactions in management of patients with LCOS.

A transient increase in intrathoracic pressure will decrease systemic venous return to the right heart, reducing right ventricle preload. Increases in intrathoracic pressure also decrease left ventricle afterload since most of the systemic vasculature is extrathoracic. Spontaneous inspiration or negative intrathoracic pressure has the opposite effects, to augment right ventricle filling and increase left ventricle afterload. Ventilation effects on right ventricle afterload (and pulmonary vascular resistance) depend primarily on lung volume, since PVR is lowest at functional residual capacity. Since the effects of intrathoracic pressure changes are opposite for the right and left ventricles, the ventilation strategy should be contingent on whether RV or LV dysfunction predominates.

Positive pressure ventilation is typically beneficial in patients with systemic ventricular dysfunction, because it results in systemic ventricular afterload reduction. Higher levels of PEEP with optimal lung recruitment may thus be hemodynamically beneficial in these patients. Tidal volumes should be maintained in the range of 8–10 mL/kg to avoid overdistension of the lungs [192]. Shorter inspiratory times may augment left ventricle filling in patients with systemic ventricular dysfunction [193]. The hemodynamic effects of any ventilatory maneuver should be carefully evaluated with respect to systemic oxygen delivery since alterations in thoracic pressure may have opposing hemodynamic effects.

Patients with RV failure are more sensitive to changes in venous return caused by increased intrathoracic pressure, especially when the right ventricle is stiff. Spontaneous inspiration enhances RV diastolic filling and overall cardiac output in these patients, so early extubation can be beneficial. Due to the detrimental effects of positive pressure ventilation on RV dynamics, alternate modes of ventilation, such as negative-pressure or high-frequency jet ventilation (HFJV) have been advocated in RV failure. Since HFJV provides a lower mean airway pressure while maintaining a similar $PaCO_2$, it may be ideally suited to patients with RV dysfunction and/or pulmonary hypertension. In postoperative Fontan patients, HFJV decreased the mean airway pressure, reduced PVR, and increased cardiac index [194]. In a similar manner, negative-pressure ventilation augments cardiac output in patients with restrictive physiology after tetralogy of Fallot repair [187,188,190]. Similar results were observed in patients with Fontan physiology [189]. Although technical challenges of negative-pressure ventilation has prevented its widespread use in postoperative cardiac surgery patients, ventilation strategies used for patients with RV failure or Fontan physiology should aim to minimize mean airway pressure while maintaining lung volume at functional residual capacity, where lung mechanics, PVR, and right ventricle afterload are optimal.

Lung Recruitment in Patients With Congenital Heart Disease

As in patients with respiratory failure, lung recruitment is also important in the management of patients with heart failure. In addition to the lung volume effects on pulmonary vascular resistance, an appropriate lung volume (i.e., FRC) also ensures optimal lung compliance and pulmonary gas exchange. Altered gas exchange in patients after Norwood palliation was ameliorated by increasing PEEP, presumably resulting in alveolar recruitment [105]. Therefore, ventilation strategies for patients with congenital heart disease should strive to maintain an adequately expanded lung, aiming for functional residual capacity.

Ventilation Effects on Pulmonary Blood Flow

Manipulation of pulmonary blood flow is often necessary in patients with congenital heart disease. Manipulation of PVR in patients with congenital heart defects has traditionally emphasized use of oxygen, carbon dioxide, and manipulation of acid–base status [195,196]. Similar to management of patients with pulmonary hypertension, ventilation strategies for patients with diminished pulmonary blood flow entail lung recruitment, supplemental inspired oxygen, hyperventilation, and alkalosis. In patients with large left-to-right shunts, including infants with single ventricle physiology, a respiratory acidosis can raise PVR, decrease systemic vascular resistance (SVR) and thus decrease pulmonary flow [197]. Respiratory acidosis can be induced either through alveolar hypoventilation or by increasing inspired CO_2 concentrations in mechanically ventilated, paralyzed patients.

In single ventricle patients manipulation of SVR has been found to be superior to manipulations in PVR; however, manipulation of PVR may be necessary in exceptional cases [198,199]. Historically data from newborns with hypoplastic left heart syndrome demonstrate inhaled CO_2 is more effective than subatmospheric oxygen to increase cerebral and/or systemic perfusion in ventilated, paralyzed patients, but it is important to note that these studies did not assess the effect of inspired CO_2 in spontaneously ventilated patients [197,200,201]. Increases in PVR may also be induced by PEEP, independent of changes in systemic vascular resistance [196]. When lung compliance is normal, PEEP increases PVR by compressing interalveolar pulmonary arterioles. Increased levels of PEEP should be used with caution, however, as this may reduce cardiac output by impeding venous return.

CONCLUSION

LCOS remains one of the most significant complications of congenital heart surgery in children. As discussed above, LCOS typically results from the combined effects of transient myocardial dysfunction and alterations in ventricular loading conditions. Residual cardiac lesions and arrhythmias increase risk for LCOS and further aggravate the underlying low output state. Recognition of LCOS after surgery is fundamental to cardiac intensive care and paramount to the prevention of associated morbidity and mortality. Monitoring of a complete targeted cardiovascular exam, venous oxygen saturation, NIRS, and serum lactate are valuable for circulatory assessment. Treatment strategies vary according to underlying etiologic factors and clinical presentation. Prompt diagnosis of residual cardiac abnormalities is imperative, especially when patients do not follow their predicted postoperative course. The mainstay of therapy, once residual structural defects have been ruled out, is optimization of preload and afterload, improvement of tissue perfusion and oxygenation, and enhancement of myocardial performance with inotrope and vasodilator agents. The modified Starling relationship may be useful to help guide hemodynamic interventions aimed to treat LCOS. In the future, innovative techniques to better assess myocardial systolic and diastolic performance and novel therapeutic agents should improve the detection and management of LCOS in postoperative cardiac surgery patients.

REFERENCES

[1] H.H. Hovels-Gurich, J.F. Vazquez-Jimenez, A. Silvestri, K. Schumacher, R. Minkenberg, J. Duchateau, B.J. Messmer, G. von Bernuth, M.C. Seghaye, Production of proinflammatory cytokines and myocardial dysfunction after arterial switch operation in neonates with transposition of the great arteries, J. Thorac. Cardiovasc. Surg. 124 (2002) 811–820.

[2] E.M. Boyle Jr., T.H. Pohlman, M.C. Johnson, E.D. Verrier, Endothelial cell injury in cardiovascular surgery: the systemic inflammatory response, Ann. Thorac. Surg. 63 (1997) 277–284.

[3] J. Butler, V.L. Pathi, R.D. Paton, R.W. Logan, K.J. MacArthur, M.P. Jamieson, J.C. Pollock, Acute-phase responses to cardiopulmonary bypass in children weighing less than 10 kilograms, Ann. Thorac. Surg. 62 (1996) 538–542.
[4] R.R. Chaturvedi, C. Lincoln, J.W. Gothard, M.H. Scallan, P.A. White, A.N. Redington, D.F. Shore, Left ventricular dysfunction after open repair of simple congenital heart defects in infants and children: quantitation with the use of a conductance catheter immediately after bypass, J. Thorac. Cardiovasc. Surg. 115 (1998) 77–83.
[5] G.V. Parr, E.H. Blackstone, J.W. Kirklin, Cardiac performance and mortality early after intracardiac surgery in infants and young children, Circulation 51 (1975) 867–874.
[6] G. Wernovsky, D. Wypij, R.A. Jonas, J.E. Mayer Jr., F.L. Hanley, P.R. Hickey, A.Z. Walsh, A.C. Chang, A.R. Castaneda, J.W. Newburger, et al., Postoperative course and hemodynamic profile after the arterial switch operation in neonates and infants. A comparison of low-flow cardiopulmonary bypass and circulatory arrest, Circulation 92 (1995) 2226–2235.
[7] S.D. Colan, E. Trowitzsch, G. Wernovsky, G.F. Sholler, S.P. Sanders, A.R. Castaneda, Myocardial performance after arterial switch operation for transposition of the great arteries with intact ventricular septum, Circulation 78 (1988) 132–141.
[8] T.M. Hoffman, G. Wernovsky, A.M. Atz, T.J. Kulik, D.P. Nelson, A.C. Chang, J.M. Bailey, A. Akbary, J.F. Kocsis, R. Kaczmarek, T.L. Spray, D.L. Wessel, Efficacy and safety of milrinone in preventing low cardiac output syndrome in infants and children after corrective surgery for congenital heart disease, Circulation 107 (2003) 996–1002.
[9] J.S. Tweddell, G.M. Hoffman, K.A. Mussatto, R.T. Fedderly, S. Berger, R.D. Jaquiss, N.S. Ghanayem, S.J. Frisbee, S.B. Litwin, Improved survival of patients undergoing palliation of hypoplastic left heart syndrome: lessons learned from 115 consecutive patients, Circulation 106 (2002) I82–I89.
[10] D.C. Bellinger, D. Wypij, K.C. Kuban, L.A. Rappaport, P.R. Hickey, G. Wernovsky, R.A. Jonas, J.W. Newburger, Developmental and neurological status of children at 4 years of age after heart surgery with hypothermic circulatory arrest or low-flow cardiopulmonary bypass, Circulation 100 (1999) 526–532.
[11] K.P. Ulate, O. Yanay, H. Jeffries, H. Baden, J.L. Di Gennaro, J. Zimmerman, An elevated low cardiac output syndrome score is associated with morbidity in infants after congenital heart surgery, Pediatr. Crit. Care Med. 18 (2017) 26–33.
[12] B. Hiemstra, R.J. Eck, F. Keus, I.C.C. van der Horst, Clinical examination for diagnosing circulatory shock, Curr. Opin. Crit. Care 23 (2017) 293–301.
[13] G. Asimakopoulos, P.L. Smith, C.P. Ratnatunga, K.M. Taylor, Lung injury and acute respiratory distress syndrome after cardiopulmonary bypass, Ann. Thorac. Surg. 68 (1999) 1107–1115.
[14] M.C. Seghaye, R.G. Grabitz, J. Duchateau, S. Busse, S. Dabritz, D. Koch, G. Alzen, H. Hornchen, B.J. Messmer, G. Von Bernuth, Inflammatory reaction and capillary leak syndrome related to cardiopulmonary bypass in neonates undergoing cardiac operations, J. Thorac. Cardiovasc. Surg. 112 (1996) 687–697.
[15] K.L. Brown, D.A. Ridout, A.P. Goldman, A. Hoskote, D.J. Penny, Risk factors for long intensive care unit stay after cardiopulmonary bypass in children, Crit. Care Med. 31 (2003) 28–33.
[16] J.E. Kist-van Holthe tot Echten, C.A. Goedvolk, M.B. Doornaar, M.M. van der Vorst, J.M. Bosman-Vermeeren, R. Brand, A.J. van der Heijden, P.H. Schoof, M.G. Hazekamp, Acute renal insufficiency and renal replacement therapy after pediatric cardiopulmonary bypass surgery, Pediatr. Cardiol. 22 (2001) 321–326.
[17] S. Dittrich, I. Dahnert, M. Vogel, B. Stiller, N.A. Haas, V. Alexi-Meskishvili, P.E. Lange, Peritoneal dialysis after infant open heart surgery: observations in 27 patients, Ann. Thorac. Surg. 68 (1999) 160–163.
[18] D. Stromberg, C.D. Fraser Jr., J.M. Sorof, K. Drescher, T.F. Feltes, Peritoneal dialysis. An adjunct to pediatric postcardiotomy fluid management, Tex. Heart Inst. J. 24 (1997) 269–277.
[19] K.L. Chan, P. Ip, C.S. Chiu, Y.F. Cheung, Peritoneal dialysis after surgery for congenital heart disease in infants and young children, Ann. Thorac. Surg. 76 (2003) 1443–1449.
[20] R.M. Giuffre, K.H. Tam, W.W. Williams, R.M. Freedom, Acute renal failure complicating pediatric cardiac surgery: a comparison of survivors and nonsurvivors following acute peritoneal dialysis, Pediatr. Cardiol. 13 (1992) 208–213.
[21] R.G. Leyh, A. Notzold, E.G. Kraatz, H.H. Sievers, A. Bernhard, Continuous venovenous haemofiltration in neonates with renal insufficiency resulting from low cardiac output syndrome after cardiac surgery, Cardiovasc. Surg. 4 (1996) 520–525.
[22] D.J. Lex, R. Toth, Z. Cserep, S.I. Alexander, T. Breuer, E. Sapi, A. Szatmari, E. Szekely, J. Gal, A. Szekely, A comparison of the systems for the identification of postoperative acute kidney injury in pediatric cardiac patients, Ann. Thorac. Surg. 97 (2014) 202–210.
[23] I. Malagon, W. Onkenhout, M. Klok, P.F. van der Poel, J.G. Bovill, M.G. Hazekamp, Gut permeability in neonates after a stage 1 Norwood procedure, Pediatr. Crit. Care Med. 6 (2005) 547–549.
[24] J.K. Stechmiller, D. Treloar, N. Allen, Gut dysfunction in critically ill patients: a review of the literature, Am. J. Crit. Care 6 (1997) 204–209.
[25] A. Hebra, M.F. Brown, R.B. Hirschl, K. McGeehin, J.A. O'Neill Jr., W.I. Norwood, A.J. Ross 3rd, Mesenteric ischemia in hypoplastic left heart syndrome, J. Pediatr. Surg. 28 (1993) 606–611.
[26] D.B. McElhinney, H.L. Hedrick, D.M. Bush, G.R. Pereira, P.W. Stafford, J.W. Gaynor, T.L. Spray, G. Wernovsky, Necrotizing enterocolitis in neonates with congenital heart disease: risk factors and outcomes, Pediatrics 106 (2000) 1080–1087.
[27] H.H. Hovels-Gurich, K. Konrad, D. Skorzenski, C. Nacken, R. Minkenberg, B.J. Messmer, M.C. Seghaye, Long-term neurodevelopmental outcome and exercise capacity after corrective surgery for tetralogy of Fallot or ventricular septal defect in infancy, Ann. Thorac. Surg. 81 (2006) 958–966.
[28] G. Miller, J.R. Tesman, J.C. Ramer, B.G. Baylen, J.L. Myers, Outcome after open-heart surgery in infants and children, J. Child Neurol. 11 (1996) 49–53.

[29] D. Wypij, J.W. Newburger, L.A. Rappaport, A.J. duPlessis, R.A. Jonas, G. Wernovsky, M. Lin, D.C. Bellinger, The effect of duration of deep hypothermic circulatory arrest in infant heart surgery on late neurodevelopment: the Boston Circulatory Arrest Trial, J. Thorac. Cardiovasc. Surg. 126 (2003) 1397–1403.

[30] D.C. Bellinger, R.A. Jonas, L.A. Rappaport, D. Wypij, G. Wernovsky, K.C. Kuban, P.D. Barnes, G.L. Holmes, P.R. Hickey, R.D. Strand, et al., Developmental and neurologic status of children after heart surgery with hypothermic circulatory arrest or low-flow cardiopulmonary bypass, N. Engl. J. Med. 332 (1995) 549–555.

[31] P.R. Hickey, Neurologic sequelae associated with deep hypothermic circulatory arrest, Ann. Thorac. Surg. 65 (1998) S65–S69 discussion S69-70, S74–S76.

[32] H.H. Hovels-Gurich, K. Konrad, M. Wiesner, R. Minkenberg, B. Herpertz-Dahlmann, B.J. Messmer, G. Von Bernuth, Long term behavioural outcome after neonatal arterial switch operation for transposition of the great arteries, Arch. Dis. Child 87 (2002) 506–510.

[33] M.Y. Naim, J.W. Gaynor, J. Chen, S.C. Nicolson, S. Fuller, T.L. Spray, D.J. Dlugos, R.R. Clancy, L.V. Costa, D.J. Licht, R. Xiao, H. Meldrum, N.S. Abend, Subclinical seizures identified by postoperative electroencephalographic monitoring are common after neonatal cardiac surgery, J. Thorac. Cardiovasc. Surg. 150 (2015) 169–178 discussion 178–180.

[34] B. Latal, G. Wohlrab, B. Brotschi, I. Beck, W. Knirsch, V. Bernet, Postoperative amplitude-integrated electroencephalography predicts four-year neurodevelopmental outcome in children with complex congenital heart disease, J. Pediatr. 178 (2016) 55–60 e1.

[35] A.J. du Plessis, Neurologic disorders, in: A.C. Chang, F.L. Hanley, G. Wernovsky, D.L. Wessel (Eds.), Pediatric Cardiac Intensive Care, 1998, pp. 369–386. Baltimore.

[36] F.A. Burrows, W.G. Williams, K.H. Teoh, A.E. Wood, J. Burns, J. Edmonds, G.A. Barker, G.A. Trusler, R.D. Weisel, Myocardial performance after repair of congenital cardiac defects in infants and children. Response to volume loading, J. Thorac. Cardiovasc. Surg. 96 (1988) 548–556.

[37] M.L. Schermerhorn, M. Tofukuji, P.R. Khoury, L. Phillips, P.R. Hickey, F.W. Sellke, J.E. Mayer Jr., D.P. Nelson, Sialyl lewis oligosaccharide preserves cardiopulmonary and endothelial function after hypothermic circulatory arrest in lambs, J. Thorac. Cardiovasc. Surg. 120 (2000) 230–237.

[38] M.L. Schermerhorn, D.P. Nelson, E.D. Blume, L. Phillips, J.E. Mayer Jr., Sialyl Lewis oligosaccharide preserves myocardial and endothelial function during cardioplegic ischemia, Ann. Thorac. Surg. 70 (2000) 890–894.

[39] A. Stamler, S.Y. Wang, D.E. Aguirre, R.G. Johnson, F.W. Sellke, Cardiopulmonary bypass alters vasomotor regulation of the skeletal muscle microcirculation, Ann. Thorac. Surg. 64 (1997) 460–465.

[40] D.L. Wessel, I. Adatia, T.M. Giglia, J.E. Thompson, T.J. Kulik, Use of inhaled nitric oxide and acetylcholine in the evaluation of pulmonary hypertension and endothelial function after cardiopulmonary bypass, Circulation 88 (1993) 2128–2138.

[41] A. Hoffman, Patterns of family extinction depend on definition and geological time scale, Nature 315 (1985) 659–662.

[42] L.A. Rhodes, G. Wernovsky, J.F. Keane, J.E. Mayer Jr., A. Shuren, C. Dindy, S.D. Colan, E.P. Walsh, Arrhythmias and intracardiac conduction after the arterial switch operation, J. Thorac. Cardiovasc. Surg. 109 (1995) 303–310.

[43] S.M. Schwartz, K.J. Anand, M.A. Portman, S. Crow, D.P. Nelson, J.J. Zimmerman, Endocrinopathies in the cardiac ICU, World J. Pediatr. Congenit. Heart Surg. 2 (2011) 400–410.

[44] R.J. Gajarski, C.B. Stefanelli, J.N. Graziano, N. Kaciroti, J.R. Charpie, D. Vazquez, Adrenocortical response in infants undergoing cardiac surgery with cardiopulmonary bypass and circulatory arrest, Pediatr. Crit. Care Med. 11 (2010) 44–51.

[45] C.L. Soto-Rivera, M.S. Agus, J.E. Sawyer, D.J. Macrae, Pediatric cardiac intensive care society 2014 consensus statement: pharmacotherapies in cardiac critical care hormone replacement therapy, Pediatr. Crit. Care Med. 17 (2016) S59–S68.

[46] K.S. Bandali, M.P. Belanger, C. Wittnich, Is hyperglycemia seen in children during cardiopulmonary bypass a result of hyperoxia? J. Thorac. Cardiovasc. Surg. 122 (2001) 753–758.

[47] G. Benzing 3rd, P.D. Francis, S. Kaplan, J.A. Helmsworth, M.A. Sperling, Glucose and insulin changes in infants and children undergoing hypothermic open-heart surgery, Am. J. Cardiol. 52 (1983) 133–136.

[48] A.R. Yates, P.C. Dyke 2nd, R. Taeed, T.M. Hoffman, J. Hayes, T.F. Feltes, C.L. Cua, Hyperglycemia is a marker for poor outcome in the postoperative pediatric cardiac patient, Pediatr. Crit. Care Med. 7 (2006) 351–355.

[49] M.S. Agus, G.M. Steil, D. Wypij, J.M. Costello, P.C. Laussen, M. Langer, J.L. Alexander, L.A. Scoppettuolo, F.A. Pigula, J.R. Charpie, R.G. Ohye, M.G. Gaies, S.S. Investigators, Tight glycemic control versus standard care after pediatric cardiac surgery, N. Engl. J. Med. 367 (2012) 1208–1219.

[50] S. de Ferranti, K. Gauvreau, P.R. Hickey, R.A. Jonas, D. Wypij, A. du Plessis, D.C. Bellinger, K. Kuban, J.W. Newburger, P.C. Laussen, Intraoperative hyperglycemia during infant cardiac surgery is not associated with adverse neurodevelopmental outcomes at 1, 4, and 8 years, Anesthesiology 100 (2004) 1345–1352.

[51] R.I. Hall, M.S. Smith, G. Rocker, The systemic inflammatory response to cardiopulmonary bypass: pathophysiological, therapeutic, and pharmacological considerations, Anesth. Analg. 85 (1997) 766–782.

[52] M. Boehne, M. Sasse, A. Karch, F. Dziuba, A. Horke, T. Kaussen, R. Mikolajczyk, P. Beerbaum, T. Jack, Systemic inflammatory response syndrome after pediatric congenital heart surgery: incidence, risk factors, and clinical outcome, J. Card Surg. 32 (2017) 116–125.

[53] M.L. Entman, C.W. Smith, Postreperfusion inflammation: a model for reaction to injury in cardiovascular disease, Cardiovasc. Res. 28 (1994) 1301–1311.

[54] W.J. Dreyer, L.H. Michael, E.E. Millman, K.L. Berens, R.S. Geske, Neutrophil sequestration and pulmonary dysfunction in a canine model of open heart surgery with cardiopulmonary bypass. Evidence for a CD18-dependent mechanism, Circulation 92 (1995) 2276–2283.

[55] W.J. Dreyer, A.R. Burns, S.C. Phillips, M.L. Lindsey, P. Jackson, G.L. Kukielka, Intercellular adhesion molecule-1 regulation in the canine lung after cardiopulmonary bypass, J. Thorac. Cardiovasc. Surg. 115 (1998) 689–698 discussion 698–699.

[56] P.M. Kilbridge, J.E. Mayer, J.W. Newburger, P.R. Hickey, A.Z. Walsh, E.J. Neufeld, Induction of intercellular adhesion molecule-1 and E-selectin mRNA in heart and skeletal muscle of pediatric patients undergoing cardiopulmonary bypass, J. Thorac. Cardiovasc. Surg. 107 (1994) 1183–1192.

[57] E.D. Blume, D.P. Nelson, K. Gauvreau, A.Z. Walsh, C. Plumb, E.J. Neufeld, P.R. Hickey, J.E. Mayer, J.W. Newburger, Soluble adhesion molecules in infants and children undergoing cardiopulmonary bypass, Circulation 96 (1997) II-352–357.

[58] E.A. Grossi, K. Kallenbach, S. Chau, C.C. Derivaux, M.G. Aguinaga, B.M. Steinberg, D. Kim, S. Iyer, M. Tayyarah, M. Artman, A.C. Galloway, S.B. Colvin, Impact of heparin bonding on pediatric cardiopulmonary bypass: a prospective randomized study, Ann. Thorac. Surg. 70 (2000) 191–196.

[59] P.R. Hansen, Role of neutrophils in myocardial ischemia and reperfusion, Circulation 91 (1995) 1872–1885.

[60] R.R. Chaturvedi, D.F. Shore, C. Lincoln, S. Mumby, M. Kemp, J. Brierly, A. Petros, J.M. Gutteridge, J. Hooper, A.N. Redington, Acute right ventricular restrictive physiology after repair of tetralogy of Fallot: association with myocardial injury and oxidative stress, Circulation 100 (1999) 1540–1547.

[61] R. Bolli, E. Marban, Molecular and cellular mechanisms of myocardial stunning, Physiol. Rev. 79 (1999) 609–634.

[62] H. Kan, M.S. Finkel, Interactions between cytokines and neurohormonal systems in the failing heart, Heart Fail. Rev. 6 (2001) 119–127.

[63] V. Stangl, G. Baumann, K. Stangl, S.B. Felix, Negative inotropic mediators released from the heart after myocardial ischaemia-reperfusion, Cardiovasc. Res. 53 (2002) 12–30.

[64] J.M. Pearl, D.P. Nelson, S.M. Schwartz, C.J. Wagner, S.M. Bauer, E.A. Setser, J.Y. Duffy, Glucocorticoids reduce ischemia-reperfusion-induced myocardial apoptosis in immature hearts, Ann. Thorac. Surg. 74 (2002) 830–836 discussion 836–837.

[65] R. Buchhorn, M. Hulpke-Wette, W. Ruschewski, R. Pregla, J. Fielitz, R. Hetzer, V. Regitz-Zagrosek, Beta-receptor downregulation in congenital heart disease: a risk factor for complications after surgical repair? Ann. Thorac. Surg. 73 (2002) 610–613.

[66] P.M. Kirshbom, S.O. Page, M.T. Jacobs, S.S. Tsui, E. Bello, R.M. Ungerleider, D.A. Schwinn, J.W. Gaynor, Cardiopulmonary bypass and circulatory arrest increase endothelin-1 production and receptor expression in the lung, J. Thorac. Cardiovasc. Surg. 113 (1997) 777–783.

[67] S.M. Schwartz, J.Y. Duffy, J.M. Pearl, D.P. Nelson, Cellular and molecular aspects of myocardial dysfunction, Crit. Care Med. 29 (2001) S214–S219.

[68] S.M. Schwartz, J.Y. Duffy, J.M. Pearl, S. Goins, C.J. Wagner, D.P. Nelson, Glucocorticoids preserve calpastatin and troponin I during cardiopulmonary bypass in immature pigs, Pediatr. Res. 54 (2003) 91–97.

[69] J.L. McDonough, D.K. Arrell, J.E. Van Eyk, Troponin I degradation and covalent complex formation accompanies myocardial ischemia/reperfusion injury, Circ. Res. 84 (1999) 9–20.

[70] J.L. McDonough, R. Labugger, W. Pickett, M.Y. Tse, S. MacKenzie, S.C. Pang, D. Atar, G. Ropchan, J.E. Van Eyk, Cardiac troponin I is modified in the myocardium of bypass patients, Circulation 103 (2001) 58–64.

[71] W.D. Gao, D. Atar, Y. Liu, N.G. Perez, A.M. Murphy, E. Marban, Role of troponin I proteolysis in the pathogenesis of stunned myocardium, Circ. Res. 80 (1997) 393–399.

[72] M.J. Davies, K. Nguyen, J.W. Gaynor, M.J. Elliott, Modified ultrafiltration improves left ventricular systolic function in infants after cardiopulmonary bypass, J. Thorac. Cardiovasc. Surg. 115 (1998) 361–369 discussion 369–370.

[73] R.R. Chaturvedi, D.F. Shore, P.A. White, M.H. Scallan, J.W. Gothard, A.N. Redington, C. Lincoln, Modified ultrafiltration improves global left ventricular systolic function after open-heart surgery in infants and children, Eur. J. Cardiothorac. Surg. 15 (1999) 742–746.

[74] P.M. Bokesch, M.B. Kapural, E.B. Mossad, M. Cavaglia, E. Appachi, J.J. Drummond-Webb, R.B. Mee, Do peritoneal catheters remove pro-inflammatory cytokines after cardiopulmonary bypass in neonates? Ann. Thorac. Surg. 70 (2000) 639–643.

[75] B.M. Steinberg, E.A. Grossi, D.S. Schwartz, D.E. McLoughlin, M. Aguinaga, C. Bizekis, J. Greenwald, A. Flisser, F.C. Spencer, A.C. Galloway, et al., Heparin bonding of bypass circuits reduces cytokine release during cardiopulmonary bypass, Ann. Thorac. Surg. 60 (1995) 525–529.

[76] T. Ozawa, K. Yoshihara, N. Koyama, Y. Watanabe, N. Shiono, Y. Takanashi, Clinical efficacy of heparin-bonded bypass circuits related to cytokine responses in children, Ann. Thorac. Surg. 69 (2000) 584–590.

[77] E. Hickey, T. Karamlou, J. You, R.M. Ungerleider, Effects of circuit miniaturization in reducing inflammatory response to infant cardiopulmonary bypass by elimination of allogeneic blood products, Ann. Thorac. Surg. 81 (2006) S2367–S2372.

[78] W.T. Mahle, E. Matthews, K.R. Kanter, B.E. Kogon, S.E. Hamrick, M.J. Strickland, Inflammatory response after neonatal cardiac surgery and its relationship to clinical outcomes, Ann. Thorac. Surg. 97 (2014) 950–956.

[79] J.M. Forbess, J.C. Ibla, H.G. Lidov, M.A. Cioffi, T. Hiramatsu, P. Laussen, T. Miura, R.A. Jonas, University of Wisconsin cerebroplegia in a piglet survival model of circulatory arrest, Ann. Thorac. Surg. 60 (1995) S494–S500.

[80] A.S. Weyrich, X.Y. Ma, D.J. Lefer, K.H. Albertine, A.M. Lefer, In vivo neutralization of P-selectin protects feline heart and endothelium in myocardial ischemia and reperfusion injury, J. Clin. Invest. 91 (1993) 2620–2629.

[81] P.J. Chai, R. Nassar, A.E. Oakeley, D.M. Craig, G. Quick Jr., J. Jaggers, S.P. Sanders, R.M. Ungerleider, P.A. Anderson, Soluble complement receptor-1 protects heart, lung, and cardiac myofilament function from cardiopulmonary bypass damage, Circulation 101 (2000) 541–546.

[82] A.J. Lodge, P.J. Chai, C.W. Daggett, R.M. Ungerleider, J. Jaggers, Methylprednisolone reduces the inflammatory response to cardiopulmonary bypass in neonatal piglets: timing of dose is important, J. Thorac. Cardiovasc. Surg. 117 (1999) 515–522.

[83] P.A. Checchia, C.L. Backer, R.A. Bronicki, H.P. Baden, S.E. Crawford, T.P. Green, C. Mavroudis, Dexamethasone reduces postoperative troponin levels in children undergoing cardiopulmonary bypass, Crit. Care Med. 31 (2003) 1742–1745.

[84] V.A. Schroeder, J.M. Pearl, S.M. Schwartz, T.P. Shanley, P.B. Manning, D.P. Nelson, Combined steroid treatment for congenital heart surgery improves oxygen delivery and reduces postbypass inflammatory mediator expression, Circulation 107 (2003) 2823–2828.

[85] R.A. Bronicki, C.L. Backer, H.P. Baden, C. Mavroudis, S.E. Crawford, T.P. Green, Dexamethasone reduces the inflammatory response to cardiopulmonary bypass in children, Ann. Thorac. Surg. 69 (2000) 1490–1495.

[86] J.R. Charpie, M.K. Dekeon, C.S. Goldberg, R.S. Mosca, E.L. Bove, T.J. Kulik, Serial blood lactate measurements predict early outcome after neonatal repair or palliation for complex congenital heart disease, J. Thorac. Cardiovasc. Surg. 120 (2000) 73–80.

[87] J.P. Gold, R.A. Jonas, P. Lang, E.M. Elixson, J.E. Mayer, A.R. Castaneda, Transthoracic intracardiac monitoring lines in pediatric surgical patients: a ten-year experience, Ann. Thorac. Surg. 42 (1986) 185–191.

[88] S. Cullen, D. Shore, A. Redington, Characterization of right ventricular diastolic performance after complete repair of tetralogy of Fallot. Restrictive physiology predicts slow postoperative recovery, Circulation 91 (1995) 1782–1789.

[89] G. Zobel, S. Rodl, B. Rigler, H. Metzler, D. Dacar, H.M. Grubbauer, A. Beitzke, Prospective evaluation of clinical scoring systems in infants and children with cardiopulmonary insufficiency after cardiac surgery, J. Cardiovasc. Surg. (Torino) 34 (1993) 333–337.

[90] T. Kanazawa, M. Egi, K. Shimizu, Y. Toda, T. Iwasaki, H. Morimatsu, Intraoperative change of lactate level is associated with postoperative outcomes in pediatric cardiac surgery patients: retrospective observational study, BMC Anesthesiol. 15 (2015) 29.

[91] K.R. Schumacher, R.A. Reichel, J.R. Vlasic, S. Yu, J. Donohue, R.J. Gajarski, J.R. Charpie, Rate of increase in serum lactate level risk-stratifies infants after surgery for congenital heart disease, J. Thorac. Cardiovasc. Surg. 148 (2014) 589–595.

[92] R.L. Alves, A.L. Aragao e Silva, N.C. Kraychete, G.O. Campos, J. Martins Mde, N.S. Modolo, Intraoperative lactate levels and postoperative complications of pediatric cardiac surgery, Paediatr. Anaesth. 22 (2012) 812–817.

[93] M. Basaran, K. Sever, E. Kafali, M. Ugurlucan, O.A. Sayin, T. Tansel, U. Alpagut, E. Dayioglu, E. Onursal, Serum lactate level has prognostic significance after pediatric cardiac surgery, J. Cardiothorac. Vasc. Anesth. 20 (2006) 43–47.

[94] F. Toraman, S. Evrenkaya, M. Yuce, N. Aksoy, H. Karabulut, Y. Bozkulak, C. Alhan, Lactic acidosis after cardiac surgery is associated with adverse outcome, Heart Surg. Forum 7 (2004) E155–E159.

[95] R. Munoz, P.C. Laussen, G. Palacio, L. Zienko, G. Piercey, D.L. Wessel, Changes in whole blood lactate levels during cardiopulmonary bypass for surgery for congenital cardiac disease: an early indicator of morbidity and mortality, J. Thorac. Cardiovasc. Surg. 119 (2000) 155–162.

[96] T. Duke, W. Butt, M. South, T.R. Karl, Early markers of major adverse events in children after cardiac operations, J. Thorac. Cardiovasc. Surg. 114 (1997) 1042–1052.

[97] L.B. Siegel, H.J. Dalton, J.H. Hertzog, R.A. Hopkins, R.L. Hannan, G.J. Hauser, Initial postoperative serum lactate levels predict survival in children after open heart surgery, Intensive Care Med. 22 (1996) 1418–1423.

[98] J.J. Ronco, J.C. Fenwick, B.R. Wiggs, P.T. Phang, J.A. Russell, M.G. Tweeddale, Oxygen consumption is independent of increases in oxygen delivery by dobutamine in septic patients who have normal or increased plasma lactate, Am. Rev. Respir. Dis. 147 (1993) 25–31.

[99] G. Buheitel, J. Scharf, M. Hofbeck, H. Singer, Estimation of cardiac index by means of the arterial and the mixed venous oxygen content and pulmonary oxygen uptake determination in the early post-operative period following surgery of congenital heart disease, Intensive Care Med. 20 (1994) 500–503.

[100] A.G. de la Rocha, J.F. Edmonds, W.G. Williams, C. Poirier, R.N. Trusler, Importance of mixed venous oxygen saturation in the care of critically ill patients, Can. J. Surg. 21 (1978) 227–229.

[101] M.D. Freed, O.S. Miettinen, A.S. Nadas, Oximetric detection of intracardiac left-to-right shunts, Br. Heart J. 42 (1979) 690–694.

[102] A.F. Rossi, H.S. Seiden, R.P. Gross, R.B. Griepp, Oxygen transport in critically ill infants after congenital heart operations, Ann. Thorac. Surg. 67 (1999) 739–744.

[103] A.F. Rossi, R.J. Sommer, A. Lotvin, R.P. Gross, L.G. Steinberg, G. Kipel, R.J. Golinko, R.B. Griepp, Usefulness of intermittent monitoring of mixed venous oxygen saturation after stage I palliation for hypoplastic left heart syndrome, Am. J. Cardiol. 73 (1994) 1118–1123.

[104] J.S. Tweddell, G.M. Hoffman, R.T. Fedderly, S. Berger, J.P. Thomas Jr., N.S. Ghanayem, M.W. Kessel, S.B. Litwin, Phenoxybenzamine improves systemic oxygen delivery after the Norwood procedure, Ann. Thorac. Surg. 67 (1999) 161–167 discussion 167–168.

[105] R. Taeed, S.M. Schwartz, J.M. Pearl, J.L. Raake, R.H. Beekman 3rd, P.B. Manning, D.P. Nelson, Unrecognized pulmonary venous desaturation early after Norwood palliation confounds Gp:Gs assessment and compromises oxygen delivery, Circulation 103 (2001) 2699–2704.

[106] G. Trittenwein, H. Pansi, B. Graf, J. Golej, G. Burda, M. Hermon, M. Marx, G. Wollenek, H. Trittenwein, A. Pollak, Proposed entry criteria for postoperative cardiac extracorporeal membrane oxygenation after pediatric open heart surgery, Artif. Organs 23 (1999) 1010–1014.

[107] G.M. Hoffman, N.S. Ghanayem, J.M. Kampine, S. Berger, K.A. Mussatto, S.B. Litwin, J.S. Tweddell, Venous saturation and the anaerobic threshold in neonates after the Norwood procedure for hypoplastic left heart syndrome, Ann. Thorac. Surg. 70 (2000) 1515–1520 discussion 1521.

[108] T.A. Tortoriello, S.A. Stayer, A.R. Mott, E.D. McKenzie, C.D. Fraser, D.B. Andropoulos, A.C. Chang, A noninvasive estimation of mixed venous oxygen saturation using near-infrared spectroscopy by cerebral oximetry in pediatric cardiac surgery patients, Paediatr. Anaesth. 15 (2005) 495–503.

[109] F.F. Jobsis, Noninvasive, infrared monitoring of cerebral and myocardial oxygen sufficiency and circulatory parameters, Science 198 (1977) 1264–1267.

[110] N. Nagdyman, T. Fleck, S. Barth, H. Abdul-Khaliq, B. Stiller, P. Ewert, M. Huebler, H. Kuppe, P.E. Lange, Relation of cerebral tissue oxygenation index to central venous oxygen saturation in children, Intensive Care Med. 30 (2004) 468–471.

[111] G. Schulz, M. Weiss, U. Bauersfeld, J. Teller, D. Haensse, H.U. Bucher, O. Baenziger, Liver tissue oxygenation as measured by near-infrared spectroscopy in the critically ill child in correlation with central venous oxygen saturation, Intensive Care Med. 28 (2002) 184–189.

[112] M. Weiss, A. Dullenkopf, A. Kolarova, G. Schulz, B. Frey, O. Baenziger, Near-infrared spectroscopic cerebral oxygenation reading in neonates and infants is associated with central venous oxygen saturation, Paediatr. Anaesth. 15 (2005) 102–109.

[113] G.K. Davis, F. Bamforth, A. Sarpal, F. Dicke, Y. Rabi, M.E. Lyon, B-type natriuretic peptide in pediatrics, Clin. Biochem. 39 (2006) 600–605.

[114] C.Y. Shih, A. Sapru, P. Oishi, A. Azakie, T.R. Karl, C. Harmon, R. Asija, I. Adatia, J.R. Fineman, Alterations in plasma B-type natriuretic peptide levels after repair of congenital heart defects: a potential perioperative marker, J. Thorac. Cardiovasc. Surg. 131 (2006) 632–638.

[115] P. Gessler, W. Knirsch, B. Schmitt, V. Rousson, A. von Eckardstein, Prognostic value of plasma N-terminal pro-brain natriuretic peptide in children with congenital heart defects and open-heart surgery, J. Pediatr. 148 (2006) 372–376.

[116] M. Cantinotti, R. Giordano, M. Scalese, S. Molinaro, F. Della Pina, S. Storti, L. Arcieri, B. Murzi, M. Marotta, V. Pak, V. Poli, G. Iervasi, S. Kutty, A. Clerico, Prognostic role of BNP in children undergoing surgery for congenital heart disease: analysis of prediction models incorporating standard risk factors, Clin. Chem. Lab. Med. 53 (2015) 1839–1846.

[117] T. Kanazawa, M. Egi, Y. Toda, K. Shimizu, K. Sugimoto, T. Iwasaki, H. Morimatsu, Perioperative brain natriuretic peptide in pediatric cardiac surgery patients: its association with postoperative outcomes, J. Cardiothorac. Vasc. Anesth. 31 (2017) 537–542.
[118] S. Nunez, A. Maisel, Comparison between mixed venous oxygen saturation and thermodilution cardiac output in monitoring patients with severe heart failure treated with milrinone and dobutamine, Am. Heart J. 135 (1998) 383–388.
[119] J. Li, I. Schulze-Neick, C. Lincoln, D. Shore, M. Scallan, A. Bush, A.N. Redington, D.J. Penny, Oxygen consumption after cardiopulmonary bypass surgery in children: determinants and implications, J. Thorac. Cardiovasc. Surg. 119 (2000) 525–533.
[120] C.F. Wippermann, R.G. Huth, F.X. Schmidt, J. Thul, M. Betancor, D. Schranz, Continuous measurement of cardiac output by the Fick principle in infants and children: comparison with the thermodilution method, Intensive Care Med. 22 (1996) 467–471.
[121] L.L. Lequier, S.R. Leonard, H. Nikaidoh, M.S. Lemler, C. Ramaciotti, Extravascular Doppler measurement of cardiac output in infants and children after operations for congenital heart disease, J. Thorac. Cardiovasc. Surg. 117 (1999) 1223–1225.
[122] J.M. Alonso-Inigo, F.J. Escriba, J.I. Carrasco, M.J. Fas, P. Argente, J.M. Galvis, J.E. Llopis, Measuring cardiac output in children undergoing cardiac catheterization: comparison between the Fick method and PRAM (pressure recording analytical method), Paediatr. Anaesth. 26 (2016) 1097–1105.
[123] J. Urbano, J. Lopez, R. Gonzalez, M.J. Solana, S.N. Fernandez, J.M. Bellon, J. Lopez-Herce, Measurement of cardiac output in children by pressure-recording analytical method, Pediatr. Cardiol. 36 (2015) 358–364.
[124] C.F. Tirotta, R.G. Lagueruela, D. Madril, E. Velis, J. Ojito, D. Monroe, D. Aguero, M. Irizarry, J. McBride, R.L. Hannan, R.P. Burke, Non-invasive cardiac output monitor validation study in pediatric cardiac surgery patients, J. Clin. Anesth. 38 (2017) 129–132.
[125] C.I. Brookes, P.A. White, A.J. Bishop, P.J. Oldershaw, A.N. Redington, N.E. Moat, Validation of a new intraoperative technique to evaluate load-independent indices of right ventricular performance in patients undergoing cardiac operations, J. Thorac. Cardiovasc. Surg. 116 (1998) 468–476.
[126] B.D. Lowes, M.A. Simon, T.O. Tsvetkova, M.R. Bristow, Inotropes in the beta-blocker era, Clin. Cardiol. 23 (2000) III11–III16.
[127] N.E. Moat, R.K. Lamb, J.C. Edwards, J. Manners, B.R. Keeton, J.L. Monro, Induced hypothermia in the management of refractory low cardiac output states following cardiac surgery in infants and children, Eur. J. Cardiothorac. Surg. 6 (1992) 579–584 discussion 585.
[128] M.J. Dalrymple-Hay, C.D. Deakin, H. Knight, J.C. Edwards, B. Keeton, A.P. Salmon, J.L. Monro, Induced hypothermia as salvage treatment for refractory cardiac failure following paediatric cardiac surgery, Eur. J. Cardiothorac. Surg. 15 (1999) 515–518.
[129] C.D. Deakin, H. Knight, J.C. Edwards, J.L. Monro, R.K. Lamb, B. Keeton, A.P. Salmon, Induced hypothermia in the postoperative management of refractory cardiac failure following paediatric cardiac surgery, Anaesthesia 53 (1998) 848–853.
[130] R.K. Freeman, P.O. Daily, W.P. Dembitsky, R.M. Adamson, R.J. Moreno-Cabral, The treatment of low cardiac output syndrome following cardiopulmonary bypass using delayed sternal closure, Am. Surg. 63 (1997) 882–884.
[131] C.A. Anderson, F. Filsoufi, L. Aklog, R.S. Farivar, J.G. Byrne, D.H. Adams, Liberal use of delayed sternal closure for postcardiotomy hemodynamic instability, Ann. Thorac. Surg. 73 (2002) 1484–1488.
[132] D.B. McElhinney, V.M. Reddy, A.J. Parry, L. Johnson, J.R. Fineman, F.L. Hanley, Management and outcomes of delayed sternal closure after cardiac surgery in neonates and infants, Crit. Care Med. 28 (2000) 1180–1184.
[133] R.S. Iyer, J.P. Jacobs, M.R. de Leval, J. Stark, M.J. Elliott, Outcomes after delayed sternal closure in pediatric heart operations: a 10-year experience, Ann. Thorac. Surg. 63 (1997) 489–491.
[134] M. Hakimi, H.L. Walters 3rd, W.W. Pinsky, M.J. Gallagher, J.M. Lyons, Delayed sternal closure after neonatal cardiac operations, J. Thorac. Cardiovasc. Surg. 107 (1994) 925–933.
[135] A. Elami, L.C. Permut, H. Laks, D.C. Drinkwater Jr., J.L. Sebastian, Cardiac decompression after operation for congenital heart disease in infancy, Ann. Thorac. Surg. 58 (1994) 1392–1396.
[136] B.H. Dorman, R.M. Sade, J.S. Burnette, H.B. Wiles, M.L. Pinosky, S.T. Reeves, B.R. Bond, F.G. Spinale, Magnesium supplementation in the prevention of arrhythmias in pediatric patients undergoing surgery for congenital heart defects, Am. Heart J. 139 (2000) 522–528.
[137] P. Raja, R.E. Hawker, A. Chaikitpinyo, S.G. Cooper, K.C. Lau, G.R. Nunn, T.B. Cartmill, G.F. Sholler, Amiodarone management of junctional ectopic tachycardia after cardiac surgery in children, Br. Heart J. 72 (1994) 261–265.
[138] K. Singh, C. Communal, D.B. Sawyer, W.S. Colucci, Adrenergic regulation of myocardial apoptosis, Cardiovasc. Res. 45 (2000) 713–719.
[139] J.M. Bailey, B.E. Miller, K.R. Kanter, S.R. Tosone, V.K. Tam, A comparison of the hemodynamic effects of amrinone and sodium nitroprusside in infants after cardiac surgery, Anesth. Analg. 84 (1997) 294–298.
[140] A.C. Chang, A.M. Atz, G. Wernovsky, R.P. Burke, D.L. Wessel, Milrinone: systemic and pulmonary hemodynamic effects in neonates after cardiac surgery, Crit. Care Med. 23 (1995) 1907–1914.
[141] J.M. Bailey, B.E. Miller, W. Lu, S.R. Tosone, K.R. Kanter, V.K. Tam, The pharmacokinetics of milrinone in pediatric patients after cardiac surgery, Anesthesiology 90 (1999) 1012–1018.
[142] S. Latifi, K. Lidsky, J.L. Blumer, Pharmacology of inotropic agents in infants and children, 12 (2000) 57–79.
[143] S.J. Lindsay, Hand-held pneumatic impact handpiece for delicate, e.g. hand engraving operation, of jewelry, has variable fuel meter and work energy supply which regulate supply of pressurized fluid and of work energy based on pressure sensor output, Derwent Innov. Index 13 (2004).
[144] C. Ramamoorthy, G.D. Anderson, G.D. Williams, A.M. Lynn, Pharmacokinetics and side effects of milrinone in infants and children after open heart surgery, Anesth. Analg. 86 (1998) 283–289.
[145] E.M. Wright, J. Skoyles, K.M. Sherry, Milrinone in the treatment of low output states following cardiac surgery, Eur. J. Anaesthesiol. Suppl. 5 (1992) 21–26.
[146] R.O. Feneck, Intravenous milrinone following cardiac surgery: I. Effects of bolus infusion followed by variable dose maintenance infusion. The European Milrinone Multicentre Trial Group, J. Cardiothorac. Vasc. Anesth. 6 (1992) 554–562.
[147] E.S. Monrad, D.S. Baim, H.S. Smith, A. Lanoue, E. Brauwald, W. Grossman, Effects of milrinone on coronary hemodynamics and myocardial energetics in patients with congestive heart failure, Circulation 71 (1985) 972–979.
[148] D.J. Lebovitz, S.T. Lawless, K.L. Weise, Fatal amrinone overdose in a pediatric patient, Crit. Care Med. 23 (1995) 977–980.

[149] M.T. Slawsky, W.S. Colucci, S.S. Gottlieb, B.H. Greenberg, E. Haeusslein, J. Hare, S. Hutchins, C.V. Leier, T.H. LeJemtel, E. Loh, J. Nicklas, D. Ogilby, B.N. Singh, W. Smith, Acute hemodynamic and clinical effects of levosimendan in patients with severe heart failure. Study Investigators, Circulation 102 (2000) 2222–2227.

[150] J.J. Nawarskas, J.R. Anderson, Levosimendan: a unique approach to the treatment of heart failure, Heart Dis. 4 (2002) 265–271.

[151] M. Turanlahti, T. Boldt, T. Palkama, S. Antila, L. Lehtonen, E. Pesonen, Pharmacokinetics of levosimendan in pediatric patients evaluated for cardiac surgery, Pediatr. Crit. Care Med. 5 (2004) 457–462.

[152] J.R. Egan, A.J. Clarke, S. Williams, A.D. Cole, J. Ayer, S. Jacobe, R.B. Chard, D.S. Winlaw, Levosimendan for low cardiac output: a pediatric experience, J. Intensive Care Med. 21 (2006) 183–187.

[153] M. Momeni, J. Rubay, A. Matta, M.T. Rennotte, F. Veyckemans, A.J. Poncelet, S. Clement de Clety, C. Anslot, R. Joomye, T. Detaille, Levosimendan in congenital cardiac surgery: a randomized, double-blind clinical trial, J. Cardiothorac. Vasc. Anesth. 25 (2011) 419–424.

[154] E. Lechner, A. Hofer, G. Leitner-Peneder, R. Freynschlag, R. Mair, R. Weinzettel, P. Rehak, H. Gombotz, Levosimendan versus milrinone in neonates and infants after corrective open-heart surgery: a pilot study, Pediatr. Crit. Care Med. 13 (2012) 542–548.

[155] Z. Ricci, C. Garisto, I. Favia, V. Vitale, L. Di Chiara, P.E. Cogo, Levosimendan infusion in newborns after corrective surgery for congenital heart disease: randomized controlled trial, Intensive Care Med. 38 (2012) 1198–1204.

[156] F.W. Holland 2nd, P.S. Brown Jr., B.D. Weintraub, R.E. Clark, Cardiopulmonary bypass and thyroid function: a "euthyroid sick syndrome", Ann. Thorac. Surg. 52 (1991) 46–50.

[157] M.A. Portman, C. Fearneyhough, X.H. Ning, B.W. Duncan, G.L. Rosenthal, F.M. Lupinetti, Triiodothyronine repletion in infants during cardiopulmonary bypass for congenital heart disease, J. Thorac. Cardiovasc. Surg. 120 (2000) 604–608.

[158] M. Bettendorf, K.G. Schmidt, J. Grulich-Henn, H.E. Ulmer, U.E. Heinrich, Tri-iodothyronine treatment in children after cardiac surgery: a double-blind, randomised, placebo-controlled study, Lancet 356 (2000) 529–534.

[159] T. Carrel, F. Eckstein, L. Englberger, R. Mury, P. Mohacsi, Thyronin treatment in adult and pediatric heart surgery: clinical experience and review of the literature, Eur. J. Heart Fail. 4 (2002) 577–582.

[160] A.S. Mackie, K.L. Booth, J.W. Newburger, K. Gauvreau, S.A. Huang, P.C. Laussen, J.A. DiNardo, P.J. del Nido, J.E. Mayer Jr., R.A. Jonas, E. McGrath, J. Elder, S.J. Roth, A randomized, double-blind, placebo-controlled pilot trial of triiodothyronine in neonatal heart surgery, J. Thorac. Cardiovasc. Surg. 130 (2005) 810–816.

[161] K. Plumpton, N.A. Haas, Identifying infants at risk of marked thyroid suppression post-cardiopulmonary bypass, Intensive Care Med. 31 (2005) 581–587.

[162] E.B. Rosenzweig, T.J. Starc, J.M. Chen, S. Cullinane, D.M. Timchak, W.M. Gersony, D.W. Landry, M.E. Galantowicz, Intravenous arginine-vasopressin in children with vasodilatory shock after cardiac surgery, Circulation 100 (1999) II182–II186.

[163] J.A. Alten, S. Borasino, R. Toms, M.A. Law, A. Moellinger, R.J. Dabal, Early initiation of arginine vasopressin infusion in neonates after complex cardiac surgery, Pediatr. Crit. Care Med. 13 (2012) 300–304.

[164] G. Papadopoulos, E. Sintou, S. Siminelakis, E. Koletsis, N.G. Baikoussis, E. Apostolakis, Perioperative infusion of low-dose of vasopressin for prevention and management of vasodilatory vasoplegic syndrome in patients undergoing coronary artery bypass grafting-A double-blind randomized study, J. Cardiothorac. Surg. 5 (2010) 17.

[165] M. Argenziano, A.F. Choudhri, M.C. Oz, E.A. Rose, C.R. Smith, D.W. Landry, A prospective randomized trial of arginine vasopressin in the treatment of vasodilatory shock after left ventricular assist device placement, Circulation 96 (1997) II-286–290.

[166] M. Argenziano, J.M. Chen, A.F. Choudhri, S. Cullinane, E. Garfein, A.D. Weinberg, C.R. Smith Jr., E.A. Rose, D.W. Landry, M.C. Oz, Management of vasodilatory shock after cardiac surgery: identification of predisposing factors and use of a novel pressor agent, J. Thorac. Cardiovasc. Surg. 116 (1998) 973–980.

[167] S. Masutani, H. Senzaki, H. Ishido, M. Taketazu, T. Matsunaga, T. Kobayashi, N. Sasaki, H. Asano, S. Kyo, Y. Yokote, Vasopressin in the treatment of vasodilatory shock in children, Pediatr. Int. 47 (2005) 132–136.

[168] D.L. Morales, D. Gregg, D.N. Helman, M.R. Williams, Y. Naka, D.W. Landry, M.C. Oz, Arginine vasopressin in the treatment of 50 patients with postcardiotomy vasodilatory shock, Ann. Thorac. Surg. 69 (2000) 102–106.

[169] D. Annane, E. Bellissant, V. Sebille, O. Lesieur, B. Mathieu, J.C. Raphael, P. Gajdos, Impaired pressor sensitivity to noradrenaline in septic shock patients with and without impaired adrenal function reserve, Br. J. Clin. Pharmacol. 46 (1998) 589–597.

[170] S. Shore, D.P. Nelson, J.M. Pearl, P.B. Manning, H. Wong, T.P. Shanley, T. Keyser, S.M. Schwartz, Usefulness of corticosteroid therapy in decreasing epinephrine requirements in critically ill infants with congenital heart disease, Am. J. Cardiol. 88 (2001) 591–594.

[171] J.P. Liu, P.J. Robinson, J.W. Funder, D. Engler, The biosynthesis and secretion of adrenocorticotropin by the ovine anterior pituitary is predominantly regulated by arginine vasopressin (AVP). Evidence that protein kinase C mediates the action of AVP, J. Biol. Chem. 265 (1990) 14136–14142.

[172] P.J. del Nido, B.W. Duncan, J.E. Mayer Jr., D.L. Wessel, R.A. LaPierre, R.A. Jonas, Left ventricular assist device improves survival in children with left ventricular dysfunction after repair of anomalous origin of the left coronary artery from the pulmonary artery, Ann. Thorac. Surg. 67 (1999) 169–172.

[173] E.V. Potapov, B. Stiller, R. Hetzer, Ventricular assist devices in children: current achievements and future perspectives, Pediatr. Transplant. 11 (2007) 241–255.

[174] S. Chen, A. Lin, E. Liu, M. Gowan, L.J. May, L.N. Doan, C.S. Almond, K. Maeda, O. Reinhartz, S.A. Hollander, D.N. Rosenthal, Outpatient outcomes of pediatric patients with left ventricular assist devices, ASAIO J. 62 (2016) 163–168.

[175] A. Jeewa, C. Manlhiot, B.W. McCrindle, G. Van Arsdell, T. Humpl, A.I. Dipchand, Outcomes with ventricular assist device versus extracorporeal membrane oxygenation as a bridge to pediatric heart transplantation, Artif. Organs 34 (2010) 1087–1091.

[176] C.D. Fraser Jr., R.D. Jaquiss, The Berlin heart EXCOR pediatric ventricular assist device: history, North American experience, and future directions, Ann. N.Y Acad. Sci. 1291 (2013) 96–105.

[177] C.S. Almond, H. Buchholz, P. Massicotte, R. Ichord, D.N. Rosenthal, K. Uzark, R.D. Jaquiss, R. Kroslowitz, M.B. Kepler, A. Lobbestael, D. Bellinger, E.D. Blume, C.D. Fraser Jr., R.H. Bartlett, R. Thiagarajan, K. Jenkins, Berlin heart EXCOR pediatric ventricular assist device Investigational Device Exemption study: study design and rationale, Am. Heart J. 162 (2011) 425–435 e6.

[178] J.M. Pearl, D.P. Nelson, S.A. Wellmann, J.L. Raake, C.J. Wagner, J.L. McNamara, J.Y. Duffy, Acute hypoxia and reoxygenation impairs exhaled nitric oxide release and pulmonary mechanics, J. Thorac. Cardiovasc. Surg. 119 (2000) 931–938.

[179] M. Beghetti, P.E. Silkoff, M. Caramori, H.M. Holtby, A.S. Slutsky, I. Adatia, Decreased exhaled nitric oxide may be a marker of cardiopulmonary bypass-induced injury, Ann. Thorac. Surg. 66 (1998) 532–534.

[180] K. Chang, Oldest Bacteria Fossils? Or are they Merely Tiny Rock Flaws? New York Times, 2002. F4.

[181] M. Friedman, S.Y. Wang, G.L. Stahl, R.G. Johnson, F.W. Sellke, Altered beta-adrenergic and cholinergic pulmonary vascular responses after total cardiopulmonary bypass, J. Appl. Physiol. 79 (1995) 1998–2006.

[182] A.M. Atz, I. Adatia, R.A. Jonas, D.L. Wessel, Inhaled nitric oxide in children with pulmonary hypertension and congenital mitral stenosis, Am. J. Cardiol. 77 (1996) 316–319.

[183] O.I. Miller, S.F. Tang, A. Keech, N.B. Pigott, E. Beller, D.S. Celermajer, Inhaled nitric oxide and prevention of pulmonary hypertension after congenital heart surgery: a randomised double-blind study, Lancet 356 (2000) 1464–1469.

[184] D.D. Ivy, J.P. Kinsella, J.W. Ziegler, S.H. Abman, Dipyridamole attenuates rebound pulmonary hypertension after inhaled nitric oxide withdrawal in postoperative congenital heart disease, J. Thorac. Cardiovasc. Surg. 115 (1998) 875–882.

[185] R.J. Barst, D. Ivy, J. Dingemanse, A. Widlitz, K. Schmitt, A. Doran, D. Bingaman, N. Nguyen, M. Gaitonde, P.L. van Giersbergen, Pharmacokinetics, safety, and efficacy of bosentan in pediatric patients with pulmonary arterial hypertension, Clin. Pharmacol. Ther. 73 (2003) 372–382.

[186] I. Schulze-Neick, D.J. Penny, M.L. Rigby, C. Morgan, A. Kelleher, P. Collins, J. Li, A. Bush, E.A. Shinebourne, A.N. Redington, L-arginine and substance P reverse the pulmonary endothelial dysfunction caused by congenital heart surgery, Circulation 100 (1999) 749–755.

[187] L.S. Shekerdemian, I. Schulze-Neick, A.N. Redington, A. Bush, D.J. Penny, Negative pressure ventilation as haemodynamic rescue following surgery for congenital heart disease, Intensive Care Med. 26 (2000) 93–96.

[188] L.S. Shekerdemian, A. Bush, D.F. Shore, C. Lincoln, A.N. Redington, Cardiorespiratory responses to negative pressure ventilation after tetralogy of Fallot repair: a hemodynamic tool for patients with a low-output state, J. Am. Coll. Cardiol. 33 (1999) 549–555.

[189] L.S. Shekerdemian, A. Bush, D.F. Shore, C. Lincoln, A.N. Redington, Cardiopulmonary interactions after Fontan operations: augmentation of cardiac output using negative pressure ventilation, Circulation 96 (1997) 3934–3942.

[190] L.S. Shekerdemian, D.F. Shore, C. Lincoln, A. Bush, A.N. Redington, Negative-pressure ventilation improves cardiac output after right heart surgery, Circulation 94 (1996) II49–II55.

[191] N.D. Bridges, J.E. Mayer Jr., J.E. Lock, R.A. Jonas, F.L. Hanley, J.F. Keane, S.B. Perry, A.R. Castaneda, Effect of baffle fenestration on outcome of the modified Fontan operation, Circulation 86 (1992) 1762–1769.

[192] I.M. Cheifetz, D.M. Craig, G. Quick, J.J. McGovern, M.L. Cannon, R.M. Ungerleider, P.K. Smith, J.N. Meliones, Increasing tidal volumes and pulmonary overdistention adversely affect pulmonary vascular mechanics and cardiac output in a pediatric swine model, Crit. Care Med. 26 (1998) 710–716.

[193] J. Meliones, K. Kocis, A.R. Bengur, A.R. Snider, Diastolic function in neonates after the arterial switch operation: effects of positive pressure ventilation and inspiratory time, Intensive Care Med. 26 (2000) 950–955.

[194] J.N. Meliones, E.L. Bove, M.K. Dekeon, J.R. Custer, F.W. Moler, L.R. Callow, N.C. Wilton, D.B. Rosen, High-frequency jet ventilation improves cardiac function after the Fontan procedure, Circulation 84 (1991) III364–III368.

[195] S. Conte, P.B. Hansen, T. Jensen, J.R. Jacobsen, M. Helvind, P. Lauridsen, G. Pettersson, Early experience with the Norwood procedure, Cardiovasc. Surg. 5 (1997) 315–319.

[196] C.J. Riordan, F. Randsbeck, J.H. Storey, W.D. Montgomery, W.P. Santamore, E.H. Austin 3rd, Effects of oxygen, positive end-expiratory pressure, and carbon dioxide on oxygen delivery in an animal model of the univentricular heart, J. Thorac. Cardiovasc. Surg. 112 (1996) 644–654.

[197] S. Tabbutt, C. Ramamoorthy, L.M. Montenegro, S.M. Durning, C.D. Kurth, J.M. Steven, R.I. Godinez, T.L. Spray, G. Wernovsky, S.C. Nicolson, Impact of inspired gas mixtures on preoperative infants with hypoplastic left heart syndrome during controlled ventilation, Circulation 104 (2001) I159–I164.

[198] Y. Naito, M. Aoki, M. Watanabe, N. Ishibashi, K. Agematsu, K. Sughimoto, T. Fujiwara, Factors affecting systemic oxygen delivery after Norwood procedure with Sano modification, Ann. Thorac. Surg. 89 (2010) 168–173.

[199] J. Li, G. Zhang, B.W. McCrindle, H. Holtby, T. Humpl, S. Cai, C.A. Caldarone, A.N. Redington, G.S. Van Arsdell, Profiles of hemodynamics and oxygen transport derived by using continuous measured oxygen consumption after the Norwood procedure, J. Thorac. Cardiovasc. Surg. 133 (2007) 441–448.

[200] C. Ramamoorthy, S. Tabbutt, C.D. Kurth, J.M. Steven, L.M. Montenegro, S. Durning, G. Wernovsky, J.W. Gaynor, T.L. Spray, S.C. Nicolson, Effects of inspired hypoxic and hypercapnic gas mixtures on cerebral oxygen saturation in neonates with univentricular heart defects, Anesthesiology 96 (2002) 283–288.

[201] S.M. Bradley, J.M. Simsic, A.M. Atz, Hemodynamic effects of inspired carbon dioxide after the Norwood procedure, Ann. Thorac. Surg. 72 (2001) 2088–2093 discussion 2093–2094.

Chapter 44

New Therapeutic Strategies in Heart Failure

Joseph W. Rossano[1], John L. Jefferies[2], William J. Dreyer[3]
[1]*Perelman School of Medicine at the University of Pennsylvania, Philadelphia, PA, United States;* [2]*Cincinnati Children's Hosptial Medical Center, Cincinnati, OH, United States;* [3]*Texas Children's Hospital, Houston, TX, United States*

INTRODUCTION

This is an exciting time for the field of pediatric heart failure. While historically there has been little improvement in overall outcomes [1,2], there is the recent suggestion that both short-term and long-term outcomes may be improving [3–5]. There are likely multiple factors that have contributed to this including the evolution and focus on pediatric heart failure as a distinct specialty within pediatric cardiology, improved medical management, and improved options for mechanical circulatory support. Moreover, there are many new promising therapies that will hopefully further improve heart failure outcomes for children in the coming decades. This chapter will focus on several of these therapies including regenerative therapy, new medications for acute and chronic therapy that are beneficial for adult heart failure patients (e.g., valsartan/sacubitril, ivabradine, serelaxin), and the next generation of ventricular assist devices (VADs).

REGENERATIVE THERAPY

The topic of regenerative medicine is discussed in more detail in Chapter 61. There is increasing interest in applying this technology to pediatric patients. The clinical investigation of stem cell therapy has been pursued for over 15 years but has not experienced wide spread use in adult heart failure and myocardial infarction patient populations secondary to recognized limitations [6,7]. There continues to be debate regarding the appropriate type of cells to use, the dose of cells delivered, the approach for delivery, and the longevity of stem cells. However, even with these ongoing debates and limited efficacy data for stem cell therapy, the topic remains aggressively investigated and continues to be a well-supported area of clinical investigation. It is estimated that the stem cell therapy market may be worth upward of $180 billion by the year 2020. Increasingly, investigators are documenting that human stem cells become dysfunctional with age. The cells become less effective at replicating as patients get older, especially over the age of 60 [8,9]. Given this information, pediatric populations may be a viable target for harvesting of stem cells as well as a population that would benefit from this therapy.

Mesenchymal cells have been increasingly used in current stem cell studies in the adult heart failure population. These cells can be harvested from the myocardium, bone marrow, or adipose tissue. One potential advantage of mesenchymal precursor cells (MPCs) is that they provoke a minimal alloimmune response that may result in increased longevity of the cells. MPCs are multipotent nonhematopoietic stem cells that can be immunoselected via monoclonal antibodies targeted to specific antigens such as stromal cell surface antigens including STRO3. STRO3 is known to isolate a group of MPCs that have significant ability to proliferate and extensive multilineage capacity [10]. Continued work in this area may allow for more selective isolation of cells that provoke minimal to no immune response and have a strong capacity to differentiate.

The optimal dosing of cells continues to be a point of interest. Many recent and ongoing studies inject ~100 million cells but there has been a wide range of delivered doses historically [6]. However, a recent study in a phase 2 study of adults with chronic heart failure compared doses of 25, 75, and 150 million cells delivered in a transendomyocardial manner [11]. Additional studies will be needed to document optimal stem cell dosing and whether this dosing is impacted by the cardiomyopathy phenotype serving as the destination for the cells. Optimal dosing in children has not been established but ongoing studies may offer insight into this issue.

A recognized limitation of stem cell therapy is the short retention time. Stem cells, regardless of type, have a finite life span ranging from a day to a few weeks. This only offers a limited opportunity to contribute to local contractility. Thus, the concept of regenerative therapy may fall out of favor over time, as the likely benefit from stem cell therapy

Heart Failure in the Child and Young Adult. http://dx.doi.org/10.1016/B978-0-12-802393-8.00044-2

does not reside in the ability to repopulate heart muscle cells in a durable manner. Increasingly, other effects of stem cell therapy are being leveraged. Most notably, recent data support the idea of the positive paracrine effects of stem cells on native myocardial cells. These favorable paracrine effects include effects on collagen deposition and ventricular remodeling, apoptosis signaling, inflammation and antioxidant formation, promotion of neovascularization, and inhibition of ongoing hypertrophy in native myocytes [12–16]. Cardiosphere-derived cells (CDCs) are groupings of cells isolated from endomyocardial biopsy that grow as self-adherent clusters when plated [17]. CDCs are known to be clonogenic and have the potential to differentiate down multiple lineage pathways [18]. The intracoronary infusion of CDCs in the CArdiosphere-Derived aUtologous stem Cells to reverse ventricular dysfunction (CADUCEUS) trial was reported as safe and was documented to increase viable myocardium by cardiac MRI in adult patients following myocardial infarction (Fig. 44.1) [19]. There are ongoing trials to further assess the value of CDC therapy in the setting of myocardial infarction as well as with end-stage heart failure in adults. There is also an ongoing study in pediatric patients assessing the potential benefit of CDC therapy. The Halt CardiomyOPathy progrEssion in Duchenne (HOPE-Duchenne) trial is a prospective, randomized study comparing CDCs added to standard cardiac care versus standard cardiac care in males with Duchenne muscular dystrophy (DMD). Given the known fibrosis burden in males with DMD and the predictable nature of decline in systolic function, subjects will be enrolled based on existing scar burden as assessed by late gadolinium enhancement on cardiac MRI [20]. Longitudinal MRI will be used to assess for changes in late gadolinium enhancement as well as systolic function over time. As cardiac complications are a significant cause of mortality in DMD, use of stem cell therapy may offer a novel opportunity to improve outcome as well as pave the way for use of this therapy in other pediatric and adolescent patients with myocardial dysfunction.

ANGIOTENSIN RECEPTOR/NEPRILYSIN INHIBITOR

Blockage of the renin–angiotensin–aldosterone system has been part of the cornerstone of heart failure management for decades. Angiotensin converting enzyme (ACE) inhibitors were the first heart failure medications associated with improved survival in prospective, randomized trials in adults with heart failure [21–25]. The landmark Cooperative North Scandinavian Enalapril Survival Study published in 1987 described a 40% improvement in mortality at 6 months in patients randomized to enalapril compared to those randomized to placebo [21]. Subsequent studies confirmed this beneficial effect in other ACE inhibitors [22–26] and also in angiotensin receptor blockers (ARBs) [27–34].

Neprilysin was first isolated in the 1970s and found to degrade natriuretic peptides and other peptides including bradykinin, angotinesin I, angiotensin II, vasoactive intestinal peptide, and substance P, though the degradation of B-type natriuretic peptide may be less than other natriuretic peptides [35,36]. Inhibition of neprilysin was subsequently found to increase levels of atrial natriuretic peptides, block activation of aldosterone, and improve diuresis and natriuresis [37–40]. Initial studies on neprilysin inhibition did not demonstrate an overall beneficial effect of these medications for blood pressure control or heart failure as the beneficial effects of increased levels of natriuretic peptides and decreased levels of aldosterone may have been countered by increases in vasoconstrictors including angiotensin II and endothelin I [41–44]. Efforts were then made to combine neprilysin inhibitors with ACE inhibitors. There were several large trials of a combined medication, omapatrilat; however, due to a higher incidence of angioedema in the omapatrilat-treated patients the drug did not obtain approval by the Food and Drug Administration (FDA) [45–47].

As ARBs result in less angioedema than ACE inhibitors, the combination of ARB with a neprilysin inhibitor could theoretically provide the best of both medications. The combination of valsartan and the neprilysin inhibitor sacubitril (LCZ696) demonstrated promising findings in hypertensive patients and patients with heart failure and preserved ventricular function [48,49]. This led to the landmark Prospective Comparison of ARNI with ACEi to Determine Impact on Global Mortality and Morbidity in Heart Failure (PARADIGM-HF) trial in which over 8000 adult heart failure with reduced ejection fraction patients were randomized to LCZ696 or enalapril [50]. The trial was stopped early after the treatment group demonstrated a significant improvement in the primary composite outcome of death from cardiovascular causes or hospitalization for heart failure (Fig. 44.2) [50]. There was also a significant improvement in overall mortality, death from cardiovascular causes, hospitalizations for heart failure, and symptoms and physical limitations from heart failure. From a safety standpoint, there was significantly more hypotension in LCZ696-treated patients, though less hyperkalemia and renal dysfunction. Angioedema was rare in both groups with no statistical difference between groups [50].

Due to the overwhelming success of LCZ696 in patients with heart failure with reduced ejection fraction, the medication received FDA approval in 2015. Subsequent studies have confirmed the benefit of LCZ696 in slowing heart failure progression and decreasing 30-day readmission after heart failure hospitalization [51,52]. Moreover, it is estimated that optimal implementation of this therapy could prevent nearly 30,000 deaths annually in the United States [53]. The ongoing PARAGON-HF study assessing the potential benefits of LCZ696 in adults with heart failure and a preserved ejection

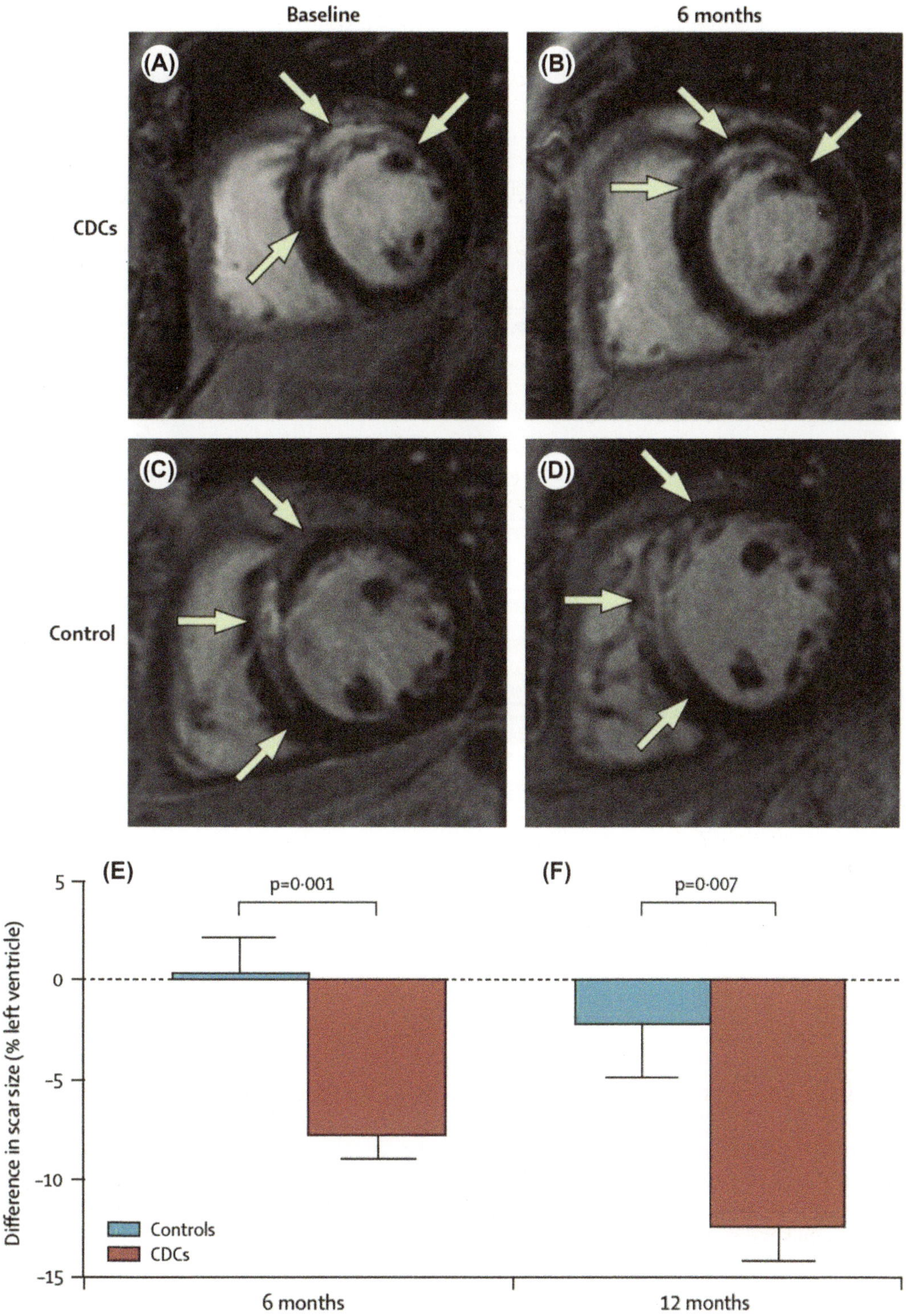

FIGURE 44.1 Short-axis MRI of heart at baseline (82 days after myocardial infarction; (A) and 6 months after CDC infusion (B) in a participant randomly allocated to receive CDCs. Short-axis MRI of heart at baseline (77 days after myocardial infarction; (C) and after 6 months (D) in a control. Infarct scar tissue (*green arrows*) is evident by areas of hyperintensity (white), whereas viable myocardium appears dark. Difference in scar size from baseline to 6 months (E) or 12 months (F). *CDC*, cardiosphere-derived cell. *(Reproduced with permission from R.R. Makkar, R.R. Smith, K. Cheng, et al., Intracoronary cardiosphere-derived cells for heart regeneration after myocardial infarction (CADUCEUS): a prospective, randomised phase 1 trial, Lancet 379 (2012) 895–904.)*

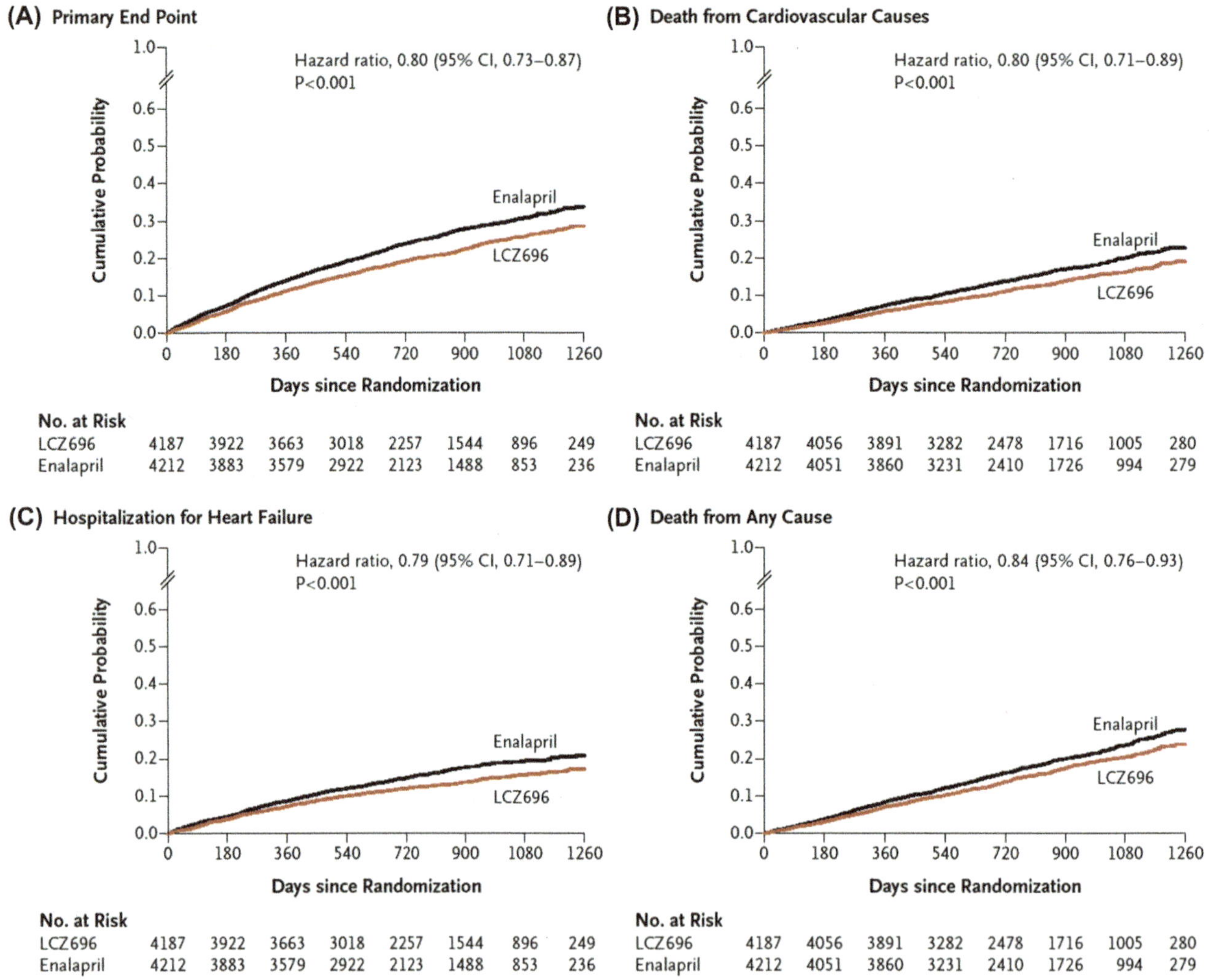

FIGURE 44.2 Kaplan–Meier curves for key study outcomes in the Prospective Comparison of Angiotensin Receptor—Neprilysin Inhibitor with Angiotensin-Converting Enzyme Inhibitor to Determine Impact on Global Mortality and Morbidity in Heart Failure Trial. Shown are estimates of the probability of the primary composite end point (death from cardiovascular causes or first hospitalization for heart failure) (Panel (A)), death from cardiovascular causes (Panel (B)), first hospitalization for heart failure (Panel (C)), and death from any cause (Panel (D)). *(Reproduced with permission from J.J. McMurray, M. Packer, A.S. Desai, et al., Angiotensin-neprilysin inhibition versus enalapril in heart failure, N. Engl. J. Med. 371 (2014) 993–1004.)*

fraction may provide some insights and novel opportunities for a growing and problematic condition [35]. Moreover, there is a prospective, randomized controlled trial of LCZ696 planned for pediatric heart failure patients in 2016.

IVABRADINE

Heart rate appears to be a predictor of clinical outcome in cardiovascular medicine and is routinely measured in patient encounters [54]. In the setting of heart failure, inadequate heart rate control can have important implications. In patients with heart failure, both resting heart rate and heart rate response to beta-blocker therapy are important predictors of outcome [55]. Given these data, therapies targeted at reducing heart rate are part of existing heart failure guidelines [56]. However, many patients fail to achieve benefit from heart rate–reducing therapies such as beta blockade. The causes for this are likely multifactorial, but some explanations may include intolerance of therapy, suboptimal dosing based on existing literature, and unique patient characteristics such as genetic traits that result in poor response to appropriately dosed therapy. This has left a gap in care that has recently been filled by a different class of drugs that can assist in lowering heart rate. Ivabradine, a selective inhibitor of the I_f current in the sinoatrial node, results in heart rate reduction and has been shown to be a drug that has benefit to adult patients with heart failure with reduced ejection fraction [57,58]. Importantly, ivabradine does not impact myocardial contractility or relaxation, cardiac conduction, or peripheral vascular resistance as seen with beta blockade [59].

Ivabradine is also known to inhibit the I_h receptors in addition to the I_f channels. These two receptors collectively are only found in the sinus node, retina, and CNS neurons [59]. However, ivabradine does not cross the blood–brain barrier so potential-expected side effects are related to bradycardia and visual changes. Ivabradine has been shown to typically result in a 10 bpm drop in heart rate, both at rest and with exercise, with the net impact on heart rate being dependent on the heart rate at baseline. The Systolic Heart failure treatment with the I_f inhibitor ivabradine Trial (SHIFT) randomized 6558 adults to either ivabradine (3268 subjects) or placebo (3290 subjects) with a composite endpoint of cardiovascular death or admission for worsening heart failure [60]. Following a median follow-up of 22.9 months, 793 (24%) of the ivabradine subjects and 937 (29%) of the placebo group met the prespecific primary endpoint of HR 0.82, (95% CI 0.75–0.9; $P<.0001$). Fewer serious adverse events were seen in the ivabradine group but symptomatic bradycardia occurred in this group more commonly. Based on results from the SHIFT trial, the US FDA approved ivabradine in 2015 for use in adult patients with stable, symptomatic heart failure with an left ventricular ejection fraction (LVEF) ≤35% who are in sinus rhythm and have a resting heart rate ≥70 bpm in the setting of either maximally tolerated doses of beta blockers or a contraindication to beta-blocker use. Ivabradine has been studied in other populations including adults with stable coronary artery disease and no evidence of heart failure and a heart rate ≥70 bpm, but ivabradine did not show a difference in outcomes when added to background therapy [61]. A subsequent study assessed subjects with coronary artery disease and evidence of systolic dysfunction (LVEF <40%), but the primary composite endpoints of cardiovascular death or admission for new-onset or worsening heart failure were not impacted by ivabradine [62]. The lack of efficacy was felt to be secondary to low heart rate at baseline. In a subset of patients who actually had heart rates ≥70 bpm, ivabradine was associated with a 30% reduction in the need for coronary revascularization and a 36% decrease in hospital admissions for myocardial infarction. The existing data in clinical trials suggest that patients with higher resting heart rates are most likely to receive benefit from treatment.

Ivabradine has been studied in other conditions where a reduction in heart rate may have favorable effects. Resting sinus tachycardia is noted frequently in patients following orthotopic heart transplantation secondary to cardiac denervation. Initial use of ivabradine compared to beta-blocker therapy revealed both to be effective with less-reported side effects in those patients treated with ivabradine [63]. Ivabradine appears to be safe and well-tolerated in adult heart transplant recipients and effective at reducing resting heart rate and improving functional class [64]. Ivabradine can be given to heart transplant patients for up to 36 months safely with continued heart-rate lowering effects and may have favorable impacts on indexed LV mass with chronic treatment [65]. Ivabradine has been used in other nontransplant cohorts with elevated heart rates. Adult patients with inappropriate sinus tachycardia have been treated with ivabradine with favorable results in lowering heart rate and an improved quality of life [66,67]. Additional preclinical studies suggest that ivabradine may have benefits over metoprolol in mouse models of heart failure undergoing mechanical unloading, which could lead to new clinical opportunities for favorable remodeling in the setting of ventricular assist device therapy [68]. There have been no controlled data generated in pediatric populations but isolated case reports exist [69,70]. Information is now being generated to study children with anticipation of a multicenter trial in the next few years [71,72].

Finally, there may be an opportunity to add ivabradine to optimal chronic oral beta-blocker therapy. There is ongoing debate in adult populations studied in clinical trials, such as those in the SHIFT study that led to the FDA approval of ivabradine, regarding optimal beta-blocker dosing. The effects of ivabradine are most beneficial in those patients with a heart rate greater than 70 bpm. Does this reflect the need simply for higher beta-blocker dosing or is there an intrinsic benefit to ivabradine in combination? Regardless, these studies have drawn attention to pulse being in important biomarker and the importance of biologic factors, such as neurohormonal activation, which promote increased heart rate. Further investigation is needed to determine whether outcomes are driven primarily by targeted beta-blocker dosing or by a cumulative reduction in heart rate [73].

SERELAXIN

Additional treatment options for acute decompensated heart failure remain an area of need. Most studies over the past decade have not met primary endpoints that likely reflect the complexity and heterogeneity of the clinical problem. Guideline-directed therapy currently relies on diuretics as first line therapy for most patients with vasodilators and inotropic support being an option for select patients. Serelaxin, a recombinant form of the naturally occurring hormone relaxin-2, is a promising drug that may offer additional treatment options in acute decompensated heart failure [74]. The drug has been studied extensively in preclinical and clinical investigation. Also, there are the results of the Pre–RELAXin in Acute Heart Failure (RELAX-AHF) trial that was a phase II study that enrolled 234 acute heart failure patients to either placebo or relaxin at prespecified doses (10, 30, 100 or 250 mcg/kg/day) for 48 h [75]. There was a noted improvement in dyspnea in the 30 mcg/kg/day group when compared to placebo ($P=.044$) without obvious safety concerns. A phase II study was also conducted in Japan, which similarly documented safety as well as a greater reduction in NT-proBNP levels in subjects receiving serelaxin compared to placebo [76].

The RELAX-AHF trial was an international, prospective, double blind, placebo controlled, phase III study comparing treatment with 48 h of intravenous serelaxin vs. placebo on top of standard of care therapy to be started within 16 h of presentation in adults with acute decompensated heart failure [77]. The primary endpoints were related to dyspnea improvement and were assessed by a change from baseline daily for 5 days using a visual analog scale and the proportion of patients having moderate or marked improvement by Likert scale in the first 24 h. Secondary endpoints included: (1) days alive and out of the hospital at day 60 and (2) cardiovascular death or readmission secondary to heart failure or renal failure before day 60. The study randomized 1161 patients to either serelaxin (n = 581) or placebo (n = 580). For the primary endpoints, there were significant changes in the visual analog scale for serelaxin compared to placebo. However, the Likert scale assessment as well as the secondary endpoints did not show a difference between treatment groups. Additional data regarding 180-day mortality were collected with the serelaxin group having fewer deaths (serelaxin 42 deaths, placebo 65 deaths; HR 0.63, 95% CI 0.42–0.93; $P = .019$). Based on these data, serelaxin was not given approval by the FDA in 2015, as the proposed filing indication was to improve the symptoms of acute HF through reduction of the rate of worsening HF, which was not adequately addressed in the initial study. However, the FDA reported no concerns with safety and was encouraged by the 180-day mortality difference. Based on the recommendations of the FDA, a subsequent study is now underway to better define outcome with serelaxin. The Efficacy, Safety, and Tolerability of Serelaxin When Added to Standard Therapy in AHF (RELAX-AHF-2) study (ClinicalTrials.gov Identifier: NCT01870778) is ongoing with the primary endpoints of: (1) time to confirmed cardiovascular death during the follow-up period of 180 days and (2) time to worsening heart failure through day 5 of treatment.

Serelaxin may also have potential benefit in patients admitted with heart failure and worsening renal function. Preclinical data suggest that serelaxin may have beneficial effects on kidney function and a concomitant decrease in collagen deposition [78]. Clinical data also suggest potential benefit. In a prospective study comparing serelaxin to placebo infusions for 20 h, creatinine clearance increased by 20% from baseline in the serelaxin group while there was a 24% decrease in the placebo group [79]. Subjects in the RELAX-AHF study experienced less worsening renal function and lower biomarkers of renal dysfunction as compared to those receiving placebo suggesting faster decongestion and a possible degree of end organ protection [80].

There is an ongoing study assessing the possible use of serelaxin in children. This phase 2, multicenter, prospective, dose escalation study will evaluate safety, tolerability, and pharmacokinetics of intravenous serelaxin in patients less than 18 years of age who are hospitalized with acute heart failure. The findings of this investigation will inform a larger study to further assess potential therapeutic benefits in children.

NEW GENERATION VENTRICULAR ASSIST DEVICE THERAPY

Any discussion of new therapeutic strategies for pediatric heart failure should include recent advances in the utilization of mechanical circulatory support.

While the use of Pediatric VADs is reviewed in detail in Chapter 53, a few comments regarding new innovation in this area are warranted here.

To date, only two pediatric VADs have been granted humanitarian device exemption (HDE) in the United States. The MicroMed HeartAssist 5 (formerly the DeBakey VAD Child; Micromed Technologies, Inc) was the first pediatric VAD granted HDE in 2004. It never gained widespread use, however, due to its large size and thromboembolic-related neurologic complications. The second device, the Berlin Heart EXCOR (Berlin Heart, Inc, Berlin, Germany) received HDE approval in December 2011 after a prospective multiinstitutional investigational device exemption trial that compared outcomes of Berlin Heart-supported patients with a propensity-score matched historical control group supported on extracorporeal membrane oxygenation (ECMO) [81]. This trial was a landmark step forward in mechanical circulatory support for pediatric patients, extending the use of an intermediate to long-term support device down to the smallest of patients. However, while the Berlin Heart was shown in trial to be superior to ECMO, it too, has been demonstrated to have a high complication rate, especially as it relates to thromboembolic stroke in small patients [82]. The extracorporeal nature of this device has also limited its usefulness.

Surgical innovation has now led to implantable continuous flow devices originally designed for adults, such as the Heartmate II (Thoratec Laboratories Corp, Pleasanton, CA) or the HeartWare HVAD (HeartWare Inc, Framingham, MA), to be placed in pediatric patients, down to a size as small as 14 kg with a BSA of 0.6 m^2 [83,84]. Not only have these devices been placed in patients with a normal biventricular circulation but also they have now been successfully utilized in patients with a so-called "failing Fontan" or failing single ventricle physiology as a bridge to cardiac transplant [85]. The advantages of these type devices are several fold. The implantable design of these devices has lead to greater ambulation and to hospital discharge of patients while being supported [86,87]. The risk of thromboembolic events with these devices has been much lower, leading to more modest anticoagulation. With a lower risk profile, physicians have been willing to support patients longer. This, in turn, has led to (1) better rehabilitation leading to shorter recovery posttransplant, (2) in some instances, a bridge to recovery of cardiac function and device explanation and (3) in a few additional cases, destination therapy.

Technology and innovation have lead the way to the dramatic changes in mechanical support of pediatric patients experienced over the last decade. Technology and innovation will again drive changes in patient management in the decade ahead. The two changes most likely to affect the way we use mechanical support are miniaturization of our implantable continuous flow devices such that they may used in our smallest of patients, even down to newborn size, and the development of wireless power-transfer technologies, which would allow for a fully implantable device.

With respect to miniaturization, as of this writing, the much anticipated National Heart, Lung and Blood Institute–sponsored trial called Pumps for Kids, Infants and Neonates (PumpKIN) remains in preclinical trials [88]. The intent of this trial is to evaluate the Infant Jarvik 2000 (Jarvik Heart Inc, New York, NY) intracorporeal continuous flow VAD in a randomized fashion with the Berlin Heart EXCOR device in children from 3 to 15 kgs. Clinical trial could begin in 2017.

With respect to wireless-transfer technology, both HeartWare and Thoratec, the two companies selling LVADs commercially that have had successful pediatric application, have announced partnerships to create a fully implantable VAD. Thoratec has collaborated with WiTricity Corp since 2010 and HeartWare has been working with Dualis MedTech since 2011 [89]. HeartWare has expressed a desire to have a wireless power-transfer VAD available within the next 5 years (personal communication, HeartWare, Inc.).

Thus it is plausible to imagine in the not-too-distant future a support device that is durable, appropriately sized for our pediatric age population, fully implantable, with a near-zero complication rate, and with long-lasting batteries and wireless charging technology. Consider this in the context of limited organ donation and a changing demographic of our patient population, with more palliated complex congenital heart disease and HLA-sensitization, and the concept of destination therapy for even our youngest of patients becomes a realistic alternative therapy.

CONCLUSION

While outcomes remain suboptimal for many children with heart failure, novel therapies including new medicines, stem cells, and the next generation of mechanical circulatory support devices are actively being investigated in children. There are several trials of these therapies either currently underway or planned to initiate in the very near future. As many of these therapies have been dramatically successful in adults, there is great hope that the improvement in survival evident in adult heart failure patients over the last several decades will also be observed in children with heart failure.

REFERENCES

[1] P.F. Kantor, J.R. Abraham, A.I. Dipchand, L.N. Benson, A.N. Redington, The impact of changing medical therapy on transplantation-free survival in pediatric dilated cardiomyopathy, J. Am. Coll. Cardiol. 55 (2010) 1377–1384.

[2] J.A. Towbin, A.M. Lowe, S.D. Colan, et al., Incidence, causes, and outcomes of dilated cardiomyopathy in children, JAMA 296 (2006) 1867–1876.

[3] C.A. Wittlieb-Weber, K.Y. Lin, T.E. Zaoutis, et al., Pediatric versus adult cardiomyopathy and heart failure-related hospitalizations: a value-based analysis, J. Card. Fail. 21 (2015) 76–82.

[4] R.K. Singh, C. Canter, L. Shi, et al., Improved transplant-free survival of children with dilated cardiomyopathy: analysis of two decades from the pediatric cardiomyopathy registry (abstract), Circulation 130 (2014) A16801.

[5] P.M. Alexander, P.E. Daubeney, A.W. Nugent, et al., Long-term outcomes of dilated cardiomyopathy diagnosed during childhood: results from a national population-based study of childhood cardiomyopathy, Circulation 128 (2013) 2039–2046.

[6] S.K. Sanganalmath, R. Bolli, Cell therapy for heart failure: a comprehensive overview of experimental and clinical studies, current challenges, and future directions, Circ. Res. 113 (2013) 810–834.

[7] D.M. Clifford, S.A. Fisher, S.J. Brunskill, et al., Stem cell treatment for acute myocardial infarction, Cochrane Database Syst. Rev. 2 (2012) CD006536.

[8] E. Sahin, R.A. Depinho, Linking functional decline of telomeres, mitochondria and stem cells during ageing, Nature 464 (2010) 520–528.

[9] D. Cesselli, A.P. Beltrami, F. D'Aurizio, et al., Effects of age and heart failure on human cardiac stem cell function, Am. J. Pathol. 179 (2011) 349–366.

[10] S. Gronthos, S. Fitter, P. Diamond, P.J. Simmons, S. Itescu, A.C. Zannettino, A novel monoclonal antibody (STRO-3) identifies an isoform of tissue nonspecific alkaline phosphatase expressed by multipotent bone marrow stromal stem cells, Stem Cells Dev. 16 (2007) 953–963.

[11] E.C. Perin, K.M. Borow, G.V. Silva, et al., A phase II dose-escalation study of allogeneic mesenchymal precursor cells in patients with ischemic or nonischemic heart failure, Circ. Res. 117 (2015) 576–584.

[12] T.P. Lozito, R.S. Tuan, Mesenchymal stem cells inhibit both endogenous and exogenous MMPs via secreted TIMPs, J. Cell Physiol. 226 (2011) 385–396.

[13] N. Bonaros, R. Rauf, D. Wolf, et al., Combined transplantation of skeletal myoblasts and angiopoietic progenitor cells reduces infarct size and apoptosis and improves cardiac function in chronic ischemic heart failure, J. Thorac. Cardiovasc. Surg. 132 (2006) 1321–1328.

[14] M. Ayatollahi, Z. Hesami, A. Jamshidzadeh, B. Gramizadeh, Antioxidant effects of bone marrow mesenchymal stem cell against carbon tetrachloride-induced oxidative damage in rat livers, Int. J. Organ Transplant. Med. 5 (2014) 166–173.

[15] T. Kinnaird, E. Stabile, M.S. Burnett, et al., Marrow-derived stromal cells express genes encoding a broad spectrum of arteriogenic cytokines and promote in vitro and in vivo arteriogenesis through paracrine mechanisms, Circ. Res. 94 (2004) 678–685.

[16] P. Farahmand, T.Y. Lai, R.D. Weisel, et al., Skeletal myoblasts preserve remote matrix architecture and global function when implanted early or late after coronary ligation into infarcted or remote myocardium, Circulation 118 (2008) S130–S137.

[17] E. Messina, L. De Angelis, G. Frati, et al., Isolation and expansion of adult cardiac stem cells from human and murine heart, Circ. Res. 95 (2004) 911–921.

[18] P.V. Johnston, T. Sasano, K. Mills, et al., Engraftment, differentiation, and functional benefits of autologous cardiosphere-derived cells in porcine ischemic cardiomyopathy, Circulation 120 (2009) 1075–1083 7 pp. following 83.

[19] R.R. Makkar, R.R. Smith, K. Cheng, et al., Intracoronary cardiosphere-derived cells for heart regeneration after myocardial infarction (CADUCEUS): a prospective, randomised phase 1 trial, Lancet 379 (2012) 895–904.

[20] A. Tandon, C.R. Villa, K.N. Hor, et al., Myocardial fibrosis burden predicts left ventricular ejection fraction and is associated with age and steroid treatment duration in duchenne muscular dystrophy, J. Am. Heart Assoc. 4 (2015).

[21] The CONSENSUS Trial Study Group, Effects of enalapril on mortality in severe congestive heart failure. Results of the Cooperative North Scandinavian Enalapril Survival Study (CONSENSUS), N. Engl. J. Med. 316 (1987) 1429–1435.

[22] J.N. Cohn, G. Johnson, S. Ziesche, et al., A comparison of enalapril with hydralazine-isosorbide dinitrate in the treatment of chronic congestive heart failure, N. Engl. J. Med. 325 (1991) 303–310.

[23] The SOLVD Investigators, Effect of enalapril on survival in patients with reduced left ventricular ejection fractions and congestive heart failure, N. Engl. J. Med. 325 (1991) 293–302.

[24] M.A. Pfeffer, E. Braunwald, L.A. Moye, The SAVE Investigators, et al., Effect of captopril on mortality and morbidity in patients with left ventricular dysfunction after myocardial infarction. Results of the survival and ventricular enlargement trial, N. Engl. J. Med. 327 (1992) 669–677.

[25] M. Packer, P.A. Poole-Wilson, P.W. Armstrong, ATLAS Study Group, et al., Comparative effects of low and high doses of the angiotensin-converting enzyme inhibitor, lisinopril, on morbidity and mortality in chronic heart failure, Circulation 100 (1999) 2312–2318.

[26] The SOLVD Investigators, Effect of enalapril on mortality and the development of heart failure in asymptomatic patients with reduced left ventricular ejection fractions, N. Engl. J. Med. 327 (1992) 685–691.

[27] D. Sharma, M. Buyse, B. Pitt, E.J. Rucinska, Losartan Heart Failure Mortality Meta-analysis Study Group, Meta-analysis of observed mortality data from all-controlled, double-blind, multiple-dose studies of losartan in heart failure, Am. J. Cardiol. 85 (2000) 187–192.

[28] G. Hamroff, S.D. Katz, D. Mancini, et al., Addition of angiotensin II receptor blockade to maximal angiotensin-converting enzyme inhibition improves exercise capacity in patients with severe congestive heart failure, Circulation 99 (1999) 990–992.

[29] M. Wong, L. Staszewsky, R. Latini, et al., Valsartan benefits left ventricular structure and function in heart failure: Val-HeFT echocardiographic study, J. Am. Coll. Cardiol. 40 (2002) 970–975.

[30] J.N. Cohn, G. Tognoni, Valsartan Heart Failure Trial I. A randomized trial of the angiotensin-receptor blocker valsartan in chronic heart failure, N. Engl. J. Med. 345 (2001) 1667–1675.

[31] A.P. Maggioni, I. Anand, S.O. Gottlieb, et al., Effects of valsartan on morbidity and mortality in patients with heart failure not receiving angiotensin-converting enzyme inhibitors, J. Am. Coll. Cardiol. 40 (2002) 1414–1421.

[32] M.A. Konstam, J.D. Neaton, K. Dickstein, et al., Effects of high-dose versus low-dose losartan on clinical outcomes in patients with heart failure (HEAAL study): a randomised, double-blind trial, Lancet 374 (2009) 1840–1848.

[33] B. Pitt, P.A. Poole-Wilson, R. Segal, et al., Effect of losartan compared with captopril on mortality in patients with symptomatic heart failure: randomised trial–the Losartan Heart Failure Survival Study ELITE II, Lancet 355 (2000) 1582–1587.

[34] B. Pitt, R. Segal, F.A. Martinez, et al., Randomised trial of losartan versus captopril in patients over 65 with heart failure (Evaluation of Losartan in the Elderly Study, ELITE), Lancet 349 (1997) 747–752.

[35] E. Braunwald, The path to an angiotensin receptor antagonist-neprilysin inhibitor in the treatment of heart failure, J. Am. Coll. Cardiol. 65 (2015) 1029–1041.

[36] L.R. Potter, Natriuretic peptide metabolism, clearance and degradation, FEBS J. 278 (2011) 1808–1817.

[37] O. Lisy, M. Jougasaki, J.A. Schirger, H.H. Chen, P.T. Barclay, J.C. Burnett Jr., Neutral endopeptidase inhibition potentiates the natriuretic actions of adrenomedullin, Am. J. Physiol. 275 (1998) F410–F414.

[38] E.J. Sybertz, P.J. Chiu, S. Vemulapalli, et al., SCH 39370, a neutral metalloendopeptidase inhibitor, potentiates biological responses to atrial natriuretic factor and lowers blood pressure in desoxycorticosterone acetate-sodium hypertensive rats, J. Pharmacol. Exp. Ther. 250 (1989) 624–631.

[39] D.B. Northridge, A.G. Jardine, C.T. Alabaster, et al., Effects of UK 69 578: a novel atriopeptidase inhibitor, Lancet 2 (1989) 591–593.

[40] F.L. Martin, T.L. Stevens, A. Cataliotti, et al., Natriuretic and antialdosterone actions of chronic oral NEP inhibition during progressive congestive heart failure, Kidney Int. 67 (2005) 1723–1730.

[41] G. McDowell, W. Coutie, C. Shaw, K.D. Buchanan, A.D. Struthers, D.P. Nicholls, The effect of the neutral endopeptidase inhibitor drug, candoxatril, on circulating levels of two of the most potent vasoactive peptides, Br. J. Clin. Pharmacol. 43 (1997) 329–332.

[42] J.G. Cleland, K. Swedberg, The International Ecadotril Multi-centre Dose-ranging Study Investigators, Lack of efficacy of neutral endopeptidase inhibitor ecadotril in heart failure, Lancet 351 (1998) 1657–1658.

[43] S. Ando, M.A. Rahman, G.C. Butler, B.L. Senn, J.S. Floras, Comparison of candoxatril and atrial natriuretic factor in healthy men. Effects on hemodynamics, sympathetic activity, heart rate variability, and endothelin, Hypertension 26 (1995) 1160–1166.

[44] C.J. Charles, E.A. Espiner, A.M. Richards, E.J. Sybertz, Endopeptidase inhibition in angiotensin-induced hypertension. Effect of SCH 39370 in sheep, Hypertension 26 (1995) 89–94.

[45] J.B. Kostis, M. Packer, H.R. Black, R. Schmieder, D. Henry, E. Levy, Omapatrilat and enalapril in patients with hypertension: the Omapatrilat Cardiovascular Treatment vs. Enalapril (OCTAVE) trial, Am. J. Hypertens. 17 (2004) 103–111.

[46] D.J. Campbell, Vasopeptidase inhibition: a double-edged sword? Hypertension 41 (2003) 383–389.

[47] M. Packer, R.M. Califf, M.A. Konstam, et al., Comparison of omapatrilat and enalapril in patients with chronic heart failure: the omapatrilat versus enalapril randomized trial of utility in reducing events (OVERTURE), Circulation 106 (2002) 920–926.

[48] S.D. Solomon, M. Zile, B. Pieske, et al., The angiotensin receptor neprilysin inhibitor LCZ696 in heart failure with preserved ejection fraction: a phase 2 double-blind randomised controlled trial, Lancet 380 (2012) 1387–1395.

[49] L.M. Ruilope, A. Dukat, M. Bohm, Y. Lacourciere, J. Gong, M.P. Lefkowitz, Blood-pressure reduction with LCZ696, a novel dual-acting inhibitor of the angiotensin II receptor and neprilysin: a randomised, double-blind, placebo-controlled, active comparator study, Lancet 375 (2010) 1255–1266.

[50] J.J. McMurray, M. Packer, A.S. Desai, et al., Angiotensin-neprilysin inhibition versus enalapril in heart failure, N. Engl. J. Med. 371 (2014) 993–1004.

[51] A.S. Desai, B.L. Claggett, M. Packer, et al., Influence of sacubitril/valsartan (LCZ696) on 30-day readmission after heart failure hospitalization, J. Am. Coll. Cardiol. 68 (2016) 241–248.

[52] M. Packer, J.J. McMurray, A.S. Desai, et al., Angiotensin receptor neprilysin inhibition compared with enalapril on the risk of clinical progression in surviving patients with heart failure, Circulation 131 (2015) 54–61.

[53] A.P. Kalogeropoulos, G.C. Fonarow, V. Georgiopoulou, G. Burkman, S. Siwamogsatham, A. Patel, S. Li, L. Papadimitriou, J. Butler. JAMA Cardiol. 1 (5) (August 1, 2016) 510–518. doi:10.1001/jamacardio.2016.1325.

[54] J.C. Tardif, Heart rate as a treatable cardiovascular risk factor, Br. Med. Bull. 90 (2009) 71–84.

[55] P. Lechat, J.S. Hulot, S. Escolano, et al., Heart rate and cardiac rhythm relationships with bisoprolol benefit in chronic heart failure in CIBIS II Trial, Circulation 103 (2001) 1428–1433.

[56] C.W. Yancy, M. Jessup, B. Bozkurt, et al., 2013 ACCF/AHA guideline for the management of heart failure: a report of the American College of cardiology Foundation/American Heart Association task force on practice guidelines, J. Am. Coll. Cardiol. 62 (2013) e147–239.

[57] D. DiFrancesco, Funny channels in the control of cardiac rhythm and mode of action of selective blockers, Pharmacol. Res. 53 (2006) 399–406.

[58] S. Sulfi, A.D. Timmis, Ivabradine – the first selective sinus node I_f channel inhibitor in the treatment of stable angina, Int. J. Clin. Pract. 60 (2006) 222–228.

[59] I. Savelieva, A.J. Camm, I f inhibition with ivabradine: electrophysiological effects and safety, Drug Saf. 31 (2008) 95–107.

[60] K. Swedberg, M. Komajda, M. Bohm, et al., Ivabradine and outcomes in chronic heart failure (SHIFT): a randomised placebo-controlled study, Lancet 376 (2010) 875–885.

[61] K. Fox, I. Ford, P.G. Steg, et al., Ivabradine in stable coronary artery disease without clinical heart failure, N. Engl. J. Med. 371 (2014) 1091–1099.

[62] K. Fox, I. Ford, P.G. Steg, M. Tendera, R. Ferrari, B. Investigators, Ivabradine for patients with stable coronary artery disease and left-ventricular systolic dysfunction (BEAUTIFUL): a randomised, double-blind, placebo-controlled trial, Lancet 372 (2008) 807–816.

[63] A.O. Doesch, S. Celik, P. Ehlermann, et al., Heart rate reduction after heart transplantation with beta-blocker versus the selective if channel antagonist ivabradine, Transplantation 84 (2007) 988–996.

[64] E. Lage-Galle, N. Romero-Rodriguez, J. Nevado-Portero, et al., Safety and effectiveness of ivabradine after cardiac transplantation, Transplant. Proc. 42 (2010) 3191–3192.

[65] A.O. Doesch, S. Mueller, C. Erbel, et al., Heart rate reduction for 36 months with ivabradine reduces left ventricular mass in cardiac allograft recipients: a long-term follow-up study, Drug Des. Dev. Ther. 7 (2013) 1323–1328.

[66] M. Annamaria, P.P. Lupo, S. Foresti, G. De Ambroggi, E. de Ruvo, L. Sciarra, R. Cappato, L. Calo, J. Interv. Card Electrophysiol. 46 (1) (June 2016) 47–53. doi:10.1007/s10840-015-0066-5 (Epub 2015 Oct 14. Review).

[67] J. Benezet-Mazuecos, J.M. Rubio, J. Farre, M.A. Quinones, P. Sanchez-Borque, E. Macia, Long-term outcomes of ivabradine in inappropriate sinus tachycardia patients: appropriate efficacy or inappropriate patients, Pacing Clin. Electrophysiol. 36 (2013) 830–836.

[68] M. Navaratnarajah, M. Ibrahim, U. Siedlecka, et al., Influence of ivabradine on reverse remodelling during mechanical unloading, Cardiovasc. Res. 97 (2013) 230–239.

[69] E. Romeo, N. Grimaldi, B. Sarubbi, et al., A pediatric case of cardiomyopathy induced by inappropriate sinus tachycardia: efficacy of ivabradine, Pediatr. Cardiol. 32 (2011) 842–845.

[70] S. Al-Ghamdi, M.I. Al-Fayyadh, R.M. Hamilton, Potential new indication for ivabradine: treatment of a patient with congenital junctional ectopic tachycardia, J. Cardiovasc. Electrophysiol. 24 (2013) 822–824.

[71] S. Peigne, F. Bouzom, K. Brendel, C. Gesson, S. Fouliard, M. Chenel, Model-based approaches for ivabradine development in paediatric population, part I: study preparation assessment, J. Pharmacokinet. Pharmacodyn. 43 (2016) 13–27.

[72] S. Peigne, S. Fouliard, S. Decourcelle, M. Chenel, Model-based approaches for ivabradine development in paediatric population, part II: PK and PK/PD assessment, J. Pharmacokinet. Pharmacodyn. 43 (2016) 29–43.

[73] D. Cullington, K.M. Goode, A.L. Clark, J.G. Cleland, Heart rate achieved or beta-blocker dose in patients with chronic heart failure: which is the better target? Eur. J. Heart Fail. 14 (2012) 737–747.

[74] K.P. Conrad, Maternal vasodilation in pregnancy: the emerging role of relaxin, Am. J. Physiol. Regul. Integr. Comp. Physiol. 301 (2011) R267–R275.

[75] J.R. Teerlink, M. Metra, G.M. Felker, et al., Relaxin for the treatment of patients with acute heart failure (Pre-RELAX-AHF): a multicentre, randomised, placebo-controlled, parallel-group, dose-finding phase IIb study, Lancet 373 (2009) 1429–1439.

[76] N. Sato, W. Takahashi, A. Hirayama, et al., Multicenter, randomized, double-blinded, placebo-controlled phase II study of serelaxin in Japanese patients with acute heart failure, Circ. J. 79 (2015) 1237–1247.

[77] J.R. Teerlink, G. Cotter, B.A. Davison, et al., Serelaxin, recombinant human relaxin-2, for treatment of acute heart failure (RELAX-AHF): a randomised, placebo-controlled trial, Lancet 381 (2013) 29–39.

[78] L.A. Danielson, A. Welford, A. Harris, Relaxin improves renal function and histology in aging Munich Wistar rats, J. Am. Soc. Nephrol. 17 (2006) 1325–1333.

[79] P. Ponikowski, V. Mitrovic, M. Ruda, et al., A randomized, double-blind, placebo-controlled, multicentre study to assess haemodynamic effects of serelaxin in patients with acute heart failure, Eur. Heart J. 35 (2014) 431–441.

[80] M. Metra, G. Cotter, B.A. Davison, et al., Effect of serelaxin on cardiac, renal, and hepatic biomarkers in the Relaxin in Acute Heart Failure (RELAX-AHF) development program: correlation with outcomes, J. Am. Coll. Cardiol. 61 (2013) 196–206.

[81] C.D. Fraser Jr., R.D. Jaquiss, D.N. Rosenthal, et al., Prospective trial of a pediatric ventricular assist device, N. Engl. J. Med. 367 (2012) 532–541.

[82] J. Conway, J. St Louis, D.L. Morales, S. Law, C. Tjossem, T. Humpl, Delineating survival outcomes in children <10 kg bridged to transplant or recovery with the Berlin Heart EXCOR Ventricular Assist Device, JACC Heart Fail. 3 (2015) 70–77.

[83] W.R. Owens, R. Bryant 3rd, W.J. Dreyer, J.F. Price, D.L. Morales, Initial clinical experience with the HeartMate II ventricular assist system in a pediatric institution, Artif. Organs 34 (2010) 600–603.

[84] E. Peng, R. Kirk, N. Wrightson, et al., An extended role of continuous flow device in pediatric mechanical circulatory support, Ann. Thorac. Surg. 102 (2016) 620–627.

[85] J.W. Rossano, R.K. Woods, S. Berger, et al., Mechanical support as failure intervention in patients with cavopulmonary shunts (MFICS): rationale and aims of a new registry of mechanical circulatory support in single ventricle patients, Congenit. Heart Dis. 8 (2013) 182–186.

[86] J. Conway, C. VanderPluym, A. Jeewa, S. Sinnadurai, A. Schubert, A. Lorts, Now how do we get them home? Outpatient care of pediatric patients on mechanical circulatory support, Pediatr. Transplant. 20 (2016) 194–202.

[87] S. Chen, A. Lin, E. Liu, et al., Outpatient outcomes of pediatric patients with left ventricular assist devices, ASAIO J. 62 (2016) 163–168.

[88] I. Adachi, S. Burki, F. Zafar, D.L. Morales, Pediatric ventricular assist devices, J. Thorac. Dis. 7 (2015) 2194–2202.

[89] M. Thibault, Another LVAD Company Joins Quest for Fully Implantable System, 2015. http://www.mddionline.com/article/another-lvad-company-joins-quest-fully-implantable-system-04-08-15.

Chapter 45

Electrophysiologic Devices in Heart Failure

Bryan Cannon, Philip Wackel
Mayo Clinic, Rochester, MN, United States

There are three ways that electrophysiology devices play a role in heart failure. The first is implantable cardioverter defibrillators (ICDs) in the prevention of sudden cardiac death. The second is chronic resynchronization therapy (CRT or biventricular pacing) in promoting more synchronous cardiac contractions to decrease heart failure symptoms. The final way is to use electronic measurements from implanted devices to attempt to predict the occurrence of or quantitate the degree of heart failure. This chapter will discuss these three modalities and their application in pediatric heart failure patients. Although devices can be very beneficial in heart failure, they are not without risks and complications. The risks and benefits of device placement must be carefully considered in heart failure patients, and frequently there are not clear cut guidelines to guide therapy.

IMPLANTABLE CARDIOVERTER DEFIBRILLATOR THERAPY

Arrhythmias are a significant concern in patients with poor ventricular function. Ventricular arrhythmias may potentially result in sudden cardiac death. While atrial arrhythmias are typically a problem only from a symptom standpoint, rapid conduction of atrial arrhythmias, especially in the presence of poor ventricular function may also result in sudden cardiac death. Although antiarrhythmic therapies may decrease the incidence of arrhythmias, the most effective therapy for decreasing the incidence of sudden cardiac death is placement of an ICD. Although criteria for ICD placement in adults with poor ventricular function are well established, pediatric data are more sparse and indications for ICD placement in young patients are more controversial.

The most likely cause of sudden cardiac death in patients with poor ventricular function is the sudden onset of a ventricular arrhythmia resulting in poor systemic perfusion. In adults, the rhythm observed in victims of out-of-hospital cardiac arrest is ventricular fibrillation in 95% of cardiac arrests who have a rhythm recorded within 4 min [1]. Although ventricular tachyarrhythmias are likely the culprit in most cases of cardiac arrest: bradycardia, electromechanical dissociation, and rapidly conducted atrial arrhythmias likely play a role in sudden death in the pediatric population.

There are two types of indications for ICD implantation. The first is an indication based on a previous resuscitated sudden cardiac death event or *secondary prevention*. Patients who have experienced one sudden death episode are at a very high risk for experiencing a second episode; and in the adult population the mortality is as high as 45% at 2 years in this population [2]. This increased risk holds true in the pediatric population with around a 40% appropriate ICD shock rate in patients with an ICD placed for secondary prevention [3]. Therefore, resuscitated sudden cardiac death episode is a Class I (definitive) indication for ICD placement in both adult and pediatric populations [4]. The second type of indication for ICD placement in *primary prevention*. In primary prevention, an ICD is implanted in patients felt to be a high risk of arrhythmias who have not yet had an aborted sudden cardiac death episode. There are less data, and therefore more controversy, over which pediatric patients need an ICD for primary prevention. The 2008 guideline recommendations for ICD implantation in the pediatric and congenital population are summarized in Table 45.1. Primary prevention ICDs were associated with appropriate therapy in 19% in 4 years of follow up in one study [5]. In this same study, the adverse event rate was 36%, and included lead failures, infection and inappropriate shocks for atrial arrhythmias or sinus tachycardia. The highest risk of an appropriate shock appears to be around the time of placement of the ICD and the risk decreases over time.

Although an ICD may be indicated in some pediatric patients as poor ventricular function creates a clinical situation where ventricular arrhythmias and sudden death can occur, it is not universally indicated in all patients. The incidence of sudden cardiac death in pediatric patients with dilated cardiomyopathy is relatively low. Initial reports showed the incidence of ventricular tachycardia to be around 6% but the incidence of sudden cardiac death was only around 1% [6]. A subsequent study from the Pediatric Cardiomyopathy Registry showed the 5-year incidence of sudden cardiac death in children with dilated cardiomyopathy to be 2.4% and 26 ICD implantations would be required to prevent one sudden death [7]. However,

Heart Failure in the Child and Young Adult. http://dx.doi.org/10.1016/B978-0-12-802393-8.00045-4

TABLE 45.1 Implantable Cardioverter Defibrillator (ICD) Indications in Children With Heart Failure

Class I: *ICD therapy is indicated in*

1. Patients who are survivors of cardiac arrest after evaluation to exclude any completely reversible causes.
2. Patients with structural heart disease and spontaneous sustained VT.
3. Patients with syncope of undetermined origin with clinically relevant sustained VT or VF induced at electrophysiological study.
4. Patients with nonischemic DCM who have an LVEF less than or equal to 35% and who are in NYHA functional Class II or III.

Class IIa: *ICD implantation is reasonable for*

1. Patients with unexplained syncope, significant LV dysfunction, and nonischemic DCM.
2. Prevention of SCD in patients with ARVD/C who have one or more risk factors for SCD.
3. Nonhospitalized patients awaiting transplantation.
4. Patients with cardiac sarcoidosis, giant cell myocarditis, or Chagas disease.

Class IIb: *ICD therapy may be considered in*

1. Patients with nonischemic heart disease who have an LVEF of less than or equal to 35% and who are in NYHA functional Class I.
2. Patients with syncope and advanced structural heart disease in whom thorough investigations have failed to define a cause.
3. Patients with a familial cardiomyopathy associated with sudden death.
4. Patients with LV noncompaction.

Class III: *ICD therapy is not indicated for*

1. Patients who do not have a reasonable expectation of survival with an acceptable functional status for at least 1 year.
2. Patients with incessant VT or VF.
3. Patients with significant psychiatric illnesses that may be aggravated by device implantation or that may preclude systematic follow-up.
4. NYHA Class IV patients with drug-refractory congestive heart failure who are not candidates for cardiac transplantation or chronic resynchronization therapy.
5. VF or VT that is amenable to surgical or catheter ablation.

LV, left ventricular; *NYHA*, New York Heart Association; *VF*, ventricular fibrillatio.
Adapted from A.E. Epstein, J.P. Dimarco, K.A. Ellenbogen, N.A. Estes 3rd, R.A. Freedman, L.S. Gettes, A.M. Gillinov, G. Gregoratos, S.C. Hammill, D.L. Hayes, M.A. Hlatky, L.K. Newby, R.L. Page, M.H. Schoenfeld, M.J. Silka, L.W. Stevenson, M.O. Sweeney, American College of Cardiology, American Heart Association Task Force on Practice Guidelines, American Association for Thoracic Surgery, Society of Thoracic Surgeons, ACC/AHA/HRS 2008 Guidelines for device-based therapy of cardiac rhythm abnormalities, Heart Rhythm 5 (6) (June 2008) e1–e62.

in children with an age at diagnosis less than 14.3 years, left ventricular posterior wall thinning and left ventricular dilation (z score >2.6), the incidence of sudden cardiac death increases to around 4%. The incidence was also significantly higher in patients on antiarrhythmic medications implying that either atrial or ventricular arrhythmias play a role in sudden death.

In the adult population, sudden cardiac death is a problem in patients awaiting heart transplantation and ICD implantation has been shown to be effective and is in fact a Class IIa indication all nonhospitalized patients awaiting heart transplantation [4]. However, in the pediatric population, ICD placement at listing for heart transplantation has not shown to reduce sudden cardiac death, all-cause mortality, or delisting [8]. It has also been shown in some studies not to be cost-effective to use prophylactic ICDs in children with dilated cardiomyopathy, poor ventricular function, and symptomatic heart failure [9]. The reason for the difference in the adult and pediatric population is very likely related to the lower sudden death rates seen in the pediatric population. However, in patients with an ischemic reason for their depressed cardiac function, the risk of sudden death may be higher (similar to the adult ischemic population) and ICD implantation may be warranted [10].

Despite their effectiveness in preventing sudden death, ICDs are not without complications. The two most common complications that occur in the pediatric population are inappropriate shocks and lead fracture. Other complications such as device or lead infection, ICD generator failure, lead dislodgement, and device or lead malfunction or recall are seen less frequently, but still play a role in clinical practice. Inappropriate shocks occur in around 20% of pediatric patients with common causes being lead failure, sinus or atrial tachycardias, and oversensing [11]. In the PLEASE study of 965 leads placed in pediatric and congenital heart disease patients, there was a 14% lead failure rate within 2 years of implant causing inappropriate shocks in 40% of patients [12]. Risk factors for lead failure included thin (<7 French) leads and patient age <8 years. Especially in the face of poor ventricular function, there is a risk of stroke following lead placement in any patient with intracardiac shunting (including a PFO) even in the presence of treatment with anticoagulants [13].

In nonhospitalized patients who need protection from the potential of sudden death from ventricular arrhythmias, a wearable automated defibrillator may serve as a viable option. This type of defibrillator is not implanted but is instead worn on the chest as a vest. The device has electrodes that contact the skin and monitor for ventricular tachycardia or fibrillation. If the device senses an abnormal ventricular rhythm, it releases gel packets in the device and then is cable of defibrillating the patient using the vest. These devices have been shown to be safe and effective in the pediatric population [14]. However, there is an incidence of inappropriate shocks in patients using this therapy. In addition, the device must be worn to be effective and compliance rates may be low in the pediatric (particularly teenage) population presumably because of the size and discomfort of the device.

Another potential option for ICD therapy is the subcutaneous ICD. These devices have been shown to be effective for terminating ventricular arrhythmias but require a higher amount of energy to convert arrhythmias than transvenous devices (average of 36.6 J for subcutaneous devices vs. 11.1 J for transvenous devices) [15]. For this reason, the subcutaneous ICD generator is over twice the size of a comparable transvenous defibrillator. Minimum size requirements for the first and second generation of devices are a weight of around 25–30 kg and age of 8–9 years. This system has the advantage of not containing any hardware within the vascular space thus eliminating the risk for venous occlusion and thromboemboli. This also greatly decreases the risk of systemic bacteremia and sepsis from a lead infection. It has the disadvantage of not being able to provide routine pacing and having a high incidence of inappropriate shocks (around 7%–13%) from oversensing of T waves and external interference, in addition to potential inappropriate shocks from sinus tachycardia or atrial arrhythmias [16]. In addition, for the detection algorithm to work properly, the patient must pass a screening procedure prior to device placement. This involves placing ECG electrodes on the chest to ensure that the patient's ECG is suitable for the device to detect ventricular arrhythmias. Up to 15% of patients will fail this screening procedure and are therefore not candidates for device placement [17].

CHRONIC RESYNCHRONIZATION THERAPY

Dyssynchronous ventricular contractions can play a significant role in the clinical symptoms of patients with heart failure, including in pediatric patients [18]. In patients with a bundle branch block, ventricular activation propagates directly through ventricular myocardium, which can be up to 4 times slower than impulses passing through the His-Purkinje system [19]. This results in dyssynchronous electrical activation and mechanical contraction causing opposing walls of the ventricle to contract out of phase reducing the efficiency of ventricular contractions.

CRT also known as biventricular pacing is used to try to promote ventricular synchrony in patients with heart failure and a wide QRS by pacing the ventricle(s) from two different sites. By causing contraction of the ventricle(s) in two different areas that are far apart from each other, CRT may serve to decrease electromechanical dyssynchrony and cause more coordinated contractions in the ventricle. Promoting more synchronous contractions by pacing has been shown to improve heart failure symptoms in adults and may decrease both mortality and hospitalization rates. However, there are limited data in pediatric patients and most of the data come from patients with underlying congenital heart disease [20–22]. Although approximately 70% of adult patients have a beneficial response, around 90% of pediatric patients symptomatically benefit from CRT. Patients with the worst function tend to have the best response, and using biventricular pacing as a bridge to transplant may have the most utility. However, there is a significant complication rate (around 20%–30%), and there have been deaths associated with the procedure.

CRT can be achieved in several different fashions. A CRT system generally involves four components: an atrial pacing lead, two ventricular pacing leads, and a CRT pulse pacemaker generator (see Fig. 45.1). In patients with a structurally normal heart, one of the ventricular leads is typically a standard transvenous pacing or ICD lead placed into the right ventricle. A second lead is then placed to pace the left ventricle. This can be achieved transvenously by placing a specially designed lead in the coronary sinus into a lateral coronary vein that is then capable of pacing the left ventricle. It is important not to pace the left ventricle endocardially directly from the left ventricular cavity (by placing a lead across a patent foramen ovale) as there is a significant risk of thromboembolic complications including stroke even if the patient is treated with anticoagulant therapy. Alternatively, if coronary sinus lead placement is not possible, it is possible to place an epicardial pacing lead on the left ventricle. If ICD functionality is needed, a standard ICD lead can be substituted for one of the ventricular leads and connected to a CRT-ICD generator (CRT-D system).

The three leads (one atrial and two ventricular) are then connected to the pacing generator. In patients in sinus rhythm, the contraction of the atrium from the patient's own sinus rhythm is sensed. The ventricles are then stimulated to contract by the ventricular pacing leads. The atrioventricular delay is typically set very short to promote pacing with synchronous contraction rather than native conduction with dyssynchronous contraction. Most devices can be programmed to pace the left ventricle and right ventricle at different times. Offsetting the timing of ventricular stimulation may create a more synchronous ventricular contraction and the process of finding the best timing for the most synchronous contraction is known as optimization. It is controversial if optimization is highly beneficial for improvement of patient symptoms, and it is also

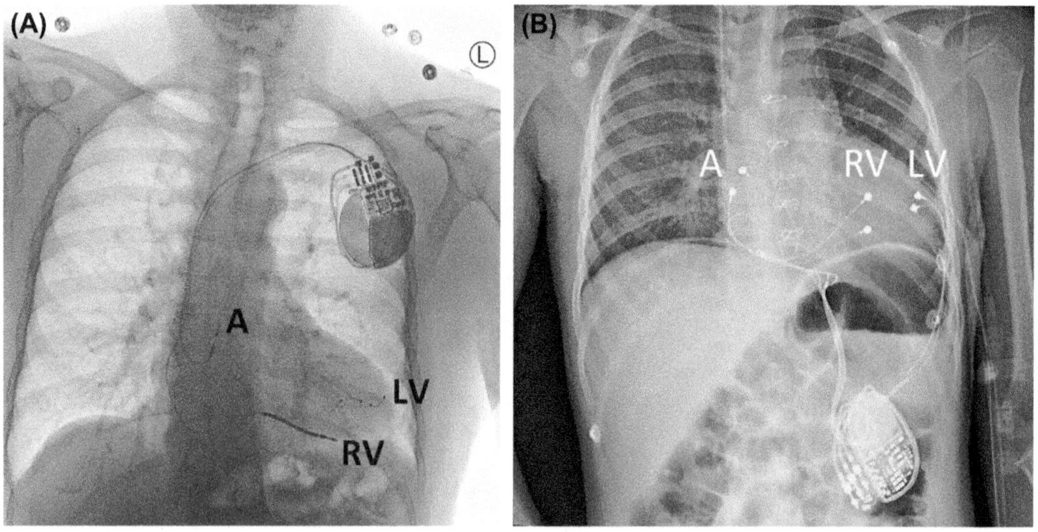

FIGURE 45.1 (A) Transvenous cardiac resynchronization therapy (CRT-D) system. (CRT system with implantable cardioverter defibrillator (ICD) capabilities). The right ventricular ICD lead is placed in a standard fashion across the tricuspid valve into the right ventricle. The left ventricular lead is placed through the coronary sinus into a small vein on the lateral aspect of the left ventricle. *A*, atrial pacing lead; *LV*, left ventricular pacing lead; *RV*, right ventricular ICD lead. (B) Epicardial CRT pacing system placed in a 6-year-old. All leads have been sewn on epicardially in the operating room through a sternotomy and then tunneled to a generator placed in the abdomen. *A*, atrial pacing lead; *LV*, left ventricular pacing lead; *RV*, right ventricular pacing lead.

controversial the best method to optimize pacemaker timing. Different centers have used echocardiograms to optimize programming including ejection fraction, strain imaging, tissue Doppler imaging, and vector velocity imaging [23]. However, determining the pacing configuration with the most narrow QRS duration on a surface ECG may be just as effective in pediatric patients and reduces the cost and time required for pacemaker optimization [24].

Guidelines for CRT therapy were published in 2012 and are listed in Table 45.2 [25]. CRT is generally only beneficial when the ejection fraction is less than 35% and is only indicated after medical therapy is optimized. CRT only improves symptoms and does not decrease the incidence of arrhythmias or increase survival. There is some evidence that CRT may be beneficial with more narrow QRS durations and in patients with a right bundle branch block pattern, but it tends to have a lower success rate in these patients and is therefore not a Class I indication. CRT is NOT recommended for patients with New York Heart Association (NYHA) Class I or II symptoms and non-left bundle branch block (LBBB) pattern with QRS duration less than 150 ms.

CRT may have a positive remodeling effect during somatic growth and may have benefits of reverse remodeling with long-term pacing. Although CRT utilizing two leads can be beneficial, synchronous left ventricular contractions can be achieved by placing a single lead in the left ventricular apex and left ventricular apical pacing should be considered in all patients undergoing epicardial pacemaker implantation. Chronic right ventricular pacing can lead to decreased left ventricular function over time and CRT may be considered as a first line therapy in patients with poor ventricular function who require right ventricular pacing >40% of the time particularly in patients with complete AV block who are paced a significant majority of the time [25].

USING DEVICE-BASED TECHNOLOGY TO PREDICT HEART FAILURE

Several different techniques have been used in pacemakers and ICDs to try to quantitate a patient's degree of heart failure and predict when a patient is going to have an episode of acute heart failure. These devices use different techniques to detect and monitor heart failure. However, this technology has limited utility in the pediatric heart failure population.

One type of system uses a wireless monitoring sensor that is implanted via cardiac catheterization in the pulmonary artery and directly measures pulmonary artery pressure. An increase in pulmonary artery pressure may precede other measures of worsening heart failure such as increased peripheral edema. The utility of these devices in the pediatric population has not been well established. In addition, there is concern about long-term difficulty in removing the device and the potential for thrombus formation and subsequent pulmonary issues related to the thrombus or emboli produced by the device, and this is particularly true in small children. A second type of system uses thoracic impedance measurements on an already implanted pacemaker or ICD to predict heart failure. Because most patients with heart failure decompensation demonstrate pulmonary congestion as a result of elevated left ventricular filling pressures, device-based diagnostics to

TABLE 45.2 Indications for Cardiac Resynchronization Therapy

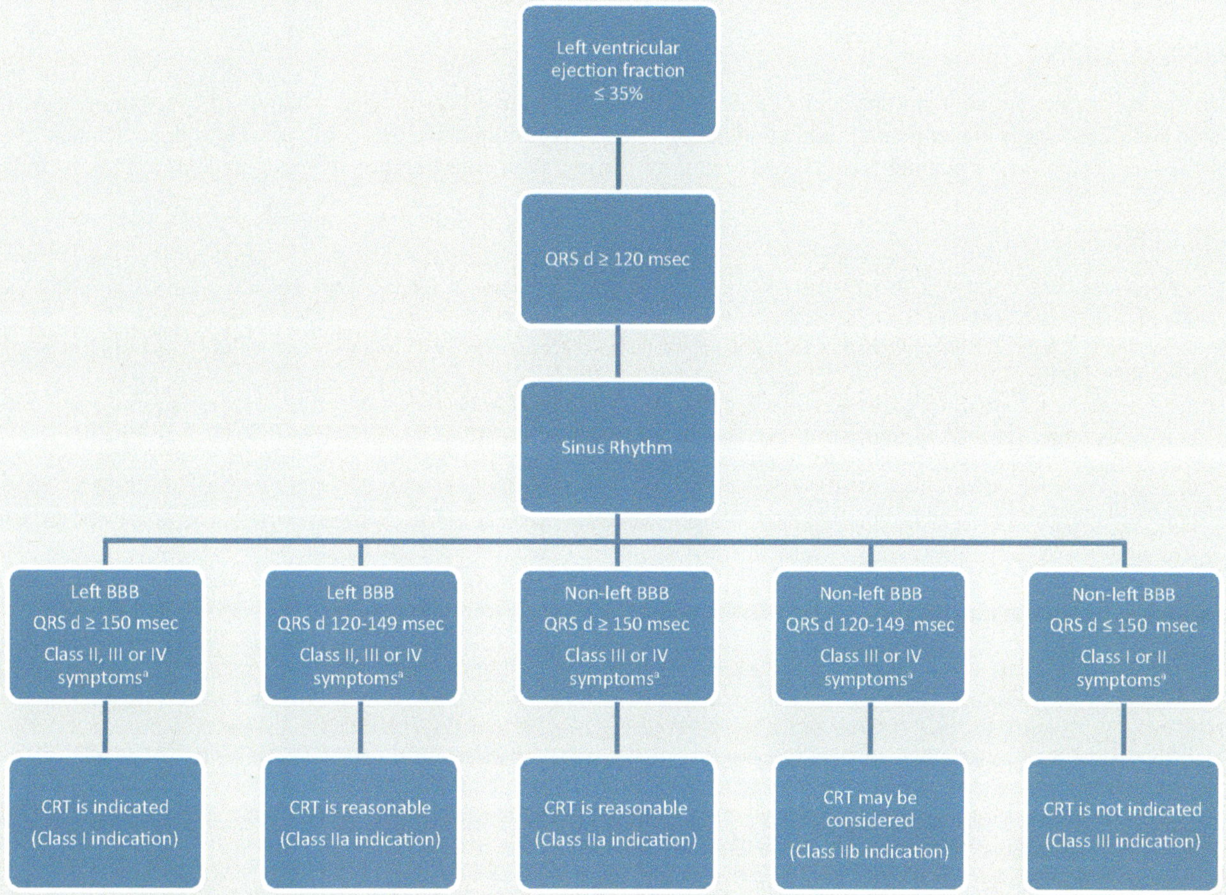

[a] New York Heart Association Symptoms on guideline directed medical therapy (GDMT).
BBB, bundle branch block, *CRT*, chronic resynchronization therapy; *ms*, milliseconds; *QRS d*, QRS duration on ECG.
Adapted from A.E. Epstein, J.P. DiMarco, K.A. Ellenbogen, N.A. Estes 3rd, R.A. Freedman, L.S. Gettes, A.M. Gillinov, G. Gregoratos, S.C. Hammill, D.L. Hayes, M.A. Hlatky, L.K. Newby, R.L. Page, M.H. Schoenfeld, M.J. Silka, L.W. Stevenson, M.O. Sweeney, American College of Cardiology Foundation, American Heart Association Task Force on Practice Guidelines, Heart Rhythm Society, 2012 ACCF/AHA/HRS focused update incorporated into the ACCF/AHA/HRS 2008 guidelines for device-based therapy of cardiac rhythm abnormalities: a report of the American College of Cardiology Foundation/American Heart Association Task Force on Practice Guidelines and the Heart Rhythm Society, Circulation 127 (3) (January 22, 2013) e283–e352.

estimate lung fluid content may provide an indirect indicator of volume status. Measurements of intrathoracic impedance can be evaluated in many ICDs and pacemakers by applying a small electric impulse between the pacing lead in the ventricle and the generator. The thoracic impedance is directly related to the overall fluid status. As the patient's lungs become congested from heart failure, intrathoracic impedance tends to decrease. Similarly, an increase in intrathoracic impedance may indicate the patient's lungs are becoming less congested. These trends can then be tracked via the ICD or pacemaker. Although the thoracic impedance is not a perfect surrogate, it can be used along with clinical symptoms to help make decisions regarding heart failure therapy. These monitoring devices may help decrease hospital admissions for heart failure [26]. The impedance trends for the ICD can be monitored by a physician remotely from the patient's home via a wireless transmission device. Although the sensitivity and positive predictive value of thoracic-based impedance measurements has relatively good correlation with clinical symptoms in adults, the accuracy in the pediatric and adult congenital population is low (sensitivity 33% and PPV ≤4.4% in one study) [27].

Changes in impedance tend to occur as early as 10–14 days in advance of clinically symptomatic heart failure and may occur before the onset of clinical symptoms. However, some data suggest this may not be a very accurate method for predicting clinically important heart failure. In a randomized prospective trial in adults (Diagnostic Outcome Trial in Heart Failure), treatment guided by routine monitoring of intrathoracic impedance did not improve clinical outcomes [28]. This may be even less accurate in children as children tend to have a higher body water composition, which may make impedance measurements less useful.

CONCLUSION

In summary, devices are an important adjunct in the treatment of pediatric heart failure. Although the incidence of device-related complications is higher than the adult population, the utility of implanted devices to prevent sudden death, improve heart failure symptoms, or monitor heart failure symptoms warrant their consideration in young patients with heart failure.

REFERENCES

[1] A.P. Hallstrom, M.S. Eisenberg, L. Bergner, The persistence of ventricular fibrillation and its implication for evaluating EMS, Emerg. Health Serv. Q. 1 (4) (1982 Summer) 41–49.

[2] M. Santini, C. Lavalle, R.P. Ricci, Primary and secondary prevention of sudden cardiac death: who should get an ICD? Heart 93 (11) (November 2007) 1478–1483.

[3] J.H. Heersche, N.A. Blom, F. van de Heuvel, C. Blank, A.G. Reimer, S.A. Clur, M. Witsenburg, A.D. ten Harkel, Implantable cardioverter defibrillator therapy for prevention of sudden cardiac death in children in The Netherlands, Pacing Clin. Electrophysiol. 33 (2) (February 2010) 179–185.

[4] A.E. Epstein, J.P. Dimarco, K.A. Ellenbogen, N.A. Estes 3rd, R.A. Freedman, L.S. Gettes, A.M. Gillinov, G. Gregoratos, S.C. Hammill, D.L. Hayes, M.A. Hlatky, L.K. Newby, R.L. Page, M.H. Schoenfeld, M.J. Silka, L.W. Stevenson, M.O. Sweeney, American College of Cardiology, American Heart Association Task Force on Practice Guidelines, American Association for Thoracic Surgery; Society of Thoracic Surgeons, ACC/AHA/HRS 2008 guidelines for device-based therapy of cardiac rhythm abnormalities, Heart Rhythm 5 (6) (June 2008) e1–62.

[5] E.S. DeWitt, J.K. Triedman, F. Cecchin, D.Y. Mah, D.J. Abrams, E.P. Walsh, K. Gauvreau, M.E. Alexander, Time dependence of risks and benefits in pediatric primary prevention implantable cardioverter-defibrillator therapy, Circ. Arrhythm. Electrophysiol. 7 (6) (December 2014) 1057–1063.

[6] V.V. Dimas, S.W. Denfield, R.A. Friedman, B.C. Cannon, J.J. Kim, E.O. Smith, S.K. Clunie, J.F. Price, J.A. Towbin, W.J. Dreyer, N.J. Kertesz, Frequency of cardiac death in children with idiopathic dilated cardiomyopathy, Am. J. Cardiol. 104 (11) (December 1, 2009) 1574–1577.

[7] E. Pahl, L.A. Sleeper, C.E. Canter, D.T. Hsu, M. Lu, S.A. Webber, S.D. Colan, P.F. Kantor, M.D. Everitt, J.A. Towbin, J.L. Jefferies, B.D. Kaufman, J.D. Wilkinson, S.E. Lipshultz, Pediatric Cardiomyopathy Registry Investigators, Incidence of and risk factors for sudden cardiac death in children with dilated cardiomyopathy: a report from the Pediatric Cardiomyopathy Registry, J. Am. Coll. Cardiol. 59 (6) (February 7, 2012) 607–615.

[8] I. El-Assaad, S.G. Al-Kindi, G.H. Oliveira, G.J. Boyle, P.F. Aziz, Implantable cardioverter-defibrillator and wait-list outcomes in pediatric patients awaiting heart transplantation, Heart Rhythm 12 (12) (December 2015) 2443–2448.

[9] B. Feingold, G. Arora, S.A. Webber, K.J. Smith, Cost-effectiveness of implantable cardioverter-defibrillators in children with dilated cardiomyopathy, J. Card. Fail. 16 (9) (September 2010) 734–741.

[10] E.K. Rhee, C.E. Canter, S. Basile, S.A. Webber, D.C. Naftel, Sudden death prior to pediatric heart transplantation: would implantable defibrillators improve outcome? J. Heart Lung Transplant. 26 (5) (May 2007) 447–452.

[11] C.I. Berul, G.F. Van Hare, N.J. Kertesz, A.M. Dubin, F. Cecchin, K.K. Collins, B.C. Cannon, M.E. Alexander, J.K. Triedman, E.P. Walsh, R.A. Friedman, Results of a multicenter retrospective implantable cardioverter-defibrillator registry of pediatric and congenital heart disease patients, J. Am. Coll. Cardiol. 51 (17) (April 29, 2008) 1685–1691.

[12] J. Atallah, C.C. Erickson, F. Cecchin, A.M. Dubin, I.H. Law, M.I. Cohen, M.J. Lapage, B.C. Cannon, T.U. Chun, V. Freedenberg, M. Gierdalski, C.I. Berul, Pediatric, Congenital Electrophysiology Society (PACES), Multi-institutional study of implantable defibrillator lead performance in children and young adults: results of the Pediatric Lead Extractability and Survival Evaluation (PLEASE) study, Circulation 127 (24) (June 18, 2013) 2393–2402.

[13] C.V. DeSimone, P.A. Friedman, A. Noheria, N.A. Patel, D.C. DeSimone, S. Bdeir, C.A. Aakre, V.R. Vaidya, J.P. Slusser, D.O. Hodge, M.J. Ackerman, A.A. Rabinstein, S.J. Asirvatham, Stroke or transient ischemic attack in patients with transvenous pacemaker or defibrillator and echocardiographically detected patent foramen ovale, Circulation 128 (13) (September 24, 2013) 1433–1441.

[14] K.K. Collins, J.N. Silva, E.K. Rhee, M.S. Schaffer, Use of a wearable automated defibrillator in children compared to young adults, Pacing Clin. Electrophysiol. 33 (9) (September 2010) 1119–1124.

[15] G.H. Bardy, W.M. Smith, M.A. Hood, I.G. Crozier, I.C. Melton, L. Jordaens, D. Theuns, R.E. Park, D.J. Wright, D.T. Connelly, S.P. Fynn, F.D. Murgatroyd, J. Sperzel, J. Neuzner, S.G. Spitzer, A.V. Ardashev, A. Oduro, L. Boersma, A.H. Maass, I.C. Van Gelder, A.A. Wilde, P.F. van Dessel, R.E. Knops, C.S. Barr, P. Lupo, R. Cappato, A.A. Grace, An entirely subcutaneous implantable cardioverter-defibrillator, N. Engl. J. Med. 363 (1) (July 1, 2010) 36–44.

[16] M.C. Burke, M.R. Gold, B.P. Knight, C.S. Barr, D.A. Theuns, L.V. Boersma, R.E. Knops, R. Weiss, A.R. Leon, J.M. Herre, M. Husby, K.M. Stein, P.D. Lambiase, Safety and efficacy of the totally subcutaneous implantable defibrillator: 2-year results from a pooled analysis of the IDE study and EFFORTLESS registry, J. Am. Coll. Cardiol. 65 (16) (April 28, 2015) 1605–1615.

[17] D.A. Randles, N.M. Hawkins, M. Shaw, A.Y. Patwala, S.J. Pettit, D.J. Wright, How many patients fulfil the surface electrocardiogram criteria for subcutaneous implantable cardioverter-defibrillator implantation? Europace 16 (7) (July 2014) 1015–1021.

[18] M.K. Friedberg, N.H. Silverman, A.M. Dubin, D.N. Rosenthal, Mechanical dyssynchrony in children with systolic dysfunction secondary to cardiomyopathy: a Doppler tissue and vector velocity imaging study, J. Am. Soc. Echocardiogr. 20 (6) (June 2007) 756–763.

[19] R.J. Myerburg, K. Milsson, H. Gelband, Physiology of canine intraventricular conduction and endocardial excitation, Circ. Res. 30 (1972) 217–243.

[20] A.M. Dubin, J. Janousek, E. Rhee, M.J. Strieper, F. Cecchin, I.H. Law, K.M. Shannon, J. Temple, E. Rosenthal, F.J. Zimmerman, A. Davis, P.P. Karpawich, A. Al Ahmad, V.L. Vetter, N.J. Kertesz, M. Shah, C. Snyder, E. Stephenson, M. Emmel, S. Sanatani, R. Kanter, A. Batra, K.K. Collins, Resynchronization therapy in pediatric and congenital heart disease patients: an international multicenter study, J. Am. Coll. Cardiol. 46 (12) (December 20, 2005) 2277–2283.

[21] J. Janousek, R.A. Gebauer, H. Abdul-Khaliq, M. Turner, L. Kornyei, O. Grollmuss, E. Rosenthal, E. Villain, A. Früh, T. Paul, N.A. Blom, J.M. Happonen, U. Bauersfeld, J.R. Jacobsen, F. van den Heuvel, T. Delhaas, J. Papagiannis, C. Trigo, Working Group for Cardiac Dysrhythmias and Electrophysiology of the Association for European Paediatric Cardiology, Cardiac resynchronisation therapy in paediatric and congenital heart disease: differential effects in various anatomical and functional substrates, Heart 95 (14) (July 2009) 1165–1171.

[22] F. Cecchin, P.A. Frangini, D.W. Brown, F. Fynn-Thompson, M.E. Alexander, J.K. Triedman, K. Gauvreau, E.P. Walsh, C.I. Berul, Cardiac resynchronization therapy (and multisite pacing) in pediatrics and congenital heart disease: five years experience in a single institution, J. Cardiovasc. Electrophysiol. 20 (1) (January 2009) 58–65.

[23] E.A. Greene, C.I. Berul, Pacing treatment for dilated cardiomyopathy: optimization of resynchronization pacing in pediatrics, Curr. Opin. Cardiol. 25 (2) (March 2010) 95–101.

[24] R. Punn, D. Hanisch, K.S. Motonaga, D.N. Rosenthal, S.R. Ceresnak, A.M. Dubin, A pilot study assessing ECG versus ECHO ventriculoventricular optimization in pediatric resynchronization patients, J. Cardiovasc. Electrophysiol. 27 (2) (February 2016) 210–216.

[25] A.E. Epstein, J.P. DiMarco, K.A. Ellenbogen, N.A. Estes 3rd, R.A. Freedman, L.S. Gettes, A.M. Gillinov, G. Gregoratos, S.C. Hammill, D.L. Hayes, M.A. Hlatky, L.K. Newby, R.L. Page, M.H. Schoenfeld, M.J. Silka, L.W. Stevenson, M.O. Sweeney, American College of Cardiology Foundation, American Heart Association Task Force on Practice Guidelines, Heart Rhythm Society, 2012 ACCF/AHA/HRS focused update incorporated into the ACCF/AHA/HRS 2008 guidelines for device-based therapy of cardiac rhythm abnormalities: a report of the American College of Cardiology Foundation/American Heart Association Task Force on Practice Guidelines and the Heart Rhythm Society, Circulation 127 (3) (January 22, 2013) e283–352.

[26] C.M. Yu, L. Wang, E. Chau, R.H. Chan, S.L. Kong, M.O. Tang, J. Christensen, R.W. Stadler, C.P. Lau, Intrathoracic impedance monitoring in patients with heart failure: correlation with fluid status and feasibility of early warning preceding hospitalization, Circulation 112 (6) (August 9, 2005) 841–848.

[27] M.J. LaPage, J. von Alvensleben, M. Dick, G. Serwer, D.J. Bradley, Utility of intrathoracic impedance monitoring in pediatric and congenital heart disease, Pacing Clin. Electrophysiol. 36 (8) (August 2013) 994–999.

[28] D.J. van Veldhuisen, F. Braunschweig, V. Conraads, I. Ford, M.R. Cowie, G. Jondeau, J. Kautzner, R.M. Aguilera, M. Lunati, C.M. Yu, B. Gerritse, M. Borggrefe, DOT-HF Investigators. Intrathoracic impedance monitoring, audible patient alerts, and outcome in patients with heart failure, Circulation 124 (16) (October 18, 2011) 1719–1726.

Chapter 46

Catheter Device Therapies for Heart Failure

Frank Ing[1,2], Patrick Sullivan[1,2], Cheryl Takao[1,2]
[1]Children's Hospital Los Angeles, Los Angeles, CA, United States; [2]University of Southern California, Los Angeles, CA, United States

Heart failure or reduced cardiac output is defined by the pathophysiologic state where the heart is unable to pump oxygen and blood to meet the body's metabolic demands. Preload, afterload, contractility, and heart rate are determinants of cardiac output. In adults, intrinsic depression in cardiac contractility from, for example, ischemic heart disease leads to congestive heart failure (CHF).

In pediatrics, while heart failure can be caused intrinsic depression of cardiac contractility, it can also be caused by structural heart defects, congenital, postsurgical, or acquired. Abnormal loading conditions placed on the heart can lead to heart failure even when contractility remains relatively normal.

Pediatric heart failure secondary to structural defects can be separated into two major groups: obstructive and volume overload lesions. Obstructive lesions include obstruction to inflow and outflow of systemic or pulmonary flow. Volume overloading lesions (or left-to-right shunts) include septal defects or any systemic-to-pulmonary arterial connection including aortopulmonary collaterals and coronary artery fistulas (CAFs). A third group of miscellaneous lesions discussed in this chapter includes valvar regurgitation, which adds a volume load on the heart, and can lead to heart failure, pericardial tamponed, and restrictive atrial septum in certain congenital heart lesions.

Diagnosis of structural heart disease has been made easier with the advances in echocardiography and other cardiac imaging modalities including CT and MRI. It is important to emphasize that not all structural heart lesions leading to heart failure can be treated by transcatheter interventions alone. Some of the lesions will require surgical intervention or a collaborative approach as in hybrid therapy.

In this chapter, we will focus on interventions that can treat certain forms of congenital or postsurgical obstructive lesions, volume loading shunts, and other miscellaneous lesions leading to or exacerbating heart failure.

OBSTRUCTION LESIONS

This group includes both right and left heart obstructive lesions and includes both inflow obstruction at the level of the atrioventricular valves and outflow obstructions at the level of the semilunar valves and along the pulmonary or systemic arterial tree.

Tricuspid Valve Stenosis

Tricuspid valve stenosis rarely is an isolated lesion in the newborn and often is accompanied by varying degrees of right ventricular hypoplasia, pulmonary stenosis or atresia, and an atrial septal defect (ASD). However, physiologically, stenosis of the tricuspid valve limits preload to the heart and impairs filling of the right ventricle and pulmonary arteries and results in poor cardiac output. It causes systemic venous congestion with jugular venous distension, ascites, and peripheral edema. In newborns, an adequate atrial communication to decompress the right atrium (RA) is necessary to allow blood flow from the RA to left atrium (LA), which results in cyanosis, but provides adequate systemic output.

Congenital tricuspid valve stenosis is rarely intervened on in the catheterization laboratory. Oftentimes these patients have concomitant right ventricular hypoplasia therefore addressing the tricuspid valve alone may not be curative. However, balloon valvuloplasty for tricuspid valve stenosis with adequate annular dimension—most commonly not only caused by rheumatic disease but also caused by pacemaker leads, carcinoid syndrome, or infection—can be performed [1,2]. Rheumatic tricuspid valve stenosis is often associated with tricuspid insufficiency and left-sided valve disease.

Heart Failure in the Child and Young Adult. http://dx.doi.org/10.1016/B978-0-12-802393-8.00046-6

Indications for surgical or catheter intervention include a symptomatic patient with severe stenosis. Severe tricuspid stenosis is defined by a Doppler mean pressure gradient >5 mmHg, pressure half-time ≥190 ms, or valve area ≤1.0 cm^2. If significant tricuspid insufficiency is also noted, or if associated left-sided valve disease requires intervention, surgical repair is recommended. Balloon valvuloplasty is indicated for isolated severe tricuspid stenosis without insufficiency [3,4]. It can also be performed in a postoperative patient with stenosis of a bioprosthetic valve in the tricuspid valve position and transcatheter valve placement can be also considered. This will be discussed later in the chapter.

Technical considerations for intervention include single or double balloon use and wire placement for stability. Often a double balloon technique is utilized for an annulus >20 mm. Wire stability typically is maintained in the distal pulmonary arteries; however, some suggest using wire position in the right ventricular apex allowing for better positioning across the valve, along its natural axis [3]. During inflation of the balloons, cardiac output decreases and blood pressures will decrease. Monitoring blood pressure during intervention is important and pressures will improve when balloons are deflated.

Newborns with tricuspid valve stenosis are likely to be born with an atrial communication, such as a patent foramen ovale (PFO) or secundum ASD. However, for those with a restrictive ASD, balloon atrial septostomy may be required. Patients with an enlarged liver dilated inferior vena cava (IVC) and RA or poor cardiac output show signs of an inadequate atrial communication.

Balloon atrial septostomy was developed initially for patients with d-transposition of the great arteries (d-TGA). This procedure now is performed in other cardiac conditions in infants with a restrictive atrial septum. The balloon is inflated in the LA and rapidly withdrawn across the defect to tear the membranous inferior margin of the septum (Fig. 46.1). Successful septostomy occurs in most infants under 1 month of age. Over that age, the septum becomes thick and tough rendering septostomy ineffective. Use of blade septostomy or cutting balloons followed by further static balloon septostomy has shown more success.

Right Heart Outflow Obstruction

Obstructive lesions to outflow of the right heart include pulmonary valve stenosis, branch pulmonary artery stenosis, and pulmonary venous obstruction. These lesions limit the blood flow to the pulmonary circulation and also results in increased loading conditions on the right ventricle. Obstructive right heart lesions lead to compensatory right ventricular hypertrophy and if not intervened on will lead to right ventricular systolic and diastolic dysfunction and ultimately right heart failure.

Pulmonary Valve Stenosis

Transcatheter therapy for pulmonary valve stenosis was first reported in 1982 and remains the treatment of choice in patients of all ages. Normal pulmonary valve anatomy includes three cusps (tricuspid) and three commissures. Stenosis can result from fusion of one or more commissures. The pulmonary valve can also have two (bicuspid) or one (unicuspid) cusp configurations. Stenosis can also be caused by annular hypoplasia or valve morphology such as thickening of the leaflets due to increase in valve spongiosa, excessive fibrosis, collagenous, myxomatous, and elastic tissue. Regardless of the etiology, significant stenosis will result in right ventricular hypertrophy and if not intervened on will develop into right ventricular failure. This can occur in infancy, often termed "critical pulmonary stenosis" or anytime during infancy, childhood as well as in adults with severe pulmonary stenosis where the right ventricle dilates, tricuspid valve annulus dilates and significant tricuspid insufficiency develops. Critical pulmonary stenosis can present in the newborn and early infancy with severe right heart failure manifesting hepatomegaly and jaundice.

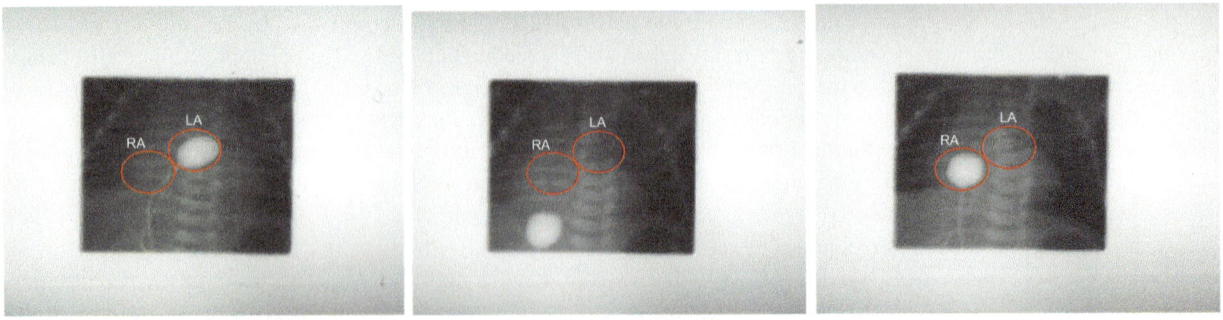

FIGURE 46.1 Balloon atrial septostomy: a rapid "jerk" of a short distance using a septostomy balloon under fluoroscopy and/or echocardiographic guidance resulted in tearing of the atrial septum in a newborn with d-TGA. It is not uncommon to see the balloon start in the left atrium (LA), then pulled fall below the diaphragm in the IVC before it "bounces" back into the right atrium (RA). *IVC*, inferior vena cava.

Indications for balloon valvuloplasty are similar to surgical indications. Mild stenosis (catheter peak systolic gradient <40 mmHg) often will remain mild over the lifetime of the patient and is well tolerated without symptoms. Class I indications for intervention include (1) A newborn with critical valvar pulmonary stenosis defined as a stenosis present at birth with cyanosis and evidence of dependence on a patent ductus arteriosus (PDA) for pulmonary blood flow; (2) Catheter peak-to-peak gradient ≥40 mmHg; or (3) Clinically significant obstruction in the presence of right ventricular dysfunction. See the current published American Heart Association (AHA) Guidelines for further indications [5].

Technical considerations for pulmonary valvuloplasty include angiographic exclusion of the right ventricle-dependent coronary circulation, balloon size selection, and careful evaluation of the subvalvar and supravalvar areas. Right ventricle angiogram is performed to evaluate any connection between the ventricular cavity and the coronary artery circulation. This is more commonly seen in patients with pulmonary atresia, however, should be evaluated in patients with critical pulmonary stenosis as well. If right ventricle to coronary connections is seen, aortic root or selective coronary angiograms should be performed to identify proximal coronary artery stenoses that indicate right ventricle-dependent coronary circulation. In such instances, once the pressure is lowered in the right ventricle by pulmonary valvuloplasty, coronary ischemia can result, and right ventricle-dependent coronary flow is a contraindication to pulmonary valvuloplasty. Once RV-dependent coronary artery circulation is excluded, the balloon diameter size selected is typically 120%–140% of the annulus diameter, which is measured on lateral projection from hinge point to hinge point. In our practice, if there is supravalvar stenosis, a conservative approach to minimize risk of pulmonary artery tear is to use a balloon 130% of the supravalvar narrowing. During balloon valvuloplasty, cardiac output will decrease with temporary occlusion of right heart output and blood pressures will decrease. After the balloon is deflated, the cardiac output improves and blood pressures will stabilize. However, careful attention to wire placement and positioning should be made to ensure blood pressures are maintained even prior to balloon valvuloplasty. Stiff wires can stent open the tricuspid valve thereby decreasing cardiac output and blood pressures. Patients with ASDs often will maintain cardiac output when the right ventricular outflow is occluded by diverting venous blood across the atrial septum to the LA. This will result in cyanosis but cardiac output and blood pressures will be somewhat maintained. Dynamic subpulmonary stenosis needs to be evaluated for after balloon valvuloplasty. When elevated right ventricular pressure is relieved, the hypertrophied ventricular infundibulum can collapse and result in severe subpulmonary obstruction leading to decreased cardiac output. This is referred to as the "suicide ventricle." Subpulmonary stenosis will regress with time; however, if it is severe, it may require beta-blockade to augment filling time, maintain adequate cardiac output, and minimize cyanosis due to persistent right-to-left shunting at the atrial level (Fig. 46.2).

Restenosis after successful balloon valvuloplasty is rare [6,7]. Pulmonary regurgitation is common, however, occurring in 10%–40% of patients [8]. Compared to surgical valvotomy, incidence, and severity of regurgitation were lower in the group treated with valvuloplasty. Although pulmonary insufficiency was felt to be well tolerated, children need to be monitored for right ventricle dilation and dysfunction at which time pulmonary valve implantation may be indicated. Dysplastic pulmonary valves commonly seen in Noonan syndrome have a lower success rate due to recoil in spite of adequate dilation. However, due to the low incidence of complications, balloon valvuloplasty is often attempted [9].

Pulmonary Valve Atresia

Pulmonary valve atresia with an intact ventricular septum is associated with varying degrees of right ventricle sizes. The right ventricle is composed of inlet, trabecular, and infundibular portions. In approximately two thirds of the patients, the right ventricle cavity is small. Often the inlet and trabecular portions are developed but in the more severe form, there is little/no infundibular portion, and there is a long distance from the outflow tract to the pulmonary artery. These patients are at higher risk for right ventricular coronary artery connections. Right ventricular-dependent coronary artery circulation will need to be evaluated for as discussed previously (Fig. 46.3). The remainder of the patients will have all three portions of the right ventricle developed and the pulmonary valve often will have three cusps but is thickened and myxomatous in appearance. In these patients the tricuspid valve orifice is increased and leaflets are abnormal with significant insufficiency. Approximately 10% will have Ebstein's anomaly of the tricuspid valve, which will often require surgical intervention.

If there is adequate size of the right ventricle and tricuspid valve and absence of right ventricular-dependent coronary circulation, transcatheter valve perforation and balloon valvuloplasty may be a good option for a membranous pulmonary atresia. Tricuspid valve size often correlates to right ventricular size therefore management is guided based on echocardiographic measurements.

Technical considerations include exclusion of RV-dependent coronary circulation and careful perforation of the pulmonary valve. Multiple techniques have been used to perforate the valve. Techniques include using the stiff end of a guidewire, transseptal needles, and radiofrequency perforation catheters or wires [10–14]. Placing a snare in the main pulmonary artery through the ductus arteriosus from the aorta provides a target for the perforation, minimizing risk of perforating the myocardium, or pulmonary artery. Patients may require an additional source of pulmonary blood flow by ductal stenting or

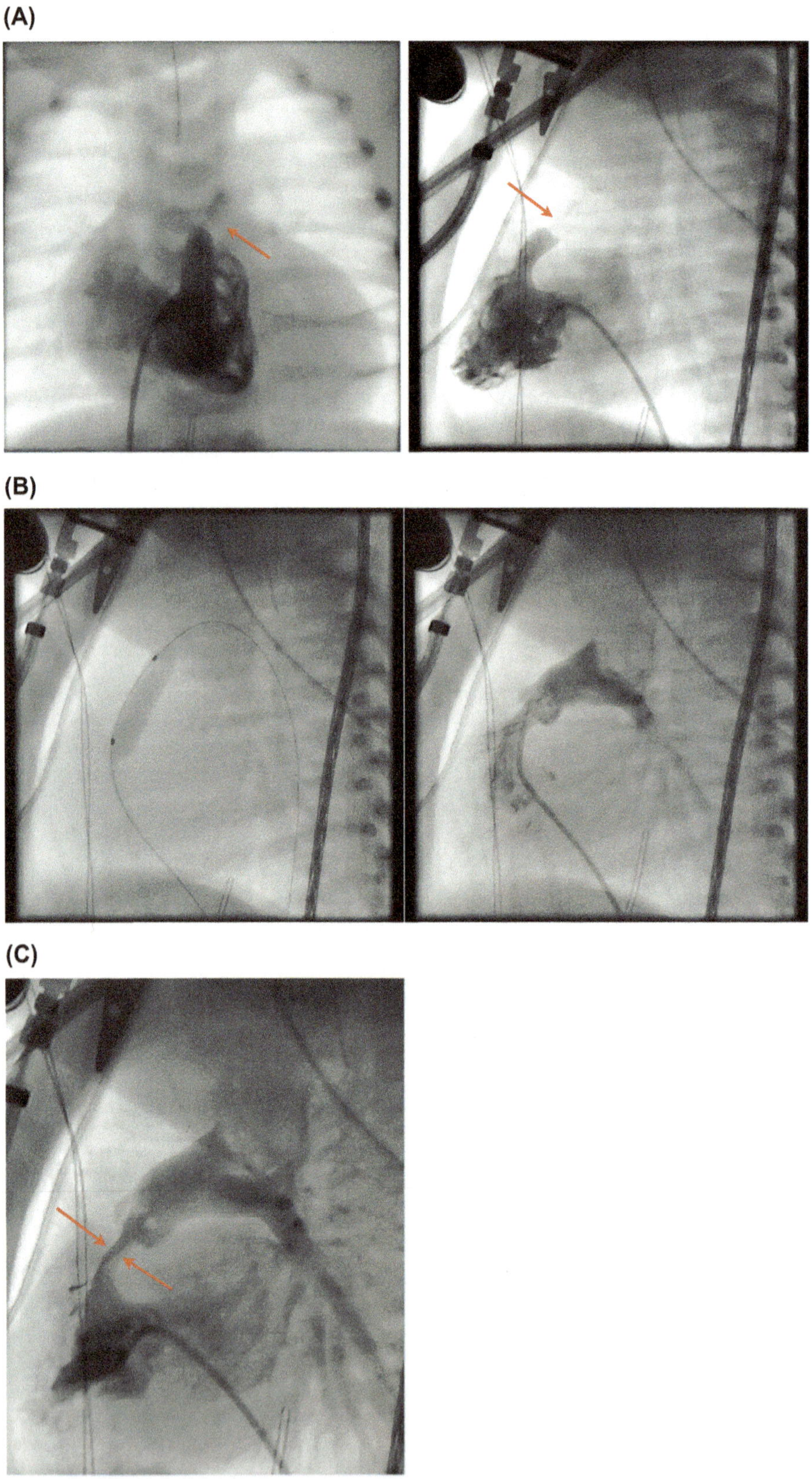

FIGURE 46.2 (A) AP and lateral projection of a neonate with severe pulmonary valve stenosis (*red arrows*). (B) Balloon valvuloplasty and angiogram showing improved flow across pulmonary valve. (C) Dynamic infundibular stenosis requiring beta-blockade.

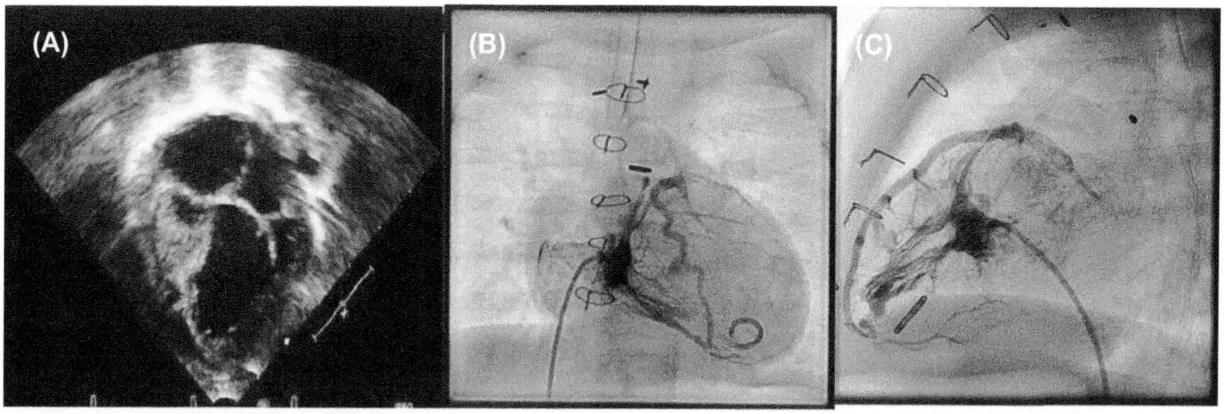

FIGURE 46.3 (A) Echocardiographic image of a severely hypoplastic right ventricle seen in pulmonary atresia with intact ventricular septum (B and C). Angiogram in the same hypoplastic right ventricle demonstrating bipartite ventricle with inlet and severely hypoplastic outlet portion of ventricle. Also right ventricle to coronary artery fistula is seen. There is right ventricle-dependent coronary circulation to the posterior descending coronary artery, precluding decompression of the right ventricle.

placement of a Blalock–Taussig shunt until right ventricular hypertrophy resolves, diastolic dysfunction improves, and RV cavity growth is adequate. This procedure needs to proceed cautiously as risks are higher than with valve stenosis. Risks include perforation of the right ventricle outflow tract or main pulmonary artery when perforating the valve. During balloon valvuloplasty, patients remain hemodynamically stable as they are receiving pulmonary blood flow through a PDA and maintain adequate cardiac output and blood pressures.

Tripartite ventricle and tricuspid valve size Z score ≥–2 has the highest chance at a two-ventricle repair. It has been shown that the right ventricle has potential to grow after the outflow tract has been opened [14,15]. Patients with tricuspid valve size Z scores between −2 and −3.5 may benefit from opening pulmonary valve with hope of a one and a half ventricle repair [16]. One and a half ventricle repair consists on a Glenn operation, which connects the superior vena cava to the right pulmonary artery (RPA), with an ASD closure. This separates the pulmonary and systemic circulations but off loads the right ventricle with the superior vena cava blood directed immediately to the pulmonary circulation.

Branch Pulmonary Artery Stenosis

Physiology

Branch pulmonary artery stenosis is commonly found in patients with congenital heart disease, occurring congenitally, or acquired postoperatively. Similar to pulmonary valvar stenosis, the chronic pressure load to the right ventricle can result in hypertrophy and eventual combination of systolic and diastolic dysfunction. Anatomically, branch pulmonary stenosis can be varied ranging from a simple discrete branch to multiple levels of stenoses involving the main branch, lobar branches, segmental branches, and subsegmental branches. They can present unilaterally or bilaterally. They can be discrete or long segment or the entire pulmonary arterial tree can be hypoplastic. The stenosis can be due to a surgical scar or a fold or twist or present congenitally in a variety of syndromes such as Alagille's or William's syndromes (Fig. 46.4).

Indications for Intervention

In general, guidelines include at least one of the following: (1) 20 mmHg gradient across a branch, (2) differential flow with less than 35% to the affected lung, and (3) RV pressure load on 2/3 systemic pressure. A relative indication includes pulmonary valve regurgitation (PR).

Interventions include angioplasty and/or stent implantation depending on a variety of factors. This is well documented in the AHA guidelines for interventions for CHD in 2011 [5].

Recommendations for Pulmonary Angioplasty

Class I

1. Pulmonary angioplasty is indicated for the treatment of significant peripheral branch pulmonary artery stenosis (see text for definition of "significant" stenosis) or for pulmonary artery stenosis in very small patients in whom primary stent implantation is not an option (Level of Evidence: B).

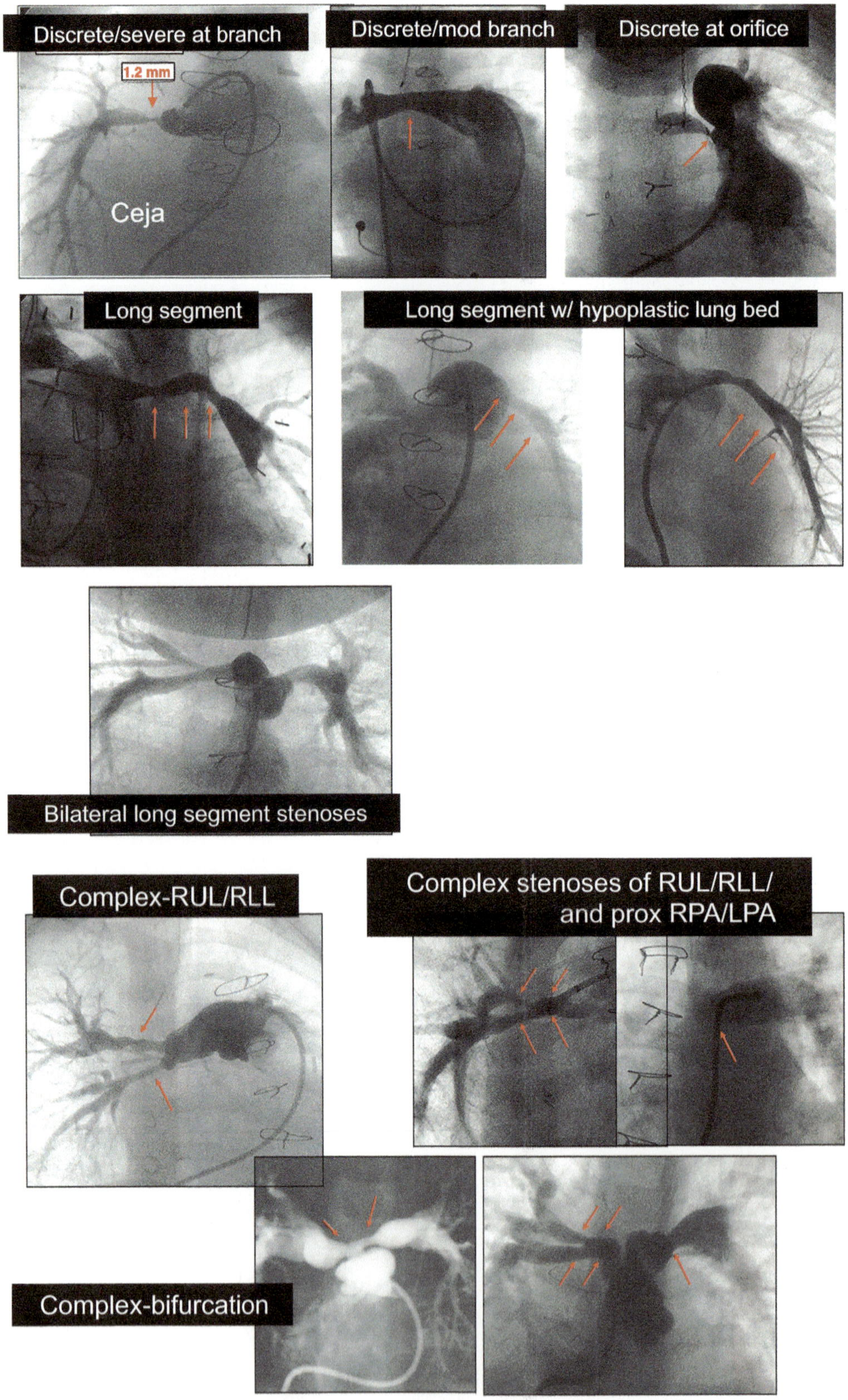

FIGURE 46.4 Diverse morphology of branch pulmonary artery stenoses.

Class IIa

1. Pulmonary angioplasty is reasonable to consider for treatment of significant distal arterial stenosis (as defined in the introduction to "Pulmonary Artery Angioplasty and Stent Placement") or for stenosis in larger, more proximal branch pulmonary arteries that do not appear to be amenable to primary stent implantation (Level of Evidence: B).

Class IIb

1. Pulmonary angioplasty may be considered for treatment of significant main pulmonary artery stenosis that results in an elevation of pressure to more than two-thirds of systemic pressure in the proximal pulmonary artery segment or in the RV (in the absence of pulmonary valve stenosis). This stenosis is usually a form of supravalvar pulmonic stenosis, which is not particularly responsive to balloon dilation alone (Level of Evidence: C).

Recommendations for Pulmonary Artery

Stent Placement

Class I

1. Primary intravascular stent implantation is indicated for the treatment of significant proximal or distal branch pulmonary artery stenosis when the vessel/patient is large enough to accommodate a stent that is capable of being dilated to the adult diameter of that vessel (Level of Evidence: B).

Class IIa

1. It is reasonable to consider pulmonary artery stent implantation in critically ill postoperative cardiac patients when it has been determined that significant branch pulmonary artery stenosis is resulting in a definite hemodynamic compromise in a patient/vessel of any size, particularly if balloon dilation is unsuccessful (Level of Evidence: B).
2. Primary intravascular stent implantation is reasonable in the treatment of significant stenosis of the main pulmonary artery segment that results in elevation of the RV pressure provided that the stent definitely will not compromise a functioning pulmonary valve and will not impinge on the pulmonary artery bifurcation (Level of Evidence: B).

Class IIb

1. It may be reasonable to implant small pulmonary artery stents that lack the potential to achieve adult size in small children as part of a cooperative surgical strategy to palliate severe branch pulmonary artery stenosis. These stents may need to be enlarged surgically or removed during a future planned operation (e.g., conduit replacement, Fontan completion) (Level of Evidence: C).

Technical Considerations

Standard techniques for stenting of pulmonary artery stenoses are well published and will not be covered here. Fig. 46.6 shows a case of stent implantation to treat a hypoplastic RPA and subsequent follow-up interventions in the process of rehabilitating the distal vessels. There is remarkable improvement in the growth of the distal small vessels poststenting (Figs. 46.5 and 46.6). It is important to note that in patients with a failing right ventricle, any stiff wires or delivery systems used can transiently cause or worsen pulmonary and/or tricuspid regurgitation resulting hypotension requiring volume and inotropic support just for the stent implant procedure. In patients with an ASD or PFO, blood pressures are usually stable but transient cyanosis from right to left shunting at the atrial level is seen during the procedure. Test balloon dilation of the stenotic vessel before stenting can be a useful test of RV reserve. Generally, when the balloon is inflated completely obstructing flow, the RV systolic pressure will rise. When the RV pressure does not rise as expected, it should be a warning sign that the RV systolic function is poor with low reserve. When severe bilateral branch pulmonary artery stenosis is found in the presence of depressed RV function, it may be advantageous to put the patient on extracorporeal membrane oxygenation prior to the intervention. Preprocedure discussion with the cardiac anesthesiologist and surgeon along with the critical care team is important to plan out the intervention as well as potential backup surgical plans and post–cath management.

Outcomes Data

Published data indicate excellent relief of RV pressure and gradient in the immediate term. However, many patients will require repeat interventions to further dilate the stented vessels to accommodate somatic growth of the child. True

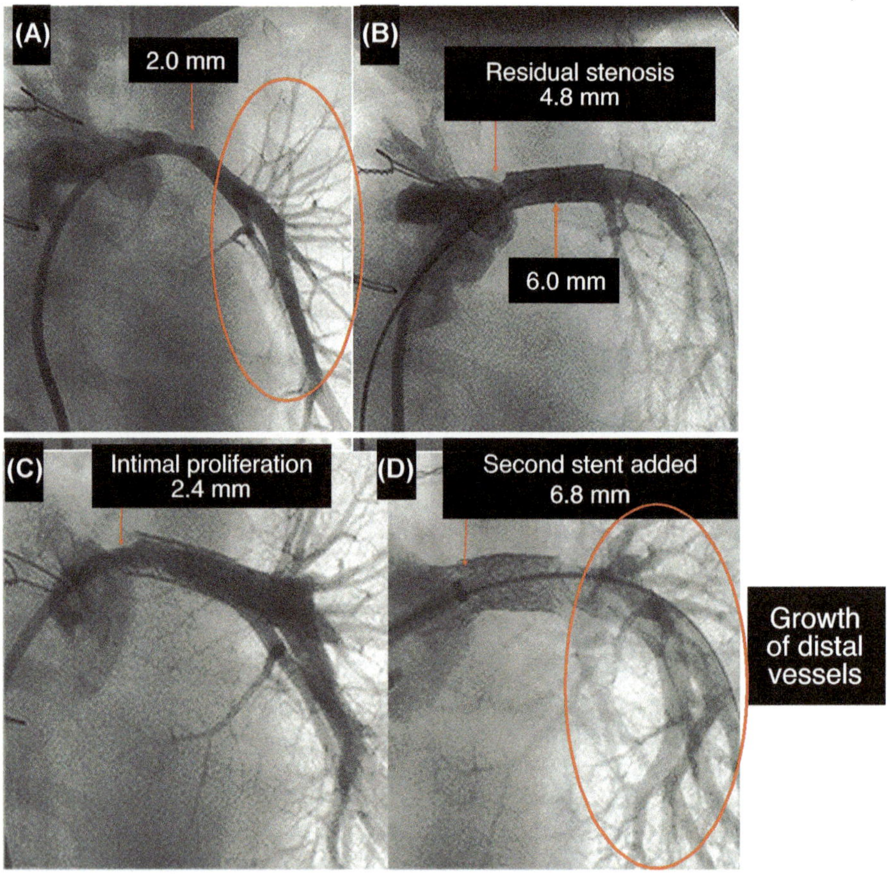

FIGURE 46.5 Severe left pulmonary artery (LPA) stenosis with a hypoplastic left pulmonary vascular bed (A). Following stenting, the diameter improves from 2 to 4.8 mm (B). At 6 months follow-up, there is in-stent intimal proliferation due to a small segment of unstented stenosis at the LPA ostium (C). An additional stent was placed at the ostium increasing the diameter from 2.4 to 6.8 mm. Notice the improvement of the distal vascular growth (D).

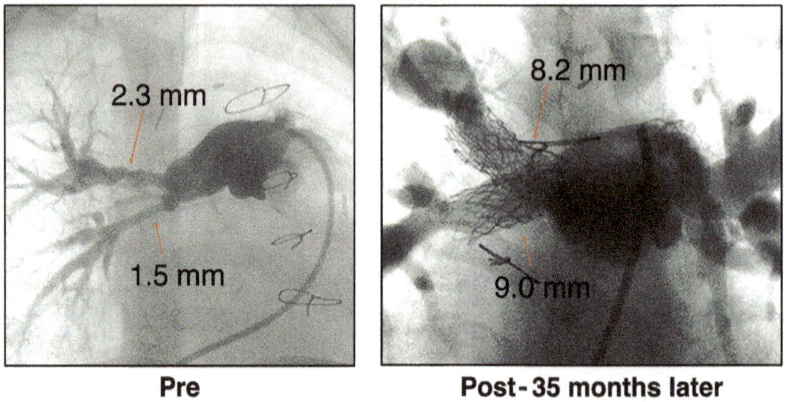

FIGURE 46.6 Complex lobar stenosis of unifocalized major aortopulmonary collateral arteries and stenting of the upper and lower lobes. After four interventions and 35 months later, there is significant enlargement of the stented vessels and distal vascular bed.

restenosis due to intimal proliferation is quite low ranging from 3% to 9% [17,18] but redilation or additional stenting can be performed successfully to maintain low RV pressures (generally ½ systemic). Redilation with additional stents appears to be easily accomplished [19,20]. In patients who require concomitant surgery such as right ventricle to pulmonary artery (RV-PA) conduit replacements, stenting can be performed in the operating room as a hybrid procedure. Law et al. reported long-term follow-up data (up to 15 years) and showed 91% of patients were in New York Heart Association (NYHA) class I and II at 13.2 ± 2.4 years poststenting. They concluded that there was long-term relief of branch pulmonary stenosis by implanted stents and that stents preserved RV function, improved quality of life, and avoided further surgery due to branch pulmonary stenosis. Figs. 46.7 and 46.8 show long-term follow-up angiograms illustrating persistent wide patency of stented pulmonary arteries.

A recent paper reviewing outcomes of stenting in the current era also showed an immediate success rate of 98% with improvement in minimal diameter from 5.1 ± 2 cm to 10.6 ± 3 cm ($P < .01$). Follow-up catheterization showed no significant change in minimal stent diameter (8.8 ± 2.6 to 7.8 ± 2.3 mm), gradient (7.7 ± 8.4 to 12.6 ± 12.2 mmHg) or right ventricular pressures (43.7 ± 9 to 47.7 ± 10.5 mmHg). 16% of patients underwent scheduled stent redilation over a period of 12 days–25 months [18].

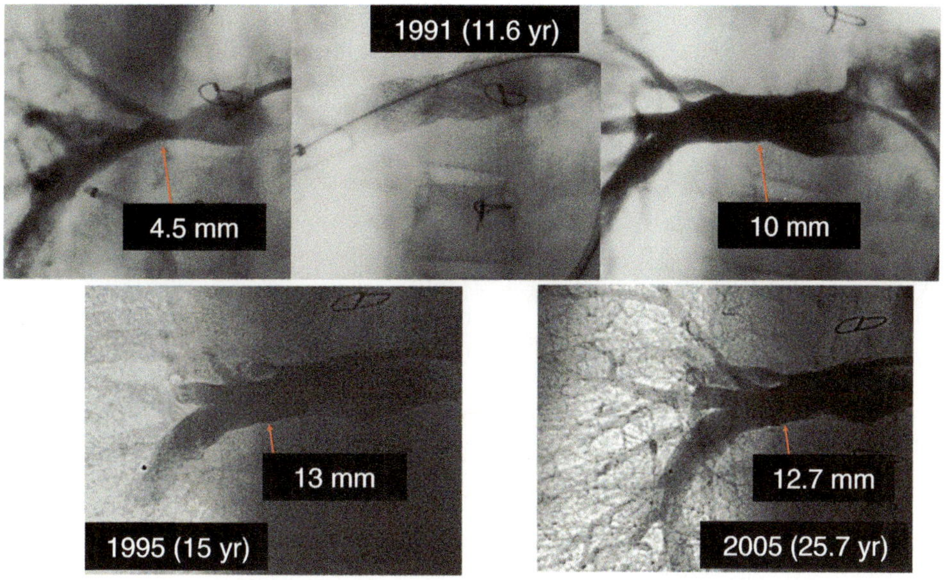

FIGURE 46.7 14-year follow-up with initial stenting in June, 1991, and last cath in January, 2005.

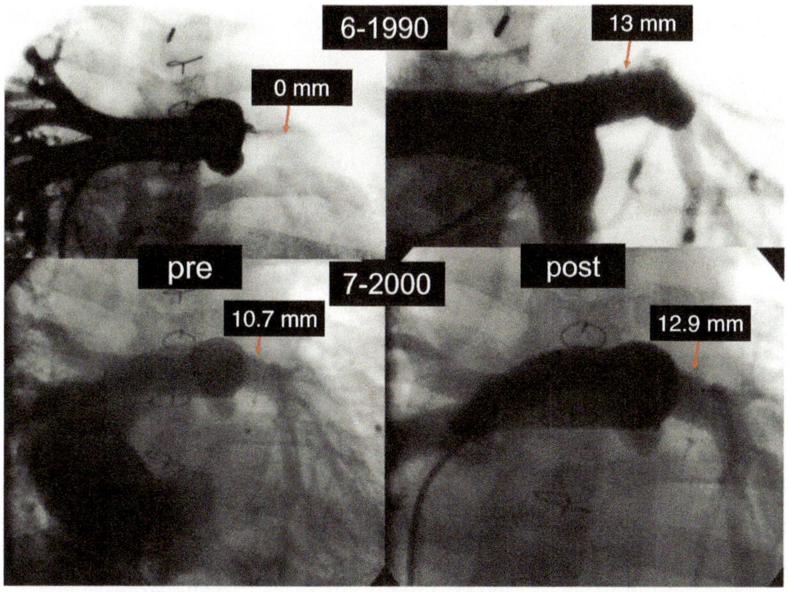

FIGURE 46.8 Hypoplastic left pulmonary artery in a Fontan patient stented in June, 1990 and last cath 10 years later in July, 2000.

Surgical reports are scant and results are poor with a recurrence rate of 35%–40% [21–27]. Angioplasty alone showed a success rate of 50%–60%, with a recurrence rate of 15% and complication rate of 6%–12% [22,28,29]. Small surgical series reported in the 2000s report outcomes that range from 100% success for surgical repair of supravalve stenosis to poor results for distal peripheral branch pulmonary stenosis [27,30–33]. In contrast, studies evaluating the effects of stent implantation report success rates as high as 90% [34–36].

Takao et al. [37] showed that upper and lower lobar branches on the side of the stented proximal branch had "catch-up" growth compared to the normal nonstented side in both single and two-ventricle patients. Interestingly, the authors noted more growth at the lobar level for two-ventricle versus single-ventricle patients.

Pulmonary Vein Obstruction

Physiology as Related to Heart Failure

Pulmonary vein stenosis can occur following surgical repair or can present congenitally. Rare cases of fibrosing mediastinitis or sarcoidosis or compression from mediastinal tumors can also result in unilateral or bilateral acquired pulmonary vein stenosis of varying degrees. Obstruction of pulmonary venous flow causes pulmonary hypertension, which can lead to RV failure over time. In bilateral cases, the pressure load can cause significant morbidity and mortality.

Indications for Intervention: American Heart Association Guidelines [5]

Class I

1. Pulmonary venous angioplasty and stenting are indicated for the management of acquired significant pulmonary vein stenosis after radiofrequency ablation procedures (Level of Evidence: C).
2. Pulmonary venous angioplasty and stenting are indicated for the management of acquired pulmonary vein stenosis after lung transplantation or for external compression due to tumors in older children and adolescents (Level of Evidence: B).

Class IIa

1. Pulmonary venous angioplasty is reasonable to consider in the management of pulmonary vein stenosis after surgical repair for anomalous pulmonary vein connections (Level of Evidence: C).

Class IIb

1. Pulmonary venous angioplasty and stenting may be considered in the management of isolated congenital pulmonary vein stenosis (Level of Evidence: C).
2. Pulmonary venous angioplasty and stenting may be considered for the management of acquired pulmonary vein stenosis after lung transplantation or for external compression due to tumors in infants and young children (Level of Evidence: C).
3. Pulmonary venous stenting may be considered for the management of postoperative pulmonary vein stenosis after surgical repair for anomalous pulmonary vein connections (Level of Evidence: C).

Technical Considerations

Angioplasty is often not adequate since recurrence is high. While it may be worthwhile to start with a surgical repair using the "sutureless technique," repeat recurrences may require stent palliation (Figs. 46.9, 46.10). Even with stents, restenosis can recur. There are preliminary data suggesting drug-eluting stents can prevent or delay restenosis. Some have advocated use of cutting balloons for angioplasty [19,20]. Technically, a transseptal puncture will be needed unless there is a PFO or ASD to permit passage of the delivery system to the LA. In general, ventricular pump failure is not an issue during pulmonary vein stenting since the delivery system does not have to pass through any valve to cause regurgitation. Thromboembolic events and occasional hypoxia are more common issues to work through during the procedure. However, in cases of bilateral pulmonary vein stenosis with severe pulmonary hypertension and RV failure, the patient can be quite sick due to the interventricular septum bowing leftward to "pancake" the left ventricle resulting in left heart failure.

Outcomes Data

In general, pulmonary vein stenosis has a high rate of restenosis and high rate of mortality regardless of surgical or transcatheter therapy (angioplasty, stents). Balasubramanian et al. reported a large series of stented pulmonary veins. 74 pulmonary veins were stented using bare metal stents, drug-eluting stents, and covered stents in 47 patients. Median age was 1.4 years. During median follow-up of 3.1 years, 21 patients died and survival was 62% at 1 year and 50% at 5 years. While acute relief of obstruction was achieved with stents, reintervention rate was 59% (32/54). Stent occlusion was found in 9 and significant in-stent stenosis in 17 [38].

Prieto et al. compared angioplasty and stenting. They reported angioplasty success and restenosis rates of 42% and 72%, respectively [39]. In contrast, stenting resulted in success and restenosis rates of 95% and 33%, respectively. In spite of reasonable immediate results, restenosis is not uncommon and repeat dilations following stenting may be needed. A few reports indicate that the stented diameter of 7–10 mm or greater may play a role in minimizing risk of restenosis [38–40]. It is not uncommon to reintervene as a bridge to lung transplant. In cases of restenosis beyond the stent and into the pulmonary parenchyma, there are little options outside of lung transplant. There are a few reports of success using drug-eluting stents.

Postsurgical Baffles and Conduits

Physiology

Various surgical baffles and conduits can experience stenosis and dysfunction over time. They include RV-PA conduits causing a combination of stenosis and regurgitation. Mustard and Senning baffles can also experience stenosis. While atrial

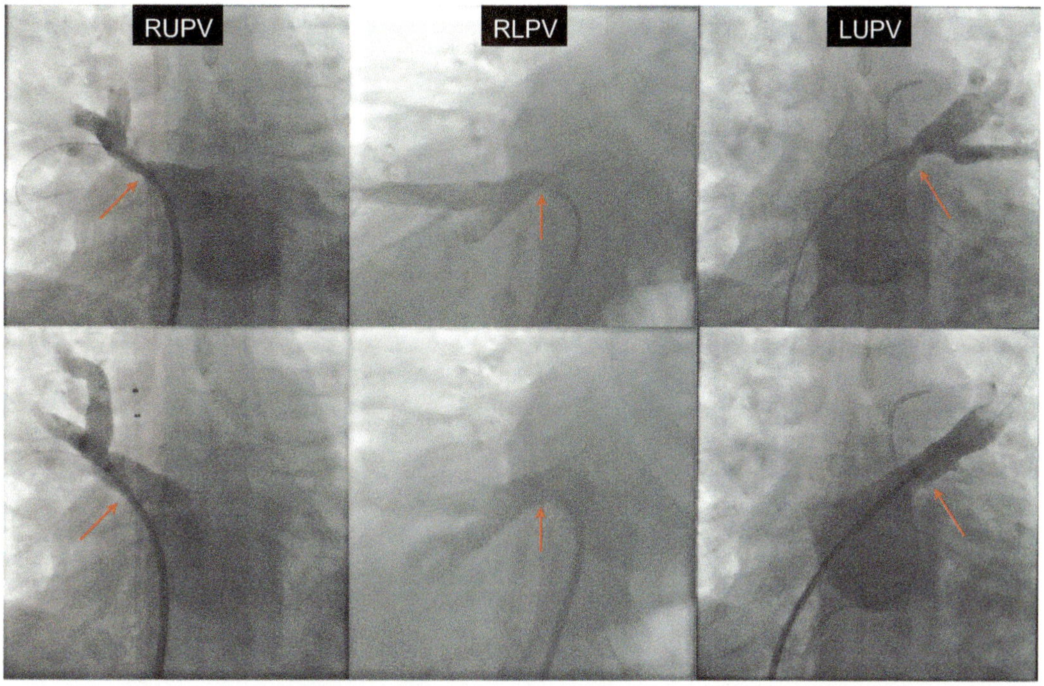

FIGURE 46.9 Bilateral pulmonary vein stenosis due to fibrosing mediastinitis causing severe pulmonary hypertension and biventricular dysfunction (top) and relief of stenoses following stent implant in the right upper pulmonary vein (RUPV), left lower pulmonary vein (RLPV), and left upper pulmonary vein (LUPV). Unfortunately, the LUPV had progressed to atresia prior to the catheterization. The patient improved from NYHA class III–IV to class II poststenting and no longer required assistant of a walker.

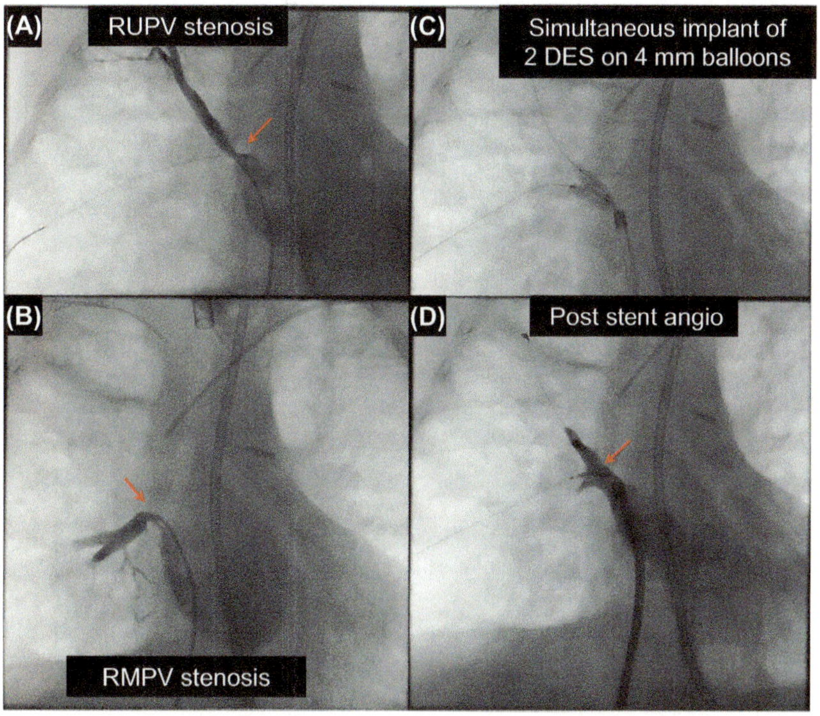

FIGURE 46.10 1-year-old, ex-26-week premature infant with chronic lung disease and combination, right upper pulmonary vein (A) and right middle pulmonary vein stenosis (B) (*red arrows*) as well and left upper pulmonary vein atresia. Pulmonary pressures were near systemic. Two drug-eluting stents (DESs) were implanted simultaneously to avoid jailing of either pulmonary veins (C). Final angiogram showing wide patency of the stenotic orifices (D). Pulmonary pressures decreased to 2/3 systemic poststenting.

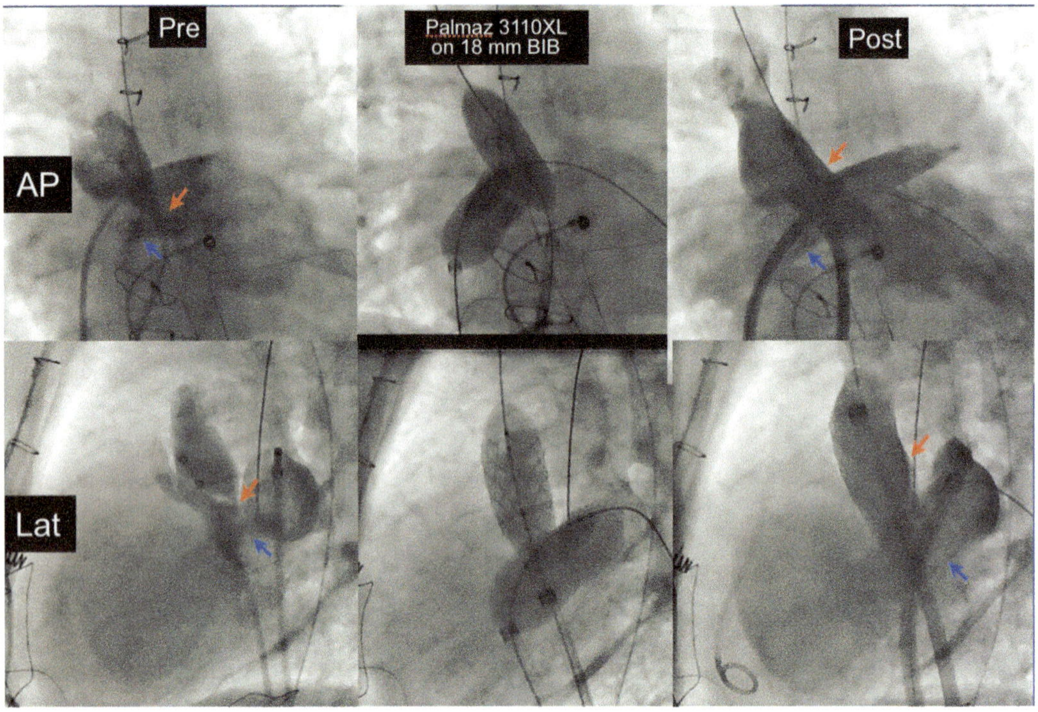

FIGURE 46.11 A patient with d-transposition of the great arteries, s/p Mustard repair presented with 3-pillow orthopnea and lower extremity pitting edema. Simultaneous injections of contrast demonstrate combination systemic venous baffle obstruction (*red arrow*) and pulmonary venous baffle obstruction (*blue arrow*) in both AP and lateral projections (left). Simultaneous stents were implanted (middle). Wide patency of both baffles is demonstrated postsimultaneous stenting (right).

baffle stenoses are usually found in older patient who underwent an atrial switch operation for d-TGA decades ago, they can still be found in younger patients who have undergone double switch operations for corrected transposition. Systemic venous baffle obstructions can lead to SVC syndrome, but the physiology of pulmonary venous baffle obstruction is similar to that of pulmonary vein obstruction. Transcatheter stenting can relieve the obstruction thereby obviating the need for further surgery. Fig. 46.11 shows a case of a patient with d-TGA status-post Mustard repair who developed a combination of a systemic and pulmonary venous baffle obstruction. She required a transseptal puncture to access to pulmonary venous baffle. The proximity of both baffle obstructions necessitated simultaneous stenting of both baffles.

Indications for Intervention [5]

Recommendation for Balloon Dilation of Right Ventricle to Pulmonary Artery Conduit Obstruction

Class IIb

1. As a palliative measure, balloon dilation of significant conduit obstruction may be indicated to relieve obstruction or to test the compliance of the obstruction before stent implantation (Level of Evidence: C).

Stent Implantation for Right Ventricle to Pulmonary Artery Conduit Obstruction

Class I

1. Primary intravascular stent implantation is indicated for the treatment of significant stenosis of an RV-to-main pulmonary artery/pulmonary artery conduit when there is a predominant and significant stenosis of the conduit, and it is believed that (1) the stent will significantly prolong the life of the conduit before further intervention becomes necessary, (2) the pulmonary regurgitation created will be tolerated better than the stenosis, and (3) the stent definitely will not impinge on the pulmonary artery bifurcation or compromise the coronary circulation by compression (Level of Evidence: B).

Technical Considerations

In Mustard/Senning baffle obstructions, it is important to understand the adjacent anatomy of the obstructed site. Multiple angiograms and simultaneous injections of both the systemic and pulmonary venous baffles may be

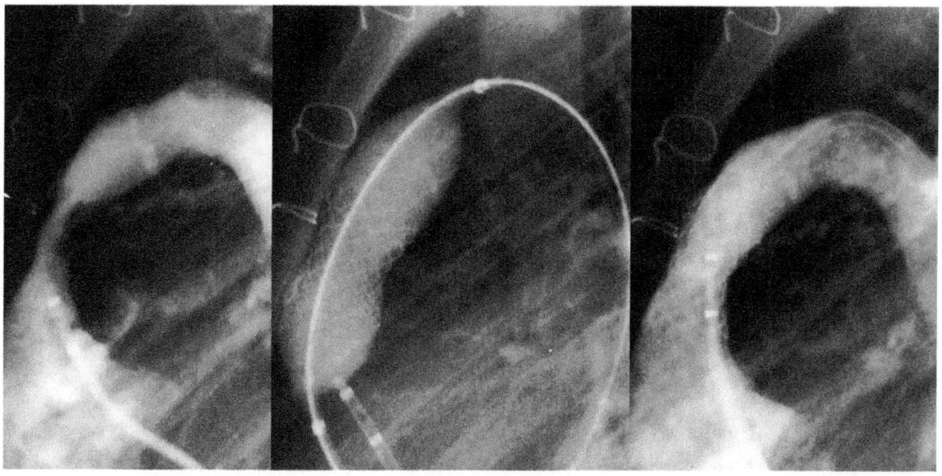

FIGURE 46.12 Right ventricle to pulmonary artery conduit stenosis (left), s/p stent implantation (middle) and wide patency postprocedure (right).

necessary to visualize the stenosis and how an implanted stent might cause compression of the adjacent baffle. Test inflations are required in some cases. Current use of MRI or CT angiography will also help. Occasionally, stents in both baffles are necessary to prevent compression of either baffle.

Transbaffle puncture: While a transseptal puncture can be technically challenging due to the stiffness and thickness of surgical baffles and prosthetic patches, it is nevertheless possible. A paper describing 18 years of experience with transseptal puncture through a variety of surgical material at the atrial septum [41] also confirms that the holes left behind after the transseptal puncture spontaneously close. Use of transesophageal echo (TEE) to guide the transseptal puncture can minimize procedural risks.

Outcomes Data

Angioplasty of RV-PA conduit in general were thought less effective compared to stenting, but use of ultrahigh pressure balloon has been shown to significantly reduce right ventricular outflow tract gradients [42]. However, conduit tears are common, occurring in 22%. Stenting of obstructed conduits have been shown to effectively and acutely relieve obstructions and can prolong the life of a conduit/homograft, but a high rate of stent fractures have also been reported on follow-up [43]. In a series of 106 obstructed conduits, angioplasty alone reduced the peak RV-PA gradient from 54.3 ± 17.4 mmHg at baseline to 46 ± 15.2 mmHg after balloon dilation alone and to 25.1 ± 11.4 mmHg with stenting (all $P < .001$) [44]. While stents can provide structural support to prevent recoil, they also result in wide open valvar insufficiency. Fortunately, conduit regurgitation can be tolerated much longer than conduit stenosis, and the current addition of transcatheter pulmonary valve implants has eliminated this problem in larger children with larger conduits. Fig. 46.12 shows a case of RV-PA conduit stenosis treated with a stent.

Left Heart Obstructive Lesions

Mitral Valve Stenosis

Mitral valve stenosis restricts blood flow from the LA to the left ventricle. Initially the LA dilates and over time the high left atrial pressure is transmitted to the pulmonary venous system. Reactive pulmonary arterial hypertension develops thereby decreasing cardiac output. Mitral valve stenosis can be divided into rheumatic or congenital. Rheumatic mitral valve stenosis is commonly due to development of thickened mitral leaflets and fused commissures. Congenital mitral stenosis involves a broad spectrum of anatomic variants. Typical congenital mitral stenosis includes thickened leaflets, shortened chordae, and decreased interchordal spaces. However, other variants include supramitral valve ring, double mitral orifices, parachute mitral valve, and hypoplastic mitral valve. Congenital mitral valve stenosis is often accompanied by hypoplastic left-sided structures and surgical intervention may be necessary when addressing additional lesions.

Balloon dilation for rheumatic mitral stenosis was first reported by Inoue in 1984 and has been extensively reported in adult literature with very good results. Balloon valvuloplasty separates the thickened valve with fused commissures. With the success of balloon dilation with rheumatic valves, this procedure was then performed with patients with congenital mitral valve stenosis. Multiple techniques have been described including the double-transseptal technique. The Inoue balloon (Toray International America) was developed for mitral valve dilations in adults and now used in older pediatric patients with congenital mitral stenosis. This requires crossing the atrial septum either through an existing ASD or by transseptal puncture. Balloon valvuloplasty of rheumatic mitral valve stenosis has good results [45–48].

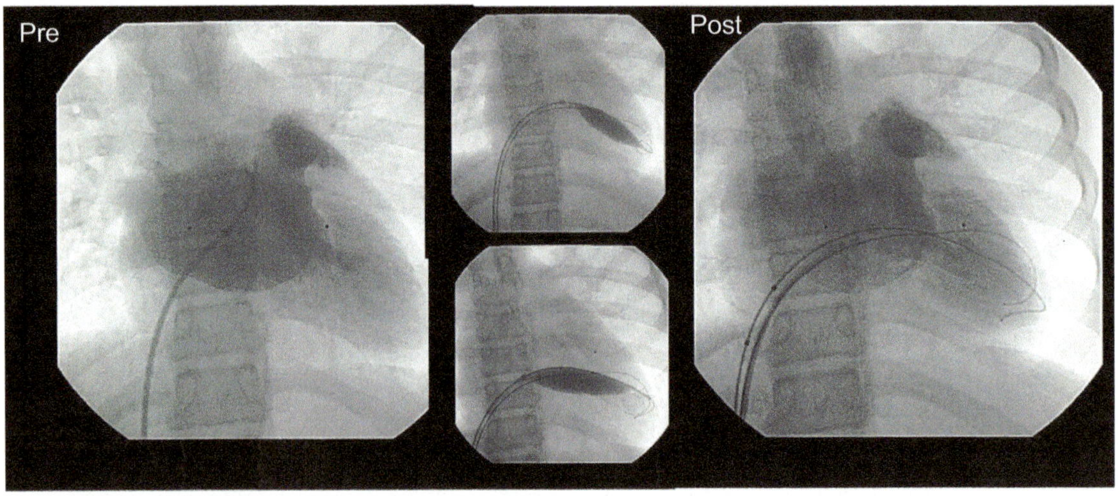

FIGURE 46.13 Mitral stenosis (left), balloon valvuloplasty with serially larger balloons (middle), and postdilation angiogram showing improved mitral valve excursion (right).

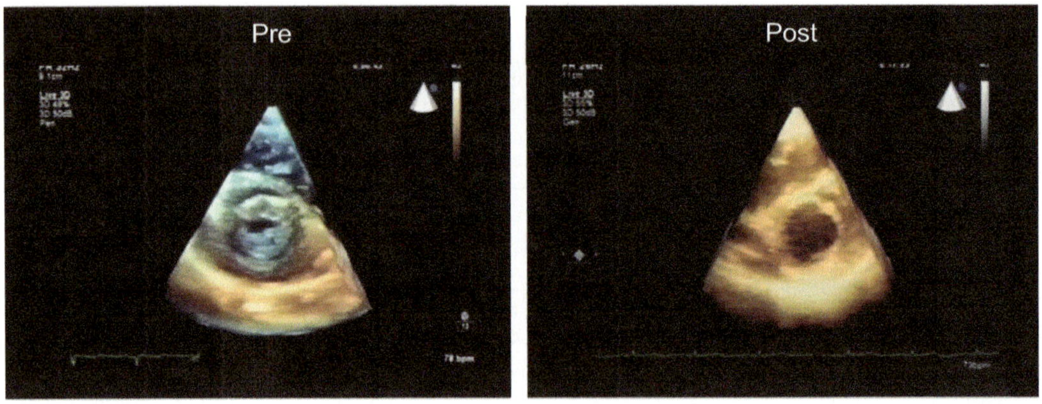

FIGURE 46.14 3-D echo showing cross-sectional area of mitral stenosis (left) and marked improvement in mitral excursion postdilation (right).

The largest study reporting balloon valvuloplasty of congenital mitral stenosis comes from Children's Hospital Boston with 64 patients [49]. Good immediate and midterm results were reported but progressive mitral regurgitation and restenosis remain a problem. Regurgitation often results from a torn mitral leaflet or chordal attachment and papillary muscle rupture. Figs. 46.13 and 46.14 show a case of congenital mitral valve stenosis successfully treated with balloon valvuloplasty using serially larger balloons. An initial mitral a-wave to left ventricular end-diastolic gradient of 19 mmHg decreased to 8 mmHg gradient. Both angiographic and 3-D echo imaging showed marked improvement in mitral valve excursion postdilation.

Classification of mitral valve stenosis include mild (mitral valve area >1.5 cm^2, mean mitral valve gradient <5 mmHg, pulmonary artery systolic pressure <30 mmHg), moderate (mitral valve area 1–1.5 cm^2, mean mitral valve gradient 5–10 mmHg, pulmonary artery systolic pressure 30–50 mmHg), and severe (mitral valve area <1 cm^2, mean valve gradient >10 mmHg, pulmonary artery systolic pressure >50 mmHg) [50].

Class I indications for intervention include symptomatic adults patients with moderate to severe rheumatic mitral stenosis and asymptomatic patients with moderate to severe rheumatic mitral stenosis with pulmonary hypertension. Class IIa indications suggest it is reasonable to treat symptomatic children ≥5 years of age with congenital mitral stenosis or restenosis who have mitral valve morphology that is favorable for balloon valvuloplasty (i.e., thickened leaflets and fused commissure). Class IIb indications state valvuloplasty may rarely be considered at centers of expertise for patients <5 years of age with congenital mitral valve stenosis with moderate to severe residual stenosis or with valve restenosis who have already undergone surgical valvuloplasty at centers with expertise in mitral valve intervention in young children; children who would otherwise undergo mitral valve replacement or when mitral valve replacement is thought to be problematic;

as a palliative measure in management of congenital moderate to severe mitral stenosis (i.e., thickened leaflets, shortened chordae, decreased interchordal spaces) [5].

Left Heart Outflow Obstruction

Obstructive left heart lesions lead to compensatory ventricular hypertrophy and eventually will lead to left ventricular dysfunction and heart failure.

Aortic Valve Stenosis

Transcatheter therapy for aortic valve stenosis was first reported in the early 1980s and has replaced open surgical valvotomy as the primary treatment of choice. Normal aortic valve anatomy includes three cusps (tricuspid) and three commissures. Stenosis can result from fusion of one or more commissures. The aortic valve can also have two cusps (bicuspid), accounting for three quarters of the patients or one cusp (unicuspid), accounting for one quarter of the patients. The valve may also be tricuspid with partial fusion of the commissures. The valve cusps are often not only thickened and immobile but may also have a normal membranous appearance. Approximately 2%–3% of individuals are reported to be born with a bicuspid aortic valve but remain without stenosis. Many of these patients will present in adulthood with stenosis secondary to calcification of the valve, typically not seen younger than 25–30 years of age. These patients will not be discussed here although transcatheter therapy continues to play a large role in their management as well.

In infants with severe valvar stenosis, the annulus is often narrow, cusps thickened and myxomatous appearing. Within a few months, the valve leaflets become thinner and more membranous in appearance, although may remain stenotic. Critical aortic stenosis in neonates typically presents with left ventricular failure and is dependent on a PDA for systemic blood flow. In infancy, severe stenosis will result initially in compensatory left ventricular hypertrophy and significant endocardial fibroelastosis may be evident. Myocardial fibrosis can occur over time and not discovered until adulthood. Fibrosis of the myocardium will lead to diastolic and systolic left heart failure.

Indications for balloon valvuloplasty are similar to surgical indications. Class I indications include newborn patients with critical valvar aortic stenosis who is ductal dependent and children with isolated valvar aortic stenosis who have depressed left ventricular systolic function regardless of valve gradient. Also, children with isolated valvar stenosis with resting peak systolic valve gradient by catheter of 50 or 40 mmHg if there are symptoms of angina, syncope or, ST-T wave changes on electrocardiography at rest or with exercise. Refer to AHA guidelines for further indications [5]. Valvuloplasty is not indicated for children with isolated valvar stenosis with resting peak systolic gradient by catheter <40 mmHg and who have no symptoms, ST-T wave changes on electrocardiogram or in patients with aortic regurgitation that warrants surgical aortic valve replacement or repair.

Technical considerations include balloon selection, evaluation for aortic insufficiency, and possible rapid ventricular pacing. A balloon to annulus diameter ratio recommended between 0.8 and 1. Using a balloon greater than this ratio increases the risk for significant aortic insufficiency. Rapid right ventricular pacing may be required to maintain balloon stability. By increasing the heart rate, the stroke volume decreases allowing the balloon to remain in good position across the valve rather than being ejected with each heartbeat. Newborn patients with critical aortic stenosis often have severe left ventricular dysfunction with poor cardiac output therefore will not require rapid ventricular pacing. Their ventricular function and cardiac output will improve somewhat immediately after valvuloplasty and over the following days to months after the procedure.

Fig. 46.15 shows a neonate with severe aortic valve stenosis as demonstrated by angiography and a significant gradient by echocardiography followed by balloon valvuloplasty via a carotid cutdown approach. Fig. 46.16 shows chest X-rays before and after balloon valvuloplasty. There is improvement in pulmonary edema and heart size postdilation.

Successful balloon valvuloplasty is defined by reduction of catheter peak systolic gradient less than 35 mmHg. Severe aortic insufficiency is uncommon. The Valvuloplasty and Angioplasty of Congenital Anomalies registry reported risk factors for suboptimal outcome defined as a residual systolic peak gradient >60 mmHg, major morbidity or mortality, included age < 3 months, higher predilation valve gradient, and a ratio or balloon-annulus diameter of <0.9, presence of unrepaired coarctation and an earlier procedure date. The optimal balloon-annulus diameter was 0.9–1.0. Larger diameter ratios were associated with higher risk of aortic regurgitation. Long-term outcome after successful balloon dilation is good, however, late stenosis and valve regurgitation eventually requires reintervention in the majority of patients [51,52]. Reintervention-free survival for newborns was 48% at 5 years. In children >6 months of age (median age 6.9 years), freedom form reintervention was 86% at 1 year, 67% at 5 years, and 46% at 12 years [53,54]. Balloon aortic valvuloplasty, while successful in the short and midterm period, has been proven to be a palliative procedure with many patients requiring repeat intervention or surgery.

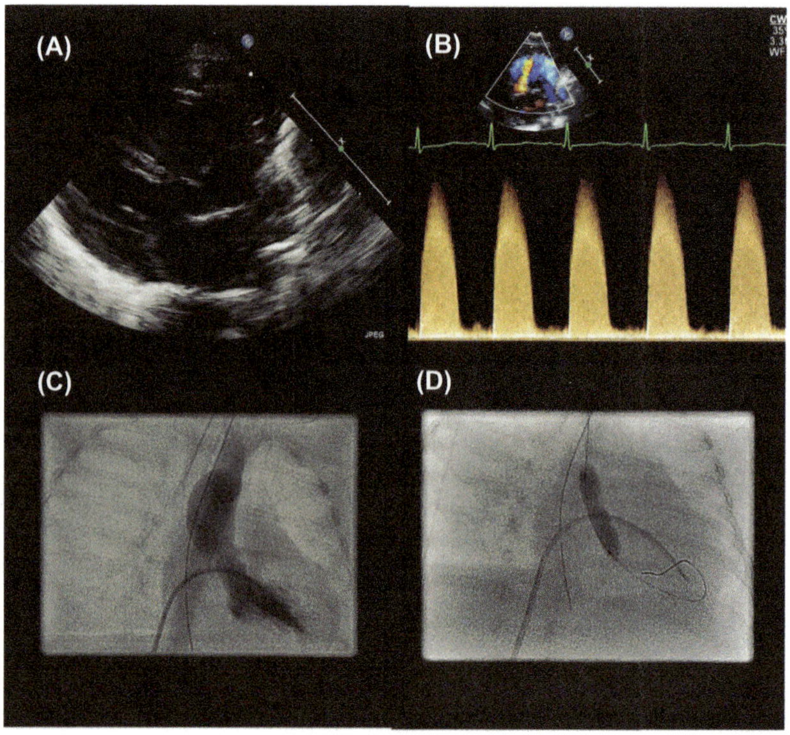

FIGURE 46.15 (A) Long axis view on echocardiogram. Bicuspid aortic valve is thickened and domes in systole. (B) Significant Doppler gradient across aortic valve. (C) Angiogram in left ventricle. The aortic valve is seen as a white lucency, noted to be thickened and doming in systole. (D) Balloon inflation at aortic valve.

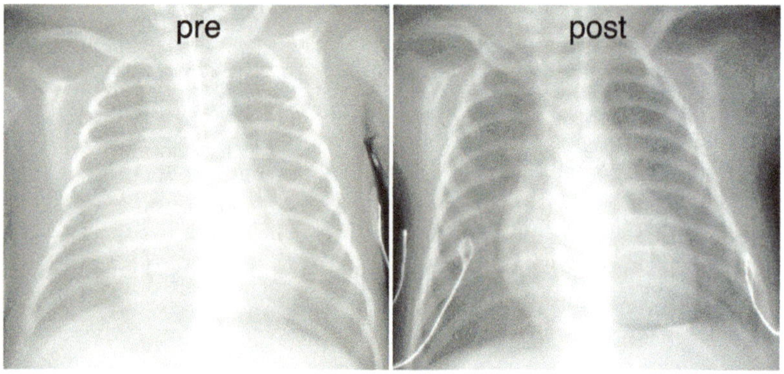

FIGURE 46.16 Comparison of heart size before and after balloon valvuloplasty. Improvement in pulmonary edema and heart size is noted postdilation.

Subvalvar aortic stenosis can result from a discrete subaortic membrane or fibromuscular ring. This type of aortic obstruction is not amenable to catheter intervention. Supravalvar aortic stenosis occurs more commonly with other anomalies. A third of these patients will have Williams syndrome or an elastin arteriopathy and is associated with stenosis of other arteries including branch pulmonary arteries, renal arteries, or head and neck arteries. Occasionally coronary artery involvement in the narrowing is seen. This lesion also requires surgical intervention.

Coarctation of the Aorta

Coarctation of the aorta accounts for 6%–8% of all cardiac defects. In patients with Turner syndrome or a bicuspid valve, the prevalence is higher. Newborn patients with severe coarctation will present with cardiogenic shock when the ductus arteriosus closes. The high afterload is a strain on the left ventricle and often newborns will present with left ventricular dysfunction. Cardiogenic shock results from inadequate perfusion of the lower body resulting in metabolic acidosis, ischemia to intestines, kidney, and liver. Older children and adults often will develop compensatory left ventricular hypertrophy and upper body hypertension. Up to 90% of the patients with isolated coarctation may die of complications of coarctation including aortic rupture, intracranial hemorrhages, hypertension, endocarditis, or heart failure if left untreated before the

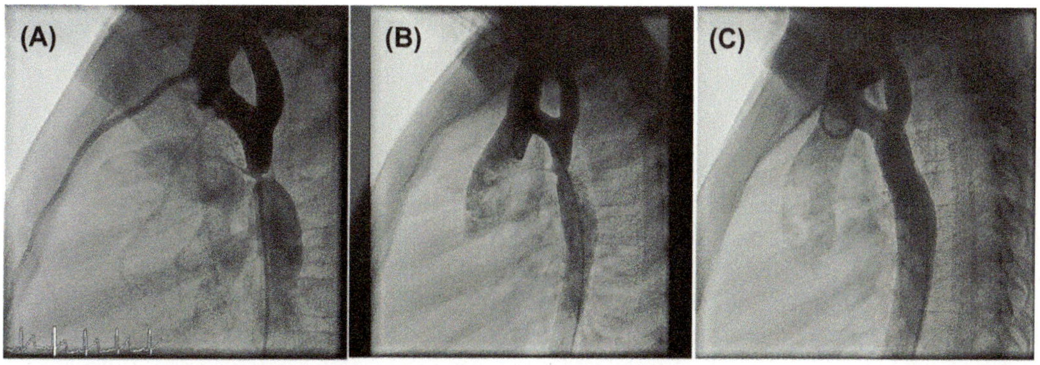

FIGURE 46.17 (A) Lateral view on angiogram demonstrating severe coarctation and a tiny patent ductus arteriosus. (B) After balloon angioplasty, coarctation is improved but mild narrowing persists. (C) After stent implantation, no residual narrowing seen.

age of 50 [55]. Newborns and infants <6 months more likely will require surgical intervention, however, balloon angioplasty and stent implantation plays a large role in recoarctation and native coarctation in older infants, children and adolescents.

Balloon angioplasty is recommended for recoarctation with a transcatheter systolic gradient of >20 mmHg and suitable anatomy irrespective of age and recoarctation with systolic gradient <20 mmHg in presence of significant collateral vessels and suitable angiographic narrowing, irrespective of age, or in patients with univentricular hearts or with significant ventricular dysfunction. Balloon angioplasty of native coarctation as a palliative measure to stabilize a patient irrespective of age when patient has severely depressed ventricular function, severe mitral insufficiency, low cardiac output, or systemic disease affected by cardiac condition. It can also be considered for native coarctation in patients >4–6 months of age with transcatheter systolic gradient >20 mmHg and suitable anatomy. Other indications are presented in more detail in the AHA guidelines [5].

Stent placement for native or recoarctation is indicated in patients with recurrent coarctation who are of sufficient size for stent placement, where the stent can be expanded to an adult size who have a transcatheter systolic gradient >20 mmHg, <20 mmHg but with systemic hypertension secondary to coarctation, long segment coarctation with gradient >20 mmHg, or when balloon angioplasty has failed in a patient with transcatheter systolic gradient >20 mmHg. Other indications are presented in more detail in the AHA guidelines [5].

Technical considerations include balloon size, femoral vessel size, and stent selection. The aorta above and below the narrowing should be measured and a balloon selected should be approximately the size of the surrounding aorta. Larger balloon sizes increase risk of aneurysm formation or dissection, with tears extending beyond the media layer. Due to lower profile balloons, concern for sheath size is only seen for smaller infants. Many balloon catheters will go through 3 or 4 Fr sheaths. For stent implantation, sheath size 1–2 Fr larger than needed for the balloon is necessary. In infants, if there are limitations due to femoral artery size, one should consider alternate access point, i.e., Carotid cutdown. In the single-ventricle patient, intervention with balloon or stent can be accomplished from the venous system in an antegrade approach. Stents that will accommodate a growing child and can be further dilated over time is currently limited to several stents. The Intrastent Max-LD (Intratherapeutics, St. Paul, MN, recently acquired by ev3, Plymouth, MN) and Palmaz stents (Johnson & Johnson Interventional Systems Co., Warren, NJ) can be further dilated to 25 mm and are good choices for the older child or teenager with adequate sized femoral arteries. The Genesis XD (Cordis/Johnson and Johnson) stent is a good choice for infants or younger children, where the stent can be mounted on a balloon as small as 6 mm and further dilated to 18–20 mm. The Valeo premounted stent (Bard Peripheral Vascular, Tempe, Arizona) can also be further dilated to 20 mm but may not have the radial strength over time. However, as the patient grows, an additional stent could be placed if necessary. One note, the Valeo stent premounted on 6–8 mm balloons will further dilate to 13 mm, not 20 mm. If one selects this stent, remounting the Valeo stent (9–10 mm) on a smaller balloon can be done. Balloon and stent implantation is typically well tolerated with inflation time 5–10 s resulting in loss of distal perfusing pressure, which recovers after balloon deflation. Fig. 46.17 compares an angiogram of a coarctation of the aorta before intervention, after angioplasty and after stenting. The best result was noted after stent implantation.

Recoarctation occurs in 5%–24% of patients after surgical arch repair. Immediate success after balloon angioplasty for recoarctation is 88%. Of those patients with immediate success, 72% had long-lasting results. The need for surgical reintervention was associated with aortic arch hypoplasia [56]. In infants less than 6 months of age, angioplasty for native coarctation is associated with a higher recurrence rate therefore surgical intervention is recommended. In infants and children with recoarctation, balloon angioplasty can avoid or delay stent implantation until the patient can accommodate stent placement. Stent implantation may be preferred in older children or adolescents for improved short-term results, however, the patients will require future procedures to further dilate the stent as the patient grows. Immediate success of stent implantation in native and recoarctation is >95% and recurrence is attributed to somatic growth at which time further dilation can be performed [57–59]. Complications of balloon angioplasty and stent implantation include aortic wall injury including aneurysm formation or dissection, arterial access site injury, cerebral vascular accidents, or peripheral emboli.

SHUNT LESIONS

Shunt lesions include ASDs, ventricular septal defects (VSDs), PDA, systemic-to-pulmonary collateral vessels (SPCs), and CAF. These lesions can lead to the development of CHF in the absence of ventricular dysfunction by resulting in significant left-to-right shunting and volume overload. As the pulmonary vascular resistance drops over the first two to 3 months after birth, left-to-right shunting increases resulting in overcirculation of the pulmonary vasculature, and pulmonary edema. At the same time, the work of the left ventricle increases to compensate and maintain cardiac output and a neurohormonal stress response is mounted [60,61] resulting in tachycardia and diaphoresis. Caloric needs increase but are not met due to tachypnea, resulting in poor feeding and failure to thrive. In the case of ASDs that are not subject to systolic driving pressures, shunting will increase as the right ventricular compliance increases relative to left ventricular compliance in early infancy. ASDs rarely result in clinical CHF but are associated with failure to thrive [62,63].

Shunt volumes are assessed along with cardiac output and pulmonary blood flow in the catheterization laboratory using the Fick principle. Flow measurements by thermodilution techniques are invalid in the presence of an intracardiac shunt. The Fick principle states that the volume of blood flow across a capillary bed can be measured by calculating the arteriovenous content difference of a substance with a constant and known rate of consumption or addition across the capillary bed. In most instances, oxygen is used as that substance. Oxygen content is directly measured ($0.03 \times pO_2 + 13.6 \times Hgb$ (g/dL) $\times SpO_2$) pre- and postcapillary bed.

Oxygen consumption (VO_2) is measured using a metabolic hood, other means of direct measurement, or, more commonly, it is assumed using published tables or equations based on age and heart rate [64]. The utility and accuracy of assumed VO_2 values in patients with congenital heart disease and children <3 years of age have been questioned and updated predictive equations have been reported [65].

In the absence of intracardiac shunts, the pulmonary arterial O_2 saturation is also the most accurate mixed venous saturation and the systemic arterial saturation is the same as the pulmonary venous saturation, making the arteriovenous O_2 content difference the same across the pulmonary and systemic capillary beds. In this situation, the pulmonary output (Qp) and the systemic output (Qs) the same and the ratio of Qp to Qs (Qp:Qs) is equal to 1. In the presence of intracardiac left-to-right shunting, the mixed venous O_2 saturation used may be the superior venous saturation or the saturation in the chamber just proximal to the shunt (i.e., the right ventricular saturation in the presence of a PDA). The pulmonary artery saturation will be higher than the mixed venous saturation in the presence of a left-to-right shunt and the AVO2 content difference will be smaller across the pulmonary vascular bed compared to the systemic vascular bed, resulting in a Qp:Qs greater than 1. The Qp:Qs ratio indicates the magnitude of the shunt in relation to cardiac output and the difference between the pulmonary and systemic flows (Qp-Qs) is the volume of the shunt. Below is a discussion of the physiology, indications for transcatheter therapy [5], technical considerations, and outcomes for shunt lesions addressed in the catheterization laboratory.

Patent Ductus Arteriosus

Physiology

In the fetus, the ductus arteriosus is large and serves as a right-to-left shunt, diverting right ventricular output away from the high-resistance pulmonary vasculature and into the systemic circulation of the lower body and placenta. Shortly after birth, the rise in systemic oxygenation and the fall in circulating prostaglandin E2 triggers constriction of the ductus, a process that typically results in the functional closure of the ductus and ultimate conversion to the ligamentum arteriosus. In an estimated 3 to 8 per 10,000 live births, the ductus fails to close, typically resulting in a left-to-right shunt that increases as the pulmonary vascular resistance drops in the first 2–3 months of life. Premature babies are particularly susceptible to persistence of the PDA and the risk is inversely related to the gestational age. In the setting of normal pulmonary vascular resistance, the degree of shunting and clinical heart failure depends on the size of the ductus and the degree of constriction that occurred before the duct failed to close. Premature infants are at greater risk of having large and unrestricted PDAs that can result in significant lung damage, pulmonary hypertension, and enough "steal" of systemic circulation to compromise organ function [66].

Indications for Transcatheter Therapy

Any patient experiencing CHF, failure to thrive, or pulmonary overcirculation, or exhibiting left heart dilation on echocardiography secondary to left-to-right shunting through a PDA meets indication for PDA occlusion or ligation (class I, level of evidence: B). The vast majority of PDAs can be occluded via transcatheter delivery of a number of devices or coils. Additionally, most would recommend occlusion of small murmur-producing PDAs that are not associated with left heart enlargement or heart failure because of the elevated endocarditis risk conferred by turbulent ductal flow and endothelial disruption (class IIa, level of evidence: C). PDA occlusion is contraindicated in patients with irreversible pulmonary hypertension (class III, level of evidence: C). Transcatheter PDA occlusion presents higher risks in small premature infants and, although there are reports of duct occlusions in premature infants as small as 870g [67], decisions about closure versus surgical ligation in such patients who have failed medical closure remain center-dependent.

Technical Considerations

PDAs can be occluded percutaneously with a variety of devices and coils depending on the anatomy and size of the ductus and the optimal delivery approach for the patient (Fig. 46.18). At the time of catheterization, a right heart sweep allows for the assessment of right heart pressures, pulmonary vascular resistance, and the volume of the shunt. An aortic angiogram is performed to assess the anatomy and the dimensions of the duct for device selection. Coils are typically reserved only for the smallest PDAs and a number of retrievable Nitinol devices are available for larger PDAs. The Amplatzer Duct Occluder (ADO; St. Jude Medical, St. Paul, MN) is the most commonly used. Its bell shape conforms nicely in the most commonly encountered type A conical ductus. For small premature infants, who more commonly have tubular shaped PDAs and who have less room in the aorta for the retention skirt of the ADO, there are a number of vascular plugs available as well as the Amplatzer Duct Occluder II (ADO II). The ADO is delivered through the right heart via antegrade venous access to the

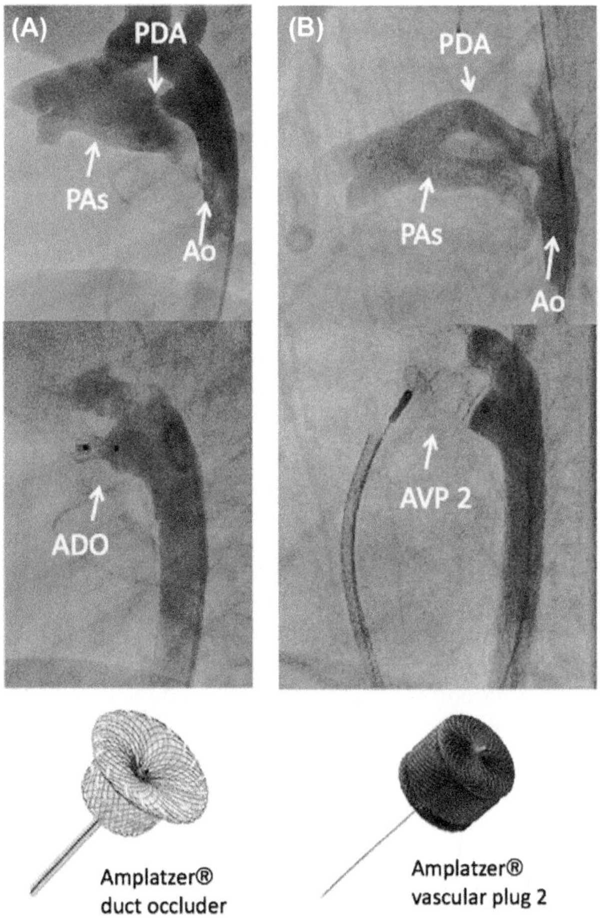

FIGURE 46.18 Device closure of patent ductus arteriosus (PDAs). (A) A moderate conical ("type A") PDA in a 15-month-old with left heart enlargement and congestive heart failure. The Amplatzer Duct Occluder is delivered and conforms well to the shape of the ductus, with the retention skirt holding the device in the large ductal aortic ampulla. After occlusion, there is no residual flow. The patient's symptoms resolved and the left heart returned to a normal size over time. (B) The Amplatzer vascular plug 2 is used to occlude a tubular ("type C") ductus in a 2.3kg premature infant in congestive heart failure. Without a conical aortic ampulla, the retention skirt of the ADO would risk aortic arch obstruction. The cylindrical AVP2 device conforms well to the shape of the ductus without obstructing the aorta. After occlusion, there is no residual flow and the patient was able to wean from mechanical ventilation and diuretic therapy. *ADO*, amplatzer duct occluder; *Ao*, aorta; *AVP*, amplatzer vascular plug; *PA*, pulmonary artery; *PDA*, patent ductus arteriosus.

ductus, while the ADO II and vascular plugs can be delivered either antegrade from the vein or retrograde from the femoral artery. Either approach is generally tolerated well in larger infants and children, but device delivery in small or premature infants can cause hypotension from valve regurgitation, heart block, and significant arrhythmias if performed antegrade, and arterial injury if delivered retrograde. These devices are retrievable using their delivery cable until they are released from the delivery cable using an unscrewing mechanism. Once a device is deployed, and before the device is released, angiography is used to assess pulmonary artery and aorta patency as well as the likelihood of device embolization after release from the delivery cable. If the device appears well seated and does not obstruct nearby vessels, it may be released and reevaluated with a postrelease angiogram. Devices that shift or embolize can typically be recaptured percutaneously using snare catheters.

Outcomes

Transcatheter PDA closure has proven to be effective and safe with appropriate patient selection. For example, in the pivotal trial for the ADO device in patient ≥6 kg and 6 months of age, the rate of successful implantation was 99% and the rate of complete PDA occlusion at 12 months was 98.6% with only a 1.3% rate of serious or major adverse events [68]. Among patients weighing less than 6 kg, a 94% rate of successful delivery and 100% rate of occlusion are reported [69]. In a study of preterm infants ≤32 weeks gestation weighing 1.2–3.9 kg, successful device placement was achieved in 46/52 (88%) of infants. Adverse events, mostly acute transient arterial injury, occurred in 33% of cases. In this study, most patients had tubular shaped PDAs and underwent occlusion with the Amplatzer Vascular Plug II and no residual shunting was appreciated at the most recent follow-up [70]. Rare complications during PDA occlusion include device embolization, obstruction of aortic or pulmonary artery flow, particularly in small infants, hemolysis, transient left ventricular dysfunction, and recanalization of the ductus.

Systemic-to-Pulmonary Collateral Vessels

Physiology

The mechanisms leading to the formation of SPCs are not well understood, but hypoxemia, diminished pulmonary blood flow, and nonpulsatility in the pulmonary arteries are thought to contribute [71]. Similar to a PDA, SPCs act as a source of left-to-right shunting from the aorta and its branches, including the brachiocephalic and chest wall arteries, to the pulmonary vasculature that, if significant in size, can lead to volume overload and CHF. SPCs often occur in association with other congenital heart malformations and have been reported in association with bronchopulmonary dysplasia. SPCs are commonly seen in palliated single-ventricle patients who have undergone Glenn anastomosis or Fontan completion. A significant left-to-right shunt in these patients volume loads the single ventricle and can raise filling and pulmonary artery pressures, worsen atrioventricular valve regurgitation, and exacerbate heart failure. In the early postoperative period, SPC flow may contribute to pleural effusions and increase the time spent on mechanical ventilation. Patients with tetralogy of Fallot and pulmonary atresia frequently have significant SPCs that provide either sole- or dual-supply pulmonary blood flow to certain segments of the lungs alongside the native pulmonary arteries. The presence of SPCs should be considered and investigated in patients with other congenital heart lesions, particularly TGA, who continue to have CHF after repair.

Indications for Transcatheter Therapy

Occlusion is indicated when SPCs are demonstrated to result in a significant left-to-right shunt in two-ventricle or single-ventricle patients with evidence of CHF, pulmonary overcirculation, pleural effusion, or protein-losing enteropathy (class I, level of evidence: B). Fontan patients may also present with life-threatening hemoptysis secondary to intrapulmonary bleeding of SPCs, which can be treated by occlusion of the collaterals. In these cases it can help to perform bronchoscopy prior to the intervention to identify the location of the bleeding vessel. It is not clear whether occlusion of SPCs is beneficial when detected on routine catheterization of clinically well patients after Glenn or Fontan surgery. The practice of occluding SPCs prior to Fontan surgery is controversial and evidence to guide decisions is sparse. Thus, there is marked variability among centers in this practice [72]. In the case of patients with tetralogy of Fallot, pulmonary atresia, and SPCs, the decision to occlude SPCs depends on the volume of shunting, the degree of cyanosis, and whether each vessel provides the sole source of pulmonary blood flow to any lung segment. SPCs should not be occluded in patients with significant cyanosis due to limited pulmonary arterial flow (class III, level of evidence: C).

Technical Considerations

The shunt volume of SPC flow typically cannot be accurately calculated using oximetric data and the Fick principle at the time of catheterization. Techniques using MRI to calculate SPC flow have been described [73] but are not widely used. Operators generally estimate shunt volumes by qualitative assessment of aortic and selective angiograms. Whether SPCs provide dual

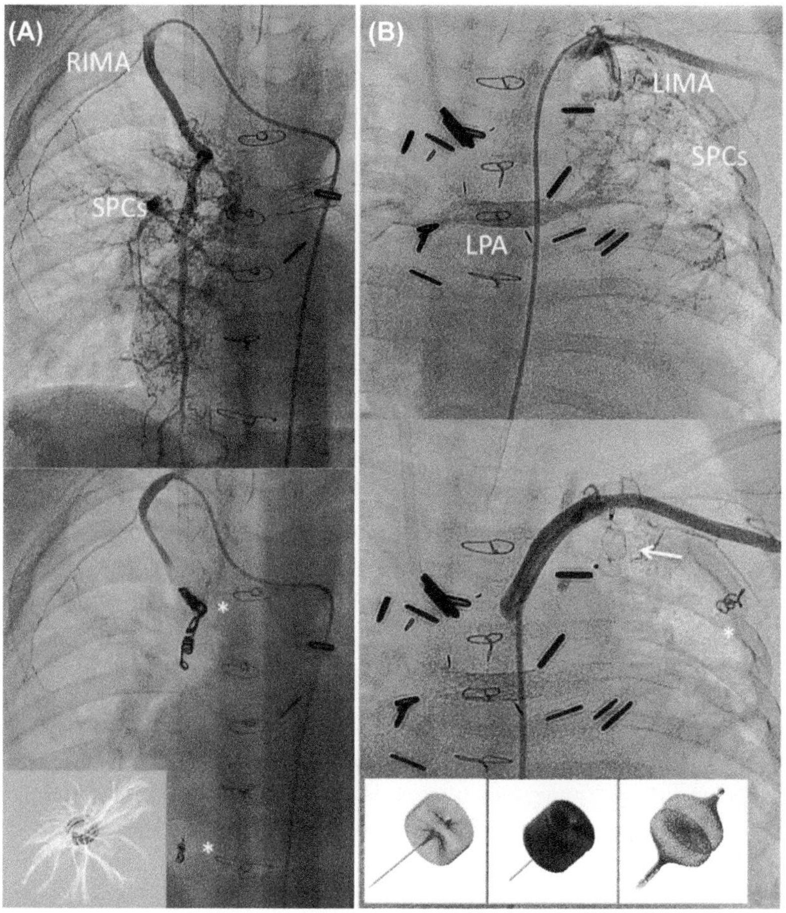

FIGURE 46.19 Coil and device occlusion of systemic-to-pulmonary collateral (SPC) vessels. (A) Selective injection into the RIMA in a single-ventricle palliated patient shows diffuse fine SPCs to the right lung (top). After placement of distal and proximal coils (*) in the RIMA, the vessel is occluded and there is no residual APC flow (bottom). Pushable coils (MReye coil from Cook Medical, Bloomington, IN is pictured in the inset) commonly have thrombogenic fibers to promote clotting and vessel occlusion. (B) Injection in the left subclavian artery shows SPC flow from the LIMA and subclavian to the left lung that backfills the stented proximal LPA (top). Pushable coils are place in the SPC from the subclavian artery (*) and a vascular plug (*arrow*) is placed in the LIMA, occluding flow (bottom). The Amplatzer Vascular Plug series (inset) provides options for device occlusion of collateral vessels. *LIMA*, left internal mammary artery; *LPA*, left pulmonary artery; *RIMA*, right internal mammary artery.

supply to lung segments in patients with tetralogy of Fallot and pulmonary atresia can be determined by selective angiography in each collateral. SPCs, however, vary widely in size, number, origin, and course. The technical approach and chance of effective occlusion depend on the anatomy, location, and distribution of the vessels. For example, a discrete medium-sized SPC from the aorta providing unnecessary dual supply to a lung segment may be easily accessed and occluded; however, diffuse innumerous tiny collateral vessels from the internal mammary arteries or other branches of the brachiocephalic arteries often seen in single-ventricle patients may require blunt aggressive occlusion along the length of the internal mammary artery, which may or may not significantly reduce the overall SPC shunting (Fig. 46.19). Generally, an attempt is made to occlude SPCs selectively and as deeply as possible to block all arterial communications with the vessel before it exits into the pulmonary circulation. Arterial access is necessary, and a number of coils and vascular plugs with small delivery systems, particulate agents, and liquids are available for SPC occlusion. Care is taken to maintain catheter position deep in the collateral during occlusion so that the occlusion device or material does not embolize into the systemic circulation.

Outcomes

Occlusions of SPCs by various techniques are relatively efficacious and safe. Coils and vascular plugs are the most commonly used means of SPC occlusion. The main risk associated with occlusions using coils and plugs is inadvertent embolization of the device into the systemic circulation. Current evidence does not demonstrate a substantial benefit from coil occlusion of SPCs in otherwise well patients undergoing Fontan surgery [72].

Coronary Artery Fistula

Physiology

CAFs are congenital or acquired communications between the coronary arteries and, most commonly, the right ventricle, RA, or pulmonary arteries, although they can communicate with other cardiac structures. The majority of these defects are small and hemodynamically insignificant. CHF may occur early in infancy if the fistula is large and results in volume

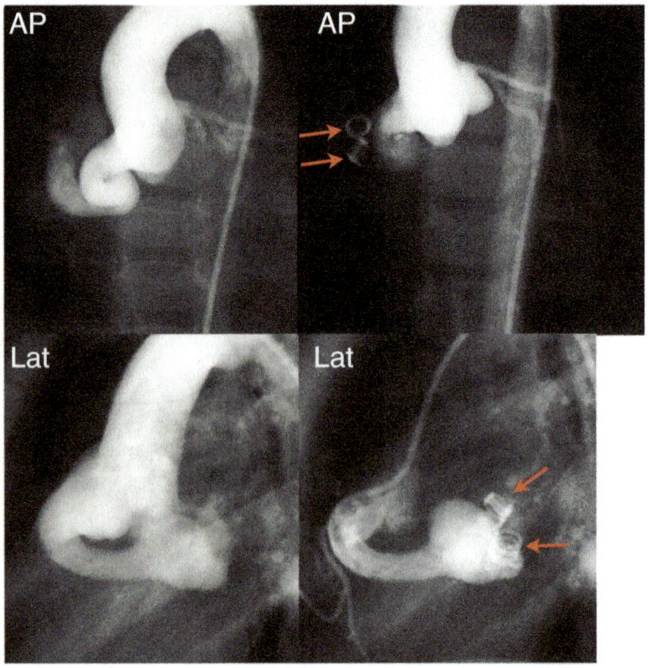

FIGURE 46.20 AP and lateral angiograms showing a large right coronary artery fistula from entering the right ventricle. The *red arrows* show two coils occluding the fistula.

overload and pulmonary overcirculation. In large shunts, there may also be coronary artery "steal" phenomenon causing ischemia distal to the fistulous connection. The affected coronary artery can dilate significantly to compensate for the shunt volume, but this can ultimately increase the risk of aneurysm, rupture, ulceration, side branch occlusion, atheroma, and calcification of the vessel. If left untreated, large CAFs can result in chronic myocardial ischemia, angina, cardiomyopathy, CHF, myocardial infarction, arrhythmia, and endocarditis.

Indications for Transcatheter Therapy

Transcatheter occlusion of CAFs is indicated in patients with symptoms of CHF or ischemia secondary to shunting at the fistula (class I, level of evidence: B). It is also reasonable to occlude moderate or large fistulas in the absence of clinical symptoms (class IIa, level of evidence: C), but it is not indicated in asymptomatic patients with small fistulas and no chamber enlargement.

Technical Considerations

The anatomy of CAFs is well characterized by selective coronary artery angiography in the catheterization lab at the time of intervention (Fig. 46.20). It is important to understand the fistula's size, origin, course, and exit location along with the number of exits, number of feeder vessels, and location of stenoses within the tract. An understanding of these features will help the operator decide the device or coil to use as well as the approach (antegrade or retrograde, need for an arteriovenous wire loop). To avoid compromising normal coronary artery flow, the fistula should be occluded as near to the exit point as possible. Coils are used most commonly in this intervention, but use of a variety of devices has been reported, including Rashkind or CardioSEAL devices, vascular plugs, PDA occlusion devices, and muscular VSD occlusion devices [74]. Some recommend test occlusion of the fistula with observation for signs of ischemia for 20–30 min before device occlusion is attempted.

Outcomes

One study reported outcomes in 39 patients evaluated for transcatheter occlusion of a CAF [75]. Occlusion devices were placed in 85% of patients and complete occlusion was documented in 82% of those who underwent occlusion. Devices were not placed in 15% of the patients because of multiple fistula drainage sites, extreme vessel tortuosity, and one intracardiac hemangioma. There were no deaths or long-term increased morbidity in this series. More recent studies have reported similar outcomes [74]. Complication rates are similar between transcatheter occlusion of CAFs and surgical ligation. Reported complications include transient ST-segment changes, arrhythmias, coronary artery spasm, device and coil embolization, fistula dissection or perforation, aneurysm thrombosis, recanalization of the fistula, and myocardial infarction.

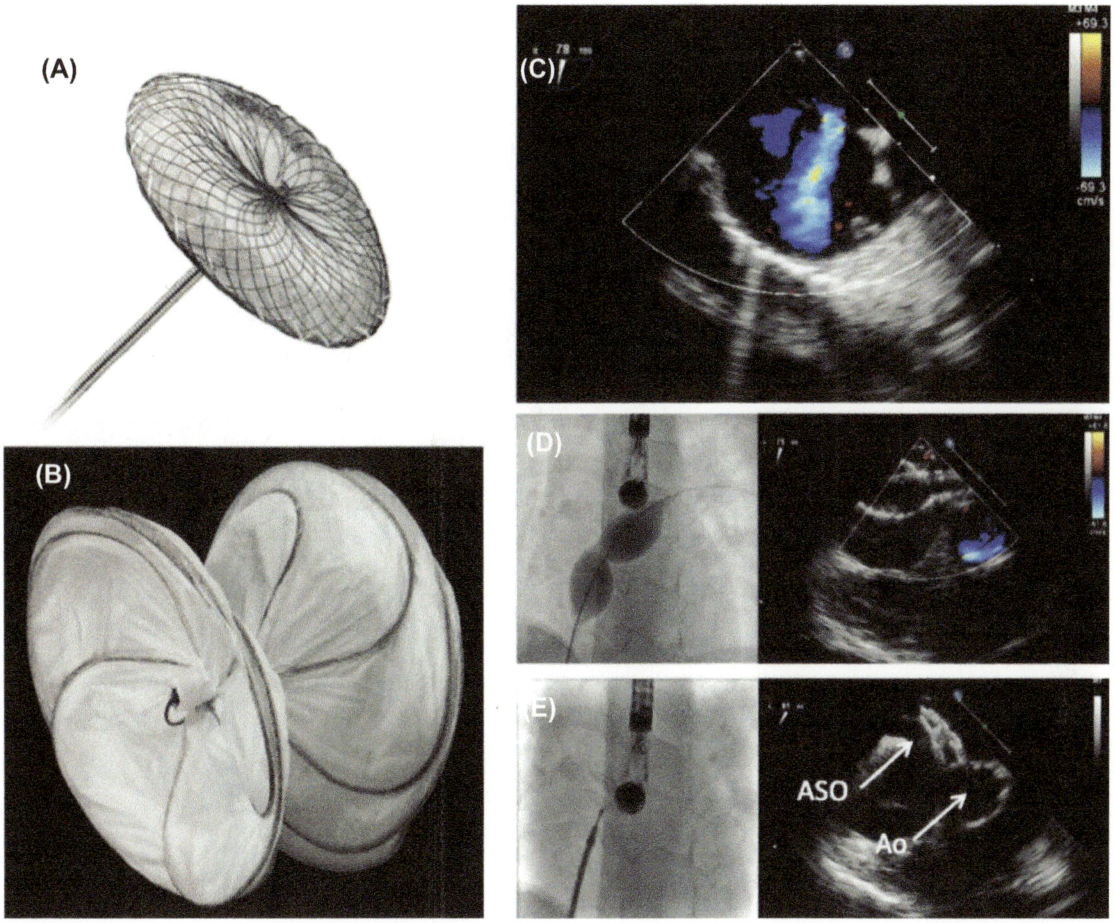

FIGURE 46.21 Device occlusion of atrial septal defects. The two available devices are pictured, (A) the Amplatzer Septal Occluder and (B) the GORE Cardioform Septal Occluder. Available devices come in a range of sizes and are designed only for occlusion of secundum defects. (C) A small secundum defect with adequate surrounding tissue rims is identified on TEE prior to occlusion. (D) A highly compliant balloon is dilated in the defect to accurately determine the defect's size both on fluoroscopy and TEE. (E) An Amplatzer device is deployed in the defect and evaluated on both fluoroscopy and TEE. Note the close proximity of the device to the aortic root on TEE. *Ao*, aorta; *ASD*, atrial septal defect; *ASO*, amplatzer septal occluder; *TEE*, transesophageal echocardiography.

Atrial Septal Defects

Physiology

ASDs are different from the other shunt lesions in that shunting is not driven by systolic pressures. Rather, shunting occurs during atrial filling and ventricular diastole, where the relative compliance of the relaxing ventricles determines the direction and volume of the shunt. Left-to-right shunting through the ASD will increase in early infancy as the compliance of the right heart increases and the right heart can become enlarged secondary to the volume overload. Although even large ASDs do not typically result in CHF in children, they can exacerbate pulmonary hypertension and chronic lung disease and are associated with failure to thrive [62,63]. Whether the failure to thrive is secondary to the shunt is debatable in many patients, however, and studies of whether catch-up growth occurs in children with failure to thrive after ASD repair or occlusion have returned mixed results [62,76,77]. If left untreated, significant atrial level shunts can ultimately result in right heart failure, arrhythmias, and pulmonary hypertension later in life.

Indications for Transcatheter Therapy

All currently available transcatheter ASD closure devices are designed to occlude secundum-type defects (Fig. 46.21). Primum defects, sinus venosus defects, and unroofed coronary sinus defects require surgical closure. Transcatheter secundum ASD closure is indicated in the presence of a hemodynamically significant shunt and suitable anatomic features (class I, level of evidence: B). A hemodynamically significant shunt is generally defined as a shunt that results in right heart enlargement, symptoms, arrhythmias, physical exam findings, or a Qp:Qs>1.5:1. Anatomic suitability is determined by the presence on preprocedure echocardiography of adequate septal tissue around the rims of the defect to hold a device securely. It is also reasonable to close secundum ASDs in patients with transient right-to-left shunting or symptomatic cyanosis who do not require the right-to-left shunt for adequate cardiac output (class 2a, level of evidence: B). There are additional class II indications for patients who have experienced or are at risk for thromboembolic events via paradoxical embolism through small atrial level defects. Closure should not be performed in patients with advanced and irreversible pulmonary vascular disease and pulmonary hypertension (class III, level of evidence: C). Generally, it is preferable to perform transcatheter ASD closure in patient weighing more than 15 kg, but closure in patients under this weight are widely reported and closure in small patients is not contraindicated.

Technical Considerations

In the United States, available ASD occlusion devices include the Amplatzer Septal Occluder (ASO; St. Jude Medical, St. Paul, MN) and the GORE CARDIOFORM Septal Occluder (GSO; W. L. Gore & Associates, Flagstaff, AZ), which has replaced the previous-generation HELEX Septal Occluder from GORE. The ASO is composed of Nitinol wire mesh encasing Dacron fabric and, when deployed, forms left and right atrial discs connected by a smaller self-centering midportion. It comes in sizes designed to close ASDs ranging from 4 to 38 mm in diameter. The GSO is composed of a nonself centering Nitinol wire frame covered with a thin expanded polytetrafluoroethylene membrane and is designed to close defects up to 17 mm in diameter.

Transcatheter ASD closure is performed using both fluoroscopy and echocardiography, either with a TEE probe or an intracardiac echo catheter. Echo imaging allows the operator to assess (1) the location, number, and size of septal defects; (2) the tissue rims used to anchor ASD closure devices, the inadequacy of which may place the patient at risk of device embolization or erosion; (3) presence of partial anomalous pulmonary venous return associated with the ASD that might necessitate surgical repair (PAPVR is noted in 2% of secundum defects [78] and can also be diagnosed on levophase of a pulmonary artery angiogram during the diagnostic catheterization); (4) the position of the device after deployment relative to tissue rims and important surrounding structures like the aortic root, atrioventricular valves, and pulmonary veins; and (5) residual shunting around the device or through separate defects Fig. 46.21.

If the defect is considered appropriate for closure, hemodynamic catheterization is performed to determine if the shunt volume and pulmonary vascular resistance are also appropriate. While some operators may base device sizing decisions on solely on preprocedure echo imaging, most prefer next to size the defect by measuring the waist of a large, highly compliant, and low-pressure balloon that is dilated carefully in the defect until no residual shunt flow is appreciated on echo (the "stop-flow diameter"). Appropriate device sizing is critical in preventing serious complications, such as device embolization and erosion. All ASD devices are delivered via venous access, preferably the femoral vein. Once the device type and size are determined, the device is delivered through a long sheath to the LA across the ASD and deployed under echo guidance using various techniques to ensure that the rims of the defect are captured. Extra care is taken to avoid perforating the left atrial wall or introducing air or thrombus into the LA during device delivery.

The deployed device remains attached to the delivery system and is retrievable if the deployment is not satisfactory. Prior to release, the rhythm is inspected on the monitor and echo is used to evaluate the device position and rim capture and to determine if there is residual shunting or impingement on any important surrounding structures, including the vena cavae, pulmonary veins, and atrioventricular valves. The positioning and movement of the device at the anterosuperior ("retro-aortic") rim, where the device may impinge on the aortic root, is inspected carefully to determine if there is concern for erosion risk. The device is released and the delivery system is withdrawn. The device is reevaluated with echo in a manner similar to postdeployment and is often retrievable using snare catheters if it embolizes after release. Patients are treated with antiplatelet agents starting a few days prior to the procedure until the device presumably is covered by endothelium approximately 6 months later.

Outcomes

Outcomes following transcatheter ASD closure have generally been excellent and are comparable to surgical closure [79,80]. The implantation success rate for the Amplatzer ASD device is approximately 96% with an early closure success rate of 95% and a late closure rate of 98% [80,81]. Implantation of the Amplatzer ASD device has a reported adverse event rate of 7.2% and a 1.6% rate of major complications, including device embolization requiring surgical removal, serious arrhythmias, and cerebral embolism [80]. Rare erosions of the device into the pericardial space and aorta have been reported. A total of 125 erosions resulting in 9 deaths were reported between 2002 and 2014 at a median time of 14 days after implantation, although 16 erosions occurred longer than 1 year after implantation [31]. The risk of erosion is estimated to be approximately 0.1% [82]. The Gore ASD device has a reported technical success rate of 85%–91%, a closure rate of 100% among devices successfully placed, and no reported major complications [83,84]. Studies of transcatheter ASD closures in patients under 10–15 kg in weight show that there may be a somewhat higher complication rate in smaller patients, but that procedural success rates are still high and improvements in pulmonary hypertension, right heart enlargement, chronic lung disease, and growth have been observed [62,63,77,85].

Ventricular Septal Defects

Physiology

VSDs can occur in the membranous septum (~80% of defects), muscular septum (~5%–20%), outlet septum (~5%), or inlet septum (~5%). Similar to other left-to-right shunt lesions, the shunt volume and resulting heart failure symptoms and pulmonary overcirculation are proportional to the effective size of the defect. Large defects will cause CHF, persistently elevated right heart pressures, pulmonary overcirculation, and failure to thrive in the first few months of life if the pulmonary vasculature relaxes normally. Smaller pressure restrictive defects, including moderate-to-large perimembranous defects partially covered by aneurismal tricuspid valve tissue, may lead to left heart volume overload as well. Multiple defects can occur in the muscular septum, in extreme cases resembling a "Swiss cheese" septum. Approximately 75% of small defects will close spontaneously in the first 2 years of life. Highly restrictive defects that persist may be benign but can lead to infective endocarditis, obstructive subaortic membranes, aortic insufficiency (if the shunt is near the valve cusp), or progressive right ventricular outflow tract obstruction.

Indications for Transcatheter Therapy

Devices are available in the United States for closure of muscular VSDs only. There is a membranous VSD Occluder device available in other countries outside of the United States. Also, a number of devices and coils have been employed off-label to close perimembranous VSDs with restrictive "windsock" tunnel formations from aneurismal tricuspid valve tissue. It is reasonable to percutaneously occlude a hemodynamically significant muscular VSD with a device in patients weighing

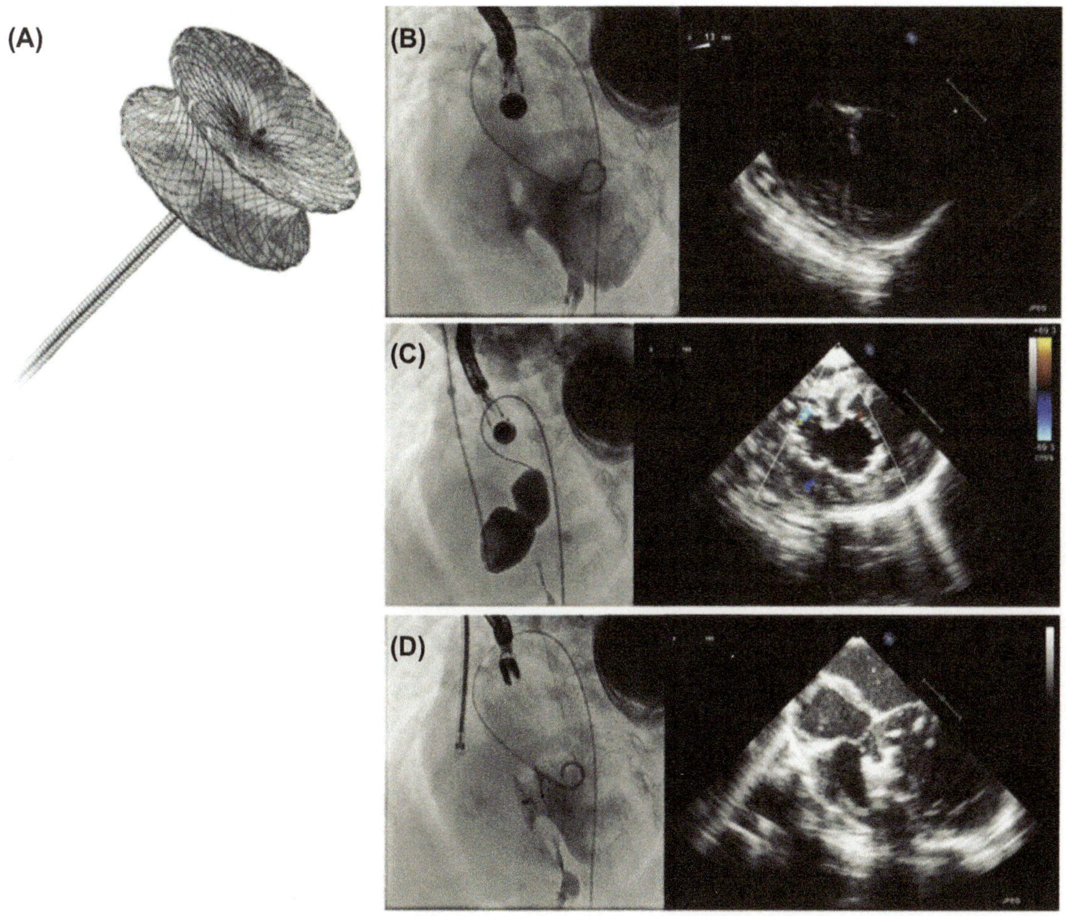

FIGURE 46.22 Device occlusion of muscular VSDs. (A) The Amplatzer Muscular VSD Occluder is the only available device designed specifically for transcatheter VSD closure. (B) A moderate midmuscular VSD is identified by left ventriculogram and transesophageal echo (TEE) in a 14-month-old patient with congestive heart failure. (C) An arteriovenous wire loop is established through the VSD from the femoral artery to the right internal jugular vein. A compliant balloon is dilated in the defect to accurately determine the size of the defect by fluoroscopy and TEE. (D) The device is delivered via the right internal jugular vein and is pictured in position after release from the delivery system. There is minimal residual shunting by angiography and no additional defects. The patient's heart failure symptoms and growth improved following closure of the defect. *TEE*, transesophageal echocardiography; *VSD*, ventricular septal defect.

more than 5 kg (class IIa; level of evidence: B). Patients weighing <5 kg or those undergoing cardiac surgery for associated lesions may be candidates for muscular VSD occlusion with a device using a periventricular open-chest hybrid approach off bypass or direct open-heart placement on bypass (class IIb; level of evidence: B). Devices should not be placed in patients with muscular defects that are too close to the atrioventricular or semilunar valves, those with irreversible pulmonary hypertension, or those in whom there is a reasonable expectation that the defect will become insignificant in size over time (class III; level of evidence: B).

Technical Considerations

In the United States, the Amplatzer Muscular VSD Occluder (St. Jude Medical, St. Paul, MN) is the only available device designed specifically for VSD closure (Fig. 46.22). This device is made of Nitinol wire with polyester mesh and has right and left ventricular discs connected by a central waist that should approximate the diameter and length of the VSD. Device sizes range from 4 to 18 mm. The Amplatzer Membranous VSD Occluder and Membranous VSD Occluder 2 (neither available in the United States) are similar in concept but have design features to better approximate the membranous septum and avoid impingement on surrounding structures.

Similar to transcatheter ASD closure, TEE is essential in evaluating the location, size, and number of defects as well as the proximity to surrounding structures such as the cardiac valves and the moderator band. TEE is also essential in evaluating device positioning and residual shunting. Transcatheter muscular and perimembranous VSD closures use a similar approach. Arterial and venous access is obtained and a hemodynamic catheterization determines the volume of the shunt and the pulmonary vascular resistance. Angulated angiograms from the left ventricle help to define the septal anatomy. The VSD is then crossed from the left ventricular side retrograde from the femoral artery and a wire is positioned in the right heart. A snare is used from the venous side to capture the wire and create an arteriovenous wire loop. A delivery sheath is then placed over the wire from the venous access site, through the right heart, and across the VSD into the left heart while the wire is secured at both ends. The wire is removed and the device, secured to its delivery cable, is delivered with care not to introduce air or thrombus to the left heart. The device is deployed across the septal defect under echo guidance and carefully evaluated prior to release from the delivery system. The membranous VSD device has asymmetric discs that must be positioned correctly with relation to the valves. These steps are repeated for each additional VSD that meets indication for closure. Similar to ASD closure, patients are placed on antiplatelet agents for 6 months until endothelialization of the device has occurred and there is no residual shunt.

In small patients (<5 kg), patients without vascular access, or those who require sternotomy or open-heart surgery for other indications, the periventricular hybrid approach to muscular VSD closure is advantageous. This procedure can be performed off bypass and avoids ventriculotomy. If the patient requires cardiopulmonary bypass to repair a separate lesion, the muscular VSD can be addressed prior to going on bypass. Under TEE or epicardial echo guidance, the surface of the heart is gently probed through the sternotomy (or subxyphoid without sternotomy using TEE) to identify the optimal location and angle of approach to directly access the VSD through the right ventricular wall. A needle is used to access the ventricle and a wire is used to cross the defect, followed by a sheath surrounded by a purse-string suture. Similar to the percutaneous approach, an appropriately sized mVSD device is delivered on its delivery cable through the sheath to the LV and deployed in the defect. In small patients, it is important to avoid damage to the LV free wall with the sheath and dilator and to make sure there is room in the LV cavity to unsheath and form the left ventricular disc. After thorough evaluation, the device is released and the sheath and delivery system are removed and the stitch tied to close the access site.

Outcomes

Prospective nonrandomized registry results from 14 tertiary US centers reported 77 muscular VSD closures using the Amplatzer muscular VSD device in patients ranging in age from 0.1 to 54 years. Devices were implanted successfully in 87% of procedures and the complete closure rate was 92% at 12 months. Major complications occurred in 10.7%, including three cerebrovascular accidents, two device embolizations, and one cardiac perforation [86]. The hybrid periventricular approach has demonstrated high procedural success rates and very rare major complications in most studies of patients presenting with mixed indications for the hybrid approach [87–90]. The risks may be higher in small patients. In one series of 24 infants <5 kg, three required conversion to surgical repair for LV perforation in one, failure to cross the defect with a wire in one, and anatomy not ultimately amenable to device closure in the other. Two patients died during the hospitalization following device implantation, one from sepsis and another likely from ventricular arrhythmia. One patient developed permanent heart block and LV outflow tract obstruction [91].

The perimembranous region has proven more difficult for device implantations given the close proximity of the defects to the aortic and tricuspid valves and the conduction system. The initial Amplatzer Membranous VSD Occluder, another Nitinol mesh device, not available in the United States, was highly successful in closing perimembranous VSDs and was widely used in the early 2000s. However, rare cases of progressive aortic and tricuspid insufficiency were reported and complete heart block was reported in ~5% of patients in most series, but as many as 22% in one study [92–94] and many centers abandoned the procedure. A 2nd-generation device, the Amplatzer Membranous VSD Occluder 2 (St. Jude Medical, St. Paul, MN), was developed to reduce the risk of heart block. This device has demonstrated a 95% rate of successful device implantation and an 83% rate of complete occlusion at most recent follow-up with no heart block or increase in aortic or tricuspid insufficiency [95]. This device is not currently available in the United States either. The off-label use of several other devices to occlude perimembranous VSDs with or without aneurismal surrounding tissue has been reported with high occlusion rates and low complication rates and no permanent heart block [96–98]. Despite the promising results for device closure of perimembranous VSDs, most centers currently prefer surgical closure for most perimembranous VSDs.

MISCELLANEOUS

Valvar Regurgitation

Physiology

PR over time leads to a volume load on the right ventricle that can lead to right heart failure. When PR is concomitant with tricuspid valve regurgitation, the volume load can be significant and cause severe RV and RA dilation. If this is coupled with any forward flow obstruction, as in pulmonary valve, conduit, or branch pulmonary artery stenosis, the effect can be additive [99,100]. Many centers have used MRI to quantify the degree of pulmonary regurgitation and right ventricular end-diastolic volume. In general, volumes of 150 cc/M2–170 cc/M2 have been deemed significant enough to indicate surgical valve replacement [101–106]. In the current era of transcatheter pulmonary valve therapy, many have continued to use this value as an indication for valve implantation. However, the Melody Transcatheter Valve (Medtronics Inc) IFU states indications include stenosis gradient >35 mmHg and/or qualitative "moderate regurgitation." Recently, the Sapien Valve (**Edwards**) has also received FDA approval for transcatheter pulmonary valve implantation. Transcatheter valve implantation techniques and outcomes are well reported in the literature [107].

Severe aortic valve regurgitation can result in low-output syndrome and LV dilation in addition to coronary artery insufficiency. Current standard of care for aortic valve replacement in pediatrics remain surgical repair or replacement. However, implantation of transcatheter valves using hybrid techniques have been reported in small infants when there were no other surgical valves available for small annuli and when the Ross procedure was not an option due to a dysfunctional pulmonary valve.

Mitral valve regurgitation will cause LA dilation and eventually pulmonary hypertension if it progresses over time.

Indications for Intervention

AHA guidelines. Aortic and mitral valve regurgitation are most commonly found in the adult population with structural heart disease and will be left for another chapter. For pulmonary valves dysfunction, indications are 35 mmHg gradient and/or moderate valve regurgitation in a patient big enough to tolerate a 22 Fr delivery system. As for tricuspid or mitral regurgitation, there are no standard guidelines for transcatheter interventions except for the combination of severe stenosis with regurgitation. It should be important to note that current commercially available transcatheter valve is FDA approved for implantation in a previously placed surgical RV-PA conduit although bioprosthetic pulmonary valves also serve well for implants.

Technical Considerations

Transcatheter valve therapy is now a standard for RV-PA conduit dysfunction, which includes both stenosis and regurgitation. For native pulmonary valves, the problem is the diameter of the outflow tracts, which is often much larger than the diameter of available transcatheter valves. Currently, there are two commercially available valves. The largest ensemble system for implanting a Melody valve is 22 mm although one can modify the delivery techniques to use a 24 mm balloon. The Edwards Sapien valve comes in 23, 26, and 29 mm diameter delivery systems. There are small series reporting the use of transcatheter valves for the tricuspid position [107–109]. The majority of these implants are in older children and adult size patients who have received surgically placed bioprosthetic valves that have become dysfunctional over time. There are also scattered reports of combined implantation of transcatheter valves in both the pulmonary and tricuspid positions [110–112]. As for the mitral valve, there are a few reports of implanting undersized transcatheter valves using hybrid techniques. These rare cases are generally reserved for the infant with severe mitral regurgitation and a mitral annulus that is too small for the smallest surgical valves (15 mm) [113–118]. Another theoretical advantage is that these undersized transcatheter valves can be further dilated as the infant grows to avoid multiple valve replacements [119].

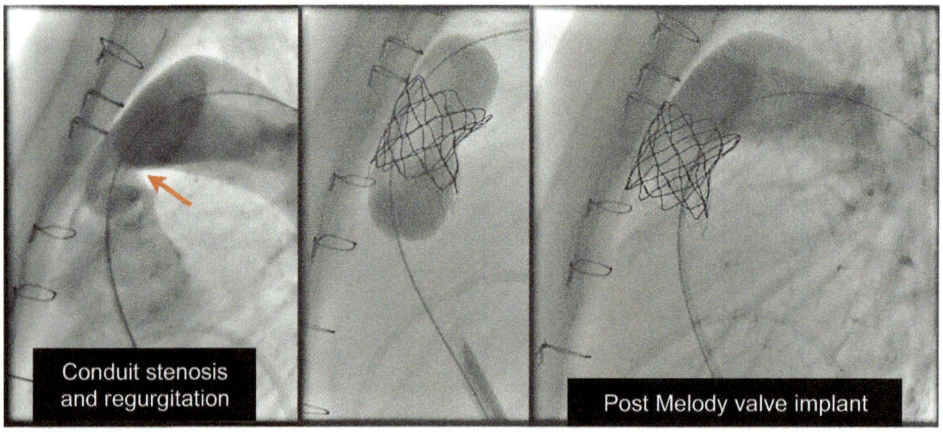

FIGURE 46.23 Right ventricle to pulmonary artery conduit with combined stenosis and regurgitation (left); Melody valve implant (middle) and post-implant angiogram demonstrating restoration of pulmonary valve function.

Outcomes Data

Pulmonary

Tricuspid-McElhinney reported from the Valve-in-Valve International Database Registry their experience with using transcatheter valves to treat tricuspid valve dysfunction [108]. Among 152 patients in whom TVIV was attempted with a Melody (n = 94) or Sapien (n = 58) valve, implantation was successful in 150, with few serious complications with significant improvement in tricuspid stenosis and/or regurgitation. Follow-up with a median of 13.3 months indicated 22 deaths, all of whom were in NYHA class III or IV. There were 10 TV reinterventions, and 3 other patients had significant recurrent TV dysfunction. 77% of patients were in NYHA class I or II ($P<.001$ vs. before TVIV). They concluded that TVIV with commercially available transcatheter prostheses is technically and clinically successful in patients of various ages across a wide range of valve sizes. While preimplantation clinical status was associated with outcome, many patients in NYHA class III or IV at baseline improved after implant. TVIV therapy should be considered a viable option for treatment of a failing tricuspid bioprosthesis. This conclusion was confirmed in a report by Aboulson et al. in which 22 patients (13 sites) with a wide age range (5–69 years) had a 91% technical success at implant [109]. 86% had severe tricuspid regurgitation and in NYHA functional class III or IV before implant. At median follow-up of 1 year, functional class improved in 70% and paravalvar leaks were found (trivial to mild) in 75%. These did not require treatment. Both Sapien and Melody valves were used. The findings of paravalvar leaks in this study may be due to the older age at implant compared to McElhinney's report. Levi et al. reported the use of the Sapien XT valve in both the pulmonary and tricuspid positions and reported an advantage of the Sapien XT's larger implantable diameters (up to 30 mm diameter) [107].

Fig. 46.23 shows an RV-PA conduit with combined stenosis and regurgitation, Melody valve implant, and restoration of pulmonary valve function postimplant.

Mitral

To date, the majority of Melody valve implants in mitral bioprostheses in CHD have been performed in infants whose mitral annulus was too small for a surgical implant. These are performed as hybrid procedures in conjunction with the cardiac surgeons. Currently, the smaller available bioprosthetic valve is 15 mm. The Melody valve has been shown to be functional when implanted in diameters as small as 10 mm and can be further dilated using transcatheter techniques as the child grows. However, in small children, the length of the valve may be an issue as it is essentially a covered stent and may cause left ventricular outflow tract obstruction. Techniques of shortening the stent by folding the edges, suturing the stent against the LV posterior wall and removing part of the covering have been described.

Additional techniques involve adding a pericardial sewing cuff for the hybrid implant and intraoperative balloon expansion once the valve is sewn in place [114].

The hybrid data are further described later in the chapter.

Emani et al. reported a series of 42 patients with a median age of 10 months (range 3 weeks–5.8 years) in whom a Melody valve was implanted using hybrid techniques in mitral, aorta, pulmonary and tricuspid positions. They conclude that the technique has acceptable short-term outcomes and the valve is amenable to further dilation as the child grows thereby reducing the number of operations over a lifetime. They also caution that additional techniques of implantation and valve modifications are needed to reduce perivalvar complications [119].

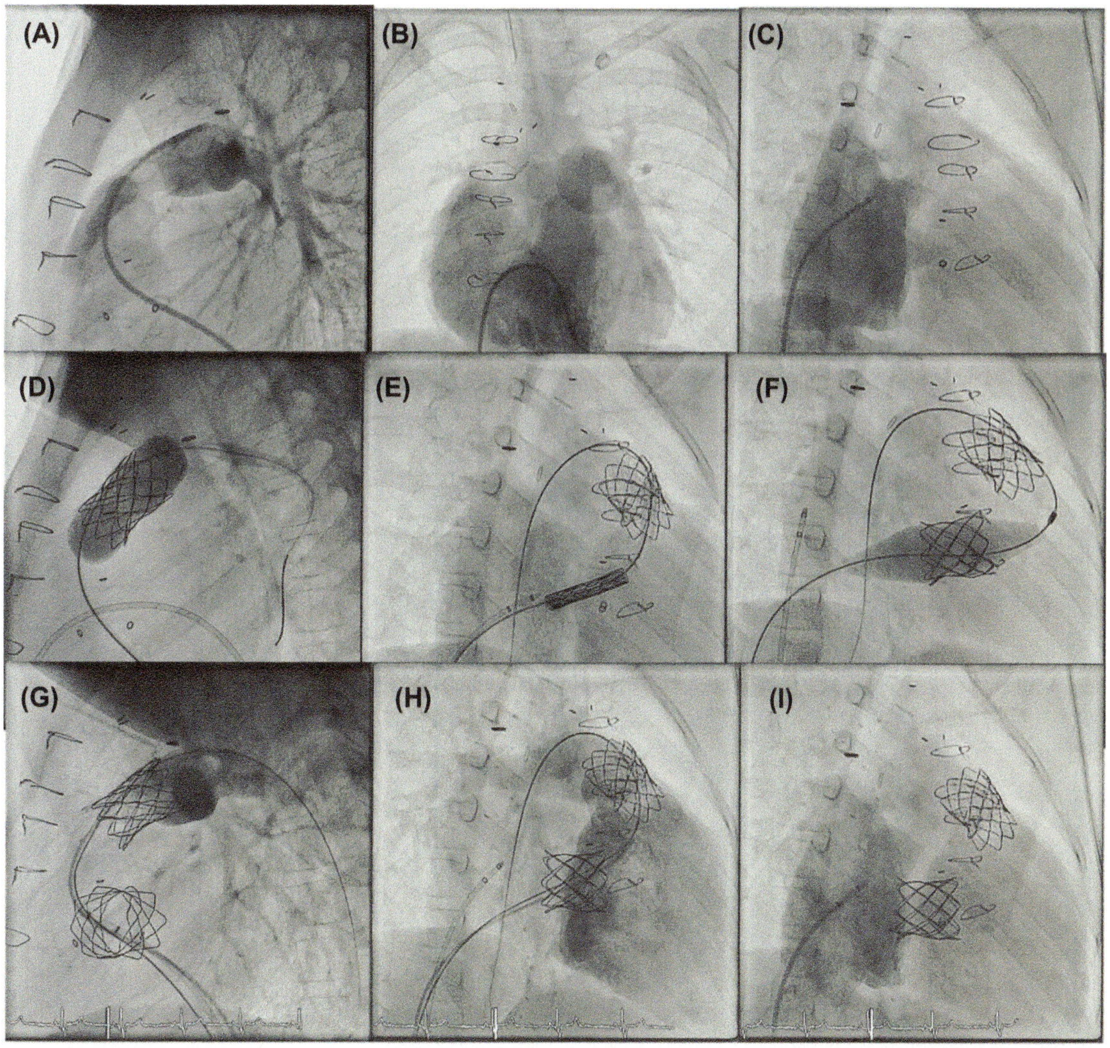

FIGURE 46.24 A double Melody valve implant in both the pulmonary and tricuspid positions. Patient has history of Ebstein's anomaly s/p pulmonary and tricuspid valve replacements presenting with a combination of significant pulmonary valve stenosis and regurgitation (A), and tricuspid valve regurgitation (B) and stenosis (C). First Melody valve was implanted into the pulmonary position (D), followed by second Melody valve implant in the tricuspid position (E and F). Pulmonary valve function is restored with elimination of regurgitation and stenosis (G), as well as restoration of tricuspid valve function with elimination of tricuspid regurgitation (H) and stenosis (I).

Aortic

Scattered case reports have demonstrated the possibility of implanting transcatheter valves in the neoaortic position in single-ventricle anatomy [117]. Since the coronary arteries come off the native aortic valve, the Melody valve can be implanted in the neoaortic regurgitant valve without compromising coronary flow. Nevertheless, balloon testing with coronary flow assessment before implant is essential.

Multivalve Implants

Several small series have reported concomitant valve implantations in both the pulmonary and tricuspid position in a single cardiac catheterization due to combined valvar dysfunction (stenosis and/or regurgitation). These patients tend to have a markedly dilated RA and right ventricular dysfunction [110–112].

Fig. 46.24 shows a series of images of a patient with a history of Ebstein's anomaly, s/p pulmonary and tricuspid valve replacements presenting with a combination of significant stenosis and regurgitation involving both the pulmonary and tricuspid valves. The RA and right ventricle are dilated and RV function was depressed. Melody valves were sequentially implanted into both the pulmonary and tricuspid positions.

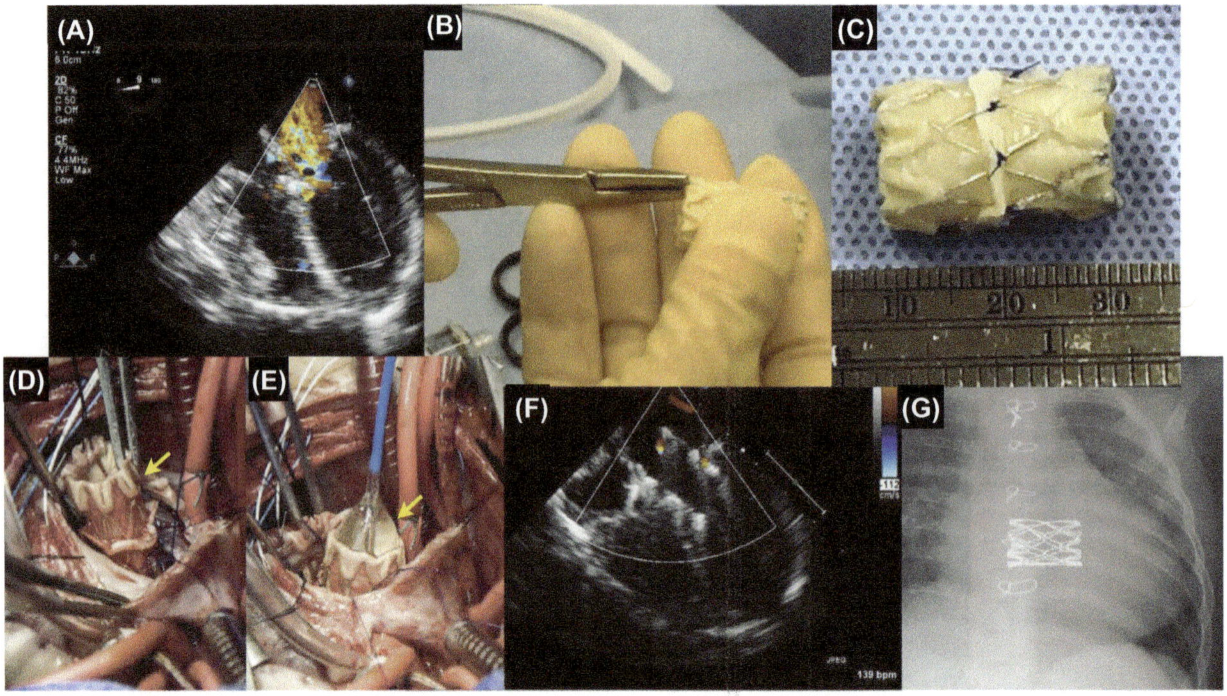

FIGURE 46.25 Hybrid implantation of a Melody valve in the mitral position was performed in a 3-month-old infant s/p AVC repair with severe mitral rerurgitation (A). Folding half a stent cell from each edge to shorten the Melody valve from 3 to 2 cm (B). Image of Melody valve prepared for implant. A pericardial cuff was hand sewn around the valve to secure the valve onto the mitral annulus (C). Surgical implantation of the valve secured with sutures placed around the pericardial cuff (D), following by balloon dilation to further expand the valve (E). Postimplant show trivial mitral regurgitation on the Melody valve (F). Final postop CXR showing the Melody valve in the mitral position (G).

Hybrid Implants

When patients are too small for transcatheter implant, successful hybrid techniques have been described, mostly from Boston Children's Hospital and a few other centers [113,114,118,120–122].

Emani et al. described a series of 42 young patients with a median age of 10 months (range, 3 weeks to 5.8 years) in whom a hybrid procedure was used to implant a Melody valve in the aortic, mitral, pulmonary, or tricuspid positions [119]. All valves remained competent with low gradients in early follow-up. At 12 months follow-up, 88% remained free from reoperation based on Kaplan–Meier analysis. 8 patients experienced central or paravalvar deterioration, 7 required reoperation for valve-related adverse outcomes, and 20 patients underwent 32 successful further balloon dilations of the implanted valve (due to somatic growth) with no significant increase in regurgitation. Six deaths occurred, three before discharge and three late. Their conclusion suggested that a surgically implanted Melody valve has acceptable short-term function and is amenable to further catheter-based enlargement as the child grows. To date, further dilation of an implanted Melody valve has been performed successfully, but longer-term follow-up is essential to determine the longevity of these valves in the systemic circulation in a growing child.

Fig. 46.25 shows implantation of a Melody valve in the mitral position using hybrid techniques in a 3-month-old infant s/p AVC repair with severe mitral rerurgitation. Due to the small size of the infant (4 kg) and concern for left ventricular obstruction, the Melody valve stent had to be shortened from 3 to 2 cm by folding half a stent cell from each edge. A pericardial cuff was hand sewn around the valve for purposed of securing the valve to the mitral annulus. Following placement of the Melody valve into the mitral annulus, balloon dilation was performed to further expand the valve. Postimplant show only trivial mitral regurgitation on the Melody valve.

Fig. 46.26 shows the same patient at 10 months follow-up. The patient had doubled her weight from 4 to 7.8 Kg. Follow-up echocardiogram showed flow turbulence across the Melody valve and the gradient had increased from 9-mmHg post-Melody valve implant to 22 mmHg. After further dilation of mitral valve in the cath lab, laminar flow was restored to the Melody valve and the residual gradient was 8 mmHg.

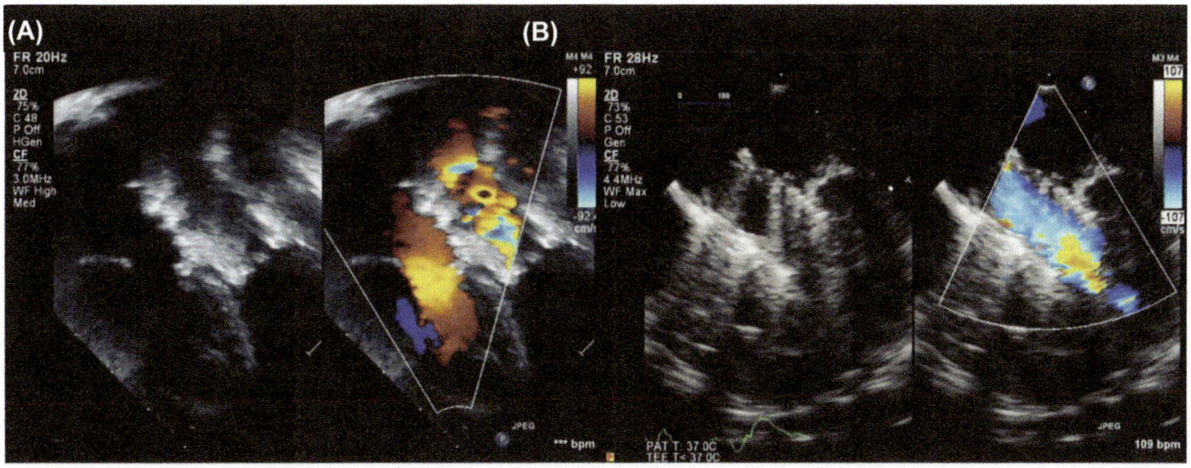

FIGURE 46.26 10 months follow-up showed the patient had double her weight from 4 to 7.8 kg. Follow-up echocardiogram showed the Melody valve gradient had increased from 9 to 22 mmHg (A). After further dilation of mitral valve in the cath lab, flow across Melody valve is now laminar (B) with a peak and mean gradient of 12 and 8 mmHg, respectively.

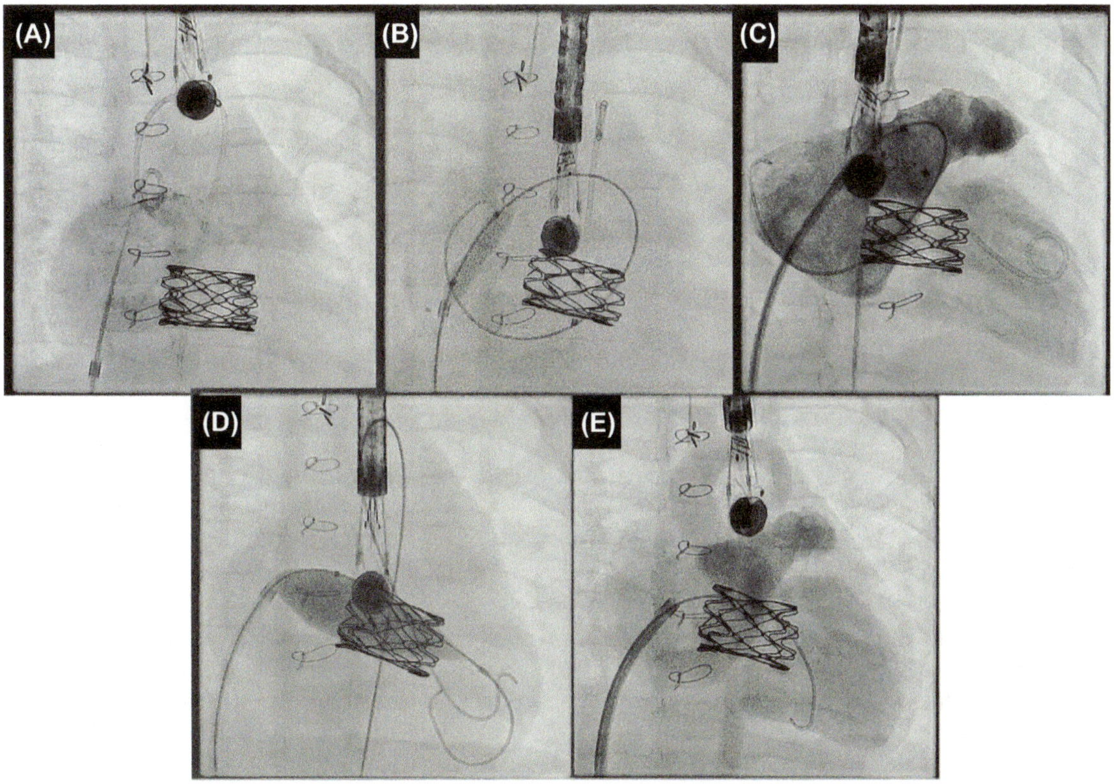

FIGURE 46.27 Fluoroscopic images of same patient in Fig. 46.26. Initial transseptal puncture to assess the left atrium. Previous atrial septal defect had been repaired with a pericardial patch (A). Balloon dilation of thickened patched septum to accommodate passage of sheath (B). Angiogram showed a dilated left atrium (LA) with restricted flow across Melody valve (C). Further dilation of Melody valve (D). Postdilation angiogram show the LA to be less dilated with more flow to LV (E).

Fig. 46.27 shows the fluoroscopic images of the further dilation in the cath lab. Initial transseptal puncture was required to assess the LA. This was a difficult procedure due to the fact that the previous ASD had been repaired with a pericardial patch, which had become thickened. Balloon dilation of the patched septum was needed to accommodate passage of the transseptal sheath. The initial angiogram showed a dilated LA with restricted flow across Melody valve. After further dilation of Melody valve, a postdilation angiogram show the LA to be less dilated with more flow to the LV (E).

Pericardial Tamponade

Physiology as Related to Heart Failure

As fluid fills the pericardial sac, the pressure–volume curve takes a logarithmic change where a small added volume results in a significant increase in pressure. Hence, tamponade can occur very quickly. Clinical signs and symptoms are well published. High index of suspicion and rapid diagnosis is key.

Indications for Intervention

Indications include impending cardiac tamponade or need for removal of pericardial fluid for diagnostic reasons. Signs and symptoms of cardiac tamponade are well documented in other publications and will not be discussed here.

Technical Considerations

Standard subxiphoid approach has been well described since the early 1900s. The technique has remained essentially unchanged except for the use of fluoroscopic guidance in the mid-1900s and echocardiographic guidance in the modern era. For effusions that are more posterior or lateral, a subxiphoid approach can pose risk of injuring the heart. In that situation, a left lateral or periapical approach may be preferable. Echocardiogram is first performed to evaluate the effusion and location of the maximal amount. As long as the echo image is not obscured by the lungs, especially on inspiration, a small needle for topical anesthesia can be used. From the left axilla or periapical region, the distance from the skin to the pericardium of often less than 2 cm in infants and children. It is not uncommon for the short numbing needle to enter the pericardial fluid. This technique using echocardiographic guidance was first reported for adult patients in the 1980s [123] and later in the pediatric population in the late 1990s.

Fig. 46.28 shows an 8-year-old presenting with viral myocarditis and a large pericardial effusion with early signs of cardiac tamponade. There is a large effusion at the left lateral region of the heart in spite of only a thin rim of effusion inferiorly by the diaphragm, which is not amenable for a standard subxiphoid approach for pericardiocentesis. Echo measurements show the distance for the needle to enter from the skin (at the anterior axillary line at the level of the nipple) to the pericardial sac is only 1.5 cm. From this area, even a 24-gauge needle used for lidocaine can enter the pericardial space. Following pericardiocentesis and drainage of the effusion, only a small amount of fluid is left in the pericardial space. With echocardiographic guidance, the wire used for placement of the drain can be seen in the pericardial sac. If the procedure is performed in the cath lab, fluoroscopy can also confirm proper placement of a pericardial drain.

Outcomes Data

The subxiphoid approach is considered to be the standard entry site for pericardiocentesis for half a century; its efficacy and safety are well recognized and outcomes will not be discussed here. However, nonstandard entry sites including left lateral and periapical approach deserve some discussion. The first description of using this approach in pediatrics was published in 1998 by Tsang et al. [124] 93/94 attempts were successfully performed in 73 patients. Seventy-two were performed in the left lateral or para-apical region using echo guidance. Others have reported equally successful procedures in infants and small children using nonstandard approaches with echo guidance [125]. In a series performed at Texas Children's Hospital from 2007 to 2009, 19 patients underwent 21 procedures using the left lateral or para-apical approach. Indications included therapeutic or diagnostic taps due to postviral, postop, leukemic pericardial effusions. The average size of the effusion was 7.8 ± 4.2 mm inferiorly and 19.3 ± 6.2 mm posterolaterally. The large discrepancy of the effusion size resulted in a decision to perform the pericardiocentesis from the left lateral or periapical approach since there was more room for needle entry. Echo guidance minimized complications of cardiac perforation. Interestingly, the depth of needle entry from skin to effusion was only 5–20 mm. Compared to the subxiphoid approach, this is a significantly shorter distance from skin to effusion. The first attempt was successful in 18/21 (85.7%) cases. Despite echo guidance, there was one major complication (LV puncture) and three minor complications (one small pneumothorax and two inadvertent entrance into the pleural space), none of which required additional intervention (unpublished data).

Restrictive Atrial Septum

Balloon atrial septostomy was developed by Rashkind in 1966 for patients with TGA to open the restrictive atrial septum and improve mixing of pulmonary venous and systemic venous blood. Patients with TGA have pulmonary and systemic

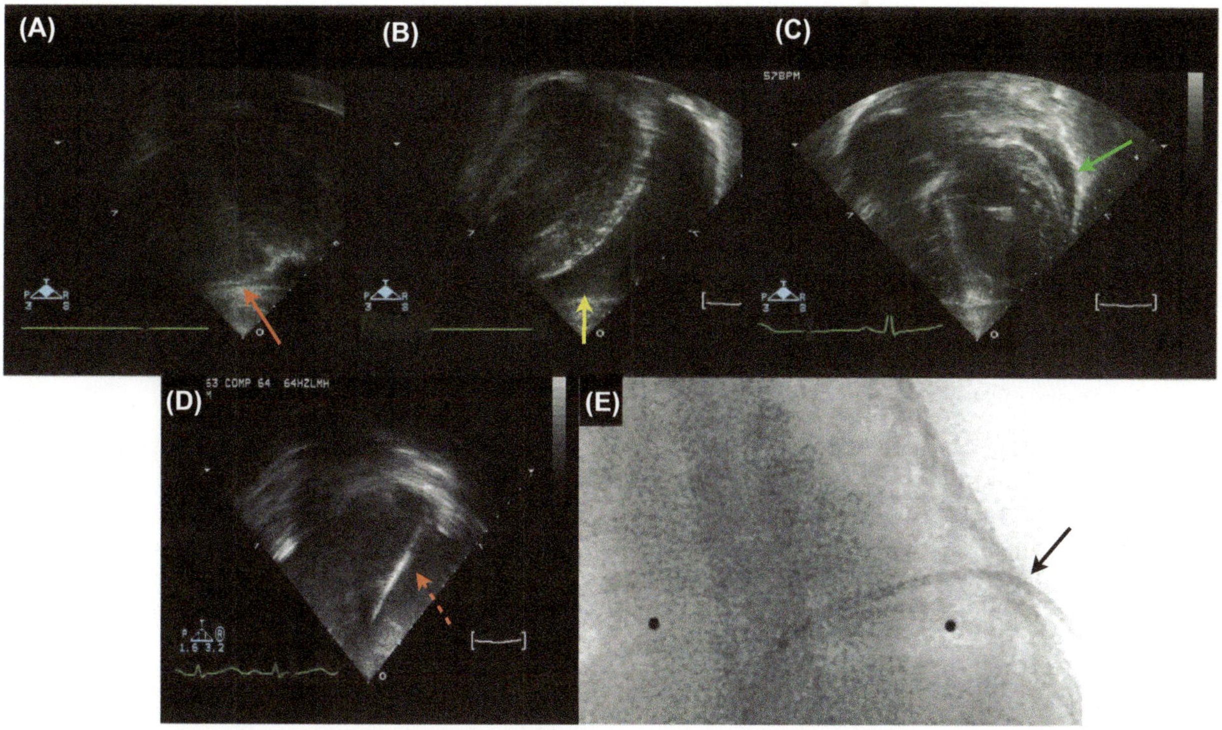

FIGURE 46.28 8-year-old with viral myocarditis and pericardial effusion and early signs of cardiac tamponade. There is only a thin rim of effusion (*red solid arrow*) inferiorly by the diaphragm (A) that is not amenable for a standard subxiphoid approach for pericardiocentesis. However, there is a large effusion at the left lateral region of the heart (B). The distance for the needle to go from the skin (at the anterior axillary line at the level of the nipple) to the pericardial sac is only 1.5cm (*yellow arrow*), which can be entered even with a 24-gauge needle used for lidocaine. (C) Postpericardiocentesis and drainage of effusion. Only a small amount of fluid is left in the pericardial space (*green arrow*). (D) Echocardiographic evidence of wire in the pericardial sac (*red dotted arrow*) in another patient. (E) Fluoroscopy of pericardial drain (*black arrow*) left in the left lateral position in another infant.

systems in parallel and an adequate ASD necessary for adequate mixing of the two systems and oxygenation. Patients with a restrictive atrial septum will have severe cyanosis but often will have adequate blood pressures. Severe cyanosis over time, however, will lead to lactic acidosis and ventricular dysfunction can develop if not intervened on. Initially the procedure was performed under fluoroscopic guidance, now more often performed using echocardiographic guidance. The 5F Miller balloon atrial septostomy catheter (Edwards Lifesciences, Irvine, CA, USA) requires a 7F introducer sheath and the dual lumen Z-5 atrioseptostomy catheter (Numed, Cornwall, ON, Canada) comes in 4F or 5F sizes, depending on the balloon diameter, and requires a 5 or 6F introducer, respectively. The Z-5 septostomy catheter can be used over a wire if it is difficult to cross the atrial septum. The balloon is inflated in the LA and rapidly withdrawn across the defect to tear the membranous inferior margin of the septum. Successful septostomy occurs in most infants under 1 month of age. Over that age, the septum is thick and tough and if septostomy was performed often results in only some stretching.

Balloon atrial septosomy is often required in less critical heart conditions as well to allow for decompression of the right heart. These include hypoplastic right heart lesions such as tricuspid atresia, tricuspid valve stenosis, and hypoplastic right ventricle with pulmonary atresia. Restriction at the atrial level will first manifest as right atrial and IVC dilation but may then lead to hepatomegaly, ascites, and peripheral edema if not intervened on. Symptoms develop over time therefore septostomy can be done in a nonemergent manner.

A severely restrictive atrial septum in hypoplastic left heart syndrome is a critical heart condition, which requires emergent intervention to open the atrial septum. In HLHS, an adequate ASD after birth is necessary to allow for egress of blood from the pulmonary veins to the right side of the heart (Fig. 46.29). Some of these patients are identified in utero and can undergo fetal intervention (Fig. 46.30) [126–128], while others will present at birth in extremis with cyanosis, metabolic acidosis and eventually poor perfusion and cardiac output. These patients often will have a very thickened atrial septum,

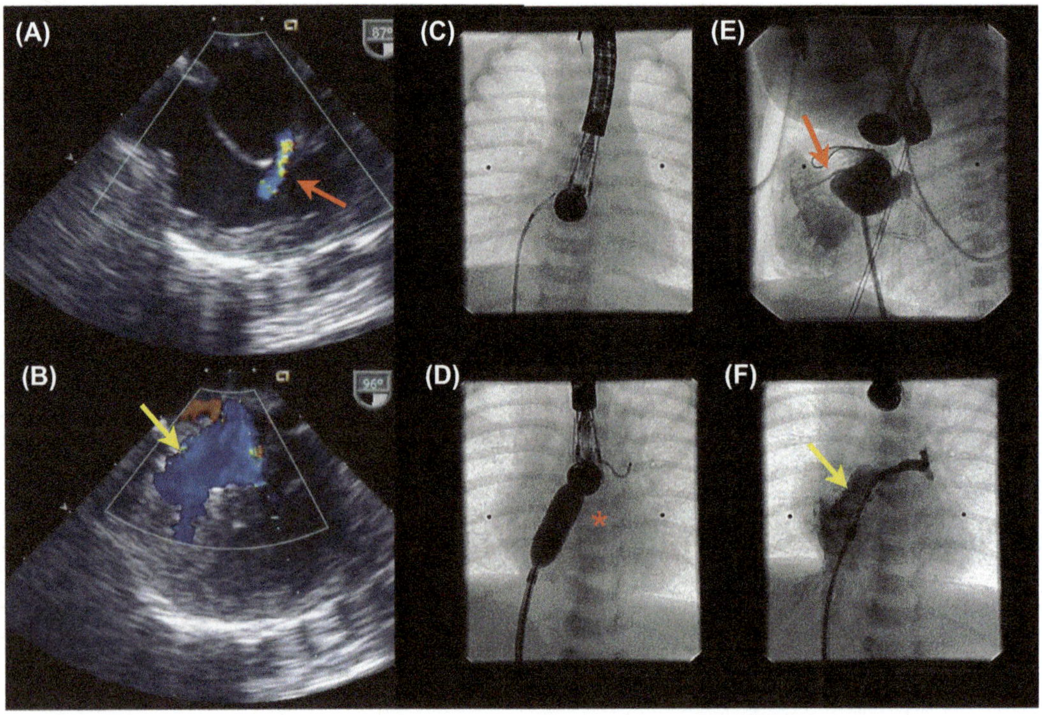

FIGURE 46.29 Newborn with hypoplastic left heart syndrome and a restrictive atrial septum and severe pulmonary edema brought to the cath lab for atrial septal stent implantation. The two left panels show echocardiogram showing a restrictive PFO (*red arrow*) shortly after birth (A) and after stent implantation (*yellow arrow*) (B). There is laminar flow through at atrial septal stent. Middle panels show perforation of the thick atrial septum using a radiofrequency wire (C) followed by stent implantation (*red asterisk*) (D). Right panels show the angiographic images of a restrictive PFO (*red arrow*) before stent implant (E) and an unrestricted atrial septum with good flow through the stent (*yellow arrow*) (F). Notice the decompressed small left atrium (LA) compared to the dilated and tense LA prior to stenting in (E). *PFO*, patent foramen ovale.

a superiorly placed ASD or atrial shunting along a channel like opening. This procedure cannot be performed at the bedside and often will require additional imaging such as fluoroscopy and transesophageal echocardiogram to cross the atrial septum. Several techniques have been described to cross the atrial septum. The existing small defect is difficult to cross due to the location and tortuosity. Creation of a new defect using either a transseptal needle, stiff end of a wire, or radiofrequency ablation may be necessary [127]. Once across the septum, balloon angioplasty, and stent implantation can be performed. These patients are highly unstable after birth requiring significant inotropic support. Despite an initial success of left atrial decompression, whether catheter or surgical intervention, these patients suffer from pulmonary hypertension and/or lymphatic congestion secondary to the long-standing in utero atrial septal obstruction. Neonatal mortality is 50% [128]. In utero intervention has been performed with an attempt to intervene prior to the pulmonary vascular changes to improve neonatal outcomes. It is yet to be seen if there is any clinical impact.

Fig. 46.29 shows echocardiographic and angiographic images of a newborn with hypoplastic left heart syndrome and a restrictive PFO before and after stent implantation. There is wide patency and laminar flow across the septum after stent implantation. Notice the LA is dilated and tense prior to the stent procedure and decompresses to a small hypoplastic chamber following stent implant.

Fig. 46.30A shows of case of fetal atrial stent implantation in a 24-week fetus with hypoplastic left heart syndrome and a restrictive atrial septum. A cannula is first introduced through the maternal abdomen, uterus, and chest into the RA and across the thick atrial septum. A 0.014″ guidewire is introduced through the cannula and positioned into the dilated pulmonary veins. Next, a coronary stent is implanted across the atrial septum. It is common to see the decompressed LA chamber to be smaller and the stent can be seen sitting in the orifice of a pulmonary vein.

Fig. 46.30B shows another similar case where the atrial stent (red arrow) is well positioned across the atrial septum.

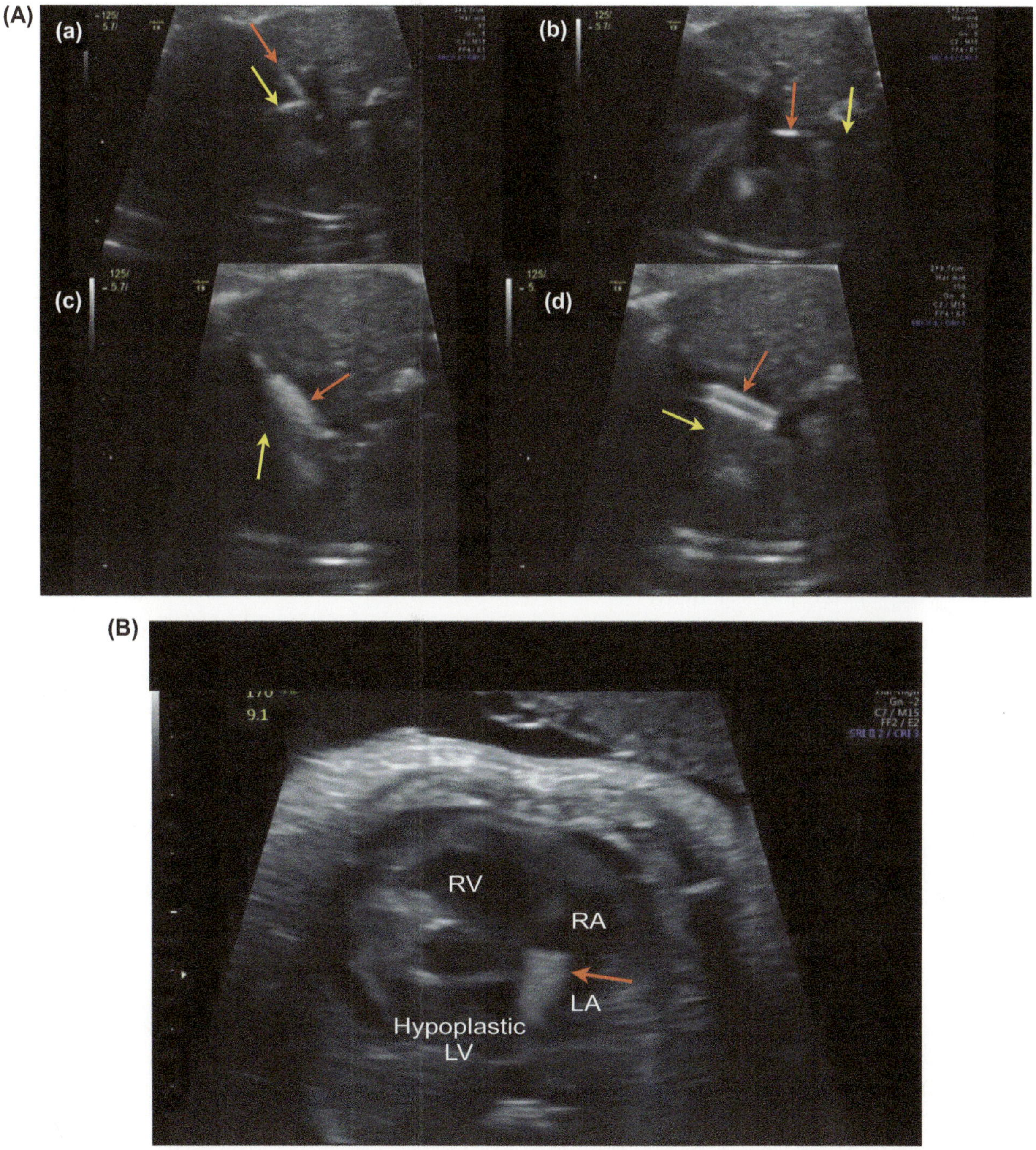

FIGURE 46.30 (A) Example of a fetal atrial stent implantation in a fetus with hypoplastic left heart syndrome and a restrictive atrial septum. Procedure was performed at 24 weeks, soon after fetal diagnosis. (a) A cannula (*red arrow*) is introduced through the maternal abdomen, uterus, and chest into the right atrium (RA) and across the thick atrial septum (*yellow arrow*). (b) A 0.014″ guidewire (*red arrow*) is introduced through the cannula into the dilated pulmonary veins (*yellow arrow*). (c) A coronary stent (*red arrow*) is implanted across the atrial septum (*yellow arrow*). (d) Stent (*red arrow*) is clearly shown positioned across the atrial septum (*yellow arrow*) with the distal end by the pulmonary vein orifice. The left atrium (LA) has decompressed and appears smaller in size. (B): In another similar case, the atrial stent (*red arrow*) is well positioned across the atrial septum relative to the four designated heart chambers.

REFERENCES

[1] J.C. Rama-Merchan, A. Arribas-Jimenez, J. Martin-Moreiras, E. Garcia-Fernandez, Pacemaker lead-related tricuspid stenosis successfully treated with percutaneous balloon valvuloplasty guided by 3D echocardiography, Cruz-Gonzalez IRev Port Cardiol. 33 (11) (November 2014) 739.e1–739.e3 Epub November 4, 2014.

[2] V. Michiels, A. Delabays, E. Eeckhout, Percutaneous balloon valvotomy for the treatment of pacemaker lead-induced tricuspid stenosis, Heart 100 (4) (February 2014) 352 Epub September 19, 2013.

[3] L.C. Orbe, N. Sobrino, R. Arcas, et al., Initial outcome of percutaneous balloon valvuloplasty in rheumatic tricuspid valve stenosis, Am. J. Cardiol. 71 (1993) 353–354E.

[4] Yeter, K. Ozlem, H. Kilic, et al., Tricuspid balloon valvuloplasty to treat tricuspid stenosis, J. Heart Valve Dis. 19 (2010) 159–160.

[5] T.F. Feltes, E. Bacha, R.H. Beekman, J.P. Cheatham, J.A. Feinstein, A.S. Gomes, Z.M. Hijazi, F.F. Ing, M. de Moor, W.R. Morrow, C.E. Mullins, K.A. Taubert, E.M. Zahn, Indications for cardiac catheterization and intervention in pediatric cardiac disease. A Scientific Statement from the American Heart Association, Circulation 123 (22) (June 7, 2011).

[6] M. Witsenburg, M. Talsma, J. Rohmer, J. Hess, Balloon valvuloplasty for valvular pulmonary stenosis in children over 6 months of age: initial results and long-term follow-up, Eur. Heart J. 14 (1993) 1657–1660.

[7] B.W. McCrindle, Independent predictors of long-term results after balloon pulmonary valvuloplasty. Valvuloplasty and Angioplasty of Congenital Anomalies (VACA) Registry Investigators, Circulation 89 (1994) 1751–1759.

[8] J. Masura, M. Burch, J.E. Deanfield, I.D. Sullivan, Five-year follow-up after balloon pulmonary valvuloplasty, J. Am. Coll. Cardiol. 21 (1993) 132–136.

[9] R. Donato, D. Di Carlo, Percutaneous balloon valvuloplasty of pulmonary valve stenosis, dysplasia, and residual stenosis after surgical valvotomy for pulmonary atresia with intact ventricular septum: long-term results, Catheter. Cardiovasc. Diagn. 19 (1990) 165–169.

[10] G. Hausdorf, I. Schulze-Neick, P.E. Lange, Radiofrequency-assisted"recon-struction"of the right ventricular outflow tract in muscular pulmonary atresia with ventricular septal defect, Br. Heart J. 69 (1993) 343–346.

[11] E. Rosenthal, S.A. Qureshi, K.C. Chan, et al., Radiofrequency-assisted balloon dilatation in patients with pulmonary valve atresia and an intact ventricular septum, Br. Heart J. 69 (1993) 347–351.

[12] R.N. Justo, D.G. Nykanen, W.G. Williams, R.M. Freedom, L.N. Benson, Transcatheter perforation of the right ventricular outflow tract as initial therapy for pulmonary valve atresia and intact ventricular septum in the newborn, Catheter. Cardiovasc. Diagn. 40 (1997) 408–413.

[13] M.A. Walsh, K.J. Lee, R. Chaturvedi, G.S. Van Arsdell, L.N. Benson, Radiofrequency perforation of the right ventricular outflow tract as a palliative strategy for pulmonary atresia with ventricular septal defect, Catheter. Cardiovasc. Interv. 69 (2007) 1015–102015.

[14] T. Humpl, B. Söderberg, B.W. McCrindle, D.G. Nykanen, R.M. Freedom, W.G. Williams, L.N. Benson, Percutaneous balloon valvotomy in pulmonary atresia with intact ventricular septum: impact on patient care, Circulation 108 (2003) 826–832 16.

[15] C. Kreutzer, R.C. Mayorquim, G.O. Kreutzer, et al., Experience with one and a half ventricle repair, J. Thorac. Cardiovasc. Surg. 117 (1999) 662–668.

[16] M. Marasini, P.F. Gorrieri, G. Tuo, et al, Long-term results of catheter-based treatment of pulmonary atresia and intact ventricular septum, Heart 95 (2009) 1520–152416.

[17] C.J. McMahon, H.G. El Said, J.A. Vincent, R.G. Grifka, M.R. Nihill, F.F. Ing, J.K. Fraley, C.E. Mullins, Refinements in the implantation of pulmonary arterial stents: impact on morbidity and mortality of the procedure over the last two decades, Cardiol. Young 12 (2002) 445–452.

[18] F.F. Ing, A. Khan, D. Kobayashi, D.J. Hagler, T.J. Forbes, Pulmonary artery stents in the recent era: immediate and intermediate follow-up, Catheter. Cardiovasc. Interv. 84 (7) (December 1, 2014) 1123–1130.

[19] A.N. Seale, P.E. Daubeney, A.G. Magee, M.L. Rigby, Pulmonary vein stenosis: initial experience with cutting balloon angioplasty, Heart 92 (2006) 815–820.

[20] A.L. Cook, L.R. Prieto, J.W. Delaney, J.F. Rhodes, Usefulness of cutting balloon angioplasty for pulmonary vein in-stent stenosis, Am. J. Cardiol. 98 (2006) 407–410.

[21] I. Luhmer, et al., Coarctation of the pulmonary artery in neonates: prevalence, diagnosis and surgical treatment, J. Thorac. Cardiovasc. Surg. 106 (1993) 889–894.

[22] C.A. Trant, M.P. O'Laughln, R.M. Ungerleider, A. Garson Jr., Pediatr. Cardiol. 18 (5) (1997) 339–344.

[23] D.C. McGoon, O.W. Kincaid, Stenosis of branch pulmonary arteries: surgical repairs, Med. Clin. N. Am. 48 (1976) 257–263.

[24] M. Barbero-Marcial, E. Atik, et al., Reconstruction of stenotic and nonconfluent pulmonary arteries simultaneously with a Blalock-Taussig shunt, J. Thorac. Cardiovasc. Surg. 95 (1988) 82–89.

[25] L.H. Cohn, J.H. Sanders Jr., J.J. Collins Jr., Surgical treatment of congenital unilateral pulmonary artery stenosis with contralateral pulmonary hypertension, Am. J. Cardiol. 38 (1976) 257–260.

[26] C.D. Fraser Jr., L.A. Latson, R.B. Mee, Surgical repair of severe bilateral branch pulmonary artery stenosis, Ann. Thorac. Surg. 59 (3) (1995) 738–740.

[27] G. Agnoletti, Y. Boudjemline, et al., Surgical reconstruction of occluded pulmonary arteries in patients with congenital heart disease: effects on pulmonary artery growth, Circulation 109 (2004) 2314–2318.

[28] A. Rothman, S.B. Perry, J.F. Keane, J.E. Lock, Early results and follow-up of balloon angioplasty for branch pulmonary artery stenoses, J. Am. Coll. Cardiol. 15 (1990) 1109–1117.

[29] J.S. Kan, W.J. Marvin Jr., J.L. Bass, A.J. Muster, J. Murphy, Balloon angioplasty-branch pulmonary artery stenosis: results from the valvuloplasty and angioplasty of congenital anomalies registry, Am. J. Cardiol. 65 (1990) 798–801.

[30] E.A. Bacha, P. Lang, J.E. Mayer, D.B. McElhinney, Connection of discontinuous pulmonary arteries in patients with superior or total cavopulmonary circulation, Ann. Thorac. Surg. 86 (6) (2008) 1948–1954.

[31] C. Stamm, I. Friehs, D. Zurakowski, A.M. Scheule, A.M. Moran, J.E. Lock, J.E. Mayer, P.J. del Nido, R.A. Jonas, Outcome after reconstruction of discontinuous pulmonary arteries, J. Thorac. Cardiovasc. Surg. 123 (2) (2002) 246–257.

[32] O.F. Dogan, M. Demircin, S. Ozkutlu, I. Pasaoglu, Surgical management of infants with isolated supravalvular pulmonary stenosis: case reports, Heart Surg. Forum 9 (4) (2006) E668–E674 Discussion E673–E674.

[33] E.A. Bacha, J. Kreutzer, Comprehensive management of branch pulmonary artery stenosis, J. Interv. Cardiol. 14 (3) (2001) 367–375.

[34] M.A. Law, P. Shamszad, A.W. Nugent, H. Justino, J.P. Breinholt, C.E. Mullins, F.F. Ing, Pulmonary artery stents: long-term followup, Catheter. Cardiovasc. Interv. 75 (2010) 757–764.

[35] I. Spadoni, S. Giusti, P. Bertolaccini, A. Maneschi, G. Kraft, M. Carminati, Long-term follow-up of stents implanted to relieve peripheral pulmonary arterial stenosis: hemodynamic findings and results of lung perfusion scanning, Cardiol. Young 9 (1999) 585–591.

[36] D. Kenny, Z. Amin, S. Slyder, Z.M. Hijazi, Medium-term outcomes for peripheral pulmonary artery stenting in adults with congenital heart disease, J. Interv. Cardiol. 24 (2011) 373–377.

[37] C.M. Takao, H. El-Said, D. Connolly, R.K. Hamzeh, F.F. Ing, Impact of stent implantation on pulmonary artery growth, Catheter. Cardiovasc. Interv. 82 (2013) 445–452.

[38] S. Balasubramanian, A.C. Marshall, K. Gauvreau, L.F. Peng, A.W. Nugent, J.E. Lock, D.B. McElhinney, Outcomes after stent implantation for the treatment of congenital and postoperative pulmonary vein stenosis in children, Circ. Cardiovasc. Interv. 5 (2012) 109–117.

[39] L.R. Prieto, P. Schoenhagen, M.J. Arruda, A. Natale, S.E. Worley, Comparison of stent versus balloon angioplasty for pulmonary vein stenosis complicating pulmonary vein isolation, J. Cardiovasc. Electrophysiol. 19 (2008) 673–678.

[40] T. Neumann, J. Sperzel, T. Dill, A. Kluge, A. Erdogan, H. Greis, J. Hansel, A. Berkowitsch, K. Kurzidim, M. Kuniss, C.W. Hamm, H.F. Pitschner, Percutaneous pulmonary vein stenting for the treatment of severe stenosis after pulmonary vein isolation, J. Cardiovasc. Electrophysiol. 16 (2005) 1180–1188.

[41] H.G. El-Said, F.F. Ing, R.G. Grifka, M.R. Nihill, C. Morris, D. Getty-Houswright, C.E. Mullins, 18-year experience with transseptal procedures through baffles, conduits, and other intra-atrial patches, Catheter. Cardiovasc. Interv. 50 (4) (2000) 434–439.

[42] H. MR, A.C. Marshall, J.E. Lock, D.B. McElhinney, Angioplasty of obstructed homograft conduits in the right ventricular outflow tract with ultra-noncompliant balloons: assessment of therapeutic efficacy and conduit tears, Circ. Cardiovasc. Interv. 6 (6) (December 2013) 671–679.

[43] L.F. Peng, D.B. McElhinney, A.W. Nugent, A.J. Powell, A.C. Marshall, E.A. Bacha, J.E. Lock, Endovascular stenting of obstructed right ventricle–to–pulmonary artery conduits a 15-year experience, Circulation 113 (2006) 2598–2605.

[44] M. Carr, L. Bergersen, A.C. Marshall, J.F. Keane, J.E. Lock, S.M. Emani, D.B. McElhinney, Bare metal stenting for obstructed small diameter homograft conduits in the right ventricular outflow tract, Catheter. Cardiovasc. Interv. 81 (1) (January 1, 2013) E44–E52.

[45] K. Inoue, T. Owaki, T. Nakamura, F. Kitamura, N. Miyamoto, Clinical application of transvenous mitral commissurotomy by a new balloon catheter, J. Thorac. Cardiovasc. Surg. 87 (1984) 394–402 17.

[46] U.U. Babic, P. Pejcic, Z. Djurisic, M. Vucinic, S.N. Grujicic, Percutaneous transarterial balloon mitral valvuloplasty: 30 months experience, Herz 13 (1988) 91–99 18.

[47] C.Y. Lee, K.W. Lau, Z.P. Ding, A. Tan, C. Chan, T.H. Koh, S. Quek, T.S. Chee, A. Ng, A. Johan, Percutaneous balloon valvuloplasty in mitral restenosis after previous surgical commissurotomy, Singap. Med. J. 36 (1995) 474–478 19.

[48] J.A. Baz, E. Pinar, A. Albarrán, J. Mauri, Spanish Society of Cardiology working group on cardiac catheterization and interventional cardiology. Spanish cardiac catheterization and coronary intervention registry: 17th official report of the Spanish Society of Cardiology working group on cardiac catheterization and interventional cardiology, Rev. Esp. Cardiol. 2008 (61) (1990–2007) 1298–1314 20.

[49] D.B. McElhinney, M.C. Sherwood, J.F. Keane, P.J. del Nido, C.S. Almond, J.E. Lock, Current management of severe congenital mitral stenosis: outcomes of transcatheter and surgical therapy in 108 infants and children, Circulation 112 (2005) 707–714 22.

[50] BW, R.A. Nishimura, P.T. O'Gara, R.A. O'Rourke, C.M. Otto, P.M. Shah, J.S. Shanewise, S.C. Smith Jr., A.K. Jacobs, C.D. Adams, J.L. Anderson, E.M. Antman, D.P. Faxon, V. Fuster, J.L. Halperin, L.F. Hiratzka, S.A. Hunt, B.W. Lytle, R. Nishimura, R.L. Page, B. Riegel, ACC/AHA 2006 guidelines for the management of patients with valvular heart disease: a report of the American College of Cardiology/American Heart Association Task Force on Practice Guidelines (writing Committee to Revise the 1998 guidelines for the management of patients with valvular heart disease), Circulation 114 (2006) e84–e23123 [published corrections appear in Circulation 121 (2010) e443 and Circulation 115 (2007) e409].

[51] B.W. McCrindle, Valvuloplasty and Angioplasty of Congenital Anomalies (VACA) Registry Investigators. Independent predictors of immediate results of percutaneous balloon aortic valvotomy in children, Am. J. Cardiol. 77 (1996) 286–293 24.

[52] A.P. Rocchini, R.H. Beekman, G. Ben Shachar, L. Benson, D. Schwartz, J.S. kan, Balloon aortic valvuloplasty: results of the valvuloplasty and angioplasty of congenital anomalies registry, Am. J. Cardiol. 65 (1990) 784–789.

[53] B.W. McCrindle, E.H. Blackstone, W.G. Williams, R. Sittiwangkul, T.L. Spray, A. Azakie, R.A. Jonas, Are outcomes of surgical versus transcatheter balloon valvotomy equivalent in neonatal critical aortic stenosis? Circulation 104 (Suppl 1) (2001) I-152–I-158 26.

[54] D.B. McElhinney, J.E. Lock, J.F. Keane, A.M. Moran, S.D. Colan, Left heart growth, function, and reintervention after balloon aortic valvuloplasty for neonatal aortic stenosis, Circulation 111 (2005) 451–458.

[55] M. Campbell, Natural history of coarctation of the aorta, Br. Heart J. 32 (1970) 633–640.

[56] A.T. Yetman, D. Nykanen, B.W. McCrindle, J. Sunnegardh, I. Adatia, R.M. Freedom, L. Benson, Balloon angioplasty of recurrent coarctation: a 12-year review, JACC 30 (3) (September 1997) 811–816.

[57] Z.R. Bulbul, E. Bruckheimer, J.C. Love, J.T. Fahey, W.E. Hellenbrand, Implantation of balloon-expandable stents for coarctation of the aorta: implantation data and short-term results, Catheter. Cardiovasc. Diagn. 39 (1996) 36–42.

[58] M.R. Ebeid, L.P. Prieto, L.A. Latson, The use of balloon expandable stents in coarctation of the aorta: short and intermediate term follow up, J. Am. Coll. Cardiol. 30 (1997) 1847–1852.

[59] M.A. Hamadan, S. Maheshwari, J.T. Fahey, W.E. Hellenbrand, Endovascular stents for coarctation of the aorta: initial results and intermediate-term follow-up, J. Am. Coll. Cardiol. 38 (2001) 1518–1523.
[60] R. Buchhorn, R.D. Ross, D. Bartmus, A. Wessel, M. Hulpke-Wette, J. Bürsch, Activity of the renin-angiotensin-aldosterone and sympathetic nervous system and their relation to hemodynamic and clinical abnormalities in infants with left-to-right shunts, Int. J. Cardiol. 78 (3) (May 2001) 225–230.
[61] R. Buchhorn, A. Hammersen, D. Bartmus, J. Bürsch, The pathogenesis of heart failure in infants with congenital heart disease, Cardiol. Young 11 (5) (September 2001) 498–504.
[62] Y. Wyss, D. Quandt, R. Weber, B. Stiasny, B. Weber, W. Knirsch, O. Kretschmar, Interventional closure of secundum type atrial septal defects in infants less than 10 kilograms: indications and procedural outcome, J. Interv. Cardiol. 29 (6) (December 2016) 646–653, http://dx.doi.org/10.1111/joic.12328. Epub September 13, 2016.
[63] K.A. Diab, Q.L. Cao, E.A. Bacha, Z.M. Hijazi, Device closure of atrial septal defects with the Amplatzer septal occluder: safety and outcome in infants, J. Thorac. Cardiovasc. Surg. 134 (4) (October 2007) 960–966.
[64] C.G. LaFarge, O.S. Miettinen, The estimation of oxygen consumption, Cardiovasc. Res. 4 (1) (January 1970) 23–30.
[65] M.D. Seckeler, R. Hirsch, R.H. Beekman 3rd, B.H. Goldstein, A new predictive equation for oxygen consumption in children and adults with congenital and acquired heart disease, Heart 101 (7) (April 2015) 517–524.
[66] S.E. Hamrick, G. Hansmann, Patent ductus arteriosus of the preterm infant, Pediatrics 125 (5) (2010) 1020–1030.
[67] E.M. Zahn, P. Nevin, C. Simmons, R. Garg, A novel technique for transcatheter patent ductus arteriosus closure in extremely preterm infants using commercially available technology, Catheter. Cardiovasc. Interv. 85 (2) (February 1, 2015) 240–248.
[68] R.H. Pass, Z. Hijazi, D.T. Hsu, V. Lewis, W.E. Hellenbrand, U.S.A. Multicenter, Amplatzer patent ductus arteriosus occlusion device trial: initial and one-year results, J. Am. Coll. Cardiol. 44 (3) (August 4, 2004) 513–519.
[69] V.V. Dimas, C. Takao, F.F. Ing, R. Mattamal, A.W. Nugent, R.G. Grifka, et al., Outcomes of transcatheter occlusion of patent ductus arteriosus in infants weighing ≤6 kg, JACC Cardiovasc. Interv. 3 (2010) 1295–1299.
[70] C.H. Backes, et al, Percutaneous patent ductus arteriosus (PDA) closure in very preterm infants: feasibility and complications, J. Am. Heart Assoc. 5 (2) (February 2016) e002923.
[71] D.B. McElhinney, V.M. Reddy, W. Tworetzky, E. Petrossian, F.L. Hanley, P. Moore, Incidence and implications of systemic to pulmonary collaterals after bidirectional cavopulmonary anastomosis, Ann. Thorac. Surg. 69 (2000) 1222–1228.
[72] P. Banka, et al., Practice variability and outcomes of coil embolization of aortopulmonary collaterals prior to Fontan completion: a report from the pediatric heart Network Fontan cross-sectional study, Am. Heart J. 162 (1) (July 2011) 125–130.
[73] T. Geva, Quantification of systemic-to-pulmonary artery collateral flow: challenges and opportunities, Circ. Cardiovasc. Imaging 5 (2012) 175–177.
[74] S.S. Wang, Z.W. Zhang, M.Y. Qian, J. Zhuang, G.H. Zeng, Transcatheter closure of coronary arterial fistula in children and adolescents, Pediatr. Int. 56 (2) (April 2014) 173–179.
[75] L.R. Armsby, J.F. Keane, M.C. Sherwood, J.M. Forbess, S.B. Perry, J.E. Lock, Management of coronary artery fistulae. Patient selection and results of transcatheter closure, J. Am. Coll. Cardiol. 39 (6) (March 20, 2002) 1026–1032.
[76] R.D. Mainwaring, H. Mirali-Akbar, J.J. Lamberti, J.W. Moore, Secundum-type atrial septal defects with failure to thrive in the first year of life, J. Card. Surg. 11 (2) (1996) 116–120.
[77] S. Bartakian, T.E. Fagan, M.S. Schaffer, J.R. Darst, Device closure of secundum atrial septal defects in children <15 kg: complication rates and indications for referral, JACC Cardiovasc. Interv. 5 (11) (2012) 1178–1184.
[78] M. Vogel, Partial anomalous pulmonary venous connection and the scimitar syndrome, in: M.A. Gatzoulis, G.D. Webb, P.E.F. Daubeney (Eds.), Diagnosis and Management of Adult Congenital Heart Disease, Churchill Livingstone, London, 2004, pp. 205–210.
[79] D.J. DiBardino, D.B. McElhinney, A.K. Kaza, J.E. Mayer Jr., Analysis of the US Food and drug Administration Manufacturer and user facility device experience database for adverse events involving amplatzer septal occluder devices and comparison with the society of thoracic surgery congenital cardiac surgery database, J. Thorac. Cardiovasc. Surg. 137 (6) (2009) 1334–1341.
[80] Z.D. Du, Z.M. Hijazi, C.S. Kleinman, N.H. Silverman, K. Larntz, Comparison between transcatheter and surgical closure of secundum atrial septal defect in children and adults: results of a multicenter nonrandomized trial, J. Am. Coll. Cardiol. 39 (11) (June 5, 2002) 1836–1844.
[81] N.J. Wilson, J. Smith, B. Prommete, C. O'Donnell, T.L. Gentles, P.N. Ruygrok, Transcatheter closure of secundum atrial septal defects with the Amplatzer septal occluder in adults and children-follow-up closure rates, degree of mitral regurgitation and evolution of arrhythmias, Heart Lung Circ. 17 (4) (2008) 318–324.
[82] D.B. McElhinney, M.D. Quartermain, D. Kenny, E. Alboliras, Z. Amin, Relative risk factors for cardiac erosion following transcatheter closure of atrial septal defects: a case-control study, Circulation 133 (18) (2016) 1738–1746.
[83] Z. Amin, Z.M. Hijazi, J.L. Bass, J.P. Cheatham, W.E. Hellenbrand, C.S. Kleinman, Erosion of Amplatzer septal occluder device after closure of secundum atrial septal defects: review of registry of complications and recommendations to minimize future risk, Catheter. Cardiovasc. Interv. 63 (4) (December 2004) 496–502.
[84] Q. de Hemptinne, E.M. Horlick, M.D. Osten, X. Millán, V.X. Tadros, M. Pighi, F. Gonzalez Barlatey, S.M. Alnasser, J. Miró, A.W. Asgar, R. Ibrahim, Initial clinical experience with the GORE® CARDIOFORM ASD occluder for transcatheter atrial septal defect closure, Catheter. Cardiovasc. Interv. (January 27, 2017), http://dx.doi.org/10.1002/ccd.26907. (Epub ahead of print).
[85] J. Grohmann, R. Höhn, T. Fleck, C. Schmoor, B. Stiller, Transcatheter closure of atrial septal defects in children and adolescents: single-center experience with the GORE® septal occluder, Catheter. Cardiovasc. Interv. 84 (6) (November 15, 2014) E51–E57, http://dx.doi.org/10.1002/ccd.25494. Epub August 6, 2014.
[86] R. Holzer, D. Balzer, Q.L. Cao, K. Lock, Z.M. Hijazi, Device closure of muscular ventricular septal defects using the Amplatzer muscular ventricular septal defect occluder: immediate and mid-term results of a U.S. registry, J. Am. Coll. Cardiol. 43 (7) (April 7, 2004) 1257–1263.

[87] C. Gan, K. Lin, Q. An, H. Tang, H. Song, R.C. Lui, K. Tao, Z. Zhuang, Y. Shi, Perventricular device closure of muscular ventricular septal defects on beating hearts: initial experience in eight children, J. Thorac. Cardiovasc. Surg. 137 (4) (April 2009) 929–933.

[88] S.L. Kang, A. Tometzki, M. Caputo, G. Morgan, A. Parry, R. Martin, Longer-term outcome of perventricular device closure of muscular ventricular septal defects in children, Catheter. Cardiovasc. Interv. 85 (6) (May 2015) 998–1005.

[89] E.A. Bacha, Q.L. Cao, M.E. Galantowicz, et al., Multicenter experience with perventricular device closure of muscular ventricular septal defects, Pediatr. Cardiol. 26 (2) (2005) 169–175.

[90] I. Haponiuk, M. Chojnicki, R. Jaworski, et al., Hybrid technique for muscular ventricular septal defect closure, J. Card. Surg. 28 (4) (2013) 453–455.

[91] B. Thakkar, N. Patel, S. Shah, V. Poptani, T. Madan, C. Shah, A. Shukla, V. Prajapati, Perventricular device closure of isolated muscular ventricular septal defect in infants: a single centre experience, Indian Heart J. 64 (6) (2012 Nov-Dec) 559–567.

[92] R. Holzer, J. de Giovanni, K.P. Walsh, et al., Transcatheter closure of perimembranous ventricular septal defects using the amplatzer membranous VSD occluder: immediate and midterm results of an international registry, Catheter. Cardiovasc. Interv. 68 (2006) 620–628.

[93] G. Butera, M. Carminati, M. Chessa, et al., Transcatheter closure of perimembranous ventricular septal defects: early and long-term results, J. Am. Coll. Cardiol. 50 (2007) 1189–1195.

[94] D. Predescu, R.R. Chaturvedi, M.K. Friedberg, L.N. Benson, A. Ozawa, K.J. Lee, Complete heart block associated with device closure of perimembranous ventricular septal defects, J. Thorac. Cardiovasc. Surg. 136 (2008) 1223–1228.

[95] A. Tzikas, R. Ibrahim, D. Velasco-Sanchez, X. Freixa, M. Alburquenque, P. Khairy, J.L. Bass, J. Ramirez, D. Aguirre, J. Miro, Transcatheter closure of perimembranous ventricular septal defect with the Amplatzer(®) membranous VSD occluder 2: initial world experience and one-year follow-up, Catheter. Cardiovasc. Interv. 83 (4) (March 1, 2014) 571–580.

[96] T.B. Polat, E. Türkmen, Transcatheter closure of ventricular septal defects using the Amplatzer Duct Occluder II device: a single-center experience, Postepy Kardiol Interwencyjnej 12 (4) (2016) 340–347.

[97] M. Kanaan, P. Ewert, F. Berger, S. Assa, S. Schubert, Follow-up of patients with interventional closure of ventricular septal defects with Amplatzer Duct Occluder II, Pediatr. Cardiol. 36 (2) (February 2015) 379–385.

[98] H.G. El Said, A. Bratincsak, B.M. Gordon, J.W. Moore, Closure of perimembranous ventricular septal defects with aneurysmal tissue using the Amplazter Duct Occluder I: lessons learned and medium term follow up, Catheter. Cardiovasc. Interv. 80 (6) (November 15, 2012) 895–903.

[99] R.R. Chaturvedi, P.J. Kilner, P.A. White, A. Bishop, R. Szwarc, A.N. Redington, Increased airway pressure and simulated branch pulmonary artery stenosis increase pulmonary regurgitation after repair of tetralogy of Fallot. Real-time analysis with a conductance catheter technique, Circulation 95 (3) (February 4, 1997) 643–649.

[100] C.J. Petit, M.J. Gillespie, M.A. Harris, T.L. Seymour, T.Y. Liu, A. Khan, J.W. Gaynor, J.J. Rome, Relief of branch pulmonary artery stenosis reduces pulmonary valve insufficiency in a swine model, J. Thorac. Cardiovasc. Surg. 138 (2) (August 2009) 382–389.

[101] J. Therrien, Y. Provost, N. Merchant, W. Williams, J. Colman, G. Webb, Optimal timing for pulmonary valve replacement in adults after tetralogy of Fallot repair, Am. J. Cardiol. 95 (2005) 779–782.

[102] C.A. Warnes, R.G. Williams, T.M. Bashore, et al., ACC/AHA guidelines for the management of the management of adults with congenital heart disease: a report of the American College of Cardiology/American Heart Association Task Force on Practice Guidelines (writing committee to develop guidelines on the management of adults with congenital heartdisease, Circulation 118 (2008) e714–e833.

[103] T. Geva, Repaired tetralogy of Fallot: the roles of cardiovascular magnetic resonance in evaluating pathophysiology and for pulmonary valve replacement decision support, J. Cardiovasc. Magn. Reson. 13 (2011) 9.

[104] T. Geva, Indications for pulmonary valve replacement in repaired tetralogy of Fallot: the quest continues, Circulation 128 (2013) 1855–1857.

[105] M. Alvarez-Fuente, E. Garrido-Lestache, L. Fernandez-Pineda, B. Romera, I. Sánchez, T. Centella, C. Abelleira, S. Villagrá, R. Tamariz, E. Barrios, M.J. Lamas, R. Gomez, M.J. Del Cerro, Timing of pulmonary valve replacement: how much can the right ventricle dilate before it looses its remodeling potential? Pediatr. Cardiol. 37 (3) (March 2016) 601–605.

[106] J.T. Tretter, M.K. Friedberg, R.M. Wald, D.B. McElhinney, Defining and refining indications for transcatheter pulmonary valve replacement in patients with repaired tetralogy of Fallot: contributions from anatomical and functional imaging, Int. J. Cardiol. 221 (October 15, 2016) 916–925.

[107] D.S. Levi, S. Sinha, M.M. Salem, J.A. Aboulhosn, Transcatheter native pulmonary valve and tricuspid valve replacement with the Sapien XT: initial experience and development of a new delivery platform, Catheter. Cardiovasc. Interv. 88 (2016) 434–443.

[108] D.B. McElhinney, A.K. Cabalka, J.A. Aboulhosn, A. Eicken, Y. Boudjemline, S. Schubert, D. Himbert, J.D. Asnes, S. Salizzoni, M.L. Bocks, J.P. Cheatham, T.S. Momenah, D.W. Kim, D. Schranz, J. Meadows, J.D.R. Thomson, B.H. Goldstein, I. Crittendon, T.E. Fagan, J.G. Webb, E. Horlick, J.W. Delaney, T.K. Jones, S. Shahanavaz, C. Moretti, M.R. Hainstock, D.P. Kenny, F. Berger, C.S. Rihal, Danny Dvir and for the valve-in-valve international database (VIVID) registry. Transcatheter tricuspid valve-in-valve implantation for theTreatment of dysfunctional surgical bioprosthetic valves. An international, multicenter registry study, Circulation 133 (2016) 1582–1593, http://dx.doi.org/10.1161/CIRCULATIONAHA.115.019353.

[109] J. Aboulhosn, A.K. Cabalka, D.S. Levi, D. Himbert, L. Testa, A. Latib, R.R. Makkar, Y. Boudjemline, D.W. Kim, J. Kefer, S. Bleiziffer, G. Kerst, D. Dvir, D.B. McElhinney, Transcatheter valve-in-ring implantation for the treatment of residual or recurrent tricuspid valve dysfunction after prior surgical repair, J. Am. Coll. Cardiol. Interv. 10 (2017) 53–63.

[110] C.J. Petit, H. Justino, F.F. Ing, Melody valve implantation in the pulmonary and tricuspid position, Catheter. Cardiovasc. Interv. 82 (2013) E944–E946.

[111] G. Dahle, K.-A. Rein, V. Bapat, Concomitant transatrial valve-in-valve in pulmonal and tricuspid position, Catheter. Cardiovasc. Interv. 86 (2015) 897–902.

[112] V.S. Mahadevan, J. Dua, A. Hoschtitzky, Combined tricuspid and pulmonic valve percutaneous replacement in a patient with a Glenn shunt, Int. J. Cardiol. 204 (2016) 128–130.

[113] I. Abdullah, F.B. Ramirez, D.B. McElhinney, J.E. Lock, P.J. del Nido, S. Emani, Modification of a stented bovine jugular vein conduit (melody valve) for surgical mitral valve replacement, Ann. Thorac. Surg. 94 (2012) e97–e98.

[114] L.G. Quinonez, R. Breitbart, W. Tworetsky, J.E. Lock, A.C. Marshall, S.M. Emani, Stented bovine jugular vein graft (Melody valve) for surgical mitral valve replacement in infants and children, J. Thorac. Cardiovasc. Surg. 148 (2014) 1443–1449.

[115] F. A1, F.R. Pluchinotta, A. Saracino, A. Giamberti, C. Arcidiacono, L. Piazza, M. Reali, G. Butera, A. Varrica, M. Carminati, Surgical mitral valve replacement with Melody valve in infants and children: the Italian experience, EuroIntervention 12 (13) (January 3, 2017), http://dx.doi.org/10.4244/EIJ-D-16-00853. pii: EIJ-D-16-00853.

[116] M.W. Cullen, A.K. Cabalka, O.O. Alli, S.V. Pislaru, P. Sorajja, V.T. Nkomo, J.F. Malouf, F. Cetta, D.J. Hagler, C.S. Rihal, Transvenous, antegrade Melody valve-in-valve implantation for bioprosthetic mitral and tricuspid valve dysfunction: a case series in children and adults, J. Am. Coll. Cardiol. Interv. 6 (2013) 598–605.

[117] M.H. Martin, P.J. Gruber, R.G. Gray, Transcatheter neoaortic valve replacement utilizing the Melody valve in hypoplastic left heart syndrome, Catheter. Cardiovasc. Interv. 85 (2015) 615–619.

[118] P.O. Myers, Preserving the V-engine shape of the left ventricle with Melody mitral valve replacement in small children, J. Thorac. Cardiovasc. Surg. 153 (2017) 151–152.

[119] S.M. Emani, B.L. Piekarski, D. Zurakowski, C.A. Baird, A.C. Marshall, J.E. Lock, P.J. del Nido, Concept of an expandable cardiac valve for surgical implantation in infants and children, J. Thorac. Cardiovasc. Surg. 152 (2016) 1514–1523.

[120] L.R. Freud, G.R. Marx, A.C. Marshall, W. Tworetzky, S.M. Emani, Assessment of the Melody valve in the mitral position in young children by echocardiography, J. Thorac. Cardiovasc. Surg. 153 (2017) 153–160.

[121] M. Hofmann, H. Dave, M. H€ubler, O. Kretschmar, Simplified surgical-hybrid Melody valve implantation for paediatric mitral valve disease, Eur. J. Cardiothorac. Surg. 47 (2015) 926–928.

[122] M. Trezzi, E. Cetrano, A. Albano, A. Carotti, Extending the limits for mitral valve replacement in low-weight infants using a stented bovine jugular vein graft, J. Thorac. Cardiovasc. Surg. 150 (2015) 729–730.

[123] J.A. Callahan, J.B. Seward, R.A. Nishimura, F.A. Miller Jr., G.S. Reeder, C. Shub, M.J. Callahan, T.T. Schattenberg, A.J. Tajik, Two-dimensional echocardiographically guided pericardiocentesis: experience in 117 consecutive patients, Am. J. Cardiol. 55 (4) (February 1, 1985) 476–479.

[124] T. TS1, E.K. El-Najdawi, J.B. Seward, D.J. Hagler, W.K. Freeman, P.W. O'Leary, Percutaneous echocardiographically guided pericardiocentesis in pediatric patients: evaluation of safety and efficacy, J. Am. Soc. Echocardiogr. 11 (11) (November 1998) 1072–1077.

[125] D. Molkara, S. Tejman-Yarden, H. El-Said, J.W. Moore, Pericardiocentesis of noncircumferential effusions using nonstandard catheter entry sites guided by echocardiography and fluoroscopy, Congenit. Heart Dis. 6 (5) (September–October 2011) 461–465.

[126] B.T. Kalish, W. Tworetzky, C.B. Benson, L. Wilkins-Haug, A. Mizrahi-Arnaud, D.B. McElhinney, J.E. Lock, A.C. Marshall, Technical challenges of atrial septal stent placement in fetuses with hypoplastic left heart syndrome and intact atrial septum, Catheter. Cardiovasc. Interv. (1) (July 1, 2014) 77–85.

[127] J.A. Glatz, S. Tabbutt, J.W. Gaynor, J.J. Rome, L. Montenegro, T.L. Spray, J. Rychik, Hypoplastic left heart syndrome with atrial level restriction in the era of prenatal diagnosis, Ann. Thorac. Surg. 84 (2007) 1633–1639.

[128] A.P. Vlahos, J.E. Lock, D.B. McElhinney, M.E. van der Velde, Hypoplastic left heart syndrome with intact or highly restrictive atrial septum: outcome after neonatal transcatheter atrial septoplasty, Circulation 109 (2004) 2326–2330.

Section IV

Cardiac Surgery and Pediatric Heart Failure

Chapter 47

Posttransplant Heart Failure

Philip T. Thrush[1], Simon Urschel[2], Elfriede Pahl[1]
[1]*Northwestern University Feinberg School of Medicine, Chicago, IL, United States;* [2]*University of Alberta, Edmonton, AB, Canada*

INTRODUCTION

Graft failure is the leading cause of death following heart transplantation (HT), regardless of time since transplant, and may manifest as either right or left ventricular failure, due to a variety of reasons [1] (Fig. 47.1). Age at transplant, as well as time since transplant, impacts the etiology of graft failure; and a thorough understanding of the varied etiologies, surveillance strategies, and treatment options is crucial to maximize survival [1,2]. The causes of acute and chronic heart failure, their evaluation, and treatment options are presented.

EARLY GRAFT FAILURE

Acute graft failure can manifest as left ventricular failure, right ventricular failure, or biventricular failure. The symptomatic presentation of graft dysfunction is a manifestation of the ventricle(s) affected, such as low cardiac output syndrome and end organ dysfunction in the setting of left ventricular dysfunction or peripheral edema and hepatic congestion in the setting of right ventricular dysfunction, and may be dependent on the specific etiology.

Etiologies

Ischemia and Reperfusion Injury

Ischemia and reperfusion injury are unavoidable consequences of HT. The donor heart is subjected to multiple insults throughout the course of procurement and the transplant, including hypothermic preservation, warm ischemia, and reperfusion of the graft. These may contribute to early graft failure and limit the longevity of the donor heart. Following brain death, there is a rapid release of catecholamines, which can contribute to myocardial ischemia, calcium overload, and altered calcium sensitivity in contractile proteins [3,4]. In addition, others have proposed that the decreased serum levels of triiodothyronine, cortisol, and insulin also contribute to decreased myocardial contractility [5]. Although hypothermic storage and transportation does significantly slow cellular metabolism, it does not completely arrest it. During this period, altered Na^+/K^+ ATPase activity leads to cellular swelling and transition to anaerobic metabolism, which result in lactic acidosis [6]. Increased ischemic time has also been shown to be a risk factor for graft failure lower mean arterial blood pressure in the first 24h following transplantation, longer postoperative mechanical ventilation, longer intensive care unit admission, and longer hospital admission [1,7]. Neonates and infants are particularly susceptible to early graft failure as reported in a multicenter study by Kaushal et al., where 16 of 92 infants transplanted under 1 year of age from 3 centers suffered severe early graft failure leading to placement on extracorporeal membrane oxygenation (ECMO), with 9 of 16 surviving to hospital discharge [8]. Finally, reperfusion results in further calcium overload and oxidative stress, which may contribute to early graft dysfunction [3,6].

Given current procurement strategies, much of the contribution of ischemia and reperfusion injury to graft failure is fixed. There have been limited animal studies which demonstrate the ability to decrease or limit the ischemia-reperfusion injury [9,10]. However, until thoroughly evaluated in human trials, minimizing ischemic time remains the best way to impact ischemia-reperfusion injury and thus graft failure.

Pulmonary Hypertension

Right ventricular failure can occur in the setting of elevated pulmonary vascular resistance (PVR) and/or pulmonary hypertension. In this situation, the donor heart, with a thin-walled right ventricle, is unable to overcome the afterload associated

Heart Failure in the Child and Young Adult. http://dx.doi.org/10.1016/B978-0-12-802393-8.00047-8

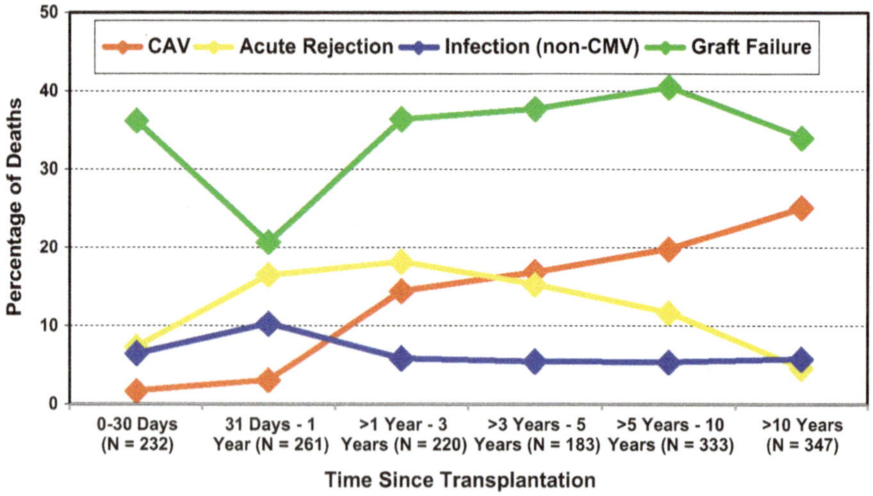

FIGURE 47.1 **Relative incidence of leading cause of death following transplantation (ISHLT Registry [1]).** Relative incidence of leading cause of death based on time since transplant for all patient deaths from January 2004 through June 2014. *CAV*, coronary allograft vasculopathy; *CMV*, cytomegalovirus.

with the elevated PVR and right ventricular pump failure ensues. Historically, a PVR >6 Woods units was used as a contraindication to HT; however, recent studies in children undergoing heart transplant have shown that elevated PVR is not a predictor of mortality despite a PVR as high as 9 Woods units [11,12]. In addition, pulmonary vasodilator testing pretransplant may allow for risk stratification, as those with unresponsive PVR are more likely to develop right ventricular failure and will benefit from additional therapy in the early posttransplant period [13].

Rejection

A mismatch of human leukocyte antigen (HLA) blood group and minor antigens between the recipient and the donor of a transplant organ inevitably results in an attempt of the recipient's immune system to attack and destroy the recognized foreign body. This reaction includes all components and pathways of the immune response; however, the mechanisms and intensity change over time and depend on many factors which impact the immune system. Consequently, diagnostic and therapeutic approaches need to be modified accordingly. Immune responses occur which are generally interactive and with redundant pathways, using cellular mechanisms (Effector T (ET) cells, Natural Killer (NK) cells, phagocytic cells), and humoral mechanisms including the innate immune response via the complement system and an adaptive specific response with production of antibodies toward antigens on the donor organ. The latter (antibody-mediated rejection, AMR) is not a mandatory part of transplant rejection and does not occur in every transplant recipient, especially not if appropriate immune suppression has been applied from early on. However, AMR never occurs as an isolated phenomenon but always includes both cellular and humoral mechanisms to cause damage to the graft and hence cannot be treated in isolation.

The HLA system differentiates two main antigen groups: HLA-class I (e.g., A, B, C) is expressed on almost all human cells (with some exceptions, e.g., Erythrocytes) and is recognized by receptors on ET and NK cells, which attack cells expressing a pattern recognized as nonself through a variety of mechanisms or attempt to induce apoptosis in the foreign or mutated cells. HLA-Class II (e.g., DR, DP, DQ) is typically expressed on antigen-presenting cells only and plays a crucial role in the activation of the adaptive immune response to produce antibodies. However, antigen-presenting capacities and consequently expression of class II HLA on the surface is found on a variety of nonlymphocyte cells including the endothelial cells of transplanted hearts explaining the importance of these antigens in the context of the development of graft vasculopathy. Similarly, blood group antigens (ABO) are expressed on many cells and tissues including the vascular wall of transplanted hearts. The gold standard for diagnosis of rejection is based on endomyocardial biopsy and is commonly reported following the revised nomenclature of the International Society of Heart and Lung Transplantation (ISHLT) [14].

Hyperacute Rejection

The term hyperacute rejection refers to a variety of different patterns all resulting in severe early primary graft dysfunction. It has been reported in the context of donor-specific antibodies (DSAs) and blood group incompatibility but also without either of these factors. The typical description includes discoloration of a vital aspect of the organ at reperfusion and/or lack of contractility or prolonged and resistant fibrillation. The presumed mechanism is a combined massive activation of the coagulation system as well as the immune system, with a key role of the innate immune response. Autopsy findings include diffuse thrombosis and hemorrhage, infiltration of macrophages, lymphocytes, as well as neutrophils, with complement deposition and disintegration of the genuine organ structure with lysis of the myocardium, apoptosis, and ischemic cell death [15].

When hyperacute rejection occurs, the situation is rarely salvageable. Unless a specific causative factor can be determined and specifically treated, while supporting the patient with mechanical circulatory support (MCS), the graft generally does not recover. Outcomes of retransplantation in a situation of early graft dysfunction are dismal with ~40% mortality in the first 4 months after retransplantation [16] and consequently will not be considered by many centers.

Fortunately, such events have become extremely rare in the recent era, probably due to appropriate organ selection and screening for donor risk factors such as preformed antibodies and improved organ preservation during the transfer and optimal clinical management of the reperfusion period.

Acute Cellular Rejection

Acute cellular rejection (ACR) is characterized by invasion of lymphocytes into the graft and graded by the number of foci of invasion and degree of associated damage to the graft tissue [14]. ET-lymphocytes and NK cells cause direct damage to the myocytes, endothelial cells, and connective tissue compartments. CD4 positive T-cells (T4) coordinate the immune attack and activate both the above-described cell-mediated graft damage (Th-1 mediated) but, if present, also B-cells (Th-2 mediated), which have been engaged with their target antigen on the graft and are activated to optimize their antibody affinity by hypersomatic mutation, differentiate into antibody-producing plasma cells, and form antigen-specific memory for future encounters [17]. The Th-2 mediated response takes approximately 3 weeks until the full and extent of optimized antibody response is developed. This explains not only why an episode of ACR may be followed by sometimes more severe and difficult to treat recurrence 2–4 weeks after the initial occurrence but also why frequency of acute rejection was found to be a strong predictor for de novo HLA-antibody production posttransplant and graft coronary allograft vasculopathy (CAV) representing chronic rejection [18,19]. The damage that the immune system causes to the graft and leading to dysfunction is mediated by a variety of effects, of which some directly target the muscle cells. The highly inflammatory milieu resulting from the cytokines secreted in the interplay of the immune cells was found to have a direct negative effect on the myocyte contractility mediated by nitric oxide [20]. A significant target of rejection is represented by endothelial cells which are not only attacked by the immune response but also actively participate in antigen presentation, production of chemokines, expression of adhesion molecules, and responsive proliferation and swelling [21]. The consequent invasion of immune cells into the vascular wall paired with the swelling and proliferation of the endothelial cells and the excretion of interstitial proteins can result in significant acute narrowing of the coronaries and consequent ischemic damage in the dependent area of perfusion [22]. This process is further aggravated by activation of the complement system and cross activation of the coagulation cascade resulting in microthrombi or occlusion of larger vessels of the coronary system [23], the latter represents a particular problem in patients with preexisting damage to the vascular wall by CAV.

The degree of cardiac dysfunction often parallels the histological degree: isolated 1R ACR in the absence of AMR is very rarely accompanied by hemodynamic compromise and was in many studies not associated with earlier CAV [18] or earlier graft loss and typically does not require specific treatment or intensified immune suppression [24]. Grade 2R ACR, with at least two foci of lymphocyte invasion and graft tissue impairment, may be associated with cardiac dysfunction but is also found in up to 15% of protocol biopsies without hemodynamic impairment or clinical concern of rejection, particularly in the first-year posttransplant [25].

In the more recent era, probably associated with more powerful baseline immune suppression and improved monitoring, the frequency of clinically unexpected ACR 2R or higher has declined to well below 10% [26,27]. A negative effect of ACR ≥2R on long-term survival was shown in a variety of studies in adult and pediatric patients [1,19]. This may partly also reflect a surrogate marker for overall less optimal immune suppression. Grade 3R ACR is almost always symptomatic and rarely found in protocol biopsies. In the recent era, it is infrequent beyond the first posttransplant month and typically associated with inappropriately low immune suppression, be it is due to nonadherence, infection, concomitant use of drugs, or substances interfering with the immune suppressant metabolism or in situations where immune suppression had to be reduced or held in the context of infection or neoplasm [28].

Antibody-Mediated Rejection

AMR results from activation of the classical pathway of the complement system by antibodies against the donor HLA present on the endothelium. These antibodies may be preformed prior to transplantation or can arise de novo after transplantation. The antigen–antibody complexes bind C1q and ultimately result in formation of the membrane attack complex, which results in the formation of pores in the myocardial cell membrane leading to an efflux of potassium and chloride ions and an influx of sodium ions and water. This ultimately results in cell lysis and death. In addition to the formation of the membrane attack complex, complement activation can promote further inflammation via endothelial activation [29], and complement fragments C3a and C5a not only have direct effects on these endothelial cells but they are also chemotactic leading to an influx of neutrophils and macrophages [30,31]. In addition to these effects of complement activation, direct linkage of HLA markers on endothelial cells by anti-HLA antibodies can result in activation of the endothelial cells and leads to growth factor production and cytokine production that further results in endothelial cell injury [32–34].

AMR has been reported in up to 20% of patients early after HT and is also a significant component of late rejection with one study in adults and children reporting 25% of cases occurring greater than 1 year after HT [35,36]. Small single center studies have demonstrated pathologic AMR in 35%–59% of pediatric heart transplant patients [37,38]. The diagnosis of AMR has transitioned from one with both pathologic and clinical criteria to a pathologic diagnosis with guidelines for the pathologic criteria outlined by ISHLT [39]. Identified risk factors for AMR include female recipient, multiparity, blood product transfusions, positive perioperative T-cell flow cytometry crossmatch, pretransplant allosensitization, MCS, and previous surgery for congenital heart disease, especially involving homograft tissue [35,40,41]. Pediatric studies have demonstrated an association between AMR, CAV, and graft failure; however, there has been no large scale analysis of the impact of patient survival following the diagnosis of AMR nor comparison to those with ACR [37,40,42]. Current therapies to treat AMR are targeted toward the removal and blockade of circulating antibodies, B-lymphocyte and plasma cell depletion, suppression of T-lymphocyte-dependent antibody responses, and inhibition of the complement cascade. These will be discussed in further detail later in this chapter.

Chronic Dysfunction

Chronic Rejection/Cardiac Allograft Vasculopathy

With the exception of genetic identity between donor and recipient or total eradication of the immune response, e.g., following lethal irradiation, some degree of immunological attack to the organ will always persist, yielding a lifelong dependency on immune suppressive therapy. The typical manifestation of chronic rejection in the transplanted heart is reflected in CAV. CAV is the result of a complex interplay of inflammatory and metabolic factors starting with early graft damage during ischemia-reperfusion injury and modified by donor organ and recipient-related aspects, infectious agents, and immune suppression [43]. Fig. 47.2 provides a schematic overview of how these factors interact and influence each other. Most relevant remain the impact of the immunological attack on the transplanted organ including degree of HLA-mismatch, particularly class 2 (HLA DR) [44], presence of antibodies [45–47], history of recurrent rejection [48], or lack of adherence to the medical regime. Interestingly, C4d deposition and specific immunologic signs of AMR may be absent in the endomyocardial biopsies, while noncomplement-mediated effects, including increased vascular wall permeability resulting in increased invasion of macrophages and lymphocytes into the vascular wall, cause progressive development of CAV [49].

CAV is less common and develops later posttransplant in children than adult patients with 1-, 3-, and 5-year angiographic incidence of moderate–severe CAV of 1%, 2%, and 5% in children compared to 15% at 5 years following transplantation in adults [50]. Recurring risk factors for CAV in many studies for are older donors, older recipients, and rejection. Furthermore, CAV is least common in children who received their transplant in the first 5 years of life [1]. The prognosis for CAV is worst in patients with signs of heart failure, either with ejection fraction <45% or with hemodynamic derangements, as shown by Kindel et al. in a recent PHTS study, and is similar to adult ISHLT registry reports [51].

Diagnostic Evaluation

There are a multitude of tools available for the evaluation of acute and chronic heart failure, including serum biomarkers, ECG, echocardiography, cardiac magnetic resonance imaging (cMRI), cardiac computed tomography (CT), cardiac catheterization, and endomyocardial biopsy.

Electrocardiography

The use of continuous ECG (telemetry) and 12-lead ECG monitoring in the early postoperative period is an ISHLT class I guideline; however, the use of ECG as a primary method for rejection surveillance in older children and adolescents is not recommended [24]. The ECG should be used to monitor for ventricular and atrial tachyarrhythmias. Although the presence of tachyarrhythmias has not been shown to correlate with rejection [52,53], the presence of new-onset Wenckebach was found to correlate with rejection or CAV in one study [52]. Vande Kappelle et al. found that children with supraventricular

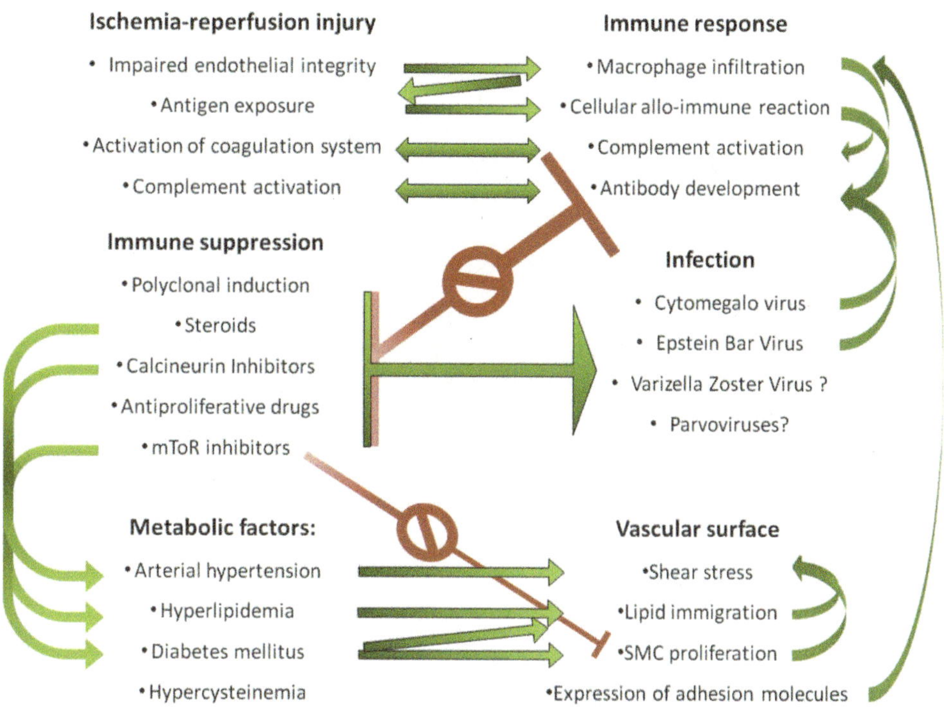

FIGURE 47.2 **Interplay of factors affecting development of graft vasculopathy.** Overview of the pathogenetic factors of coronary allograft vasculopathy (CAV) and their interaction: *Green arrows* symbolize enhancing effects and *red bars* inhibition. I/R-injury includes damage to the endothelium facilitating macrophage invasion and leading to exposure of graft antigens and activation of the complement system. This triggers an early response of the adaptive immune system, which is enhanced if preformed graft-specific antibodies are present but also yields their development if no appropriate immune suppression is introduced. Adverse effects of the immune suppressants include enhancement of constitutional factors of atherosclerosis and increased risk for infections with negative impact on CAV. Viral infections under immune suppression may enhance antibody production and have additional direct effects on endothelium integrity. Formation of plaques in the vessel perpetuates itself through increasing shear stress and further disturbance of the endothelial integrity and subsequently enhanced immune response. mTOR inhibitors have antiproliferative effects on small muscle cell delaying the progression of graft vasculopathy. *(Modified version published in K.R. Schumacher, R.J. Gajarski, S. Urschel, Pediatric coronary allograft vasculopathy–a review of pathogenesis and risk factors, Congenit. Heart Dis. 7 (2012) 312–323.)*

tachyarrhythmias were more likely to develop CAV [54]. In the setting of current immunosuppression, reduced QRS complex voltage is now rare except for severe cases of rejection [55].

Pacemaker implantation and the use of intramyocardial electrocardiograms to monitor for changes in myocardial impedance have been used to assess for early signs of rejection with promising results in both canine models and in human studies [56–58]. While this novel use of a permanent implantable pacemaker appears to be a relatively reliable method of screening for rejection, it does impact the ability to obtain cMRI on these patients in the future unless newer MRI-compatible devices and leads are placed. As such, it may not be warranted for all patients, but it could be considered for those patients already undergoing device implantation.

Echocardiography

Echocardiography is the primary mode of evaluation of graft performance following HT. Echocardiographic protocols vary but often involve imaging multiple times in the first weeks following transplant, including a transesophageal echocardiogram in the operating room prior after removal from cardiopulmonary bypass. Typical evaluation of left ventricular systolic performance includes ejection fraction and shortening fraction. Evaluation of the right ventricular systolic function may include tricuspid annular plane systolic excursion or right ventricular fractional area of change. In addition to assessment for systolic graft failure, diastolic graft failure should also be assessed, including tricuspid and mitral valve inflow Doppler interrogation and tissue Doppler index evaluation, as diastolic dysfunction is often seen in the early posttransplant period and may be a manifestation of rejection. Other echocardiographic measures, including speckle tracking and a novel tissue Doppler assessment of global left ventricular relaxation, have also been shown to correlate with rejection and systolic failure; however, their use has not become routine [59,60].

Serum Biomarkers

Several serum biomarkers have been evaluated in the pediatric heart transplant population, most commonly B-type natriuretic peptide (BNP) and N-terminus proBNP (NT-proBNP). These biomarkers ideally could provide a noninvasive method to quickly and accurately guide medical decision-making and monitor patients for graft failure. BNP has been shown to gradually plateau 3–4 months after transplant [61,62]. Unfortunately, the data regarding BNP to screen for graft failure/rejection are mixed for suitability as a useful biomarker [62–65].

The utility of NT-proBNP to identify graft failure/rejection has been met with results similar to BNP; the benefit of NT-proBNP is that it has a longer half-life but this has not proven to have better diagnostic utility in clinical studies [66–68].

While these biomarkers show promise, current ISHLT guidelines do not recommend routine screening for allograft rejection using these biomarkers, nor troponins, C-reactive protein, or systemic inflammatory markers [24].

Novel approaches, including detection of donor cell-free DNA, have not been thoroughly evaluated in pediatric populations but show promise for noninvasive assessment of graft failure. Recent studies have demonstrated that circulating donor cell-free DNA is elevated in the setting of allograft rejection and injury [69–71]. While this science is novel, at its current stage of investigation, it is not able to differentiate between ACR and AMR, but it may provide a noninvasive measure of reassurance combined with additional allograft measure and relegate the endomyocardial biopsy to those patients with elevated circulating levels of cell-free DNA for further characterization of graft injury or failure.

Invasive Evaluation

Hemodynamic Assessment

Initial assessment of intracardiac hemodynamics can be accomplished in the immediate postoperative setting either via right atrial intracardiac catheters or central venous catheters, which allow for central venous pressure monitoring. This can also allow for estimation of right ventricular and pulmonary pressures to help guide therapies directed at lowering PVR, if persistently elevated posttransplantation.

Endomyocardial Biopsy

Endomyocardial biopsy remains the gold standard for evaluation of rejection following heart transplant and, to date, is the only method that allows one to differentiate ACR from AMR in the failing graft. Endomyocardial biopsy has been shown to be safe with an overall adverse event rate, including transient heart block, tricuspid valve injury, and right bundle branch block, of 0.3% in one study [72] and a 0.1% risk of cardiac perforation in another study [73]. However, there remains wide variation in the use of endomyocardial biopsy with fewer biopsies performed in infants compared to adolescents, and international centers perform significantly fewer biopsies compared to centers within the United States [74].

Coronary Angiography

Coronary angiography remains the most commonly used evaluation for CAV, and the current ISHLT grading scheme for CAV is based on angiographic results (the percent narrowing in main coronary arteries and branch vessels augmented by functional classification) [75]. However, recent data from the Pediatric Heart Transplant study found that less than 50% of pediatric patients undergo routine annual coronary angiography for CAV surveillance [50]. Newer imaging techniques, such as intravascular ultrasound (IVUS) and optical coherence tomography (OCT), provide better anatomic and luminal detail of vessels in children with CAV. Various IVUS measurements, including intimal thickness and intimal index, have been shown to correlate age at transplant, time from transplant, and rejection (especially with hemodynamic compromise) [76]. OCT has shown that patients with high grade cellular rejection had increased intimal thickening with macrophage infiltration [77] and that OCT-identified microchannels, suggestive of neovascularization, correlated with intimal thickness [78]. Unfortunately, a recent study has shown that characteristic OCT-identified lesions were rare in late survivors of pediatric heart transplant [79]. Currently, neither of these imaging modalities is routinely performed in most pediatric centers.

Advanced Imaging

Computed Tomography

While data regarding the use of CT angiography in the pediatric heart transplant population are limited, there are a fair amount of data using CT angiography for coronary artery evaluation in other pediatric populations, including Kawasaki disease and congenital heart disease. Limitations include ionizing radiation as well as spatial and temporal relationships that are affected by patient movement and heart rate. The latter of which can make gating difficult without pharmacologic intervention to decrease the heart rate to more optimal ranges. In adult studies, the negative predictive value approaches >99% for obstructive lesions with >50% stenosis which may make CT angiography an excellent screening test for CAV in certain patients [80].

Cardiac Magnetic Resonance Imaging

The utility of cMRI continues to evolve in the evaluation of heart failure and heart transplant recipients. In the failing graft, cMRI yields excellent evaluation of function and anatomic abnormalities, such as anastomotic stenosis, and can also provide additional information specific to rejection and CAV assessment. T2 relaxation time (a measure of myocardial edema) has been shown to be higher in patients with higher grades of rejection [81]. In addition, T2 relaxation time, combined with right ventricular end-diastolic volume index, has a high sensitivity and negative predictive value for predicting biopsy-proven rejection (ACR grade 2R and higher or AMR) [82]. Late gadolinium enhancement (LGE) has been shown to correlate with the presence and prevalence of CAV [83,84] as well as with maximal intimal wall thickness on IVUS in a small pediatric series [85]. However, LGE appears to have less utility in screening for acute rejection [86,87].

Therapy

The treatment of systolic and diastolic dysfunction associated with graft failure follows typical management strategies, including the use of inotropic support, enteral heart failure medications, and diuretics, as outlined in other chapters of this textbook. This section is focused on the specific management of the failing graft posttransplantation, including acute right ventricular failure secondary to elevated PVR, treatment of rejection, and management and prevention of CAV.

Right Ventricular Failure Secondary to Elevated Pulmonary Vascular Resistance

In patients with elevated PVR prior to transplant, preemptive therapy with pulmonary vasodilators can be beneficial. Preemptive use of inhaled nitric oxide has been shown to decrease the incidence of right ventricular failure postoperatively [13]. Patients routinely are treated with milrinone, a phosphodiesterase 3 inhibitor, in the immediate postoperative period for a multitude of reasons, including inotropy and lusitropy. However, an additional benefit is smooth muscle relaxation and pulmonary vasodilation, which is beneficial in the setting of increased PVR.

In addition, sildenafil, a selective phosphodiesterase 5 inhibitor, has been shown to be effective in the treatment of patients with elevated PVR posttransplantation. Its use in this population has demonstrated decreased systolic and mean pulmonary artery pressures, decreased transpulmonary gradient, and decreased indexed PVR, as well as safe administration and the ability to transition patients off inhaled or intravenous pulmonary vasodilators [88]. Additional therapeutic agents such as bosentan, an endothelin receptor antagonist, and treprostinil, a prostacyclin analog, are potential adjunctive or alternative therapies for right ventricular failure. Bosentan has been shown to effectively decrease PVR pretransplantation resulting in similar transplant outcomes compared to patients with low PVR [89]. There is a paucity of data regarding the use of treprostinil in patients either awaiting or undergoing HT. While it has been used safely in the pediatric patient population for pulmonary arterial hypertension, there are minimal data to guide its use in this population following transplantation.

Acute Cellular Rejection Management

Whenever acute functional deterioration of the transplanted heart is going along with a clinical or diagnostic suspicion of ACR, therapy should be initiated immediately [24]. The risk of rapid deterioration and development of potentially life-threatening arrhythmia is high and does not permit significant delay of treatment. Histological features of ACR typically remain detectable for 12–24 h after a first steroid pulse [90] and signs of AMR including C4d deposition even beyond that; consequently, therapy can be initiated even while planning and awaiting the endomyocardial biopsy results. The sensitivity of the biopsy is estimated at 90% if 4 adequate pieces are obtained, leaving 10% of ACR biopsy negative, hence whenever there is a strong clinical suspicion, a full course of rejection therapy should be completed.

Careful assessment of the circumstances in which ACR occurs is essential: dose and level of maintenance immune suppression, possible nonadherence or intake of interfering medications or substances, reasons for impaired intestinal absorption, concomitant infections or flare of viral infections, particularly cytomegalovirus was described to trigger ACR while HLA-antibody levels may secondarily increase in presence of a flare of EBV infection. In any case of AMR after the first year or in absence of clear causative events, HLA-antibody screening is recommended. Therapeutic choices are directed by the clinical presentation and the histological findings and outlined in Table 47.1. ACR 1R was not associated with impaired long-term outcome and does not require pulse therapy or augmentation of maintenance

TABLE 47.1 Typical Approach to Isolated ACR in Absence of DSA or Histological Signs of AMR

Histology	Clinical Signs of Rejection	Hemodynamic Compromise	DSA	Therapy Options
1R	no	no	no	none
2R	no	no	no	Oral steroid pulse
				Adaption of maintenance IS
2R	yes	yes or no	no	IV steroid pulse
3R	yes or no	yes or no	no	ATG
1R/2R/3R	yes	yes	no	Reserve therapies
				Intensified search for antibodies
				ex juvantibus AMR therapy

ACR, acute cellular rejection; *AMR*, antibody-mediated rejection; *DSA*, donor-specific antibody.

immunosuppression [91]. ACR 3R independent of hemodynamic compromise and any degree of ACR or AMR with hemodynamic compromise should always trigger pulse steroid therapy followed by increased maintenance therapy. For ACR 2R with no or mild impairment of the graft, a reduced pulse with oral steroids or simply optimization of the maintenance therapy can be sufficient.

The first-line drug of choice is typically intravenous methylprednisolone 10 mg/kg once daily for 3–5 days or, for mild or asymptomatic cases, 2 mg/kg of prednisone or prednisolone once daily may represent an alternative. The effect of successful pulse therapy is usually visible within 24–48 h of treatment initiation with improvement of systolic function and mitral regurgitation, reduction of effusion and swelling in the echocardiogram, normalization of conduction and repolarization abnormalities, and clinical improvement. If no improvement can be detected by the end of the steroid pulse or relapse shortly after discontinuation is observed, a second high dose pulse can be considered and should be administered parenterally.

Alternatively or as a next step of escalation, polyclonal induction agents (Antithymocyte globulins: e.g., Thymoglobulin, ATGAM, MALG) can be used in similar dosage as for primary induction (1.5 mg/kg/day as continuous intravenous infusion or divided into 1–2 doses/d). Effect and dose can be monitored by lymphocyte count (target 0.2–0.4 per mL), CD3 T-cell count (target <100 per μL), or absolute CD3 T-cell count (<25 cells/mm^3) [92]. Further escalation includes anti-CD52 (alemtuzumab/Campath-1H), cyclophosphamide, photopheresis, or total body irradiation, with the latter mostly considered obsolete given the exorbitant risk of lethal infections. The diagnostic focus in ACR recalcitrant to pulse therapy has to be on potential concomitant AMR (see below) and consideration of the therapeutic steps outlined in that section. In any case of ACR therapy that exceeds oral pulse steroid, infectious prophylaxis, at least for *pneumocystis* pneumonia, should be reinitiated [93]. Most centers will transiently adapt the maintenance immune suppression (e.g., increase calcineurin inhibitor target by 10%–20%, maintain prednisone at 0.1 mg/kg/day, or replace mycophenolate with an mToR inhibitor).

ACR ≥2R or with hemodynamic compromise that has clinically resolved should always trigger a follow-up biopsy 2–4 weeks after therapy to confirm complete remission [24]. Since development of de novo HLA antibodies is commonly triggered by ACR, screening is recommended also for patients that were previously nonsensitized or free of DSA.

Antibody-Mediated Rejection Management

Therapies for AMR are aimed at interrupting various points in the process of rejection, including removal of circulating antibodies, inhibition of circulating antibodies, suppression of the T-lymphocyte antibody response, suppression of B-lymphocytes, depletion of plasma cells, and inhibition of the complement cascade. Although there is consensus that AMR with allograft dysfunction should be treated aggressively, there is no agreement regarding the treatment of asymptomatic AMR without dysfunction. In addition, there is neither consensus nor standardization regarding the optimal treatment for AMR in pediatric heart transplant recipients. Recommended surveillance strategies exist and various treatment options include T-lymphocyte suppression using steroids, antithymocyte globulin, and calcineurin inhibitors, mTOR inhibitors, as well as mycophenolate mofetil, plasmapheresis, Intravenous immunoglobulin (IVIG), rituximab, bortezomib, and eculizumab in multimodal combination approaches [94].

Plasmapheresis is utilized to remove circulating antibodies but does not inhibit antibody production. While the use of plasmapheresis has been described for the treatment of AMR since 1992 [95,96], there is no consensus regarding the duration or frequency of plasmapheresis. In practice, this may be used in isolation but is frequently employed with other therapies, to remove circulating antibodies, enhance the therapeutic target of bortezomib, or both.

IVIG is often utilized to inhibit remaining circulating antibodies due to its immunomodulatory effects including blockade of Fc receptors, complement inhibition, downregulation of B-lymphocyte receptors, and inhibition of both T- and B-lymphocytes. Not only does IVIG contain antibodies against various cytokines but it may also decrease the synthesis of cytokines [40]. In addition, in a recent survey regarding treatment of AMR, IVIG was one of the most frequently utilized therapies and was recommended for initial treatment along with steroids and plasmapheresis [97].

T-lymphocyte stimulation is necessary for B-cell activation, and thus suppression of T-lymphocytes can be used as adjuncts in the treatment of AMR to indirectly inhibit B-lymphocyte activation and production of high-affinity antibodies. The addition or augmentation of the aforementioned therapies is common in treating mixed rejection.

Rituximab, a monoclonal antibody directed against CD20+ B-lymphocytes, results in suppression and elimination of B-lymphocytes due to antibody-dependent cell cytotoxicity and induction of apoptosis via CD20 cellular cross-linking; limited studies have evaluated rituximab for the treatment of AMR and suggested it may be beneficial [98,99]. However, optimal dosing strategies for rituximab in pediatric HT patients with AMR are unknown, thus lymphoma dosing strategies are typically used. There is one report of successful use of low-dose rituximab to treat AMR [100]. Unfortunately, the utility of rituximab may be limited in the treatment of AMR due to its target; as B-lymphocytes differentiate into plasma cells, the expression of CD20 on the surface of the lymphocyte is lost, and thus rituximab is ineffective in suppressing plasma cells.

Newer therapies for the treatment of AMR include bortezomib and eculizumab. Bortezomib is a proteasome inhibitor which leads to cell cycle arrest and apoptosis of plasma cells and has been shown to be effective in the treatment of AMR in both pediatric kidney and heart transplant patients in small case series [101,102]. Given the limitations of rituximab as B-lymphocytes differentiate, some have advocated that initial treatment with both rituximab and bortezomib is reasonable initial management for AMR [101]. Eculizumab, a humanized monoclonal antibody directed against C5, prevents conversion of C5 into C5a and C5b and, thus, prevents formation of the membrane attack complex; studies have shown efficacy for AMR in renal transplant patients [103,104] and one lung transplant patient with hyperacute AMR [105]. However, neither of these agents has been widely used in the treatment of AMR for pediatric heart transplant patients.

Mechanical Circulatory Support

For the patient who experiences graft failure, regardless of etiology, and is unable to maintain adequate tissue and organ perfusion despite maximal pharmacologic and ventilator support, MCS may provide the last therapeutic option to bridge the patient to recovery or, rarely, retransplantation. This includes ECMO and ventricular assist devices. The decision to support a patient with MCS is multifactorial and important factors include the etiology of graft failure, likelihood of recovery, time from initial transplantation, retransplant candidacy, and patient/family consent. In a recent study of 203 pediatric patients undergoing HT with postoperative graft failure, 29 required ECMO support, and 62% of these patients survived to hospital discharge [106]. Survival was 75% and 53% for those with rejection/allograft vasculopathy and primary graft failure groups, respectively [106]. In addition, the need for MCS while listed for retransplantation is predictive of mortality while waiting for retransplantation [8,107].

Long-Term Adjuvant Therapies for Prevention of Coronary Allograft Vasculopathy

As outlined above, CAV is a multifactorial process that does not only involve the immune response but is also exacerbated by traditional contributing metabolic factors that cause typical atherosclerosis. Thus, regular assessment and consultation with a dietitian and physiotherapist may be beneficial to reinforce appropriate diet and physical exercise. Urinalysis and blood pressure need to be monitored regularly and elevated blood pressures medically controlled. HBa1C as a marker for subclinical diabetes should be annually assessed, as a recent UNOS registry analysis identified new-onset diabetes mellitus in 8% of pediatric heart transplant recipients, 77% of which were insulin-dependent [108]. Lipid profiles should be obtained regularly, and statins may be beneficial in pediatric patients and are standard of care in adult heart recipients. In adults randomized controlled trials have shown that the use of statins did not only improve the lipid profile but also reduce the incidence of ACR in the first year [109], a finding that was confirmed in smaller pediatric studies [110,111]. A recent PHTS registry analysis could not confirm a benefit of statins on survival and CAV [112]. However, statins were only given to less than 50% of the patients which is likely reflective of a selective group of patients for which the treating physicians assumed a higher risk profile.

The antiproliferative capacities of mToR inhibitors are not only limited to leukocytes but also include endothelial cells of the coronary arteries. This theoretical benefit on reduced incidence of CAV was recently shown in several studies in adult patients replacing MMF with sirolimus or everolimus in a dual combination with a CNI. Clinical data on potential benefits in childhood are not yet available.

CONCLUSION

Graft failure remains the greatest limitation to survival after pediatric HT. In the perioperative period, causes include primary graft failure, pulmonary hypertension, and ischemia-reperfusion injury with hyperacute rejection occurring rarely in the modern era. Late graft failure can be a manifestation of rejection, in particular if patients have been nonadherent or may be due to allograft vasculopathy. Immunologic, as well as heart failure, therapies, including MCS, may be beneficial for rescue; however, mortality is high in severe cases.

REFERENCES

[1] A.I. Dipchand, J.W. Rossano, L.B. Edwards, A.Y. Kucheryavaya, C. Benden, S. Goldfarb, B.J. Levvey, L.H. Lund, B. Meiser, R.D. Yusen, J. Stehlik, The registry of the international society for heart and lung transplantation: eighteenth official pediatric heart transplantation report-2015; focus theme: early graft failure, J. Heart Lung Transplant. 34 (2015) 1233–1243.

[2] J.M. Karamichalis, S.D. Miyamoto, D.N. Campbell, J. Smith, K.K. McFann, S. Clark, B. Pietra, M.B. Mitchell, Pediatric cardiac retransplant: differing patterns of primary graft failure by age at first transplant, J. Thorac. Cardiovasc. Surg. 141 (2011) 223–230.

[3] M.S. Jahania, T.W. Mullett, J.A. Sanchez, P. Narayan, R.D. Lasley, R.M. Mentzer Jr., Acute allograft failure in thoracic organ transplantation, J. Card. Surg. 15 (2000) 122–128.

[4] J.B. Ryan, M. Hicks, J.R. Cropper, S.R. Garlick, S.H. Kesteven, M.K. Wilson, M.P. Feneley, P.S. Macdonald, Functional evidence of reversible ischemic injury immediately after the sympathetic storm associated with experimental brain death, J. Heart Lung Transplant. 22 (2003) 922–928.

[5] D. Novitzky, D.K. Cooper, J.D. Rosendale, H.M. Kauffman, Hormonal therapy of the brain-dead organ donor: experimental and clinical studies, Transplantation 82 (2006) 1396–1401.

[6] M. Hicks, A. Hing, L. Gao, J. Ryan, P.S. Macdonald, Organ preservation, Methods Mol. Biol. 333 (2006) 331–374.

[7] W. Rodrigues, M. Carr, D. Ridout, K. Carter, S.L. Hulme, J. Simmonds, M. Elliott, A. Hoskote, M. Burch, K.L. Brown, Total donor ischemic time: relationship to early hemodynamics and intensive care morbidity in pediatric cardiac transplant recipients, Pediatr. Crit. Care Med. 12 (2011) 660–666.

[8] S. Kaushal, K.L. Matthews, X. Garcia, B. Wehman, E. Riddle, Z. Ying, R. Nubani, C.E. Canter, W.R. Morrow, C.B. Huddleston, C.L. Backer, E. Pahl, A multicenter study of primary graft failure after infant heart transplantation: impact of extracorporeal membrane oxygenation on outcomes, Pediatr. Transplant. 18 (2014) 72–78.

[9] S.O. Syrjala, A.I. Nykanen, R. Tuuminen, A. Raissadati, M.A. Keranen, R. Arnaudova, R. Krebs, G.Y. Koh, K. Alitalo, K.B. Lemstrom, Donor heart treatment with comp-ang1 limits ischemia-reperfusion injury and rejection of cardiac allografts, Am. J. Transplant. 15 (2015) 2075–2084.

[10] S.O. Syrjala, R. Tuuminen, A.I. Nykanen, A. Raissadati, A. Dashkevich, M.A. Keranen, R. Arnaudova, R. Krebs, C.C. Leow, P. Saharinen, K. Alitalo, K.B. Lemstrom, Angiopoietin-2 inhibition prevents transplant ischemia-reperfusion injury and chronic rejection in rat cardiac allografts, Am. J. Transplant. 14 (2014) 1096–1108.

[11] M.E. Richmond, Y.M. Law, B.B. Das, M.D. Everitt, M. Kukreja, D.C. Naftel, M.S. Kemna, H.T. Henderson, K. Beddows, F.J. Fricker, W.T. Mahle, Elevated pre-transplant pulmonary vascular resistance is not associated with mortality in children without congenital heart disease: a multicenter study, J. Heart Lung Transplant. 34 (2015) 448–456.

[12] P. Chiu, J.M. Schaffer, A.Y. Sheikh, R. Ha, O. Reinhartz, R. Mainwaring, B.A. Reitz, Elevated pretransplant pulmonary vascular resistance index does not predict mortality after isolated orthotopic heart transplantation in children: a retrospective analysis of the unos database, Pediatr. Transplant. 19 (2015) 623–633.

[13] G. Ofori-Amanfo, D. Hsu, J.M. Lamour, S. Mital, M.L. O'Byrne, A.J. Smerling, J.M. Chen, R. Mosca, L.J. Addonizio, Heart transplantation in children with markedly elevated pulmonary vascular resistance: impact of right ventricular failure on outcome, J. Heart Lung Transplant. 30 (2011) 659–666.

[14] S. Stewart, G.L. Winters, M.C. Fishbein, H.D. Tazelaar, J. Kobashigawa, J. Abrams, C.B. Andersen, A. Angelini, G.J. Berry, M.M. Burke, A.J. Demetris, E. Hammond, S. Itescu, C.C. Marboe, B. McManus, E.F. Reed, N.L. Reinsmoen, E.R. Rodriguez, A.G. Rose, M. Rose, N. Suciu-Focia, A. Zeevi, M.E. Billingham, Revision of the 1990 working formulation for the standardization of nomenclature in the diagnosis of heart rejection, J. Heart Lung Transplant. 24 (2005) 1710–1720.

[15] A.G. Rose, D.K. Cooper, P.A. Human, H. Reichenspurner, B. Reichart, Histopathology of hyperacute rejection of the heart: experimental and clinical observations in allografts and xenografts, J. Heart Lung Transplant. 10 (1991) 223–234.

[16] A.I. Dipchand, L.B. Edwards, A.Y. Kucheryavaya, C. Benden, F. Dobbels, B.J. Levvey, L.H. Lund, B. Meiser, R.D. Yusen, J. Stehlik, The registry of the international society for heart and lung transplantation: seventeenth official pediatric heart transplantation report–2014; focus theme: retransplantation, J. Heart Lung Transplant. 33 (2014) 985–995.

[17] T.W. LeBien, T.F. Tedder, B lymphocytes: how they develop and function, 112 (2008) 1570–1580.

[18] S.C. Stoica, F. Cafferty, M. Pauriah, C.J. Taylor, L.D. Sharples, J. Wallwork, S.R. Large, J. Parameshwar, The cumulative effect of acute rejection on development of cardiac allograft vasculopathy, J. Heart Lung Transplant. 25 (2006) 420–425.

[19] H.P. Brunner-La Rocca, G. Sutsch, J. Schneider, F. Follath, W. Kiowski, Natural course of moderate cardiac allograft rejection (international society for heart transplantation grade 2) early and late after transplantation, Circulation 94 (1996) 1334–1338.

[20] M.S. Finkel, C.V. Oddis, T.D. Jacob, S.C. Watkins, B.G. Hattler, R.L. Simmons, Negative inotropic effects of cytokines on the heart mediated by nitric oxide, Science 257 (1992) 387–389.

[21] D.M. Leppink, D.K. Bishop, D.D. Sedmak, M.L. Henry, R.M. Ferguson, P.R. Streeter, E.C. Butcher, C.G. Orosz, Inducible expression of an endothelial cell antigen on murine myocardial vasculature in association with interstitial cellular infiltration, Transplantation 48 (1989) 874–877.

[22] W.H. Barry, Mechanisms of immune-mediated myocyte injury, Circulation 89 (1994) 2421–2432.

[23] S.L. Houser, K. Kuwaki, C. Knosalla, F.J. Dor, B. Gollackner, J. Cheng, A. Shimizu, H.J. Schuurman, D.K. Cooper, Thrombotic microangiopathy and graft arteriopathy in pig hearts following transplantation into baboons, Xenotransplantation 11 (2004) 416–425.

[24] M.R. Costanzo, A. Dipchand, R. Starling, A. Anderson, M. Chan, S. Desai, S. Fedson, P. Fisher, G. Gonzales-Stawinski, L. Martinelli, D. McGiffin, J. Smith, D. Taylor, B. Meiser, S. Webber, D. Baran, M. Carboni, T. Dengler, D. Feldman, M. Frigerio, A. Kfoury, D. Kim, J. Kobashigawa, M. Shullo, J. Stehlik, J. Teuteberg, P. Uber, A. Zuckermann, S. Hunt, M. Burch, G. Bhat, C. Canter, R. Chinnock, M. Crespo-Leiro, R. Delgado, F. Dobbels, K. Grady, W. Kao, J. Lamour, G. Parry, J. Patel, D. Pini, J. Towbin, G. Wolfel, D. Delgado, H. Eisen, L. Goldberg, J. Hosenpud, M. Johnson, A. Keogh, C. Lewis, J. O'Connell, J. Rogers, H. Ross, S. Russell, J. Vanhaecke, The international society of heart and lung transplantation guidelines for the care of heart transplant recipients, J. Heart Lung Transplant. 29 (2010) 914–956.

[25] A.E. Lammers, P. Roberts, K.L. Brown, M. Fenton, P. Rees, N.J. Sebire, M. Burch, Acute rejection after paediatric heart transplantation: far less common and less severe, Transpl. Int. 23 (2010) 38–46.

[26] K.B. Shah, M.P. Flattery, M.C. Smallfield, G. Merinar, D.G. Tang, E.H. Sheldon, L.R. Thacker, V. Kasirajan, R.H. Cooke, M.L. Hess, Surveillance endomyocardial biopsy in the modern era produces low diagnostic yield for cardiac allograft rejection, Transplantation 99 (2015) e75–80.

[27] R.K. Ameduri, J. Zheng, K.B. Schechtman, T.M. Hoffman, R.J. Gajarski, R. Chinnock, D.C. Naftel, J.K. Kirklin, A.I. Dipchand, C.E. Canter, Has late rejection decreased in pediatric heart transplantation in the current era? A multi-institutional study, J. Heart Lung Transplant. 31 (2012) 980–986.

[28] M.D. Everitt, E. Pahl, K.B. Schechtman, J. Zheng, J.M. Ringewald, T. L'Ecuyer, D.C. Naftel, J.K. Kirklin, E.D. Blume, E.A. Bullock, C.E. Canter, Rejection with hemodynamic compromise in the current era of pediatric heart transplantation: a multi-institutional study, J. Heart Lung Transplant. 30 (2011) 282–288.

[29] K.S. Kilgore, E. Schmid, T.P. Shanley, C.M. Flory, V. Maheswari, N.L. Tramontini, H. Cohen, P.A. Ward, H.P. Friedl, J.S. Warren, Sublytic concentrations of the membrane attack complex of complement induce endothelial interleukin-8 and monocyte chemoattractant protein-1 through nuclear factor-kappa b activation, Am. J. Pathol. 150 (1997) 2019–2031.

[30] K. Murata, W.M. Baldwin 3rd, Mechanisms of complement activation, c4d deposition, and their contribution to the pathogenesis of antibody-mediated rejection, Transplant. Rev. (Orl.) 23 (2009) 139–150.

[31] R. Snyderman, M.C. Pike, D. McCarley, L. Lang, Quantification of mouse macrophage chemotaxis in vitro: role of c5 for the production of chemotactic activity, Infect. Immun. 11 (1975) 488–492.

[32] J.D. Smith, C. Lawson, M.H. Yacoub, M.L. Rose, Activation of nf-kappa b in human endothelial cells induced by monoclonal and allospecific hla antibodies, Int. Immunol. 12 (2000) 563–571.

[33] P.D. Hughes, S.J. Cohney, Modifiers of complement activation for prevention of antibody-mediated injury to allografts, Curr. Opin. Organ Transplant. 16 (2011) 425–433.

[34] F.M. Naemi, V. Carter, J.A. Kirby, S. Ali, Anti-donor hla class i antibodies: pathways to endothelial cell activation and cell-mediated allograft rejection, Transplantation 96 (2013) 258–266.

[35] P.J. Michaels, M.L. Espejo, J. Kobashigawa, J.C. Alejos, C. Burch, S. Takemoto, E.F. Reed, M.C. Fishbein, Humoral rejection in cardiac transplantation: risk factors, hemodynamic consequences and relationship to transplant coronary artery disease, J. Heart Lung Transplant. 22 (2003) 58–69.

[36] G.W. Wu, J.A. Kobashigawa, M.C. Fishbein, J.K. Patel, M.M. Kittleson, E.F. Reed, K.K. Kiyosaki, A. Ardehali, Asymptomatic antibody-mediated rejection after heart transplantation predicts poor outcomes, J. Heart Lung Transplant. 28 (2009) 417–422.

[37] M.D. Everitt, M.E. Hammond, G.L. Snow, J. Stehlik, M.P. Revelo, D.V. Miller, A.K. Kaza, D. Budge, R. Alharethi, K.M. Molina, A.G. Kfoury, Biopsy-diagnosed antibody-mediated rejection based on the proposed international society for heart and lung transplantation working formulation is associated with adverse cardiovascular outcomes after pediatric heart transplant, J. Heart Lung Transplant. 31 (2012) 686–693.

[38] T.W. Casarez, G. Perens, R.J. Williams, E. Kutay, M.C. Fishbein, E.F. Reed, J.C. Alejos, D.S. Levi, Humoral rejection in pediatric orthotopic heart transplantation, J. Heart Lung Transplant. 26 (2007) 114–119.

[39] G.J. Berry, M.M. Burke, C. Andersen, P. Bruneval, M. Fedrigo, M.C. Fishbein, M. Goddard, E.H. Hammond, O. Leone, C. Marboe, D. Miller, D. Neil, D. Rassl, M.P. Revelo, A. Rice, E. Rene Rodriguez, S. Stewart, C.D. Tan, G.L. Winters, L. West, M.R. Mehra, A. Angelini, The 2013 international society for heart and lung transplantation working formulation for the standardization of nomenclature in the pathologic diagnosis of antibody-mediated rejection in heart transplantation, J. Heart Lung Transplant. 32 (2013) 1147–1162.

[40] N. Nair, T. Ball, P.A. Uber, M.R. Mehra, Current and future challenges in therapy for antibody-mediated rejection, J. Heart Lung Transplant. 30 (2011) 612–617.

[41] A. Brand, Immunological aspects of blood transfusions, Transpl. Immunol. 10 (2002) 183–190.

[42] A.G. Kfoury, M.E. Hammond, G.L. Snow, S.G. Drakos, J. Stehlik, P.W. Fisher, B.B. Reid, M.D. Everitt, F.M. Bader, D.G. Renlund, Cardiovascular mortality among heart transplant recipients with asymptomatic antibody-mediated or stable mixed cellular and antibody-mediated rejection, J. Heart Lung Transplant. 28 (2009) 781–784.

[43] K.R. Schumacher, R.J. Gajarski, S. Urschel, Pediatric coronary allograft vasculopathy–a review of pathogenesis and risk factors, Congenit. Heart Dis. 7 (2012) 312–323.

[44] I. Kaczmarek, M.A. Deutsch, M.E. Rohrer, A. Beiras-Fernandez, J. Groetzner, S. Daebritz, M. Schmoeckel, M. Spannagl, B. Meiser, B. Reichart, Hla-dr matching improves survival after heart transplantation: is it time to change allocation policies? J. Heart Lung Transplant. 25 (2006) 1057–1062.

[45] I. Kaczmarek, M.A. Deutsch, T. Kauke, A. Beiras-Fernandez, M. Schmoeckel, C. Vicol, R. Sodian, B. Reichart, M. Spannagl, P. Ueberfuhr, Donor-specific hla alloantibodies: long-term impact on cardiac allograft vasculopathy and mortality after heart transplant, Exp. Clin. Transplant. 6 (2008) 229–235.

[46] R. Frank, M.R. Molina, L.R. Goldberg, J.W. Wald, M. Kamoun, P. Lal, Circulating donor-specific anti-human leukocyte antigen antibodies and complement c4d deposition are associated with the development of cardiac allograft vasculopathy, Am. J. Clin. Pathol. 142 (2014) 809–815.

[47] A. Tran, D. Fixler, R. Huang, T. Meza, C. Lacelle, B.B. Das, Donor-specific hla alloantibodies: impact on cardiac allograft vasculopathy, rejection, and survival after pediatric heart transplantation, J. Heart Lung Transplant 35 (2016) 87–91.

[48] M.R. Mehra, P.A. Uber, W.E. Uber, R.L. Scott, M.H. Park, Allosensitization in heart transplantation: implications and management strategies, Curr. Opin. Cardiol. 18 (2003) 153–158.

[49] F. Li, M.E. Atz, E.F. Reed, Human leukocyte antigen antibodies in chronic transplant vasculopathy-mechanisms and pathways, Curr. Opin. Immunol. 21 (2009) 557–562.

[50] E. Pahl, D.C. Naftel, M.A. Kuhn, R.E. Shaddy, W.R. Morrow, C.E. Canter, J. Kirklin, The impact and outcome of transplant coronary artery disease in a pediatric population: a 9-year multi-institutional study, J. Heart Lung Transplant. 24 (2005) 645–651.

[51] S.J. Kindel, Y.M. Law, C. Chin, M. Burch, J.K. Kirklin, D.C. Naftel, E. Pruitt, M.P. Carboni, A. Arens, A.M. Atz, W.J. Dreyer, W.T. Mahle, E. Pahl, Improved detection of cardiac allograft vasculopathy: a multi-institutional analysis of functional parameters in pediatric heart transplant recipients, J. Am. Coll. Cardiol. 66 (2015) 547–557.

[52] N.J. Kertesz, J.A. Towbin, S. Clunie, A.L. Fenrich, R.A. Friedman, D.L. Kearney, W.J. Dreyer, J.F. Price, B. Radovancevic, S.W. Denfield, Long-term follow-up of arrhythmias in pediatric orthotopic heart transplant recipients: incidence and correlation with rejection, J. Heart Lung Transplant. 22 (2003) 889–893.

[53] M.J. LaPage, E.K. Rhee, C.E. Canter, Tachyarrhythmias after pediatric heart transplantation, J. Heart Lung Transplant. 29 (2010) 273–277.

[54] R.P. Vande Kappelle, K. Gambetta, B.J. Deal, C.L. Backer, C.L. Sullivan, E. Pahl, Late sinus and atrial tachycardia after pediatric heart transplantation might predict poor outcome, Pediatr. Cardiol. 31 (2010) 643–649.

[55] L. Hoskova, I. Malek, R. Krausova, M. Podzimkova, J. Pirk, [electrocardiographic changes after heart transplantation], Vnitrni lekarstvi 48 (Suppl. 1) (2002) 72–75.

[56] C. Knosalla, O. Grauhan, J. Muller, R. Pfitzmann, E. Fietze, T. Cohnert, H.D. Volk, R. Hetzer, Intramyocardial electrogram recordings (imeg) for diagnosis of cellular and humoral mediated cardiac allograft rejection, Ann. Thorac. Cardiovasc. Surg. 6 (2000) 89–94.

[57] Y.X. Jia, X. Meng, L.B. Sun, J. Han, Y.T. Chen, Using intramyocardial electrograms combined with other noninvasive methods for monitoring acute rejection following human heart transplantation, Chin. Med. J. 122 (2009) 136–139.

[58] R. Hetzer, E.V. Potapov, J. Muller, M. Loebe, M. Hummel, Y. Weng, H. Warnecke, P.E. Lange, Daily noninvasive rejection monitoring improves long-term survival in pediatric heart transplantation, Ann. Thorac. Surg. 66 (1998) 1343–1349.

[59] S. Buddhe, M.E. Richmond, J. Gilbreth, W.W. Lai, Longitudinal strain by speckle tracking echocardiography in pediatric heart transplant recipients, Congenit. Heart Dis. 10 (2015) 362–370.

[60] L.E. Hernandez, C.W. Shepard, J. Menk, V.C. Lilliam, R.K. Ameduri, Global left ventricular relaxation: a novel tissue doppler index of acute rejection in pediatric heart transplantation, J. Heart Lung Transplant. 34 (2015) 1190–1197.

[61] J.D. Sparks, U. Boston, P. Eghtesady, C.E. Canter, B-type natriuretic peptide trends after pediatric heart transplantation, Pediatr. Transplant. 18 (2014) 477–484.

[62] J.W. Rossano, S.W. Denfield, J.J. Kim, J.F. Price, J.L. Jefferies, J.A. Decker, E.O. Smith, S.K. Clunie, J.A. Towbin, W.J. Dreyer, B-type natriuretic peptide is a sensitive screening test for acute rejection in pediatric heart transplant patients, J. Heart Lung Transplant. 27 (2008) 649–654.

[63] C.L. Lindblade, D.S. Chun, R.K. Darragh, R.L. Caldwell, D.J. Murphy, M.S. Schamberger, Value of plasma b-type natriuretic peptide as a marker for rejection in pediatric heart transplant recipients, Am. J. Cardiol. 95 (2005) 909–911.

[64] E.K. Hall, A.C. Glatz, M.D. Quartermain, C. Ravishankar, B. Kaufman, M.S. Cohen, B.D. Hanna, D.J. Goldberg, Brain-type natriuretic peptide correlates with right heart pressures in a cross section of pediatric heart transplant patients, Pediatr. Transplant. 15 (2011) 70–74.

[65] M. Bramlet, R. Moore, D. Murphy, R. Caldwell, R. Darragh, M. Schamberger, Increase of b-type natriuretic peptide from baseline increases the risk of death or retransplant in pediatric cardiac transplant patients, midterm results, Congenit. Heart Dis. 5 (2010) 297–302.

[66] A.K. Dyer, A.P. Barnes, D.E. Fixler, T.K. Shah, D.L. Sutcliffe, I. Hashim, M.H. Drazner, J.A. de Lemos, Use of a highly sensitive assay for cardiac troponin t and n-terminal pro-brain natriuretic peptide to diagnose acute rejection in pediatric cardiac transplant recipients, Am. Heart J. 163 (2012) 595–600.

[67] K.R. Knecht, M.L. Alexander, C.J. Swearingen, E.A. Frazier, Ntprobnp as a marker of rejection in pediatric heart transplant recipients, Pediatr. Transplant. 16 (2012) 335–339.

[68] L.C. Battes, K. Caliskan, D. Rizopoulos, A.A. Constantinescu, J.L. Robertus, M. Akkerhuis, O.C. Manintveld, E. Boersma, I. Kardys, Repeated measurements of nt-pro-b-type natriuretic peptide, troponin t or c-reactive protein do not predict future allograft rejection in heart transplant recipients, Transplantation 99 (2015) 580–585.

[69] J. Beck, M. Oellerich, U. Schulz, V. Schauerte, L. Reinhard, U. Fuchs, C. Knabbe, A. Zittermann, C. Olbricht, J.F. Gummert, M. Shipkova, I. Birschmann, E. Wieland, E. Schutz, Donor-derived cell-free DNA is a novel universal biomarker for allograft rejection in solid organ transplantation, Transplant. Proc. 47 (2015) 2400–2403.

[70] M. Oellerich, P. Walson, J. Beck, J. Schmitz, O. Kollmar, E. Schutz, Cell free DNA as a marker of transplant graft injury (liquid biopsy), Ther. Drug Monit 38 (Suppl. 1) (2016) S75–S79.

[71] K.P. Daly, Emerging science in paediatric heart transplantation: donor allocation, biomarkers, and the quest for evidence-based medicine, Cardiol. Young 25 (Suppl. 2) (2015) 117–123.

[72] K.P. Daly, A.C. Marshall, J.A. Vincent, W.A. Zuckerman, T.M. Hoffman, C.E. Canter, E.D. Blume, L. Bergersen, Endomyocardial biopsy and selective coronary angiography are low-risk procedures in pediatric heart transplant recipients: results of a multicenter experience, J. Heart Lung Transplant. 31 (2012) 398–409.

[73] S.G. Pophal, G. Sigfusson, K.L. Booth, S.A. Bacanu, S.A. Webber, J.A. Ettedgui, W.H. Neches, S.C. Park, Complications of endomyocardial biopsy in children, J. Am. Coll. Cardiol. 34 (1999) 2105–2110.

[74] J. Godown, M.T. Harris, J. Burger, D.A. Dodd, Variation in the use of surveillance endomyocardial biopsy among pediatric heart transplant centers over time, Pediatr. Transplant. 19 (2015) 612–617.

[75] M.R. Mehra, M.G. Crespo-Leiro, A. Dipchand, S.M. Ensminger, N.E. Hiemann, J.A. Kobashigawa, J. Madsen, J. Parameshwar, R.C. Starling, P.A. Uber, International society for heart and lung transplantation working formulation of a standardized nomenclature for cardiac allograft vasculopathy-2010, J. Heart Lung Transplant. 29 (2010) 717–727.

[76] R.T. Nicolas, H.W. Kort, D.T. Balzer, K. Trinkaus, C.L. Dent, R. Hirsch, C.E. Canter, Surveillance for transplant coronary artery disease in infant, child and adolescent heart transplant recipients: an intravascular ultrasound study, J. Heart Lung Transplant. 25 (2006) 921–927.

[77] L. Dong, A. Maehara, T.M. Nazif, A.T. Pollack, S. Saito, L.E. Rabbani, M.A. Apfelbaum, K. Dalton, J.W. Moses, U.P. Jorde, K. Xu, G.S. Mintz, D.M. Mancini, G. Weisz, Optical coherence tomographic evaluation of transplant coronary artery vasculopathy with correlation to cellular rejection, Circ. Cardiovasc. Interv. 7 (2014) 199–206.

[78] Y. Ichibori, T. Ohtani, D. Nakatani, K. Tachibana, O. Yamaguchi, K. Toda, T. Akasaka, N. Fukushima, Y. Sawa, I. Komuro, J. Kotani, Y. Sakata, Optical coherence tomography and intravascular ultrasound evaluation of cardiac allograft vasculopathy with and without intimal neovascularization, Eur. Heart J. Cardiovasc. Imaging 17 (2016) 51–58.

[79] F. Tomai, L. De Luca, A. Petrolini, L. Di Vito, A.S. Ghini, P. Corvo, G. De Persio, F. Parisi, G. Pongiglione, M. Giulia Gagliardi, F. Prati, Optical coherence tomography for characterization of cardiac allograft vasculopathy in late survivors of pediatric heart transplantation, J. Heart Lung Transplant 35 (2016) 74–79.

[80] B. Gupta, D. Jacob, R. Thompson, Imaging in patients after cardiac transplantation and in patients with ventricular assist devices, J. Nucl. Cardiol. 22 (2015) 617–638.

[81] P.Y. Marie, J.P. Carteaux, J.M. Escanye, O. Claudon, N. David, S. Mattei, N. Hassan, N. Danchin, G. Karcher, A. Bertrand, J.P. Villemot, Detection and prediction of acute heart transplant rejection with the myocardial t2 determination provided by a black-blood magnetic resonance imaging sequence, J. Heart Lung Transplant. 20 (2001) 193–194.

[82] C.R. Butler, A. Savu, J.A. Bakal, M. Toma, R. Thompson, K. Chow, H. Wang, D.H. Kim, M. Mengel, M. Haykowsky, G.J. Pearson, P. Kaul, I. Paterson, Correlation of cardiovascular magnetic resonance imaging findings and endomyocardial biopsy results in patients undergoing screening for heart transplant rejection, J. Heart Lung Transplant. 34 (2015) 643–650.

[83] H. Steen, C. Merten, S. Refle, R. Klingenberg, T. Dengler, E. Giannitsis, H.A. Katus, Prevalence of different gadolinium enhancement patterns in patients after heart transplantation, J. Am. Coll. Cardiol. 52 (2008) 1160–1167.

[84] C.A. Miller, J. Sarma, J.H. Naish, N. Yonan, S.G. Williams, S.M. Shaw, D. Clark, K. Pearce, M. Stout, R. Potluri, A. Borg, G. Coutts, S. Chowdhary, G.P. McCann, G.J. Parker, S.G. Ray, M. Schmitt, Multiparametric cardiovascular magnetic resonance assessment of cardiac allograft vasculopathy, J. Am. Coll. Cardiol. 63 (2014) 799–808.

[85] T. Hussain, M. Fenton, S.A. Peel, A.J. Wiethoff, A. Taylor, V. Muthurangu, R. Razavi, R.M. Botnar, M. Burch, G.F. Greil, Detection and grading of coronary allograft vasculopathy in children with contrast-enhanced magnetic resonance imaging of the coronary vessel wall, Circ. Cardiovasc. Imaging 6 (2013) 91–98.

[86] C. Krieghoff, M.J. Barten, L. Hildebrand, M. Grothoff, L. Lehmkuhl, C. Lucke, C. Andres, S. Nitzsche, F. Riese, M. Struber, F.W. Mohr, M. Gutberlet, Assessment of sub-clinical acute cellular rejection after heart transplantation: comparison of cardiac magnetic resonance imaging and endomyocardial biopsy, Eur. Radiol. 24 (2014) 2360–2371.

[87] E. Simsek, S. Nalbantgil, N. Ceylan, M. Zoghi, H.S. Kemal, C. Engin, T. Yagdi, M. Ozbaran, Diagnostic performance of late gadolinium enhancement in the assessment of acute cellular rejection after heart transplantation, Anatol. J. Cardiol 16 (2016) 113–118.

[88] R.K. Singh, M.E. Richmond, W.A. Zuckerman, T.M. Lee, T.B. Giblin, R. Rodriguez, J.M. Chen, L.J. Addonizio, The use of oral sildenafil for management of right ventricular dysfunction after pediatric heart transplantation, Am. J. Transplant. 14 (2014) 453–458.

[89] F. Perez-Villa, M. Farrero, M. Cardona, M.A. Castel, I. Tatjer, D. Penela, I. Vallejos, Bosentan in heart transplantation candidates with severe pulmonary hypertension: efficacy, safety and outcome after transplantation, Clin. Transplant. 27 (2013) 25–31.

[90] M.S. Sweeney, M.P. Macris, O.H. Frazier, J.T. Sinnott, M. Peric, H.A. McAllister Jr., The treatment of advanced cardiac allograft rejection, Ann. Thorac. Surg. 46 (1988) 378–381.

[91] G.L. Winters, E. Loh, F.J. Schoen, Natural history of focal moderate cardiac allograft rejection. Is treatment warranted? Circulation 91 (1995) 1975–1980.

[92] P.T. Thrush, J.G. Gossett, J.M. Costello, K.L. Matthews, R. Nubani, H. Bhagat, C.L. Backer, E. Pahl, Role for immune monitoring to tailor induction prophylaxis in pediatric heart recipients, Pediatr. Transplant. 18 (2014) 79–86.

[93] E.H. Wang, N. Partovi, R.D. Levy, R.J. Shapiro, E.M. Yoshida, E.D. Greanya, Pneumocystis pneumonia in solid organ transplant recipients: not yet an infection of the past, Transpl. Infect. Dis. 14 (2012) 519–525.

[94] S. Chih, A. Chruscinski, H.J. Ross, K. Tinckam, J. Butany, V. Rao, Antibody-mediated rejection: an evolving entity in heart transplantation, J. Transplant. 2012 (2012) 210210.

[95] J. Partanen, M.S. Nieminen, L. Krogerus, A.L. Harjula, S. Mattila, Heart transplant rejection treated with plasmapheresis, J. Heart Lung Transplant. 11 (1992) 301–305.

[96] M. Malafa, M.C. Mancini, J.L. Myles, A. Gohara, J.M. Dickinson, T.E. Walsh, Successful treatment of acute humoral rejection in a heart transplant patient, J. Heart Lung Transplant. 11 (1992) 486–491.

[97] S. Chih, K.J. Tinckam, H.J. Ross, A survey of current practice for antibody-mediated rejection in heart transplantation, Am. J. Transplant. 13 (2013) 1069–1074.

[98] H.E. Garrett Jr., K. Groshart, D. Duvall-Seaman, D. Combs, R. Suggs, Treatment of humoral rejection with rituximab, Ann. Thorac. Surg. 74 (2002) 1240–1242.

[99] D.A. Baran, S. Lubitz, S. Alvi, J.T. Fallon, S. Kaplan, I. Galin, R. Correa, M.C. Courtney, M. Chan, D. Spielvogel, S.L. Lansman, A.L. Gass, Refractory humoral cardiac allograft rejection successfully treated with a single dose of rituximab, Transplant. Proc. 36 (2004) 3164–3166.

[100] A. Aggarwal, J. Pyle, J. Hamilton, G. Bhat, Low-dose rituximab therapy for antibody-mediated rejection in a highly sensitized heart-transplant recipient, Tex. Heart Inst. J. 39 (2012) 901–905.

[101] W.R. Morrow, E.A. Frazier, W.T. Mahle, T.O. Harville, S.E. Pye, K.R. Knecht, E.L. Howard, R.N. Smith, R.L. Saylors, X. Garcia, R.D. Jaquiss, E.S. Woodle, Rapid reduction in donor-specific anti-human leukocyte antigen antibodies and reversal of antibody-mediated rejection with bortezomib in pediatric heart transplant patients, Transplantation 93 (2012) 319–324.

[102] E.S. Woodle, R.C. Walsh, R.R. Alloway, A. Girnita, P. Brailey, Proteasome inhibitor therapy for antibody-mediated rejection, Pediatr. Transplant. 15 (2011) 548–556.

[103] H. Wang, J. Arp, W. Liu, S.J. Faas, J. Jiang, D.R. Gies, S. Ramcharran, B. Garcia, R. Zhong, R.P. Rother, Inhibition of terminal complement components in presensitized transplant recipients prevents antibody-mediated rejection leading to long-term graft survival and accommodation, J. Immunol. 179 (2007) 4451–4463.

[104] M.D. Stegall, T. Diwan, S. Raghavaiah, L.D. Cornell, J. Burns, P.G. Dean, F.G. Cosio, M.J. Gandhi, W. Kremers, J.M. Gloor, Terminal complement inhibition decreases antibody-mediated rejection in sensitized renal transplant recipients, Am. J. Transplant. 11 (2011) 2405–2413.

[105] K.L. Dawson, A. Parulekar, H. Seethamraju, Treatment of hyperacute antibody-mediated lung allograft rejection with eculizumab, J. Heart Lung Transplant. 31 (2012) 1325–1326.

[106] J.A. Su, R.B. Kelly, T. Grogan, D. Elashoff, J.C. Alejos, Extracorporeal membrane oxygenation support after pediatric orthotopic heart transplantation, Pediatr. Transplant. 19 (2015) 68–75.

[107] M.J. Bock, K. Nguyen, S. Malerba, K. Harrison, E. Bagiella, B.D. Gelb, S.P. Pinney, I.D. Lytrivi, Pediatric cardiac retransplantation: waitlist mortality stratified by age and era, J. Heart Lung Transplant. 34 (2015) 530–537.

[108] S. Sehgal, M.J. Bock, H.L. Palac, J.G. Gossett, B.S. Marino, C.L. Backer, E. Pahl, New onset diabetes mellitus after heart transplant in children, J. Heart Lung Transplant. 34 (2015) S325.

[109] J.A. Kobashigawa, Statins in solid organ transplantation: is there an immunosuppressive effect? Am. J. Transplant. 4 (2004) 1013–1018.

[110] W.T. Mahle, R.N. Vincent, A.M. Berg, K.R. Kanter, Pravastatin therapy is associated with reduction in coronary allograft vasculopathy in pediatric heart transplantation, J. Heart Lung Transplant. 24 (2005) 63–66.

[111] C. Chin, S.S. Lukito, J. Shek, D. Bernstein, S.B. Perry, Prevention of pediatric graft coronary artery disease: Atorvastatin, Pediatr. Transplant. 12 (2008) 442–446.

[112] S.C. Greenway, R. Butts, D.C. Naftel, E. Pruitt, J.K. Kirklin, I. Larsen, S. Urschel, K. Knecht, Y. Law, Statin therapy is not associated with improved outcomes after heart transplantation in children and adolescents, J. Heart Lung Transplant. (2015) 34.

Chapter 48

Surgical Management of the Failing Systemic Ventricle

Jack Wallen[1], James S. Tweddell[1,2]

[1]Cincinnati Children's Hospital Medical Center, Cincinnati, OH, United States; [2]University of Cincinnati, Cincinnati, OH, United States

INTRODUCTION

Heart failure (HF) is a complex physiologic phenomenon that, prior to the modern era, was poorly understood despite being widely recognized. The typical symptoms of dyspnea, cachexia, and edema were known in antiquity and were a portent of death. Today, it is recognized as a progressive clinical syndrome with a variety of etiologies and pathophysiologies and is becoming better understood at a molecular level. Compared to older patients, HF in children and young adults not only includes many of the same diagnoses but also the sequelae of complex congenital heart disease. Many of these are rare conditions and defy a simple classification system. All of congenital heart surgery may be considered as treatment for or prevention of HF. In this chapter, we will focus on emerging surgical strategies for the systemic right ventricle, the failing Fontan, and the borderline left ventricle.

THE SYSTEMIC RIGHT VENTRICLE

The right ventricle is the systemic or subaortic ventricle among patients with congenitally corrected transposition of the great vessels (discordant connections at both the atrioventricular and ventriculoarterial junctions) and among patients who have undergone atrial level correction of transposition of the great vessels (ventriculoarterial discordance). Conditions in which the right ventricle serves as the systemic pumping chamber are commonly complicated by the development of right ventricular failure and tricuspid valve regurgitation. The left ventricle is a highly preserved in vertebrate evolution and is well suited for the prolonged pressure work of the systemic circulation. The right ventricle is a more recent evolutionary adaptation of the bulbus cordis and is better suited to serve as a low pressure, volume pump [1]. The anatomic differences between the left and right ventricles have been summarized by Van Praagh and colleagues (Table 48.1) [2]. The right ventricle differs from the left ventricle in both anatomy and geometry. Whereas the LV has three layers of myofibrils, the RV has only two [3]. The compact myocardium (stratum compactum) of the left ventricle is much thicker in relation to the spongy myocardium (stratum spongiosum) in the right ventricle. The atrioventricular valves have important differences. There are two papillary muscles attaching the mitral valve chords to the left ventricle free wall without attachment to the septum. In contrast, the papillary muscles of the right ventricle are multiple and small with both septal and free wall attachments. The attachments of the tricuspid valve to both the septum and free wall may predispose the tricuspid valve to the development of regurgitation with right ventricular dilatation. Indeed, tricuspid regurgitation and failure of the systemic right ventricle occur together [4–6]. The overall frequency of HF in a cohort of 188 adult patients with systemic right ventricles or single ventricle was 32% [7]. Interestingly, when analyzed according to anatomy, the frequencies were 22% in patients with TGA palliated with a Mustard operation, 32.3% for patients with ccTGA, and 40% for patients with a Fontan procedure. Mortality among symptomatic patients was 47.1% versus 5% among asymptomatic patients. Norozi et al. also found a higher incidence of HF in patients with TGA and atrial correction (30.8%) and single ventricle (47.1%) [8]. Placing the RV in the subaortic position increases the risk of systolic ventricular dysfunction.

Survival to adulthood for patients with a systemic right ventricle is about 80% with similar survival between those ccTGA and those after the atrial level switch operation for D-TGA [9]. Medical therapy generally mirrors that of treatment of acquired HF with little evidence of success [3]. Surgical strategies may be directed at the tricuspid valve, pulmonary artery banding including retraining of the left ventricle and resynchronization therapy.

Heart Failure in the Child and Young Adult. http://dx.doi.org/10.1016/B978-0-12-802393-8.00048-X

TABLE 48.1

Characteristic	Left Ventricle	Right Ventricle
Cavity	Cylindric	Crescentic
Contraction patter	Concentric	Bellows-like
Inlet and outlet valves	Close proximity	Distant
Coronary artery supply	Two coronary arteries	One coronary artery
Developmental origin	Primitive ventricle	Bulbus cordis
Atrioventricular valve	Closure for circular orifice	Closure for crescentic orifice
Papillary muscles	Two large papillary muscles	Multiple small papillary muscles

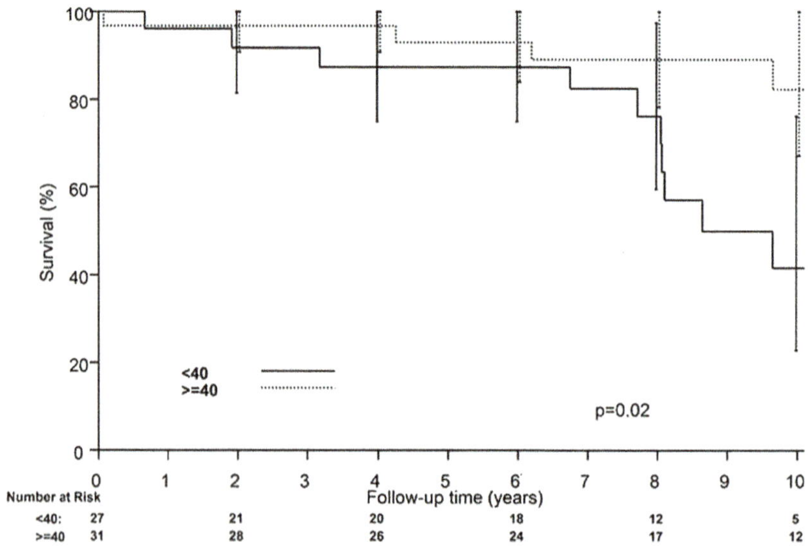

FIGURE 48.1 Survival after tricuspid valve replacement among patients with congenitally corrected transposition stratified by preoperative systemic right ventricular ejection fraction (EF). Poor systemic right ventricular EF was a risk factor for mortality. *Reproduced with permission from: F.P. Mongeon, H.M. Connolly, J.A. Dearani, Z. Li, C.A. Warnes, Congenitally corrected transposition of the great arteries ventricular function at the time of systemic atrioventricular valve replacement predicts long-term ventricular function, J. Am. Coll. Cardiol. 57 (20) (2011) 2008–2017.*

Tricuspid Valve Surgery

Tricuspid valve regurgitation results in excess volume loading of the systemic right ventricular dysfunction and accelerates development of dysfunction. Surgery directed at the TV should eliminate excess volume loading and stabilize RV function and therefore improve long-term outcome [10]. Tricuspid repair for the patient with a systemic RV is technically difficult. The intermediate outcomes are unsatisfactory and fail to achieve long-term tricuspid valve competence [11]. Therefore tricuspid valve replacement is recommended over repair. Significant RV dysfunction (ejection fraction (EF) <40%) at the time of tricuspid valve replacement is an important risk factor for survival and persistent dysfunction and TV replacement should be considered before RV dysfunction develops (Fig. 48.1) [12].

Pulmonary Artery Banding for the Failing Systemic Right Ventricle

Pulmonary artery banding may be used in the traditional way in neonates and infants with ccTGA and D-TGA with a ventricular septal defect (VSD) for relief of congestive HF and prevention of pulmonary artery hypertension in advance of definitive repair. It is also applied to children, teenagers, and adults with systemic right ventricles without a significant VSD to improve tricuspid valve function and retrain the left ventricle. The technique was initially pioneered in hopes of retraining the left ventricle in anticipation of anatomic repair, but it became apparent that by increasing afterload to the morphologic LV, the interventricular septum is shifted toward the RV and results in better coaptation of the tricuspid valve. The pulmonary artery band applies afterload to the morphologic left ventricle and care must be taken to avoid inducing pulmonary ventricular failure, including close monitoring of hemodynamics and intraoperative echo while the band is applied [1,13].

The pressure in the morphologic LV is raised to 50%–75% of systemic pressure while monitoring the central venous pressure and mitral valve by echo. Elevation of central venous pressure or the development of mitral regurgitation would suggest the band is too tight and should be loosened. Some groups have experimented with dilatable PABs that would allow for catheter dilatation to allow the band to be loosened as patients grow.

The results with anatomic repair following left ventricular retraining are mixed and patients who have undergone retraining are at increased risk of mortality [14]. Different techniques of retraining have been suggested without an obviously superior method [13,15]. Older age, greater than 12 years, appears to be an important factor predicting the inability to retrain the LV and achieve a durable anatomic repair. Reports have shown that maintenance of the pulmonary artery banding resulted in sustained improvement in RV function and tricuspid regurgitation [16,17]. These data suggest that banding alone may be a reasonable end point, particularly for the patient >12 years of age for whom banding has resulted in improvement in TR and stabilization of RV function.

Cardiac Resynchronization Therapy

Cardiac resynchronization therapy (CRT) is well established as an effective treatment for adults with symptomatic morphologic left ventricular failure that is refractory to medical therapy [18]. The efficacy of CRT in CHD patients with HF is less clear [19–21]. Despite these differences, there are reports of reductions in QRS duration of 19%–24%, increases in LVEF of 26%–52%, and improved New York Heart Association (NYHA) functional classification in children with failing morphologic LV [22–24]. The proportion of nonresponders in these studies ranged from 12% to 16%, which is generally lower than that reported in studies in adults.

As anticipated the response to CRT in CHD patients is dependent on systemic ventricular morphology. In a retrospective analysis of 20 patients with QRS duration >130 ms who underwent CRT, responses were compared in three groups: systemic LV, systemic RV, and biventricular repairs [25]. Overall, systemic ventricular end-diastolic volume index (EDVI), plasma B-type natriuretic peptide levels, and NYHA class improved with CRT by 6 months following device implantation. However, although QRS duration was significantly reduced in all three morphologic groups, no improvement in EDVI or ventricular EF was seen in those with a systemic RV. Other groups have also shown a reduced response to CRT in patients with systemic RV compared with systemic LV [23,24,26]. Dubin et al. found that CRT was associated with a 13% increase in EF in 14 of 17 patients with systemic RVs, which is comparable to the (nonsignificant) 14% increase seen by Sakaguchi and colleagues [22,25]. All these studies suffer the limitations of small size and retrospective analysis. Recommendations for optimal placement of CRT pacing leads in systemic RV patients have recently been made [27]. The reason(s) for the diminished benefit of CRT in CHD patients with systemic RV are unclear but may be related to generally older age in the patients with systemic RV at the time of device implantation. Furthermore, alterations in the pattern of ventricular contraction in the systemic RV compared with the normal RV have been found, suggesting an adaptive change in contractile elements to the systemic load [28].

THE FAILING FONTAN

Since the original description of the procedure in 1971, surgical creation of a Fontan circulation has undergone several modifications. Originally described for the repair of tricuspid atresia, The Fontan operation involved the creation of an atriopulmonary (AP) connection by isolating the right atrial chamber by closing the atrial septal defect and the tricuspid valve. It became evident that the atrium did not become "ventricularized" and serve as a pumping chamber following this operation. Since this initial description, two major surgical modifications have been introduced; the lateral tunnel technique and the extracardiac conduit (Fig. 48.2). These modifications are based on the hydrodynamic studies of deLeval that showed that greater efficiency and the lowest energy loss was achieved with a Fontan circuit of uniform caliber with minimal acute angles [29]. Significantly better 15-year survival following lateral tunnel (94%) versus classic Fontan (81%) procedures has been reported [30]. More recent analysis of registry data of 1006 patients who underwent a Fontan procedure showed Kaplan–Meier estimates of survival at 15, 20, and 25 years were 93%, 90%, and 83%, respectively [31]. Pundi et al. recently published follow-up data of 1052 patients who underwent a Fontan operation at the Mayo Clinic between 1973 and 2012 [32]. Overall 10-, 20-, and 30-year survival was 74%, 61%, and 43%, respectively. This represents remarkable progress compared with the 26% 1-year mortality reported in the first generation of tricuspid atresia patients undergoing this procedure [33]. When survival data were broken down by type of Fontan procedure performed (AP connection, lateral tunnel, extracardiac conduit), a significant benefit was seen in those patients receiving an extracardiac conduit (Fig. 48.3) [32].

The original selection criteria for a Fontan procedure in patients with tricuspid atresia were defined by Choussat and Fontan and became known as the "10 commandments" (Table 48.2) [34]. Current selection criteria include competent,

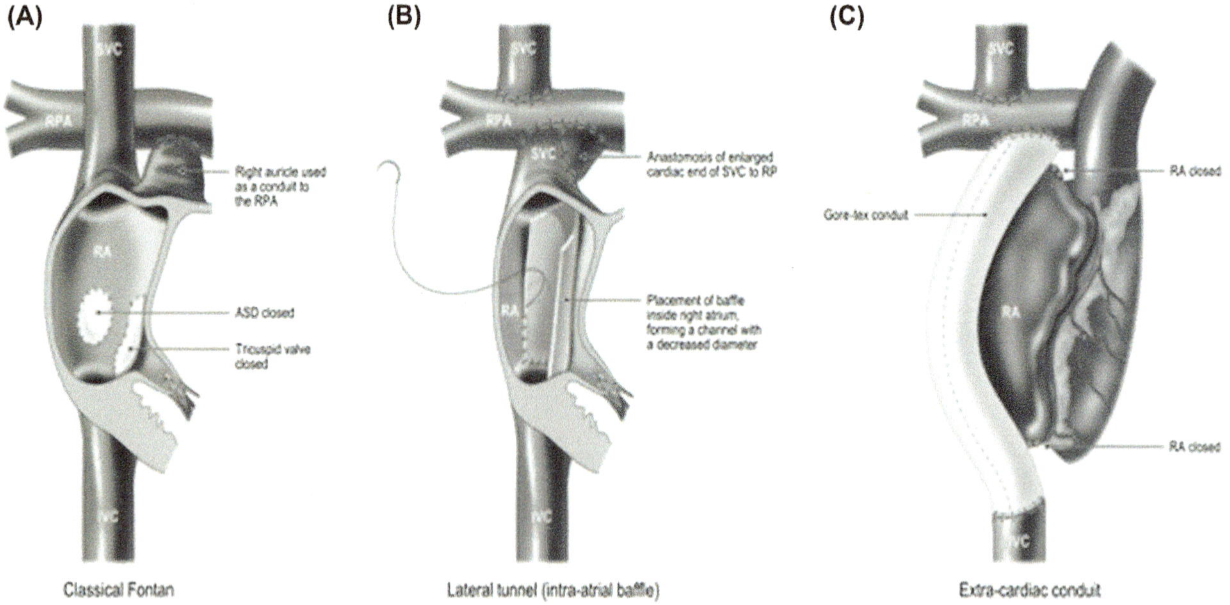

FIGURE 48.2 Types of Fontan procedures. (A) Atriopulmonary connection, (B) lateral tunnel, (C) extracardiac conduit. *Reproduced with permission from: Y. d'Udekem, A.J. Iyengar, A.D. Cochrane, et al., The Fontan procedure: contemporary techniques have improved long-term outcomes, Circulation 116 (11 Suppl.) (2007) I157–I164.*

FIGURE 48.3 Survival by Fontan procedure performed. *Reproduced with permission from: K.N. Pundi, J.N. Johnson, J.A. Dearani, et al., 40-Year follow-up after the Fontan operation: long-term outcomes of 1,052 patients, J. Am. Coll. Cardiol. 66 (15) (2015) 1700–1710.*

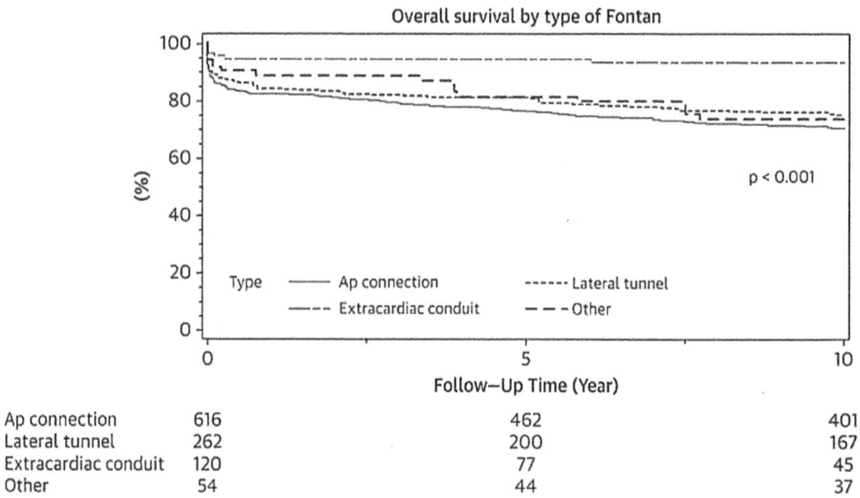

TABLE 48.2 "10 Commandments" for Fontan Suitability
Age > 4 years
Sinus rhythm
Normal systemic venous return
Normal right atrial volume
Low mean pulmonary artery pressure (≤15 mmHg)
Pulmonary resistance <4 WU/m²
Adequate pulmonary artery size (PA/Ao ratio > 0.75)
Normal left-ventricular function (ejection fraction ≥60%)
Competent mitral valve
No distortion of pulmonary artery following BT shunt

nonstenotic, or repairable AV valve; good ventricular function with unobstructed ventricular outflow; and a satisfactory pulmonary vascular bed; nonstenotic pulmonary arteries; normal pulmonary vascular resistance (PVR) (less than 2.5 WU/m^2) and unobstructed pulmonary venous return [35].

Fontan Physiology

The goal of the Fontan circulation is to provide adequate pulmonary blood flow and systemic ventricular preload, despite bypass of the subpulmonary ventricle without a significant elevation in venous pressures. By separating the systemic and pulmonary venous circulations, cyanosis is relieved and ventricular volume load is reduced. Complications are related to elevations in venous pressure, venous congestion, and reduced cardiac output. These complications can manifest as

- Early and late mortality
- Exercise intolerance
- Cardiomegaly
- Ventricular dysfunction/HF
- Rhythm/conduction disturbances
- Hepatomegaly
- Protein-losing enteropathy (PLE)
- Plastic bronchitis
- Venous thrombi/thromboembolism
- Ascites
- Peripheral edema

Exercise capacity in Fontan patients, measured by peak oxygen consumption (VO_2) at a mean age of 14 years, is reduced to 65% of that predicted for age and gender [36]. With increasing age through adolescence and into adulthood, exercise capacity will fall even farther, by approximately 2.6% per year [37]. A fall in peak VO_2 to approximately 50% predicted correlates with the development of symptoms of HF in adult congenital heart patients, implying that Fontan patients can expect to reach this critical value in their 20s [38].

The Failing Fontan

The benefits of palliating patients with a Fontan procedure are well established. Despite the impressive survival outcomes reported during long-term follow-up, at its core the Fontan circulation is hemodynamically imperfect. While cyanosis is eliminated by redirecting systemic venous return directly to the pulmonary circulation, without the benefit of a prepulmonary ventricle, this passive flow leads to greatly elevated central venous pressures, in the region of 10–15 mmHg. This passive flow also results in a restricted return to the systemic ventricle, dramatically reducing preload. This is associated with a reduced cardiac output in Fontan patients compared with patients with two functional ventricles [39]. Preload is determined by transpulmonary flow, which in turn is determined by the transpulmonary gradient and PVR.

$$\text{TPG} = \text{mean PA pressure} - \text{LA pressure}$$

$$\text{PVR} = 80 \times \frac{\text{TPG}}{\text{CO}}$$

PVR is expressed in Wood units (1 WU = 1 mmHg min/L = 80 dyne s/cm^5); CO, cardiac output.

Numerous lines of evidence support the idea that PVR is the major determinant of cardiac output in Fontan patients. For example, negative pressure ventilation increased cardiac index by approximately 40% compared with positive pressure ventilation in Fontan patients [40]. Fenestration of the Fontan conduit, allowing a fraction of the venous return to bypass the pulmonary vascular bend particularly when PVR may be elevated, significantly improved CO [41,42].

Long-Term Sequelae of Fontan Circulation

The palliative, rather than curative, nature of the Fontan operation has long been recognized [43]. Fontan palliation has been a significant surgical success since its inception, with excellent survival in the modern era. Nevertheless, long-term consequences are well recognized and represent a significant source of hospitalization. Regular follow-up with a team experienced in the care of complex CHD, specifically single-ventricle physiology, is mandatory, particularly for potentially reversible causes of Fontan failure. The American Heart Association recommends that the Fontan patient should be evaluated for the following [44]:

- Ventricular dysfunction
- Arrhythmias
- Fontan pathway thrombus
- Inflow/outflow obstruction
- PLE
- Valve dysfunction
- Residual right-to-left shunts
- Elevated systemic vascular resistance
- Elevated systemic venous pressure
- Plastic bronchitis

An in-depth discussion of the medical management of these patients is beyond the scope of this chapter but may involve ACE inhibitors, β-blockers, diuretics, and digoxin. Currently, there are no guidelines that specifically address the problem of HF in patients with CHD, and the efficacy of standard HF management strategies in these select patients is unknown. As stated recently by the American Heart association "...extrapolation from HF data and guidelines in adult acquired heart disease requires that we assume that the mechanisms, surrogate end points, and responses to therapy are sufficiently similar in CHD, which may not be the case" [44].

Treatment of Late Complications Following Single Ventricle Palliation

Protein-Losing Enteropathy

Enteric loss of serum proteins, including albumin, immunoglobulins, and clotting factors, is characteristic of PLE. The resultant hypoproteinemia leads to peripheral edema, ascites, pleural effusions, diarrhea, malabsorption, and cachexia. First reported in a 7-year-old patient 1-year after Fontan operation, the incidence of PLE ranges from 3.7% to 15% [45–48]. Risk factors for PLE include non-LV anatomy for single ventricles, prolonged hospital stay, postoperative renal failure, and prolonged cardiopulmonary bypass times [47,49]. Historically, PLE has been a much feared complication, with a median survival following diagnosis of 5 years [32,46]. However, analysis of a cohort of 42 Fontan patients with PLE operated in the current era (1992–2010) found survival rates of 88% and 72% at 5 and 10 years, respectively [50]. Aggressive surgical and interventional management of these patients may account for the improved survival following diagnosis. PLE is an independent predictor of death associated with HF in these patients [51]. Factors associated with worse outcome following a diagnosis of PLE include elevated Fontan pressures (>15 mmHg), NYHA class > II, elevated PVR and elevated serum creatinine, EF <55%, low cardiac index, and low mixed venous saturations.

Symptoms of PLE develop when the intestinal loss of proteins exceeds the synthetic capacity of the patient. A multifactorial mechanism for PLE has been proposed: Fontan physiology results in a chronic state of reduced cardiac index, with an increase in mesenteric vascular resistance and venous congestion and resultant diminished perfusion. This, coupled with the chronic inflammatory state seen in patients with HF, results in the release of proinflammatory mediators (including TNF-α), which activates matrix-metalloprotienases leading to the removal of membrane proteins, including the glycosaminoglycan heparan sulfate [52,53]. This alters the membrane integrity of enterocytes and leads to intestinal protein leak. Interestingly, a possible genetic predisposition to developing PLE has been observed [53].

Medical management of PLE should focus on dietary modifications, the management of HF, and relief of symptoms [50,54,55]. Diets should be sodium restricted, low-fat, high protein, and high medium-triglycerides. Periodic supplementation with intravenous albumin may be required for severe protein loss. Medical management alone of Fontan patients with PLE resulted in symptomatic improvement in 47% [50]. Virtually all patients should receive treatment for edema using diuretics. Angiotensin converting enzyme inhibitors and/or angiotensin receptor blockers, corticosteroids, and the enteric-specific steroid budesonide are also useful. Pulmonary vasodilators such as sildenafil and bosentan have also been effective. Octreotide is a somatostatin analogue shown to reduce lymphatic flow and has been used successfully to treat PLE in a small case series (n = 3) of Fontan patients [56]. Subcutaneous unfractionated heparin has been investigated for symptomatic improvement and elevation in serum protein [57,58].

Arrhythmias

Late arrhythmias have been documented in 11%–52% of Fontan patients [48,59–63]. Arrhythmias are a significant contributor to morbidity. Atrial tachyarrhythmias predominate, with intraatrial reentrant tachycardia (IART) the most frequent, occurring in up to 40% of Fontan patients by 25 years [64]. IART refers to any macro reentrant atrial arrhythmia, including typical atrial flutter. The management of these arrhythmias is difficult and may involve catheter ablation, a surgical maze procedure, and device therapy [65]. The etiology of these arrhythmias is likely multifactorial, involving sinus node dysfunction, the presence of atrial suture lines, and elevated atrial pressures in the Fontan circulation. These factors may be mitigated in patients who received an extracardiac conduit procedure, which reduces the number of atrial suture lines and lowers atrial pressures compared with the lateral tunnel procedure. However, in a recent multicenter retrospective cohort study of 1271 of patients who underwent a Fontan procedure (669 extracardiac, 602 lateral tunnel), no difference was found in the incidence of late (>30 days) arrhythmia [66]. There was a higher incidence of early (<30 days) bradyarrhythmias in the extracardiac (11%) versus lateral tunnel (4%) groups. Apart from surgical issues, underlying conduction abnormalities, primarily macroreentrant, and AV nodal reentry have been identified as potential mechanisms for these tachyarrhythmias [67]. A number of risk factors for the development of supraventricular tachycardia have been identified in these patients, including AP Fontan, low functional status, sinus node dysfunction, and nonsustained atrial tachycardia [64,68–70]. Interestingly, the risk of developing IART after the Fontan procedure is biphasic, with increased risk in the first 2 years following the procedure, followed by a decline from years 4 to 6, then rising steadily [68].

Medical management should be the first line of therapy for patients with arrhythmias. Radiofrequency ablation has been used to treat these patients, with complete or partial procedural success in 87.5% [67]. Of these, 50% eventually had recurrence of their arrhythmia within 18 months of the ablation. Others have observed similar high rates of recurrence following ablation in Fontan patients [71,72]. Patients with atrial tachyarrhythmias reported symptoms including palpitations (62%), fatigue (44%), dyspnea (23%), edema (21%), presyncope (21%), and syncope (3%) [69]. These patients were also more likely to have HF and atrial thrombus.

Surgical Management of the Failing Fontan

The term "Failing Fontan" refers to the clinical scenario that includes rhythm disturbances, constitutional effects (exercise intolerance, growth failure), thrombosis in the Fontan circuit, cirrhosis, ascites, PLE, plastic bronchitis, and ventricular failure. Systemic ventricular failure occurs in up to 40% of adult Fontan patients [7]. There are three widely accepted surgical options for management of this condition: Fontan takedown, Fontan conversion, and cardiac transplantation. Mechanical circulatory support for the failing Fontan is also an option, whether in the form of ECMO or VAD support [73]. This topic is discussed in detail elsewhere in this textbook.

Fontan Takedown

Catastrophic acute failure of the Fontan circulation requiring takedown is a rare event in the current era [30,74,75]. Referred to as early Fontan failure, this involves a postoperative state characterized by systemic malperfusion, elevated Fontan circuit pressures, and large volume requirements, which is unresponsive to inotropic support and carries a high risk for mortality. When recognized, rescue options include either ECMO support or surgical Fontan takedown to an intermediate palliative circulatory state (systemic-pulmonary arterial shunt and bidirectional Glenn).

High mortality rates have been reported following Fontan takedown. The Boston group reported on 53 patients who underwent Fontan takedown from 1979 to 2006 of whom 43 underwent takedown within 1 month of Fontan creation [76]. The most common indications for takedown were high PVR leading to elevated Fontan pressure/low cardiac output, PA obstruction/hypoplasia, and persistent pleural or pericardial effusions or ascites. Early (<30 day) mortality among the 53 patients was 45%. Other risk factors for early death following Fontan takedown included circulation other than bidirectional Glenn prior to Fontan creation, AP connection, fenestrated Fontan, and systemic RV. Of the survivors, 66% ultimately underwent recreation of the Fontan circulation at a median 4.6 years (range, 0.6–13.1 years) after takedown. Three quarters of patients who received a redo Fontan had medical or technical factors that likely contributed to their initial Fontan failure, most commonly PA stenosis or discontinuity. Three patients underwent cardiac transplantation for persistent ventricular dysfunction. In a small series of 14 patients that underwent Fontan takedown between 1980 and 2007 at Royal Children's Hospital, Melbourne, hospital mortality was 36% [77]. Compared with the overall cohort of Fontan patients, those who underwent takedown had pre-Fontan PA pressures that were 14% higher (13.8 vs. 12.1 mmHg). There were no late deaths or cardiac transplants, and only two survivors later underwent ECC Fontan creation. Overall, these studies suggest that Fontan takedown in cases of early failure is a rare event that is associated with significant risk despite surgical intervention. However, Fontan takedown does serve to stabilize the circulation of a certain group of patients and does not preclude the possibility of future recreation of a Fontan circulation, particularly in patients with readily correctible factors that contributed to early Fontan failure.

Fontan Conversion

An AP anastomosis is associated with late complications including atrial dilation, thrombus, and arrhythmias, leading to reduced cardiac output and decreased quality of life. Development of the total cavopulmonary connection (lateral tunnel and extracardiac conduit Fontan) has superseded the classic technique. Laks and colleagues developed the Fontan conversion procedure and reported on the outcome of three patients with AP Fontan with atrial tachyarrhythmias unresponsive to medical therapy who were surgically converted to a lateral tunnel Fontan circulation [78]. This operation resulted in marked clinical improvement in a majority of patients [79,80]. Intraoperative electrophysiology mapping and cryoablation of arrhythmia circuits was added to Fontan conversion surgery [81]. While early reports of Fontan conversion had mixed results with some centers reporting mortality as high as 33% and high arrhythmia recurrence with refinement of indications and technique results have improved and current midterm results are encouraging. Several institutions report 5-year survival >90% and 10-year survival >80% [78,82–90]. It is evident that Fontan conversion is associated with acceptable risk and provides functional improvement in patients who undergo this procedure when combined with antiarrhythmia procedures [91,92].

Patient selection for Fontan conversion is crucial to optimizing outcome. The Mayo Clinic analyzed the outcomes of 70 patients who underwent conversion of AP Fontan from 1994 to 2011 and found a 14% mortality rate [93]. Multivariate analysis showed that only age greater than 27 years, male sex, lack of antiarrhythmia surgery, and AV valve regurgitation were predictive of death. Deal et al. found right ventricular morphology, ascites, PLE, prolonged CPB time, and biatrial arrhythmia operation to be independent risk factors for cardiac death or transplantation in their series of 140 Fontan conversions [90]. Cardiopulmonary exercise testing has been shown to be predictive of perioperative survival following Fontan conversion, with baseline peak VO_2 less than 14 mL/kg/min an independent predictor of death, along with male sex, age greater than 25, and AV valve regurgitation [94]. Van Melle et al. reported the outcome of 225 failing Fontan patients who underwent either takedown (n = 38), conversion (n = 137), or transplantation (n = 50) surgery at 22 European centers [95]. Kaplan–Meier survival estimates showed no difference between transplant and conversion patients ($P = .13$) but decreased ventricular function was an independent risk factor for poor outcome in the conversion group. These findings suggest that Fontan conversion is most likely to be successful in patients with preserved single ventricle function and that delaying Fontan conversion surgery until the onset of organ dysfunction is detrimental to the outcome.

Cardiac Resynchronization Therapy

CRT was discussed earlier as a surgical treatment for the failing systemic right ventricle and is well established as an effective treatment for adults with symptomatic HF that is refractory to medical therapy, who have both left ventricular dysfunction and dyssynchrony secondary to left bundle-branch block (LBBB). CRT is recommended for patients with systolic dysfunction (LVEF ≤35%), sinus rhythm, LBBB pattern with QRS duration ≥150 ms, and NYHA class II, III, or ambulatory IV symptoms on guideline directed medical therapy [18]. CRT is not recommended for patients with no or minimal symptoms and non-LBBB pattern with QRS duration <150 ms or for those in whom survival of less than 1 year is expected.

The efficacy of CRT in CHD patients with HF is less clear, due to the variety of cardiomyopathies found in the pediatric population (e.g., associated with CHD, noncompaction, muscular dystrophy, etc.) and because the incidence of LBBB pattern in these patients is rare [19–21]. Despite these differences, studies of the effects of CRT in children have reported significant reductions in QRS duration of 19%–24%, increases in LVEF of 26%–52%, and improved NYHA functional classification [22–24]. The proportion of nonresponders in these studies ranged from 12% to 16%, which is generally lower than that reported in studies in adults. High-quality studies identifying patients with congenital heart disease and HF who should receive CRT are not available, and the benefit of CRT among patients with a failed Fontan is isolated to case reports [96–99]. Nevertheless, single-ventricle dysfunction with a prolonged QRS duration would seem to be a reasonable indication for a trial of multisite pacing. The potential benefits must be balanced against the technical challenges in complex and fragile patients with multiple prior surgeries and abnormal native conduction pathways that make precise lead placement challenging.

Cardiac Transplantation for Failing Fontan

Indications for OHT include patients with refractory severe HF who will not benefit from further medical or surgical intervention, and patients with normal ventricular function but with PLE or plastic bronchitis despite optimal medical/surgical therapy [73]. The International Society for Heart Lung Transplantation advised that congenital heart disease patients be listed for heart transplant if they have "...certain anatomic and physiologic conditions with or without associated ventricular dysfunction. These conditions may include... persistent protein-losing enteropathy and/or plastic bronchitis associated with CHD despite optimal medical-surgical therapy…" [100,101]. Analysis of the UNOS database shows that the number of adults with CHD who undergo heart transplant has risen steadily over time [102].

The prevalence of heart transplant among adult patients with congenital heart disease has increased 41% since 1999 [103]. This patient population represents a unique challenge to the cardiac transplant team; patients have typically undergone prior cardiac surgeries (often multiple) and have been exposed to blood products resulting in the presence of human leukocyte antigen antibodies and a high PRA. These factors increase both the risk and complexity of transplant surgery, can affect the length of time on a transplant waiting list, and make the management of these patients afterward more difficult. Transplantation in the patient with a failing Fontan circulation is typically indicated for the presence of PLE, plastic bronchitis, and HF.

Fontan patients are at greater risk for early and ongoing mortality following heart transplantation. The results of studies of outcome of transplantation for the Fontan procedure are summarized in Table 48.3 [104]. Early mortality in multiinstitutional studies is between 10% and 20%. This contrasts sharply with the 94.4% 30-day survival seen in two-ventricle patients undergoing cardiac transplantation for HF [105]. 1 and 5-year survival is lower in Fontan patients undergoing heart transplant compared with other CHD patients (non-Fontan 83% and 74% vs. 71% and 60% Fontan, respectively, $P=.006$) [106]. Compared with other CHD patients who received a transplant, the survival in Fontan patients is significantly worse (Fig. 48.4). A number of risk factors for mortality following transplantation have been identified. The most common cause of death in Fontan patients was infection (30%), followed by early graft failure (17%), and rejection (13%) [107]. Other factors that have been identified as risk factors for posttransplant mortality include early Fontan failure, PLE, Fontan obstruction, earlier era of transplant, renal failure, pretransplant ECMO, and pretransplant mechanical ventilation [108–111]. The presence of PLE combined with the use of posttransplant immunosuppression likely accounts for the finding that infection is a significant cause of postoperative death in this group of patients.

There may be room for cautious optimism, Davies et al. retrospectively compared the outcomes of primary cardiac transplantation of 43 Fontan patients with 129 with other forms of CHD (TGA, tetralogy of Fallot, pulmonary atresia, pulmonary stenosis, tricuspid atresia, HLHS) [112]. The mean interval between the Fontan procedure and transplantation was 8.6 years (range, 6 days to 24.5 years). While earlier mortality was higher in the Fontan group late mortality was similar between the Fontan group and those with other forms of CHD, suggesting that if anatomic barriers, physiologic and immunologic challenges can be overcome the results of transplantation may be satisfactory. The benefits of cardiac

TABLE 48.3 Outcomes Following Cardiac Transplantation in Failing Fontan Patients

	Author	N	Early Mortality	5-Year Survival
Single-center	Davies et al. [112]	43	25%	58.7%
	Backer et al. [110]	22	23%	66%
	Jayakumar et al. [114]	24	38%	57%
	Lamour et al. [125]	8	38%	60%
	Petko et al. [126]	9	44%	50%[a]
	Michielon et al. [105]	6	67%	68%
	Bhama et al. [127]	5	60%	N/A
	Kanter [113]	9	11%	70.8%
	Mitchell et al. [128]	14	7%	N/A
	Gamba et al. [129]	14	14%	77%
Multicenter	Bernstein et al. [107]	70	20% (6 months)	68%
	Lamour et al. [106]	107	≈20%	60%
	Kovach et al. [111]	194	≈13%	N/A
	Michielon et al. [108]	61	18.3%	73%

Only those patients with failing Fontan physiology who underwent cardiac transplantation are included.
[a]*Late interval not specified.*
Modified from D.C. Mauchley, M.B. Mitchell, Transplantation in the fontan patient, Semin. Thorac. Cardiovasc. Surg. Pediatr. Card. Surg. Annu. 18 (1) (2015) 7–16.

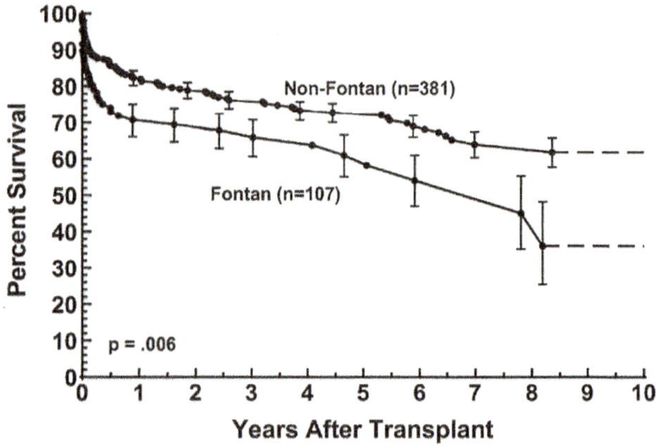

FIGURE 48.4 Posttransplant survival in Fontan versus non-Fontan CHD patients. *Reproduced with permission from: J.M. Lamour, K.R. Kanter, D.C. Naftel, et al., The effect of age, diagnosis, and previous surgery in children and adults undergoing heart transplantation for congenital heart disease, J. Am. Coll. Cardiol. 54 (2) (2009) 160–165.*

transplantation in patients with failing Fontan physiology can be dramatic. In those patients that survived the early post-transplant period, resolution of PLE was seen in more than 85% [107,110,113,114]. Michielon et al. showed that the greatest survival benefit of cardiac transplant occurred in patients with late (>2 years after Fontan procedure) failure and poor ventricular function, in whom the 5-year survival exceeded 90% [108].

THE BORDERLINE LEFT VENTRICLE

The challenging long-term outlook for the individual palliated with a Fontan has been the motivation to test the boundaries of achieving a two-ventricle circulation among a subgroup of patients with small left-sided structures such as nonapex forming left ventricle with coarctation, Shone complex and right dominant unbalanced atrioventricular septal defect. In contrast to the patient with right heart hypoplasia such pulmonary atresia with intact septum where the decision concerning candidacy for a 2-ventricle repair is routinely deferred past the newborn period, for the patient with left heart hypoplasia, especially with arch hypoplasia with ductal-dependent systemic blood flow, neonatal palliation is necessary and incorrect choices concerning candidacy for two-ventricle repair are associated with increased mortality [115]. Decision-making can be challenging as the potential dimension of the left-sided structures is difficult to determine in the face of a volume loaded right ventricle [116–119]. Primary repair of infants with borderline LV undergoing endocardial fibroelastosis (EFE) resection has been reported [120]. The EFE results in diastolic dysfunction (Fig. 48.5). The results were excellent in this group of patients but it is noteworthy that the median follow-up is less than 3 years and the patients had mild LV hypoplasia suggesting that proper selection is important to success. Postnatal improvement in diastolic function and the potential for catch-up growth have motivated a strategy of staged biventricular conversion.

A subset of patients with hypoplastic left heart structures who underwent single ventricle palliation may be eligible for later biventricular conversion and a potential improvement in long-term outcome. Risk factors for poor long-term outcomes following single-ventricle repair include genetic syndromes, tricuspid regurgitation, right ventricular dysfunction, and elevated PVR. Biventricular conversion involves takedown of the aortopulmonary anastomosis and reestablishing separate systemic and pulmonary circulations. This may require aortic arch reconstruction and a Rastelli-type baffle with a pulmonary artery conduit. Additional procedures may include aortic or mitral valve repair, closure of atrial septal defects, and resection of EFE. Determining which patients are suitable for biventricular conversion is complex. Several scoring systems have been developed to determine which neonates with borderline hypoplastic left heart structures are candidates for initial biventricular repair, but these do not apply to patients already palliated to a single ventricle physiology [121]. Factors that must be assessed in making the decision to pursue biventricular conversion following single-ventricle repair include the size and function of left-sided structures, typically based on echocardiography and cardiac MRI. The presence of a small mitral valve and/or EFE must be approached with caution but may possibly be addressed at the time of surgery. Preoperative cardiac catheterization is important to evaluate left atrial pressures, which will rise on establishing biventricular physiology. The optimal timing of conversion in suitable candidates is unclear.

Boston Children's Hospital retrospectively analyzed the outcome of biventricular conversion in 28 patients initially palliated with single-ventricle repair [122]. Reconstruction of the aorta involved direct anastomosis (with or without patch enlargement) or the Ross procedure, while right ventricular outflow was established using homograft conduits or direct anastomosis of the pulmonary artery. Caval reanastomosis to the right atrium was established. Median postoperative ICU stay was 18 days (range, 3 days to 2.9 years), and ECMO support was required in 11%. Median age at conversion was 42 months (range, 4–95 months) but tended to be younger in those with unbalanced complete atrioventricular canal defect

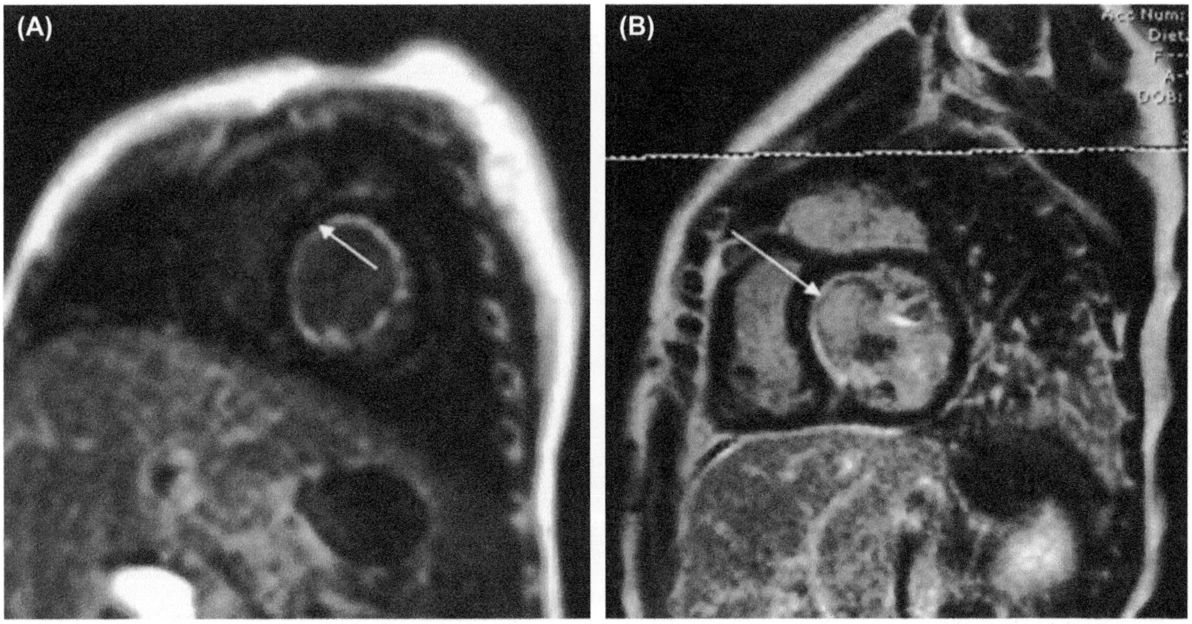

FIGURE 48.5 Endocardial fibroelastosis (EFE) results in diastolic dysfunction. MRI images depicting circumferential EFE before LV rehabilitation (A) and residual EFE along the interventricular septum on follow-up MRI (B). *Reproduced with permission from: S.M. Emani, E.A. Bacha, D.B. McElhinney, et al., Primary left ventricular rehabilitation is effective in maintaining two-ventricle physiology in the borderline left heart, J. Thorac. Cardiovasc. Surg. 138 (6) (2009) 1276–1282.*

(median, 11.3 months) versus those with HLHS (median age 46.5 months). After median follow-up of 31.7 months, survival was 89.3%, while 61% required either catheter-based or surgical reintervention. Left-ventricular volume increased significantly compared with the preconversion volumes. Long-term outcomes are required to determine the utility of biventricular conversion in these patients.

The hybrid approach to HLHS, maintenance of ductal patency with a stent, atrial septal defect creation, and branch pulmonary artery banding, results in relief of prostaglandin-dependent systemic circulation and control of pulmonary blood flow has the same as the Norwood procedure without the use of cardiopulmonary bypass [123]. Patients with small left-sided heart structures may be initially palliated with the hybrid procedure and if adequate growth of left heart structures occurs, these patients can undergo biventricular repair, which involves the repair of any intracardiac defects such as VSDs, arterial switch as needed, enlargement of LVOT (e.g., Ross Konno), and reconstruction of the RVOT. This strategy has been pursued by the group in Geissen, Germany, who reported on 40 patients undergoing biventricular repair following initial hybrid palliation [124]. They reported significant growth of left-sided structures (aortic and mitral valve diameters, ratio of LV to RV length) following the hybrid procedure. Median survival in this cohort was 7.9 years; the mortality rate following biventricular conversion was 10%.

Strategies for management of the borderline LV remain are isolated to single institution experience with small patient groups with a broad spectrum of primary diagnoses. The publications are single armed uncontrolled case series and follow-up is short. In addition, to a high rate of reintervention, there are long-term issues related to persistent diastolic dysfunction with poor exercise tolerance and most concerning pulmonary hypertension that may make the patients high risk for heart transplantation. Given the small numbers encountered even at large centers, high-quality multiinstitutional studies will be necessary to define the selection criteria and techniques to achieve the optimal outcome for the individual with a borderline LV.

CONCLUSION

HF in children resulting from congenital heart disease represents a major health care burden. Again, all of congenital heart surgery may be considered as treatment for or prevention of HF. In this chapter we have focused on emerging surgical strategies for the systemic right ventricle, the failing Fontan and the borderline left ventricle. Improvement in outcome for this patient population will depend on ongoing research to identify the causes of structural heart disease and myocardial dysfunction at the cellular and tissue level. In addition, while we work to identify the mechanisms of the cause of CHD we need to obtain more complete and better patient level data to help us guide our therapies and identify new strategies.

REFERENCES

[1] B.W. Duncan, R.B. Mee, Management of the failing systemic right ventricle, Semin. Thorac. Cardiovasc. Surg. 17 (2) (2005) 160–169.

[2] R. Van Praagh, W.K. Jung, The arterial switch operation in transposition of the great arteries: anatomic indications and contraindications, Thorac. Cardiovasc. Surg. 39 (Suppl. 2) (1991) 138–150.

[3] S.L. Roche, A.N. Redington, The failing right ventricle in congenital heart disease, Can. J. Cardiol. 29 (7) (2013) 768–778.

[4] J.M. Rutledge, M.R. Nihill, C.D. Fraser, O.E. Smith, C.J. McMahon, L.I. Bezold, Outcome of 121 patients with congenitally corrected transposition of the great arteries, Pediatr. Cardiol. 23 (2) (2002) 137–145.

[5] P. Moons, M. Gewillig, T. Sluysmans, et al., Long term outcome up to 30 years after the Mustard or Senning operation: a nationwide multicentre study in Belgium, Heart 90 (3) (2004) 307–313.

[6] C.A. Kral Kollars, S. Gelehrter, E.L. Bove, G. Ensing, Effects of morphologic left ventricular pressure on right ventricular geometry and tricuspid valve regurgitation in patients with congenitally corrected transposition of the great arteries, Am. J. Cardiol. 105 (5) (2010) 735–739.

[7] S. Piran, G. Veldtman, S. Siu, G.D. Webb, P.P. Liu, Heart failure and ventricular dysfunction in patients with single or systemic right ventricles, Circulation 105 (10) (2002) 1189–1194.

[8] K. Norozi, A. Wessel, V. Alpers, et al., Incidence and risk distribution of heart failure in adolescents and adults with congenital heart disease after cardiac surgery, Am. J. Cardiol. 97 (8) (2006) 1238–1243.

[9] R. Dobson, M. Danton, W. Nicola, W. Hamish, The natural and unnatural history of the systemic right ventricle in adult survivors, J. Thorac. Cardiovasc. Surg. 145 (6) (2013) 1493–1501 Discussion 1501–1493.

[10] A.A. Filippov, P.J. Del Nido, N.V. Vasilyev, Management of systemic right ventricular failure in patients with congenitally corrected transposition of the great arteries, Circulation 134 (17) (2016) 1293–1302.

[11] S. Talwar, T. Ahmed, A. Saxena, S.S. Kothari, R. Juneja, B. Airan, Morphology, surgical techniques, and outcomes in patients above 15 years undergoing surgery for congenitally corrected transposition of great arteries, World J. Pediatr. Congenit. Heart Surg. 4 (3) (2013) 271–277.

[12] F.P. Mongeon, H.M. Connolly, J.A. Dearani, Z. Li, C.A. Warnes, Congenitally corrected transposition of the great arteries ventricular function at the time of systemic atrioventricular valve replacement predicts long-term ventricular function, J. Am. Coll. Cardiol. 57 (20) (2011) 2008–2017.

[13] D.S. Winlaw, S.P. McGuirk, C. Balmer, et al., Intention-to-treat analysis of pulmonary artery banding in conditions with a morphological right ventricle in the systemic circulation with a view to anatomic biventricular repair, Circulation 111 (4) (2005) 405–411.

[14] D.W. Quinn, S.P. McGuirk, C. Metha, et al., The morphologic left ventricle that requires training by means of pulmonary artery banding before the double-switch procedure for congenitally corrected transposition of the great arteries is at risk of late dysfunction, J. Thorac. Cardiovasc. Surg. 135 (5) (2008) 1137–1144 1144 e1131–1132.

[15] P.A. Zartner, M.B. Schneider, B. Asfour, V. Hraska, Enhanced left ventricular training in corrected transposition of the great arteries by increasing the preload, Eur. J. Cardiothorac. Surg. 49 (6) (2016) 1571–1576.

[16] B. Cools, S.C. Brown, J. Louw, R. Heying, B. Meyns, M. Gewillig, Pulmonary artery banding as 'open end' palliation of systemic right ventricles: an interim analysis, Eur. J. Cardiothorac. Surg. 41 (4) (2012) 913–918.

[17] K. Ma, H. Gao, Z. Hua, et al., Palliative pulmonary artery banding versus anatomic correction for congenitally corrected transposition of the great arteries with regressed morphologic left ventricle: long-term results from a single center, J. Thorac. Cardiovasc. Surg. 148 (4) (2014) 1566–1571.

[18] C.M. Tracy, A.E. Epstein, D. Darbar, et al., 2012 ACCF/AHA/HRS focused update of the 2008 guidelines for device-based therapy of cardiac rhythm abnormalities: a report of the American College of Cardiology Foundation/American heart association task force on practice guidelines, Heart Rhythm. 9 (10) (2012) 1737–1753.

[19] M.I. Cohen, Heart Failure Summit Review: cardiac re-synchronisation therapy in the failing heart, Cardiol. Young 25 (Suppl. 2) (2015) 124–130.

[20] I. Puggia, M. Merlo, G. Barbati, et al., Natural history of dilated cardiomyopathy in children, J. Am. Heart Assoc. 5 (7) (2016).

[21] O. Schiller, N. Dham, E.A. Greene, D.M. Heath, M.E. Alexander, C.I. Berul, Pediatric dilated cardiomyopathy patients do not meet traditional cardiac resynchronization criteria, J. Cardiovasc. Electrophysiol. 26 (8) (2015) 885–889.

[22] A.M. Dubin, J. Janousek, E. Rhee, et al., Resynchronization therapy in pediatric and congenital heart disease patients: an international multicenter study, J. Am. Coll. Cardiol. 46 (12) (2005) 2277–2283.

[23] J. Janousek, R.A. Gebauer, H. Abdul-Khaliq, et al., Cardiac resynchronisation therapy in paediatric and congenital heart disease: differential effects in various anatomical and functional substrates, Heart 95 (14) (2009) 1165–1171.

[24] F. Cecchin, P.A. Frangini, D.W. Brown, et al., Cardiac resynchronization therapy (and multisite pacing) in pediatrics and congenital heart disease: five years experience in a single institution, J. Cardiovasc. Electrophysiol. 20 (1) (2009) 58–65.

[25] H. Sakaguchi, A. Miyazaki, O. Yamada, et al., Cardiac resynchronization therapy for various systemic ventricular morphologies in patients with congenital heart disease, Circ. J. 79 (3) (2015) 649–655.

[26] J. Janousek, Cardiac resynchronisation in congenital heart disease, Heart 95 (11) (2009) 940–947.

[27] A. Miyazaki, H. Sakaguchi, K. Kagisaki, et al., Optimal pacing sites for cardiac resynchronization therapy for patients with a systemic right ventricle with or without a rudimentary left ventricle, Europace 18 (1) (2016) 100–112.

[28] E. Pettersen, T. Helle-Valle, T. Edvardsen, et al., Contraction pattern of the systemic right ventricle shift from longitudinal to circumferential shortening and absent global ventricular torsion, J. Am. Coll. Cardiol. 49 (25) (2007) 2450–2456.

[29] M.R. de Leval, P. Kilner, M. Gewillig, C. Bull, Total cavopulmonary connection: a logical alternative to atriopulmonary connection for complex Fontan operations. Experimental studies and early clinical experience, J. Thorac. Cardiovasc. Surg. 96 (5) (1988) 682–695.

[30] Y. d'Udekem, A.J. Iyengar, A.D. Cochrane, et al., The Fontan procedure: contemporary techniques have improved long-term outcomes, Circulation 116 (11 Suppl.) (2007) I157–I164.

[31] Y. d'Udekem, A.J. Iyengar, J.C. Galati, et al., Redefining expectations of long-term survival after the Fontan procedure: twenty-five years of follow-up from the entire population of Australia and New Zealand, Circulation 130 (11 Suppl. 1) (2014) S32–S38.
[32] K.N. Pundi, J.N. Johnson, J.A. Dearani, et al., 40-Year follow-up after the fontan operation: long-term outcomes of 1,052 patients, J. Am. Coll. Cardiol. 66 (15) (2015) 1700–1710.
[33] D.A. Girod, F. Fontan, C. Deville, J. Ottenkamp, A. Choussat, Long-term results after the Fontan operation for tricuspid atresia, Circulation 75 (3) (1987) 605–610.
[34] A. choussat, F. Fontan, F. Besse, F. Vallot, A. Chauve, H. Bricaud, Selection criteria for Fontan's procedure, in: R.H. Anderson, E. Shinebourne (Eds.), Paediatric Cardiology, Churchill Livingston, Edinburgh, 1978, pp. 559–566.
[35] M. Gewillig, The Fontan circulation, Heart 91 (6) (2005) 839–846.
[36] S.M. Paridon, P.D. Mitchell, S.D. Colan, et al., A cross-sectional study of exercise performance during the first 2 decades of life after the Fontan operation, J. Am. Coll. Cardiol. 52 (2) (2008) 99–107.
[37] A. Giardini, A. Hager, C. Pace Napoleone, F.M. Picchio, Natural history of exercise capacity after the Fontan operation: a longitudinal study, Ann. Thorac. Surg. 85 (3) (2008) 818–821.
[38] G.P. Diller, K. Dimopoulos, D. Okonko, et al., Exercise intolerance in adult congenital heart disease: comparative severity, correlates, and prognostic implication, Circulation 112 (6) (2005) 828–835.
[39] M. Gewillig, S.C. Brown, The Fontan circulation after 45 years: update in physiology, Heart 102 (14) (2016) 1081–1086.
[40] L.S. Shekerdemian, A. Bush, D.F. Shore, C. Lincoln, A.N. Redington, Cardiopulmonary interactions after Fontan operations: augmentation of cardiac output using negative pressure ventilation, Circulation 96 (11) (1997) 3934–3942.
[41] N.D. Bridges, J.E. Lock, A.R. Castaneda, Baffle fenestration with subsequent transcatheter closure. Modification of the Fontan operation for patients at increased risk, Circulation 82 (5) (1990) 1681–1689.
[42] J. Kreutzer, J.E. Lock, R.A. Jonas, J.F. Keane, Transcatheter fenestration dilation and/or creation in postoperative Fontan patients, Am. J. Cardiol. 79 (2) (1997) 228–232.
[43] F. Fontan, J.W. Kirklin, G. Fernandez, et al., Outcome after a "perfect" Fontan operation, Circulation 81 (5) (1990) 1520–1536.
[44] K.K. Stout, C.S. Broberg, W.M. Book, et al., Chronic heart failure in congenital heart disease: a scientific statement from the American Heart Association, Circulation 133 (8) (2016) 770–801.
[45] G. Crupi, G. Locatelli, R. Tiraboschi, M. Villani, M. De Tommasi, L. Parenzan, Protein-losing enteropathy after Fontan operation for tricuspid atresia (imperforate tricuspid valve), Thorac. Cardiovasc. Surg. 28 (5) (1980) 359–363.
[46] L. Mertens, D.J. Hagler, U. Sauer, J. Somerville, M. Gewillig, Protein-losing enteropathy after the Fontan operation: an international multicenter study. PLE study group, J. Thorac. Cardiovasc. Surg. 115 (5) (1998) 1063–1073.
[47] R.H. Feldt, D.J. Driscoll, K.P. Offord, et al., Protein-losing enteropathy after the Fontan operation, J. Thorac. Cardiovasc. Surg. 112 (3) (1996) 672–680.
[48] D.J. Driscoll, K.P. Offord, R.H. Feldt, H.V. Schaff, F.J. Puga, G.K. Danielson, Five- to fifteen-year follow-up after Fontan operation, Circulation 85 (2) (1992) 469–496.
[49] A.J. Powell, K. Gauvreau, K.J. Jenkins, E.D. Blume, J.E. Mayer, J.E. Lock, Perioperative risk factors for development of protein-losing enteropathy following a Fontan procedure, Am. J. Cardiol. 88 (10) (2001) 1206–1209.
[50] A.S. John, J.A. Johnson, M. Khan, D.J. Driscoll, C.A. Warnes, F. Cetta, Clinical outcomes and improved survival in patients with protein-losing enteropathy after the Fontan operation, J. Am. Coll. Cardiol. 64 (1) (2014) 54–62.
[51] P. Khairy, S.M. Fernandes, J.E. Mayer Jr., et al., Long-term survival, modes of death, and predictors of mortality in patients with Fontan surgery, Circulation 117 (1) (2008) 85–92.
[52] A.M. Ostrow, H. Freeze, J. Rychik, Protein-losing enteropathy after fontan operation: investigations into possible pathophysiologic mechanisms, Ann. Thorac. Surg. 82 (2) (2006) 695–700.
[53] L. Bode, H.H. Freeze, Applied glycoproteomics–approaches to study genetic-environmental collisions causing protein-losing enteropathy, Biochim. Biophys. Acta 1760 (4) (2006) 547–559.
[54] L. Lastinger, A.N. Zaidi, The adult with a fontan: a panacea without a cure? Review of long-term complications, Circ. J. 77 (11) (2013) 2672–2681.
[55] J.N. Johnson, D.J. Driscoll, P.W. O'Leary, Protein-losing enteropathy and the Fontan operation, Nutr. Clin. Pract. 27 (3) (2012) 375–384.
[56] A.S. John, S.D. Phillips, D.J. Driscoll, C.A. Warnes, F. Cetta, The use of octreotide to successfully treat protein-losing enteropathy following the Fontan operation, Congenit. Heart Dis. 6 (6) (2011) 653–656.
[57] J.P. Donnelly, A. Rosenthal, V.P. Castle, R.D. Holmes, Reversal of protein-losing enteropathy with heparin therapy in three patients with univentricular hearts and Fontan palliation, J. Pediatr. 130 (3) (1997) 474–478.
[58] L. Ryerson, C. Goldberg, A. Rosenthal, A. Armstrong, Usefulness of heparin therapy in protein-losing enteropathy associated with single ventricle palliation, Am. J. Cardiol. 101 (2) (2008) 248–251.
[59] H.M. Burkhart, J.A. Dearani, D.D. Mair, et al., The modified Fontan procedure: early and late results in 132 adult patients, J. Thorac. Cardiovasc. Surg. 125 (6) (2003) 1252–1259.
[60] D.D. Mair, F.J. Puga, G.K. Danielson, Late functional status of survivors of the Fontan procedure performed during the 1970s, Circulation 86 (5 Suppl.) (1992) II106–109.
[61] M.I. Cohen, G. Wernovsky, V.L. Vetter, et al., Sinus node function after a systematically staged Fontan procedure, Circulation 98 (19 Suppl.) (1998) II352–II358 Discussion II358–II359.
[62] T.L. Gentles, K. Gauvreau, J.E. Mayer Jr., et al., Functional outcome after the Fontan operation: factors influencing late morbidity, J. Thorac. Cardiovasc. Surg. 114 (3) (1997) 392–403 Discussion 404–395.

[63] M.A. Gatzoulis, M.D. Munk, W.G. Williams, G.D. Webb, Definitive palliation with cavopulmonary or aortopulmonary shunts for adults with single ventricle physiology, Heart 83 (1) (2000) 51–57.
[64] M.K. Song, E.J. Bae, B.S. Kwon, et al., Intra-atrial reentrant tachycardia in adult patients after Fontan operation, Int. J. Cardiol. 187 (2015) 157–163.
[65] P.J. Kannankeril, F.A. Fish, Management of intra-atrial reentrant tachycardia, Curr. Opin. Cardiol. 20 (2) (2005) 89–93.
[66] S. Balaji, A. Daga, D.J. Bradley, et al., An international multicenter study comparing arrhythmia prevalence between the intracardiac lateral tunnel and the extracardiac conduit type of Fontan operations, J. Thorac. Cardiovasc. Surg. 148 (2) (2014) 576–581.
[67] R. Correa, E.D. Sherwin, J. Kovach, et al., Mechanism and ablation of arrhythmia following total cavopulmonary connection, Circ. Arrhythm. Electrophysiol. 8 (2) (2015) 318–325.
[68] E.A. Stephenson, M. Lu, C.I. Berul, et al., Arrhythmias in a contemporary fontan cohort: prevalence and clinical associations in a multicenter cross-sectional study, J. Am. Coll. Cardiol. 56 (11) (2010) 890–896.
[69] A. Ghai, L. Harris, D.A. Harrison, G.D. Webb, S.C. Siu, Outcomes of late atrial tachyarrhythmias in adults after the Fontan operation, J. Am. Coll. Cardiol. 37 (2) (2001) 585–592.
[70] S.B. Fishberger, G. Wernovsky, T.L. Gentles, et al., Factors that influence the development of atrial flutter after the Fontan operation, J. Thorac. Cardiovasc. Surg. 113 (1) (1997) 80–86.
[71] J.M. Kalman, G.F. VanHare, J.E. Olgin, L.A. Saxon, S.I. Stark, M.D. Lesh, Ablation of 'incisional' reentrant atrial tachycardia complicating surgery for congenital heart disease. Use of entrainment to define a critical isthmus of conduction, Circulation 93 (3) (1996) 502–512.
[72] J.K. Triedman, M.E. Alexander, B.A. Love, et al., Influence of patient factors and ablative technologies on outcomes of radiofrequency ablation of intra-atrial re-entrant tachycardia in patients with congenital heart disease, J. Am. Coll. Cardiol. 39 (11) (2002) 1827–1835.
[73] H.J. Ross, Y. Law, W.M. Book, et al., Transplantation and mechanical circulatory support in congenital heart disease: a scientific statement from the American Heart Association, Circulation 133 (8) (2016) 802–820.
[74] J.S. Tweddell, M. Nersesian, K.A. Mussatto, et al., Fontan palliation in the modern era: factors impacting mortality and morbidity, Ann. Thorac. Surg. 88 (4) (2009) 1291–1299.
[75] M.O. Murphy, A.C. Glatz, D.J. Goldberg, et al., Management of early Fontan failure: a single-institution experience, Eur. J. Cardiothorac. Surg. 46 (3) (2014) 458–464 Discussion 464.
[76] C.S. Almond, J.E. Mayer Jr., R.R. Thiagarajan, E.D. Blume, P.J. del Nido, D.B. McElhinney, Outcome after Fontan failure and takedown to an intermediate palliative circulation, Ann. Thorac. Surg. 84 (3) (2007) 880–887.
[77] A.J. Iyengar, C.P. Brizard, I.E. Konstantinov, Y. d'Udekem, The option of taking down the Fontan circulation: the Melbourne experience, J. Thorac. Cardiovasc. Surg. 139 (5) (2010) 1346–1348.
[78] J.M. Kao, J.C. Alejos, P.W. Grant, R.G. Williams, K.M. Shannon, H. Laks, Conversion of atriopulmonary to cavopulmonary anastomosis in management of late arrhythmias and atrial thrombosis, Ann. Thorac. Surg. 58 (5) (1994) 1510–1514.
[79] J. Kreutzer, J.F. Keane, J.E. Lock, et al., Conversion of modified Fontan procedure to lateral atrial tunnel cavopulmonary anastomosis, J. Thorac. Cardiovasc. Surg. 111 (6) (1996) 1169–1176.
[80] D.A. Vitullo, S.Y. DeLeon, T.E. Berry, et al., Clinical improvement after revision in Fontan patients, Ann. Thorac. Surg. 61 (6) (1996) 1797–1804.
[81] C. Mavroudis, C.L. Backer, B.J. Deal, C.L. Johnsrude, Fontan conversion to cavopulmonary connection and arrhythmia circuit cryoblation, J. Thorac. Cardiovasc. Surg. 115 (3) (1998) 547–556.
[82] S. Balaji, T.B. Johnson, R.M. Sade, C.L. Case, P.C. Gillette, Management of atrial flutter after the Fontan procedure, J. Am. Coll. Cardiol. 23 (5) (1994) 1209–1215.
[83] D.B. McElhinney, V.M. Reddy, P. Moore, F.L. Hanley, Revision of previous Fontan connections to extracardiac or intraatrial conduit cavopulmonary anastomosis, Ann. Thorac. Surg. 62 (5) (1996) 1276–1282 Discussion 1283.
[84] J.A. van Son, F.W. Mohr, J. Hambsch, P. Schneider, H. Hess, G.S. Haas, Conversion of atriopulmonary or lateral atrial tunnel cavopulmonary anastomosis to extracardiac conduit Fontan modification, Eur. J. Cardiothorac. Surg. 15 (2) (1999) 150–157 Discussion 157–158.
[85] A.M. Sheikh, A.T. Tang, K. Roman, et al., The failing Fontan circulation: successful conversion of atriopulmonary connections, J. Thorac. Cardiovasc. Surg. 128 (1) (2004) 60–66.
[86] S. Weinstein, C. Cua, D. Chan, J.T. Davis, Outcome of symptomatic patients undergoing extracardiac Fontan conversion and cryoablation, J. Thorac. Cardiovasc. Surg. 126 (2) (2003) 529–536.
[87] W.H. Kim, H.G. Lim, J.R. Lee, et al., Fontan conversion with arrhythmia surgery, Eur. J. Cardiothorac. Surg. 27 (2) (2005) 250–257.
[88] W.S. Jang, W.H. Kim, K. Choi, et al., The mid-term surgical results of Fontan conversion with antiarrhythmia surgery, Eur. J. Cardiothorac. Surg. 45 (5) (2014) 922–927.
[89] H.K. Park, H.J. Shin, Y.H. Park, Outcomes of Fontan conversion for failing Fontan circulation: mid-term results, Interact. Cardiovasc. Thorac. Surg. 23 (1) (2016) 14–17.
[90] B.J. Deal, J.M. Costello, G. Webster, S. Tsao, C.L. Backer, C. Mavroudis, Intermediate-term outcome of 140 consecutive Fontan conversions with arrhythmia operations, Ann. Thorac. Surg. 101 (2) (2016) 717–724.
[91] C.A. Warnes, R.G. Williams, T.M. Bashore, et al., ACC/AHA 2008 guidelines for the management of adults with congenital heart disease: a report of the American College of Cardiology/American Heart Association task force on practice guidelines (writing committee to develop guidelines on the management of adults with congenital heart disease). Developed in collaboration with the American Society of echocardiography, Heart Rhythm Society, International Society for Adult Congenital Heart Disease, Society for Cardiovascular Angiography and Interventions, and Society of Thoracic Surgeons, J. Am. Coll. Cardiol. 52 (23) (2008) e143–263.

[92] C.K. Silversides, O. Salehian, E. Oechslin, et al., Canadian Cardiovascular Society 2009 Consensus Conference on the management of adults with congenital heart disease: complex congenital cardiac lesions, Can. J. Cardiol. 26 (3) (2010) e98–117.

[93] S.M. Said, H.M. Burkhart, H.V. Schaff, et al., Fontan conversion: identifying the high-risk patient, Ann. Thorac. Surg. 97 (6) (2014) 2115–2121 Discussion 2121–2112.

[94] A.C. Egbe, H.M. Connolly, J.A. Dearani, et al., When is the right time for Fontan conversion? The role of cardiopulmonary exercise test, Int. J. Cardiol. 220 (2016) 564–568.

[95] J.P. van Melle, D. Wolff, J. Horer, et al., Surgical options after Fontan failure, Heart 102 (14) (2016) 1127–1133.

[96] D. Takeuchi, S. Asagai, K. Ishihara, T. Nakanishi, Successful Fontan conversion combined with cardiac resynchronization therapy for a case of failing Fontan circulation with ventricular dysfunction, Eur. J. Cardiothorac. Surg. 46 (5) (2014) 913–915.

[97] Y. Enomoto, M. Aoki, Y. Nakamura, I. Hagino, T. Fujiwara, H. Nakajima, Successful Fontan completion after cardiac resynchronization therapy, Circulation 125 (19) (2012) e655–658.

[98] T. Higaki, C. Kondo, H. Tomimatsu, et al., Asynchronous contraction of the 2 ventricles caused by ventricular pacing after a Fontan-type operation in a patient with a biventricular heart, Int. J. Cardiol. 150 (3) (2011) e116–e118.

[99] V. Sojak, U. Mazic, M. Cesen, J. Schrader, N. Danojevic, Cardiac resynchronization therapy for the failing Fontan patient, Ann. Thorac. Surg. 85 (6) (2008) 2136–2138.

[100] M.R. Mehra, C.E. Canter, M.M. Hannan, et al., The 2016 International Society for Heart Lung Transplantation listing criteria for heart transplantation: a 10-year update, J. Heart Lung Transplant. 35 (1) (2016) 1–23.

[101] C.E. Canter, R.E. Shaddy, D. Bernstein, et al., Indications for heart transplantation in pediatric heart disease: a scientific statement from the American Heart Association Council on cardiovascular disease in the young; the councils on clinical cardiology, cardiovascular nursing, and cardiovascular surgery and anesthesia; and the quality of care and outcomes research interdisciplinary working group, Circulation 115 (5) (2007) 658–676.

[102] N.D. Patel, E.S. Weiss, J.G. Allen, et al., Heart transplantation for adults with congenital heart disease: analysis of the United network for organ sharing database, Ann. Thorac. Surg. 88 (3) (2009) 814–821 Discussion 821–812.

[103] T. Karamlou, J. Hirsch, K. Welke, et al., A United Network for Organ Sharing analysis of heart transplantation in adults with congenital heart disease: outcomes and factors associated with mortality and retransplantation, J. Thorac. Cardiovasc. Surg. 140 (1) (2010) 161–168.

[104] D.C. Mauchley, M.B. Mitchell, Transplantation in the fontan patient, Semin. Thorac. Cardiovasc. Surg. Pediatr. Card. Surg. Annu. 18 (1) (2015) 7–16.

[105] G. Michielon, F. Parisi, D. Di Carlo, et al., Orthotopic heart transplantation for failing single ventricle physiology, Eur. J. Cardiothorac. Surg. 24 (4) (2003) 502–510 Discussion 510.

[106] J.M. Lamour, K.R. Kanter, D.C. Naftel, et al., The effect of age, diagnosis, and previous surgery in children and adults undergoing heart transplantation for congenital heart disease, J. Am. Coll. Cardiol. 54 (2) (2009) 160–165.

[107] D. Bernstein, D. Naftel, C. Chin, et al., Outcome of listing for cardiac transplantation for failed Fontan: a multi-institutional study, Circulation 114 (4) (2006) 273–280.

[108] G. Michielon, J.P. van Melle, D. Wolff, et al., Favourable mid-term outcome after heart transplantation for late Fontan failure, Eur. J. Cardiothorac. Surg. 47 (4) (2015) 665–671.

[109] R.R. Davies, J.M. Chen, R.S. Mosca, The Fontan procedure: evolution in technique; attendant imperfections and transplantation for "failure", Semin. Thorac. Cardiovasc. Surg. Pediatr. Card. Surg. Annu. 14 (1) (2011) 55–66.

[110] C.L. Backer, H.M. Russell, E. Pahl, et al., Heart transplantation for the failing Fontan, Ann. Thorac. Surg. 96 (4) (2013) 1413–1419.

[111] J.R. Kovach, D.C. Naftel, F.B. Pearce, et al., Comparison of risk factors and outcomes for pediatric patients listed for heart transplantation after bidirectional Glenn and after Fontan: an analysis from the Pediatric Heart Transplant Study, J. Heart Lung Transplant. 31 (2) (2012) 133–139.

[112] R.R. Davies, R.A. Sorabella, J. Yang, R.S. Mosca, J.M. Chen, J.M. Quaegebeur, Outcomes after transplantation for "failed" Fontan: a single-institution experience, J. Thorac. Cardiovasc. Surg. 143 (5) (2012) 1183–1192 e1184.

[113] K.R. Kanter, Heart transplantation in children after a fontan procedure: better than people think, Semin. Thorac. Cardiovasc. Surg. Pediatr. Card. Surg. Annu. 19 (1) (2016) 44–49.

[114] K.A. Jayakumar, L.J. Addonizio, M.R. Kichuk-Chrisant, et al., Cardiac transplantation after the fontan or Glenn procedure, J. Am. Coll. Cardiol. 44 (10) (2004) 2065–2072.

[115] E.J. Hickey, C.A. Caldarone, E.H. Blackstone, et al., Critical left ventricular outflow tract obstruction: the disproportionate impact of biventricular repair in borderline cases, J. Thorac. Cardiovasc. Surg. 134 (6) (2007) 1429–1436 Discussion 1436–1427.

[116] L.L. Minich, L.Y. Tani, J.A. Hawkins, R.E. Shaddy, Possibility of postnatal left ventricular growth in selected infants with non-apex-forming left ventricles, Am. Heart J. 133 (5) (1997) 570–574.

[117] C.I. Tchervenkov, S.A. Tahta, L.C. Jutras, M.J. Beland, Biventricular repair in neonates with hypoplastic left heart complex, Ann. Thorac. Surg. 66 (4) (1998) 1350–1357.

[118] J.A. van Son, C.K. Phoon, N.H. Silverman, G.S. Haas, Predicting feasibility of biventricular repair of right-dominant unbalanced atrioventricular canal, Ann. Thorac. Surg. 63 (6) (1997) 1657–1663.

[119] L. Grosse-Wortmann, T.J. Yun, O. Al-Radi, et al., Borderline hypoplasia of the left ventricle in neonates: insights for decision-making from functional assessment with magnetic resonance imaging, J. Thorac. Cardiovasc. Surg. 136 (6) (2008) 1429–1436.

[120] S.M. Emani, E.A. Bacha, D.B. McElhinney, et al., Primary left ventricular rehabilitation is effective in maintaining two-ventricle physiology in the borderline left heart, J. Thorac. Cardiovasc. Surg. 138 (6) (2009) 1276–1282.

[121] C.R. Mart, A.W. Eckhauser, Development of an echocardiographic scoring system to predict biventricular repair in neonatal hypoplastic left heart complex, Pediatr. Cardiol. 35 (8) (2014) 1456–1466.

[122] B.T. Kalish, P. Banka, T. Lafranchi, W. Tworetzky, P. Del Nido, S.M. Emani, Biventricular conversion after single ventricle palliation in patients with small left heart structures: short-term outcomes, Ann. Thorac. Surg. 96 (4) (2013) 1406–1412.

[123] J.L. Gibbs, C. Wren, K.G. Watterson, S. Hunter, J.R. Hamilton, Stenting of the arterial duct combined with banding of the pulmonary arteries and atrial septectomy or septostomy: a new approach to palliation for the hypoplastic left heart syndrome, Br. Heart J. 69 (6) (1993) 551–555.

[124] C. Yerebakan, J. Murray, K. Valeske, et al., Long-term results of biventricular repair after initial Giessen hybrid approach for hypoplastic left heart variants, J. Thorac. Cardiovasc. Surg. 149 (4) (2015) 1112–1120 Discussion 1120-1112 e1112.

[125] J.M. Lamour, L.J. Addonizio, M.E. Galantowicz, et al., Outcome after orthotopic cardiac transplantation in adults with congenital heart disease, Circulation 100 (19 Suppl.) (1999) II200–205.

[126] M. Petko, R.J. Myung, G. Wernovsky, et al., Surgical reinterventions following the Fontan procedure, Eur. J. Cardiothorac. Surg. 24 (2) (2003) 255–259.

[127] J.K. Bhama, J. Shulman, C.A. Bermudez, et al., Heart transplantation for adults with congenital heart disease: results in the modern era, J. Heart Lung Transplant. 32 (5) (2013) 499–504.

[128] M.B. Mitchell, D.N. Campbell, D. Ivy, et al., Evidence of pulmonary vascular disease after heart transplantation for Fontan circulation failure, J. Thorac. Cardiovasc. Surg. 128 (5) (2004) 693–702.

[129] A. Gamba, M. Merlo, R. Fiocchi, et al., Heart transplantation in patients with previous Fontan operations, J. Thorac. Cardiovasc. Surg. 127 (2) (2004) 555–562.

Chapter 49

Valve Interventions in the Young Adult With Heart Failure

Ralf J. Holzer[1,4], Hussam Suradi[2,3], Ziyad M. Hijazi[1,4]

[1]NewYork-Presbyterian Hospital – Weill Cornell Medical Center, New York, NY, United States; [2]St. Mary Medical Center/Community Healthcare System, Hobart, IN, United States; [3]Rush University Medical Center, Chicago, IL, United States; [4]Weill Cornell Medical College, New York, NY, United States

INTRODUCTION

Heart failure as a result of stenotic valvar heart disease in the young adult is rare. In general, congenitally stenotic valves, whether in arterial or atrioventricular position, do not cause heart failure early in the disease process and, as such, are usually intervened on well before this would manifest itself in deteriorating ventricular function and associated symptoms of congestive heart failure. In fact, even if the disease process were allowed to continue without attempts at therapeutic transcatheter or surgical intervention, it is much more likely for a patient to present with (exercise-induced) arrhythmias rather than symptoms of congestive cardiac failure. Exceptions are neonates with critical aortic stenosis or neonates with critical pulmonary valve stenosis, the latter being much less commonly a cause of reduced ventricular function than the former. Another exception is pediatric patients and young adults with fulminant rheumatic heart disease who may present with a combination of rheumatic myocarditis and (mitral) valve disease.

In contrast to congenitally stenotic valves, symptoms of heart failure and reduced ventricular function with a volume loaded ventricle are much more common though in the presence of moderate–severe regurgitation of either arterial or atrioventricular valves, usually in patients who have undergone previous surgical or transcatheter interventions for congenital heart disease. However, with exception of percutaneous pulmonary valve implantation, therapeutic transcatheter interventions are limited in patients with regurgitant lesions, and cardiothoracic surgery is the most commonly used treatment modality. With the emergence of transcatheter aortic valve implantation for the adult patient with calcific aortic valve stenosis, this technology may eventually become an option for the older pediatric patient or young adult with a combination of aortic valve stenosis and regurgitation and heart failure, but, at this point and time, this treatment strategy has not been established for this patient population [1].

This section therefore focuses on transcatheter interventions for neonates and infants that present with heart failure and (critical) aortic or pulmonary valve stenosis, patients with congenital heart disease that undergo percutaneous pulmonary valve implantation, as well as patients with mitral valve stenosis.

BALLOON AORTIC VALVULOPLASTY

Patient Selection

For the usual patient with a stenotic aortic valve and normal ventricular function, the decision on when to refer a patient for balloon aortic valvuloplasty is often a difficult one. A variety of factors need to be taken into consideration, such as clinical data (symptoms, exercise tolerance), echo data (mean and peak instantaneous Doppler gradients, ventricular function, presence of left ventricular hypertrophy, valve morphology, preexisting aortic insufficiency, associated lesions), and others (EKG, exercise test data including echo gradients with exercise). Valvar and ventricular morphology are extremely important in a disease that ranges from a neonate with critical aortic valve stenosis and borderline-sized left ventricle (LV), to an infant with a dysplastic unicusp aortic valve, to an older child with a well-formed stenotic tricuspid valve with fused commissures [2,3].

However, while most of the above factors are also important in a neonate with critical aortic valve stenosis, the indication to intervene is usually absolute, with critical aortic valve stenosis with depressed ventricular function in a neonate

Heart Failure in the Child and Young Adult. http://dx.doi.org/10.1016/B978-0-12-802393-8.00049-1

representing probably one of the few true emergencies for the congenital interventional cardiologist. Patients that present with this condition usually deteriorate despite aggressive conservative management, and the only therapy to improve the condition is to perform an emergent balloon aortic valvuloplasty to relief the critical obstruction. The current American Heart Association (AHA) recommendations for balloon aortic valvuloplasty list as class I indication for balloon aortic valvuloplasty the newborns with critical duct-dependent aortic stenosis and aortic stenosis in the presence of poor left ventricular systolic function [4]. In the presence of poor ventricular function, systolic Doppler gradients become meaningless and a low gradient should not deter from intervening on a severely stenotic aortic valve. Surgical valvotomy is an option in centers with outstanding surgical results, but, in general, the transcatheter approach is the preferred primary mode of therapy in the vast majority of patients and centers.

Procedural Background

Balloon aortic valvuloplasty has been a core therapeutic transcatheter intervention for congenital aortic valve stenosis for several decades, with one of the earliest series reported by Lababidi as far back as 1984 [5]. The emergence of transcatheter aortic valve implantation in adults over the last decade has created a renewed interest for balloon aortic valvuloplasty not just for adults with acquired calcific aortic valve stenosis but also for patients with congenital aortic valve stenosis. One of the main concerns of this procedure has always been the potential for creating significant aortic insufficiency, and historically studies have demonstrated results of balloon aortic valvuloplasty to be similar to those achieved by surgery, with a lesser morbidity. Polimenakos and colleagues reported a freedom from aortic valve replacement after surgical intervention of 72% at 10 years and 60% at 18 years [6], which is similar to results reported by Brown and colleagues with a freedom from aortic valve replacement of 79% at 10 years and 53% at 20 years [7]. Several other studies have demonstrated comparable results [8,9]. However, some recent surgical series advocate that newer surgical techniques may be able to achieve superior result when compared to transcatheter balloon aortic valvuloplasty results [10]. Whether those surgical results can be reproduced by all centers remains to be seen and for now and for most centers, balloon aortic valvuloplasty is still the most commonly performed initial procedure for patients with congenital aortic valve stenosis of all ages. However, each center has to evaluate and compare individual surgical and transcatheter results, to decide on the best approach specific to institutional outcomes for different patients' sizes.

Procedural Technique

Wherever feasible, the procedure should be performed using as little anesthetic agents as possible, to avoid its impact on blood pressure and valve gradient. Furthermore, it is important to try to keep the same conditions throughout the procedure, to better allow comparisons of pre-and postprocedure gradients and cardiac output. In patients with critical aortic valve stenosis and very poor left ventricular function, operators may want to consider performing the procedure with extracorporeal membrane oxygenation support or at least with support on standby in the catheterization laboratory [11].

All procedures should include a full left heart catheterization and an aortogram. However, a left ventricular angiogram should be avoided in patients with poor left ventricular function. Hemodynamic evaluation should ideally not only include the baseline valvar gradient but also evaluate the cardiac output, document the left ventricular end-diastolic pressure (LVEDP), and record the presence of any aortic arch gradient. The best angles for the aortogram are a straight lateral projection, as well as a 25-degree left anterior oblique (LAO), and 25-degree cranial angulation on the frontal tubes. A right anterior oblique caudal projection can also be helpful. The aortogram serves two main purposes: to document the preexisting angiographic degree of aortic insufficiency and measuring the maximum valve annulus size at the hinge points. In patients with depressed ventricular function, it may be useful to perform an aortogram prior to trying to cross the aortic valve, especially if one can expect greater difficulties in doing so. That way, the degree of regurgitation can be documented without a wire across the aortic valve. In addition, the jet of negative washout above the valve gives the operator a reasonable idea on the appropriate direction of catheter and wire to cross the valve. In fact, in patients that tolerate the procedure poorly, a quick approach is needed and rather than spending time performing a complete hemodynamic evaluation. In these circumstances, an aortogram should be performed to decide on the appropriate balloon diameter and the balloon prepped and ready to use prior to any attempts at crossing the valve. That way, if needed, valvuloplasty can be performed immediately after crossing the valve.

Crossing the aortic valve is usually the most difficult aspect of the procedure. Whichever technique is used, a soft wire should be utilized to do so as using a stiff wire has the potential of crossing in a nonintended position and if not recognized, this can lead to avulsion of the aortic valve leaflet with balloon inflation [12]. There are essentially three ways to cross the

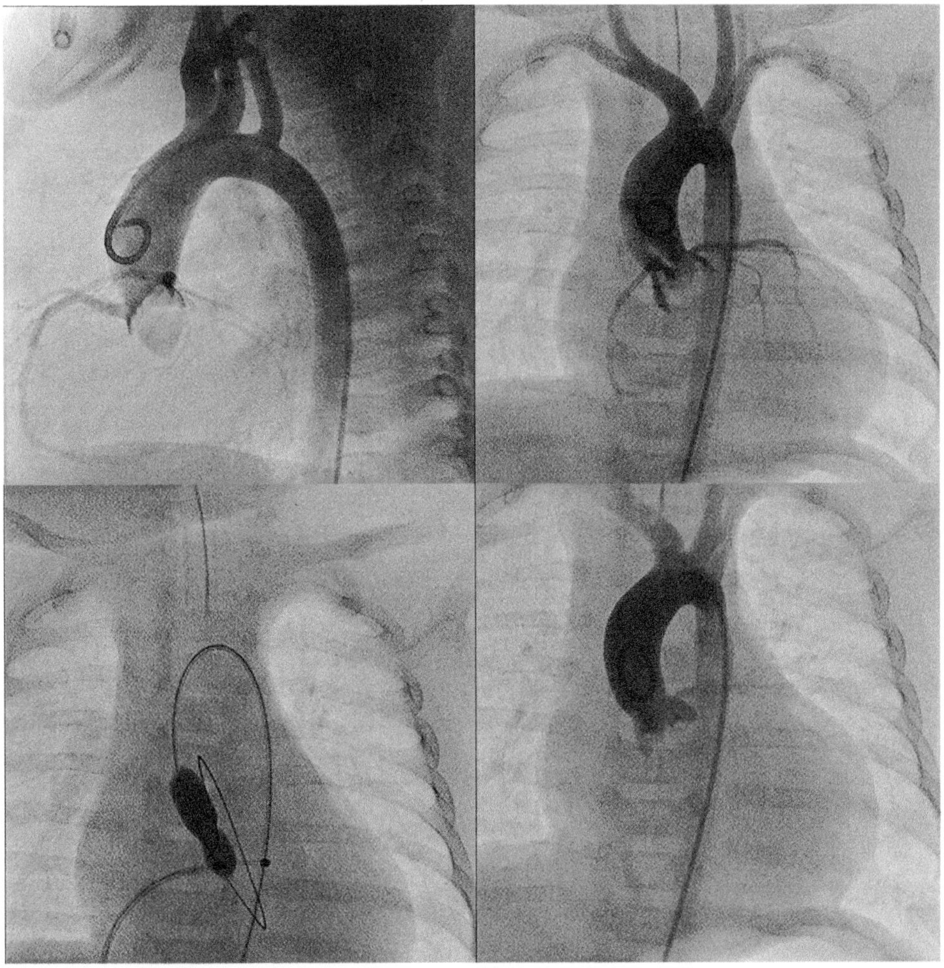

FIGURE 49.1 **Balloon aortic valvuloplasty.** Balloon aortic valvuloplasty in a 3-month infant with severe congenital aortic valve stenosis. Top left and right: aortogram profiling the doming aortic valve annulus. A negative washout can be seen from the jet egressing through the valve leaflets. Bottom left: balloon inflation centered across the aortic valve with concomitant rapid right ventricular pacing. Bottom right: aortogram after balloon valvuloplasty documenting absence of aortic insufficiency.

valve, each having advantages and disadvantages: a retrograde approach from the femoral artery, an antegrade approach through the atrial septum and LV, and a Hybrid approach with carotid cut down.

The retrograde approach is the one most commonly used (Fig. 49.1). It requires placing a femoral arterial sheath that accommodates the size of the balloon. Even though this has the potential to create femoral arterial injury, the availability of low profile balloons and smaller sheaths usually does not create a significant problem even in small infants and neonates [13]. However, crossing the aortic valve can be a little more cumbersome using this technique. While a variety of catheters can be used, a Judkins left coronary catheter often points toward the opening of the aortic valve and works well in the majority of patients. In smaller patients, a 0.014″ coronary wire with a floppy tip and reasonably stiff body can be used to cross the valve and depending on the wire and chosen balloon, it can also be used for the valvuloplasty itself, thereby not requiring any catheter or wire exchanges.

Crossing the valve using an antegrade approach through the atrial septum and LV is usually not an appropriate approach in patients with reduced ventricular function, as too much manipulation need to be performed within the LV, irrespective of the additional risk of creating injury to the mitral valve apparatus with balloon inflation [14].

Performing valvuloplasty using a carotid cut down is technically probably the easiest way to perform balloon aortic valvuloplasty, and the suitability of this technique has been well-documented [15]. It is probably the ideal approach in a neonate with critical aortic valve stenosis on an infant with poor left ventricular function. It requires cooperation from the surgical team, and a sheath is usually inserted through a purse string in the carotid artery. This is a great technique for very small infants, as it avoids the use of a femoral arterial sheath and crossing the valve is usually much easier than using a retrograde approach, thereby making the procedure quicker and safer for the patient [16]. If the tip of the sheath is pointing to or within the ascending aorta, a hand injection is often sufficient to outline the valve and assess the degree of aortic insufficiency. A 0.014″ coronary wire can be advanced through the sheath and usually directly crosses the valve and is curved within the LV. Other Hybrid approaches that have been described include a transaortic as well as a transapical approach [17–19].

If a valve is very difficult to cross, ideally a catheter or wire should be maintained across the valve until valvuloplasty is performed to avoid having to recross the aortic valve. Hemodynamic evaluation is fairly straight forward if the patient has a patent foramen ovale (PFO), which is present in virtually all patients with critical aortic valve stenosis. In the (rare) absence of a PFO and when the valve has been difficult to cross in smaller children, a helpful technique is to advance a catheter that takes a 0.035″ wire over the coronary wire that is positioned in the LV, but to keep the position of the catheter just above the valve. One can then buddy a 0.014″ pressure wire next to the coronary wire and position it also within the LV. With the help of a Tuohy-Borst adapter simultaneous pressure recordings can be obtained in LV and ascending aorta, thereby avoiding catheter and wire exchanges to obtain a pressure gradient and at the same time maintaining wire position across the valve throughout. In infants, the coronary wire used to cross the aortic valve is usually a suitable wire for the valvuloplasty itself as it can be looped within the LV with the tip often pointing back to the aortic valve, thereby providing a good stability for the valvuloplasty itself. In all patients, once the valve has been crossed, it is important to control and maintain the wire position continuously, as it can easily be ejected from the LV into the ascending aorta.

One of the main concerns after balloon aortic valvuloplasty is the degree of aortic regurgitation, which may result in the need for surgical valve repair or replacement. For this very reason, a conservative approach when choosing the initial balloon size is advisable. The chosen balloon size should be about 80%–90% of the valve annulus. The smaller the child, especially in neonates and infants, the less adequate surgical options are available to address significant aortic regurgitation. For this reason, it is advisable to use initially a balloon size at the lower end of the acceptable range. Reintervening in a neonate after 3 months because of recurrent or residual aortic valve stenosis is much preferred to being overly aggressive during the first procedure, with a significant risk of undesirable degrees of aortic insufficiency. As to the balloon choice, ideally a fairly long compliant balloon (3 cm in neonates/infants) should be used as it provides greater stability, and sufficient length of the balloon will be positioned in the LV as well as the ascending aorta. A long balloon aids in limiting some of the "shear" trauma to the valve created by balloon movement during inflation. Provided the valve annulus was appropriately captured, repeat balloon inflation should be avoided as this always risks of creating more regurgitation to the aortic valve.

Stabilizing the balloon across the valve is important, not only to capture the valve and avoid having to perform repeat inflations but also to minimize the forward movement of the deflated (and less smooth) balloon across the aortic valve and the shear stress created with it. Methods of cardiac output control, such as rapid right ventricular pacing, are helpful in the older child with normal left ventricular function [20–22]. However, while it is an excellent tool for balloon stabilization, it is probably not a good idea to use this technique in patients with depressed left ventricular function, especially in neonates with critical aortic stenosis, as this can lead to arrhythmias that may not be easily converted back after pacing is discontinued.

Balloon inflations should generally be performed rapidly but controlled to limit the time the left ventricular outflow tract is obstructed, with blood pressure being recorded throughout the procedure. Usually a transient drop in systemic blood pressure can be observed, occasionally combined with transient bradycardia, but this usually resolves fairly quickly after balloon deflation. The operator should observe the balloon carefully for disappearance of the waist and maintenance of position during inflation. The operator should try to maintain balloon position by having one hand at the balloon catheter close to the sheath, while operating the inflation device with the other hand.

After each balloon inflation, the valvar gradient as well as the degree of aortic insufficiency is reevaluated. However, in neonates with critical aortic valve stenosis and/or patients with reduced ventricular function, the gradient may not change a lot after valvuloplasty. In fact, opening of the valve may lead to improvement in left ventricular systolic function and potentially even an increase in the systolic gradient. For that reason, single balloon inflation with a balloon of about 80% the valve annulus is all that should be initially performed in these patients, irrespective of the degree of aortic insufficiency. Aortic valve surgery in the neonatal period or infancy has limited options available, and given the higher risks and poorer outcomes, the purpose of early transcatheter interventions in this group of patients is not necessarily a long-term palliation, but an intervention that removes the acute risks related to aortic valve stenosis while at the same time meticulously avoiding the potential need for surgery. It is much more preferable to reintervene after 3 months for recurrent aortic valve stenosis if there is no significant aortic insufficiency, than upsizing the balloon by 1 mm to get a better gradient reduction, only to create significant aortic insufficiency, which then requires an early Ross or other cardiac surgical procedure.

Ideally, the degree of aortic insufficiency should be assessed in the cath lab not only by angiography but also by echocardiography. A high power injection very close to the aortic valve can make the degree of aortic insufficiency appear worse than it is, especially in neonates and infants. One has to remember that the aortic valve is under physiologic conditions not exposed to those high inflation pressures that are generally being used for an aortogram. At the opposite end of the spectrum, injecting a little to high within the aorta may not reveal the true degree of aortic insufficiency. To identify any changes, it is therefore important to use the same injection parameters and same catheter position that was used for the prevalvuloplasty angiogram. However, while the degree of aortic insufficiency is important, it does not necessarily immediately tell you whether this will be clinically tolerated for a longer period of time. The effect of aortic insufficiency on LV function and volume may not be immediately apparent at the time of cardiac catheterization or even the day after the procedure. A stiff LV with diastolic dysfunction may not dilate notably until any ventricular hypertrophy has improved.

Outcomes

The expected long-term outcome from balloon aortic valvuloplasty is fundamentally different from balloon pulmonary valvuloplasty, with results usually being of a palliative nature, with many patients requiring either transcatheter or surgical reinterventions. Brown and colleagues from Boston Children's hospital reported on the long-term outcome after balloon aortic valvuloplasty, identifying a 47% chance of requiring surgical aortic valve replacement within 20 years of valvuloplasty, and 73% chance of any type of reintervention (whether transcatheter or surgical) [7]. The Boston data suggest that the gradient reduction may be at least as important as the degree of aortic insufficiency after intervention. In fact, the odds of requiring surgical aortic valve replacement were higher if the residual gradient was more than 35 mmHg with only mild aortic insufficiency, as opposed to patients who had a gradient reduction to less than 35 mmHg but with moderate to severe aortic insufficiency [7].

Balloon aortic valvuloplasty is generally a fairly safe procedure. Recent multicenter data from the Congenital Cardiac Catheterization Project on Outcomes (C3PO) registry documented no procedural mortality, with an incidence of higher severity adverse events of 10%, which is similar to other larger series [23,24]. The only risk factor associated with an increased risk for high severity adverse events was neonatal status, and as such, operators need to be aware of the increased risk of performing this procedure in neonates with critical aortic valve stenosis. Procedural success in achieving a gradient reduction to 35 mmHg or less was 71%. Independent factors associated with procedural success were first time intervention, nonprostaglandin dependent, and isolated aortic valve stenosis with absence of aortic regurgitation. Other studies have documented the presence of reduced left ventricular function in neonates to be associated with a higher risk for future interventions [25]. Given the larger experience with balloon aortic valvuloplasty, some centers have utilized standardized clinical assessment and management plans for this group of patients, documenting improved results when compared to matched, historical controls [26].

BALLOON PULMONARY VALVULOPLASTY

Patient Selection

In general, congenital pulmonary valve stenosis is usually intervened on well before ventricular function deteriorates, and, as such, a clinical presentation with cardiac failure is a very rare occurrence. Furthermore, even neonates with critical pulmonary valve stenosis usually have preserved right ventricular function. The "critical" does not refer to an emergent need for intervention or poor right ventricular function, but instead to the fact that blood flow across the pulmonary valve is limited to a "critical" degree, thereby requiring an additional source of pulmonary blood supply until balloon pulmonary valvuloplasty has been performed. This also applies to patients with pulmonary valve atresia and intact ventricular septum, who usually have a hypoplastic right ventricle (RV) with the need for additional pulmonary blood flow, but usually do not present with reduced ventricular function and cardiac failure.

Very occasionally, intervening for pulmonary valve stenosis may be deferred, such as in an extremely premature patient with pulmonary valve stenosis and multiple associated anomalies. This can occasionally lead to deterioration in right ventricular function, which is one of the few clinical circumstances when we see a patient with cardiac failure and congenital pulmonary valve stenosis. Similar to balloon aortic valvuloplasty, the current AHA recommendations for balloon pulmonary valvuloplasty list as class I indications among others the presence of critical (duct-dependent) pulmonary valve stenosis as, a peak-to-peak catheter or peak instantaneous echo gradient of more than 40 mmHg, or clinically significant stenosis in the presence of RV dysfunction [4]. In contrast to critical aortic valve stenosis, pulmonary valve stenosis associated with right ventricular dysfunction or critical pulmonary valve stenosis are usually not emergent indications to intervene.

Procedural Technique

The procedure can be performed under general anesthesia or deep sedation, but as with aortic valvuloplasty, it is important to maintain a steady state throughout the procedure, to allow an adequate comparison of hemodynamic results before and after the intervention. All procedures are usually performed using femoral venous access, and an arterial line is placed for monitoring throughout the procedure. A Hybrid subxiphoid approach can be considered in very small premature infants, as it has the advantage of avoiding any prolonged catheter manipulation or wire loops within a dysfunctional RV [27].

A basic right heart catheterization is performed, documenting the valvar (and sub/supravalvar) peak systolic gradients as well as the right ventricular pressure in relation to the systemic arterial pressure. A pressure wire can be useful to document any supravalvar or subvalvar gradients. However, prior to valvuloplasty, right ventricular pressures are usually elevated, thereby expanding the right ventricular outflow tract (RVOT) and frequently masking the presence of any subvalvar obstruction.

Once all hemodynamic data are obtained, the right ventricular angiogram is performed using usually cranial angulations on the frontal tube with some degree of LAO, as well as a straight lateral projection. This usually documents the valve morphology, thickness of the valve, presence of sub/supravalvar narrowing, as well as allowing measuring the size of the valve annulus at the hinge points. In patients with diminished right ventricular function or severe valvar stenosis in the absence of an arterial duct, crossing the pulmonary valve to obtain direct pressure recordings may be poorly tolerated and therefore in those circumstances, right ventricular and systemic arterial pressures may be all that is being obtained prior to performing a right ventricular angiogram. This allows having the appropriately sized balloon catheter prepped and ready, so that valvuloplasty can be performed immediately if hemodynamic instability is encountered when crossing the valve (Fig. 49.2).

The choice of the wire used for valvuloplasty depends on the balloon type that is being used, but for neonates and infants, in general a 0.014″ coronary wire will be sufficient to allow tracking of the balloon, while avoiding the wire loop creating too much tension to the RV and tricuspid valve apparatus. This is important because in the presence of reduced right ventricular function, splinting the tricuspid valve through the use of a very stiff wire may lead to a detrimental drop in cardiac output. The initial balloon diameter chosen should be about 1.2–1.3 times the size of the pulmonary valve annulus [28]. Choosing a smaller balloon may lead to an inadequate result, while larger balloons in excess of 1.4 times the annulus risk potential vascular injury and a higher degree of pulmonary insufficiency. In contrast to balloon aortic valvuloplasty where the ascending aorta usually provides plenty of room to use a long balloon for better stability, the useable length of the balloon in patients with pulmonary valve stenosis is usually limited by the bifurcation to the branch pulmonary arteries. One should avoid having the shoulders of the balloon reaching into the pulmonary branches, as this may lead to the balloon milking backward during inflation. Furthermore, choosing a balloon that is too long may have the balloon impact and potentially damage the tricuspid valve apparatus. Therefore, whenever feasible, crossing the tricuspid valve using a balloon wedge catheter virtually guarantees that the wire does not traverse through the tricuspid valve chordal apparatus. This, however, may not always be feasible in all patients, in particular in neonates and infants, and in those circumstances the operator needs to watch very carefully when the balloon is being advanced. Any holdup at the tricuspid valve apparatus could suggest that chordae may have been crossed and in those situations, it is important to consider removing and repositioning the guide wire.

In small patients with typical nondysplastic pulmonary valve stenosis, using a compliant balloon for the initial inflation, such as Tyshak II (NuMED, Hopkinton, New York), is usually appropriate and limits the sheath size that is required. The balloon inflation should be quick but controlled. It is best to position two-thirds of the balloon length above the valve and then pulling back slightly on the catheter during balloon inflation once the valve is captured to maintain position of the balloon and avoid it milking distally to the valve. Balloon inflation is usually associated with a drop in blood pressure and/or drop in systemic oxygen saturations if a PFO is present. In patients with reduced right ventricular function, a balloon with quick deflation characteristics should be considered to limit the amount of hemodynamic instability. The balloon inflation needs to be watched carefully for disappearance of the waist and in contrast to aortic valvuloplasty, the inflation is usually repeated to confirm that any residual waist disappears at low inflation pressures. If a waist cannot be abolished using an adequately sized a low-pressure compliant balloon, then the use of a less compliant higher pressure balloon of the same size should be considered as the next step.

After use of each balloon size, the hemodynamic results should be assessed. It is also a good practice to perform a right ventricular angiogram to assess for any damage caused by the balloon inflation.

What is considered to be an adequate result has evolved over time. Parameters that have been used include the residual peak-to-peak valvar gradient, the relative reduction of the peak-to-peak gradient, as well as the relative reduction of the RV to systemic arterial pressure ratio. However, in patients with reduced right ventricular function, gradient reduction may

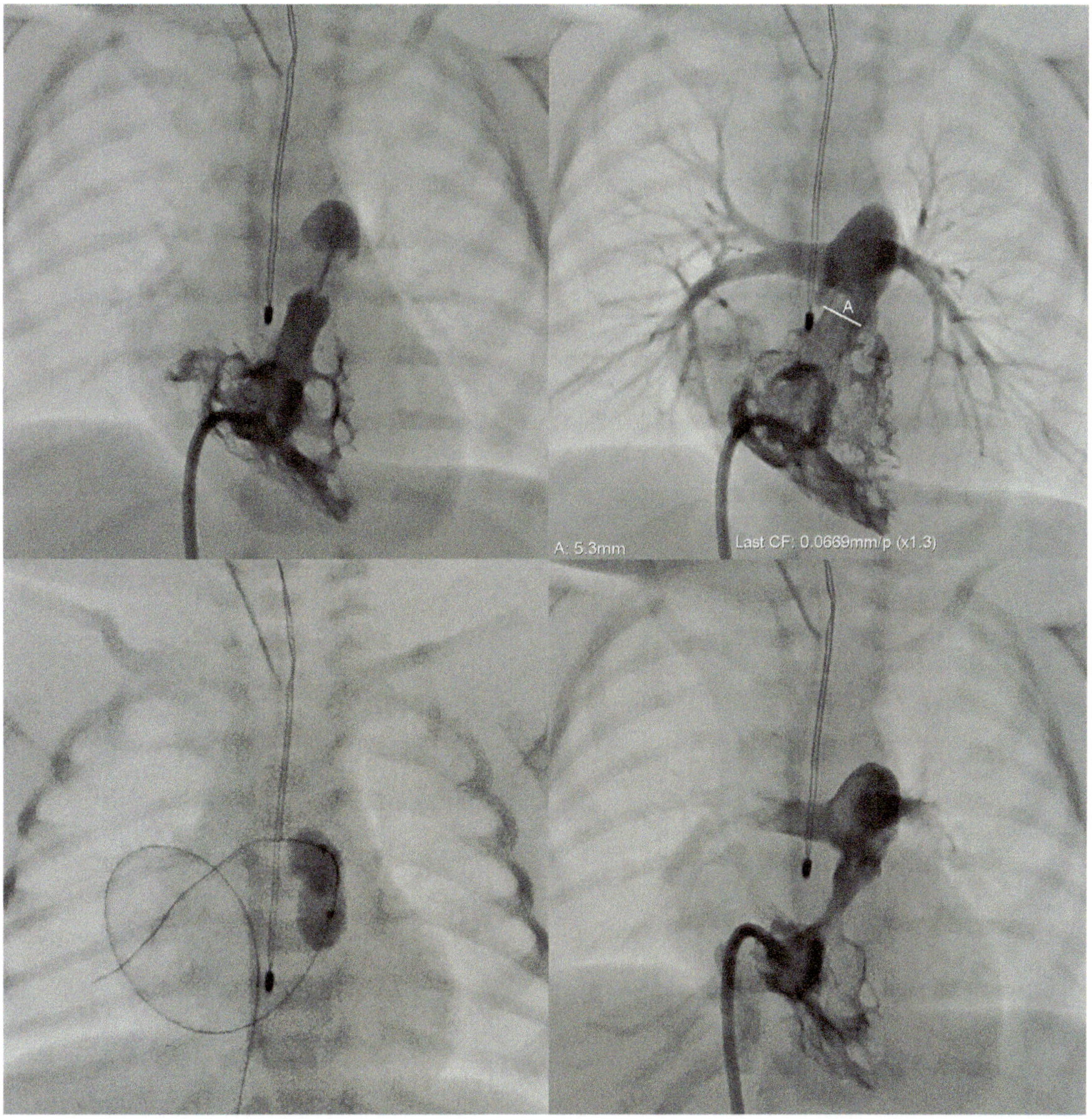

FIGURE 49.2 **Balloon pulmonary valvuloplasty.** Balloon pulmonary valvuloplasty in a 2-day-old infant with critical pulmonary valve stenosis. Top left: right ventricular (RV) angiogram documenting a severely stenotic valve with a narrow jet of contrast. Top right: pulmonary valve annulus measuring 5.3 mm. Bottom left: balloon pulmonary valvuloplasty using a 7 mm×2 cm Tyshak II balloon. Bottom right: RV angio after valvuloplasty documenting a degree of subpulmonary narrowing.

be meaningless, and if function does improve, the residual gradient after valvuloplasty may be even higher than the gradient at baseline. However, in contrast to valvuloplasty in patients with critical aortic valve stenosis, gradients are reevaluated and repeat intervention performed accordingly (if criteria are met). The Valvuloplasty and Angioplasty of Congenital Anomalies registry considered a residual gradient of less than 35 mmHg as an adequate result [28]. However, given that current AHA recommendations list a peak-to-peak gradient of just 40 mmHg as an indication for pulmonary valvuloplasty, it is probably more appropriate to aim for a residual valvar gradient of less than 25 mmHg, or ideally less than 10 mmHg in patients with isolated nondysplastic valvar stenosis beyond the neonatal period. Holzer and colleagues reported on the results of the C3PO registry and used a composite measure of either a valvar gradient reduction to less than 25 mmHg, a relative gradient reduction by 50%, or a relative reduction of the RV to systemic pressure ration by 50% as a measure of an adequate outcome [29]. If the residual gradient between main pulmonary artery and RV is more than expected or does not meet the criteria of a satisfactory outcome, it is important to assess for the presence of any subvalvar narrowing (Fig. 49.2). This can be easily accomplished with the use of a pressure wire. Subvalvar gradients usually manifest themselves after the valve has been opened with the balloon, but the infundibular hypertrophy has been well-documented to regress over time.

Subpulmonary gradients after valvuloplasty are particularly common in adults with long-standing congenital pulmonary valve stenosis and have been reported to be present in more than 40% of patients, even though the vast majority of these gradients regress over time [30,31]. If an adequate result has not been achieved with a given balloon size, the next larger balloon should be used, usually not exceeding 1.4 times the size of the valve annulus.

Outcomes of Balloon Pulmonary Valvuloplasty

Results of balloon pulmonary valvuloplasty are usually excellent. The C3PO registry documented acute procedural success in 77% of cases. Independent risk factors for procedural failure were the presence of a genetic syndrome, complex 2-ventricle anatomy, presence of supravalvar pulmonary stenosis, a hemodynamic vulnerability score of 2 or more, and the need for balloon inflation above 8 atm [29]. Out of more than 290 patients within the C3PO registry, no patient died as a result of the procedure, and the incidence of higher severity adverse events was less than 3%. There were only two level 4 adverse events, both of an electrophysiological nature.

Studies have documented a need for reintervention (surgical or transcatheter) for residual or recurrent pulmonary valve stenosis in about 5%–10% of patients within 10 years of the initial intervention [32,33]. Several studies have documented the presence of a dysplastic pulmonary valve, frequently associated with a genetic syndrome such as Noonan's, to be associated with a lower procedural success, with an adequate result being achieved in less than 50% of patients [29,34]. The long-term impact of pulmonary regurgitation after balloon pulmonary valvuloplasty is unknown. However, while it is unclear how many patients may require transcatheter or surgical pulmonary valve replacement at some future point after pulmonary valvuloplasty, for the majority of patients one can likely expect a lasting long-term result without the need for transcatheter or surgical reintervention. One recent study on 53 patients that underwent balloon pulmonary valvuloplasty found 58% of patients with grade II and 31% of patients with grade III pulmonary insufficiency after a median follow-up of 15 years, with no patient so far having required pulmonary valve replacement [35].

TRANSCATHETER PULMONARY VALVE IMPLANTATION

Patient Selection

Transcatheter pulmonary valve implantation is usually a procedure performed in patients that have previously undergone palliation or repair of congenital heart disease, such as tetralogy of Fallot. While the aim of selecting patients is to perform transcatheter pulmonary valve implantation prior to the right ventricular function deteriorating, there are still many patients that for a variety of reasons get referred late and in whom right ventricular dysfunction with exercise intolerance and symptoms of cardiac failure are already present. This is even more common in patients with predominant pulmonary regurgitation, or pulmonary regurgitation combined with pulmonary stenosis, rather than isolated stenosis of the RVOT, pulmonary valve, or conduit.

Appropriate patient selection for pulmonary valve replacement is crucial, and the guidelines for both surgical as well as transcatheter pulmonary valve replacement have continued to evolve over the last decade [36–40]. In general, it is recommended to use a composite measure of clinical data (symptoms, exercise capacity, presence of arrhythmias), EKG and echo data, and MRI-based data elements such as right ventricular end-diastolic volume index (≥150 mL/m^2), right ventricular end-systolic volume index (>80 mL/m^2), pulmonary regurgitant fraction (≥40%), and right ventricular function (ejection fraction <40%) [41,42]. Pulmonary valve replacement should ideally be performed before right ventricular function declines.

Until a valve that is suitable for treating patients with a native RVOT is widely commercially available, the standard approach to transcatheter pulmonary valve implantation is presently limited to implantation diameters of about 18 up to 29 mm. While implantation of transcatheter valves have been performed in selected patients with repaired tetralogy of Fallot and native/patched RVOT [43–46], in general, the standard approach requires either a bioprosthetic valve or an RVPA (right ventricle to pulmonary artery) conduit of at least 18 mm in diameter. When selecting patients with a bioprosthetic valve, it is important to consider the type of prosthetic valves, due to variations of the inner valvar diameter in comparison to the labeled diameter of the valve. Furthermore, one has to be aware that the transcatheter valve itself will further reduce the effective internal diameter within a bioprosthetic valve, which is especially important when considering valve implantation into bioprosthetic valves with a diameter at the lower end of the implantation range.

Weight is not necessarily a limiting factor when considering patients for percutaneous pulmonary valve implantation and has been reported in patients as little as 13.8 with results very similar to those seen in larger patients [47]. When discussing therapeutic options, one should consider a periventricular subxiphoid approach in patients with a low weight or a potentially difficult percutaneous approach [48–50].

Selecting the appropriate center and operator to perform these highly specialized procedures is just as important as selecting the right patient. Recent published guidelines recommended a case volume of at least 150 congenital and/or structural cases per center, and 50 congenital and/or structural interventional cases per operator [51]. Procedures should be performed in a center with an adult congenital program (≥25 cardiac surgical case/year), or be associated with a congenital or structural cardiac surgical program (≥100 cardiac surgical cases/year).

Procedural Background

Phillip Bonhoeffer, MD performed the first transcatheter pulmonary valve replacement in a human in 2000 and since then, several thousand procedures have been performed worldwide [36,52]. Patient selection, institutional and operator requirements, conduit fractures, the risk of endocarditis, and prevention of coronary compressions are only some of the challenges that have been seen as a result of these procedures [51].

At present, the two commercially available valves approved for transcatheter pulmonary valve replacement include the Melody valve (Medtronic, Minneapolis, Minnesota, United States) and the Sapien valve (Edwards Lifescience, Irvine, California, United States), and details of the valve design and basic implantation technique have been described previously [52–54]. The Melody valve consists of a bovine jugular venous valve, which is sutured within an 8-zig, 28 mm Covered Cheatham Platinum stents (Fig. 49.3). The valve is implanted using the 22Fr Ensemble delivery system, which allows the valve to be mounted on a BiB balloon with a diameter of either 18, 20, or 22 mm. The Melody valve is available in two sizes, one that can be implanted up to 20 mm (TPV20) and one that can be implanted up to a diameter of 22 mm (TPV22).

In contrast to the Melody valve, the Edwards valve was originally developed for use in aortic valve position, and the first successful implantation in pulmonary position was reported in 2006 [54]. The Edwards Sapien valve is a bovine pericardial tissue valve mounted within a stainless steel stent with a height of 14.6–16 mm [55]. Due to the limited height of the valve, prestenting is required for safe delivery. The valve is available in diameters of 23 and 26 mm (Fig. 49.4), with a new model

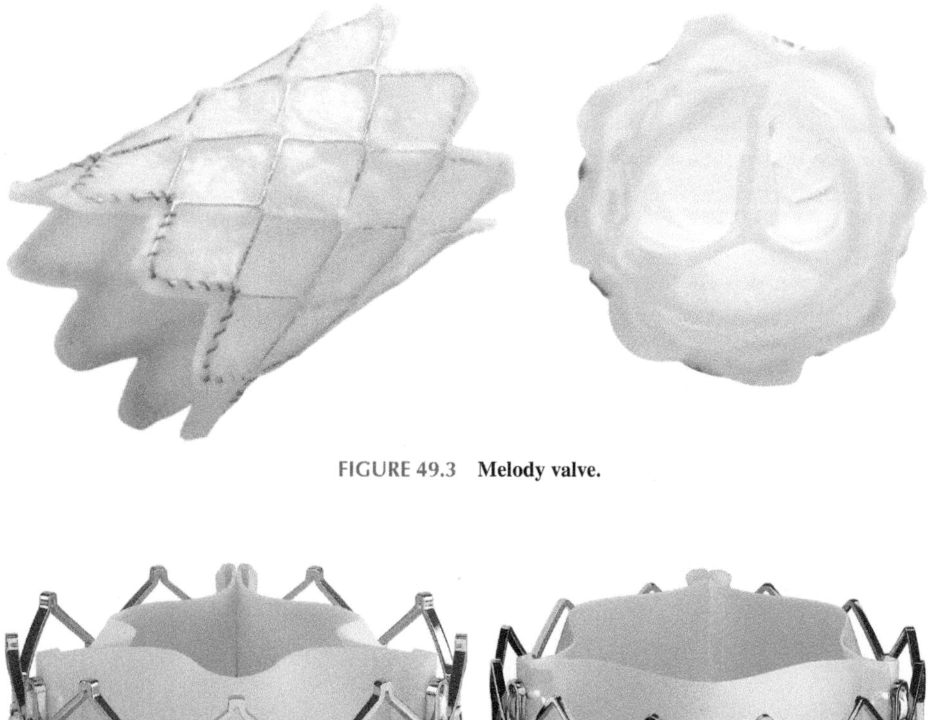

FIGURE 49.3 **Melody valve.**

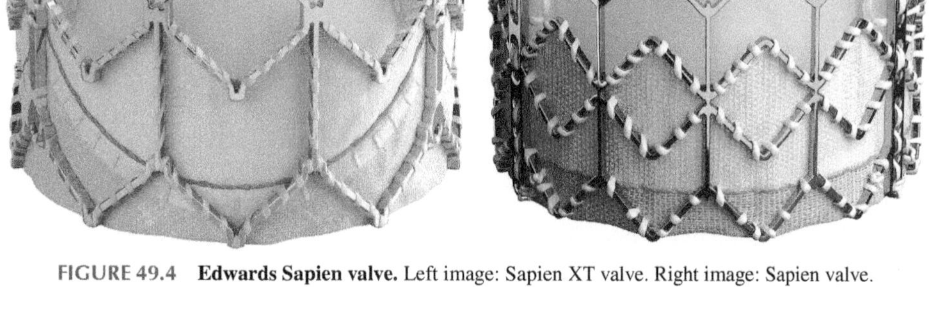

FIGURE 49.4 **Edwards Sapien valve.** Left image: Sapien XT valve. Right image: Sapien valve.

(Sapien XT, not approved in the United States) being available in diameters of 23, 26, and 29 mm. The Edwards Sapien valve is delivered using the 22-24Fr Retroflex delivery system, while the newer Sapien XT valve only requires an 18-19Fr introducer.

Patients with repaired tetralogy of Fallot and native/patched RVOT are for the most part not suitable candidates for the Edwards Sapien or Melody valves. However, a variety of recent animal and human research is focused on developing suitable transcatheter valves for this patient population [56–60].

Procedural Technique

The basic technique of transcatheter pulmonary valve implantation of the Melody and Edwards Sapien valves, using the Ensemble and the Retroflex delivery systems, has been well described and is the same, whether a patient has reduced right ventricular function (as many have) or not [52–54].

The anatomy of the main and branch pulmonary arteries should be well know from preprocedure MRI and/or CT scans, but it is nevertheless beneficial in the cath lab to obtain a rotational angiography to choose the best angles for valve/stent deployment and the relationship of MPA/conduit to the branch pulmonary arteries. This is ideally performed using a Multitrack catheter under rapid right ventricular pacing—the wire is best positioned in the left pulmonary artery, unless there is a specific need to treat any right pulmonary artery stenosis in the same setting. It is helpful to use (and precurve) a stiff wire that could also be utilized for subsequent balloon angioplasty or stent placement. Once a rotational angiography has been obtained, a biplane angiography should be performed within the MPA/Conduit/RVOT. Angles should be chosen using the aid of the reconstructed 3-dimensional (3D) rotational images, but for most patients, maximum cranial angulation on the frontal tubes, and straight lateral projection on the lateral tubes are the angles needed to open and profile the MPA/conduit. Measurements should be obtained, using the smallest and largest diameters of the MPA/conduit, as well as the distance from RVOT to PA bifurcation.

At this stage, it is important to evaluate the coronary arteries, and the operator should have at least some idea of the likelihood of potential coronary problems based on the diagnosis and previous procedures (e.g., arterial switch, single coronary artery), as well as baseline data from MRI and/or CT. Coronary compression can be identified in as much as 5% of cases during test balloon inflation, with potentially catastrophic consequences if not recognized prior to proceeding with valve implantation [61]. A baseline aortogram can be useful for comparison but is not absolutely essential. Coronary evaluation is performed by placing a very compliant balloon with diluted contrast (~20%) across the conduit, while simultaneously performing an aortogram in the ascending aorta using a projection that ideally shows the axial circumference of the balloon (usually LAO and caudal on the frontal tubes), as well as a straight lateral projection (Fig. 49.5). The balloon is inflated with a very low pressure, as the purpose is not to perform an angioplasty, but to just get an initial impression of the proximity of coronary branches to the position where later the stented valve would be placed. A sufficient distance between the inflated balloon and the coronary arteries only implies that there is no risk of coronary compression, if the balloon is fully inflated to the desired diameter of valve implantation because scar and other tissue surrounding the MPA/conduit can shift and move outward sufficiently to cause coronary problems. Therefore coronary evaluation may need to be repeated once a

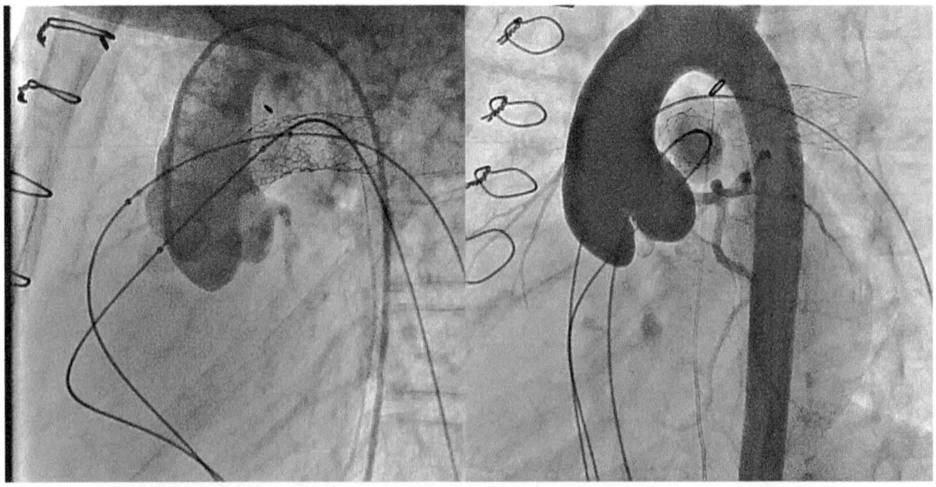

FIGURE 49.5 **Coronary evaluation prior to pulmonary valve implantation.** 17-year-old patient with a distal stenosis of a dysfunctional RVPA conduit, and bilateral pulmonary artery stents. Coronary evaluation (aortogram) during double-balloon inflation in right pulmonary artery and left pulmonary artery (no evidence of coronary compression). *RVPA*, right ventricle to pulmonary artery.

larger-diameter high-pressure balloon angioplasty of the conduit is being performed that approximates the diameter of the intended valve implantation. Equally, if an aortogram does not provide appropriate coronary imaging, the operator will have to consider selective coronary angiography.

At this point it becomes important to perform a very gradual staged angioplasty and evaluation of the conduit, with the hope that if a dissection occurs, it will be small and contained by scar tissue, rather than leading to a catastrophic injury. Even though conduit dissections occur in as much as 6% of cases, the majority is usually contained. The main risk factor for a conduit dissection has—not surprisingly—been identified as a very elevated RVOT baseline gradient [62]. A gradual expansion is best facilitated by using a high-pressure balloon with a diameter of no more than 125% of the stenotic area and no more than the diameter of the intended valve implantation. Angiographies are essential prior to upsizing the balloon gradually up to the intended diameter of valve implantation. If a conduit dissection is identified, then implantation of a covered stent is the treatment of choice. For this purpose, it is crucial to have all equipment available and ready that may be needed if a catastrophic injury were to occur. This includes a long sheath, as well as the covered stent ideally premounted over an appropriately sized balloon. If a problem does occur, this is not the time to realize that the required equipment is not available, or to waste important time gathering the needed equipment.

Once angioplasty of the conduit has been performed up to the intended diameter of valve implantation, the operator should consider prestenting of the conduit. Irrespective of the degree of stenosis, this is a necessary prerequisite for implantation of the Edwards Sapien valve due to the short stent height, to create a suitable landing zone. For most patients undergoing Melody valve implantation within a conduit (not a bioprosthetic valve), prestenting is equally required to reduce the incidence of stent fractures, which have been reported in as much as 25% of cases over a median follow-up of 30 month [63]. Large diameter stents that are suitable for prestenting include the Palmaz XL stents (Cordis, Fremont, California) as well as the Andra stent XXL (Andramed, Reutlingen, Germany). The operator should also document and play close attention to the balloon deflation, as it will show whether there is still residual dynamic compression of the stent. If the difference in diameters between balloon inflation and deflation is more than 0.5 mm, then adding additional stents should be considered to reduce the chance of stent fractures of the Melody valve stent. It is also important to also adjust the camera angles to document whether a circular shape of the stents is being maintained after balloon deflation, the lack of which has been significantly associated with the risk of stent fractures [64]. The results from the US Melody valve trial documented a freedom from diagnosis of stent fracture of 77% at 14 month, and 60% at 30 month. On multivariate analysis, prestenting, presence of a previous stent, or implantation within a prosthetic valve were associated with a longer freedom from stent fracture, while a compressed conduit, severely obstructed RVOT, or position directly behind the anterior chest wall had the opposite effect [63].

Once the conduit has been adequately prestented, valve implantation is performed according to the previously described techniques [52–54]. Advancing the delivery system across the landing zone can be tricky for both valve types. On occasions this can be aided by gently adjusting the wire position and/or (quickly) buckling the entire assembly within the right atrium (Fig. 49.6). As a last-resort bailout, operators can consider pulling back the stiff wire that may allow the assembly to pop forward once the stiff wire is pulled back and then this could be replaced with a softer glide wire. This, however, is only a last-resort bailout technique and should only be considered if the operator is in a situation where the valve is in suboptimal position for deployment and cannot be pulled back or recaptured. If needed, the Melody valve can be implanted using a 24 mm BiB balloon and a standard 22Fr delivery sheath, which is technically more challenging than using the more flexible Ensemble delivery system. However, it is not associated with any significant pulmonary insufficiency [65]. If the Melody valve needs to be implanted in a distal conduit stenosis, a Flower-Blossom technique or the use of a stent implanted into a branch pulmonary artery (jailing the other branch with subsequent strut breakage) can be utilized (Fig. 49.6) [66,67]. For very short conduits, the Melody valve can be folded and still utilized with the Ensemble delivery system [68,69].

If needed, the Melody valve can be implanted at 24 mm using a standard BiB balloon and a long sheath, even though the Sapien valve is usually the better option for larger implantation diameters [65]. Even though the presently available transcatheter valves were not designed to be implanted in patients with repaired tetralogy of Fallot and a native/patched RVOT, it can be considered in selected patients [43–46]. Boudjemline and colleagues described technical modifications that may be helpful, such as implantation of multiple coaxial stents to reduce the diameter ("Russian Doll Technique"), or anchoring multiple overlapping stents in one of the branch pulmonary arteries to create a landing zone [44].

Following valve implantation and a final hemodynamic and angiographic evaluation, intracardiac echocardiography should be performed, which has been shown to be an excellent tool to evaluate leaflet mobility and degree of regurgitation directly after valve implantation (Fig. 49.7) [70,71]. In addition, documenting the stent in various cine projections at the end of the procedure is a good practice and can provide reference data that can be useful for subsequent follow-up.

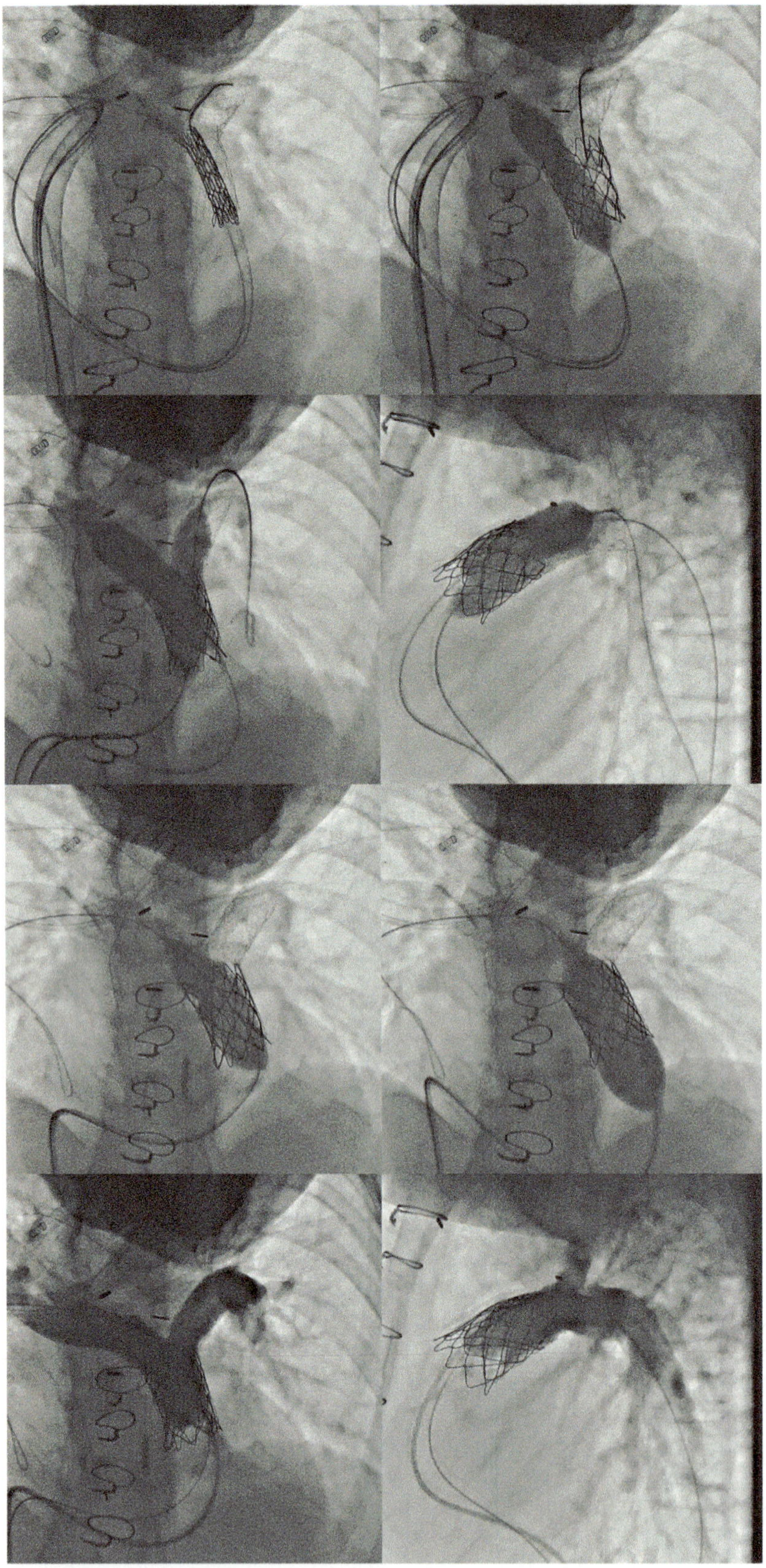

FIGURE 49.6 **Melody valve implantation using a Flower-Blossom Technique.** 17-year-old patient with a distal stenosis of a dysfunctional RVPA conduit and bilateral pulmonary artery stents. After presenting with a Palmaz XL stent using a Flower-Blossom technique, the same technique was utilized for Melody valve implantation. Top left: Melody valve positioned on two 12mm×4cm ZMedII balloons, initially positioned using a 22Fr long sheath (now in RA). The RPA wire had to be exchanged to an 0.035″ angled glide wire and the LPA wire pulled back with the sheath retracted to the RA to allow the valve to be freed from the in situ XL stent and to be appropriately positioned distally. Top right: expansion of the Melody valve on two 12mm×4cm ZMedII balloons—the LPA balloon unintentionally did not have any contrast and is only faintly visible (but the distal marker can be noted). Second row: double-balloon angioplasty of the Melody valve using a 14mm×4cm ZMedII balloon to the RPA and a 12mm×4cm ZMedII balloon to the LPA. Third row: expansion of the Melody valve using a single 20mm×3cm ZMedII balloon—note the positioning of the balloon at the beginning of the inflation (left) and at the end (right) clearly documenting that mounting the Melody on a single larger balloon would have led to the valve being implanted significantly within the RVOT, due to the limitations by the distal smaller diameter stents in the branch PAs. Bottom row: angiography after Melody valve implantation documenting no significant pulmonary insufficiency and no residual angiographic narrowing. *LPA*, left pulmonary artery; *PAs*, pulmonary arteries; *RPA*, right pulmonary artery; *RVOT*, right ventricular outflow tract; *RVPA*, right ventricle to pulmonary artery.

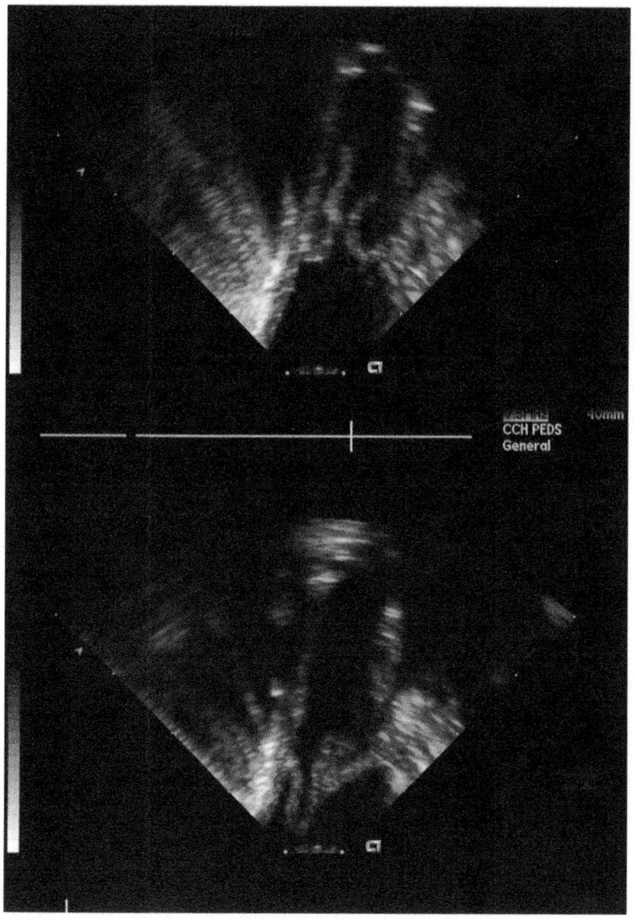

FIGURE 49.7 **Intracardiac echocardiography for evaluation of the pulmonary valve.** Baseline intracardiac echocardiography prior to considering Melody valve implantation. Top image: leaflets of the CoreMatrix conduit opening into the conduit (systole). Bottom image: the leaflets prolapsing into the right ventricular outflow tract.

Outcome

In general, the outcome of transcatheter pulmonary valve implantation has been good with results comparable if not superior to surgical pulmonary valve implantation. Recent surgical results have documented the in-hospital mortality rate and rate of major adverse events after surgical pulmonary valve replacement to be 0.9% and 2.2% using the STS congenital heart surgery database, and 4.1% and 20.9% using the STS adult cardiac surgery database [72]. In another recent study, the 5, 10, and 15-year freedom from pulmonary valve reintervention after surgical valve replacement in patients with repaired tetralogy of Fallot has been reported to be 97%, 85%, and 75% [73]. A Metaanalysis of results after surgical pulmonary valve replacement reported an early mortality of 2.1% and a later mortality of 0.5% per patient-year, with a redo rate for pulmonary valve replacement of 1.9% per patient-year [74].

While long-term data are still lacking, short-term data on transcatheter pulmonary valve implantation are encouraging. In general procedural mortality to discharge is rare, and most studies report do not report any acute procedural mortality [53]. Using data from the original US IDE trial, Cheatham and colleagues reported a 5-year freedom from reintervention and explantation of 76% and 92%, with conduit prestenting and a lower discharge RVOT gradient being associated with a longer freedom from reintervention [75]. Over a median follow-up of 4.5 years almost all patients were in New York Heart Association (NYHA) class I or II. Data from the Italian Society of Cardiology documented early major complications in 11% and freedom from valve failure over a median follow-up of 30 months of 81.4% [76].

Very similar results to the Melody valve were seen with the Edwards valve, with Faza and colleagues reporting no significant difference in immediate residual gradients and no difference in pulmonary insufficiency on follow-up when comparing the two transcatheter valve implantations [77]. Stent fracture though does not appear to be a problem after implantation of the Edwards Sapien valve [78].

Some of the most common major complications after transcatheter valve implantation include pulmonary hemorrhage as a result of the use of the stiff guide wires, as well as valve malposition or migration. Less frequently reported complications include hyperacute flash pulmonary edema, cardiomyopathy, as well as melody valve erosion into the ascending aorta [79–82].

Melody valve endocarditis, while usually not an acute procedural problem, has been reported to be a significant concern on follow-up of these patients, with abrupt Aspirin discontinuation and unprotected additional procedures being significant risk factors for Melody valve endocarditis [83–87]. McElhinney and colleagues reported an annualized rate of a first episode of infective endocarditis of 2.4% and freedom from transcatheter pulmonary valve–related endocarditis of 97% at 4 years [86].

TRANSCATHETER TREATMENT FOR RHEUMATIC MITRAL VALVE STENOSIS

Background

Rheumatic heart disease continues to be endemic in developing countries where isolated mitral valve stenosis (MS) occurs in 40% of affected patients. On the other hand, the incidence of MS continues to decrease in industrialized countries probably due to improved hygienic standards and routine use of antibiotics for acute pharyngitis [88,89]. Rheumatic fever is caused by beta-hemolytic group A streptococcus that leads to the formation of antibodies, which attack valve tissues due to cross-reactivity with some heart valve components leading to valvular injury. Nearly all cases of rheumatic MS involve commissural fusion along with thickening and restricted mobility of the mitral leaflets. The chordae tendineae are typically involved as well with variable degrees of fibrosis, thickening, shortening, and calcification.

The normal mitral valve area (MVA) is typically 4.0–5.0 cm^2 with symptoms usually developing with a valve area less than 2.5 cm^2. Obstruction of the blood flow across the mitral valve results in an increase in the pressure within the left atrium, pulmonary vasculature, and right side of the heart. The LV is typically spared in isolated mitral stenosis with no effect on its size or function. Presenting symptoms may vary depending on the severity of MS. Symptoms may include exertional dyspnea, hemoptysis, and chest pain. Any situation that increases cardiac output or causes tachycardia can markedly increase the transmitral pressure gradient precipitating symptoms. It is important to note that many patients with severe MS may not manifest any symptoms because of the slow progression of the disease accompanied by the gradual reduction in activity. The chronic rise in left atrial pressure ultimately leads to atrial dilatation and fibrillation and along with this comes the sequela of atrial thrombi formation. Additionally, chronic pulmonary hypertension may eventually lead to right heart failure manifesting with peripheral edema and hepatomegaly.

Patient Selection

The goal of management of MS is to control symptoms and to prevent the complications of mitral stenosis. Percutaneous mitral balloon valvuloplasty (PMBV) is an important therapeutic tool in treating rheumatic mitral stenosis by improving the valve orifice through splitting of the fused mitral commissures. In patients with favorable valve morphology the procedure can be performed with a high success rate (>90%), low complication rate (<3%), and a sustained improvement in 80%–90% over a 3–7 year follow-up period [90]. To yield good outcome, patients selected for PMBV should meet both clinical and anatomical criteria. The 2014 ACC/AHA guidelines for valvular heart disease give a Class I recommendation for PMBV in symptomatic patients with severe mitral stenosis (MVA ≤1.5 cm^2 (Stage D)) in the presence of favorable anatomy [91]. It may also be considered for symptomatic patients with MVA >1.5 cm^2 if there is evidence of hemodynamically significant MS during exercise (Class IIb). PMBV is particularly useful in treating the symptomatic pregnant woman with critical mitral stenosis and refractory heart failure with fewer fetal and neonatal complications compared to surgical commissurotomy [92]. It can also be a lifesaving procedure in patients with severe mitral stenosis who have suboptimal valve anatomy and are not candidates for surgery.

Asymptomatic patients should also be considered for PMBV when they develop pulmonary hypertension (pulmonary artery systolic pressure >50 mmHg at rest or >60 mmHg with exercise) (Class IIa) or new-onset atrial fibrillation (Class IIb), as these conditions reflect the severity of underlying valvular disease.

In addition to meeting clinical indications, patients have to fulfill several anatomical criteria to qualify for PMBV. Favorable valve morphology is fundamental in predicting immediate outcome and follow-up results of PMBV. Currently, the echocardiographic score described by Wilkins is the most widely used and validated method for the evaluation of the morphologic characteristics of the mitral valve apparatus. This score grades the morphologic features of the mitral valve that include leaflet mobility, leaflet thickening, valve calcification, and subvalvular thickening, each of which is graded in a 0–4 scale (Table 49.1) [93]. An echocardiographic score ≤8 is considered the optimal cut-off point to predict a favorable outcome to PMBV; however, patients with higher echocardiographic score (>8) should not be excluded as these patients require individualized approach. It is also critical to ensure that significant mitral regurgitation is excluded; nevertheless, PMBV may be carried out in selected patients with moderate mitral regurgitation if the risk of surgery is high. Additionally, mitral valvuloplasty should not be carried out in the presence of left atrial appendage thrombus because of the risk of thrombus dislodgement during the procedure.

TABLE 49.1 Echocardiographic Score System of the Mitral Valve

Characteristic	Score	Description
Leaflet mobility	1	Highly mobile valve with only leaflet tips restricted
	2	Mid and base leaflet portions have normal mobility
	3	Valve continues to move forward in diastole, mainly at base
	4	No or minimal forward movement of leaflets in diastole
Leaflet thickening	1	Leaflets near normal in thickness (4–5 mm)
	2	Mid leaflets normal, thickening of margins (5–8 mm)
	3	Entire leaflet thickening (5–8 mm)
	4	Considerable thickening of entire leaflet (>8–19 mm)
Leaflet calcification	1	A single area of increased echo brightness
	2	Scattered areas of brightness confined to leaflet margins
	3	Brightness extending into the midportion of leaflets
	4	Extensive brightness throughout the leaflet
Subvalvular thickening	1	Minimal thickening just below the mitral leaflets
	2	Thickening of chordae extending up to one-third of chordal length
	3	Thickening extending to the distal third of the chordae
	4	Extensive thickening and shortening of chordae extending to the papillary muscles

Adapted from Abascal, Wilkins, prediction of successful outcome in 130 patients undergoing percutaneous balloon mitral valvotomy.

Procedural Background

The idea of balloon dilatation of the mitral valve was first introduced in 1984 by Dr. Kanji Inoue, a Japanese cardiac surgeon, who developed a technique as a logical extension of surgical closed commissurotomy using a balloon made of strong yet pliant rubber [94]. This balloon functions by changing its shape in three stages, depending on the extent of inflation (see below). This initial work set the stage for the first human percutaneous transseptal mitral balloon valvuloplasty to be performed in India by Dr. James Lock using cylindrically shaped balloon [95]. Soon thereafter, in 1985, Drs. Igor Palacios and Peter Block performed the first US human PMBV at Massachusetts General Hospital in Boston. Subsequently, the idea of a double-balloon technique was introduced from Saudi Arabia as a potential alternative method for balloon commissurotomy [96]. The double balloon required that two guide wires be positioned in the left ventricular apex, through which two floating balloon catheters are then advanced across the mitral valve orifice. Although this technique is effective, it is more technically demanding with similar efficacy when compared with the single Inoue balloon [97]. Today, PMBV using Inoue balloon has largely replaced surgical mitral valvulotomy and is the treatment of choice for patients with rheumatic mitral stenosis with favorable anatomy in most parts of the world.

Procedural Technique

Prior to considering any patient for transcatheter intervention for a stenotic mitral valve, it is important to have detailed and accurate echocardiographic data available, including 3D echocardiography if available. Furthermore, echocardiographic guidance is crucial during the procedure to be able to evaluate the mitral valve continuously. Hemodynamic and echocardiographic assessments need to be performed in the catheterization laboratory at baseline and after each valvuloplasty.

Mitral valvuloplasty is usually performed using an antegrade femoral venous approach through the atrial septum. Variety of techniques have been described of which the Inoue balloon is the most widely used. Other techniques include the passage of two balloons through two large transseptal sheaths, the passage of two balloons over separate guide wires without long sheaths and without the need for specific dilation of the septum, as well as a double-balloon technique using a Multitrack system over a single guide wire (NuMED, Hopkinton, New York) [98]. These techniques are seldom used nowadays.

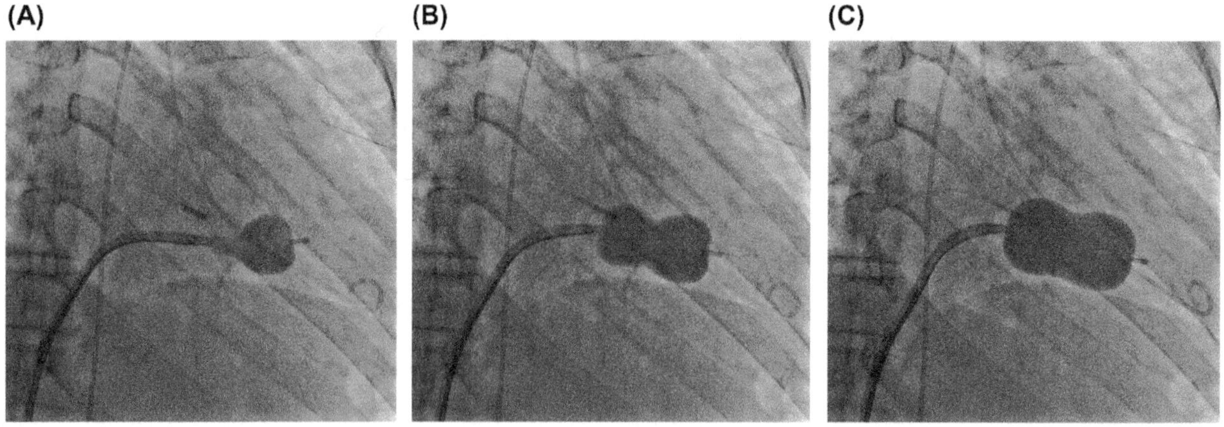

FIGURE 49.8 **The Inoue balloon.** Percutaneous balloon mitral valvuloplasty using the Inoue technique. (A–C) Sequential inflation of the Inoue balloon across the mitral valve.

The Inoue balloon (Toray Industries, Houston, Texas) is a custom-made hourglass-shaped balloon that specifically facilitates balloon valvuloplasty using a single balloon technique without the use of a guide wire in the LV. Its use has demonstrated success in treating rheumatic MS [94]. The balloon has three distinct parts, each with a specific elasticity, enabling them to be inflated sequentially, which allows fast and stable positioning across the valve. The Inoue balloon is available in three sizes (26, 28, and 30 mm); each size can be varied by up to 4 mm as needed.

Following transseptal access into the left atrium, a stiff guide wire is inserted in the left atrium followed by predilatation of the atrial septum using the provided 14 French dilator. A balloon catheter selected according to the patient's height is then advanced into the left atrium (26 mm in very small patients or children, 28 mm in patients shorter than 180 cm, and 30 mm in patients taller than 180 cm). After insertion of the stylet, the distal portion of the balloon is inflated slightly to act as a floating balloon when crossing the mitral valve. Once in the LV, the distal portion is further inflated then pulled back into the mitral orifice. Inflation then occurs in the proximal portion and finally in the central part of the balloon until the central waist disappears at full inflation (Fig. 49.8 A–C). It is recommended that the first inflation occurs initially 4 mm below the maximal balloon size, and the balloon size is then increased in 1 mm increments as needed. The end of the procedure is dictated by achieving an adequate valve area or worsening in the degree of mitral regurgitation.

When using a double-balloon technique, the left atrium is entered and one or two separate transseptal punctures are made. Exchange wires are manipulated from the right atrium through previously positioned catheters or long sheaths across the septum, across the mitral valve, and into the LV with the "transition" and floppy portions of the wires looped in the ventricle. It is important to remember that if a guide wire is to be used for balloon dilation, a balloon-tipped end-hole catheter should be initially directed from the left atrium across the mitral valve to lessen the chance of crossing between chordal attachments. Once the wires are in place, either the two long sheath/dilator sets or the two separate "uncovered" balloons are passed over the wires into the left atrium. The balloons are advanced and positioned across the mitral valve. The sheaths are withdrawn off the balloons, and the balloons are simultaneously inflated. Again, longer balloons (5–6 cm in older children and adolescents) help to stabilize during inflation. The sum of the two balloon diameters equals the measured or estimated maximal normal mitral valve diameter for a patient of that particular body size. The two balloons allow an adequate total balloon diameter for the much larger mitral annulus without causing injury to the entry veins or atrial septum during balloon passage. As with any interventional catheterization, these patients require anticoagulation with heparin.

Procedural complications are low and occur more frequently in patients with echo score >8, supporting the importance of appropriate patient selection. The failure rates range from 1% to 17% and are mainly related to the steep learning curve. Procedural mortality is uncommon with main causes related to left ventricular perforation or the poor health condition of the patient. Severe mitral regurgitation is the most worrisome complication and occurs in 2%–10% of patients as a result of noncommissural leaflet tearing [90,99]. The incidence of hemopericardium varies from 0.5% to 12%, and systemic embolism is encountered in 0.5%–5% of cases. Overall, the rate of procedural complications is directly related to operator experience with fewer complications in centers with high number of procedures [100].

Outcome

Successful mitral valvuloplasty for rheumatic mitral stenosis usually provides immediate hemodynamic improvement with increase in valve area, rapid reduction in left atrial pressure, and gradual improvement in pulmonary arterial pressure and pulmonary vascular resistance. The most widely accepted definition for an ideal result is a final valve area >1.5 cm^2 in the absence of more than +2 mitral regurgitation.

Typically if the initial valvuloplasty is successful, the survival rate is excellent with improvement in functional status and infrequent need for secondary intervention. The United States National Heart, Lung, and Blood Institute (NHLBI) Balloon Valvuloplasty Registry evaluated 736 patients over the age of 18 who were followed for 4 years; the survival rate and event-free survival (freedom from death, mitral valve surgery, or repeat PMBV) were 84% and 60%, respectively [101]. Multivariate predictors of mortality in this registry were functional NYHA class IV, higher echocardiography valve score, and higher postprocedural pulmonary artery systolic and LVEDP. The incidence of restenosis following successful valvuloplasty is usually low. In a study of 912 patients followed for a median of 12 years following PMBV, 38% of patients required reintervention, surgery was performed in 266 patients and repeat balloon valvuloplasty in 85 patients. The cardiovascular survival for the population who underwent repeat valvuloplasty was 60% at 10 years [102]. These data support the concept that PMBV is an effective therapy for MS and that a repeat valvuloplasty may allow further delay in surgery. Clinical outcomes following PMBV have been compared with outcomes following surgical commissurotomy in several randomized trials [103–106]. The outcome after PMBV was as good as or even better than after surgery in patients who are candidates for valvuloplasty.

REFERENCES

[1] B.S. Hasan, D.B. McElhinney, D.W. Brown, et al., Short-term performance of the transcatheter Melody valve in high-pressure hemodynamic environments in the pulmonary and systemic circulations, Circ. Cardiovasc. Interv. 4 (6) (December 1, 2011) 615–620.

[2] N. Wilson, Aortic valve morphology is associated with outcomes following balloon valvuloplasty for congenital aortic stenosis: reflection on morphological retrospection aids selection for interventional rejection, Catheter. Cardiovasc. Interv. 81 (1) (January 1, 2013) 96.

[3] S.A. Maskatia, H. Justino, F.F. Ing, M.A. Crystal, R.J. Mattamal, C.J. Petit, Aortic valve morphology is associated with outcomes following balloon valvuloplasty for congenital aortic stenosis, Catheter. Cardiovasc. Interv. 81 (1) (January 1, 2013) 90–95.

[4] T.F. Feltes, E. Bacha, R.H. Beekman 3rd, et al., Indications for cardiac catheterization and intervention in pediatric cardiac disease: a scientific statement from the American Heart Association, Circulation 123 (22) (June 7, 2011) 2607–2652.

[5] Z. Lababidi, J.R. Wu, J.T. Walls, Percutaneous balloon aortic valvuloplasty: results in 23 patients, Am. J. Cardiol. 53 (1) (January 1, 1984) 194–197.

[6] A.C. Polimenakos, S. Sathanandam, C. Elzein, M.J. Barth, R.S. Higgins, M.N. Ilbawi, Aortic cusp extension valvuloplasty with or without tricuspidization in children and adolescents: long-term results and freedom from aortic valve replacement, J. Thorac. Cardiovasc. Surg. 139 (4) (April 2010) 933–941 discussion 941.

[7] D.W. Brown, A.E. Dipilato, E.C. Chong, J.E. Lock, D.B. McElhinney, Aortic valve reinterventions after balloon aortic valvuloplasty for congenital aortic stenosis intermediate and late follow-up, J. Am. Coll. Cardiol. 56 (21) (November 16, 2010) 1740–1749.

[8] S.M. Prijic, V.A. Vukomanovic, M.S. Stajevic, et al., Balloon dilation and surgical valvotomy comparison in non-critical congenital aortic valve stenosis, Pediatr. Cardiol. 36 (3) (March 2015) 616–624.

[9] S.A. Maskatia, F.F. Ing, H. Justino, et al., Twenty-five year experience with balloon aortic valvuloplasty for congenital aortic stenosis, Am. J. Cardiol. 108 (7) (October 1, 2011) 1024–1028.

[10] J.W. Brown, M.D. Rodefeld, M. Ruzmetov, O. Eltayeb, O. Yurdakok, M.W. Turrentine, Surgical valvuloplasty versus balloon aortic dilation for congenital aortic stenosis: are evidence-based outcomes relevant? Ann. Thorac. Surg. 94 (1) (July 2012) 146–153 discussion 153–145.

[11] S. Deo, K.L. Greason, R. Gulati, A.S. Jaffe, D.R. Holmes, Balloon aortic valvuloplasty under temporary mechanical circulatory support as a bridge to aortic valve replacement in a patient with hemodynamic failure secondary to critical aortic valve stenosis, Heart Surg. Forum 15 (3) (June 2012) E177–E179.

[12] S. Hadjimiltiades, A. Ziakas, G. Kazinakis, C. Nikolaidou, K. Anastasiadis, H. Karvounis, Avulsion of an aortic cusp during aortic balloon valvuloplasty, JACC 8 (2) (February 2015) e15–e16.

[13] D.W. Kim, A.A. Raviele, R.N. Vincent, Use of a 3 French system for balloon aortic valvuloplasty in infants, Catheter. Cardiovasc. Interv. 66 (2) (October 2005) 254–257.

[14] A. Akin, H.H. Aykan, T. Karagoz, Antegrade balloon valvuloplasty for critical aortic stenosis in a premature neonate weighing 1100 g, Turk. J. Pediatr. 56 (1) (January–February 2014) 115–117.

[15] S. Patel, A.P. Saini, A. Nair, H.S. Weber, Transcarotid balloon valvuloplasty in neonates and small infants with critical aortic valve stenosis utilizing continuous transesophageal echocardiographic guidance: a 22 year single center experience from the cath lab to the bedside, Catheter. Cardiovasc. Interv. 86 (5) (November 2015) 821–827.

[16] R.I. Rossi, J.L. Manica, R. Petraco, M. Scott, L. Piazza, P.M. Machado, Balloon aortic valvuloplasty for congenital aortic stenosis using the femoral and the carotid artery approach: a 16-year experience from a single center, Catheter. Cardiovasc. Interv. 78 (1) (July 1, 2011) 84–90.

[17] A. Baykan, M. Argun, S.S. Sezer, H. Ceyran, N. Narin, Transapical aortic balloon valvuloplasty in a 6-year-old child with unsuccessful retrograde approach, Cardiol. Young 23 (1) (February 2013) 129–131.

[18] X.B. Pan, F.W. Zhang, S.S. Hu, et al., Hybrid balloon valvuloplasty through the ascending aorta via median sternotomy in infants with severe congenital valvular aortic stenosis: feasibility of a new method dagger, Eur. J. Cardiothorac. Surg. 47 (6) (June 2015) 1003–1005.

[19] N. Maschietto, V. Vida, O. Milanesi, Transapical aortic balloon valvuloplasty in a 890-gram infant: hybrid is better!, Catheter. Cardiovasc. Interv. 77 (1) (January 1, 2011) 112–114.

[20] I. Daehnert, C. Rotzsch, M. Wiener, P. Schneider, Rapid right ventricular pacing is an alternative to adenosine in catheter interventional procedures for congenital heart disease, Heart 90 (9) (2004) 1047–1050.

[21] C. Witzke, C.W. Don, R.J. Cubeddu, et al., Impact of rapid ventricular pacing during percutaneous balloon aortic valvuloplasty in patients with critical aortic stenosis: should we be using it? Catheter. Cardiovasc. Interv. 75 (3) (February 15, 2010) 444–452.

[22] S.D. Gupta, S. Das, T. Ghose, A. Sarkar, A. Goswami, S. Kundu, Controlled transient respiratory arrest along with rapid right ventricular pacing for improving balloon stability during balloon valvuloplasty in pediatric patients with congenital aortic stenosis–a retrospective case series analysis, Ann. Card. Anaesth. 13 (3) (September–December 2010) 236–240.

[23] A. Torres, J.A. Vincent, A. Everett, et al., Balloon valvuloplasty for congenital aortic stenosis: multi-center safety and efficacy outcome assessment, Catheter. Cardiovasc. Interv. 86 (5) (November 2015) 808–820.

[24] P. Ewert, H. Bertram, J. Breuer, et al., Balloon valvuloplasty in the treatment of congenital aortic valve stenosis–a retrospective multicenter survey of more than 1000 patients, Int. J. Cardiol. 149 (2) (June 2, 2011) 182–185.

[25] C.J. Petit, F.F. Ing, R. Mattamal, R.H. Pignatelli, C.E. Mullins, H. Justino, Diminished left ventricular function is associated with poor mid-term outcomes in neonates after balloon aortic valvuloplasty, Catheter. Cardiovasc. Interv. 80 (7) (December 1, 2012) 1190–1199.

[26] D. Porras, D.W. Brown, R. Rathod, et al., Acute outcomes after introduction of a standardized clinical assessment and management plan (SCAMP) for balloon aortic valvuloplasty in congenital aortic stenosis, Congenit. Heart Dis. 9 (4) (July–August 2014) 316–325.

[27] R.J. Holzer, M. Sisk, A. Phillips, Hybrid balloon pulmonary valvuloplasty in a 700-g infant: thinking outside the box, Catheter. Cardiovasc. Interv. 72 (1) (July 1, 2008) 93–96.

[28] B.W. McCrindle, Independent predictors of long-term results after balloon pulmonary valvuloplasty. Valvuloplasty and Angioplasty of Congenital Anomalies (VACA) Registry Investigators, Circulation 89 (4) (April 1994) 1751–1759.

[29] R.J. Holzer, K. Gauvreau, J. Kreutzer, et al., Safety and efficacy of balloon pulmonary valvuloplasty: a multicenter experience, Catheter. Cardiovasc. Interv. 80 (4) (October 1, 2012) 663–672.

[30] M.E. Fawzy, W. Hassan, B.M. Fadel, et al., Long-term results (up to 17 years) of pulmonary balloon valvuloplasty in adults and its effects on concomitant severe infundibular stenosis and tricuspid regurgitation, Am. Heart J. 153 (3) (March 2007) 433–438.

[31] M.E. Fawzy, O. Galal, B. Dunn, A. Shaikh, R. Sriram, C.M. Duran, Regression of infundibular pulmonary stenosis after successful balloon pulmonary valvuloplasty in adults, Catheter. Cardiovasc. Diagn. 21 (2) (October 1990) 77–81.

[32] M. Jarrar, F. Betbout, M.B. Farhat, et al., Long-term invasive and noninvasive results of percutaneous balloon pulmonary valvuloplasty in children, adolescents, and adults, Am. Heart J. 138 (5 Pt 1) (1999) 950–954.

[33] P.S. Rao, O. Galal, M. Patnana, S.H. Buck, A.D. Wilson, Results of three to 10 year follow up of balloon dilatation of the pulmonary valve, Heart 80 (6) (1998) 591–595.

[34] P. Stanger, S.C. Cassidy, D.A. Girod, J.S. Kan, Z. Lababidi, S.R. Shapiro, Balloon pulmonary valvuloplasty: results of the Valvuloplasty and Angioplasty of Congenital Anomalies Registry, Am. J. Cardiol. 65 (11) (1990) 775–783.

[35] R. Merino-Ingelmo, J. Santos-de Soto, F. Coserria-Sanchez, A. Descalzo-Senoran, I. Valverde-Perez, Long-term results of percutaneous balloon valvuloplasty in pulmonary valve stenosis in the pediatric population, Revista espanola de cardiologia 67 (5) (May 2014) 374–379.

[36] M.L. O'Byrne, A.C. Glatz, L. Mercer-Rosa, et al., Trends in pulmonary valve replacement in children and adults with tetralogy of fallot, Am. J. Cardiol. 115 (1) (January 1, 2015) 118–124.

[37] M.A. Quail, A. Frigiola, A. Giardini, et al., Impact of pulmonary valve replacement in tetralogy of Fallot with pulmonary regurgitation: a comparison of intervention and nonintervention, Ann. Thorac. Surg. 94 (5) (November 2012) 1619–1626.

[38] H. Baumgartner, P. Bonhoeffer, N.M. De Groot, et al., ESC Guidelines for the management of grown-up congenital heart disease (new version 2010), Eur. Heart J. 31 (23) (December 2010) 2915–2957.

[39] C.K. Silversides, M. Kiess, L. Beauchesne, et al., Canadian Cardiovascular Society 2009 Consensus Conference on the management of adults with congenital heart disease: outflow tract obstruction, coarctation of the aorta, tetralogy of Fallot, Ebstein anomaly and Marfan's syndrome, Can. J. Cardiol. 26 (3) (March 2010) e80–97.

[40] C.A. Warnes, R.G. Williams, T.M. Bashore, et al., ACC/AHA 2008 Guidelines for the Management of Adults with Congenital Heart Disease: a report of the American College of Cardiology/American Heart Association Task Force on Practice Guidelines (writing committee to develop guidelines on the management of adults with congenital heart disease), Circulation 118 (23) (December 2, 2008) e714–833.

[41] C. Lee, Y.M. Kim, C.H. Lee, et al., Outcomes of pulmonary valve replacement in 170 patients with chronic pulmonary regurgitation after relief of right ventricular outflow tract obstruction: implications for optimal timing of pulmonary valve replacement, J. Am. Coll. Cardiol. 60 (11) (September 11, 2012) 1005–1014.

[42] D.W. Brown, D.B. McElhinney, P.A. Araoz, et al., Reliability and accuracy of echocardiographic right heart evaluation in the U.S. Melody Valve Investigational Trial, J. Am. Soc. Echocardiogr. 25 (4) (April 2012) 383–392 e384.

[43] J.J. Meadows, P.M. Moore, D.P. Berman, et al., Use and performance of the Melody Transcatheter Pulmonary Valve in native and postsurgical, nonconduit right ventricular outflow tracts, Circ. Cardiovasc. Interv. 7 (3) (June 2014) 374–380.

[44] Y. Boudjemline, G. Brugada, I. Van-Aerschot, et al., Outcomes and safety of transcatheter pulmonary valve replacement in patients with large patched right ventricular outflow tracts, Arch. Cardiovasc. Dis. 105 (8–9) (August–September 2012) 404–413.

[45] P. Guccione, O. Milanesi, Z.M. Hijazi, G. Pongiglione, Transcatheter pulmonary valve implantation in native pulmonary outflow tract using the Edwards SAPIEN transcatheter heart valve, Eur. J. Cardiothorac. Surg. 41 (5) (May 2012) 1192–1194.

[46] R.A. Bertels, N.A. Blom, M.J. Schalij, Edwards SAPIEN transcatheter heart valve in native pulmonary valve position, Heart 96 (9) (May 2010) 661.

[47] D.P. Berman, D.B. McElhinney, J.A. Vincent, W.E. Hellenbrand, E.M. Zahn, Feasibility and short-term outcomes of percutaneous transcatheter pulmonary valve replacement in small (<30 kg) children with dysfunctional right ventricular outflow tract conduits, Circ. Cardiovasc. Interv. 7 (2) (April 2014) 142–148.

[48] N. Holoshitz, M.N. Ilbawi, Z. Amin, Perventricular Melody valve implantation in a 12 kg child, Catheter. Cardiovasc. Interv. 82 (5) (November 1, 2013) 824–827.

[49] K.E. Simpson, C.B. Huddleston, S. Foerster, R. Nicholas, D. Balzer, Successful subxyphoid hybrid approach for placement of a Melody percutaneous pulmonary valve, Catheter. Cardiovasc. Interv. 78 (1) (July 1, 2011) 108–111.

[50] R.J. Cubeddu, Z.M. Hijazi, Bailout perventricular pulmonary valve implantation following failed percutaneous attempt using the Edwards Sapien transcatheter heart valve, Catheter. Cardiovasc. Interv. 77 (2) (February 1, 2011) 276–280.

[51] Z.M. Hijazi, C.E. Ruiz, E. Zahn, et al., SCAI/AATS/ACC/STS operator and institutional requirements for transcatheter valve repair and replacement, part III: pulmonic valve, J. Am. Coll. Cardiol. 65 (23) (June 16, 2015) 2556–2563.

[52] P. Bonhoeffer, Y. Boudjemline, Z. Saliba, et al., Percutaneous replacement of pulmonary valve in a right-ventricle to pulmonary-artery prosthetic conduit with valve dysfunction, Lancet 356 (9239) (2000) 1403–1405.

[53] E.M. Zahn, W.E. Hellenbrand, J.E. Lock, D.B. McElhinney, Implantation of the melody transcatheter pulmonary valve in patients with a dysfunctional right ventricular outflow tract conduit early results from the u.s. Clinical trial, J. Am. Coll. Cardiol. 54 (18) (October 27, 2009) 1722–1729.

[54] F. Garay, J. Webb, Z.M. Hijazi, Percutaneous replacement of pulmonary valve using the Edwards-Cribier percutaneous heart valve: first report in a human patient, Catheter. Cardiovasc. Interv. 67 (5) (May 2006) 659–662.

[55] D. Kenny, Z.M. Hijazi, S. Kar, et al., Percutaneous implantation of the Edwards SAPIEN transcatheter heart valve for conduit failure in the pulmonary position: early phase 1 results from an international multicenter clinical trial, J. Am. Coll. Cardiol. 58 (21) (November 15, 2011) 2248–2256.

[56] Y. Boudjemline, S. Schievano, C. Bonnet, et al., Off-pump replacement of the pulmonary valve in large right ventricular outflow tracts: a hybrid approach, J. Thorac. Cardiovasc. Surg. 129 (4) (April 2005) 831–837.

[57] T. Attmann, R. Quaden, T. Jahnke, et al., Percutaneous pulmonary valve replacement: 3-month evaluation of self-expanding valved stents, Ann. Thorac. Surg. 82 (2) (August 2006) 708–713.

[58] G.J. Zong, Y. Bai, Y.W. Qin, et al., [Transcatheter pulmonary valve replacement in sheep: 6-month evaluation of self-expanding valved stents], Zhonghua Xin Xue Guan Bing Za Zhi 36 (2) (February 2008) 151–155.

[59] Y. Boudjemline, G. Agnoletti, D. Bonnet, D. Sidi, P. Bonhoeffer, Percutaneous pulmonary valve replacement in a large right ventricular outflow tract: an experimental study, J. Am. Coll. Cardiol. 43 (6) (March 17, 2004) 1082–1087.

[60] Q.L. Cao, D. Kenny, D. Zhou, et al., Early clinical experience with a novel self-expanding percutaneous stent-valve in the native right ventricular outflow tract, Catheter. Cardiovasc. Interv. 84 (7) (December 1, 2014) 1131–1137.

[61] B.H. Morray, D.B. McElhinney, J.P. Cheatham, et al., Risk of coronary artery compression among patients referred for transcatheter pulmonary valve implantation: a multicenter experience, Circ. Cardiovasc. Interv. 6 (5) (October 1, 2013) 535–542.

[62] R.N. Bishnoi, T.K. Jones, J. Kreutzer, R.E. Ringel, NuMED Covered Cheatham-Platinum Stent for the treatment or prevention of right ventricular outflow tract conduit disruption during transcatheter pulmonary valve replacement, Catheter. Cardiovasc. Interv. 85 (3) (February 15, 2015) 421–427.

[63] D.B. McElhinney, J.P. Cheatham, T.K. Jones, et al., Stent fracture, valve dysfunction, and right ventricular outflow tract reintervention after transcatheter pulmonary valve implantation: patient-related and procedural risk factors in the US Melody Valve Trial, Circ. Cardiovasc. Interv. 4 (6) (December 1, 2011) 602–614.

[64] D. Cosentino, M.A. Quail, G. Pennati, et al., Geometrical and stress analysis of factors associated with stent fracture after melody percutaneous pulmonary valve implantation, Circ. Cardiovasc. Interv. 7 (4) (August 2014) 510–517.

[65] S.L. Cheatham, R.J. Holzer, J.L. Chisolm, J.P. Cheatham, The Medtronic Melody(R) transcatheter pulmonary valve implanted at 24-mm diameter–it works, Catheter. Cardiovasc. Interv. 82 (5) (November 1, 2013) 816–823.

[66] C. Wilhelm, J. Swinning, M. Sisk, R. Holzer, Melody valve implantation using a double-balloon "Flower-Blossom" technique, Congenit. Cardiol. Today 8 (2014) 1–8.

[67] R. Violini, U. Vairo, Z.M. Hijazi, Stent strut breakage using high-pressure balloons for bifurcation stenting and subsequent percutaneous pulmonary valve replacement using the Edwards Sapien THV, Catheter. Cardiovasc. Interv. 82 (5) (November 1, 2013) 834–837.

[68] Z. Jalal, S. Malekzadeh-Milani, M. Hofbeck, K. Al Najashi, J.B. Thambo, Y. Boudjemline, A new percutaneous pulmonary valve implantation technique for complex right ventricular outflow tracts: the "folded melody valve", Catheter. Cardiovasc. Interv. 85 (4) (March 2015) 604–610.

[69] S. Malekzadeh-Milani, M. Patel, Y. Boudjemline, Folded Melody valve technique for complex right ventricular outflow tract, EuroIntervention 9 (10) (February 2014) 1237–1240.

[70] S.M. Awad, S.A. Masood, I. Gonzalez, et al., The use of intracardiac echocardiography during percutaneous pulmonary valve replacement, Pediatr. Cardiol. 36 (1) (January 2015) 76–83.

[71] M. Chessa, G. Butera, M. Carminati, Intracardiac echocardiography during percutaneous pulmonary valve replacement, Eur. Heart J. 29 (23) (December 2008) 2908.

[72] A.D. Khanna, K.D. Hill, S.K. Pasquali, et al., Benchmark outcomes for pulmonary valve replacement using the Society of Thoracic Surgeons Databases, Ann. Thorac. Surg. (May 22, 2015).

[73] A. Sabate Rotes, B.W. Eidem, H.M. Connolly, et al., Long-term follow-up after pulmonary valve replacement in repaired tetralogy of Fallot, Am. J. Cardiol. 114 (6) (September 15, 2014) 901–908.

[74] E.W. Cheung, W.H. Wong, Y.F. Cheung, Meta-analysis of pulmonary valve replacement after operative repair of tetralogy of fallot, Am. J. Cardiol. 106 (4) (August 15, 2010) 552–557.

[75] J.P. Cheatham, W.E. Hellenbrand, E.M. Zahn, et al., Clinical and hemodynamic outcomes up to 7 years after transcatheter pulmonary valve replacement in the US Melody Valve Investigational Device Exemption Trial, Circulation 131 (22) (June 2, 2015) 1960–1970.

[76] G. Butera, O. Milanesi, I. Spadoni, et al., Melody transcatheter pulmonary valve implantation. Results from the registry of the Italian Society of Pediatric Cardiology, Catheter. Cardiovasc. Interv. 81 (2) (February 2013) 310–316.

[77] N. Faza, D. Kenny, C. Kavinsky, Z. Amin, M. Heitschmidt, Z.M. Hijazi, Single-center comparative outcomes of the Edwards SAPIEN and Medtronic Melody transcatheter heart valves in the pulmonary position, Catheter. Cardiovasc. Interv. 82 (4) (October 1, 2013) E535–E541.
[78] R.H. Boone, J.G. Webb, E. Horlick, et al., Transcatheter pulmonary valve implantation using the Edwards SAPIEN transcatheter heart valve, Catheter. Cardiovasc. Interv. 75 (2) (February 1, 2010) 286–294.
[79] G. Alsulami, M. Patel, S. Malekzadeh-Milani, D. Bonnet, Y. Boudjemline, Hyperacute flash pulmonary oedema after transcatheter pulmonary valve implantation: the melody of an overwhelmed left ventricle, Arch. Cardiovasc. Dis. 107 (4) (April 2014) 219–224.
[80] E.O. Aregullin, R. Garg, D. Berman, Takotsubo cardiomyopathy after transcatheter Edwards Sapien pulmonary valve placement in a patient with tetralogy of Fallot, Pediatr. Cardiol. 34 (8) (2013) 1972–1975.
[81] N.W. Taggart, D.J. Hagler, H.M. Connolly, Melody valve erosion into the ascending aorta, Congenit. Heart Dis. 8 (2) (March–April 2013) E64.
[82] D. Kenny, N. Holoshitz, D. Turner, Z.M. Hijazi, Aortopulmonary fistula after transcatheter pulmonary valve replacement, Circ. Cardiovasc. Interv. 6 (6) (December 2013) e67–e68.
[83] J. Villafane, G.H. Baker, E.H. Austin 3rd, S. Miller, L. Peng, R. Beekman 3rd, Melody pulmonary valve bacterial endocarditis: experience in four pediatric patients and a review of the literature, Catheter. Cardiovasc. Interv. 84 (2) (August 1, 2014) 212–218.
[84] S. Malekzadeh-Milani, M. Ladouceur, M. Patel, et al., Incidence and predictors of Melody(R) valve endocarditis: a prospective study, Arch. Cardiovasc. Dis. 108 (2) (February 2015) 97–106.
[85] H. Schneider, M. Vogt, R. Boekenkamp, et al., Melody transcatheter valve: histopathology and clinical implications of nine explanted devices, Int. J. Cardiol. 189 (June 15, 2015) 124–131.
[86] D.B. McElhinney, L.N. Benson, A. Eicken, J. Kreutzer, R.F. Padera, E.M. Zahn, Infective endocarditis after transcatheter pulmonary valve replacement using the Melody valve: combined results of 3 prospective North American and European studies, Circ. Cardiovasc. Interv. 6 (3) (June 2013) 292–300.
[87] G. Cheung, N. Vejlstrup, N. Ihlemann, et al., Infective endocarditis following percutaneous pulmonary valve replacement: diagnostic challenges and application of intra-cardiac echocardiography, Int. J. Cardiol. 169 (6) (November 30, 2013) 425–429.
[88] L. Gordis, The virtual disappearance of rheumatic fever in the United States: lessons in the rise and fall of disease. T. Duckett Jones memorial lecture, Circulation 72 (6) (December 1985) 1155–1162.
[89] C.Y. Miyake, K. Gauvreau, L.Y. Tani, R.P. Sundel, J.W. Newburger, Characteristics of children discharged from hospitals in the United States in 2000 with the diagnosis of acute rheumatic fever, Pediatrics 120 (3) (September 2007) 503–508.
[90] B. Iung, A. Nicoud-Houel, O. Fondard, et al., Temporal trends in percutaneous mitral commissurotomy over a 15-year period, Eur. Heart J. 25 (8) (April 2004) 701–707.
[91] R.A. Nishimura, C.M. Otto, R.O. Bonow, et al., 2014 AHA/ACC guideline for the management of patients with valvular heart disease: a report of the American College of Cardiology/American Heart Association Task Force on Practice Guidelines, J. Am. Coll. Cardiol. 63 (22) (June 10, 2014) e57–e185.
[92] J.A. de Souza, E.E. Martinez Jr., J.A. Ambrose, et al., Percutaneous balloon mitral valvuloplasty in comparison with open mitral valve commissurotomy for mitral stenosis during pregnancy, J. Am. Coll. Cardiol. 37 (3) (March 1, 2001) 900–903.
[93] G.T. Wilkins, A.E. Weyman, V.M. Abascal, P.C. Block, I.F. Palacios, Percutaneous balloon dilatation of the mitral valve: an analysis of echocardiographic variables related to outcome and the mechanism of dilatation, Br. Heart J. 60 (4) (October 1988) 299–308.
[94] K. Inoue, T. Owaki, T. Nakamura, F. Kitamura, N. Miyamoto, Clinical application of transvenous mitral commissurotomy by a new balloon catheter, J. Thorac. Cardiovasc. Surg. 87 (3) (March 1984) 394–402.
[95] J.E. Lock, M. Khalilullah, S. Shrivastava, V. Bahl, J.F. Keane, Percutaneous catheter commissurotomy in rheumatic mitral stenosis, N. Engl. J. Med. 313 (24) (December 12, 1985) 1515–1518.
[96] M. Al Zaibag, P.A. Ribeiro, S. Al Kasab, M.R. Al Fagih, Percutaneous double-balloon mitral valvotomy for rheumatic mitral-valve stenosis, Lancet 1 (8484) (April 5, 1986) 757–761.
[97] C.S. Rihal, D.R. Holmes Jr., Percutaneous balloon mitral valvuloplasty: issues involved in comparing techniques, Catheter. Cardiovasc. Diagn. (Suppl. 2) (1994) 35–41.
[98] P. Bonhoeffer, J.F. Piechaud, D. Sidi, et al., Mitral dilatation with the multi-track system: an alternative approach, Catheter. Cardiovasc. Diagn. 36 (2) (1995) 189–193.
[99] E. Marijon, B. Iung, A.O. Mocumbi, et al., What are the differences in presentation of candidates for percutaneous mitral commissurotomy across the world and do they influence the results of the procedure? Arch. Cardiovasc. Dis. 101 (10) (October 2008) 611–617.
[100] D.S. Baim, Grossman's cardiac catheterization, angiography and intervention, 7 (2006).
[101] L.S. Dean, M. Mickel, R. Bonan, et al., Four-year follow-up of patients undergoing percutaneous balloon mitral commissurotomy. A report from the National Heart, Lung, and Blood Institute Balloon Valvuloplasty Registry, J. Am. Coll. Cardiol. 28 (6) (November 15, 1996) 1452–1457.
[102] C. Bouleti, B. Iung, D. Himbert, et al., Reinterventions after percutaneous mitral commissurotomy during long-term follow-up, up to 20 years: the role of repeat percutaneous mitral commissurotomy, Eur. Heart J. 34 (25) (July 2013) 1923–1930.
[103] J.J. Patel, D. Shama, A.S. Mitha, et al., Balloon valvuloplasty versus closed commissurotomy for pliable mitral stenosis: a prospective hemodynamic study, J. Am. Coll. Cardiol. 18 (5) (November 1, 1991) 1318–1322.
[104] Z.G. Turi, V.P. Reyes, B.S. Raju, et al., Percutaneous balloon versus surgical closed commissurotomy for mitral stenosis. A prospective, randomized trial, Circulation 83 (4) (April 1991) 1179–1185.
[105] V.P. Reyes, B.S. Raju, J. Wynne, et al., Percutaneous balloon valvuloplasty compared with open surgical commissurotomy for mitral stenosis, N. Engl. J. Med. 331 (15) (October 13, 1994) 961–967.
[106] M. Ben Farhat, M. Ayari, F. Maatouk, et al., Percutaneous balloon versus surgical closed and open mitral commissurotomy: seven-year follow-up results of a randomized trial, Circulation 97 (3) (January 27, 1998) 245–250.

Chapter 50

Principles of Mechanical Cardiopulmonary Support

Tim Maul[1], Angela Lorts[2], Peter Wearden[1], Jennifer L. Conway[3]

[1]*Nemours Children's Hospital, Orlando, FL, United States;* [2]*Cincinnati Children's Hospital Medical Center, Cincinnati, OH, United States;* [3]*University of Alberta, Edmonton, AB, Canada*

INTRODUCTION

Since the introduction of cardiopulmonary bypass in 1953, the field of cardiac surgery and mechanical circulatory support (MCS) has made significant progress, particularly within the last 20 years. We are entering an era where destination therapy, recently approved for adult devices, is now being considered for adolescents [1]. While most of this technology has been developed for use in the adult population, the principles of pump mechanics and the end goal of cardiopulmonary support, oxygen delivery via the circulation of blood, are the same no matter what the size of the patient is. Understanding how blood pumps work and the various conditions that can alter pump mechanics is essential requirement for optimal patient management.

PHYSICS OF VENTRICULAR ASSIST DEVICES

Movement of blood around the body for the purposes of MCS can be performed using a variety of technologies ranging from the relatively noninvasive (e.g., external compression of legs to promote venous return) to percutaneous applications (e.g., intraaortic balloon pumps (IABPs), paracorporeal ventricular assist devices (VADs), and extracorporeal membrane oxygenation (ECMO)), and finally to devices placed via invasive surgical procedures (e.g., left ventricular assist devices (LVADs), total artificial heart (TAH)). In general, the various MCS pumps can be broken down into two basic categories: pulsatile or continuous, examples of which are depicted in Fig. 50.1.

PULSATILE DEVICES

A pulsatile device attempts to recreate the natural movement of the blood, which is pumped by the four-chambered heart. They were among the first types of VADs to be clinically utilized due to their relatively simple mechanical properties, ease of development, and the initial belief that pulsatility was required for normal physiologic function of end organs and that its absence could result in pathologic remodeling. Pulsatile systems belonging to the volume displacement category of pumps generally require a valve or occlusive system to ensure the proper forward flow of blood. Valves can be mechanical, homografts, or xenografts. The presence of these artificial valves, as well as the required reservoirs, promotes turbulence and stasis leading to coagulation and is likely one of the major sources of thrombotic complications [5]. In the case of a roller pump set to pulsatile mode, the rollers that propel the blood forward provide the necessary occlusion; therefore negating the need for additional valves. Occasionally, the natural valves in the body are utilized in the process of pump operation. For example, the IABP relies on a competent aortic valve to ensure that the volume displaced by the balloon is directed away from the heart and not back into the left ventricle.

When utilizing a pulsatile device, there is a peak velocity and flow driving blood forward through the vascular tree into the capillaries, followed by drop in pressure and flow until the next cycle. If the pump (balloon) is positioned in the large capacitance arteries (i.e., aorta), a certain amount of energy is stored in the wall for release as the pressure decreases to continue driving flow forward. Depending on the category of pump and the timing of the pulse, there can be a zero velocity state in the capillaries or a time-varying continuous forward flow. The key to understanding the differences in the true blood flow rate in a pulsatile system compared to a continuous system relies on the integration of the volumetric flow over each cycle. In general, pulsatile systems create 30% more forward flow for a given mean pressure than their continuous

Heart Failure in the Child and Young Adult. http://dx.doi.org/10.1016/B978-0-12-802393-8.00050-8

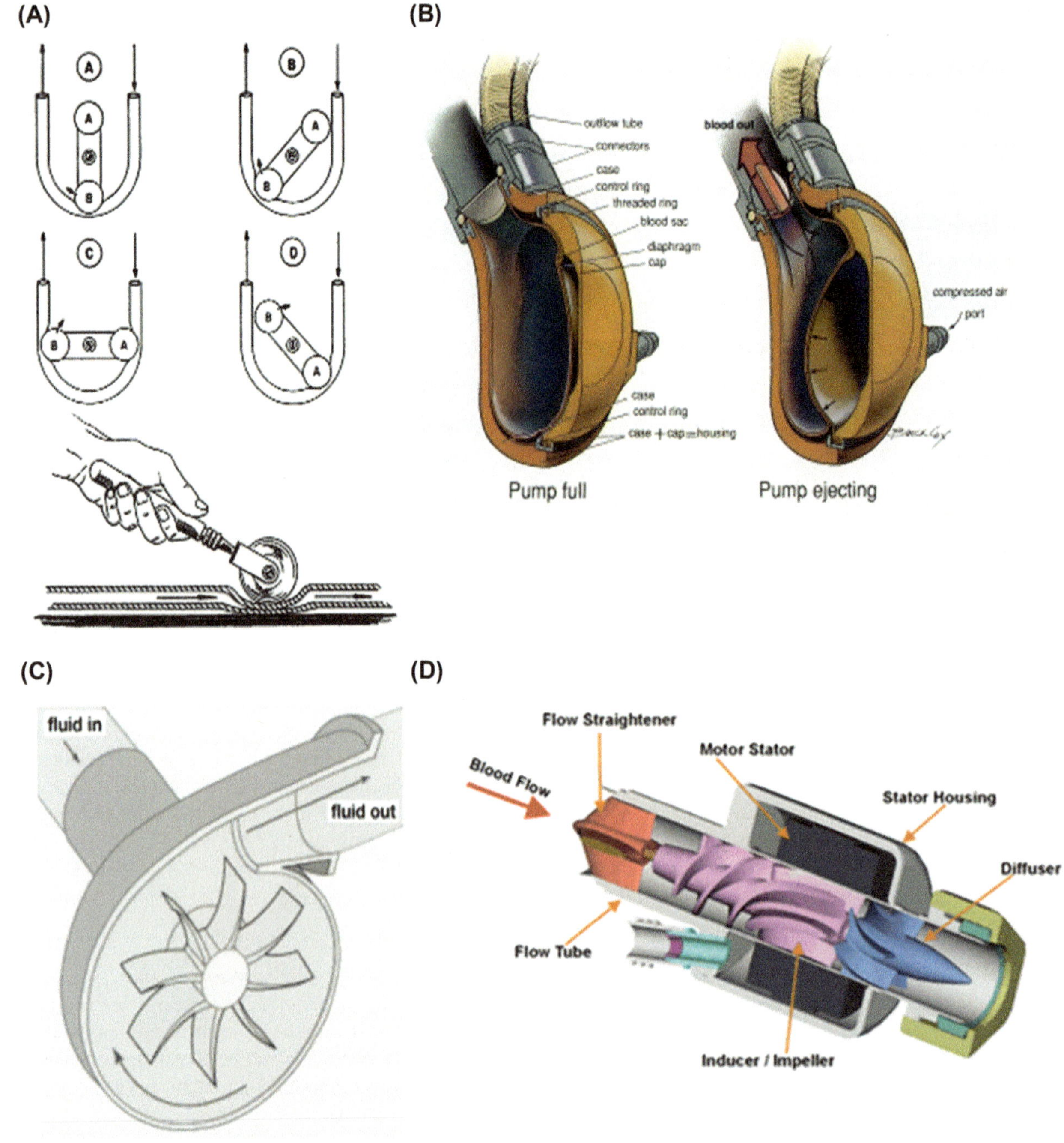

FIGURE 50.1 Overview of the available pumping mechanisms. (A–B) are volume displacement pumps. (C–D) are pressure-generating pumps. (A) A roller pump squeezes blood along a piece of tubing. This pump is generally run in a continuous mode (steady RPM) but could be run in a pulsatile fashion by varying the RPM of the rollers. (B) Pierce–Donachy style volume displacement pump that uses a blood sac inside a solid housing to propel blood past valves using pneumatic pressure applied to the exterior of the blood sac. Some versions of this pump have fill and empty sensing technology to accurately calculate volumetric flow rate. Filling and emptying can be assisted by the vacuum and driving pneumatic pressures. (C) A centrifugal pump uses a spinning impeller to create a low pressure vortex in the center of the device, which is redirected orthogonally in the circumferential direction toward the fluid outlet. The impeller can sit on a traditional bearing, hydrodynamic bearing, or be magnetically levitated. This pump type can be operated continuously or in a pulsatile fashion. Fluid flow rates are very sensitive to preload and afterload. (D) An axial flow pump that uses a spinning impeller to induce fluid rotation along the same axis of the entrance and exit from the device. These pumps typically have flow straighteners at the inlet and outlet to recover pressure losses from secondary flows. The impeller can be supported by standard bearings or magnetically levitated. It can also be operated in a continuous or pulsatile fashion. *(A) Reproduced from R.C. Stofer, A Technique for Extracorporeal Circulation, Charles C. Thomas, Springfield, IL, 1968, p. 22. (B) Reproduced from B. Bogue, A. Messer (Eds.), The Penn State Heart Pump, American Society of Mechanical Engineers, 1990. https://www.asme.org/wwwasmeorg/media/ResourceFiles/AboutASME/Who%20We%20Are/Engineering%20History/Landmarks/142-Pierce-Donachy-Ventricular-Assist-Device.pdf. (D) Adapted from Clinical Trials, University of Southern California, Department of Cardiothoracic Surgery. http://www.cts.usc.edu/clinicaltrials-debakeyvad.html.*

flow counterparts because of the peak pressure being higher than the mean and the energy storage and recapture in the elastic arteries [6]. It is for this reason that pulsatile devices are routinely reported to have better perfusion than continuous flow devices when experiments are conducted at equal mean pressures. To date, there is very little evidence from a tissue remodeling standpoint that provides evidence that pulsatile flow is an absolute prerequisite for proper organ function [7].

CONTINUOUS FLOW DEVICES

Continuous flow devices provide a relatively constant forward flow of blood through the device during the entire cardiac cycle. This is accomplished by maintaining a constant speed of either the roller heads in the case of a volume displacement pump or the impeller in the case of a pressure-generating pump. The use of a continuous flow pump opens greater engineering design options for miniaturization because a smaller pump with a faster spinning impeller can generate as much flow as a larger impeller spinning slowly, or, in the case of a pulsatile pump, a blood sac being pumped at a set rate. Continuous flow devices generally do not contain valves, which makes them more attractive from a thrombotic standpoint [5,6], and the flow of blood is nearly always forward except in certain instances of pressure-generating pumps. Despite their designation as "continuous flow," most patients with continuous flow devices do not exhibit a complete lack of pulsatility. This is due to the fact that these devices generally operate in parallel with the heart itself; therefore any native cardiac output will be superimposed on the flow coming from the MCS device, thus creating a modified pulsatile flow pattern. In the instances of left MCS where the heart is too weak to pump, a continuous flow pump might keep the aortic valve from opening, leading to blood stagnation on the leaflets and a potential for thrombosis. Further, aortic leaflets that are constantly in the closed state have been documented to fuse together, increasing the risk of aortic insufficiency and complications associated with this morbidity [8].

VOLUME DISPLACEMENT PUMPS

Volume displacement pumps were the first developed pumps for both cardiopulmonary bypass, left heart assist devices, and MCS devices. They are mechanically much easier to create, to understand conceptually, and to monitor. Volume displacement is accomplished via a pure mechanical–fluid interaction as seen in the roller pump and the Heart Mate XVE and the Novacor LVADs, or an intermediate gas as seen in the IABP, Jarvik TAH, Syncardia TAH, and Pierce–Donachy styled pumps, including the Berlin Heart EXCOR. In essence, with each stroke, a specific volume of blood is displaced from a holding chamber. Optimal operation of these devices will always produce the same amount of volume displaced per stroke or revolution, thus making flow rate calculation straightforward. Because blood is an incompressible medium, this also means that provided there is sufficient mechanical force generation on the part of the device, the blood will flow in and out of the device regardless of the pressures of afterload or preload. In the case of high afterload, this can create enormous strain on the pump, associated peripheral tubing, and the cellular elements in the blood. Restrictions in the outflow of these devices have been reported to create acquired von Willebrand's disease due to shear [9,10] and hemolysis [11]. Volume displacement pumps tend to be much larger than pressure-generating devices that provide the same cardiac output because their mechanics require suitable reservoirs of volume to be pumped in addition to the mechanical hardware required for pumping. Volume displacement pumps that use compressed gas to provide the force for blood displacement also require large controllers to contain the requisite compressors (air or other gases) for generating the necessary pressures. Most volume displacement pumps are pulsatile, with the exception of the roller pump, which is for all intents and purposes continuous.

PRESSURE-GENERATING PUMPS

Pressure-generating pumps are the newest types of MCS devices and have been developed through advances in mechanical design and computational fluid dynamics. These are more mechanically complicated in terms of sensors, controllers, and general equipment but are more compact and easily implantable than their volume displacement counterparts. Pressure-generating pumps are also more difficult to conceptually understand and monitor total volumetric flow rate because they do not consistently produce the same amount of volumetric flow. Unlike volume displacement pumps these pumps are sensitive to both preload and afterload at any given pump speed.

A pressure-driven pump uses a moving series of blades attached to central mass, called an impeller, to act as an Archimedes screw and produce a specific rotational velocity of a fluid. This rotational velocity creates a pressure gradient across the pump, and it is this pressure gradient that drives the flow of the fluid from high to low pressure. The pressure gradients are highly dependent on the density and viscosity of the fluid. The ultimate flow rate of the fluid is dependent on the preload and afterload pressures (or resistance) on the pump, and it is the afterload that can ultimately induce retrograde flow in a pressure-generating pump that does not generate sufficient pressure to overcome it. For pressure-generating pumps operating in pulsatile mode, the automatic adjustment of the impeller speed provides the pulsatile flow and pressure in the body; but the flow is almost always continuously forward without interruption or reversal unless there is a greater pressure at the outlet of the pump than is generated by the lower speed of the pump at the bottom of the cycle, causing blood to flow backward through the pump. This mechanism of blood flow can be achieved by axial or centrifugal pumps.

The flow path of the blood through the device generally classifies it as centrifugal or axial. Centrifugal pumps utilize the principles of centripetal motion to bring fluid in on one 3D axis and exit the fluid on an orthogonal axis. Axial pumps bring the fluid in and exit the fluid along the same general axis. Although these pump designs achieve the same goal, there are some differences between axial and centrifugal pumps including response to preload and afterload. Centrifugal pumps are typically more sensitive to preload and afterload when compared to axial pumps. In fact, the pressure difference (dP) between the inlet and outlet of a centrifugal pump is always the same for a given impeller rotation, regardless of the flow rate, but the dP for an axial pump is actually different depending on the flow rate. Further, axial pumps generally do not have a linear relationship between power and blood flow over the entire operating range of the device, which is the reason that the flow estimators often fail to report a flow rate when the pump enters into these nonlinear ranges [12]. Table 50.1 highlights some of the key features of these pumps with respect to their operation and under various preload and afterload conditions.

There are several characteristics of these types of pumps that are highly important when the fluid to be pumped is blood. Smaller blood pumps are obviously desirable, but they must also be biocompatible. Shear stress imparted on the blood by the blade tips of the impeller and in various parts of the pump can activate and damage blood elements. Of particular concern are red cells that can be ruptured at shear rates of $1500\,s^{-1}$ [13] and therefore no longer function as oxygen carriers. In addition, platelets can be activated to aggregate at shear rates over $5000\,s^{-1}$ and will deposit on surfaces at much lower shear rates ($<500\,s^{-1}$) [14]. Although these thresholds provide easy design points for reference, cellular activation and destruction is actually a shear magnitude and time-dependent process. An amalgamation of many research studies on this topic presented by Leverett et al. [15] shows that threshold curves can be created, which offer a design envelope for all blood elements (Fig. 50.2).

Another factor that can affect the biocompatibility is pump efficiency. Pump efficiency is determined by how much energy imparted to the spinning impeller goes toward creating forward flow in the blood. Pumps that are inefficient tend to generate vortices and heat, which can lead to blood coagulation and damage [16]. Pump efficiencies are ultimately determined by the pump type, the size of the pump, the rotational speed, and the gaps between the blades on the impeller that impart flow and the wall of the device. Smaller pumps are much less efficient because the blade size relative to the gap size tends to shrink due to limits of physical construction. These factors explain why the efficiency of centrifugal pumps is generally higher than axial pumps and in theory should have improved biocompatibility.

THE PHYSICS OF OXYGENATORS IN CARDIOPULMONARY SYSTEMS

A key component of cardiopulmonary assist or replacement systems is the ability to simulate function of the lungs. In essence, they have the ability to provide diffusion of oxygen into the blood and carbon dioxide out of the blood. The development of oxygenators has a rich history going back to the 1700s that has been outlined in several excellent papers [17–19].

TABLE 50.1 General Characteristics of Pressure-Generating Pumps

	Axial Pumps			Centrifugal Pumps		
	dP	**Power**	**Flow**	**dP**	**Power**	**Flow**
Decreased preload RHF, hypovolemia, inlet restriction/suction	↑↑	↑ or ↓	↓	–	↓↓	↓↓
Increased afterload restricted outlet, SVR increase	↑↑	↑ or ↓	↓	–	↓↓	↓↓
Decreased afterload low SVR	↓↓	↑ or ↓	↑	–	↑↑	↑↑

RHF, right heart failure; *SVR*, systemic vascular resistance.
Adapted from N. Moazami, K. Fukamachi, M. Kobayashi, N.G. Smedira, K.J. Hoercher, A. Massiello, et al., Axial and centrifugal continuous-flow rotary pumps: a translation from pump mechanics to clinical practice, J. Heart Lung Transplant. 32 (1) (2013) 1–11.

One of the challenges of creating an oxygenator is the interface between the blood and gas phases. The larger the physical barrier, the more resistance there is to diffusion across the barrier, and therefore the less total diffusion can occur. Likewise, the larger the thickness of the fluid layers in contact with the interface, the greater the resistance to diffusion. Elimination of the barrier would at first glance appear to be the simplest solution, which was the approach of many early oxygenators, but was not without significant potential for blood damage [18]. Silicone membranes provided one of the first semipermeable barriers to blood and air, which permitted sufficient diffusion for a clinically applicable oxygenator.

At baseline, all oxygenators are required to provide at least 250 mL O_2/min, which is the baseline metabolism of an adult at 5 L/min cardiac output. However, manufacturing of silicone membranes was limited to thicknesses around 100 μm because of the mechanical strength and rupture potential; thus there was a finite membrane resistance that limited gas transfer [20]. The largest breakthrough came with the advent of the microporous hollow fiber oxygenator. These are fibers of a polymer, initially made from polypropylene (PP), that have a diameter of approximately 100 μm and a thickness of approximately 10 μm. The key to these fibers, though, is that the walls are porous, with pore sizes on the order of 30 nm. Because of the hydrophobic nature of the PP fiber, the surface tension of the water in the plasma is great enough to prevent fluid from entering the pores; thus creating a stable, infinitely thin air–blood interface. Hollow fiber oxygenators were two times more efficient than their silicone membrane counterparts [20], which permitted smaller oxygenators to be created (both in surface area and subsequently priming volume). Movement of blood around the outside of the fibers (while the gas flows inside the fiber) creates a mixing phenomenon and a more efficient transfer profile. Thus fiber diameter, distance between fibers, total number of fibers, and the path length of the blood through the oxygenator determine the total transfer in these oxygenators. Oxygenators with a long path length have longer time in contact with the blood and can transfer more oxygen per volume, requiring smaller surface areas but are more resistant to blood flow (higher inlet pressures). Short path oxygenators allow the blood to pass quickly past the fibers in a short distance and therefore require higher surface area and have less resistance (lower inlet pressure and total surface drop) [21–25].

This technology was perfectly suitable for cardiopulmonary bypass where the blood was in contact with the oxygenator for several hours before the patient's lungs can take over function. With the advent of ECMO and patients being supported much longer, the Achilles heel of PP hollow fibers became apparent. Over the course of blood contact with these fibers, plasma proteins are deposited. The presence of these amphiphilic proteins (or lipids as was often the case) would break the surface tension on the pores and allow plasma to enter the inside of the fibers [23,26,27]. The pores in these oxygenators were too small for the cellular element, but the presence of plasma in the gas phase drastically reduced the efficiency of the oxygenator. The efficiency was reduced because the gas had to diffuse through the liquid inside the fiber, to get to the outside of the fiber where

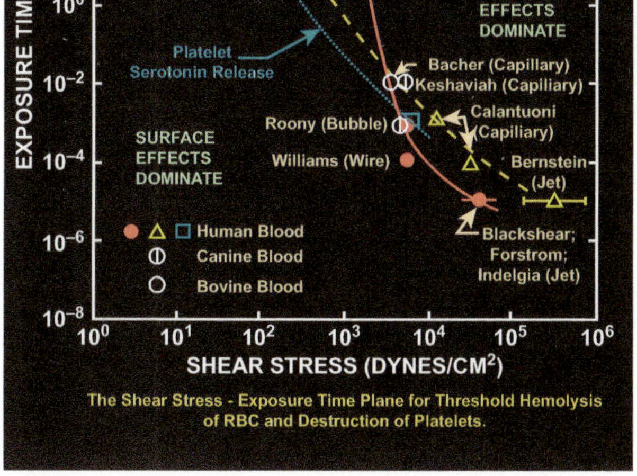

FIGURE 50.2 The so-called "Leverett curve" depicts the time and shear stress-dependent damage to red cells, platelets, and white cells on one graph. Areas left of the isolines are believed to be safe and primarily influenced by the artificial surface these blood elements are exposed to, while the area to the right of the curves indicates that the damage is primarily from the shear stress. MCS device design and operation should take great care to attempt to operate in the left side of the curves at all times and illustrates why operating adult-sized devices at lower flow rates with equivalent motor speeds through the use of narrowed grafts or throttles can actually do more damage than would be expected from operation at adult flow rates because it keeps the same shear stress but increases the residence time of the blood in the device. *(Adapted from L.B. Leverett, Red blood cell damage by shear stress, Biophys. J. 12 (3) (March 1972) 257–273.)*

the red cells are streaming past. The clinical sign that this was occurring was a large amount of yellow foam pouring out of the gas vents of these oxygenators, which necessitated the oxygenator to be changed for a new one.

To prevent plasma infiltration in long-term applications, an asymmetric (narrowing) or blind (closed) pore is needed [20,26,28]. However, this would require a polymer with moderately good diffusional characteristics since the gases would need to diffuse into the bulk of a polymer that could still be manufactured into a hollow fiber strand. Polymethylpentene (PMP) was thus chosen to replace PP in these long-term cardiopulmonary bypass applications. The efficiency of PMP is less than the microporous PP [29], but through creative fiber orientations and oxygenator design, oxygenators that meet the demands of patients were created that enabled ECMO patients to remain on a single oxygenator for upward of 60 days or longer before other biocompatibility issues would require their changeout [26].

It is important to note, as well, that both PMP and PP do transmit water vapor in addition to oxygen and carbon dioxide because of the specific, but low solubility of the polymers in water. The water vapor, which comes from the blood at 37°C, results in condensation on the inside of the fibers. This condensation can work just like the plasma leakage in the PP failure to limit gas exchange, particularly CO_2, because its diffusional gradient is much lower than O_2. The carrying away of water vapor is not inconsequential and can add up to over a 1 L of water per day depending on temperature of the blood, fluid pressure in the oxygenator, and gas flow rate. Several mathematical relationships have been generated to compute the insensible losses through an oxygenator [30,31].

GENERAL HEMODYNAMIC PRINCIPLES OF VENTRICULAR ASSIST DEVICES

VADs can be necessary to support the pulmonary circulation, systemic circulation, or in a minority of cases both circulations. For the pulmonary circulation, the most common cannulation strategy includes an inflow cannula to the right atrium and an outflow cannula to the pulmonary artery. For the systemic circulation the inflow cannula may be placed in the left atrium but is more commonly in the left ventricular (LV) apex. For LV support the outflow cannula is placed in the ascending aorta. Despite the system that is utilized, either temporary or durable support or continuous or pulsatile, the concepts of cannulation are similar. Peak flow rates usually range from 2.5 to 7.0 L/min depending on the system used. The goal cardiac index for children is often >2.4 L/min/m^2. The optimal cardiac index needed should be determined based on hemodynamic parameters (i.e., mixed venous saturations, end organ function, etc.). Flow rates, cannulation strategy, and circuit configuration have major impacts on the cardiac output achieved, but many other factors do play into the support that can be provided. Other patient-related factors that change cannulation strategies and maximum flow include patient size, cardiac diagnosis, the degree of recovery following unloading, right-sided function when only the LV is supported, systemic and pulmonary afterload, baseline heart rate, and arrhythmias.

In pediatrics, patient size and cardiac diagnosis are major factors in determining the type of device to be used and the cannulation strategy that would be best. In small patients, with a body surface area <1.0 m^2, the only VADs that may be considered as options are typically a temporary centrifugal pump or a Berlin EXCOR. The Berlin pump size that will allow for the optimal stroke volume is determined by the patient size and the rate that the device will safely pump at. An example of when cardiac diagnosis is very important in regard to cannulation strategy is in restrictive cardiomyopathy. If the ventricular cavity is small at baseline, unloading the heart may lead to contraction of the myocardium around the cannula leading to inflow obstruction. Children with restrictive physiology may be best supported with atrial cannulation.

With isolated LV support, the right ventricular performance must be maintained to fill the VAD. When the right ventricle begins to fail the VAD will not get optimal preload and systemic output will be compromised. Perioperative support of the right ventricle is often necessary and may consist of pulmonary vasodilators and inotropes. In addition, maintaining the lungs at functional residual capacity will prevent further increases in pulmonary vascular reactivity. Controlling bleeding to avoid massive volumes of blood product administration will likely also help with right ventricular function postoperatively. In addition, avoiding beta blockers in the immediate postoperative period may prevent right ventricular deterioration.

Systemic afterload effects all VAD types but to different extremes. The pulsatile pumps' function will be suboptimal in the face of high afterload, but is much less affected compared to continuous flow devices. The continuous flow devices, especially the centrifugal pumps, are extremely sensitive to afterload. The device flow will decline with increasing afterload. Poorly controlled blood pressure is a risk factor for embolic stroke in adults on durable continuous flow VADS, but it is unclear if this is true for children [32]. Blood pressure control is vital and oftentimes requires the addition of multiple medications to keep the pressures within goal. Heart rate and rhythm may be important if only the left ventricle is supported. If biventricular support is supplied the rhythm and rate will not change the hemodynamics.

There are an increasing number of VAD options for treating children with acute and chronic heart failure. The options vary depending on the size of the patient and the etiology of the heart failure. Despite changes in pump dynamics and cannulation strategies all of the devices are dependent on preload and afterload to some extent. The pump does not function in isolation, and optimal output is dependent on multiple device and patient factors.

CONCLUSION

MCS in the pediatric population can be provided by a number of different pumps with different underlying physical principles. Regardless of pump design, the ultimate goal is to provide adequate oxygen delivery, via circulatory support. It is imperative for clinicians to understand how the various systems work, along with their strengths and weaknesses, to achieve optimal hemodynamics and minimize support-related adverse events.

REFERENCES

[1] D.S. Char, S.S. Lee, A.A. Ikoku, D. Rosenthal, D. Magnus, Can destination therapy be implemented in children with heart failure? A study of provider perceptions, Pediatr. Transplant. (2016) (Epub ahead of print).
[2] R.C. Stofer, A Technique for Extracorporeal Circulation, Charles C. Thomas, Springfield, IL, 1968, p. 22.
[3] B. Bogue, A. Messer (Eds.), The Penn State Heart Pump, American Society of Mechanical Engineers, 1990. https://www.asme.org/wwwasmeorg/media/ResourceFiles/AboutASME/Who%20We%20Are/Engineering%20History/Landmarks/142-Pierce-Donachy-Ventricular-Assist-Device.pdf.
[4] Clinical Trials, University of Southern California, Department of Cardiothoracic Surgery. http://www.cts.usc.edu/clinicaltrials-debakeyvad.html.
[5] W.R. Wagner, P.C. Johnson, R.L. Kormos, B.P. Griffith, Evaluation of bioprosthetic valve-associated thrombus in ventricular assist device patients, Circulation 88 (5 Pt. 1) (1993) 2023–2029.
[6] Y. Nose, K. Kawahito, T. Nakazawa, Can we develop a nonpulsatile permanent rotary blood pump? Yes, we can, Artif. Organs 20 (6) (1996) 467–474.
[7] F. Sansone, E. Zingarelli, R. Flocco, G.M. Dato, F. Parisi, G. Punta, et al., Pulsed or continuous flow in long-term assist devices: a debated topic, Transplant. Rev. (Orlando Fla) 26 (4) (2012) 241–245.
[8] K. May-Newman, L. Enriquez-Almaguer, P. Posuwattanakul, W. Dembitsky, Biomechanics of the aortic valve in the continuous flow VAD-assisted heart, ASAIO J. 56 (4) (2010) 301–308.
[9] S. Crow, C. Milano, L. Joyce, D. Chen, G. Arepally, D. Bowles, et al., Comparative analysis of von Willebrand factor profiles in pulsatile and continuous left ventricular assist device recipients, ASAIO J. 56 (5) (2010) 441–445.
[10] J.P. Costello, Y.A. Diab, M. Philippe-Auguste, M.B. Jones, V. Shankar, K.D. Friedman, et al., Acquired von Willebrand syndrome in a child following Berlin Heart EXCOR Pediatric ventricular assist device implantation: case report and concise literature review, World J. Pediatr. Congenit. Heart Surg. 5 (4) (2014) 592–598.
[11] Z. Xu, M. Yang, X. Wang, Z. Wang, The influence of different operating conditions on the blood damage of a pulsatile ventricular assist device, ASAIO J. 61 (6) (2015) 656–663.
[12] N. Moazami, K. Fukamachi, M. Kobayashi, N.G. Smedira, K.J. Hoercher, A. Massiello, et al., Axial and centrifugal continuous-flow rotary pumps: a translation from pump mechanics to clinical practice, J. Heart Lung Transplant. 32 (1) (2013) 1–11.
[13] T. Yasuda, A. Funakubo, Y. Fukui, An investigation of blood damage induced by static pressure during shear-rate conditions, Artif. Organs 26 (1) (2002) 27–31.
[14] M.A. Navitsky, J.O. Taylor, A.B. Smith, M.J. Slattery, S. Deutsch, C.A. Siedlecki, et al., Platelet adhesion to polyurethane urea under pulsatile flow conditions, Artif. Organs 38 (12) (2014) 1046–1053.
[15] L.B. Leverett, Red blood cell damage by shear stress, Biophys. J. 12 (3) (March 1972) 257–273.
[16] K.A. Dasse, B. Gellman, M.V. Kameneva, J.R. Woolley, C.A. Johnson, T. Gempp, et al., Assessment of hydraulic performance and biocompatibility of a MagLev centrifugal pump system designed for pediatric cardiac or cardiopulmonary support, ASAIO J. 53 (6) (2007) 771–777.
[17] M.W. Lim, The history of extracorporeal oxygenators, Anaesthesia 61 (10) (2006) 984–995.
[18] A.H. Stammers, Historical aspects of cardiopulmonary bypass: from antiquity to acceptance, J. Cardiothorac. Vasc. Anesth. 11 (3) (1997) 266–274.
[19] R.A. DeWall, The evolution of the helical reservoir pump-oxygenator system at the University of Minnesota, Ann. Thorac. Surg. 76 (6) (2003) S2210–S2215.
[20] W. Federspiel, K. Henchir, Lung, artificial: basic principles and current applications, in: Encyclopedia of Biomaterials and Biomedical Engineering: LZ: Informa Healthcare, 2004, p. 910.
[21] J. Schaadt, Fiber manufacturing, membrane classification, and winding technologies associated with membrane oxygenators, J. Extra Corpor. Technol. 30 (1) (1998) 30–34.
[22] R.B. Hirschl, Devices, in: J.B. Zwischenberger, R.H. Bartlett (Eds.), ECMO: Extracoporeal Cadiopulmonary Support in Critical Care, Extracoporeal Life Support Organization, Ann Arbor, MI, 1995, pp. 159–190.
[23] J.A. Wegner, Oxygenator anatomy and function, J. Cardiothorac. Vasc. Anesth. 11 (3) (1997) 275–281.
[24] P. Galletti, C. Colton, Artificial lungs and blood-gas exchange devices, in: J.D. Bronzino (Ed.), The Biomedical Engineering Handbook, CRC Press: IEEE Press, Boca Raton, 1995, pp. 1879–1897.
[25] L. Mockros, K. Cook, Engineering Design of Thoracic Artificial Lungs. The Artificial Lung, Landes Biosciences Publishers, Austin, 2002, pp. 33–64.

[26] J.M. Toomasian, R.J. Schreiner, D.E. Meyer, M.E. Schmidt, S.E. Hagan, G.W. Griffith, et al., A polymethylpentene fiber gas exchanger for long-term extracorporeal life support, ASAIO J. 51 (4) (2005) 390–397.

[27] H.J. Eash, H.M. Jones, B.G. Hattler, W.J. Federspiel, Evaluation of plasma resistant hollow fiber membranes for artificial lungs, ASAIO J. 50 (5) (2004) 491–497.

[28] K. Eya, E. Tatsumi, Y. Taenaka, Y. Takewa, Y. Wakisaka, K. Toda, et al., Development of a membrane oxygenator for long-term respiratory support and its experimental evaluation in prolonged ECMO, ASAIO J. 42 (5) (1996) M832–M836.

[29] O.A. Osipov, Gas permeability of polymer films for use in membrane oxygenators, Biomed. Eng. (NY) 7 (1) (1973) 19–21.

[30] L.L. Chang, O.Y. Tam, M.C. Kwan, H.P. Shum, K.C. Chan, W.W. Yan, Insensible water loss through adult extracorporeal membrane oxygenation circuit: an in vitro study, ASAIO J. 60 (5) (2014) 508–512.

[31] D. Lawson, D. Holt, Insensible water loss from the Jostra Quadrox D oxygenator: an in vitro study, Perfusion 22 (6) (2007) 407–410.

[32] S.S. Najjar, M.S. Slaughter, F.D. Pagani, R.C. Starling, E.C. McGee, P. Eckman, A.J. Tatooles, N. Moazami, R.L. Kormos, D.R. Hathaway, K.B. Najarian, G. Bhat, K.D. Aaronson, S.W. Boyce, HVAD Bridge to Transplant ADVANCE Trial Investigators. An analysis of pump thrombus events in patients in the HeartWare ADVANCE bridge to transplant and continued access protocol trial, J. Heart Lung Transplant. 33 (1) (January 2014) 23–34, http://dx.doi.org/10.1016/j.healun.2013.12.001. (Epub December 12, 2013).

Chapter 51

Short-Term Mechanical Cardiopulmonary Support Devices

Ryan R. Davies[1,2], David L.S. Morales[3]

[1]*Nemours/A.I. duPont Hospital for Children, Wilmington, DE, United States;* [2]*Thomas Jefferson University, Philadelphia, PA, United States;* [3]*The University of Cincinnati, Cincinnati, OH, United States*

INTRODUCTION

The advent of successful mechanical cardiopulmonary support (MCS) in children has ushered in profound changes in the management of pediatric heart failure over the past 15 years. While attention has often been focused on the Berlin Heart EXCOR (which remains the only device specifically approved for use in children) [1], improvements in short-term devices have also had a dramatic impact. Historically, extracorporeal membrane oxygenation (ECMO) provided the only option for mechanical support in children with heart failure. While the ability to provide full cardiopulmonary support continues to make ECMO a viable option for temporary support, an increasing number of ventricular assist devices (VADs) are now available in sizes appropriate for many children. A thorough understanding of the devices available, their indications and contraindications, and technical nuances is critical to successful outcomes when managing children with heart failure refractory to medical management.

GOALS OF SHORT-TERM MECHANICAL CARDIOPULMONARY SUPPORT

The goal of all short-term devices in pediatric heart failure is to provide temporary mechanical support of the acutely failing heart until support is no longer required. Terms such as "bridge-to-recovery," "bridge-to-decision," and "bridge-to-bridge" have been used to describe the potential end points, but there is significant overlap and patients may move from one expected end point to another [2]. Independent of the long-term expected end point, the goals of short-term MCS, include: maintenance of adequate systemic tissue perfusion, stabilization and recovery of renal and hepatic function, myocardial unloading, stabilization of a patient in cardiogenic shock, and/or at times, respiratory support in patients with severe pulmonary edema.

Short-term devices have several potential advantages over the immediate implantation of a more durable device, especially in patients with cardiogenic shock or cardiac arrest:

1. Initiation of mechanical support can occur rapidly often without use of cardiopulmonary bypass (CPB).
2. Total cardiopulmonary support can be obtained through the use of ECMO, mitigating the consequences of severe pulmonary edema.
3. Explanation of temporary devices is usually easier.
4. Where no durable device is required, costs may be lowered [3].
5. Implantation of a durable device in patients subsequently determined not to be transplant candidates may complicate subsequent care decisions [4].
6. Use of temporary devices may enable easier anticoagulation management, recovery from shock with improvement of end-organ function, and mitigation of the resultant systemic inflammatory response prior to durable device implantation.

On the other hand, short-term devices often limit patient mobility and potential for rehabilitation.

INDICATIONS FOR SHORT-TERM MECHANICAL CARDIOPULMONARY SUPPORT

Among patients with heart failure, the general indication for the use of short-term MCS devices is the failure of maximal medical therapy. However, the definition of "maximal" in this context may vary significantly depending on the experience of the institution and heart failure team. In addition, because of the salutary effects of mechanical support on ventricular

Heart Failure in the Child and Young Adult. http://dx.doi.org/10.1016/B978-0-12-802393-8.00051-X

work and oxygen demand [5], early initiation of mechanical support results in better outcomes in most circumstances. In particular, using mechanical support at the earliest signs of end-organ insufficiency and avoiding MCS initiation during cardiogenic shock wherever possible, results in better patient outcomes.

Preoperative Stabilization Prior to Cardiac Surgery

Patients with undiagnosed congenital heart disease may present with symptoms of cardiogenic shock or severe cyanosis. Although some patients may benefit from rapid surgical repair or palliation, delayed diagnosis is associated with higher postoperative mortality [6]. In many patients, preoperative stabilization may enable resolution of pulmonary, renal, or other end-organ dysfunction and optimize patients for surgical repair [7]. The inability to wean from ECMO at the termination of the surgical repair predicts a high mortality; possibly because of the presence of residual lesions, irreversible preoperative end-organ injury, or that the patient required ECMO for an etiology other than the pathophysiology of their congenital heart defect (e.g., sepsis) [7]. Because of the multiorgan dysfunction (i.e., lungs) frequently present in preoperative patients with unrepaired congenital heart disease, the fact that the instability is usually not caused by isolated ventricular dysfunction, and the challenges of supporting especially unrepaired congenital heart disease patients on VADS, ECMO is the preferred modality for short-term MCS prior to surgical repair.

Postcardiotomy Low Cardiac Output Syndrome and Inability to Wean From Cardiopulmonary Bypass

In children, the most common indication for the use of short-term MCS is the patient who cannot be weaned from CPB or develops postoperative low cardiac output syndrome following cardiac surgery. In these patients, cardiac dysfunction is often temporary, resulting from a combination of myocardial inflammation and edema after prolonged CPB, myocardial stunning due to periods of myocardial ischemia during surgery, and anatomic or physiologic factors, such as shunt-dependent pulmonary circulation with resulting diastolic run-off, which place the heart at additional risk for ischemia [8]. Short-term circulatory support preserves end-organ function and enables recovery of stunned myocardium, resolution of myocardial edema with consequent improvement in diastolic function, and stabilization of volume status. Intraoperative identification of patients likely to survive postoperative ECMO is difficult, but it is clear that later initiation (in the intensive care unit) and a higher incidence of ECMO complications result in worse outcomes [9]. Long-term outcomes among hospital survivors are similar to patients not requiring ECMO [10].

Where postcardiotomy dysfunction is related to an intraoperative complication such as a coronary artery occlusion, the myocardial injury may not be recoverable. However, it is often difficult to determine in the intraoperative or immediate postoperative period the extent of injury and the potential for recovery. The use of short-term MCS in these patients enables a full assessment of the cardiac function after providing time for resolution of the temporary factors described above. In patients with adequate (if not complete) recovery of cardiac function, weaning of support is possible, while conversion to a more durable device may be performed in those who cannot be weaned from the short-term device. It is important to note, however, that the use of postcardiotomy ECMO after unsuccessful palliation of CHD to bridge to a long-term VAD has poor outcomes, with mortality exceeding 70% especially in infants (Fig. 51.1) [11]. Therefore, with increased experience with short-term VADs, ECMO use should be avoided for patients with isolated cardiac failure.

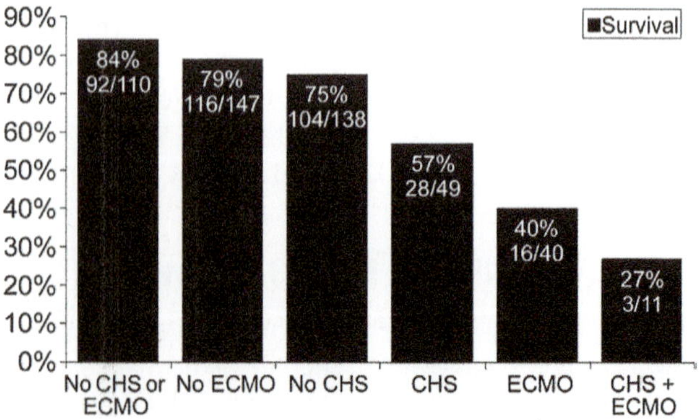

FIGURE 51.1 The effect of survival by cogential heart surgery (CHS) and extracorporeal membrane oxygenation (ECMO) before ventricular assist device implantation.

Myocarditis and Dilated Cardiomyopathy

As with postcardiotomy dysfunction, recovery potential is often unclear at presentation among children with acute fulminant myocarditis and dilated cardiomyopathy. Patients with acute fulminant myocarditis may proceed to full ventricular recovery or to dilated cardiomyopathy with end-stage heart failure requiring transplantation [12,13]. Data from the Pediatric Cardiomyopathy Registry suggest that as many of 70% of patients with presumed or biopsy-proven myocarditis (and 25% of those with idiopathic dilated cardiomyopathy) may eventually have normalization of ventricular function [14]. While this suggests relatively good long-term prognosis among those with myocarditis, it also demonstrates the imprecision of initial diagnostic categories and the potential for eventual recovery among a significant proportion of patients.

Medical therapies, including steroids and intravenous immunoglobulins continue to be used, but their efficacy remains in doubt. The use of VADs and ECMO was instituted predominantly as a salvage procedure among patients with fulminant failure and cardiogenic shock. However, as familiarity with short-term VADs increases the use of this type of MCS is occurring earlier so that end-organ damage can be avoided and the patient can be well supported during the inflammatory storm of fulminant myocarditis. In these patients, mechanical support can often prolong survival and enable effective bridge-to-recovery or transplantation. The timing of recovery is highly variable. In adults it has even been seen beyond 1 year of mechanical circulatory support [15], although recovery is usually more rapid, occurring commonly within 10 days and rarely beyond 40 [12]. In children, the timing of recovery often mirrors the time course of the child becoming ill. Fulminant myocarditis with a rapid progression of a few days from healthy to requiring support can usually be expected to subside and the child recover in several days as opposed to subacute myocarditis with a several week history of worsening symptoms, which will take weeks to months to recover and in general has less of a chance of recovery. The potential for recovery and its time course suggest that many of these patients are ideal candidates for short-term mechanical circulatory support devices.

In addition to providing effective end-organ perfusion in patients with acute, refractory cardiogenic shock, mechanical support may have salutary effects on myocardial function and recovery. The beneficial effects on myocardial and myocyte remodeling are well documented, although rates of myocardial recovery sufficient to result in device explanation after long-term support remain small [16]. In the short-term, however, mechanical circulatory support decreases myocardial oxygen demand and may lessen ongoing myocardial ischemia and injury [5]. Fulminant myocarditis is an inflammatory storm causing myocardial edema and dysfunction and temporary VAD support merely supports the circulation until that the inflammation resolves, thus LV decompression is less important. This process usual is less than 14 days if recovery is to happen quickly. Recovery in subacute myocarditis or dilated cardiomyopathy is a different process of myocardial reverse remodeling, not just the receding of inflammation, which does benefit from LV decompression is a much longer process. It is important to note that venoarterial ECMO alone does not provide effective left ventricular decompression because while providing minimal volume unloading it increases the afterload on the failing heart [5]. Insertion of a left ventricular or left atrial vent provides better ventricular unloading [5] but requires more complex procedures (see below).

Despite this downside, ECMO remains the most commonly used modality at initial presentation for patients with acute fulminant myocarditis [13], predominantly because many patients will present with significant respiratory compromise due to pulmonary edema. Overall success rates with ECMO in pediatric fulminant myocarditis are excellent with hospital discharge rates between 60% and 80% [13]. Longer-term support on ECMO (>2 weeks) is associated with higher complication rates and a lower likelihood of survival [13,17].

Short-term VADs, including the Thoratec CentriMag/PediMag or Maquet Rotaflow or the percutaneous devices designed for adults, provide an important alternative to ongoing ECMO support (or conversion to a durable device). In addition, in patients presenting without the need for mechanical ventilation and without severe pulmonary edema, these devices may provide optimal initial support. Less data exist on this strategy not only because most children with fulminant myocarditis present with compromised respiratory gas exchange but also because of the historically lower familiarity with mechanical circulatory support among pediatric providers. The use of short-term VADs rather than ECMO has become more common as devices improve and provider familiarity increases. The use of mechanical circulatory support in patients with acute fulminant myocarditis is associated with excellent outcomes, with survival exceeding 80% [18,19].

The decision to implant a short-term or more durable device is based predominantly on the perceived likelihood of recovery. While durable devices such as the Berlin Heart or Heartware HVAD have been explanted following myocardial recovery [20], the financial costs as well as the complexity of the explant procedure are higher with durable than with short-term devices. One can often implant and explant short-term VADs without going onto CPB. The efficiency of placing the device and the minimal trauma to the heart makes it ideal for the early and quick initiation of circulatory support in an acutely ill patient. Generally, patients with longer-standing (if incompletely recognized) signs and symptoms of chronic heart failure are less likely to have recovery of cardiac function, although in patients who have not had maximal medical therapy initiated, symptomatic improvement may occur and transplantation may be importantly delayed even where it is thought to be inevitable.

In patients with myocarditis or acute presentations with dilated cardiomyopathy, fulminant cardiac failure and refractory cardiogenic shock provide obvious indications for the institution of mechanical support. However, in the absence of these, the indications differ widely between institutions. To some extent this is the result of differences in familiarity with the devices, specific device availability, and outcomes following support initiation.

Consideration for implanting a short-term VAD in children, should also take into account the variable device complications rates based on patient size [21]. Due to variability in coagulation function [22] and the necessity for lower flows, smaller patients appear to be at higher risk for thromboembolic complications in all forms of extracorporeal support. Conversely, the immature neonatal brain appears to be at higher risk for bleeding and anticoagulation may be difficult to maintain within the narrow therapeutic window in pediatric patients, resulting in higher hemorrhagic stroke risk as well. However, as the field of temporary pediatric VADs is maturing, many centers have found that it may be easier to manage anticoagulation during the inflammatory period of early acute heart failure using a temporary rather than a long-term VAD.

It is important to note that the use of ECMO continues to be associated with high posttransplant mortality [23]. The impact of short-term VADs on posttransplant outcomes is less clear. While analysis of the UNOS dataset suggests that extracorporeal VADs are associated with higher posttransplant mortality [23], more recent single-institutional studies demonstrate that outcomes comparable to patients not requiring VADs are achievable [24]. Downsides of temporary devices (depending on implant technique) may include decreased mobility and an increased need for mechanical ventilation; when combined with pretransplant deconditioning, these may result in more morbidity in the peritransplant period. Therefore, consideration should be given to initial support with a longer-term device when implantation is more elective, or to conversion to a more durable device once a patient has stabilized and the chance of myocardial function is low (i.e., an acute on chronic process).

Extracorporeal Cardiopulmonary Resuscitation

The use of mechanical support among patients with cardiac arrest refractory to standard medical advanced cardiac life support protocols has been increasing [25]. Among patients requiring more than 10 min of cardiopulmonary resuscitation (CPR), the use of extracorporeal CPR (E-CPR) results in improved likelihood of survival to discharge (40% vs. 27%) and discharge with a favorable neurological outcome (27% vs. 18%) compared to conventional CPR (C-CPR) [25]. However, poor outcomes continue to occur in a large proportion of patients. Contraindications to the use of E-CPR are relative, but include unwitnessed arrest, no-flow times exceeding 5 min, and low-flow times exceeding 100 min. Little data exist to guide candidate selection, but consideration should be given to underlying medical conditions, cardiac anatomy/physiology, and the likelihood that an acute, reversible event (rather than progression of underlying disease) resulted in cardiac arrest. Children with cardiac diagnoses appear to have better outcomes with E-CPR than those with noncardiac diagnoses resulting in arrest [25], with some series reporting survival to discharge exceeding 75% [26]. However some cardiac diagnoses are associated with worst E-CPR outcomes such as Glenn physiology since peripheral cannulation is inadequate to support these circulations or restrictive cardiomyopathy with a small ventricular cavity since CPR in these patients is often inadequate. The optimal timing of E-CPR initiation remains unclear. Historically, E-CPR support times beyond 20 min in children have been considered futile [25], but that is no longer the case. Survivors occur following 45–60 min of C-CPR prior to E-CPR initiation, and outcomes do not appear worse with resuscitation longer than 30 min [27]. However, depending on provider and resource availability, there may be a significant delay between ECMO team activation and initiation of E-CPR support. Therefore, relatively early initiation of a rapidly deployable team is important to successful outcomes.

Posttransplant Cardiac Graft Failure

Early Primary Graft Dysfunction

Early graft dysfunction after cardiac transplant is a multifactorial problem; contributing factors include elevated pulmonary vascular resistance, prolonged donor allograft ischemic times, and increased volume load in patients with CHD and extensive pulmonary collaterals. With myocardial unloading and preservation of end-organ and coronary perfusion, allograft function is likely to recover; therefore, this is an ideal use for short-term mechanical circulatory support. Both ECMO and temporary VADs have been used. For patients with right ventricular failure associated with elevated pulmonary vascular resistance, support with either a short-term RVAD or ECMO allows for gradual loading of the donor heart following recovery from the effects of brain death and organ ischemia [28].

ECMO eliminates the need to identify which ventricle is failing as well as the management challenges posed by balancing right and left ventricular flows to prevent pulmonary vascular congestion while on support. However, in a series of

28 patients supported by ECMO for early graft dysfunction, mortality was high (13%, 46.4%) [29]. Similar results have been obtained by others [30,31]. While predictors of survival following ECMO initiation have not been identified, patients undergoing emergent cannulation in the ICU had an increased incidence of neurologic injury [29]. Results in adults also suggest that early institution of support, prior to the onset of end-organ failure is associated with better outcomes [26]. "Elective" cannulation of patients with marginal cardiac output or significant pulmonary collateralization prior to leaving the operating room should be considered. While ECMO provides an option when pulmonary failure occurs in concert with graft failure, selective ventricular support with a short-term VAD should be preferred as in postcardiotomy failure. Unless the function of the left ventricle is unclear, right ventricular failure can often be managed with an isolated short-term RVAD. Long-term outcomes among hospital survivors are excellent, although few patients who do not recover and are not decannulated from ECMO within 4 days survive [29].

It is notable that adult centers have identified an increased incidence of primary graft dysfunction in recent years associated with the transition to long-term support with continuous flow VADs [32]. As pediatric use of longer-term, continuous flow VADs increases, a similar trend may occur with pediatric transplantation, and there may be an increased need for postoperative mechanical support.

Late Acute Rejection

Patients presenting with refractory cardiogenic shock as the result of acute rejection remote from cardiac transplantation are likely to recover following antirejection therapy but may need short-term mechanical circulatory support during the treatment period. Percutaneous devices are ideally suited to this support because they avoid a sternotomy, which both carries its own complications and adds to the potential complications in someone who may eventually need retransplantation. When support is initiated prior to cardiogenic shock, temporary VAD support via a sternotomy may offer the most stable ventricular support in these patients. Initiation of support via a left thoracotomy with left atrial and descending aortic cannulation provides another option for isolated left ventricular support in patients with multiple previous sternotomies. Unfortunately, patients with acute rejection episodes often need biventricular support. ECMO has historically been the mainstay treatment in these patients because it enables biventricular support with a single device via percutaneous access. However, where devices and expertise are available, percutaneous biventricular VADs provide an important option. In these cases, support of the left ventricle is usually achieved via an Impella. Right ventricular support can be obtained by percutaneous placement of an outflow cannula into the pulmonary artery (often a long venous cannula is effective in this position), and one or more venous cannulae within the right atrium for VAD inflow [33]. Mechanical support is then provided using an extracorporeal pump. The TandemHeart device can also be used in similar fashion; however, patients have to be kept very still to avoid cannulation migration [30]. Case reports of percutaneous support of children with episodes of rejection have noted good outcomes with durations of support usually around 1 week [33]. A larger series from Texas Children's Hospital, demonstrated that traditional cannulation with predominantly left ventricular support (using left atrial cannulation) also had good outcomes with five out seven patients surviving to hospital discharge [34].

EXTRACORPOREAL MEMBRANE OXYGENATOR

General Considerations

Historically, ECMO was the only choice for short-term mechanical support of children with heart failure refractory to maximal medical therapy. Due in part to the extensive historical experience and continued familiarity among pediatric practitioners, it continues to be the first-line choice for pediatric mechanical support at many institutions [35]. The oxygenator provides some advantages over other methods of support in that where biventricular (or single ventricular) support is required; ECMO enables simplified support strategies and the use of peripheral cannulation. Among patients presenting late or diagnosed only at the onset of cardiogenic shock, ECMO can provide cardiopulmonary support while pulmonary dysfunction as the result of volume overload and elevated left ventricular end-diastolic pressure improves. However, with the many options for short-term VAD devices available, ECMO should be reserved for cases in which the pulmonary support component is necessary, rather than as a default strategy in all patients.

Cannulation Strategies

The flexibility provided by ECMO provides one of its most important advantages over other mechanical support techniques. Therefore, multiple cannulation strategies have been used and customization of the cannulation strategy to the patient is an important component of successful ECMO support. Arterial cannulation sites include: central aortic, carotid artery, femoral artery, and less commonly the subclavian artery. Venous drainage may be obtained from the internal jugular vein, femoral veins, or centrally from the right atrium. Each site has advantages and disadvantages, which should inform cannulation decisions.

Central Cannulation

Central cannulation is widely used among postcardiotomy patients because the sternum has often been recently opened (or remains open) following cardiac surgery; so there is little disadvantage to its use. Among other patients, there may be a reluctance (particularly among noncardiac surgical providers less familiar with mediansternotomy) to use central cannulation. However, it has important advantages. Where the patient has had a recent mediansternotomy or has a virgin mediastinum, central initiation of ECMO can be performed rapidly, usually in less than 10 min from prepping in our experience. In addition, for patients in cardiac arrest, internal cardiac massage can often be continued with few interruptions during the cannulation. Venous drainage is improved and higher flow rates are obtainable than through other techniques. Central access also enables easy placement of a surgical left ventricular or atrial drain, which improves ventricular decompression and may improve the likelihood of recovery, especially for postcardiotomy ventricular dysfunction (see below). These vents, especially when placed in a left atrial position, also often accelerate recovery of the lungs. Perhaps the primary disadvantage is the need for a mediansternotomy itself. This may result in increased bleeding risk: meticulous hemostasis, a low threshold to reexplore for any increase in bleeding, and avoidance over anticoagulation (especially in infants) are important in the successful use of central cannulation. Patients with a history of previous sternotomies may be challenging to safely and expeditiously cannulate; need for a reoperative sternotomy provides a relative contraindication to the use of central cannulation. However, given its many advantages, central cannulation is our preferred method of ECMO cannulation in most patients.

Peripheral Cannulation

Arterial Cannulation Sites

Carotid Artery. Among noncardiac pediatric providers, peripheral neck cannulation is the most common method for initiation of ECMO support. Due to the smaller size of other peripheral arteries in children—especially neonates—the carotid artery is often the only artery through which reliable full-flow support can be obtained. While neck cannulation can be performed rapidly, among patients undergoing CPR, it often necessitates frequent pauses in compressions to enable dissection and vascular access. Also, unlike central cannulation where cannula size is not limited and can be upsized if collaterals exist, peripheral cannulation often limits cannula size and may limit the ability to achieve full flow, especially where left-to-right shunting is present. The primary disadvantage of carotid artery cannulation remains the occlusion of distal flow in the carotid artery during cannulation and support. The impact of this remains controversial. However, among patients with fulminant heart failure, cardiogenic shock, hemodynamic instability, and CPR, who are already at risk for hypoxic-ischemic brain injury, reliance on collateral flow for cerebral perfusion is suboptimal. A recent review of ELSO data identified carotid artery cannulation as associated with a higher incidence of neurologic events [36]. Reconstruction of the carotid artery does not appear to have a direct impact on neurologic outcomes, although late outcomes among older adult survivors with only a single patent carotid artery are not available. Given the potential disadvantages of carotid artery cannulation it may be best reserved for use among neonates and infants with a history of previous sternotomy in whom central cannulation requires a reoperative sternotomy.

Femoral Artery. The femoral artery remains the most common cannulation site for ECMO support in older children (greater than approximately 20 kg) and young adults. In older children without a complex past-medical history, the femoral artery is usually large enough to provide full cardiac output support. Although in patients with complex past-medical history, especially CHD, where the femoral artery may have been accessed multiple times, it may not be as reliable. Femoral artery cannulation allows for rapid institution of ECMO support and in patients receiving CPR does not usually require many pauses in cardiac compressions. It may be performed either openly or percutaneously depending on operator experience, available cannulae, and patient anatomy. There are two important disadvantages. First, where there is native cardiac function and ventricular ejection, the poorly oxygenated blood from the patient's ventricle will be directed into the coronary arteries and left carotid artery. Thus, it may be necessary to forego reduction in mechanical ventilator support to maintain oxygen delivery to these organs, and the heart and brain are less likely to benefit from the enhanced oxygen delivery from the circuit. Second, appropriately sized arterial cannulae may completely obstruct distal femoral arterial flow. While rarely a problem during cardiac surgical procedures using femoral arterial CPB, when support duration exceeds 24 h, there is an increasing risk of distal limb ischemia, which may lead to limb loss [37].

Several techniques have been described to augment flow distal to the femoral artery cannula, including posterior tibial cannulation [38], insertion of an antegrade perfusion catheter in the femoral artery [39], or cannulation through a side-arm graft rather than directly into the artery [40]. These techniques may be used selectively where distal perfusion appears compromised during support or routinely in all patients cannulated via the femoral artery.

Because femoral cannulation is often being performed emergently, our preference is to initially cannulate through the most expeditious technique (usually either open or percutaneous direct arterial cannulation) and initiate ECMO support. We then proceed to evaluate the relative merits of each distal limb perfusion technique and choose the most appropriate technique for each patient. Usually, our preference is to proceed with dissection of the contralateral groin and anastomosis of a 6–10mm wove dacron side-arm graft to the contralateral femoral artery. Notably, placing the side-arm at a 30–45degrees angle (directed proximally) may prevent some of the distal limb swelling sometimes observed (as has been described with subclavian artery cannulation [41]). The side-arm graft is then cannulated and ECMO support is transitioned to this artery. The original cannula is removed and the cannulation site repaired to reestablish distal flow. The primary downside of this technique is that it is time-consuming and may not be appropriate depending on patient condition; in such situations, use of an antegrade perfusion catheter placed distally on the femoral artery ipsilateral to the initial cannulation may be more expeditious.

Subclavian Artery. Although rarely used, the subclavian artery has several advantages when used for long-term ECMO support. In contrast to femoral artery cannulation it delivers highly oxygenated blood to the brain and proximal aorta. Also, patients can often be extubated and mobilized. Although only of suitable size in larger patients, it should be considered in young adults as an alternative to other cannulation sites when prolonged ECMO support may be required.

Venous Cannulation Sites

Internal Jugular Vein. Optimal location for venous access is often dependent on a combination of patient size and needed flow rates. In smaller patients, especially neonates, the internal jugular vein is the only peripheral vein of appropriate size to provide near full flow. In larger patients, the shorter cannula length and easier positioning of the tip within the right atrium often enable higher flows than a similar diameter femoral venous cannula. As with subclavian arterial cannulation, venous cannulation in the neck allows for mobilization in these patients as well.

Femoral Vein. The femoral vein is often chosen for venous drainage during ECMO support in larger patients. Access can be obtained rapidly at the same time as femoral arterial access. In patients receiving CPR, compressions may not need to be paused as they often do for internal jugular cannulation. While long cannulas can be placed from the femoral vein into the right atrium, drainage is often suboptimal, both as a result of cannula length and the potential for positional kinking and drainage obstruction as the cannula passes through the pelvis and into the inferior vena cava. For these reasons, we often find that femoral venous cannulation is useful for initial support, but a second cannula (either in the contralateral groin or in the internal jugular vein) is often required to obtain full flow.

Summary of Cannulation Strategies

We have found that familiarity with the advantages and disadvantages of all of these cannulation strategies enables a flexible approach to the institution of ECMO. By customizing the approach to each patient, appropriate MCS can be provided expeditiously and then subsequently optimized. Wherever the cannulae are placed, meticulous attention to hemostasis is critical. Bleeding treated with additional blood products and lowering of anticoagulation goals (particularly heparin activity levels) often results in a deleterious cascade with early oxygenator failure and circuit thrombosis [42]. We have found that patients can be supported by ECMO without circuit or oxygenator change for 30–60days when a low threshold for reexploration and achievement of surgical hemostasis is combined with a circuit with low thrombogenic potential.

Left Ventricular/Left Atrial Venting

Use of venoarterial ECMO for support of the acutely failing left ventricle does not provide ventricular offloading; in fact, without left atrial or ventricular decompression, the left ventricle remains pressure loaded and under significant strain [5]. Because of the perceived benefits of ventricular unloading in improving myocardial recovery, left ventricular or atrial venting has been advocated by some [43]. However, decompression of the left atrium or ventricle remains controversial. Some institutions report reasonable recovery and weaning rates without the use of left-sided vents, and the use of left-sided vents was relatively uncommon in pediatric patients with myocarditis as of 2010 [17,44].

Some of the confusion or controversy surrounding this issue may be the result of the rarity of left ventricular decompression and poor understanding of the indications for left-sided decompression. While left-atrial decompression may improve unloading, it is not equivalent to left-ventricular decompression [5]. On the other hand, atrial venting may better assist in the more rapid resolution of pulmonary edema. Therefore, the indication for ECMO initiation guides optimal vent placement.

In postcardiotomy heart failure, complete left ventricular unloading is an important component of recovery. This can only be achieved via placement of a left ventricular vent (either via the mitral valve or directly into the apex) [5]. On the other hand, left atrial decompression can often be obtained more readily and is ideal for fulminant myocarditis where resolution of pulmonary edema is the primary goal of left-sided vent placement.

Percutaneous methods in patients with peripheral cannulation include balloon atrial septostomy or placement of a percutaneous left atrial drainage catheter. Unfortunately, percutaneous vents are often relatively small and prone to clotting; balloon atrial septostomy requires subsequent atrial septal device closure following myocardial recovery. One of the authors has used a percutaneous, balloon-directed venous cannula placed into the pulmonary artery to achieve left-sided decompression. Therefore, we feel none of these methods are as effective as direct left atrial or ventricular cannulation. Despite the theoretical benefits of left-sided decompression, no definitive data exist demonstrating improved outcomes, so practice continues to vary based on individual and institutional preference.

Shunts and the Patent Ductus

Strategies for dealing with left-to-right arterial level shunts (most commonly the patent ductus arteriosus or surgically created Blalock–Taussig shunts) vary between institutions. The flow through a shunt may be a significant component of the total flow provided by the ECMO circuit [45]. While this might argue for occlusion of the shunt during initiation of ECMO, Jaggers et al. identified a higher mortality (100% vs. 20%, $P=.05$) among patients in whom the shunt was occluded during support [46]. There is concern that complete shunt occlusion may result in pulmonary ischemia and severe ischemia-reperfusion injury when the shunt is reopened prior to ECMO weaning [46]. However, we prefer a strategy used by other centers in which the shunt is partially occluded [47,48], this preserves some delivery of oxygen to the lungs while minimizing the potential for pulmonary overcirculation and "steal" from systemic perfusion. When the shunt is left partially open and even more so when left completely open, mechanical support will require higher flows than the standard systemic cardiac output based on patient size. These strategies, therefore, rely on central cannulation because cannulae and cannulation sites should allow for flows as high as 200cc/kg/min with adequate drainage and without excessive arterial pressure.

Ambulatory ECMO and Extracorporeal VAD Support

One of the downsides of short-term MCS remains the frequent need to maintain patients mechanically ventilated and sedated, either for pain control and respiratory mechanics (where central cannulation with an open sternum is present), or to maintain effective drainage (where movement may result in kinking of peripherally inserted cannulae, particularly in the femoral vessels). Cannulation strategies designed to enable liberation from mechanical ventilation and ambulation mitigate some of this downside and enable early mobilization with a potentially lower risk of infection and pneumonia. Although one of the authors' centers has extubated neonatal patients on venoarterial ECMO via neck vessels to enable spontaneous ventilation and feeding in a manner similar to reported in the literature [49], these techniques are likely to be of highly circumscribed utility in smaller, younger patients who are less able to cooperate with instructions. However, in appropriate adolescents, ECMO cannulation via a combination of subclavian arterial and internal jugular venous access may enable rapid mobilization [41]. Similarly, temporary biventricular support can be provided in adolescents using standard CPB cannulae brought out through the skin and connected to a CentriMag or other centrifugal extracorporeal pump [50]. Doubling-up of purse strings and adequate internal fixation of the cannulae is critical to maintain safety [50]. More recently, the use of Berlin Heart EXCOR cannulae connected to a temporary centrifugal pump (often a Thoratec CentriMag/PediMag or Rotaflow) has become an increasingly common strategy. This technique mitigates the risks of dislodgement associated with standard CPB cannulae but does come at the cost of a slightly more complex explant procedure in cases of myocardial recovery. In patients requiring support for longer than 7days, this may decrease the risks associated with maintenance of a temporary support device and minimize the need to convert to a more durable device in patients with a continued high likelihood of recovery.

SPECIFIC DEVICES

Extracorporeal Membrane Oxygenation Pumps and Circuits

The choice of pumps and specific circuits is highly variable across institutions. While centrifugal pumps are becoming increasingly common for ECMO support across the pediatric age and weight range, there remain advantages to the use of roller pumps, especially for neonatal support. In postcardiotomy patients, the use of roller pumps may enable rapid transition on and off CPB without replacing oxygenators or circuits (by cutting in a reservoir). In addition, flow rates are less variable with alterations from the planned flow clearly identified with an alarm and pump shut down in response to pressure measurements outside the set range. Because centrifugal pumps are preload and afterload dependent, the flow is likely to vary more frequently with physiologic alterations in the patient. Especially in smaller patients, at lower flows, this may result in variability in delivered systemic perfusion as well as flow variability and a risk of thrombosis (personal communication). Overall, centrifugal pumps may have a higher incidence of ECMO-related complications [51]. Despite these potential advantages of roller pumps, there has been an increasing use of centrifugal pumps at most ECMO centers driven predominantly by the potential for smaller prime volumes, increasing availability, ease of bedside monitoring, and the lower maintenance requirements. Whichever pump is used, recognition of the advantages, disadvantages, and potential complications is essential to optimizing outcomes.

Ventricular Assist Devices

Although ECMO has traditionally been the mainstay of short-term mechanical support in pediatrics, several recent trends have resulted in the increasing adoption of VADs. These include: the availability of progressively smaller pumps designed primarily for adults but adaptable to children, increasing familiarity among pediatric practitioners with the potential advantages of mechanical support without an oxygenator, and improved management of anticoagulation as part of the approval process for the Berlin Heart EXCOR device in children, including subsequent modifications. Therefore, in the absence of cardiogenic shock, severe pulmonary edema resulting in respiratory failure, or anatomic contraindications to VAD therapy, short-term VADs should generally be preferred over ECMO for support of the patient with heart failure.

Cannulation Strategies

Without the oxygenator, cannulation strategies for support using VADs are more limited. Generally, the inflow cannula is either placed directly into the ventricle or into the atrium. As noted above, left atrial cannulation may be preferred in inflammatory states with significant pulmonary disease (such as fulminant myocarditis). While cannulation between the right pulmonary veins immediately posterior to Sondergaard's groove is an option, cannulation via the left atrial appendage may be more optimal. Because the left atrium is often quite dilated and lays lateral and slightly anterior to the main pulmonary artery, it is relatively easy to place a side-biting clamp on the appendage, followed by a purse string for rapid and consistent cannulation without the need for CPB. It is important that the cannula used be a wire-reinforced bullet-type cannula that can be shaped with a significant curve to slip around the dilated left ventricle and into a position just above the mitral valve. Appropriate position within the body of the left atrium should be confirmed via echocardiography because leaving the cannula tip within the appendage results in poor drainage, inadequate flow, and continued high left atrial pressures.

For support of the left ventricle from a noninflammatory etiology, ventricular cannulation at the apex is usually preferred. It has important advantages including improved left ventricular offloading and minimization of stasis within the ventricular cavity, especially if prolonged support is anticipated [52]. Although these advantages may be less important with short-term devices. While left atrial cannulation does avoid a ventriculotomy, apical ventriculotomy does not appear to affect long-term ventricular function significantly if myocardial recovery and decannulation occur [53]. Restrictive/hypertrophic cardiomyopathy patients are an important subset where apical cannulation may not be effective because of intraventricular restriction of blood flow and poor inflow the device. In these cases, myectomy or excision of the atrioventricular valve may provide adequate drainage, but atrial cannulation is often used with success.

Short-Term Ventricular Assist Devices Suitable for Use in Children

Centrifugal Pumps

In the current era, short-term mechanical circulatory support is primarily obtained with centrifugal pumps. Standard extracorporeal surgically implanted pumps include the Thoratec CentriMag/PediMag (Fig. 51.2), Sorin Revolution, and the Maquet Rotaflow. While different in minor technical aspects, there is little data to support significantly different outcomes between manufacturers. Data on the use of short-term centrifugal pumps in children are only just beginning to accumulate. Individual cases and case series have been published, but the largest series to date includes only 33 uses of short-term continuous flow devices [54]. In that single-institution experience, 67% of patients supported with these devices survived to discharge [54]. This represents excellent outcomes in critically ill patients, 45% of whom were on ECMO prior to support [54]. Patients were supported for a median of 12 days with the longest run of 75 days; significant complications occurred,

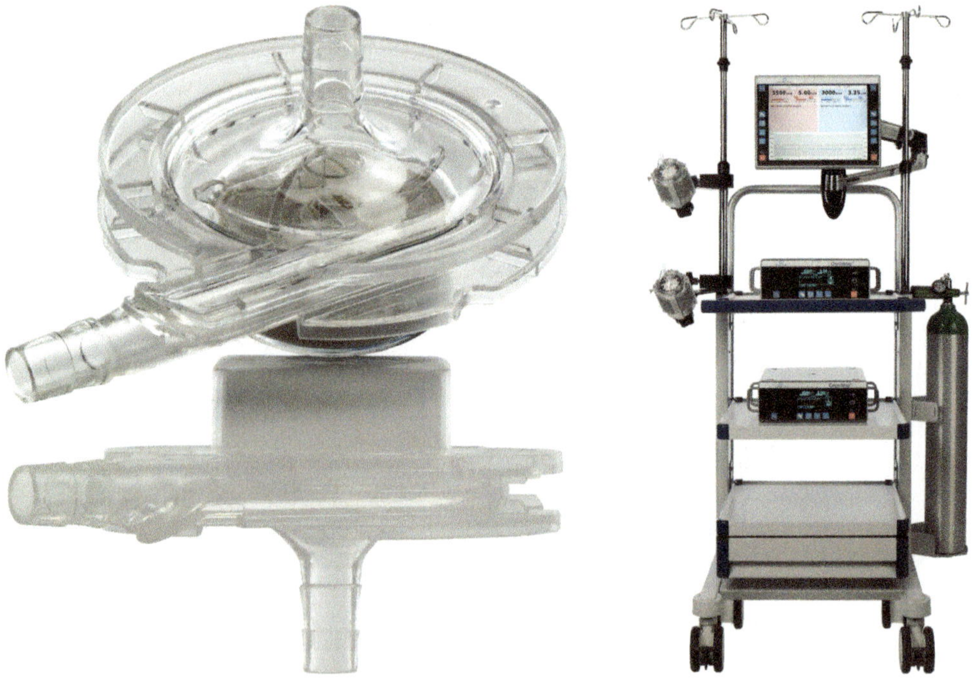

FIGURE 51.2

including neurologic events in six and reexploration for bleeding in eight [54]. Outcomes included recovery, conversion to a durable device, and transplantation off the short-term device [54]. Unfortunately, the heterogeneity of the population limits the specific conclusions. More recent data from Pedimacs reports consistent results in a multiinstitutional series of 49 patients supported with temporary VADs; positive outcomes were identified in 75% [55]. Although the devices have been used to support single ventricle patients at all stages of palliation [56–58], and other forms of congenital heart disease, as well as patients with dilated or restrictive cardiomyopathy [54,56,57,59–61], experience is limited such that there is little to data to guide decision-making regarding either implantation or patient management.

Impella

The Abiomed Impella series of devices are left ventricular support devices intended predominantly for percutaneous arterial insertion. Three sizes are available, which results in maximum flows of 2.5 (Impella 2.5), 4 (Impella CP), or 5 (Impella 5.0) liters per minute. The Impella 5.0 is available in two versions, one designed for percutaneous access, the other for direct placement through the aorta. All of the pumps are microaxial, catheter-mounted pumps intended for retrograde placement across the aortic valve such that the pump inflow is in the left ventricular outflow tract and the pump outflow is located in the ascending aorta (Fig. 51.3). Because of the size limitations of the Impella pump, it is suitable only for patients with BSA > $1.3\,m^2$; as such there is little specific data on outcomes in children beyond case reports of its successful use [62].

TandemHeart

The CardiacAssist TandemHeart pVAD is another continuous flow device initially designed for percutaneous implantation into adults, but seeing some increased use among pediatric practitioners. The traditional implantation of the TandemHeart is performed in the catheterization laboratory and involved venous access to the right atrium with the inflow cannula placed across the septum into the left atrium using a transseptal puncture. Arterial outflow was through percutaneous arterial insertion (usually in the femoral artery). This enables rapid initiation of left ventricular support during cardiac catheterization procedures. Among larger children, percutaneous insertion provides for rapid initiation of mechanical support without need for a sternotomy. The authors have personal experience with using this device on adolescents and found that the positioning of the LA cannula is quite tenuous in this cohort. Minimal manipulation (i.e., movement to get a CXR) can often cause migration and the need for cannula repositioning. Modifications of this device have enabled the pump alone to be used as an extracorporeal pump for infants and children requiring short-term support [63]. This may provide an option for centers without availability of more commonly used pediatric VADs.

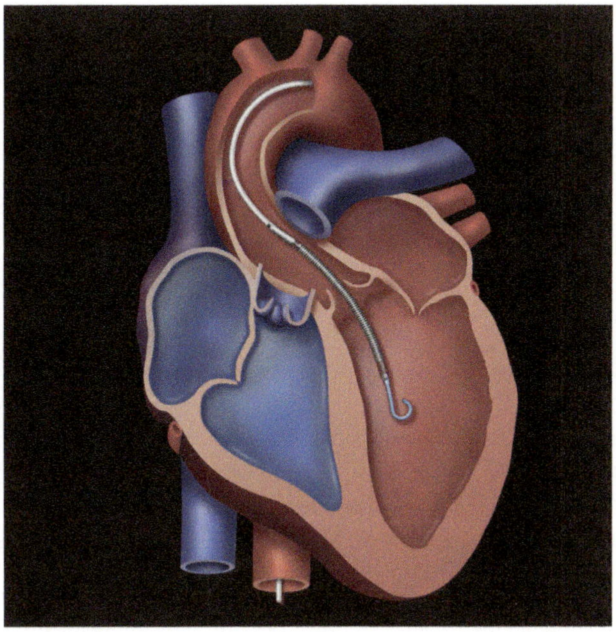

FIGURE 51.3

OTHER CONSIDERATIONS

Infants/Neonates

Mechanical circulatory support in infants and neonates is made particularly challenging due to a combination of higher thrombogenic risk at lower flows, altered coagulation cascades in infancy, and the limited number of devices available. For these reasons, as well as the high incidence of congenital heart disease and single ventricular heart failure, ECMO remains a common method of support in this age group. However, for infants and neonates requiring only temporary support for myocarditis or for those presenting without congenital heart disease whose etiology is not known, short-term VAD support is an effective strategy that can avoid many of the issues with ECMO support. While the Berlin Heart EXCOR provides a medium to long-term solution for ventricular assist, it has poor outcomes in this population [64].

Several series of short-term mechanical support include infants and neonates, but there are fewer that include results specific to this population [54]. Recovery following device implantation for dilated cardiomyopathy has been reported, but thromboembolic complications occurred in three out of seven patients less than 1 year old, and no child was supported beyond 22 days [53]. We do not recommend short-term VAD support for patients with dilated cardiomyopathy unless it is acute support of the circulation until diagnosis is made or for resuscitation of a patient in INTERMACS 1 heart failure (cardiogenic shock). Short-term VAD support should be used only to stabilize the patient without committing to the more involved procedure of implanting a long-term device. Here, the short-term VAD serves simply as a bridge to a long-term device The Berlin Heart EXCOR has been used for short-term support, but mortality rates exceed 50% in many series [21,54,65–67]. The assumption is that current continuous flow VADs may have better outcomes; data specific to small patients to validate this assumption continue to grow but remain insufficient at this time.

Because of the high-risk of complications in this population, indications for mechanical circulatory support are generally narrower. While renal or hepatic dysfunction despite maximal medical therapy remains an important indication for the VAD implantation, mechanical ventilation with significant inotropic support usually precedes implantation of a short-term device.

Congenital Heart Disease

Mechanical circulatory support of the patients with congenital heart disease (CHD) may be complicated by several factors. Because of this, a full assessment of cardiac anatomy and physiology is required prior to support initiation [68]. Among the important challenges are: residual intracardiac shunts that may result in hypoxemia following systemic ventricular decompression in patients with two ventricles, atrial baffles or systemic right ventricles that may alter positioning of inflow cannulae or impede drainage, and the presence of collateral vessels that may necessitate higher than usual flows and better than usual drainage. Single ventricle patients have an additional set of challenges related to balancing systemic and pulmonary outflow, characterizing whether cardiac failure is the result of ventricular dysfunction or pulmonary circuit failure, and identifying appropriate sites for drainage. Because support with ECMO eliminates many of these issues, it remains a common method of short-term support in patients with CHD. Short-term support among patients with CHD is most commonly related to perioperative management surrounding cardiac surgery. However, patients with progressive heart failure may require short-term support in the setting of acute decompensation or arrhythmias resulting sudden death. More interestingly, based on the poor experience with the Berlin Heart in supporting children (especially infants) with single ventricle physiology [69,70], there is increasing interest in the use of "short-term" devices as longer-term continuous flow support. This may provide an important improvement in outcomes while we await implantable devices sized for neonates and infants.

CONCLUSION

Pediatric patients have been the beneficiary of the recent improvements in function and reductions in size of mechanical circulatory support devices. ECMO continues to be an important support strategy, particularly in patients with acute biventricular failure, severe pulmonary edema, or congenital heart disease. However, pediatric practitioners are becoming more familiar with the use of short-term VADs. In specific applications, especially patients with myocarditis, short-term VADs may provide a lower complication profile and improve the likelihood of recovery or successful bridge-to-transplant. Also, like our adult colleagues, we are moving away from long-term VAD implantation in patients with cardiogenic shock (INTERMACS 1) because of suboptimal outcomes and have started to use short-term VADs as an efficient way to resuscitate these patients, with the expectation of improving their outcomes from long-term VAD support. New devices and innovative approaches to temporary mechanical support continue to improve the options for children with medically refractory heart failure. A flexible approach to the individual patient is required to optimize mechanical support and outcomes in this challenging population.

REFERENCES

[1] C.D. Fraser, R.D.B. Jaquiss, D.N. Rosenthal, T. Humpl, C.E. Canter, E.H. Blackstone, D.C. Naftel, R.N. Ichord, L. Bomgaars, J.S. Tweddell, M.P. Massicotte, M.W. Turrentine, G.A. Cohen, E.J. Devaney, F.B. Pearce, K.E. Carberry, R. Kroslowitz, C.S. Almond, Berlin Heart Study Investigators, Prospective trial of a pediatric ventricular assist device, N. Engl. J. Med. 367 (2012) 532–541.

[2] J.J. Teuteberg, G.C. Stewart, M. Jessup, R.L. Kormos, B. Sun, O.H. Frazier, D.C. Naftel, L.W. Stevenson, Implant strategies change over time and impact outcomes: insights from the INTERMACS (interagency registry for mechanically assisted circulatory support), JCHF 1 (2013) 369–378.

[3] R. Stretch, C.M. Sauer, D.D. Yuh, P. Bonde, National trends in the utilization of short-term mechanical circulatory support: incidence, outcomes, and cost analysis, J. Am. Coll. Cardiol. 64 (2014) 1407–1415.

[4] J.W. Rossano, T.M. Hoffman, J.L. Jefferies, A. Lorts, R.E. Kirsch, R.R. Thiagarajan, Clinical issues and controversies in heart failure and transplantation, World J. Pediatr. Congenit. Heart Surg. 7 (2016) 63–71.

[5] D. Burkhoff, G. Sayer, D. Doshi, N. Uriel, Hemodynamics of mechanical circulatory support, J. Am. Coll. Cardiol. 66 (2015) 2663–2674.

[6] K.L. Brown, D.A. Ridout, A. Hoskote, L. Verhulst, M. Ricci, C. Bull, Delayed diagnosis of congenital heart disease worsens preoperative condition and outcome of surgery in neonates, Heart 92 (2006) 1298–1302.

[7] V. Bautista-Hernandez, R.R. Thiagarajan, F. Fynn-Thompson, S.K. Rajagopal, D.E. Nento, V. Yarlagadda, S.A. Teele, C.K. Allan, S.M. Emani, P.C. Laussen, F.A. Pigula, E.A. Bacha, Preoperative extracorporeal membrane oxygenation as a bridge to cardiac surgery in children with congenital heart disease, Ann. Thorac. Surg. 88 (2009) 1306–1311.

[8] D.L. Wessel, Managing low cardiac output syndrome after congenital heart surgery, Crit. Care Med. 29 (2001) S220–S230.

[9] E.D. Sherwin, K. Gauvreau, M.A. Scheurer, P.T. Rycus, J.W. Salvin, M.C. Almodovar, F. Fynn-Thompson, R.R. Thiagarajan, Extracorporeal membrane oxygenation after stage 1 palliation for hypoplastic left heart syndrome, J. Thorac. Cardiovasc. Surg. 144 (2012) 1337–1343.

[10] B. Alsoufi, M. Wolf, P. Botha, B. Kogon, C. McCracken, A. Ehrlich, K. Kanter, S. Deshpande, Late outcomes of infants supported by extracorporeal membrane oxygenation following the Norwood operation, World J. Pediatr. Congenit. Heart Surg. 6 (2015) 9–17.

[11] D.L.S. Morales, F. Zafar, J.W. Rossano, J.D. Salazar, J.L. Jefferies, D.E. Graves, J.S. Heinle, C.D. Fraser, Use of ventricular assist devices in children across the United States: analysis of 7.5 million pediatric hospitalizations, Ann. Thorac. Surg. 90 (2010) 1313–1318 discussion 1318–9.

[12] R. Hetzer, F. Kaufmann, E.M. Delmo Walter, Paediatric mechanical circulatory support with Berlin Heart EXCOR: development and outcome of a 23-year experience, Eur. J. Cardiothorac. Surg. (2016) ezw011.

[13] C.E. Canter, K.E. Simpson, K.P. Simpson, Diagnosis and treatment of myocarditis in children in the current era, Circulation 129 (2014) 115–128.

[14] S.R. Foerster, C.E. Canter, A. Cinar, L.A. Sleeper, S.A. Webber, E. Pahl, P.F. Kantor, J.A. Alvarez, S.D. Colan, J.L. Jefferies, J.M. Lamour, R. Margossian, J.E. Messere, P.G. Rusconi, R.E. Shaddy, J.A. Towbin, J.D. Wilkinson, S.E. Lipshultz, Ventricular remodeling and survival are more favorable for myocarditis than for idiopathic dilated cardiomyopathy in childhood: an outcomes study from the pediatric cardiomyopathy registry, Circ. Heart Fail. 3 (2010) 689–697.

[15] S. Pan, B. Aksut, O.E. Wever-Pinzon, S.D. Rao, A.P. Levin, A.R. Garan, J.A. Fried, K. Takeda, T. Hiroo, M. Yuzefpolskaya, N. Uriel, U.P. Jorde, D.M. Mancini, Y. Naka, P.C. Colombo, V.K. Topkara, Incidence and predictors of myocardial recovery on long-term left ventricular assist device support: results from the united network for organ sharing database, J. Heart Lung Transplant. 34 (2015) 1624–1629.

[16] D.L. Mann, P.M. Barger, D. Burkhoff, Myocardial recovery and the failing heart: myth, magic, or molecular target?(Internet), J. Am. Coll. Cardiol. 60 (2012) 2465–2472. Available from: http://content.onlinejacc.org/article.aspx?articleid=1389697.

[17] S.K. Rajagopal, C.S. Almond, P.C. Laussen, P.T. Rycus, D. Wypij, R.R. Thiagarajan, Extracorporeal membrane oxygenation for the support of infants, children, and young adults with acute myocarditis: a review of the extracorporeal life support organization registry(Internet), Crit. Care Med. 38 (2010) 382–387. Available from: http://content.wkhealth.com/linkback/openurl?sid=WKPTLP:landingpage&an=00003246-201002000-00003.

[18] I. Wilmot, D.L.S. Morales, J.F. Price, J.W. Rossano, J.J. Kim, J.A. Decker, M.C. McGarry, S.W. Denfield, W.J. Dreyer, J.A. Towbin, J.L. Jefferies, Effectiveness of mechanical circulatory support in children with acute fulminant and persistent myocarditis, J. Card. Fail. 17 (2011) 487–494.

[19] B.W. Duncan, D.J. Bohn, A.M. Atz, J.W. French, P.C. Laussen, D.L. Wessel, Mechanical circulatory support for the treatment of children with acute fulminant myocarditis, J. Thorac. Cardiovasc. Surg. 122 (2001) 440–448.

[20] R. Kirk, E. Peng, A. Woods, J. Flett, T. Hewitt, M. Griselli, S. Schueler, N. Wrightson, A. Hasan, Successful HeartWare bridge to recovery in a 3-year old: a game changer? Ann. Thorac. Surg. 101 (2016) 1984–1987.

[21] J. Conway, J. St Louis, D.L.S. Morales, S. Law, C. Tjossem, T. Humpl, Delineating survival outcomes in children <10kg bridged to transplant or recovery with the Berlin Heart EXCOR Ventricular Assist Device, JCHF 3 (2015) 70–77.

[22] T.M. Giglia, M.P. Massicotte, J.S. Tweddell, R.J. Barst, M. Bauman, C.C. Erickson, T.F. Feltes, E. Foster, K. Hinoki, R.N. Ichord, J. Kreutzer, B.W. McCrindle, J.W. Newburger, S. Tabbutt, J.L. Todd, C.L. Webb, American Heart Association Congenital Heart Defects Committee of the Council on Cardiovascular Disease in the Young, Council on Cardiovascular and Stroke Nursing, Council on Epidemiology and Prevention, and Stroke Council, Prevention and treatment of thrombosis in pediatric and congenital heart disease: a scientific statement from the American Heart Association(Internet), Circulation 128 (2013) 2622–2703. Available from: http://circ.ahajournals.org/cgi/doi/10.1161/01.cir.0000436140.77832.7a.

[23] R.R. Davies, S. Haldeman, M.A. McCulloch, C. Pizarro, Ventricular assist devices as a bridge-to-transplant improve early post-transplant outcomes in children, J. Heart Lung Transplant. 33 (2014) 704–712.

[24] C. Villa, R. Rizwan, F. Zafar, A. Lorts, D.L.S. Morales, Bridging children to transplant with short term VADs does not affect post-transplant mortality, J. Heart 35 (2016) S351.

[25] J.J. Lasa, R.S. Rogers, R. Localio, J. Shults, T. Raymond, M. Gaies, R. Thiagarajan, P.C. Laussen, T. Kilbaugh, R.A. Berg, V. Nadkarni, A. Topjian, Extracorporeal-cardiopulmonary resuscitation (E-CPR) during pediatric in-hospital cardiopulmonary arrest is associated with improved survival to discharge: a report from the American Heart Association's get with the Guidelines® - resuscitation registry (GWTG-R), Circulation 133 (2015) 165–176.

[26] C. Chrysostomou, V.O. Morell, B.A. Kuch, E. O'Malley, R. Munoz, P.D. Wearden, Short- and intermediate-term survival after extracorporeal membrane oxygenation in children with cardiac disease, J. Thorac. Cardiovasc. Surg. 146 (2013) 317–325.

[27] D.A. Kane, R.R. Thiagarajan, D. Wypij, M.A. Scheurer, F. Fynn-Thompson, S. Emani, P.J. del Nido, P. Betit, P.C. Laussen, Rapid-response extracorporeal membrane oxygenation to support cardiopulmonary resuscitation in children with cardiac disease, Circulation 122 (2010) S241–S248.

[28] A. Hoskote, C. Carter, P. Rees, M. Elliott, M. Burch, K. Brown, Acute right ventricular failure after pediatric cardiac transplant: predictors and long-term outcome in current era of transplantation medicine, J. Thorac. Cardiovasc. Surg. 139 (2010) 146–153.

[29] C. Tissot, S. Buckvold, C.M. Phelps, D.D. Ivy, D.N. Campbell, M.B. Mitchell, S.O. da Cruz, B.A. Pietra, S.D. Miyamoto, Outcome of extracorporeal membrane oxygenation for early primary graft failure after pediatric heart transplantation, J. Am. Coll. Cardiol. 54 (2009) 730–737.

[30] J.A. Su, R.B. Kelly, T. Grogan, D. Elashoff, J.C. Alejos, Extracorporeal membrane oxygenation support after pediatric orthotopic heart transplantation, Pediatr. Transplant. (2014) (n/a–n/a).

[31] K. Fenton, S.A. Webber, D. Danford, S.K. Gandhi, J. Periera, F. Pigula, Long-term survival after pediatric cardiac transplantation and postoperative ECMO support, Ann. Thorac. Surg. 76 (2003) 843–846 discussion 847.

[32] J. Kobashigawa, A. Zuckermann, P. Macdonald, P. Leprince, F. Esmailian, M. LuuMBBS, D. Mancini, J. Patel, R. Razi, H. Reichenspurner, J. Segovia, N. Smedira, J. Stehlik, F. Wagner, Participants OBOTCC, Report from a consensus conference on primary graft dysfunction after cardiac transplantation, J. Heart Lung Transplant. (2014) 1–48.

[33] H. Takayama, Y. Naka, S.K. Kodali, J.A. Vincent, L.J. Addonizio, U.P. Jorde, M.R. Williams, A novel approach to percutaneous right-ventricular mechanical support(Internet), Eur. J. Cardiothorac. Surg. 41 (2012) 423–426. Available from: http://ejcts.oxfordjournals.org/content/41/2/423.full.

[34] I. Adachi, F.A. Guzmán-Pruneda, M.S. Khan, E.D. McKenzie, C.D. Fraser, Ventricular assist device in children with cardiac graft failure, ASAIO J. 61 (2015) 729–730.

[35] J.L. Jefferies, D.L. Morales, Mechanical circulatory support in children: bridge to transplant versus recovery, Curr. Heart Fail. Rep. 9 (2012) 236–243.

[36] S.A. Teele, J.W. Salvin, C.S. Barrett, P.T. Rycus, F. Fynn-Thompson, P.C. Laussen, R.R. Thiagarajan, The association of carotid artery cannulation and neurologic injury in pediatric patients supported with venoarterial extracorporeal membrane oxygenation, Pediatr. Crit. Care Med. 15 (2014) 355–361.

[37] J.W. Gander, J.C. Fisher, A.R. Reichstein, E.R. Gross, G. Aspelund, W. Middlesworth, C.J. Stolar, Limb ischemia after common femoral artery cannulation for venoarterial extracorporeal membrane oxygenation: an unresolved problem, J. Pediatr. Surg. 45 (2010) 2136–2140.

[38] D.J. Spurlock, J.M. Toomasian, M.A. Romano, E. Cooley, R.H. Bartlett, J.W. Haft, A simple technique to prevent limb ischemia during veno-arterial ECMO using the femoral artery: the posterior tibial approach, Perfusion 27 (2012) 141–145.

[39] M.J. Haley, J.C. Fisher, A.R. Ruiz-Elizalde, C.J.H. Stolar, N.J. Morrissey, W. Middlesworth, Percutaneous distal perfusion of the lower extremity after femoral cannulation for venoarterial extracorporeal membrane oxygenation in a small child, J. Pediatr. Surg. 44 (2009) 437–440.

[40] K.W. Jackson, J. Timpa, R.B. McIlwain, C. O'Meara, J.K. Kirklin, S. Borasino, J.A. Alten, Side-arm grafts for femoral extracorporeal membrane oxygenation cannulation, Ann. Thorac. Surg. 94 (2012) e111–e112.

[41] M. Biscotti, M. Bacchetta, The "Sport Model": extracorporeal membrane oxygenation using the subclavian artery, Ann. Thorac. Surg. 98 (2014) 1487–1489.

[42] K. Irby, C.J. Swearingen, J.W. Byrnes, J. Bryant, P. Prodhan, R.T. Fiser, Unfractionated heparin activity measured by anti-factor Xa levels is associated with the need for ECMO circuit/membrane oxygenator change: a retrospective pediatric study, Pediatr. Crit. Care Med. 15 (2014) e175–e182.

[43] D.F. Hacking, D. Best, Y. d'Udekem, C.P. Brizard, I.E. Konstantinov, J. Millar, W. Butt, Elective decompression of the left ventricle in pediatric patients may reduce the duration of venoarterial extracorporeal membrane oxygenation, Artif. Organs 39 (2015) 319–326.

[44] T.-H. Kim, C. Lim, P. Il, D.J. Kim, Y. Jung, K.-H. Park, Prognosis in the patients with prolonged extracorporeal membrane oxygenation, Korean J. Thorac. Cardiovasc. Surg. 45 (2012) 236–241.

[45] R.B. Tanke, A.F. van Heijst, J.H.G.M. Klaessens, O. Daniëls, C. Festen, Measurement of the ductal L-R shunt during extracorporeal membrane oxygenation in the lamb, J. Pediatr. Surg. 39 (2004) 43–47.

[46] J.J. Jaggers, J.M. Forbess, A.S. Shah, J.N. Meliones, P.M. Kirshbom, C.E. Miller, R.M. Ungerleider, Extracorporeal membrane oxygenation for infant postcardiotomy support: significance of shunt management, Ann. Thorac. Surg. 69 (2000) 1476–1483.

[47] A. Aharon, D.C. Drinkwater, K. Churchwell, S. Quisling, V. Reddy, M. Taylor, S. Hix, K. Christian, J. Pietsch, J. Deshpande, J. Kambam, T.P. Graham, P. Chang, Extracorporeal membrane oxygenation in children after repair of congenital cardiac lesions, Ann. Thorac. Surg. 72 (2001) 2095–2101 discussion 2101–2.

[48] T.K.S. Kumar, D. Zurakowski, H. Dalton, S. Talwar, A. Allard-Picou, L.F. Duebener, P. Sinha, A. Moulick, Extracorporeal membrane oxygenation in postcardiotomy patients: factors influencing outcome, J. Thorac. Cardiovasc. Surg. 140 (2010) 330–336.e2.

[49] F. Schmidt, T. Jack, M. Sasse, T. Kaussen, H. Bertram, A. Horke, K. Seidemann, P. Beerbaum, H. Koeditz, "Awake veno-arterial extracorporeal membrane oxygenation" in pediatric cardiogenic shock: a single-center experience, Pediatr. Cardiol. 36 (2015) 1647–1656.

[50] H. Takayama, J.M. Chen, U.P. Jorde, Y. Naka, Implantation technique of the CentriMag biventricular assist device allowing ambulatory rehabilitation, Interact. Cardiovasc. Thorac. Surg. 12 (2011) 110–111.

[51] C.S. Barrett, J.J. Jaggers, E.F. Cook, D.A. Graham, V.V. Yarlagadda, S.A. Teele, C.S. Almond, S.L. Bratton, J.D. Seeger, H.J. Dalton, P.T. Rycus, P.C. Laussen, R.R. Thiagarajan, Pediatric ECMO outcomes: comparison of centrifugal versus roller blood pumps using propensity score matching, ASAIO J. 59 (2013) 145–151.

[52] D.B. Sims, H. Takayama, N. Uriel, L.D. Gillam, Y. Naka, U.P. Jorde, Ventricular assist device-associated thrombus, Circulation 124 (2011) e197–e198.

[53] H. Zimmerman, D. Covington, R. Smith, C. Inaht, B. Barber, J. Copeland, Recovery of dilated cardiomyopathies in infants and children using left ventricular assist devices, ASAIO J. 1 (2010).

[54] J. Conway, M. Al-Aklabi, D. Granoski, S. Islam, L. Ryerson, V. Anand, G. Guerra, A.S. Mackie, I. Rebeyka, H. Buchholz, Supporting pediatric patients with short-term continuous-flow devices, J. Heart Lung Transpl. 35 (2016) 603–609.

[55] A. Lorts, R.R. Davies, J.C. Alejos, K.R. Kanter, J.G. Gossett, R.S. Cantor, I. Adachi, Utilization and outcomes of temporary ventricular assist devices in children: a report from the pediatric interagency registry for mechanical circulatory support (pedimacs), J. Heart Lung Transplant. 35 (2016) S45–S46.

[56] A.K. Lal, S. Chen, K. Maeda, A. McCammond, D.N. Rosenthal, O. Reinhartz, J. Yeh, Successful bridge to transplant with a continuous flow ventricular assist device in a single ventricle patient with an aortopulmonary shunt, ASAIO J. 60 (2014) 119–121.

[57] E.M. Darling, D. Kaemmer, D.S. Lawson, J.J. Jaggers, R.M. Ungerleider, Use of ECMO without the oxygenator to provide ventricular support after Norwood Stage I procedures, Ann. Thorac. Surg. 71 (2001) 735–736.

[58] C.J. VanderPluym, N.S. Khoo, I.M. Rebeyka, H. Buchholz, Unique case of total artificial cardiac support in failed Fontan circulation after cardiectomy: is continuous flow better than pulsatile flow? J. Thorac. Cardiovasc. Surg. 145 (2013) e62–e63.

[59] C.J. VanderPluym, I.M. Rebeyka, D.B. Ross, H. Buchholz, The use of ventricular assist devices in pediatric patients with univentricular hearts, J. Thorac. Cardiovasc. Surg. 141 (2011) 588–590.

[60] R. Gerrah, K. Charette, J.M. Chen, The first successful use of the Levitronix PediMag ventricular support device as a biventricular bridge to transplant in an infant, J. Thorac. Cardiovasc. Surg. 142 (2011) 1282–1283.

[61] J.M. Chen, M.E. Richmond, H. Takayama, L. Gilmore, A. Garcia, L.J. Addonizio, A decade of pediatric mechanical circulatory support before and after cardiac transplantation, J. Thorac. Cardiovasc. Surg. 143 (2012) 344–351.

[62] J.G. Andrade, H. Al-Saloos, A. Jeewa, G.G.S. Sandor, A. Cheung, Facilitated cardiac recovery in fulminant myocarditis: pediatric use of the Impella LP 5.0 pump, J. Heart Lung Transplant. 29 (2010) 96–97.

[63] M.C. Monge, B.T. Kulat, O. Eltayeb, S. Balasubramanya, A.E. Sarwark, N.R. Zingle, S.T. Moss, M.A. Moga, J.G. Gossett, E. Pahl, J.M. Costello, C.L. Backer, Novel modifications of a ventricular assist device for infants and children(Internet), Ann. Thorac. Surg. 102 (2016) 147–153. Available from: http://linkinghub.elsevier.com/retrieve/pii/S0003497516303733.

[64] C.S. Almond, D.L. Morales, E.H. Blackstone, M.W. Turrentine, M. Imamura, M.P. Massicotte, L.C. Jordan, E.J. Devaney, C. Ravishankar, K.R. Kanter, R. Kroslowitz, C. Tjossem, L. Thuita, G.A. Cohen, H. Buchholz, J.D. St Louis, K. Nguyen, R.A. Niebler, H.L. Walters, B. Reemtsen, P.D. Wearden, O. Reinhartz, K.J. Guleserian, M.B. Mitchell, M.S. Bleiweis, C.E. Canter, T. Humpl, Berlin Heart EXCOR pediatric ventricular assist device for bridge to heart transplantation in US children, Circulation 127 (2013) 1702–1711.

[65] R. Hetzer, M. Loebe, Y. Weng, B. Stiller, E. Hennig, V. Alexi-Meskishvili, P.E. Lange, Circulatory support with pneumatic paracorporeal ventricular assist device in infants and children, Ann. Thorac. Surg. 66 (1998) 1498–1506.

[66] D.L.S. Morales, C.S.D. Almond, R.D.B. Jaquiss, D.N. Rosenthal, D.C. Naftel, M.P. Massicotte, T. Humpl, M.W. Turrentine, J.S. Tweddell, G.A. Cohen, R. Kroslowitz, E.J. Devaney, C.E. Canter, F. Fynn-Thompson, O. Reinhartz, M. Imamura, N.S. Ghanayem, H. Buchholz, S. Furness, R. Mazor, S.K. Gandhi, C.D. Fraser, Bridging children of all sizes to cardiac transplantation: the initial multicenter North American experience with the Berlin Heart EXCOR ventricular assist device, J. Heart Lung Transplant. 30 (2011) 1–8.

[67] S.C. Malaisrie, M.P. Pelletier, J.J. Yun, K. Sharma, T.A. Timek, D.N. Rosenthal, G.E. Wright, R.C. Robbins, B.A. Reitz, Pneumatic paracorporeal ventricular assist device in infants and children: initial Stanford experience, J. Heart Lung Transplant. 27 (2008) 173–177.

[68] H.J. Ross, Y. Law, W.M. Book, C.S. Broberg, L. Burchill, F. Cecchin, J.M. Chen, D. Delgado, K. Dimopoulos, M.D. Everitt, M. Gatzoulis, L. Harris, D.T. Hsu, J.T. Kuvin, C.M. Martin, A.M. Murphy, G. Singh, T.L. Spray, K.K. Stout, Transplantation and mechanical circulatory support in congenital heart disease a scientific statement from the American Heart Association, Circulation 133 (2016) 802–820.

[69] S. Weinstein, R. Bello, C. Pizarro, F. Fynn-Thompson, J. Kirklin, K. Guleserian, R. Woods, C. Tjossem, R. Kroslowitz, P. Friedmann, R. Jaquiss, The use of the Berlin Heart EXCOR in patients with functional single ventricle, J. Thorac. Cardiovasc. Surg. 147 (2014) 697–705.

[70] F. De Rita, A. Hasan, S. Haynes, D. Crossland, R. Kirk, L. Ferguson, E. Peng, M. Griselli, Mechanical cardiac support in children with congenital heart disease with intention to bridge to heart transplantation, Eur. J. Cardiothorac. Surg. 46 (2014) 656–662 discussion 662.

Chapter 52

Decision-Making in Ventricular Assist Device Support in Pediatric Advanced Heart Failure Patients

Christina J. VanderPluym, Francis Fynn-Thompson, Elizabeth D. Blume
Boston Children's Hospital, Boston, MA, United States

INTRODUCTION

Ventricular assist device (VAD) support for children has advanced tremendously in the last 5 years. This is attributable to the adoption of newer generation intracorporeal devices, originally intended for use in adults, but small enough for children. Having access to additional VAD options has opened the door to new indications of VAD use in children beyond just bridge to transplant. Today, bridge to decision, bridge to transplant candidacy, destination therapy, and potentially bridge to recovery are all established and viable therapeutic strategies. However, as the field grows, with ever more device options and support strategies, we are faced with more decisions to reconcile. Initially the looming question was "who needs a VAD" but now we also need to address a myriad of other considerations that are a direct result of the burgeoning growth in device options and applications. In this chapter, we will address the decisions that face the pediatric heart failure cardiologist in supporting the advanced heart failure patient from VAD evaluation to implantation and beyond (Fig. 52.1).

DECISION #1: DOES THE PATIENT NEED A VENTRICULAR ASSIST DEVICE?

The first most fundamental question is *who needs a VAD*? The answer to this is not so simple and has changed dramatically over the last 10 years. Prior to the availability of pediatric VAD options, extracorporeal membrane oxygenation (ECMO) was the cornerstone of mechanical circulatory support. Its ease of use, rapidity of implantation, and applicability to all patient sizes made it the first and only choice for cardiopulmonary support. However, the high risk of adverse events, such as stroke and bleeding, restricted the use of ECMO to children in cardiac crisis and prevented its adoption as a long-term support strategy. As such, the answer to the question "who needs a VAD?" 15 years ago would have been a child in severe cardiogenic shock who is thought to recover within a few days to weeks with short-term cardiopulmonary support. Today we would describe this patient profile as Interagency Registry for Mechanically Assisted Circulatory Support (INTERMACS) level 1 or 2. The INTERMACS scale was developed with seven levels of clinical severity based on hemodynamic profile and degree of end-organ dysfunction [1]. INTERMACS 1 denotes the most critically ill, the "crash and burn" profile, with hemodynamic instability in spite of escalating catecholamines and/or mechanical ventilation, and hypoperfusion of target organs. INTERMACS 2 characterizes the patient "*sliding on inotropes*," with rapid deterioration of renal function, nutrition state, and/or other end-organ function despite intravenous inotropic support. Moving across the INTERMACS levels, patient profiles begin to resemble the ambulatory heart failure patient, with little to no physical limitations. The INTERMACS scale has demonstrated robust prognostic value in predicting mortality and postoperative complications following VAD support in adults [2,3]. In adults, there has been a steady migration away from implanting INTERMACS profile 1 patients toward earlier implantation in INTERMACS 2, 3, and even 4 patients [4,5]. This shift in implantation threshold has been mirrored in pediatrics over the last few years due to the advent of more VAD options for children. The Berlin Heart EXCOR gained widespread popularity as an alternative to ECMO in Europe and was later approved by the Food and Drug Administration in the United States as a pediatric-specific VAD for bridge to transplantation in 2011 [6,7]. While the US Investigational Device Exemption (IDE) trial demonstrated superiority of the EXCOR VAD to ECMO with higher survival rates, there remained an unacceptably high risk of infection, bleeding, and stroke [7]. As such, the decision to place a child on Berlin Heart support needs to be rigorously considered, accepting the risk of catastrophic adverse events against further deterioration or death without VAD support. In the last 5 years, the evolution of VAD design has allowed a

Heart Failure in the Child and Young Adult. http://dx.doi.org/10.1016/B978-0-12-802393-8.00052-1

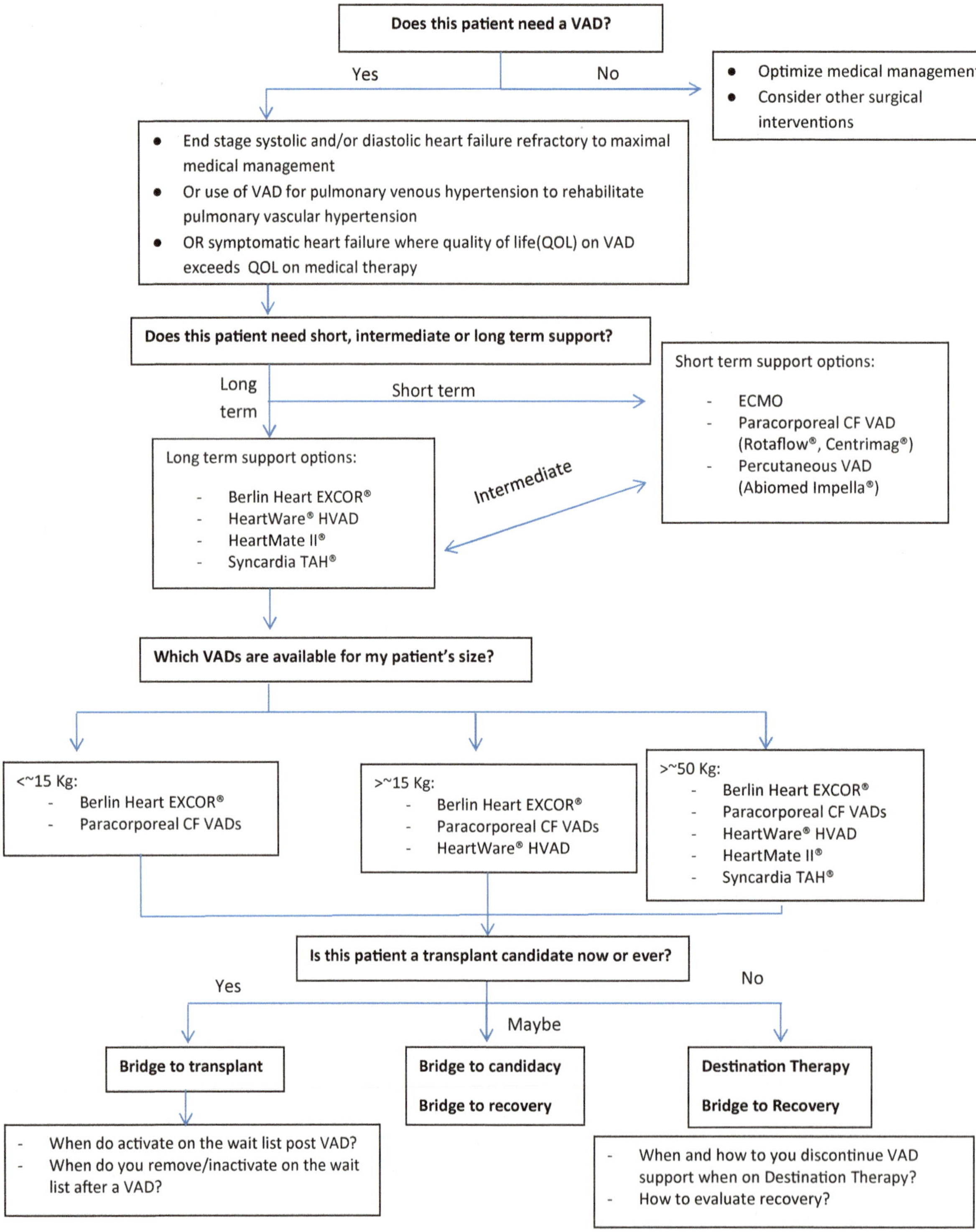

FIGURE 52.1 Decision making for ventricular assist device (VAD) support in children.

lower threshold for VAD implantation. The advent of continuous flow (CF) devices designed and labeled for use in adults such as the HeartWare HVAD (HeartWare Inc. Frammingham, MA) and the HeartMate II (Thoratec Inc, Pleasanton, Ca) have crossed over to the pediatric population [8–12]. Now, larger children (generally >15 kg) and adolescents can utilize this device technology and benefit from its lower adverse event profile as compared to the Berlin Heart EXCOR and other paracorporeal devices. Additionally the intracorporeal design of the CF devices allows for outpatient management, which was previously not possible with the Berlin Heart or ECMO [9,13,14]. The improvements in VAD design and performance are reflected in improved patient outcomes, not only in terms of survival but also in terms of improved quality of life. As such, with currently available VAD options, the advanced heart failure child may be much less critically ill to warrant a VAD as compared to years ago. In years to come, we anticipate that the answer to the question "who needs a VAD" will continue to evolve to reflect improvements in VAD technology and patient outcomes on VAD support.

DECISION #2: DOES THIS PATIENT NEED SHORT-, LONG-, OR INDETERMINATE-TERM SUPPORT?

Once it is decided a patient warrants VAD support, the next consideration is what type of support will best address the needs of the patient. Underlying diagnosis and clinical presentation generally dictates the anticipated duration of support. A previously well teenager with myocarditis and acute deterioration of left ventricular systolic function would benefit from the least invasive temporary mechanical circulatory support strategy as a bridge to recovery. On the other hand, a child with progressive left ventricular dilation and dysfunction in the setting of known genetic cardiomyopathy would require a long-term VAD option as a bridge to transplantation. In most cases, the cardiologist has a preexisting relationship with the patient and anticipates a time when VAD support may be needed. However, in some situations, a patient not known the cardiologist may present from home or an outside hospital with severe left and/or right ventricular dysfunction of unclear etiology. Despite exhaustive investigation, it may not be clear what is the cause and course of the dysfunction. This makes it especially challenging in determining what support strategy to use. In these situations of uncertainty, one could advocate to use the least invasive mechanical circulatory support option that will provide the most comprehensive hemodynamic stability as a bridge to decision-waiting and watching for stabilization, recovery, or further deterioration. Options include: ECMO, percutaneous MCS (Tandem Heart, Abiomed Impella), or paracorporeal CF VADs (Centrimag, Rotaflow). The downside of these short-term devices is that in most situations, they require the patient to be heavily sedated and/or paralyzed during support due to the tenuous nature of peripheral cannulation. The upside of these device options is that they can be implanted with ease and removed at the bedside in most cases once there is hemodynamic and echocardiographic evidence of recovery. Others advocate that going straight to a durable VAD is best because it obviates the need for reoperation and transitioning to another MCS device should there be no recovery. In addition, going straight to a durable VAD (such as the Berlin Heart or HeartWare; size permitting) allows for early extubation, mobilization, and rehabilitation of the patient, which improves the ability to evaluate patients for recovery or transplantation. With growing experience in implanting, supporting, and removing durable devices such as HeartWare, there may be a shift in practice tendencies toward using these devices for short-term support (days to weeks to months) in situations where the clinical course is unknown and unpredictable because it allows the patient more options going forward. Ultimately, a patient on HeartWare support could to bridged to recovery or transplantation, or could remain on the device for an indeterminate amount of time (destination therapy) should transplantation be contraindicated. The same cannot be said for the Berlin Heart or other paracorporeal VADs, as these devices cannot currently be managed as outpatients and as such, should not be offered as destination therapy if there is no foreseeable way to be discharged from the hospital. Patient's size and anatomy will dictate which long-term VADs can be used.

DECISION #3: WHAT VENTRICULAR ASSIST DEVICES CAN BE USED BASED ON THE PATIENT'S SIZE AND ANATOMY?

VAD options for children are still quite limited as compared to the armamentarium of devices available to adults (Fig. 52.2). Paracorporeal support devices such Berlin Heart can be used to accommodate all patient sizes from infants to adults, with multiple cannulae and pump sizes (Fig. 52.2). The use of paracorporeal CF devices, such as the Rotaflow and Pedimag/Centrimag, with Berlin Heart cannula can also be fitted to patients of all sizes depending on the size of inflow and outflow cannula used [15].

The feasibility of implanting intracorporeal CF devices (HeartWare and HeartMate II) is dependent on the size of the patient and the ventricle. While there is no formal size limitation to use of the HeartWare device, clinical practice has suggested a lowest weight range of 12–15 kg to allow significant cardiothoracic space to house the pump [9]. In this smaller size range, it is generally not possible to close the pericardium around the pump, and instead the pericardial space and left pleural space are left open. An additional consideration is the size of the inflow cannula. For the HeartWare device, the inflow cannula is 25 mm in length, thus the dimension of the ventricle must exceed the inflow length. Preoperative imaging using echocardiography, computer topography (CT), and/or cardiac magnetic resonance imaging (cMRI) is vital to ensure that the end-systole dimension is sufficient to accommodate the inflow cannula and prevent obstruction by adjacent tissue (mitral valve apparatus or leaflets, posterior wall of the left ventricle, trabeculations, etc.). Virtual "fit" studies can be completed using CT 3-dimensional (3-D) reconstruction of the cardiothoracic space to ensure that it is large enough to permit

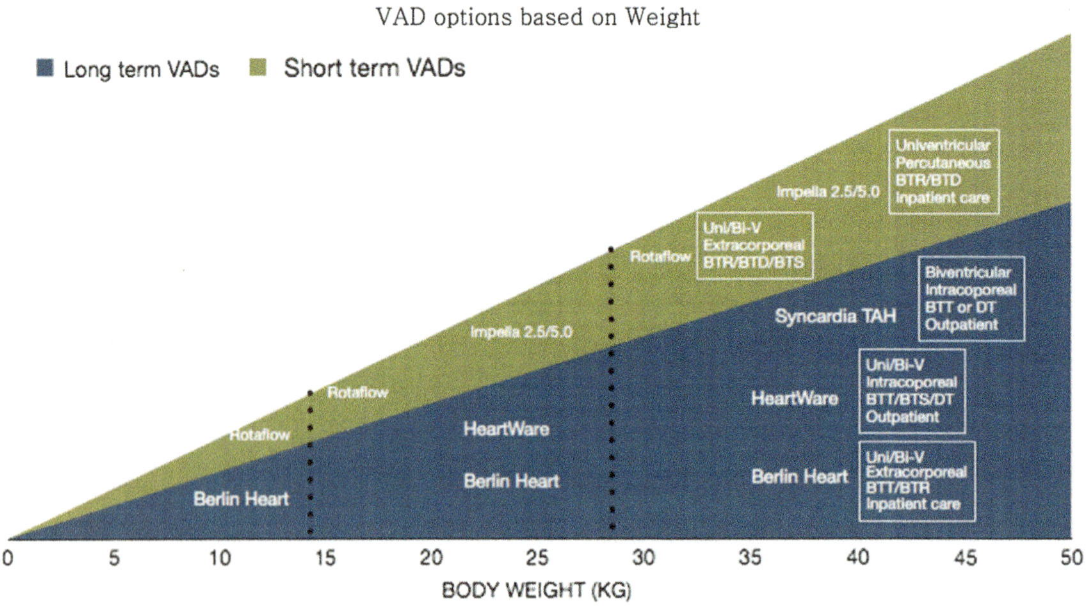

FIGURE 52.2 Ventricular assist device (VAD) options for children. *BDT*, bridge to decision; *BTR*, bridge to recovery; *BTS*, bridge to suitability; *BTT*, bridge to transplant; *DT*, destination therapy.

chest closure. While this imaging can help to assess whether the pump can physically be placed in chest, it will not account for the changes in ventricular size and geometry following unloading with the VAD, which may significantly decrease the size of the ventricle and result in inflow cannula obstruction.

The HeartWare device was designed for use in adult patients, with a recommended speed of operation of 2400–3600 RPM. This speed in a small child would result in complete collapse of the ventricle and inevitable inflow obstruction. To overcome this obstacle, the outflow graft of the HeartWare can be restricted using clips. Restricting the outflow graft increases the afterload to the centrifugal pump, thus allowing the pump to run at higher speeds, while not completely decompress the ventricle. The advantage of running the pump within its recommended speeds of operation (~2400–3600 RPM) is that it protects against *retrograde flow* through the pump. Retrograde flow occurs when the pump is operating at the lowest margin of its speed continuum (~1800–2000 RPM), where in effect, the propeller of the pump is rotating but not generating any forward flow. In this setting, there could be backward flow from the aorta through the valveless pump back into the ventricle with increase in afterload conditions resulting in volume load to the dysfunctional ventricle.

For larger children and adolescents who require biventricular support, the Total Artificial Heart (TAH) Syncardia can be used. The original Syncardia TAH consists of two 70 cc pneumatically driven pulsatile flow pumps that replace the entire heart within the chest, with externalized cannula connected to the driving unit. The 70 cc Syncardia was generally too large for use in children and adolescents due to the need for ~10 cm in anterior to posterior dimension at the level of vertebrae T-10. To accommodate a smaller patient population, the 50 cc Syncardia TAH was developed for a recommended body surface area of >1.2 m^2. Imaging "fit" studies using 3-D CT programs are paramount in preoperative planning to account for variable cardiothoracic dimensions and anatomical variants such as scoliosis [16].

DECISION #4: IS THIS VENTRICULAR ASSIST DEVICE RECIPIENT A TRANSPLANT CANDIDATE NOW OR IN THE FUTURE?

Not all transplant candidates are VAD candidates and not all VAD candidates are transplant candidates. As such, separate evaluation for transplant candidacy should be completed in parallel to VAD evaluation.

There are three possible scenarios to consider:

1. *Bridge to transplant*: Currently listed for transplantation but due to progressive deterioration or instability needs a VAD. Does this patient remain listed throughout the surgical and postsurgical recovery time period or should they be inactivated pending some clearly defined criteria of recovery/normalization of end-organ function?
2. *Bridge to candidacy*: Not listed for transplant currently, with VAD implantation to improve candidacy for transplantation by improving end-organ function, or decreasing pulmonary vascular resistance, or allowing more time for ongoing

transplant evaluation and observation. What criteria are needed to determine transplant candidacy after VAD implantation? How long do you wait before listing for transplant after VAD implantation?

3. *Destination Therapy*: May or may not have been listed for heart transplant at time of VAD implantation, but due to one or many contraindications or complications, cannot undergo transplantation now, or at any time in the future, and therefore will remain on VAD support indefinitely. What VAD complications or VAD-related factors would deem a patient no longer a transplant candidate?

These three scenarios lead to the following decisions:

DECISION #5: WHEN SHOULD A VENTRICULAR ASSIST DEVICE RECIPIENT BE *LISTED OR REACTIVATED FOR TRANSPLANT*?

The optimal timing of listing for transplant after VAD implantation varies from institution to institution and also depends on the type of VAD being used for support. Currently in the United States, children supported with a VAD are at the highest priority for transplant (UNOS status 1A) throughout their listing period, which differs from the adult listing criteria that gives VAD-supported patients 1 month of time as 1A and then they are downgraded to 1B. This strategy of organ allocation is intended to decrease wait list times for children who may be most at risk of death or significant morbidity while on device support. However, there is significant variability in the adverse event profiles for different types of VADs, with a much higher rate of thrombotic and hemorrhagic neurological events in children supported on paracorporeal devices such as the Berlin Heart EXCOR as compared to the newer generation intracorporeal CF VADs such as HeartWare and HeartMate II. Data from the PediMACS have shown very low adverse event rate in the CF-VAD implant group compared to pulsatile VADs [12]. These device-specific risks taken in conjunction with patient-specific factors may prompt centers to list a patient on Berlin Heart support sooner than a similar patient on intracorporeal CF-VAD support. In light of the encouraging outcomes with CF-VAD support in children, it is reasonable to wait a period of time after VAD implant to allow for recovery of end-organ function, adequate rehabilitation, and quiescence of any inflammation that can occur after cardiopulmonary bypass exposure [12,17]. This period of time also allows for the assessment of any potential for myocardial recovery (including the histologic review of the myocardial core removed at the time of implant) that may result in device explant and potentially obviate the need for heart transplantation.

Ultimately, the decision to list for transplantation must take into consideration the overall benefits of improved cardiac output and optimal rehabilitation of an end-stage heart failure patient versus the risk of VAD-related complications and thus is most often done on a case-by-case basis.

DECISION #6: WHEN SHOULD A VENTRICULAR ASSIST DEVICE RECIPIENT BE *REMOVED FROM THE TRANSPLANT LIST*?

To answer this question simply: a VAD recipient should be removed from the transplant list when he/she is either *too sick* to survive to hospital discharge posttransplant *or* when he/she is *too well* to require heart transplant.

There are a myriad of clinical factors that may conspire to adversely impact a patient's ability to survive transplantation after VAD support. These include: severe renal failure thought to worsen rather than improve with transplantation, significant pulmonary embolism, nonreactive pulmonary hypertension, catastrophic hemorrhagic or ischemic cerebrovascular event, high allosensitization, systemic viral, bacterial, or fungal infection thought to be fatal with immunosuppressive therapy. Each center, provider, patient, and family will have a different threshold in what risks they would find acceptable in continuing to pursue transplantation. As such, it is imperative that prior to VAD implantation, a comprehensive discussion is undertaken with the patient (age permitting), family, care givers, and invested providers to review criteria that would dictate removal from the wait list and what options of care are then available. Walking through these scenarios will help facilitate the often difficult discussions surrounding end of life wishes and expectations as well as establish the possibility of destination therapy. As stated earlier, a caveat to destination therapy is that the device is compatible with outpatient management and ideally home discharge. Currently only the intracorporeal CF VADs (HeartWare and HeartMate II) permit home discharge, and a result destination therapy is generally not offered for paracorporeal devices. Knowing that certain VADs have no feasible long-term option as destination therapy dramatically impacts the decision to remove a patient from the wait list. Thus, as with many of the decisions that we face in the long journey of VAD support, each case is individualized based on the complex constellation of patient-, device-, and center-specific factors [18].

The patient population is "too well" for transplantation while on VAD support is poorly defined in the literature [19]. Currently, less than 1% of VADs in pediatric patients are explanted due to recovery and less is known on the number of these children removed from the wait list. There have been cases of severe cardiac dysfunction (related to infection, chemotoxic agents) that have shown complete recovery with mechanical circulatory support permitting explanation of the pump as well as deactivation from the transplant wait list [15,20,21]. A more common scenario in the adult field of long-term VAD support is that of patients requesting to stay on the VAD support rather than undergo transplantation, with its associated perioperative and long-term risk factors. This decision is heavily dependent on the patient's subjective feeling of their quality of life on device support versus their anticipated quality of life after heart transplantation.

DECISION #7: IN WHAT CIRCUMSTANCES CAN OR SHOULD VENTRICULAR ASSIST DEVICE SUPPORT BE DISCONTINUED?

Discontinuing medical support in any form—be it nutritional, ventilatory, or circulatory—is an immensely challenging decision and one that neither patient, parents, or providers feel they should ever have to make. When introducing a medical intervention as invasive as VAD support, it is paramount to discuss end of life expectations as early in the VAD evaluation process as possible, and ideally before implantation. The goal of having a frank discussion about end of life and quality of life before VAD implantation is to understand and harmonize the expectations of what VAD support entails with the patient, family, and providers. By walking through "best case" and "worse case" scenarios of VAD support both in the short term and long term with the patient (age permitting), family, and the VAD care team, allows all involved parties to identify their individual thresholds of care. These thresholds are subjective limits to care that in the most simplistic terms denotes the point where the medical intervention is imposing more harm (be it physical or emotional) to the patient and their care team than benefit derived from it. Because every person has different and possibly fluctuating thresholds, it is paramount to have open and frequent discussions about more futile and nonfutile circumstances that would prompt *evaluation* for VAD discontinuation. Note the term *evaluation*, as the decision to withdraw VAD support is not made hastily but rather warrants the same comprehensive assessment as did the initial decision to implant the VAD. Through a multidisciplinary team that incorporates the primary cardiologist, VAD team, psychiatry, social work, other involved subspecialty teams, family, and patient, the request to withdraw care is reviewed. Reasons for discontinuation of VAD support can fall into two categories: futile and nonfutile circumstances. Futile circumstances entails complications that are severe and will either dramatically impair quality of life or are life limiting/threatening regardless of the ongoing VAD support. Examples include: irreversible coma or vegetative state due to cerebrovascular events, cardiogenic shock, overwhelming infections refractory to antimicrobial therapy, multiple organ failure, refractory hypoxia, or catastrophic device failure [22,23]. In these circumstances, discontinuation of VAD support is equivalent with allowing natural death when there is an onset of new lethal pathophysiology notwithstanding the functioning of the VAD itself. Nonfutile circumstances are defined as VAD discontinuation requested by the patient or family for psychosocial reasons and/or quality of life. These reasons may be as impactful on a patient's existence as are the nonfutile issues but are more difficult to reconcile because of the ethical and legal principles surrounding discontinuation of life-sustaining therapies for the reason of "they just do not want it anymore." That said, there is growing experience with concept of compassionate deactivation (CD), where life-sustaining therapies (including VAD support) withdraw at the request of an adult patient or his/her surrogate who perceives the burden of the therapy outweighs the benefits. While the CD has been extensively discussed and evaluated in the adult population for a variety of disease states and therapies, there is scarce literature for children and a notable absence of guideline for pediatric mechanical circulatory support. The concept of CD in children is complicated by the fact that for most children decision-making is by parents or other altruistic surrogate, and that informed consent and patient assent are variable by patient age and capacity. As such, approaches to CD that work in adults may not be feasible in the pediatric population. That said, in recent years many useful documents have emerged to guide patient, families, and providers through end of life decision-making. These documents are directed to addressing active discussion around preparedness planning ("walking through worst and best case scenarios") as well as interdisciplinary checklists for VAD deactivation to ensure the least traumatic death experience for all involved parties. While none of the documents are specifically tailored to the pediatric population, they all highlight the need for clear communication of expectations with all members of the care team, family, and patient. With expanding use of VAD support in the pediatric population, we foresee the evolution and development of VAD-centric palliative care as part of the multidisciplinary advanced heart failure team.

REFERENCES

[1] L.W. Stevenson, F.D. Pagani, J.B. Young, et al., INTERMACS profiles of advanced heart failure: the current picture, J. Heart Lung Transplant. 28 (6) (2009) 535–541, http://dx.doi.org/10.1016/j.healun.2009.02.015.

[2] A.C. Alba, V. Rao, J. Ivanov, H.J. Ross, D.H. Delgado, Usefulness of the INTERMACS scale to predict outcomes after mechanical assist device implantation, J. Heart Lung Transplant. 28 (8) (2009) 827–833, http://dx.doi.org/10.1016/j.healun.2009.04.033.

[3] E. Barge-Caballero, J. Segovia-Cubero, L. Almenar-Bonet, et al., Preoperative INTERMACS profiles determine postoperative outcomes in critically ill patients undergoing emergency heart transplantation analysis of the Spanish national heart transplant registry, Circ. Heart Fail. 6 (4) (2013) 763–772, http://dx.doi.org/10.1161/CIRCHEARTFAILURE.112.000237.

[4] J.K. Kirklin, D.C. Naftel, F.D. Pagani, et al., Sixth INTERMACS annual report: a 10,000-patient database, J. Heart Lung Transplant. 33 (6) (2014) 555–564, http://dx.doi.org/10.1016/j.healun.2014.04.010.

[5] J.K. Kirklin, D.C. Naftel, F.D. Pagani, et al., Seventh INTERMACS annual report: 15,000 patients and counting, J. Heart Lung Transplant. 34 (12) (2015) 1495–1504, http://dx.doi.org/10.1016/j.healun.2015.10.003.

[6] C.S. Almond, D.L. Morales, E.H. Blackstone, et al., Berlin heart EXCOR pediatric ventricular assist device for bridge to heart transplantation in US children, Circulation 127 (16) (2013) 1702–1711, http://dx.doi.org/10.1161/CIRCULATIONAHA.112.000685.

[7] C.D. Fraser, R.D.B. Jaquiss, D.N. Rosenthal, et al., Prospective trial of a pediatric ventricular assist device, N. Engl. J. Med. 367 (6) (2012) 532–541, http://dx.doi.org/10.1056/NEJMoa1014164.

[8] O. Miera, E.V. Potapov, M. Redlin, et al., First experiences with the heartware ventricular assist system in children, Ann. Thorac. Surg. 91 (4) (2011) 1256–1260, http://dx.doi.org/10.1016/j.athoracsur.2010.12.013.

[9] O. Miera, R. Kirk, H. Buchholz, et al., A multicenter study of the HeartWare ventricular assist device in small children, J. Heart Lung Transplant. (2016), http://dx.doi.org/10.1016/j.healun.2016.01.019.

[10] M.A. Padalino, T. Bottio, V. Tarzia, et al., HeartWare ventricular assist device as bridge to transplant in children and adolescents, Artif. Organs 38 (5) (2014) 418–422, http://dx.doi.org/10.1111/aor.12185.

[11] O. Balciotlu, S. Erkul, F. Ayik, et al., First successful experience with the heartware assist device in child in Turkey, Cardiovasc. Ther. 29 (2012) 30. https://doi.org/10.1111/1755-5922.12011_1.

[12] J.W. Rossano, A. Lorts, C.J. VanderPluym, et al., Outcomes of pediatric patients supported with continuous-flow ventricular assist devices: a report from the pediatric interagency registry for mechanical circulatory support (PediMACS), J. Heart Lung Transplant. (2016), http://dx.doi.org/10.1016/j.healun.2016.01.1228.

[13] J. Conway, C. Vanderpluym, A. Jeewa, S. Sinnadurai, A. Schubert, A. Lorts, Now how do we get them home? Outpatient care of pediatric patients on mechanical circulatory support, Pediatr. Transplant. 20 (2) (2016) 194–202, http://dx.doi.org/10.1111/petr.12674.

[14] M. Schweiger, C. Vanderpluym, A. Jeewa, et al., Outpatient management of intra-corporeal left ventricular assist device system in children: a multi-center experience, Am. J. Transplant. 15 (2) (2015) 453–460, http://dx.doi.org/10.1111/ajt.13003.

[15] P.C. Kouretas, A.K. Kaza, P.T. Burch, et al., Experience with the levitronix centrimag in the pediatric population as a bridge to decision and recovery, Artif. Organs 33 (11) (2009) 1002–1004, http://dx.doi.org/10.1111/j.1525-1594.2009.00952.x.

[16] B. Zhang, T. Masuzawa, E. Tatsumi, et al., Three-dimensional thoracic modeling for an anatomical compatibility study of the implantable total artificial heart, Artif. Organs 23 (3) (1999) 229–234, http://dx.doi.org/10.1046/j.1525-1594.1999.06313.x.

[17] A.G. Cabrera, K.S. Sundareswaran, A.X. Samayoa, et al., Outcomes of pediatric patients supported by the HeartMate II left ventricular assist device in the United States, J. Heart Lung Transplant. 32 (11) (2013) 1107–1113, http://dx.doi.org/10.1016/j.healun.2013.07.012.

[18] C.J. VanderPluym, E.D. Blume, The role of continuous flow ventricular assist device for destination therapy in children: can it work or is it a bridge too far? Prog. Pediatr. Cardiol. 40 (2016) 25–27, http://dx.doi.org/10.1016/j.ppedcard.2016.01.008.

[19] C. Vanderpluym, D.A. Graham, C.S. Almond, E.D. Blume, C.E. Milliren, T.P. Singh, Survival in patients removed from the heart transplant waiting list before receiving a transplant, J. Heart Lung Transplant. 33 (3) (2014) 261–269, http://dx.doi.org/10.1016/j.healun.2013.12.010.

[20] C.L.S. George, R.K. Ameduri, R.C. Reed, K.B. Dummer, D.M. Overman, J.D. St Louis, Long-term use of ventricular assist device as a bridge to recovery in acute fulminant myocarditis, Ann. Thorac. Surg. 95 (3) (2013), http://dx.doi.org/10.1016/j.athoracsur.2012.09.036.

[21] A.W. Lowry, I. Adachi, I.D. Gregoric, A. Jeewa, D.L.S. Morales, The potential to avoid heart transplantation in children: outpatient bridge to recovery with an intracorporeal continuous-flow left ventricular assist device in a 14-year-old, Congenit. Heart Dis. 7 (6) (2012), http://dx.doi.org/10.1111/j.1747-0803.2012.00659.x.

[22] M.Y. Rady, J.L. Verheijde, Ethical challenges with deactivation of durable mechanical circulatory support at the end of life: left ventricular assist devices and total artificial hearts, J. Intensive Care Med. 29 (1) (2012) 3–12, http://dx.doi.org/10.1177/0885066611432415.

[23] V.D. Lachman, Left ventricular assist device deactivation: ethical issues, MEDSURG Nurs. 20 (2) (2011) 98–100. http://ezproxy.usherbrooke.ca/login?url=https://search.ebscohost.com/login.aspx?direct=true&db=a9h&AN=59598836&site=ehost-live.

Chapter 53

Long-Term Ventricular Assist Devices in Children

Iki Adachi, Sarah Burki, Charles D. Fraser
Texas Children's Hospital, Houston, TX, United States

INTRODUCTION

There has been a substantial advancement over the last decade in the field of ventricular assist device (VAD). In the adult community, VAD therapy is now considered to be the standard care for intractable heart failure [1]. By contrast, the use of VAD support has not been popularized until relatively recently in the pediatric world. Given the increasing number of children with severe heart failure [2], however, long-term VAD support for children has rapidly been gaining an increasing attention. Ongoing miniaturization of implantable continuous-flow devices further accelerates this trend. The era of pediatric long-term VAD support has finally begun. In this chapter, we will review options for long-term VAD support in children, with a particular focus on patient/device selection and challenges unique to pediatric population.

CANDIDATE SELECTION

At present, no standardized candidate selection criteria have been established for pediatric VAD support. In general, VAD therapy is considered when the potential benefits of VAD outweigh the risks involved. In the old era where the risk profiles of VAD support was extremely high, VAD support was offered only when the patient was in extremis. This has completely changed especially in the adult population, favoring earlier initiation of VAD support since the traditional approach with VAD placement in an extreme situation has clearly been demonstrated to result in poor outcome. The Fifth Interagency Registry for Mechanically Assisted Circulatory Support (INTERMACS) report found that preoperative clinical status of a VAD candidate has a substantial impact on postimplant outcomes [3]. There are ongoing discussions about expanding the indication for VAD support even to less sick patients (i.e., INTERMACS profile 4 to 7) who would not have been offered VAD support in the past [4,5]. Since the optimal timing for VAD initiation is closely associated with risk profiles of VAD support, it would continue to change as devices and clinical management improve.

Pediatric physicians, contrary to adult physicians, tend to be more conservative when evaluating indications for VAD use in children. This is particularly true for small children, who can only be supported with pulsatile, paracorporeal VADs (e.g., Berlin Heart EXCOR; Berlin Heart Inc., The Woodlands, TX; Fig. 53.1) that are associated with significantly higher risk profiles than implantable, continuous-flow devices [6]. Pulsatile VADs present a challenge to clinicians with respect to determining the optimal timeframe within which to initiate VAD therapy. As waiting too long to implant VAD sharply increases the risk of mortality, initiating VAD support too soon may unnecessarily expose the patient to the risk of device-related complications. The appropriate timeframe for VAD implantation is, therefore, debatable and dependent on multiple variables [7]. As with all interventions, a practitioner's individual threshold in deciding whether to provide or withhold an invasive and potentially high risk therapy such as VAD implantation is influenced by the degree of confidence in that modality to consistently produce positive outcomes. Since the risk to benefit ratio is largely determined by the patient's clinical status, institutional experience, and type of devices available, the decision needs be made on a case-by-case basis by an experienced multidisciplinary team.

At Texas Children's Hospital, the application of the Berlin Heart EXCOR is considered when the patient is critically ill with cardiogenic shock or end-organ injury (INTERMACS profile 1 or 2) [8]. In fact, the vast majority of patients that undergo Berlin EXCOR implantation at our center are already on temporary mechanical circulatory support (i.e., extracorporeal membrane oxygenation (ECMO) or short-term VAD) or mechanically ventilated. A similar trend is seen in a multicenter study described by Almond and colleagues [9]. In this study involving 204 patients from 47 centers in North America, >50% of patients who underwent EXCOR implantation were at INTERMACS profile 1, and 40% were on ECMO

Heart Failure in the Child and Young Adult. http://dx.doi.org/10.1016/B978-0-12-802393-8.00053-3

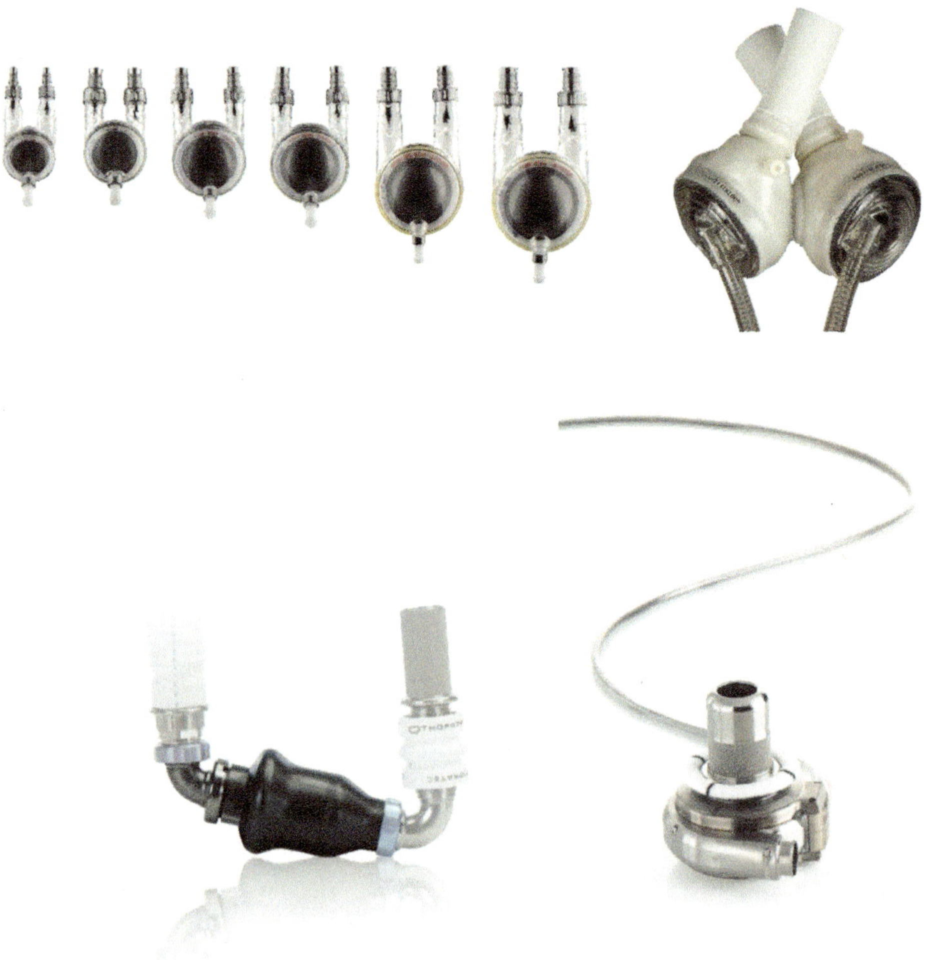

FIGURE 53.1 Long-term devices currently available. *Left upper; EXCOR (Berlin Heart Inc., The Woodlands, Texas), Right upper; Total Artificial Heart (Syncardia, Inc., Tucson, Arizona), Left lower; HVAD (HeartWare Inc., Framingham, Massachusetts), Right lower; HeartMate II (St. Jude Medical, Inc., St. Paul, Minnesota).*

support at the time of EXCOR implantation. VAD implantation at such an advanced stage is certainly a reflection of the high risk nature of VAD support with the currently available pulsatile pump system, which prevents pediatric clinicians from early initiation of VAD support.

This is the background of the ongoing enthusiasm for the use of continuous-flow VADs [e.g., HeartMate II (St. Jude Medical, Inc., St. Paul, Minnesota) or HVAD (HeartWare Inc., Framingham, Massachusetts), Fig 53.1] in pediatric patients. At Texas Children's Hospital, VAD support with a continuous-flow device is typically initiated at INTERMACS profile 2 or 3. Since these implantable VADs are designed for adult patients, there are still hesitations among our team in early initiation of support particularly in small children due to a concern for patient-device size mismatch that may have a significant negative impact on outcome. Miera and associates recently published a multicenter study regarding the use of HeartWare HVAD in children with a body surface area of 1.0 or less [10]. In this study involving 13 patients from 4 major pediatric heart centers worldwide (Berlin, Germany; Newcastle upon Tyne, United Kingdom; Boston, United States; and Edmonton, Canada), 23% of patients were on ECMO support and 30% were mechanically ventilated at the time of HVAD placement. These data have suggested that even at prominent pediatric centers worldwide, the initiation of continuous-flow VAD support is at much more advanced stage comparing to the standard adult practice.

Another challenge unique to the pediatric population is congenital heart disease. Congenitally malformed hearts have anatomic variations that pose technical challenges in placement of VAD. Examples would include abnormal location and size of the aorta and anomalous origin of coronary arteries. These anatomical variations may affect where the outflow cannula can be safely placed. Location and shape of the systemic ventricle has an important relevance in inflow cannula insertion. Since many of the implantable VADs [e.g., HeartMate II, INCOR (Berlin Heart, Inc.), HeartAssist 5 (ReliantHeart Inc.,

Houston, Texas)] are designed to fit a heart with normal anatomy (*d*-looping ventricle with levocardia), these devices are not suitable for hearts with abnormal ventricular configuration. Previous surgical palliation may jeopardize the provision of VAD placement even more due to further anatomic and circulatory physiologic disarrangement. Systemic-to-pulmonary artery shunts, disconnected vena cava and pulmonary artery after the Glenn or Fontan operations, and Damus–Kaye–Stansel anastomosis would be examples. In addition, full assessment of patient's social and familial situation needs to be conducted prior to VAD implantation. This is particularly important when considering the use of an implantable continuous-flow VAD. Ensuring a reliable home environment is extremely important for successful outpatient management of children with ongoing VAD support.

Device Selection and Management

As discussed earlier, we prefer to use an implantable continuous-flow device when feasible due to lower risk profiles and potential for home discharge. The selection of device to be implanted is primarily dependent on the patient's body size and the need for biventricular support. There has been an ongoing discussion regarding what would be the lower limit for adult-size implantable continuous-flow devices. Our experience at Texas Children's Hospital [11] and others [10,12] have suggested that the lower limit for the HVAD would be somewhere at around a body surface area of $0.7\,m^2$, provided that left ventricular assist device (LVAD) support is all that is needed. However, in a situation where BiVAD support is necessary, size constraint becomes stricter. The chest cavity must be much larger to accommodate two implantable VADs. The Berlin EXCOR is therefore the device of choice in children with a small body surface area (i.e., $\leq 0.7\,m^2$) or in those who will likely need BiVAD support but are not large enough to accommodate two implantable VADs [13]. It must be emphasized, however, that most children with severe heart failure can be supported with LVAD only. This is despite the fact that the right ventricular (RV) function often looks significantly depressed on echocardiography prior to VAD implantation. Once the left ventricle (LV) is decompressed with VAD support, the pulmonary artery pressure falls, subsequently reducing afterload on the RV. LVAD support alone is oftentimes adequate if RV failure is secondary to LV failure. Studies have previously been conducted to predict the need for BiVAD support. Predictors for the need of BiVAD support include preoperative high central venous pressure, preoperative intubation, and severe tricuspid regurgitation [14,15]. One of the most significant limitations of these studies is that they have not fully considered intraoperative factors, which would have the most direct impact on the RV function in the acute postoperative period. The cardiopulmonary bypass strategy and the need for aortic cross-clamp directly affect postoperative RV function and, hence, the need for BiVAD support. Some pediatric centers have a policy of routinely using BiVAD support for the majority of patients [16]. It is our opinion that BiVAD should be reserved only when absolutely necessary. Previous studies have consistently shown BiVAD support to be associated with worse outcomes compared to that with LVAD alone [17]. Our practice is that unless the RV has an intrinsic myocardial dysfunction (e.g., myocardial ischemia with transplant coronary vasculopathy), every effort will be made to support with an LVAD alone. If RV function is not adequate to sustain the LVAD physiology intraoperatively, we will use a temporary RV support to see if there is a chance of recovery in RV function before completely committing to BiVAD support with durable devices.

With isolated LVAD physiology, it is the native RV that determines overall systemic cardiac output. An LVAD can flow only the amount it receives from the RV through the pulmonary circulation provided that there is no intracardiac shunting or aortic insufficiency.

In patients with isolated LVAD support, therefore, the focus of postoperative care is directed at enhancing RV cardiac output. The basic principle of preventing right heart failure on LVAD is to support the RV pharmacologically and to minimize pulmonary vascular resistance while maintaining adequate preload to the right heart. Although echocardiography is a useful tool to assess RV function, its findings alone may not suffice. What is clinically important is whether the performance of the RV is sufficient enough to fill the LVAD adequately or not. It is not uncommon to see decent filling of the LVAD in the face of echocardiographic evidence of severe RV dysfunction. With an extracorporeal, pulsatile pump, such as the Berlin Heart EXCOR, direct visual assessment of the pump's filling status is the most direct indicator of right heart cardiac output.

Also important is a balanced position of the ventricular septum. While excessive LVAD setting may cause leftward deviation of the ventricular septum and resultant worsening in tricuspid valve regurgitation and globally impaired RV contractility [18], insufficient LVAD setting also needs to be avoided. Unlike the native heart, there is no cross talk between the two ventricles in this setting since the status of the LV is artificially modulated by the LVAD. Although echocardiography is a useful tool to look at the configuration of the ventricular septum, it can be done only sporadically, and hence, its usefulness is limited in the acute postoperative period where hemodynamics change drastically time to time. In our experience, the best approach to ensure the optimal balance between the two ventricles is to continuously monitor pressures of both atria.

By comparing the filling pressures of the two ventricles (represented by the left and right atrial pressures), one can easily maintain the balanced configuration as represented by nearly equivalent atrial pressures. Table 53.1 summarizes suggested medical actions for different types of hemodynamic conditions.

Surgical Considerations

When implanting adult-size VADs in children, there is an inherent issue related to the "patient-device" size mismatch. Negative impact of the size mismatch on survival has clearly been demonstrated [19]. Since Berlin Heart EXCOR has several different sizes of pumps and cannulas, size mismatch can be avoidable in most circumstances with this system. However, if attempting at using the adult continuous-flow VAD in children, size mismatch issue is inevitable. This has been becoming more critical in the current era where there is a clear trend toward using adult VADs in smaller children. Careful consideration should be given, therefore, to avoid or lessen the issues inherently associated with the patient-device size mismatch.

In our opinion, the most crucial is an accurate placement of the inflow cannula to ensuring successful long-term VAD support in children. Placement of a VAD in a small ventricular cavity in children requires technical preciseness. Even adult hearts with a smaller ventricular chamber, such as seen in restrictive cardiomyopathy, possess limited tolerance for minor technical imperfections [20]. In the interest of avoiding inflow-related issues such as pump suctioning against the ventricular septum or pump thrombosis, the inflow cannula should be placed with a particular attention to its angle relative to the ventricular septum. Based on extensive experience with the HeartMate II, the axis of the inflow cannula (and hence the relationship of the inflow relative to the ventricular septum) is believed to have an impact on the incidence of pump thrombosis [21]. Ideal configuration is that the axis of the inflow cannula lies parallel to the septum rather than perpendicularly. One could argue that the lessons learned from the HeartMate II may not necessarily be applicable to the HVAD due to different device technology and specification. However, it is our belief that the basic principle of inflow cannula angle relative to the septum should hold true regardless of device type.

Owing to its miniaturized design, the HVAD is now increasingly being used in the pediatric population [10,11,22–24]. It does not seem that the angle of the inflow cannula with HVAD has received as much attention as the HeartMate II. The HVAD inflow cannula is often found to spontaneously situate itself in a horizontal plane (i.e., perpendicularly to the interventricular septum; Fig. 53.2) when implanted in the standard way, so-called intrapericardial placement, as recommended by the manufacturer. A group at Texas Heart Institute has recognized this occurrence and advocated modifying the implantation technique by inserting the inflow cannula through the diaphragmatic surface of the LV instead of the apex [25], so as to achieve a more vertical orientation of the inflow cannula. Our approach at Texas Children's Hospital [11] shares the basic concept of making the inflow cannula in a vertical orientation. The major difference between the two modifications is the location of the inflow insertion. We use the LV apex as an insertion point as in the usual manner. Then, we gently and purposefully relocate the LV apex medially and caudally by placing the HVAD pump housing in a small pocket created on the left hemidiaphragm. With this maneuver, the tip of the inflow cannula sits in a vertical plane, satisfying the requirement that it virtually lie parallel to the interventricular septum (Fig. 53.2). Anecdotal evidence and experiential wisdom may warrant this extra effort, especially when using HVAD in small hearts. In our experience with 20 patients with HVAD support, we experienced pump thrombosis in one patient. At the time of this occurrence, the patient was suffering from hemorrhagic pancreatitis and gastrointestinal bleeding, for which her anticoagulation had been held for more than a week. No other patient in our series experienced pump thrombosis. The calculated pump thrombosis rate in our series is 0.11 event per patient year. By contrast, the pump thrombosis was seen more often in the multicenter study mentioned earlier [10]; 3 out of 13 patients had pump thrombosis, with nearly a sevenfold difference in the event rate: 0.70 event per patient year. Further investigation will be necessary to clarify if the inflow angle has a clinical impact on outcome in the pediatric population.

In comparison to the infradiaphragmatic approach by Texas Heart group, our approach may have some theoretical advantages. Since our approach involves relocation of the LV apex away from the left chest cavity, the left lower lobe of the lung would have more space to expand.

TABLE 53.1 Postimplant Hemodynamic Assessment Based on Bilateral Atrial Pressure Monitoring

	Elevated Left Atrial Pressure	Decreased Left Atrial Pressure
Elevated right atrial pressure	Increased intravascular volume	Right heart failure, or inappropriately high LVAD setting
Decreased right atrial pressure	Inappropriately low LVAD setting	Diminished intravascular volume

LVAD, left ventricular assist device.

In fact, left lower lobe atelectasis is a very common finding in patients with severe cardiomegaly. Persistently atelectatic lung can be a nidus for infection. If the cardiac mass is relocated more medially (i.e., cardiac mass is moved away from the left chest cavity), the left lung would expand properly (Fig. 53.2). More critical is the potential distortion or interruption of coronary blood supply with the sutures for a sewing ring. Given the size of the sewing ring, coronary branches around the coring site will inevitably be sacrificed if placed on small hearts. It would be less detrimental to coronary perfusion if such coronary compromise occurs at its terminal lesion (i.e., cardiac apex) rather than at its middle portion (i.e., diaphragmatic surface of the LV wall at the middle of the posterior descending coronary).

Anticoagulation

There are wide variations in anticoagulation strategies among practitioners and institutions. What is described here is an overview of our strategy at Texas Children's Hospital. In most of cases, we use heparin bridge before starting vitamin K antagonist and antiplatelet agents. Some centers utilize bivalirudin, a direct thrombin inhibitor, as a second-line agent [26], but we do not have experience with this medication. When administering heparin infusion for the long-term VAD, we primarily manage based on heparin assay, with a goal of 0.3–0.5 (U/mL). Activated partial thromboplastin time is also monitored. Oftentimes, these numbers fluctuate considerably and are not always consistent with each other. It is important not to focus on just a single marker and rather the clinicians should look at the entire picture. It is critically important to tailor the target level of anticoagulation according to the risk of bleeding at that moment. For instance, the bleeding risk is substantially higher in the acute postoperative setting. Our approach is that we initiate heparin drip with a lower goal and then gradually uptitrate as the bleeding risk decreases over time. We maintain antithrombin III level of 80 or higher so that heparin can take effect. We also try to maintain fibrinogen level within normal range, but this is often difficult. In the acute postoperative period, fibrinogen level tends to be elevated as a reflection of systemic inflammation. Since hyperfibrinosis can lead to hypercoagulable state, suppression of fibrinogen production with steroids may be considered if the level is excessive (typically >600) [27]. The basic principle of anticoagulation for VAD is maintenance of underlying coagulation profiles as normal as possible. In the past, we used to use thromboelastography to evaluate the underlying coagulation status. We now prefer to use Rotem (Tem Systems, Inc., Durham, North Carolina).

Once the patient resumes stable enteral feeding, we start vitamin K antagonist and antiplatelet agents. The Berlin Heart EXCOR is more challenging than other implantable VADs in terms of anticoagulation due to its higher tendency for clot

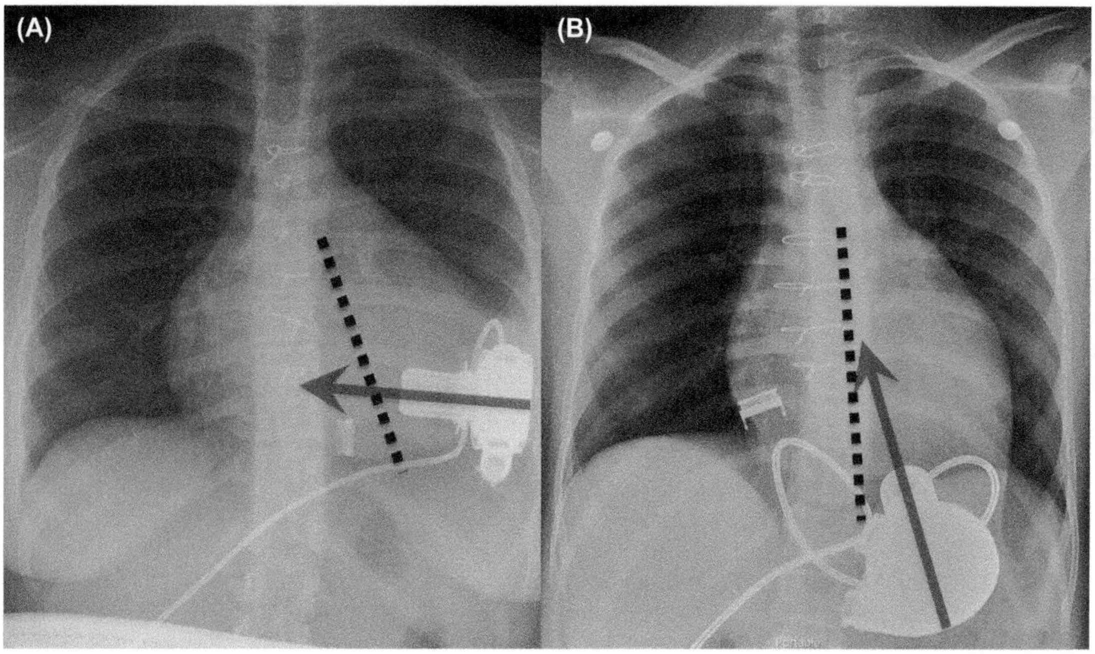

FIGURE 53.2 Relationship of the inflow cannula relative to the ventricular septum. Postoperative chest X-rays with the standard intrapericardial technique (panel A) and with the modified technique at Texas Children's Hospital (panel B). A *dotted line* represents an imaginary line of the interventricular septum. Note the difference in the relationship of the inflow cannula relative to the ventricular septum. With the modified technique, the inflow cannula lies in a more parallel orientation relative to the ventricular septum. The left lower lobe is well expanded with the modified technique since the device does not occupy the space in the pleural cavity. *Image copyright Texas Children's Hospital 2016.*

formation. Although the standard anticoagulation protocol for the Berlin EXCOR (so-called Edmonton protocol) [28] involves the use of low-molecular weight heparin in infants (<12-months-old), it is our practice to administer vitamin K agonist for all age groups. Clinicians are often placed in a dilemma of two mutually related complications, i.e., bleeding and thrombotic complications. The safety margin between the two complications can be slim. For example, when a patient has severe inflammation with extremely high fibrinogen level, the requirement for heparin drip is substantially increased. In such a situation, the risk of bleeding is high even if measured heparin assay level (or other markers) is not very elevated. The clinical team often has to err on the side of one complication over the other, depending on the clinical scenario. One of the advantages of paracorporeal pulsatile devices is that the pump can be visually examined and easily replaced if necessary. When therapeutic level of anticoagulation cannot be achieved without excessive amount of anticoagulants, the clinicians may have to accept subtherapeutic level to avoid bleeding complications while being aware of possible development of pump fibrin/thrombus, which may require pump exchange. Such a "permissive underanticoagulation" strategy is feasible with the pulsatile pump system owing to the ease of pump replacement.

CHALLENGING PATIENT POPULATION

There are certain group of patients that represent significant challenges in VAD support.

Failing Univentricular Physiology

This is certainly the most challenging group due to complex anatomy and physiology. Given the palliative nature of the univentricular palliations, pessimism exists that all the univentricular patients including those who have completed Fontan operation will eventually fail. Nevertheless, experience in VAD support for univentricular circulation is currently limited and the outcome remains suboptimal. In reviewing the outcomes of Berlin EXCOR VAD during the IDE trial, Weinstein et al. found that survival was significantly worse in univentricular cohort compared to those with biventricular physiology (42% vs. 73%) [29]. The most striking finding is significant difference in survival depending on at which stage of univentricular palliations the Berlin EXCOR was implanted. Comparing to dismal outcome (11% survival) in stage I palliation group, the survival with VAD support for Stage II (58%) and III (60%) are more favorable. These numbers are in fact superior to what has previously been reported on outcome of ECMO support for univentricular physiology [Stage II (41%) [30] and Stage III (35%) [31]]. To improve the outcome further, attention may need to be given to the type of VAD used. Horne et al. have described the superiority of continuous-flow VAD over to pulsatile VAD in univentricular physiology [32]. Pulsatile VAD decompresses the failing systemic ventricle only during pump diastole. Continuous decompression could be advantageous in univentricular circulation that lacks a subpulmonary ventricle. There have been several reports describing successful use of an implantable continuous-flow VAD in larger children with failing Fontan circulation [33,34]. As Fontan circulation can fail for multiple reasons, such as systolic or diastolic dysfunction of the heart, elevated pulmonary vascular resistance, and a combination of these [32], careful determination of the exact cause of circulatory failure is necessary. If systolic dysfunction is the predominant cause of circulatory failure, it is likely that VAD support for the failing systemic ventricle would significantly improve hemodynamics.

In contrast, the use of an implantable continuous-flow VAD in failing Glenn circulation is even more limited. To our knowledge, the report we have published is the only one currently available [35]. This would certainly reflect the fact that most of children with failing Glenn physiology would be too small to accommodate an adult implantable VAD. We expect that, however, with ongoing miniaturization of devices, implantable continuous-flow VAD will soon become the mainstay of VAD support for failing Glenn physiology.

Neonate and Small Infants

Neonates and small infants represent a challenge in VAD support. In a multicenter study on Berlin EXCOR VAD [36], Conway et al. reviewed outcomes specifically in small children weighing less than 10 kg in weight. In general, the outcome of this patient population is less favorable; successful outcome achieved only in 57% versus 83% in ≥10 kg. In particular, outcome in children of <5 kg was extremely poor; successful outcome was achieved only in 27%. Congenital heart disease was more common in children weighing <5 kg than in those weighing 5 to <10 kg (39% vs. 20%; $P<.04$). INTERMACS profile 1 at VAD implant tended to be more frequent (67% vs. 47%, respectively; $P<.06$). The difference in basic demographics would have been contributing, at least in part, to the difference in outcomes. One may wonder, nonetheless, there could be an additional factor that had led to such a poor outcome in children weighing <5 kg. We believe the patient-device size mismatch might have played a role. Even the smallest 10 mL pump may be excessive for such small children. Excessive pump size relative to the patient size may cause stasis resulting from slow pump rate, which is a risk for pump thrombosis.

Certainly, there is a definitive need to improve outcomes in this high risk subset of small children. The application of a centrifugal pump, such as PediMag [St. Jude Medical] and Rotaflow [Maquet Cardiovascular, LLC, Wayne, New Jersey] (Fig. 53.3) [37], instead of EXCOR pulsatile pump, may alleviate pump size matching issue. The fact that a centrifugal pump is, in general, less thrombogenic than a pulsatile pump, particularly at a low flow state, would favor this approach. The potential benefits of this approach remain theoretical, however, at this time due to little clinical experience.

Another potential alternative is the use of pulmonary artery banding. Initially reported from Germany by Schranz et al. [38,39] and later confirmed by our group [40], pulmonary artery banding improves overall hemodynamics in selected infant with dilated cardiomyopathy. The exact mechanism of hemodynamic improvement remains unclear. It has been suggested that leftward shift of the ventricular septum by increasing RV afterload may decrease the degree of mitral regurgitation and increase systemic cardiac output. One thing to be emphasized is that placement of pulmonary artery band would not necessarily preclude future performance of VAD support. Pulmonary artery band may serve as a temporizing measure until a suitable organ becomes available for heart transplantation. Even if the patient deteriorates with pulmonary artery band and requires placement of VAD, delaying the need for a VAD can be beneficial if somatic growth is achieved while on pulmonary artery band. In fact, with this strategy, the RV is preconditioned with pulmonary artery band, which would be favorable for LVAD physiology [40]. More study is necessary to better understand how pulmonary artery band improves circulation and who would be the best candidates for this strategy.

Chronic Graft Dysfunction

Three decades have passed since pediatric heart transplantation became a clinical reality [41]. Not surprisingly, many of previous transplant pediatric recipients now return with medically resistant chronic graft dysfunction. This group of patients also represents a challenging population for several reasons. In particular, the fact that these patients are immunologically compromised due to immunosuppression puts them at increased risk of infectious complications with VAD support [42]. The Total Artificial Heart (Syncardia, Inc., Tucson, Arizona; Fig. 53.1) presents an alternate option in these circumstances since cardiectomy, as a part of the implantation procedure, makes it possible to discontinue immunosuppression [43]. There used to be a significant size constraint with this system since only a large pump (70 mL) was available previously. A smaller pump (50 mL), however, has recently become available. It is hoped that this new system would widen its applicability in the pediatric population. A clinical trial with the 50 mL pump has begun in both adults and children [44].

FUTURE PERSPECTIVE

Newer Generation of Adult Devices

There are several adult devices that would have significant potential for pediatric application. These would include the HeartMate 3 (St. Jude; Fig. 53.4) and the MVAD (HeartWare, Inc.; Fig. 53.4). The HeartMate 3 has a magnetically levitated rotor in a pump housing. This feature is expected to result in less mechanical stress to the rotor as well as to the blood. The HeartMate 3 is also equipped with another unique technology with which the device can generate artificial pulse. Such

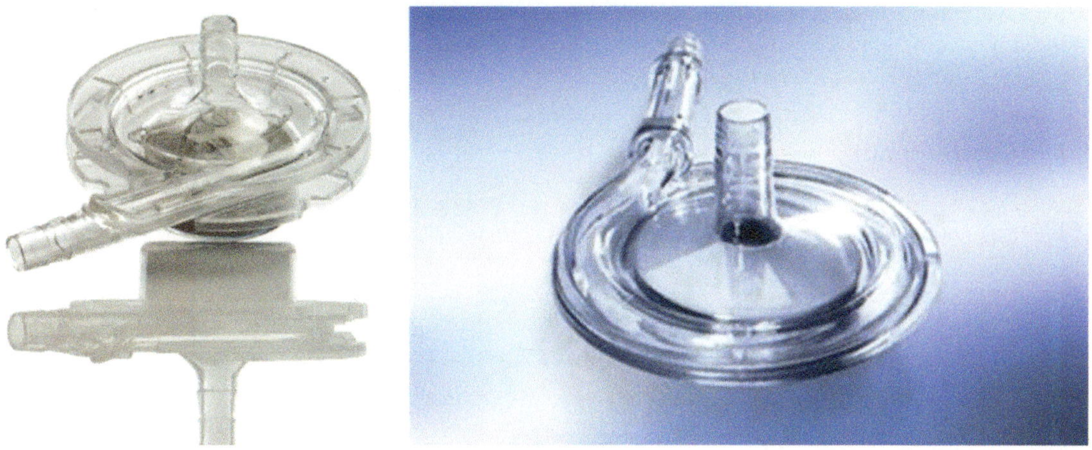

FIGURE 53.3 Extracorporeal centrifugal devices currently available. *Left; Pedimag (St. Jude Medical, Inc., St. Paul, Minnesota), Right; Rotaflow (Maquet Cardiovascular, LLC, Wayne, New Jersey).*

artificial pulsation may decrease the incidence of clinical adverse events such as gastrointestinal bleeding. The HeartMate 3 has been tested in the CE Mark clinical trial and its US trial is underway [45].

The MVAD pump may be even more promising for pediatric patients owing to its compact design. This device may have the potential to drastically change the outlook of pediatric VAD field. MVAD Advantage CE Trial started in 2015 [46]. This is a multicenter, prospective, nonrandomized, single-arm trial to enroll 70 patients at 11 sites in the United Kingdom, Austria, Australia, France, and Germany. Owing to its significantly smaller design, the MVAD pump may become the first implantable VAD that gains widespread acceptance in small children with a body surface area of 1.0 or less.

Development of Pediatric-Specific Continuous-Flow Device

The serious need for pediatric-specific VADs, particularly designed for small children, has long been recognized. In 2004, the US government, through the National Heart, Lung, and Blood Institute, awarded 5-year contracts totaling $23 million to 5 groups developing pediatric-specific mechanical circulatory support devices [47]. In 2010, the National Heart, Lung, and Blood Institute launched the PumpKIN (Pumps for Kids, Infants, and Neonates) program to continue work on some of the most promising devices with the goal of translation to clinical use [48]. The only device remaining in this program is the Infant Jarvik (Jarvik Heart, Inc., New York, NY). Development of a pediatric-specific VAD is an especially challenging task since the pump must meet the essential criteria required for adult VADs without increased blood damage using tiny blood flow channels and very thin and precise device components. The initial approach taken was to scale down the adult Jarvik

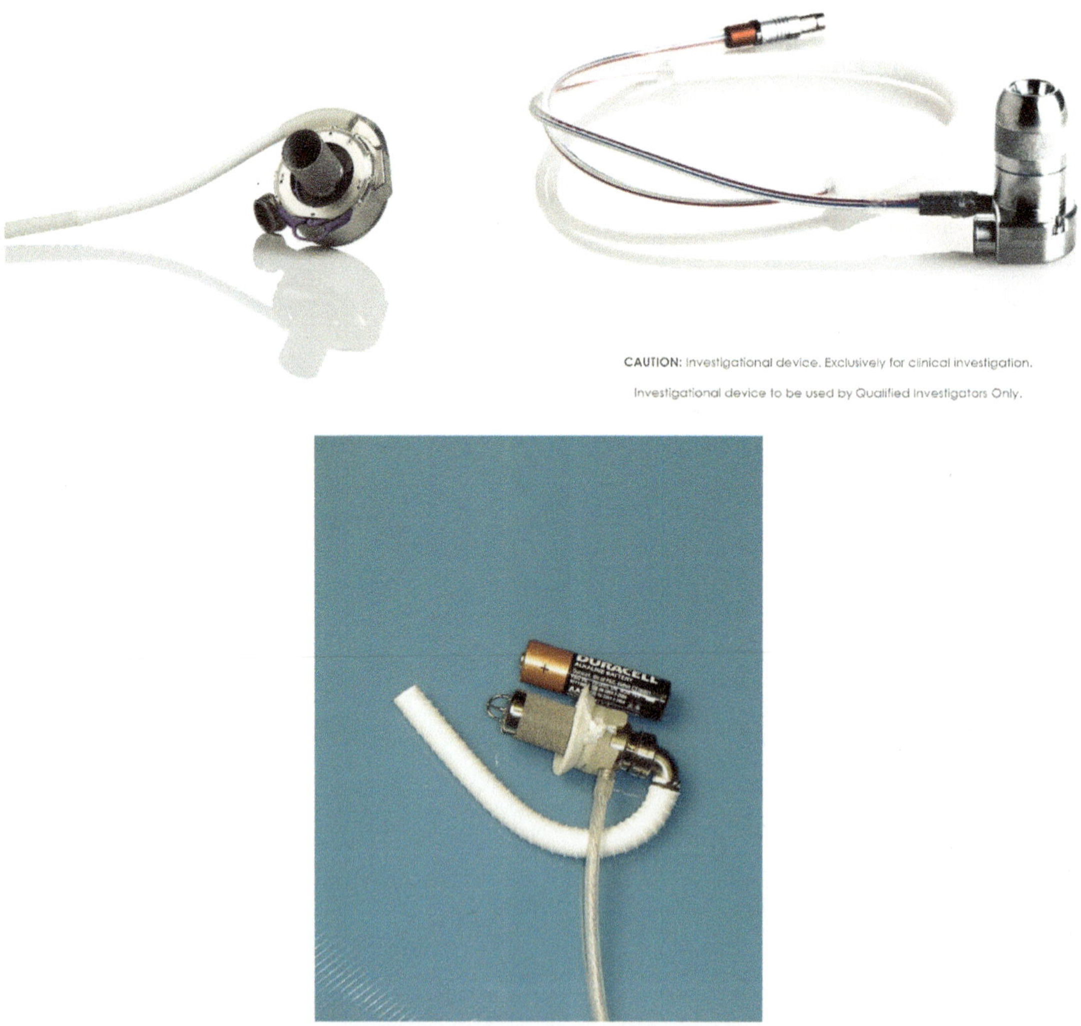

FIGURE 53.4 Newer generation of long-term devices. *Left upper; HeartMate 3 (St. Jude Medical, Inc., St. Paul, Minnesota), Right upper; MVAD (HeartWare Inc., Framingham, Massachusetts), Lower; Infant Jarvik 2015 (Jarvik Heart, Inc. New York, New York).*

2000, which has been successfully used in the clinical setting. This approach, however, failed in animal implants because of thrombosis of the pin bearings, resulting in the rotor to seize up and stop. Success could not be achieved until the new cone bearing was developed. With this cone bearing, the 11 mm outer diameter infant Jarvik 2000 was tested in an animal model. This pump was clinically used in a few cases in Europe. The outcomes have not been reported but were not overly successful (personal communication). More importantly, however, the most significant issue with this pump was significant hemolysis. In Vitro Normalized Index of Hemolysis was over 1.00 g/100L. Although the pump function seemed adequate in an acute animal model [49], the animals were in poor condition when VAD support duration was extended. This is why the FDA did not grant approval to initiate the PumpKIN clinical trial.

Significant effort was made to optimize pump design with bench hemolysis tests. The Normalized Index of Hemolysis was decreased from ~1.00 down to 0.4 g/100L. The cone bearing contact points were identified as the source of hemolysis at pump speeds over 20,000 rpm but also showed minimal hemolysis below 20,000 rpm. To achieve adequate flow and pressure with <20,000 rpm, the pump outer diameter was increased to 15 mm. The new version of the pump was renamed the Infant Jarvik 2015 (Fig. 53.4). We are now, in collaboration with a team at Texas Heart Institute, conducting in vivo testing with a chronic animal model, using 20–30 kg Barbado sheep. Of note, hemolysis has been minimal with this model. The study was completed in May 2016 and the data were submitted to FDA for approval to initiate the clinical trial.

CONCLUSION

Long-term VAD support has become an integral part of clinical management in children with severe congestive heart failure. Appropriate selection of patients and devices is a key to successful outcome. Since this field is rapidly changing, it is crucial to have an updated information on the outcomes of currently available device and the status of newer devices on the horizon. Introduction of miniaturized implantable continuous-flow VADs may drastically change the outlook of pediatric VAD support.

REFERENCES

[1] M.R. Mehra, M.J. Domanski, Should left ventricular assist device should be standard of care for patients with refractory heart failure who are not transplantation candidates?: left ventricular assist devices should be considered standard of care for patients with refractory heart failure who are not transplantation candidates, Circulation 126 (25) (2012) 3081–3087.

[2] J.W. Rossano, J.J. Kim, J.A. Decker, J.F. Price, F. Zafar, D.E. Graves, et al., Prevalence, morbidity, and mortality of heart failure-related hospitalizations in children in the United States: a population-based study, J. Card. Fail. 18 (6) (2012) 459–470.

[3] J.K. Kirklin, D.C. Naftel, R.L. Kormos, L.W. Stevenson, F.D. Pagani, M.A. Miller, et al., Fifth INTERMACS annual report: risk factor analysis from more than 6,000 mechanical circulatory support patients, J. Heart Lung Transplant. 32 (2) (2013) 141–156.

[4] A. Barbone, D. Pini, F. Rega, D. Ornaghi, E. Vitali, B. Meyns, Circulatory support in elderly chronic heart failure patients using the CircuLite(R) Synergy(R) system, Eur. J. Card. Thorac. Surg. 44 (2) (2013) 207–212 discussion 12.

[5] B. Meyns, S. Klotz, A. Simon, W. Droogne, F. Rega, B. Griffith, et al., Proof of concept: hemodynamic response to long-term partial ventricular support with the synergy pocket micro-pump, J. Am. Coll. Cardiol. 54 (1) (2009) 79–86.

[6] C.D. Fraser Jr., R.D. Jaquiss, D.N. Rosenthal, T. Humpl, C.E. Canter, E.H. Blackstone, et al., Prospective trial of a pediatric ventricular assist device, N. Engl. J. Med. 367 (6) (2012) 532–541.

[7] I. Adachi, C.D. Fraser Jr., Berlin heart EXCOR food and drug administration investigational device exemption trial, Semin. Thorac. Cardiovasc. Surg. 25 (2) (2013) 100–106.

[8] L.W. Stevenson, F.D. Pagani, J.B. Young, M. Jessup, L. Miller, R.L. Kormos, et al., INTERMACS profiles of advanced heart failure: the current picture, J. Heart Lung Transplant. 28 (6) (2009) 535–541.

[9] C.S. Almond, D.L. Morales, E.H. Blackstone, M.W. Turrentine, M. Imamura, M.P. Massicotte, et al., Berlin heart EXCOR pediatric ventricular assist device for bridge to heart transplantation in US children, Circulation 127 (16) (2013) 1702–1711.

[10] O. Miera, R. Kirk, H. Buchholz, K.R.L. Schmitt, C. VanderPluym, I.M. Rebeyka, et al., A multicenter study of the HeartWare HVAD ventricular assist device in small children, J. Heart Lung Transplant. (2016).

[11] I. Adachi, F.A. Guzman-Pruneda, A. Jeewa, C.D. Fraser Jr., E. Dean McKenzie, A modified implantation technique of the HeartWare ventricular assist device for pediatric patients, J. Heart Lung Transplant. 34 (1) (2015) 134–136.

[12] O. Miera, E.V. Potapov, M. Redlin, A. Stepanenko, F. Berger, R. Hetzer, et al., First experiences with the HeartWare ventricular assist system in children, Ann. Thorac. Surg. 91 (4) (2011) 1256–1260.

[13] B. Stiller, I. Adachi, C.D. Fraser Jr., Pediatric ventricular assist devices, Pediatr. Crit. Care Med. 14 (5 Suppl. 1) (2013) S20–S26.

[14] P. Atluri, A.B. Goldstone, A.S. Fairman, J.W. MacArthur, Y. Shudo, J.E. Cohen, et al., Predicting right ventricular failure in the modern, continuous flow left ventricular assist device era, Ann. Thorac. Surg. 96 (3) (2013) 857–863 discussion 63–64.

[15] J.R. Fitzpatrick 3rd, J.R. Frederick, V.M. Hsu, E.D. Kozin, M.L. O'Hara, E. Howell, et al., Risk score derived from pre-operative data analysis predicts the need for biventricular mechanical circulatory support, J. Heart Lung Transplant. 27 (12) (2008) 1286–1292.

[16] J.R. Miller, D.J. Epstein, M.C. Henn, T. Guthrie, R.B. Schuessler, K.E. Simpson, et al., Early biventricular assist device use in children: a single-center review of 31 patients, ASAIO J. 61 (6) (2015) 688–694.

[17] D.L. Morales, C.S. Almond, R.D. Jaquiss, D.N. Rosenthal, D.C. Naftel, M.P. Massicotte, et al., Bridging children of all sizes to cardiac transplantation: the initial multicenter North American experience with the Berlin Heart EXCOR ventricular assist device, J. Heart Lung Transplant. 30 (1) (2011) 1–8.

[18] W.P.J.D.L. Dembitsky, Right heart dysfunction, in: D.L. Joyce, L.D. Joyce, M. Loebe (Eds.), Mechanical Circulatory Support: Principles and Applications, McGraw Hill Medical, 2012.

[19] E.D. Blume, D.C. Naftel, H.J. Bastardi, B.W. Duncan, J.K. Kirklin, S.A. Webber, et al., Outcomes of children bridged to heart transplantation with ventricular assist devices: a multi-institutional study, Circulation 113 (19) (2006) 2313–2319.

[20] J.K. Kirklin, D.C. Naftel, R.L. Kormos, F.D. Pagani, S.L. Myers, L.W. Stevenson, et al., Interagency registry for mechanically assisted circulatory support (INTERMACS) analysis of pump thrombosis in the HeartMate II left ventricular assist device, J. Heart Lung Transplant. 33 (1) (2014) 12–22.

[21] S. Taghavi, C. Ward, S.N. Jayarajan, J. Gaughan, L.M. Wilson, A.A. Mangi, Surgical technique influences HeartMate II left ventricular assist device thrombosis, Ann. Thorac. Surg. 96 (4) (2013) 1259–1265.

[22] M.L. Stein, J. Yeh, O. Reinhartz, D.N. Rosenthal, B.D. Kaufman, C.S. Almond, et al., HeartWare HVAD for biventricular support in children and adolescents: the Stanford Experience, ASAIO J. (2016).

[23] G. Ferro, R. Murthy, D. Williams, V.A. Sebastian, J.M. Forbess, K.J. Guleserian, Early outcomes with HeartWare HVAD as bridge to transplant in children: a single institution experience, Artif. Organs 40 (1) (2016) 85–89.

[24] J. Sparks, D. Epstein, S. Baltagi, M.E. Mehegan, K.E. Simpson, C.E. Canter, et al., Continuous flow device support in children using the HeartWare HVAD: 1,000 Days of lessons learned from a single center experience, ASAIO J. 61 (5) (2015) 569–573.

[25] I.D. Gregoric, W.E. Cohn, O.H. Frazier, Diaphragmatic implantation of the HeartWare ventricular assist device, J. Heart Lung Transplant. 30 (4) (2011) 467–470.

[26] J.M. Rutledge, S. Chakravarti, M.P. Massicotte, H. Buchholz, D.B. Ross, U. Joashi, Antithrombotic strategies in children receiving long-term Berlin Heart EXCOR ventricular assist device therapy, J. Heart Lung Transplant. 32 (5) (2013) 569–573.

[27] J.W. Byrnes, P. Prodhan, B.A. Williams, M.L. Schmitz, M.M. Moss, U. Dyamenahalli, et al., Incremental reduction in the incidence of stroke in children supported with the Berlin EXCOR ventricular assist device, Ann. Thorac. Surg. 96 (5) (2013) 1727–1733.

[28] C.S. Almond, H. Buchholz, P. Massicotte, R. Ichord, D.N. Rosenthal, K. Uzark, et al., Berlin Heart EXCOR Pediatric ventricular assist device Investigational Device Exemption study: study design and rationale, Am. Heart J. 162 (3) (2011) 425–435.e6.

[29] S. Weinstein, R. Bello, C. Pizarro, F. Fynn-Thompson, J. Kirklin, K. Guleserian, et al., The use of the Berlin Heart EXCOR in patients with functional single ventricle, J. Thorac. Cardiovasc. Surg. 147 (2) (2014) 697–704 discussion -5.

[30] M. Jolley, R.R. Thiagarajan, C.S. Barrett, J.W. Salvin, D.S. Cooper, P.T. Rycus, et al., Extracorporeal membrane oxygenation in patients undergoing superior cavopulmonary anastomosis, J. Thorac. Cardiovasc. Surg. 148 (4) (2014) 1512–1518.

[31] K.L. Rood, S.A. Teele, C.S. Barrett, J.W. Salvin, P.T. Rycus, F. Fynn-Thompson, et al., Extracorporeal membrane oxygenation support after the Fontan operation, J. Thorac. Cardiovasc. Surg. 142 (3) (2011) 504–510.

[32] D. Horne, J. Conway, I.M. Rebeyka, H. Buchholz, Mechanical circulatory support in univentricular hearts: current management, Semin. Thorac. Cardiovasc. Surg. Pediatr. Card. Surg. Annu. 18 (1) (2015) 17–24.

[33] D.L. Morales, I. Adachi, J.S. Heinle, C.D. Fraser Jr., A new era: use of an intracorporeal systemic ventricular assist device to support a patient with a failing Fontan circulation, J. Thorac. Cardiovasc. Surg. 142 (3) (2011) e138–e140.

[34] R.A. Niebler, N.S. Ghanayem, T.K. Shah, A. De La Rosa Bobke, S. Zangwill, C. Brosig, et al., Use of a HeartWare ventricular assist device in a patient with failed Fontan circulation, Ann. Thorac. Surg. 97 (4) (2014) e115–e116.

[35] I. Adachi, A. Jeewa, S. Burki, E.D. McKenzie, C.D. Fraser Jr., Outpatient management of a child with bidirectional Glenn shunts supported with implantable continuous-flow ventricular assist device, J. Heart Lung Transplant. 35 (5) (2016) 688–690.

[36] J. Conway, J. St Louis, D.L.S. Morales, S. Law, C. Tjossem, T. Humpl, Delineating survival outcomes in children <10 kg bridged to transplant or recovery with the Berlin heart EXCOR ventricular assist device, JACC 3 (1) (2015) 70–77.

[37] A.P. Maat, R.J. van Thiel, M. Dalinghaus, A.J. Bogers, Connecting the Centrimag Levitronix pump to Berlin Heart Excor cannulae; a new approach to bridge to bridge, J. Heart Lung Transplant. 27 (1) (2008) 112–115.

[38] D. Schranz, S. Rupp, M. Muller, D. Schmidt, A. Bauer, K. Valeske, et al., Pulmonary artery banding in infants and young children with left ventricular dilated cardiomyopathy: a novel therapeutic strategy before heart transplantation, J. Heart Lung Transplant. 32 (5) (2013) 475–481.

[39] S. Recla, B. Steinbrenner, D. Schranz, Medical therapy in dilated cardiomyopathy and pulmonary arterial banding in children, J. Heart Lung Transplant. 32 (10) (2013) 1045–1046.

[40] J.F. Goldberg, T.P. Vesel, A. Jeewa, I. Adachi, Pulmonary artery band reduces left atrial pressure in dilated cardiomyopathy, Ann. Thorac. Surg. 100 (2) (2015) e35–e36.

[41] R.E. Chinnock, L.L. Bailey, Heart transplantation for congenital heart disease in the first year of life, Curr. Cardiol. Rev. 7 (2) (2011) 72–84.

[42] I. Adachi, F.A. Guzman-Pruneda, M.S. Khan, E.D. McKenzie, C.D. Fraser Jr., Ventricular assist device in children with cardiac graft failure, ASAIO J. 61 (6) (2015) 729–730.

[43] T.D. Ryan, J.L. Jefferies, F. Zafar, A. Lorts, D.L. Morales, The evolving role of the total artificial heart in the management of end-stage congenital heart disease and adolescents, ASAIO J. 61 (1) (2015) 8–14.

[44] FDA Approves Investigational Study for New Smaller SynCardia Total Artificial Heart. Available from: http://www.syncardia.com/2015-multimedia-releases/fda-approves-investigational-study-for-smaller-syncardia-total-artificial-heart/itemid-1750.html.

[45] The MOMENTUM 3 U.S. Clinical Trial. Available from: http://www.thoratec.com/vad-trials-outcomes/ongoing-clinical-trials/hmiii-usa.aspx.

[46] HeartWare Inc. Clinical Trials. Available from: http://www.heartware.com/clinicians/clinical-trials.

[47] J.T. Baldwin, H.S. Borovetz, B.W. Duncan, M.J. Gartner, R.K. Jarvik, W.J. Weiss, et al., The national heart, lung, and blood Institute pediatric circulatory support program, Circulation 113 (1) (2006) 147–155.

[48] J.T. Baldwin, H.S. Borovetz, B.W. Duncan, M.J. Gartner, R.K. Jarvik, W.J. Weiss, The national heart, lung, and blood Institute pediatric circulatory support program: a summary of the 5-year experience, Circulation 123 (11) (2011) 1233–1240.

[49] X. Wei, T. Li, S. Li, H. Sung Son, P. Sanchez, S. Niu, et al., Pre-clinical evaluation of the infant Jarvik 2000 heart in a neonate piglet model, J. Heart Lung Transplant. 32 (1) (2013) 112–119.

Chapter 54

Adult Experience With Long Term Devices

James K. Kirklin[1], Francis D. Pagani[2]

[1]*University of Alabama at Birmingham, Birmingham, AL, United States;* [2]*University of Michigan, Ann Arbor, MI, United States*

INTRODUCTION

As mechanical circulatory support (MCS) therapies are increasingly applied to the pediatric population, many concepts and lessons from the adult experience (especially with continuous flow devices) are relevant to the care of children and adolescents with advanced heart failure. The importance of MCS in the pediatric population was embraced at the national level with the creation in 2012, of the US national registry for Pediatric Mechanical Assisted Circulatory Support, which was initiated as a component of the National Heart, Lung, and Blood Institute (NHLBI)-funded Interagency Registry for Mechanically Assisted Circulatory Support (INTERMACS). In the current era, continuous flow left ventricular assist devices (LVADs) account for >95% of durable MCS device implants. This chapter will review concepts and experiences with continuous flow technology in the adult population that are particularly relevant to applications in pediatric patients.

STRATEGY

Since the first clinical introduction of continuous flow technology in the early 1990s [1,2], the goal of industry and the medical community has been long-term MCS. As far back as 1992, the Institute of Medicine concluded in their report of the Total Artificial Heart project, that "Because of the patients' total dependence on the device and because problems can occur at any time, clinical trial patients…and other MCS patients should be followed, through a registry, for the remainder of their lives…" [3]. Over the past decade, the Federal Government and NHLBI have sought information on longer-term outcomes through the INTERMACS registry [4]. Following approval of the Heartmate II (HMII; Abbott Laboratories, Abbott Park, IL), (an axial design, continuous flow LVAD) by the US Food and Drug Administration (FDA) in 2008 and its subsequent approval for long-term destination therapy (DT) in 2010, the proportion of patients in the United States implanted as DT has progressively increased, from 28% in 2011 to 45% in 2014 [5].

As the experience with DT LVAD therapy evolves and the shortage of available donor hearts for transplantation continues, practitioners ponder about patient groups on the transplant waiting lists who might be better served with long-term MCS. An analysis of the INTERMACS database in 2012 [6] suggested that optimal candidates for MCS DT (about 20% of stable DT patients) experienced 2-year survival essentially equivalent to heart transplantation, supporting an ongoing dialog of this future direction in therapies for advanced heart failure.

In the group of adult ventricular assist device (VAD) patients awaiting heart transplantation (bridge-to-transplant therapy, or BTT), the expected waiting time often exceeds a year, with only about 30% undergoing heart transplantation within 12 months (Fig. 54.1) [5]. Thus, decisions regarding donor heart quality suitable for a stable VAD patient remain challenging. Certainly, the risk of transplant hospital mortality following VAD support remains low if the donor heart is optimal. However, the wisdom of pursuing transplantation with a "marginal donor" heart in a stable VAD has been questioned. A multiinstitutional analysis by Fudim et al. reported reduced early and late graft survival in that circumstance [7].

Another area of evolving management strategy relates to patients who are present in INTERMACS Patient Profile Level 1 (critical cardiogenic shock) (Table 54.1) [4]. INTERMACS analyses have consistently demonstrated an increased risk of death after durable MCS device implant for patients in Level 1 [5]. To mitigate this increased risk, alternative strategies have evolved that utilize support with a temporary MCS device designed to stabilize hemodynamics and facilitate recovery of end-organ function prior to proceeding with durable MCS device implant. Whether this approach is more cost-effective and increases the net saving of lives remains unproven. These risk mitigation strategies have resulted in fewer patients receiving MCS device implants with Level 1 in recent years.

Heart Failure in the Child and Young Adult. http://dx.doi.org/10.1016/B978-0-12-802393-8.00054-5

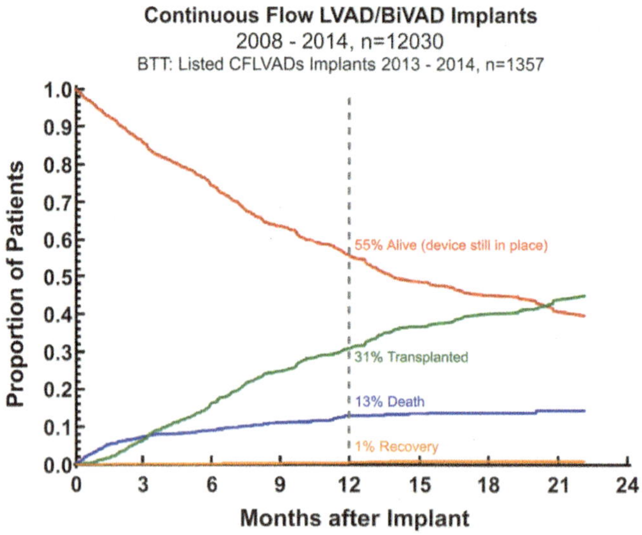

FIGURE 54.1 Competing outcomes depiction for continuous-flow left ventricular assist devices (CFLVADs) that were implanted with the bridge-to-transplant (BTT) strategy. Note that the sum of the proportion of patients with each outcome event equals 1 at each time-point. *BiVAD*, biventricular assist device; *LVAD*, Left ventricular assist device. *(Reproduced with permission, J.K. Kirklin, D.C. Naftel, F.D. Pagani, R.L. Kormos, S. Myers, M.A. Acker, J. Rogers, M.S. Slaughter, L.W. Stevenson, Pump thrombosis in the Thoratec HeartMate II device: an update analysis of the INTERMACS Registry, J. Heart Lung Transplant. 34 (12) (December 31, 2015) 1515–1526.)*

TABLE 54.1 INTERMACS Patient Profile Level (Pre-MCS Device Implant)

1. Critical cardiogenic shock
2. Progressive decline
3. Stable but inotrope dependent
4. Recurrent advanced HF
5. Exertion intolerant
6. Exertion limited
7. Advanced NYHA III

HF, heart failure; *INTERMACS*, Interagency Registry for Mechanically Assisted Circulatory Support; *MCS*, mechanical circulatory support; *NYHA*, New York Heart Association Classification.
Reproduced with permission J.K. Kirklin, D.C. Naftel, L.W. Stevenson, R.L. Kormos, F,D. Pagani, M.A. Miller, K. Ulisney, J.B. Young, INTERMACS database for durable devices for circulatory support: first annual report, J. Heart Lung Transplant. 27 (10) (October 31, 2008) 1065–1072.

PHYSIOLOGY: ISSUES OF PULSATILITY

Controversy exists about the importance of pulsatility for organ perfusion. Pulse pressure is defined as the difference between the maximum systolic and minimum diastolic aortic pressures [8]. Pulsatility index is another parameter used to assess pulsatility and is defined as the difference between maximum and minimum blood flow velocity [9], normalized to the average velocity. A number of investigators have used these and other hemodynamic energy parameters to assess the effectiveness of continuous flow pumps in providing "physiologic" perfusion of the microcirculation [10]. At the capillary/cellular level, pulsatility is characterized by sheer stress (the stress or forces are parallel to the surface of the material, in this case the vascular wall) and pulse pressure, which induce specific cellular signaling pathways. In the microcirculation, these pathways are largely regulated through the vascular endothelium [10]. The cyclical changes in sheer stress associated with pulsatile flow induce endothelial responses, which directly affect systemic vascular resistance [10]. Nonpulsatile (or reduced pulsatile) flow impairs endothelial-dependent vascular relaxation and constriction [11], related in part to reduced nitric oxide production. Impaired cyclical vasoconstriction has been correlated with increased smooth muscle proliferation, increased apoptosis, and reduced vascular smooth muscle cell contractile protein expression [11]. Other studies have associated nonpulsatile flow with elevated oxidated stress, a proinflammatory state, and arterial remodeling [12,13]. These chronic changes in systemic vascular resistance induce decreased vascular reactivity after 6 weeks of nonpulsatile circulatory support in an experimental model [14]. These observations may in part explain the common occurrence of circulatory vasoplegia at the time of cardiac transplantation following a prolonged period of continuous flow MCS.

Experimental studies have generated conflicting conclusions about which organs are most affected by prolonged nonpulsatile or minimally pulsatile flow. Chronic nonpulsatile flow appears to provide a reduction in microcirculation in the gastrointestinal (GI) organs and the liver; whereas perfusion to the brain and kidney appears relatively unaffected [15–17]. The general perception that pulsatile flow is negligible at the capillary level may be inaccurate, suggesting that microcirculatory flow patterns differ between pulsatile and continuous flow support [18].

Despite these experimental findings and the ongoing debate, the clinical function of all major organ systems are generally similarly supported by both pulsatile and continuous flow durable MCS systems [18]. The major clinical impact appears to relate to the susceptibility to bleeding in the GI tract and the brain.

CURRENT DEVICES: BASIC-ENGINEERING CONCEPTS

The most frequently utilized durable MCS devices for adults include the HeartMate II, HVAD (Medtronic Inc., Minneapolis, MN), and HeartMate 3 (HM3; Abbott Laboratories, Abbott Park, IL). All three devices are continuous flow pumps but utilize different flow designs and suspension mechanisms of the internal impeller. The HMII utilizes an axial pump design that incorporates an internal bearing (mechanical pivot design) for impeller suspension and support. The HM3 and HVAD are centrifugal designs but differ in levitation mechanism of the internal impeller. The HVAD utilizes a combination of hydrodynamic (fluid forces) and magnetic suspension while the HM3 utilizes a fully magnetically levitated impeller design. An additional design feature of the HM3 pump is a fixed artificial pulse every 2 s elicited by changes in pump speed thought to prevent areas of stasis in the pumping chamber.

SURGICAL TECHNIQUES IN EVOLUTION

Median Sternotomy Approach

The standard surgical approach to device implantation of durable MCS devices is a median sternotomy, reflecting the flexibility offered for the vast majority of cardiac operations using cardiopulmonary bypass.

Particularly in the presence of previous cardiac surgery (a known risk factor for postimplant mortality), exposure through a prior sternotomy carries the complexities of a dilated, hypokinetic right ventricle often adherent to the back of the sternum, extensive dissection necessary to expose the apex of the left ventricle, and the often diffuse mediastinal bleeding postimplant that requires administration of multiple clothing factors/blood products. The resultant milieu sets the stage for at least temporary increase in pulmonary vascular resistance and the propensity for further depression of an already myopathic right ventricle.

Lateral Thoracotomy Approach

Even without prior cardiac surgery, avoiding a sternotomy may reduce intrapericardial adhesions and potentially simplify a subsequent transplant operation or pump exchange procedure. These issues have provided the impetus for the development of nonsternotomy approaches [19]. The anterolateral thoracotomy approach has been primarily applied to the HVAD [20,21]. Although the geometric dimensions are less favorable with the HMII, successful limited access approaches with this device have also been reported [22,23]. The basic features include a limited anterolateral left thoracotomy to expose the left ventricular apex and either a tunneling maneuver to pass the graft to the ascending aorta (or rarely the right subclavian artery), or exposure of the left subclavian (less commonly the descending thoracic aorta or supraceliac aorta) for outflow implantation. If the ascending aorta is selected, a partial upper sternotomy to the level of the manubrium or high right anterior thoracotomy exposes the right lateral aspect of the ascending aorta. The outflow graft can either be tunneled anterior to the right ventricle, or the graft can course along the diaphragmatic surface (with the addition of a counter incision just to the right of the xyphoid) and then tunneled through the right pleural space to reach the ascending aorta. Alternatively, the graft can be tunneled through the anterior mediastinum [21].

Various approaches have been employed for circulatory support during implantation, ranging from full cardiopulmonary bypass to off-pump techniques. Most commonly, left femoral artery and vein are utilized for cannulation, although right axillary artery and ascending aortic cannulation are alternative approaches. If the ascending aorta is used for graft implantation, deairing is facilitated by placing a catheter in the ascending aorta.

If the outflow graft is connected to the descending aorta [21,24], the potential may exist for increased stasis in the aortic root and subsequent clot formation. Maltais et al. have recommended adjusting the pump speed to allow frequent aortic valve opening and washing of the aortic root to minimize the risk of clot formation [21].

To date, rigorous information is lacking demonstrating a clear benefit of nonsternotomy approaches in terms of survival, postoperative blood product utilization, and length of hospital stay [16]. However, early reports from the HVAD Lateral Thoracotomy trial (an observational postmarket study conducted through the INTERMACS registry) suggest no detrimental impact of the lateral thoracotomy approach. Importantly, this study required the outflow graft be anastomosed to the ascending aorta. Alternative sites for anastomosis of the outflow graft, such at the axillary artery or thoracic descending aorta, were not evaluated in this study. (Unpublished date, ISHLT Annual Meeting, San Diego, April 2017).

Inflow Cannula Positioning

With an increased observed incidence of pump thrombosis in the HMII over the past 4 years [14,25,26], attention has focused on surgical details, which might contribute to pump thrombosis. An inadequately sized pocket and a more acute angle of the inflow cannula are associated with a higher incidence of pump thrombosis [27]. Whatever device is implanted, the inflow cannula should be parallel to the interventricular septum and directed toward the mitral valve orifice.

SURVIVAL

Dramatic improvement in survival with durable MCS devices has occurred with the current generation of continuous flow LVADs. In the current era [5], 1 and 2-year survival with CF pumps has improved to 80% at 1 year and 70% at 2 years (Fig. 54.2) [5]. The early risk of death merges with a gradually increasing late hazard at about 6 months.

Causes of Death

In the era of continuous flow MCS, the major causes/modes of early mortality are neurologic events, right heart failure, and multiorgan system failure (Fig. 54.3) [5]. In the later phase, neurologic events and infection are most common causes of death, with persistent right heart failure (RHF) and multiorgan failure accounting for about 20% of late deaths (after first year). Among patients with neurologic events, intracerebral hemorrhage is the predominant cause of neurologic death.

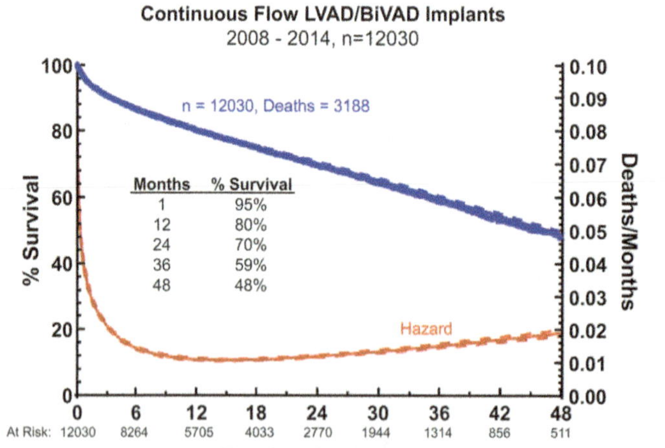

FIGURE 54.2 Parametric survival curve and associated hazard function with the 70% confidence limit for survival after implantation of a continuous-flow left ventricular assist device (LVAD) or biventricular assist device (BiVAD). The number of patients at risk during each time interval is indicated below. *(Reproduced with permission, J.K. Kirklin, D.C. Naftel, F.D. Pagani, R.L. Kormos, S. Myers, M.A. Acker, J. Rogers, M.S. Slaughter, L.W. Stevenson, Pump thrombosis in the Thoratec HeartMate II device: an update analysis of the INTERMACS Registry, J. Heart Lung Transplant. 34 (12) (December 31, 2015) 1515–1526.)*

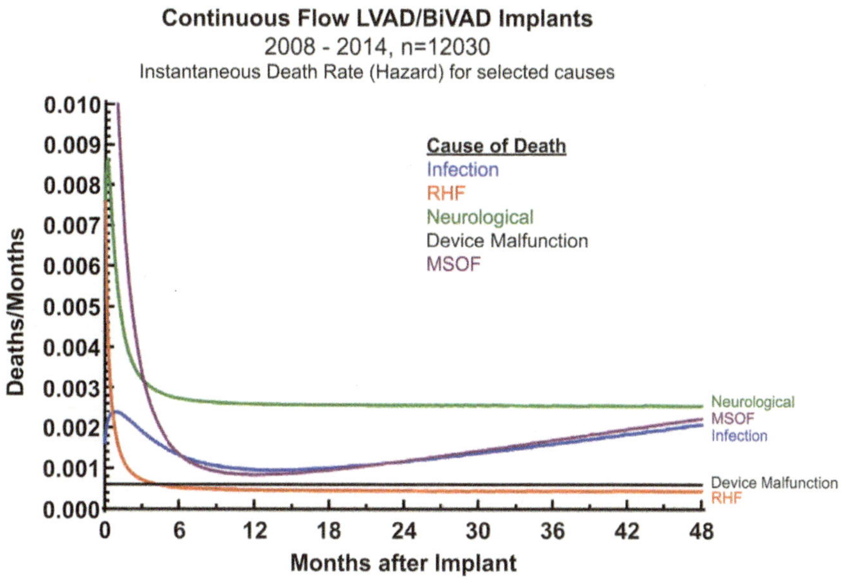

FIGURE 54.3 Hazard function curves indicating the instantaneous risk of death over time for the major causes/modes of death. *BiVAD*, biventricular assist device; *LVAD*, Left ventricular assist device; *MSOF*, multisystem organ failure; *RHF*, right heart failure. *(Reproduced with permission, J.K. Kirklin, D.C. Naftel, F.D. Pagani, R.L. Kormos, S. Myers, M.A. Acker, J. Rogers, M.S. Slaughter, L.W. Stevenson, Pump thrombosis in the Thoratec HeartMate II device: an update analysis of the INTERMACS Registry, J. Heart Lung Transplant. 34 (12) (December 31, 2015) 1515–1526.)*

RISK FACTORS

Not surprisingly, the expected survival is heavily dependent on the patient risk profile and other factors. By multivariable analysis, a variety of demographic variables, cardiac, and noncardiac clinical factors, and surgical complexities affect the expected survival (Table 54.2) [5]. A few of the risk factors are highlighted below.

Age and Patient Profile

Older age is a risk factor during the early phase and is particularly evident in patients above 65 years (Fig. 54.4) [5]. This is noteworthy, since in the current era, nearly 50% of patients receiving durable MCS devices are age 60 and over [5]. Severity of Illness is a risk factor for early mortality. Patients undergoing implantation as INTERMACS Level I or II carry an increased early risk compared to all other INTERMACS Levels [5].

Renal Dysfunction

Among noncardiac subsystems, renal dysfunction dominates as a risk factor (Table 54.2) [5]. When renal dysfunction requires dialysis prior to implant, the early risk is especially high. Despite the importance of renal dysfunction as a risk factor, improved cardiac output with VAD implantation is associated with improved renal function among survivors with moderate or severe preoperative renal dysfunction. Although renal dysfunction usually does not completely normalize, significant improvement is noted out to 2 years following VAD implant [28].

Right Heart Failure

Signs of severe right ventricular dysfunction are a powerful predictor of reduced early and late survival. Risk factors that are directly linked to right ventricular dysfunction include elevated bilirubin and high right atrial pressure [5]. When RHF is severe enough to require biventricular support, expected mortality by 6 months approaches 40% (Fig. 54.5) [5]. A multitude of VADs have been applied to right ventricular support. Among durable continuous flow devices, the HVAD has been most frequently utilized [29]. A multitude of temporary MCS devices have been used for right ventricular support, both pulsatile and continuous. In addition, novel percutaneous MCS systems have been developed for temporary right ventricular support [30,31].

TABLE 54.2 Adult Primary CF LVADs and BiVAD Implants: April 2008 to December 2014 (n = 12,030)

	Early Hazard	
Risk Factors for Death	**Hazard Ratio**	***P*-Value**
Demographic		
Age (older)	1.03	<0.0001
Female	1.32	<0.0001
BMI (higher)	1.10	<0.0001
Clinical Status		
History of stroke	1. 33	0.03
Ventilator	1.25	0.02
ICD	1.30	0.0001
INTERMACS Level 1	1.55	<0.0001
INTERMACS Level 2	1.37	<0.0001
Destination therapy	1.23	<0.0001
Noncardiac Systems		
Albumin (lower)	1.14	0.0007
Creatinine (higher)	1.06	0.04
Dialysis	2.34	<0.0001
BUN (higher)	1.05	<0.0001
Right Heart Dysfunction		
Right atrial pressure (higher)	1.13	0.0004
RVAD in same operation	2.57	<0.0001
Bilirubin (higher)	1.48	<0.0001
Surgical Complexities		
History of cardiac surgery	1.24	0.003
History of CABG	1.17	0.04
Concomitant cardiac surgery	1.26	<0.0001

BiVAD, biventricular assist device; *BMI*, body mass index; *BUN*, blood urea nitrogen; *CABG*, coronary artery bypass graft; *CF*, continuous flow; *ICD*, implantable cardioverter-defibrillator; *LVAD*, left ventricular assist device; *NYHA*, New York Heart Association; *RVAD*, right ventricular assist device.
Modified from J.K. Kirklin, D.C. Naftel, F.D. Pagani, R.L. Kormos, S. Myers, M.A. Acker, J. Rogers, M.S. Slaughter, L.W. Stevenson, Pump thrombosis in the Thoratec HeartMate II device: an update analysis of the INTERMACS Registry, J. Heart Lung Transplant. 34 (12) (December 31, 2015) 1515–1526.

Valvular Regurgitation

Despite the somewhat reduced survival for LVAD implants with concomitant aortic valve procedures [32,33], the general consensus among experienced VAD surgeons and cardiologists is that moderate or severe aortic insufficiency at time of implant is an indication for aortic valve repair, closure, or replacement [34]. Although the optimal surgical therapy for aortic regurgitation in this setting remains controversial, a large multiinstitutional analysis suggested that complete aortic valve closure was an independent risk factor for mortality compared to either aortic valve repair (including placement of a suture through the midpoint of each cusp to eliminate central incompetence) or replacement [34]. Although repair is associated with greater residual aortic insufficiency than replacement, prosthetic valves pose special challenges in LVAD patients. Bioprosthetic valve leaflets have a tendency to undergo fusion if the aortic does not regularly open. Mechanical valves pose

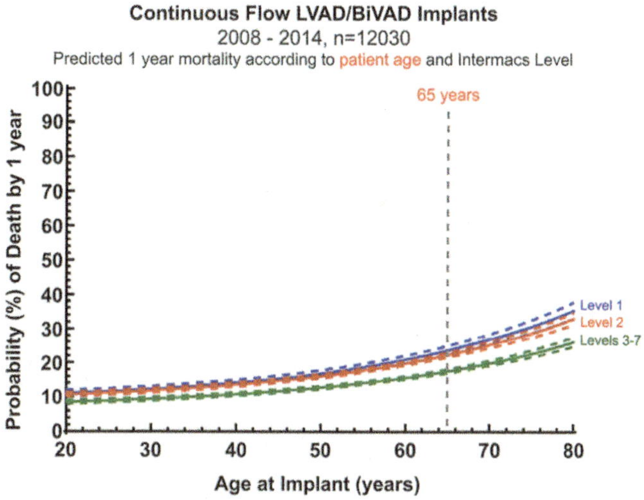

FIGURE 54.4 Nomogram depicting the solution to the multivariable equation for death by 1 year, depicting the interaction between patient age and INTERMACS level. *BiVAD*, biventricular assist device; *INTERMACS*, Interagency Registry for Mechanically Assisted Circulatory Support; *LVAD*, Left ventricular assist device. *(Reproduced with permission, J.K. Kirklin, D.C. Naftel, F.D. Pagani, R.L. Kormos, S. Myers, M.A. Acker, J. Rogers, M.S. Slaughter, L.W. Stevenson, Pump thrombosis in the Thoratec HeartMate II device: an update analysis of the INTERMACS Registry, J. Heart Lung Transplant. 34 (12) (December 31, 2015) 1515–1526.)*

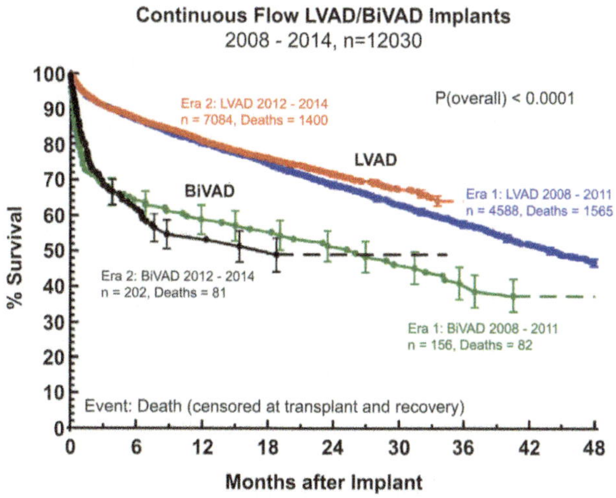

FIGURE 54.5 Actuarial survival curve for continuous-flow LVADs and BiVADs, stratified by era. The error bars indicate 1 SE. *BiVAD*, biventricular assist device; *LVAD*, left ventricular assist device. *(Reproduced with permission, J.K. Kirklin, D.C. Naftel, F.D. Pagani, R.L. Kormos, S. Myers, M.A. Acker, J. Rogers, M.S. Slaughter, L.W. Stevenson, Pump thrombosis in the Thoratec HeartMate II device: an update analysis of the INTERMACS Registry, J. Heart Lung Transplant. 34 (12) (December 31, 2015) 1515–1526.)*

a significant risk of thromboembolic complications secondary to the obligatory aortic root stasis [35]. Mechanical aortic valve prostheses should probably be replaced with a bioprosthetic valve at the time of LVAD implant.

In contrast to moderate-to-severe aortic insufficiency, unrepaired **mitral valve regurgitation** (moderate-to-severe vs. none-to-moderate) has not been identified as a risk factor for reduced survival after LVAD implant [29].

The advantages of repairing severe **tricuspid regurgitation** have been debated. Although conclusive evidence is lacking for a survival benefit of repairing moderate to severe tricuspid regurgitation, several studies suggest that repair of TR facilitates recovery after LVAD implantation [36].

Frailty

Although difficult to measure, frailty is emerging as an important predictor of poor survival following LVAD implant [37,38]. Various models have been used to describe and define frailty. The phenotype model defines frailty as the presence of three of five of the following traits: unintentional weight loss, self-reported exhaustion, low energy expenditure, slow gait speed and weak grip strength. The cumulative deficit model calculates a deficit index from a long list of variables describing symptoms, abnormal lab values, disease states, and disabilities. Each method has its supports and critics, and some experts have focused on simple measures such as handgrip strength and other basic screening tools.

Although the best definition remains challenging, additional studies are necessary to identify strategies to reverse the frailty condition in advanced heart failure and what degrees of frailty are amendable to reversal with MCS rather than simply using it as a marker for poor post-VAD outcomes.

MAJOR ADVERSE EVENTS WITH CONTINUOUS FLOW TECHNOLOGY

Major adverse events after LVAD implant constitute the greatest barrier to more widespread application of these life-saving devices.

Pump Thrombosis

All continuous flow pumps currently approved for clinical use have a propensity for fibrin and clot deposition in the absence of effective anticoagulation, and at times even with adequate anticoagulation. Multiinstitutional studies of the HMII suggest about an 8% risk of pump thrombosis within the first 6 months [5]. The possibility that centrifugal flow pumps have a reduced tendency for pump thrombosis compared to axial flow pumps remains unresolved. However, in a recent clinical trial, the HM3 pump appears to have a particularly low tendency for pump thrombus formation [38].

An analysis of pump thrombosis in the HVAD underscored the need for adequate anticoagulation. One multiinstitutional study identified an INR less than 2 and aspirin dose of 81 mg or less as risk factors for pump thrombosis [39].

Increasing hemolysis is generally considered a harbinger of progressive fibrin deposition within the pump [40]. Patients with lactate dehydrogenase (LDH) levels above 2.5× the upper limits of the reference range for LDH or approximately 600 IU/L are more likely to experience pump exchange or death due to pump thrombosis. Similarly, a plasma-free hemoglobin >60 mg/dL in association with clinical signs of hemolysis is significantly correlated with pump thrombosis within 6 months [41]. Other INTERMACS studies identified higher LDH during the first month following device implant as a significant predictor of subsequent pump thrombosis, with a cumulative risk of 20% by 6 months if the peak LDH at 1 month exceeded 600 IU/L [5].

Treatment of pump thrombosis includes medical therapy with heparin, glycoprotein 2b/3a inhibitors, tissue plasminogen activator, or pump exchange. Reliable data for medical therapy are not available, since the diagnosis of pump thrombosis is often presumptive. However, the success of medical therapy particularly when applied early in the process has been estimated at 50% but may differ between different types of pumps [39]. Surgical therapy requires pump exchange, which, for the HMII, usually is limited to the pump itself but may include the inflow cannula and/or the outflow graft if they are suspected to be the site or source of thrombus generation. For the HMII, a significant number of pump exchanges can be accomplished through a limited subcostal or transcostal incision assisted with a short period of cardiopulmonary bypass via femoral cannulation. The HVAD more frequently requires a full sternotomy for device exchange.

The mortality associated with pump thrombosis is estimated at 25% within 3 months [26]. Following pump exchange for thrombosis, 1-year mortality approaches 30% and increases with each subsequent need for pump exchange [5].

De-Novo Aortic Insufficiency and Aortic Valve Cusp Fusion

Several studies have documented a greater propensity for progressive aortic insufficiency as well as cusp fusion with continuous flow support compared to pulsatile flow pumps, especially in the absence of aortic valve opening [42]. The aortic insufficiency may relate to the constant and elevated transvalvar pressure gradient and increased average strain on the aortic leaflets that results in progressive aortic valve fusion and leaflet remodeling in the presence of continuous flow circulatory support [43,44].

Gastrointestinal Bleeding and Arteriovenous Malformations

The higher incidence of GI bleeding during continuous flow compared to pulsatile support has been well documented [45]. The decrease in pulse pressure has been linked to arteriovenous malformations within the GI tract, as has also been reported with aortic stenosis [46,47]. The higher sheer stress in the microcirculation associated with continuous flow support has been hypothesized to break down the co-coagulant molecule von Willebrand factor [48].

Neurologic Events

A major stroke can be a devastating event during LVAD support, destroying any benefit in quality of life achieved by the device implant. Neurologic events are generally categorized as hemorrhagic strokes (the most commonly fatal), ischemic (thromboembolic) strokes, and transient ischemic attacks. The freedom from any neurologic event is approximately 90% at 1 year [24], and (by multivariable analysis) is not related to INTERMACS level at implant or the presence of atrial fibrillation. The only significant risk factor is older age [27]. Since the clinical introduction of continuous flow pumps in the United States in 2008, these stroke rates with continuous flow pumps have decreased from 0.26 events per patient year in 2008–10 to 0.1 events per patient year in 2011–13 [49]. Recent data from the ENDURANCE and ENDURANCE Supplement Pivotal trials evaluating performance of the HVAD compared to the HMII for DT indication have identified a higher risk of stroke for the HVAD. The ENDURANCE Supplement trial importantly demonstrated the role of blood pressure management and treatment of hypertension as an important management strategy in mitigating stroke risk for the HVAD [50,51].

Right Heart Failure

The failing right ventricle presents one of the greatest obstacles to long-term successful left ventricular support. Even when right ventricular failure is controlled early postimplant, the potential for clinically important chronic right ventricular failure exists, more as a persisting condition (occasionally requiring continuous intravenous inotropic support) rather than a discreet event. Although not yet rigorously studied, chronic elevation of right atrial pressure undoubtedly adversely impacts hepatic function, renal reserves, functional capacity, health-related quality of life, and ultimately survival.

When evaluating patients for RHF during follow-up and planning management strategies, it should be noted that right heart failure is not always present from the time of implant. A European analysis emphasized the variability of patient hemodynamic parameters early postimplant in those that develop RHF more than 3 months later [52]. Predictive scoring models for the development of RHF have only been modestly useful [53].

MYOCARDIAL RECOVERY

Support of the left ventricle with a VAD routinely induces favorable changes (reverse remodeling) in the damaging remodeling process of advanced heart failure. Despite the frequency of documented improvement in structure and function with chronic MCS, recovery sufficient for successful device explanation following myocardial recovery or remission has been uncommon.

Reverse Remodeling and the Myocyte Milieu

Chronic ventricular unloading with an LVAD, typically to a partial extent, reduces the myocyte defects of hypertrophy, alterations in contractile properties, beta adrenergic desensitization, and myocyte death [54]. Reduction of wall stress reduces oxidative stress and decreases the generation of proinflammatory cytokines such as tumor necrosis factor and interleukin I, as well as hypertrophic signaling pathways [55].

The reduction of mechanical stretch during MCS results in restoration of collagen networks within the extracellular matrix, which in turn promotes improvement in ventricular geometry [56,57]. Despite this improvement in the collagen networks, data are conflicting regarding whether VAD support results in an increase or decrease in interstitial fibrosis [58–60]. Patients who can be weaned and explanted within 6 months of the original VAD implant have a higher likelihood of long-term heart failure remission [61].

Alterations in myocyte structure and contractile function are at least partially reversible during LVAD support [57,62]. Documented reversal of heart failure induced sarcomeric disarray, restoration of membrane-associated proteins, and improved myocyte function has been observed during VAD support [63,64].

During ventricular support, these cellular and extracellular processes contribute to reduction of left ventricular end diastolic dimension, reduced left ventricular volume, reduction in left ventricular sphericity, and a shift of the left ventricular end diastolic pressure–volume relationship toward normal [55].

Recovery Sufficient for Explanation

Despite the nearly uniform presence of reverse remodeling during support, less than 10% of patients with dilated cardiomyopathy undergo explanation for recovery [28,65], and fewer with ischemic cardiomyopathy [66,67]. The highest rates of

TABLE 54.3 Criteria for Left Ventricular Assist Device Explantation Due to Myocardial Recovery

Echocardiography	LV end-diastolic diameter (LVEDD) ≤55 mm
	LV ejection fraction (LVEF) ≥45%
	Stable pre-explant LVEF after maximum improvement
	Stable pre-explant LVEDD after maximum improvement and during the final off pump
	Stable stroke volume (SV) during the final off-pump trial
	Systolic wall motion peak velocity (Sm) ≥8 cm/s, stable after maximum improvement and during the final off-pump trial
	No or less than grade II regurgitation at mitral and/or aortic valve
	No RV dilation (RVOT diameter<35 mm, end-diastolic short/long axis ratio<0.6)
	No or maximum grade II regurgitation of the mitral or aortic valves
RH Catheterization	Cardiac index (CI) >2.6 L/min/m²
	Pulmonary capillary wedge pressure <14 mmHg
	Right atrial pressure (mean) <12 mmHg
	Mean atrial pressure >65 mmHg
Electrocardiography	Sinus rhythm
	Heart rate (HR) 90 bpm or less
	No more than 25% HR increase during off-pump trials

RWT_{ED} = [interventricular septum thickness + posterior wall thickness]/LVEDD. A product of time velocity integral measured with pulsed-wave Doppler at the LV outflow tract (LVOT) and cross-sectional area of the LVOT.
Modified from M. Dandel, C. Knosalla, R. Hetzer, Contribution of ventricular assist devices to the recovery of failing hearts: a review and the Berlin Heart Center Experience, Eur. J. Heart Fail. 16 (3) (March 1, 2014) 248–263.

recovery have been reported in younger patients with more rapid onset of heart failure [55] and for acute inflammatory states such as fulminant myocarditis, in which the onset of symptoms to cardiogenic shock usually occurs within a week [68].

From the compendium of available studies and large clinical experience, it is evident that reverse remodeling is necessary but not sufficient for myocardial recovery. Partial reversible of the remodeling process does not usually translate into the normalization of myocardial structure or function. The hallmarks of nonreversibility and the markers for successful recovery have not been elucidated. However, when the criteria for explanation have been fulfilled in experienced centers, long-term heart failure remission with freedom from death or heart transplantation have been generally good, particularly in patients with nonischemic chronic cardiomyopathy, for whom 5-year survival exceeds 70% [54]. A typical algorithm for hemodynamic evaluation during VAD weaning, in preparation for explanation, is shown in Table 54.3 [54].

INSIGHTS FROM RECENT CLINICAL TRIALS

The potential contribution of device design to improving adverse event profiles has been explored in a recent series of prospective, randomized control trials.

ENDURANCE was a prospective, multicenter, randomized clinical trial evaluating performance of the HVAD compared to the HMII for patients receiving durable MCS for DT indication [50]. The trial enrolled 446 patients who were assigned, in a 2:1 ratio, to the HVAD (n=297) or HMII (n=148). The primary endpoint was survival at 2 years, free from disabling stroke or device removal for malfunction or failure. Results from ENDURANCE demonstrated noninferiority of the HVAD with respect to the HMII device for the primary endpoint (55% vs. 57.4%, respectively). Overall survival at 2 years was not different (60.2% for the HVAD vs. 67.6% for the HMII, P=.17). Despite similar survival, the devices differed substantially in adverse event profile. More patients who received the HMII experienced device malfunction or device failure requiring replacement (16.2% vs. 8.8%), while more patients who received the HVAD experienced a stroke (29.7% vs. 12.1%).

With increasing experience with the HVAD, subsequent analyses identified hypertension as a major contributor to both hemorrhagic and ischemic stroke [69]. As a consequence, the US FDA required a supplemental trial of the HVAD to examine the relationship between hypertension and stroke. The ENDURANCE supplemental trial was a prospective, multicenter, randomized clinical trial evaluating performance of the HVAD compared to the HMII for patients receiving durable MCS for DT indication. (Milano, unpublished data, ISHLT Annual Meeting, San Diego, April 2017) The trial enrolled 465 patients who were assigned, in a 2:1 ratio, to the HVAD (n=308) or HMII (n=157). The primary endpoint was the incidence of neurologic injury at 12 months between HVAD and HMII. ENDURANCE Supplemental trial required that all patients receiving the HVAD take their blood pressure twice daily documented in a diary for the first 3 months of support and continue this protocol beyond 3 months until the blood pressure consistently remained within the recommended range. Recommended blood pressure values were defined as a mean arterial press of less than 85 mmHg using an automated cuff method or less than 90 mmHg using a Doppler and cuff method. Overall incidence of neurological injury at 1 year was 14.7% in the HVAD and 12.1% in the HMII (not significant with respect to noninferiority; i.e., study did not meet the primary endpoint). However, examination of the secondary endpoint of survival at 2 years free from disabling stroke or device removal for malfunction or failure demonstrated the HVAD to be statistically superior to the HMII, 76.4% versus 66.9% (P=.035). The major difference in outcome was the higher need for device exchange in HMII. Overall survival at 1 year was 818% and 80.3% for the HVAD and HMII (P=.71). Overall, there was a 50% reduction in rate of hemorrhagic stroke with HVAD when results of the ENDURANCE supplemental trial were compared to ENDURANCE, suggesting that blood pressure management is effective in reducing stroke.

The novel design features of the HM3 were recently evaluated against the HMII in a multicenter prospective randomized clinical trial, MOMENTUM 3 [38]. The primary endpoint of the trial was a composite of survival free of disabling stroke or survival free of reoperation to replace or remove the device at 6 months after implantation. Of 294 patients, 152 were assigned to the HM3 pump and 142 to the HMII. The primary endpoint was achieved in 86.2% of the HM3 group and was superior to that of the HMII, 76.8% (P=.001). There were no significant between difference in the rates of death or disabling stroke, but reoperation for pump malfunction was less frequent in the HM3 compared to the HMII, 0.7% versus 7.7% (P=.002). Suspected or confirmed pump thrombosis occurred in 0.0% of the patients in the HM3 group and 10.1% of the HMII group. These early results of the MOMENTUTUM 3 trial suggest that critical design features of the HM3 pump, including full magnetic levitation of the internal impeller with wider gaps between impeller and pump housing and artificial pulse, may enhance resistance to pump thrombosis.

QUALITY OF LIFE

On average, most quality of life (QOL) metrics are improved after implantation of durable CF pumps. The general EQ-5D Visual Analog Scale score usually improves dramatically, with persistence in that improvement out to 2 years [5]. Measures of self-care and the ability to engage in usual activities show similar sustained improvement. Older patients experience as good or better improvement than younger patients and sicker patients see the greatest benefit [70].

As MCS therapy is expanded to the ambulatory heart failure population, QOL will become as important as absolute survival. Future studies are needed to quantify the impact of adverse events and their sequelae on life satisfaction during extended support. Prevention and improved management of these complications are critical to the success of MCS therapy in the advanced heart failure domain.

REFERENCES

[1] C.M. Burnett, J.D. Vega, B. Radovancevic, J.L. Lonquist, S. Birovilev, M.S. Sweeney, J.M. Duncan, O.H. Fraier, Improved survival after hemopump insertion in patients experiencing postcardiotomy cardiogenic shock during cardiopulmonary bypass, ASAIO J. 36 (3) (July 1, 1990) M626–M628.

[2] R.K. Wampler, O.H. Frazier, A.M. Lansing, R.W. Smalling, J.M. Nicklas, S.J. Phillips, R.A. Guyton, L.A. Golding, Treatment of cardiogenic shock with the Hemopump left ventricular assist device, Ann. Thorac. Surg. 52 (3) (September 1, 1991) 506–513.

[3] S. Perry, Report from the US Institute of Medicine (IOM), Int. J. Technol. Assess. Health Care 8 (02) (March 1, 1992) 371.

[4] J.K. Kirklin, D.C. Naftel, L.W. Stevenson, R.L. Kormos, F.D. Pagani, M.A. Miller, K. Ulisney, J.B. Young, INTERMACS database for durable devices for circulatory support: first annual report, J. Heart Lung Transplant. 27 (10) (October 31, 2008) 1065–1072.

[5] J.K. Kirklin, D.C. Naftel, F.D. Pagani, R.L. Kormos, S. Myers, M.A. Acker, J. Rogers, M.S. Slaughter, L.W. Stevenson, Pump thrombosis in the Thoratec HeartMate II device: an update analysis of the INTERMACS Registry, J. Heart Lung Transplant. 34 (12) (December 31, 2015) 1515–1526.

[6] J.K. Kirklin, D.C. Naftel, F.D. Pagani, R.L. Kormos, L. Stevenson, M. Miller, J.B. Young, Long-term mechanical circulatory support (destination therapy): on track to compete with heart transplantation? J. Thorac. Cardiovasc. Surg. 144 (3) (September 30, 2012) 584–603.

[7] M. Fudim, M.E. Davis, C. Jenkins, C.L. Brown, M.A. Wigger, J.M. Stulak, S. Maltais, N. Haglund, Marginal donor use in patients undergoing heart transplantation with left ventricular assist device explantation, Ann. Thorac. Surg. 100 (6) (December 31, 2015) 2117–2126.

[8] A. Ündar, T. Masai, O.H. Frazier, C.D. Fraser Jr., Pulsatile and nonpulsatile flows can be quantified in terms of energy equivalent pressure during cardiopulmonary bypass for direct comparisons, ASAIO J. 45 (6) (November 1, 1999) 610–614.

[9] B. Voss, M. Krane, C. Jung, G. Brockmann, S. Braun, T. Günther, R. Lange, R. Bauernschmitt, Cardiopulmonary bypass with physiological flow and pressure curves: pulse is unnecessary!, Eur. J. Cardio Thorac. Surg. 37 (1) (January 1, 2010) 223–232.

[10] T. Nakano, R. Tominaga, S. Morita, M. Masuda, I. Nagano, K.I. Imasaka, H. Yasui, Impacts of pulsatile systemic circulation on endothelium-derived nitric oxide release in anesthetized dogs, Ann. Thorac. Surg. 72 (1) (July 31, 2001) 156–162.

[11] T. Thacher, V. Gambillara, R. Da Silva, G. Montorzi, N. Stergiopulos, P. Silacci, Oscillatory shear stress and reduced compliance impair vascular functions, Clin. Hemorheol. Microcirc. 37 (1–2) (January 1, 2007) 121–130.

[12] G. Montorzi, P. Silacci, M. Zulliger, N. Stergiopulos, Functional, mechanical and geometrical adaptation of the arterial wall of a non-axisymmetric artery in vitro, J. Hyperten. 22 (2) (February 1, 2004) 339–347.

[13] V. Gambillara, T. Thacher, P. Silacci, N. Stergiopulos, Effects of reduced cyclic stretch on vascular smooth muscle cell function of pig carotids perfused ex vivo, Am. J. Hypertens. 21 (4) (April 1, 2008) 425–431.

[14] T. Nishinaka, E. Tatsumi, T. Nishimura, K. Shioya, H. Ohnishi, Y. Taenaka, H. Takano, Change in vasoconstrictive function during prolonged non-pulsatile left heart bypass, Artif. Organs 25 (5) (May 1, 2001) 371–375.

[15] Y. Orime, M. Shiono, K.I. Nakata, M. Hata, A. Sezai, H. Yamada, M. Iida, S. Kashiwazaki, M. Nemoto, J.I. Kinoshita, T. Kojima, The role of pulsatility in end-organ microcirculation after cardiogenic shock, ASAIO J. 42 (5) (September 1, 1996) M724–M728.

[16] A. Sezai, M. Shiono, Y. Orime, K.I. Nakata, M. Hata, M. Iida, S. Kashiwazaki, J.I. Kinoshita, M. Nemoto, T. Koujima, M. Furuichi, Major organ function under mechanical support: comparative studies of pulsatile and nonpulsatile circulation, Artif. Organs 23 (3) (March 1, 1999) 280–285.

[17] K. Eya, E. Tuzun, J. Conger, H.K. Chee, D. Byler, C. Nojiri, O.H. Frazier, K. Kadipasaoglu, Effect of pump flow mode of novel left ventricular assist device upon end organ perfusion in dogs with doxorubicin induced heart failure, ASAIO J. 51 (1) (January 1, 2005) 41–49.

[18] F. Kamdar, A. Boyle, K. Liao, M. Colvin-adams, L. Joyce, R. John, Effects of centrifugal, axial, and pulsatile left ventricular assist device support on end-organ function in heart failure patients, J. Heart Lung Transplant. 28 (4) (April 30, 2009) 352–359.

[19] S.V. Rojas, M. Avsar, J.S. Hanke, Z. Khalpey, S. Maltais, A. Haverich, J.D. Schmitto, Minimally invasive ventricular assist device surgery, Artif. Organs 39 (6) (June 1, 2015) 473–479.

[20] J.D. Schmitto, U. Molitoris, A. Haverich, M. Strueber, Implantation of a centrifugal pump as a left ventricular assist device through a novel, minimized approach: upper hemisternotomy combined with anterolateral thoracotomy, J. Thorac. Cardiovasc. Surg. 143 (2) (February 29, 2012) 511–513.

[21] S. Maltais, M.E. Davis, N. Haglund, Minimally invasive and alternative approaches for long-term LVAD placement: the Vanderbilt strategy, Ann. Cardiothorac. Surg. 3 (6) (October 21, 2014) 563–569.

[22] I.D. Gregoric, S. La Francesca, T. Myers, W. Cohn, P. Loyalka, B. Kar, C. Gemmato, O.H. Frazier, A less invasive approach to axial flow pump insertion, J. Heart Lung Transplant. 27 (4) (April 30, 2008) 423–426.

[23] A.C. Anyanwu, Technique for less invasive implantation of Heartmate II left ventricular assist device without median sternotomy, Semin. Thorac. Cardiovasc. Surg. 23 (3) (November 30, 2011) 241–244 WB Saunders.

[24] R. Umakanthan, N.A. Haglund, J.M. Stulak, L.D. Joyce, R. Ahmad, M.E. Keebler, S. Maltais, Left thoracotomy HeartWare implantation with outflow graft anastomosis to the descending aorta: a simplified bridge for patients with multiple previous sternotomies, ASAIO J. 59 (6) (November 2013) 664.

[25] J.K. Kirklin, D.C. Naftel, R.L. Kormos, F.D. Pagani, S.L. Myers, L.W. Stevenson, M.A. Acker, D.L. Goldstein, S.C. Silvestry, C.A. Milano, J.T. Baldwin, Interagency registry for mechanically assisted circulatory support (INTERMACS) analysis of pump thrombosis in the HeartMate II left ventricular assist device, J. Heart Lung Transplant. 33 (1) (January 31, 2014) 12–22.

[26] N.G. Smedira, E.H. Blackstone, J. Ehrlinger, L. Thuita, C.D. Pierce, N. Moazami, R.C. Starling, Current risks of HeartMate II pump thrombosis: non-parametric analysis of interagency registry for mechanically assisted circulatory support data, J. Heart Lung Transplant. 34 (12) (December 31, 2015) 1527–1534.

[27] S. Taghavi, C. Ward, S.N. Jayarajan, J. Gaughan, L.M. Wilson, A.A. Mangi, Surgical technique influences HeartMate II left ventricular assist device thrombosis, Ann. Thorac. Surg. 96 (4) (October 31, 2013) 1259–1265.

[28] J.K. Kirklin, D.C. Naftel, R.L. Kormos, L.W. Stevenson, F.D. Pagani, M.A. Miller, J.T. Baldwin, J.B. Young, Fifth INTERMACS annual report: risk factor analysis from more than 6,000 mechanical circulatory support patients, J. Heart Lung Transplant. 32 (2) (February 28, 2013) 141–156.

[29] J.M. Stulak, V. Tchantchaleishvili, N.A. Haglund, M.E. Davis, J.A. Schirger, J.A. Cowger, P. Shah, K.D. Aaronson, F.D. Pagani, S. Maltais, Uncorrected pre-operative mitral valve regurgitation is not associated with adverse outcomes after continuous-flow left ventricular assist device implantation, J. Heart Lung Transplant. 34 (5) (May 31, 2015) 718–723.

[30] M.B. Anderson, J. Goldstein, C. Milano, L.D. Morris, R.L. Kormos, J. Bhama, N.K. Kapur, A. Bansal, J. Garcia, J.N. Baker, S. Silvestry, Benefits of a novel percutaneous ventricular assist device for right heart failure: the prospective RECOVER RIGHT study of the impella RP device, J. Heart Lung Transplant. 34 (12) (December 31, 2015) 1549–1560.

[31] H. Takayama, Y. Naka, S.K. Kodali, J.A. Vincent, L.J. Addonizio, U.P. Jorde, M.R. Williams, A novel approach to percutaneous right-ventricular mechanical support, Eur. J. Cardio Thorac. Surg. 41 (2) (February 1, 2012) 423–426.

[32] R. John, Y. Naka, S.J. Park, C. Sai-Sudhakar, C. Salerno, K.S. Sundareswaran, D.J. Farrar, C.A. Milano, Impact of concurrent surgical valve procedures in patients receiving continuous-flow devices, J. Thorac. Cardiovasc. Surg. 147 (2) (February 28, 2014) 581–589.

[33] J.D. Pal, C.T. Klodell, R. John, F.D. Pagani, J.G. Rogers, D.J. Farrar, C.A. Milano, Low operative mortality with implantation of a continuous-flow left ventricular assist device and impact of concurrent cardiac procedures, Circulation 120 (11 Suppl. 1) (September 15, 2009) S215–S219.

[34] J.O. Robertson, D.C. Naftel, S.L. Myers, S. Prasad, G.D. Mertz, A. Itoh, F.D. Pagani, J.K. Kirklin, S.C. Silvestry, Concomitant aortic valve procedures in patients undergoing implantation of continuous-flow left ventricular assist devices: an INTERMACS database analysis, J. Heart Lung Transplant. 34 (6) (June 30, 2015) 797–805.

[35] V. Rao, J.P. Slater, N.M. Edwards, Y. Naka, M.C. Oz, Surgical management of valvular disease in patients requiring left ventricular assist device support, Ann. Thorac. Surg. 71 (5) (May 31, 2001) 1448–1453.
[36] V. Piacentino, C.D. Troupes, A.M. Ganapathi, L.J. Blue, G.B. Mackensen, M. Swaminathan, G.M. Felker, M. Stafford-Smith, A.J. Lodge, J.G. Rogers, C.A. Milano, Clinical impact of concomitant tricuspid valve procedures during left ventricular assist device implantation, Ann. Thorac. Surg. 92 (4) (October 31, 2011) 1414–1419.
[37] S.M. Dunlay, S.J. Park, L.D. Joyce, R.C. Daly, J.M. Stulak, S.M. McNallan, V.L. Roger, S.S. Kushwaha, Frailty and outcomes after implantation of left ventricular assist device as destination therapy, J. Heart Lung Transplant. 33 (4) (April 30, 2014) 359–365.
[38] M.R. Mehra, Y. Naka, N. Uriel, D.J. Goldstein, J.C. Cleveland Jr., P.C. Colombo, M.N. Walsh, C.A. Milano, C.B. Patel, U.P. Jorde, F.D. Pagani, A fully magnetically levitated circulatory pump for advanced heart failure, N. Engl. J. Med. 376 (5) (2017) 440–450.
[39] S.S. Najjar, M.S. Slaughter, F.D. Pagani, R.C. Starling, E.C. McGee, P. Eckman, A.J. Tatooles, N. Moazami, R.L. Kormos, D.R. Hathaway, K.B. Najarian, An analysis of pump thrombus events in patients in the HeartWare ADVANCE bridge to transplant and continued access protocol trial, J. Heart Lung Transplant. 33 (1) (January 31, 2014) 23–34.
[40] J.A. Cowger, M.A. Romano, P. Shah, N. Shah, V. Mehta, J.W. Haft, K.D. Aaronson, F.D. Pagani, Hemolysis: a harbinger of adverse outcome after left ventricular assist device implant, J. Heart Lung Transplant. 33 (1) (January 31, 2014) 35–43.
[41] J.N. Katz, B.C. Jensen, P.P. Chang, S.L. Myers, F.D. Pagani, J.K. Kirklin, A multicenter analysis of clinical hemolysis in patients supported with durable, long-term left ventricular assist device therapy, J. Heart Lung Transplant. 34 (5) (May 31, 2015) 701–709.
[42] M. Hatano, K. Kinugawa, T. Shiga, N. Kato, M. Endo, M. Hisagi, T. Nishimura, A. Yao, Y. Hirata, S. Kyo, M. Ono, Less frequent opening of the aortic valve and a continuous flow pump are risk factors for postoperative onset of aortic insufficiency in patients with a left ventricular assist device, Circ. J. 75 (5) (2011) 1147–1155.
[43] K. May-Newman, L. Enriquez-Almaguer, P. Posuwattanakul, W. Dembitsky, Biomechanics of the aortic valve in the continuous flow VAD-assisted heart, ASAIO J. 56 (4) (July 1, 2010) 301–308.
[44] J.O. Mudd, J.D. Cuda, M. Halushka, K.A. Soderlund, J.V. Conte, S.D. Russell, Fusion of aortic valve commissures in patients supported by a continuous axial flow left ventricular assist device, J. Heart Lung Transplant. 27 (12) (December 31, 2008) 1269–1274.
[45] G.V. Letsou, N. Shah, I.D. Gregoric, T.J. Myers, R. Delgado, O.H. Frazier, Gastrointestinal bleeding from arteriovenous malformations in patients supported by the Jarvik 2000 axial-flow left ventricular assist device, J. Heart Lung Transplant. 24 (1) (January 31, 2005) 105–109.
[46] D.R. Stern, J. Kazam, P. Edwards, S. Maybaum, R.A. Bello, D.A. D'Alessandro, D.J. Goldstein, Increased incidence of gastrointestinal bleeding following implantation of the HeartMate II LVAD, J. Card. Surg. 25 (3) (May 1, 2010) 352–356.
[47] E.C. Heyde, Gastrointestinal bleeding in aortic stenosis, N. Engl. J. Med. 259 (1958) 196.
[48] N. Uriel, S.W. Pak, U.P. Jorde, B. Jude, S. Susen, A. Vincentelli, P.V. Ennezat, S. Cappleman, Y. Naka, D. Mancini, Acquired von Willebrand syndrome after continuous-flow mechanical device support contributes to a high prevalence of bleeding during long-term support and at the time of transplantation, J. Am. Coll. Cardiol. 56 (15) (October 5, 2010) 1207–1213.
[49] B. Sileshi, N.A. Haglund, M.E. Davis, N.M. Tricarico, J.M. Stulak, Z. Khalpey, M.R. Danter, R. Deegan, J. Kennedy, M.E. Keebler, S. Maltais, In-hospital outcomes of a minimally invasive off-pump left thoracotomy approach using a centrifugal continuous-flow left ventricular assist device, J. Heart Lung Transplant. 34 (1) (January 31, 2015) 107–112.
[50] J.G. Rogers, F.D. Pagani, A.J. Tatooles, G. Bhat, M.S. Slaughter, E.J. Birks, S.W. Boyce, S.S. Najjar, V. Jeevanandam, A.S. Anderson, I.D. Gregoric, Intrapericardial left ventricular assist device for advanced heart failure, N. Engl. J. Med. 376 (5) (February 2, 2017) 451–460.
[51] S.J. Park, C.A. Milano, A.J. Tatooles, J.G. Rogers, R.M. Adamson, D.E. Steidley, G.A. Ewald, K.S. Sundareswaran, D.J. Farrar, M.S. Slaughter, Outcomes in advanced heart failure patients with left ventricular assist devices for destination therapy, Circ. Heart Fail. 111 (January 1, 2012).
[52] C.J. Kapelios, C. Charitos, E. Kaldara, K. Malliaras, E. Nana, C. Pantsios, E. Repasos, M. Tsamatsoulis, S. Toumanidis, J.N. Nanas, Late-onset right ventricular dysfunction after mechanical support by a continuous-flow left ventricular assist device, J. Heart Lung Transplant. 34 (12) (December 31, 2015) 1604–1610.
[53] A.P. Kalogeropoulos, A. Kelkar, J.F. Weinberger, A.A. Morris, V.V. Georgiopoulou, D.W. Markham, J. Butler, J.D. Vega, A.L. Smith, Validation of clinical scores for right ventricular failure prediction after implantation of continuous-flow left ventricular assist devices, J. Heart Lung Transplant. 34 (12) (December 31, 2015) 1595–1603.
[54] M. Dandel, C. Knosalla, R. Hetzer, Contribution of ventricular assist devices to the recovery of failing hearts: a review and the Berlin Heart Center Experience, Eur. J. Heart Fail. 16 (3) (March 1, 2014) 248–263.
[55] D.L. Mann, P.M. Barger, D. Burkhoff, Myocardial recovery and the failing heart: myth, magic, or molecular target? J. Am. Coll. Cardiol. 60 (24) (December 18, 2012) 2465–2472.
[56] J.L. Hall, D.R. Fermin, E.J. Birks, P.J. Barton, M. Slaughter, P. Eckman, H.A. Baba, J. Wohlschlaeger, L.W. Miller, Clinical, molecular, and genomic changes in response to a left ventricular assist device, J. Am. Coll. Cardiol. 57 (6) (February 8, 2011) 641–652.
[57] A.V. Ambardekar, J.S. Walker, L.A. Walker, J.C. Cleveland, B.D. Lowes, P.M. Buttrick, Incomplete recovery of myocyte contractile function despite improvement of myocardial architecture with left ventricular assist device support clinical perspective, Circ. Heart Fail. 4 (4) (July 1, 2011) 425–432.
[58] S. Saito, G. Matsumiya, T. Sakaguchi, S. Miyagawa, T. Yamauchi, T. Kuratani, Y. Sawa, Cardiac fibrosis and cellular hypertrophy decrease the degree of reverse remodeling and improvement in cardiac function during left ventricular assist, J. Heart Lung Transplant. 29 (6) (June 30, 2010) 672–679.
[59] S.G. Drakos, A.G. Kfoury, E.H. Hammond, B.B. Reid, M.P. Revelo, B.Y. Rasmusson, K.J. Whitehead, M.E. Salama, C.H. Selzman, J. Stehlik, S.E. Clayson, Impact of mechanical unloading on microvasculature and associated central remodeling features of the failing human heart, J. Am. Coll. Cardiol. 56 (5) (July 27, 2010) 382–391.

[60] H. Muranaka, A. Marui, M. Tsukashita, J. Wang, J. Nakano, T. Ikeda, R. Sakata, Prolonged mechanical unloading preserves myocardial contractility but impairs relaxation in rat heart of dilated cardiomyopathy accompanied by myocardial stiffness and apoptosis, J. Thorac. Cardiovasc. Surg. 140 (4) (October 31, 2010) 916–922.

[61] M. Dandel, Y. Weng, H. Siniawski, E. Potapov, H.B. Lehmkuhl, R. Hetzer, Long-term results in patients with idiopathic dilated cardiomyopathy after weaning from left ventricular assist devices, Circulation 112 (9 Suppl.) (August 30, 2005) 1–37.

[62] H.A. Baba, J. Wohlschlaeger, Morphological and molecular changes of the myocardium after left ventricular mechanical support, J. Mol. Cell Cardiol. 45 (4) (October 31, 2008) S1–S2.

[63] N. Latif, M.H. Yacoub, R. George, P.J. Barton, E.J. Birks, Changes in sarcomeric and non-sarcomeric cytoskeletal proteins and focal adhesion molecules during clinical myocardial recovery after left ventricular assist device support, J. Heart Lung Transplant. 26 (3) (March 31, 2007) 230–235.

[64] E.J. Birks, J.L. Hall, P.J. Barton, S. Grindle, N. Latif, J.P. Hardy, J.E. Rider, N.R. Banner, A. Khaghani, L.W. Miller, M.H. Yacoub, Gene profiling changes in cytoskeletal proteins during clinical recovery after left ventricular–assist device support, Circulation 112 (9 Suppl.) (August 30, 2005) I-57.

[65] M. Dandel, Y. Weng, H. Siniawski, E. Potapov, T. Krabatsch, H.B. Lehmkuhl, T. Drews, C. Knosalla, R. Hetzer, Pre-explant stability of unloading-promoted cardiac improvement predicts outcome after weaning from ventricular assist devices, Circulation 126 (11 Suppl. 1) (September 11, 2012) S9–S19.

[66] S. Maybaum, D. Mancini, S. Xydas, R.C. Starling, K. Aaronson, F.D. Pagani, L.W. Miller, K. Margulies, S. McRee, O.H. Frazier, G. Torre-Amione, Cardiac improvement during mechanical circulatory support, Circulation 115 (19) (May 15, 2007) 2497–2505.

[67] M. Dandel, Y. Weng, H. Siniawski, E. Potapov, T. Drews, H.B. Lehmkuhl, C. Knosalla, R. Hetzer, Prediction of cardiac stability after weaning from left ventricular assist devices in patients with idiopathic dilated cardiomyopathy, Circulation 118 (14 Suppl. 1) (September 30, 2008) S94–S105.

[68] P. Atluri, B.W. Ullery, J.L. Howard, W. Hiesinger, J.R. Fitzpatrick, M. Jessup, M.A. Acker, R.J. Morris, Y.J. Woo, Rapid onset of fulminant myocarditis portends a favorable prognosis and ability to bridge mechanical support to recovery, J. Card. Fail. 16 (8) (August 31, 2010) S51.

[69] J.J. Teuteberg, M.S. Slaughter, J.G. Rogers, E.C. McGee, F.D. Pagani, R. Gordon, E. Rame, M. Acker, R.L. Kormos, C. Salerno, T.P. Schleeter, The HVAD left ventricular assist device: risk factors for neurological events and risk mitigation strategies, JACC 3 (10) (October 31, 2015) 818–828.

[70] K.L. Grady, D.C. Naftel, S. Myers, M.A. Dew, G. Weidner, J.A. Spertus, K. Idrissi, H.B. Lee, E.C. McGee, J.K. Kirklin, Change in health-related quality of life from before to after destination therapy mechanical circulatory support is similar for older and younger patients: analyses from INTERMACS, J. Heart Lung Transplant. 34 (2) (February 28, 2015) 213–221.

FURTHER READING

[1] A. Baba, P. Dobsak, I. Saito, T. Isoyama, K. Takiura, Y. Abe, T. Chinzei, J. Vasku, K. Imachi, Microcirculation of the bulbar conjunctiva in the goat implanted with a total artificial heart: effects of pulsatile and nonpulsatile flow, ASAIO J. 50 (4) (July 1, 2004) 321–327.

[2] F. Dobbels, O. Mauthner, K. Milisen, Frailty in left ventricular assist device destination therapy: putting a new motor in a rickety old car running out of gas? J. Heart Lung Transplant. 33 (4) (April 1, 2014) 347–349.

Chapter 55

Future of Mechanical Circulatory Support Devices in Children and Young Adults

David L. Sutcliffe, Robert D.B. Jacquiss
University of Texas Southwestern Medical Center, Dallas, TX, United States

HISTORY OF VENTRICULAR ASSIST DEVICE THERAPY

Mechanical circulatory support has revolutionized heart failure management for adult and pediatric patients alike. Though the field has been marked by near continuous technologic advances, its origins are undoubtedly inauspicious. First performed in 1966, Dr. Michael Debakey described the use of an extracorporeal, pulsatile device to support the circulation of a 37-year-old woman for a mere 10 days [1]. However, it was not until the early 1990s that the use of ventricular assist device (VAD) technology became routine with the FDA approval of the HeartMate IP left ventricular assist system (LVAS) (Fig. 55.1A). This and other similar first generation VADs utilized pneumatically driven, pulsatile pumps to offload the failing ventricle and provide adequate blood flow to reverse the unrelenting course of end-stage heart failure.

Driven by the needs of a rapidly growing population of adult heart failure patients that vastly exceeded the availability of donor hearts for transplantation, the use of VAD support expanded throughout the 1990s [2]. This culminated with the landmark REMATCH trial that showed clear superiority of "mechanical" management of end-stage heart disease by left ventricular assist device (LVAD) therapy as compared to optimal medical therapy [3]. This study demonstrated the advantage of the more invasive, expensive, and profitable LVAD approach to end-stage heart failure. This demonstration, combined with the demographics of the large and expanding patient pool, suggested a clear return on investment for companies bold enough to develop better technology. It was by this drive that second and third generation VADs (Fig. 55.1B–D) were developed, and a transition from pulsatile to continuous flow pumps was solidified with clear evidence of the superiority of continuous flow devices [4–6].

With widespread application of this novel approach to heart failure management, the need for careful and rigorous analysis of the longitudinal outcomes of this expensive technology was obvious. Based on recommendations by the National Institute of Medicine that "...patients be followed in a registry...," funding was provided for such a registry by the National Institutes of Health, the Food and Drug Administration, and the Centers for Medicaid and Medicare Services [7]. Thus was born the Interagency Registry for Mechanical Circulatory Support (INTERMACS) with enrollment beginning on June 23, 2006 [8]. This registry continues to serve as an event-driven database to define VAD outcomes and provide a medium with which to improve the quality of device therapy across centers. It grew to an enrollment of over 15,000 patients by 2015, and it has provided the construct by which VAD therapy and management has evolved [9].

PEDIATRIC VENTRICULAR ASSIST DEVICE THERAPY: A BEGINNING

As with adults, the pediatric heart failure population has rapidly grown over the past two decades. Though the sheer volume of end-stage heart disease in pediatric patients, an estimated 12,000–35,000 patients annually, is dwarfed by that of adults; the per patient repercussions of the disease are much more broad reaching [10]. Lost years of productivity in pediatric patients and economic consequences affecting both patient and parent lead to a much greater overall cost of heart failure in pediatrics. However, it has long been realized that the rising need for definitive heart failure treatment outstrips the donor supply. As evidenced by plateaued international transplant volumes that approximate organ availability, heart transplantation remains the gold standard for the management of end-stage heart disease but is a therapy available to only some of the larger number who could benefit [11]. Historically the gap between supply and demand was filled through the use of extracorporeal membrane oxygenator (ECMO) support. However, the temporal limitations and attendant morbidity of such support have long been realized [12,13]. As VAD therapy demonstrated reproducible efficacy in adult heart failure management, attempts

Heart Failure in the Child and Young Adult. http://dx.doi.org/10.1016/B978-0-12-802393-8.00055-7

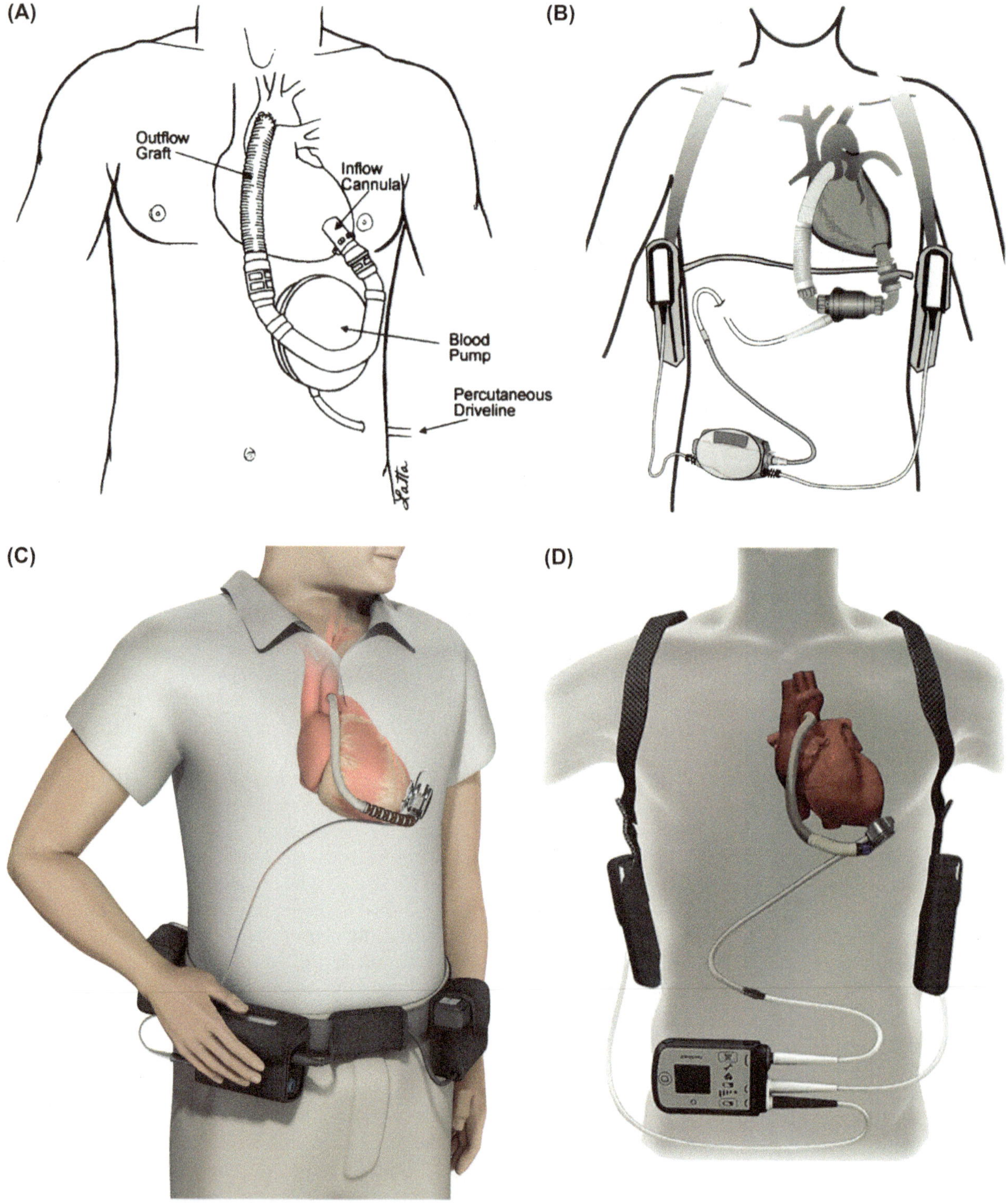

FIGURE 55.1 Over the history of ventricular assist device support, devices have gone through multiple generations of design: (A) the HeartMate IP LVAS represented the first generation pulsatile devices; (B) the HeartMate II marked the transition to second generation continuous flow pumps; (C) the HeartWare and (D) HeartMate 3 represent the current era of fully magnetically levitated devices.

were made to adapt adult-intended devices for use in pediatric patients. First described in 1989, VAD therapy offered adult-size pediatric patients an opportunity for improved waitlist survival through a then-novel bridge to transplant (BTT) [14].

Early successes in pediatric VAD therapy led to its increased use internationally [15–18]. Despite the progression of technology toward continuous flow devices in adults, however, none were suitable for small patients, leaving pediatric heart failure patients to first generation technology. Among the multitude of pulsatile device options available, a single device gained prominence in pediatric VAD support, the Berlin EXCOR VAD. Driven not only by its proven success and versatility in LVAD and biventricular assist device (BiVAD)-capable support but also by its available pump sizes ranging from 10 to 60mL stroke volume (Fig. 55.2), this pneumatically driven device became the most commonly chosen for pediatric VAD support. Therefore with enrollment beginning in 2007 and the study culminating in a landmark publication in 2012, the first and only prospective trial in pediatric VAD support compared the use of Berlin EXCOR VAD to ECMO support as BTT [19]. The investigators in this trial showed a clear and undeniable survival advantage for patients supported with VAD therapy (Fig. 55.3), paving the way for the Berlin Heart Pediatric VAD to become FDA approved through Humanitarian Device Exemption for pediatric BTT. Since its FDA approval, the Berlin Heart has gained wider acceptance for a variety of support ranging from LVAD to BiVAD to systemic VAD in the setting of congenital heart disease (CHD) and single ventricle physiology. The extension of VAD therapy to the pediatric population eventually grew to such an extent as to justify the creation of PediMACS, the pediatric counterpart of INTERMACS.

For many years, the Berlin EXCOR was the mainstay of pediatric support, but this support had its clear limitations. Patients were committed to prolonged hospital admissions while awaiting heart transplantation, and device support was accompanied by a regrettably high rate of adverse events including bleeding, infection, and stroke ranging from 40% to 50%. Meanwhile adult patients enjoyed the use of second generation devices with corresponding adverse event profiles that were a fraction of that seen in pulsatile devices. This changed with the development of third generation, intrapericardial devices and specifically the HeartWare Ventricular Assist System. Owing to its compact design and light weight, children as young as 7 years and with body surface area as small as $0.7\,m^2$ were able undergo successful support with durable continuous flow VADs [20]. As had

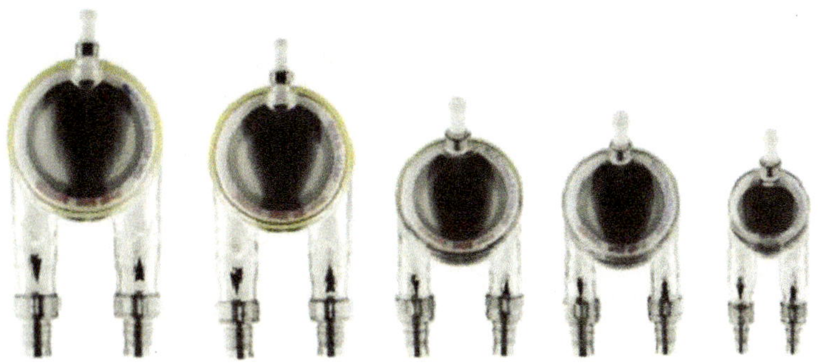

FIGURE 55.2 The Berlin EXCOR Pediatric ventricular assist device (VAD) provided great versatility in device support with the ability to function as an LVAD, systemic VAD, or BiVADs in a variety of sizes ranging from 10 to 60mL stroke volumes.

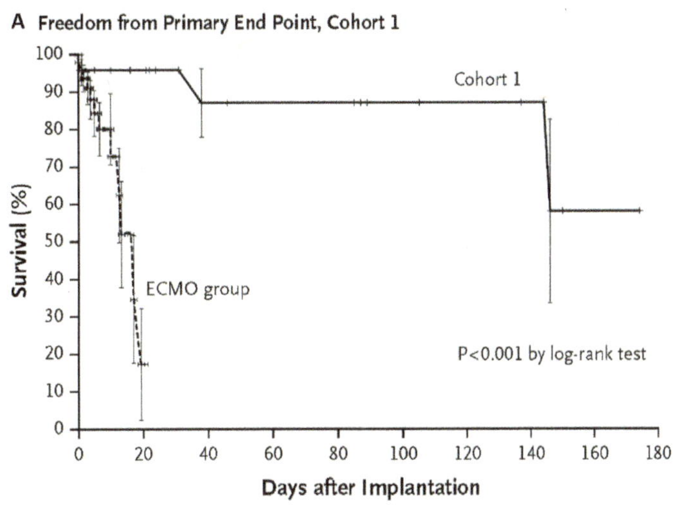

FIGURE 55.3 The first and only prospective trial in pediatric ventricular assist device (VAD) support showed clear survival benefit for patients supported by the Berlin EXCOR Pediatric VAD over those supported by extracorporeal membrane oxygenator (ECMO).

long been the case for all VADs prior to the FDA approval of the Berlin Heart, HeartWare device usage remains off label in pediatrics and in patients outside the prescribed size restrictions of body surface area greater than 1.5 m^2.

Therefore similar to the drive in adult device support to provide a medium for studying device outcomes and for improvement in management strategies, the PediMACS registry was created as a mirror to the established adult INTERMACS registry. Patient enrollment began on September 12, 2012, and the first annual report published in 2016 described an enrollment of 200 patients with 86% achieving either transplantation or living on device at 6 months postimplant (Fig. 55.4) [21]. Subsequent reports from the PediMACS registry have shed light in various areas of VAD support. Rosenthal et al., for example, provided insight into adverse events suffered by VAD supported patients. The authors showed the majority of events occurred predominantly in the first 3 months with bleeding, device malfunction, infection, and stroke occurring most commonly. They additionally demonstrated that adverse events occurred with a much greater frequency in pulsatile than continuous flow devices [22]. In the midst of these findings, Rossano et al. using the PediMACS registry defined the population of pediatric patients undergoing support with continuous flow devices [23]. They described a population that was, as would be expected, older and larger given the size restrictions for most durable continuous flow devices. They additionally showed these patients enjoyed superior 6-month survival compared to the overall PediMACS population (92% vs. 81%), and they showed fewer adverse events in this group supported with continuous flow. Clearly the rich data sets of this registry have only begun to pay analytic dividends.

PEDIATRIC VENTRICULAR ASSIST DEVICE SUPPORT: REFINING THE SELECTION

Though technological advances will certainly continue to advance the field of mechanical circulatory support therapy, improvements in both quality and safety of device support hinges on further refinements in the selection process. Improved selection applies to patient evaluation as it pertains to the constraints of mechanical support as well as to the array of devices available to the VAD team. Issues of patient selection relate to the degree of clinical instability determining appropriate timing for support; variations in patient coagulation factors as they relate to age, genetics, and underlying cause and chronicity of heart failure; and patient anatomic factors requiring adaptations of traditional support strategies to name a few.

Traditionally centers have relied on their own experiences to guide patterns of practice, however, resources such as INTERMACS and PediMACS have allowed these practices to be further optimized. Perhaps the most valuable resource that has come from these registries has been the INTERMACS and PediMACS profiles by which patients are categorized prior to device implantation (Table 55.1). These profiles have normalized the description of patients' clinical statuses, and they have allowed for risk stratification in so much as showing increased risk of postimplant mortality in Profile 1 patients [9,21]. Though not intrinsically related to PediMACS profile, development of end-organ dysfunction has also long been considered a risk for negative outcomes. This finding has even led to the consideration of preimplant mechanical support including ECMO to normalize the acute shock state [24]. Though timing of device support remains a controversial and challenging issue, it has been increasingly clear that delaying to high-level INTERMACS/PediMACS profiles only results in poor outcomes.

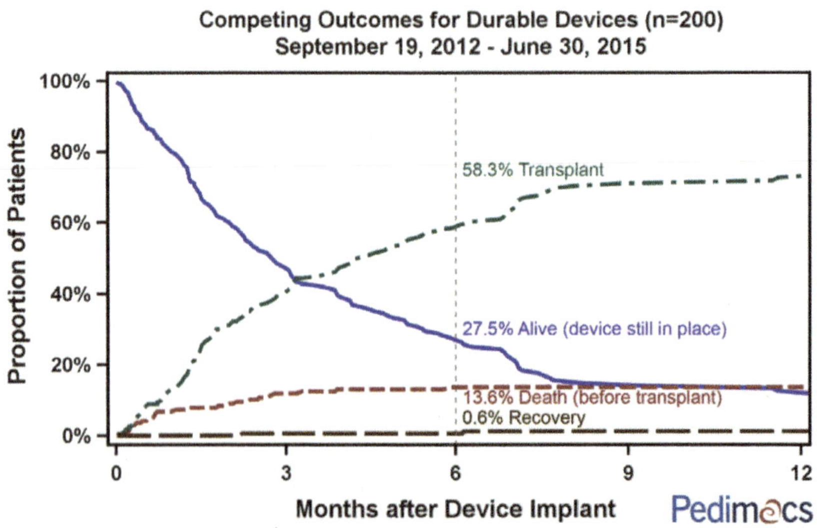

FIGURE 55.4 The PediMACS first annual report provided encouraging results with over 86% of patients achieving positive outcomes by 6 months postdevice support.

Additionally challenging patient factors in the pediatric population include the immaturity of the hemostatic system most notably in the youngest of patients. With the majority of VAD adverse events relating to the management of anticoagulation in both adults and pediatric patients, the quest for device hemocompatability has been an important but elusive one. This pursuit becomes increasingly difficult given the realization that pediatric patients exhibit dramatic differences in platelet function and reactivity, coagulation factor concentration, and factor activities related to thrombus formation and breakdown across the broad range of ages [25,26]. Further complicating the matter is that whether in the setting of myocarditis or chronic heart failure, patients generally present in an inflamed state. The result is an increasingly unpredictable hemostatic system prior to and following VAD surgery [27,28]. Though no consensus regarding anticoagulation management has been reached among pediatric centers, efforts are well underway to establish standard practices. Future multiinstitutional studies will undoubtedly include strategies to avoid heparin contamination of blood samples, types of coagulation lab testing performed, and both number and targets of medications selected for ideal management.

Even in the setting of optimal anticoagulation management, device selection in pediatric patients remains a continuously evolving practice. Though adult-size pediatric patients often enjoy the benefits of adult-intended technology, anatomic considerations weigh heavily in the selection process of both candidates and devices. Long thought to be a challenge facing predominantly pediatric cardiologists and cardiothoracic surgeons, CHD has grown to an estimated 2.4 million affected individuals in the United States alone with more affected adults than children [29]. Given that a significant percentage of CHD interventions are palliative in nature, the natural history often ends in heart failure of varying etiologies. Therefore device selection as well as device orientation in both pediatric and adult CHD is a practice in engineering and creativity. Historically outcomes in device support of CHD patients have unfortunately been marred by the outcomes seen in single ventricle support. In this population, survival to transplant or recovery has been a third of that seen in patients with a biventricular circulation. Given the anatomic limitations present in single ventricle heart disease, patients have long been relegated to extracorporeal pulsatile devices with higher rates of complications and mortality [30,31]. Only recently has an increasing shift toward utilizing durable continuous flow devices been seen, but this has largely been reserved for adult-sized patients with late failure, while heart failure in early stages of palliation continue to have limited options [32–34]. To combat the limitations of first generation devices in the setting of smaller sized and single ventricle patients, emerging trends have shown an increased utilization of temporary devices for durable support [32,35,36]. Though many of the shortcomings experienced with early era devices including cannula length, infection risks, and bleeding risks persist, initial results have been encouraging at the ability to safely support such tenuous patient populations.

PEDIATRIC VENTRICULAR ASSIST DEVICE SUPPORT: THE FUTURE OF DEVICES AND DEVICE MANAGEMENT

Over the history of mechanical support in pediatrics, innovation has been largely through device adaptation as opposed to device design. Despite the rising number of affected patients, financial barriers to pursuing pediatric-focused device design have been insurmountable. In light of this limitation, the US FDA and the Office of Orphan Products Development committed over $20 million to the development of pediatric circulatory support devices to five contractors in the Spring

TABLE 55.1 Interagency Registry for Mechanical Circulatory Support (INTERMACS) Profile Definitions Have Provided a Framework by Which Patient Clinical Status at Implant Can Translate Into Risk Stratification

INTERMACS Level	Definition
1	Critical cardiogenic shock
2	Progressive decline
3	Stable but inotrope-dependent
4	Resting symptoms
5	Exertion intolerant
6	Exertion limited
7	Advanced modified Ross/NYHA Class III

NYHA, New York Heart Association.

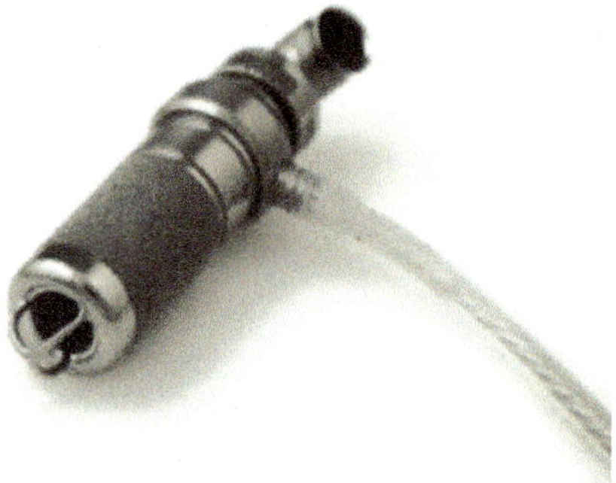

FIGURE 55.5 The Jarvik 2015 represents the first intracorporeal device designed for small children, and it is the focus of the upcoming Pumps for Kids, Infants, and Neonates (PumpKIN) trial.

of 2004 [37]. This landmark commitment provided hope for a future in which pediatric patients would enjoy the benefits of pediatric-focused support. Device designs chosen in the initial development program included the PediaFlow Pediatric VAD, the PediPump, Ension's Pediatric Cardiopulmonary Assist System (next-generation ECMO), the Jarvik 2000, and the Penn State Pediatric VAD. Though four of these five devices failed to progress to full clinical trials, the Jarvik 2000 was selected to proceed to the Pumps for Kids, Infants, and Neonates (PumpKIN) trial. The trial design included 1:1 randomization to either the infant Jarvik or the FDA approved Pediatric Berlin Heart.

Despite the need for modifications to combat complications with hemolysis in animal trials, the redesigned Jarvik 2015 (Fig. 55.5) and the PumpKIN trial stand poised in 2017 to enroll the first patients [38]. Though the trial is designed to support patients as small as 8 kg, expectations are that the device could safely extend into the most vulnerable of pediatric patients weighing <5 kg. In addition to the benefit of the novel device design in the trial, PumpKIN will provide a standardization of anticoagulation management in both the Berlin as well as the Jarvik cohorts.

Device design benefiting small pediatric patients has been a focus of federal funding; however, devices designed to support the many anatomic variations seen in pediatric and adult CHD remain a smaller scale endeavor. Of specific interest has been the development of a Fontan Assist Device designed to support the failed cavopulmonary circulation in palliated single ventricle physiology. To date, this field has remained more theoretic than clinical with the majority of successes occurring in computational modeling and early device design [39–42]. Some centers, alternatively, have elected to manage these "end-stage Fontan" patients with the use of Total Artificial Heart (TAH) VAD support [43]. Though the feasibility of such an undertaking is clear, the outcomes for such patients are certainly clouded. As reported by Vanderpluym et al. in their analysis of the INTERMACS registry, the subgroup of adult congenital heart disease (ACHD) patients requiring biventricular or TAH support had significantly worse survival than both ACHD and non-ACHD patients supported with a systemic VAD or LVAD alone. Whether or not Fontan assist devices will become the eventual "fourth stage" of univentricular palliation is unclear [44]. What is clear, however, is that the need for donor organs in this growing population will far surpass the available supply in the near future.

As device support and management strategies have led to increasingly positive clinical outcomes, pediatric VAD support is poised to enter a new age where bridge to recovery and even destination therapy (DT) become a distinct reality. Historically, myocardial recovery with VAD support and subsequent device explant in pediatrics has been relegated to case reports. However, recent evidence as shown by Weia et al. has begun to define the molecular changes that occur in the unloaded pediatric heart and may promote reverse of pathologic remodeling [45]. Though the relatively small volume of pediatric supported patients across the county has allowed for only preliminary assessment of these molecular pathways, the theoretical regenerative capacity of the pediatric heart provides the perfect substrate for use of molecular study to predict or even induce recovery.

Though recovery or heart transplantation is not a possibility for all patients, certain subgroups in pediatrics may benefit from mechanical support focused primarily on improved length and quality of life. DT in pediatric heart failure has not yet become standard practice; however, experiences in patient populations such as muscular dystrophy with end-stage heart disease have served as an initial exposure [46–48]. Additional populations that represent ideal candidates for DT include patients with end-stage heart disease related to on-going oncologic therapies or severe systemic disease that pose risk to a potential donor heart. Prior to the acceptance and increased use of DT in children, pediatric heart failure physicians will inevitably have to undergo a culture shift. Definitions of "successful VAD support" will require reassessment and revision with a transition of goals from improved waitlist survival to improved quality of life.

CONCLUSION

Pediatric VAD therapy has grown with the rising numbers of pediatric heart failure patients, and it has revolutionized the care of pediatric end-stage heart disease. From its historic foundation in the Berlin Heart to its potential future in the Jarvik 2015, VAD therapy has led to improved patient outcomes despite the many challenges intrinsic to supporting pediatric patients. With the next era of VAD therapy on the horizon, be it Fontan assist devices, device-promoted cardiac recovery, or DT; the face of pediatric heart failure management will undoubtedly change with improving quantity, quality, and support for patients.

REFERENCES

[1] M.E. DeBakey, Left ventricular bypass pump for cardiac assistance. Clinical experience, Am. J. Cardiol. 27 (1) (1971) 3–11.

[2] E.J. Benjamin, et al., Heart disease and stroke statistics-2017 update: a report from the American Heart Association, Circulation 135 (10) (2017) e146–e603.

[3] E.A. Rose, et al., Long-term use of a left ventricular assist device for end-stage heart failure, N. Engl. J. Med. 345 (20) (2001) 1435–1443.

[4] M.S. Slaughter, et al., Advanced heart failure treated with continuous-flow left ventricular assist device, N. Engl. J. Med. 361 (23) (2009) 2241–2251.

[5] M.R. Mehra, et al., A fully magnetically levitated circulatory pump for advanced heart failure, N. Engl. J. Med. 376 (5) (2017) 440–450.

[6] J.G. Rogers, et al., Intrapericardial left ventricular assist device for advanced heart failure, N. Engl. J. Med. 376 (5) (2017) 451–460.

[7] W.L. Holman, Interagency registry for mechanically assisted circulatory support (INTERMACS): what have we learned and what will we learn? Circulation 126 (11) (2012) 1401–1406.

[8] J.K. Kirklin, et al., INTERMACS database for durable devices for circulatory support: first annual report, J. Heart Lung Transplant. 27 (10) (2008) 1065–1072.

[9] J.K. Kirklin, et al., Seventh INTERMACS annual report: 15,000 patients and counting, J. Heart Lung Transplant. 34 (12) (2015) 1495–1504.

[10] D.T. Hsu, G.D. Pearson, Heart failure in children: part I: history, etiology, and pathophysiology, Circ. Heart Fail. 2 (1) (2009) 63–70.

[11] J.W. Rossano, et al., The registry of the International Society for heart and lung transplantation: nineteenth pediatric heart transplantation report-2016; focus theme: primary diagnostic indications for transplant, J. Heart Lung Transplant. 35 (10) (2016) 1185–1195.

[12] C.S. Almond, et al., Extracorporeal membrane oxygenation for bridge to heart transplantation among children in the United States: analysis of data from the organ procurement and transplant network and extracorporeal life support organization registry, Circulation 123 (25) (2011) 2975–2984.

[13] A.I. Dipchand, et al., Extracorporeal membrane oxygenation as a bridge to pediatric heart transplantation: effect on post-listing and post-transplantation outcomes, Circ. Heart Fail. 8 (5) (2015) 960–969.

[14] O.H. Frazier, et al., Use of a left ventricular assist device as a bridge to transplantation in a pediatric patient, Tex. Heart Inst. J. 16 (1) (1989) 46–50.

[15] B. Stiller, et al., Heart transplantation in children after mechanical circulatory support with pulsatile pneumatic assist device, J. Heart Lung Transplant. 22 (11) (2003) 1201–1208.

[16] F.A. Arabia, et al., Pediatric bridge to heart transplantation: application of the Berlin Heart, Medos and Thoratec ventricular assist devices, J. Heart Lung Transplant. 25 (1) (2006) 16–21.

[17] R. Hetzer, et al., Improvement in survival after mechanical circulatory support with pneumatic pulsatile ventricular assist devices in pediatric patients, Ann. Thorac. Surg. 82 (3) (2006) 917–924, discussion 924–925.

[18] E.D. Blume, et al., Outcomes of children bridged to heart transplantation with ventricular assist devices: a multi-institutional study, Circulation 113 (19) (2006) 2313–2319.

[19] C.D. Fraser Jr., et al., Prospective trial of a pediatric ventricular assist device, N. Engl. J. Med. 367 (6) (2012) 532–541.

[20] O. Miera, et al., First experiences with the HeartWare ventricular assist system in children, Ann. Thorac. Surg. 91 (4) (2011) 1256–1260.

[21] E.D. Blume, et al., Outcomes of children implanted with ventricular assist devices in the United States: first analysis of the pediatric interagency registry for mechanical circulatory support (PediMACS), J. Heart Lung Transplant. 35 (5) (2016) 578–584.

[22] D.N. Rosenthal, et al., Adverse events in children implanted with ventricular assist devices in the United States: data from the pediatric interagency registry for mechanical circulatory support (PediMACS), J. Heart Lung Transplant. 35 (5) (2016) 569–577.

[23] J.W. Rossano, et al., Outcomes of pediatric patients supported with continuous-flow ventricular assist devices: a report from the pediatric interagency registry for mechanical circulatory support (PediMACS), J. Heart Lung Transplant. 35 (5) (2016) 585–590.

[24] J. Riebandt, et al., Preoperative patient optimization using extracorporeal life support improves outcomes of INTERMACS Level I patients receiving a permanent ventricular assist device, Eur. J. Cardiothorac. Surg. 46 (3) (2014) 486–492, discussion 492.

[25] P. Massicotte, et al., Ventricular assist device thrombosis: mind your P's &Q's-Pumps, patients, and pills, J. Thorac. Cardiovasc. Surg. 153 (6) (2017) 1503–1506.

[26] E.J. Favaloro, G. Lippi, Translational aspects of developmental hemostasis: infants and children are not miniature adults and even adults may be different, Ann. Transl. Med. 5 (10) (2017) 212.

[27] X. Yu, et al., The profile of the systemic inflammatory response in children undergoing ventricular assist device support, Interact. Cardiovasc. Thorac. Surg. 15 (3) (2012) 426–431.

[28] J.W. Byrnes, et al., Steroid therapy attenuates acute phase reactant response among children on ventricular assist device support, Ann. Thorac. Surg. 99 (4) (2015) 1392–1398.

[29] S.M. Gilboa, et al., Congenital heart defects in the United States: estimating the magnitude of the affected population in 2010, Circulation 134 (2) (2016) 101–109.

[30] S. Weinstein, et al., The use of the Berlin Heart EXCOR in patients with functional single ventricle, J. Thorac. Cardiovasc. Surg. 147 (2) (2014) 697–704, discussion 704–705.

[31] D.L. Morales, et al., Berlin Heart EXCOR use in patients with congenital heart disease, J. Heart Lung Transplant. (February 8, 2017) pii:S1053-2498(17)31350-5.

[32] M.C. Monge, et al., Successful bridge-to-transplant of functionally univentricular patients with a modified continuous-flow ventricular assist device, Artif. Organs 41 (1) (2017) 25–31.

[33] B.R. Imielski, et al., HeartWare ventricular assist device implantation in patients with Fontan physiology, Artif. Organs 41 (1) (2017) 40–46.

[34] C.J. VanderPluym, et al., Outcomes following implantation of mechanical circulatory support in adults with congenital heart disease: an analysis of the Interagency Registry for Mechanically Assisted Circulatory Support (INTERMACS), J. Heart Lung Transplant. (March 7, 2017). pii:S1053–2498(17)31682-0.

[35] J. Conway, et al., Delineating survival outcomes in children <10 kg bridged to transplant or recovery with the Berlin Heart EXCOR ventricular assist device, JACC Heart Fail. 3 (1) (2015) 70–77.

[36] T.K. B, et al., Modified TandemHeart ventricular assist device for infant and pediatric circulatory support, Ann. Thorac. Surg. 98 (4) (2014) 1437–1441.

[37] J.T. Baldwin, et al., The national heart, lung, and blood institute pediatric circulatory support program: a summary of the 5-year experience, Circulation 123 (11) (2011) 1233–1240.

[38] J.T. Baldwin, et al., Closing in on the PumpKIN trial of the Jarvik 2015 ventricular assist device, Semin. Thorac. Cardiovasc. Surg. Pediatr. Card Surg. Annu. 20 (2017) 9–15.

[39] J.L. Bruse, et al., Statistical shape modeling for cavopulmonary assist device development: variability of vascular graft geometry and implications for hemodynamics, J. Med. Device 11 (2) (2017).

[40] P.L. Hsu, et al., A numerical simulation comparing a cavopulmonary assist device and VA ECMO for failing Fontan support, ASAIO J. 63 (5) (September/October 2017) 604–612.

[41] M. Tree, et al., In vitro examination of the HeartWare CircuLite ventricular assist device in the Fontan connection, ASAIO J. 63 (4) (2017) 482–489.

[42] S. Shimizu, et al., Partial cavopulmonary assist from the inferior vena cava to the pulmonary artery improves hemodynamics in failing Fontan circulation: a theoretical analysis, J. Physiol. Sci. 66 (3) (2016) 249–255.

[43] J.W. Rossano, et al., Successful use of the total artificial heart in the failing Fontan circulation, Ann. Thorac. Surg. 97 (4) (2014) 1438–1440.

[44] R.D. Jaquiss, H. Aziz, Is four stage management the future of univentricular hearts? Destination therapy in the young, Semin. Thorac. Cardiovasc. Surg. Pediatr. Card Surg. Annu. 19 (1) (2016) 50–54.

[45] B.C. Weia, I. Adachi, J.G. Jacot, Clinical and molecular comparison of pediatric and adult reverse remodeling with ventricular assist devices, Artif. Organs 39 (8) (2015) 691–700.

[46] G. Perri, et al., Left ventricular assist device as destination therapy in cardiac end-stage dystrophinopathies: midterm results, J. Thorac. Cardiovasc. Surg. 153 (3) (2017) 669–674.

[47] N.J. Purkey, et al., Long-term pediatric ventricular assist device therapy: a case report of 2100+ days of support, ASAIO J. (February 9, 2017) (Epub ahead of print).

[48] T.D. Ryan, et al., Implantation of the HeartMate II and HeartWare left ventricular assist devices in patients with duchenne muscular dystrophy: lessons learned from the first applications, ASAIO J. 60 (2) (2014) 246–248.

Section V

Special Topics

Chapter 56

Genetic Testing

Ana Morales[1,2], Ray Hershberger[1,2]

[1]*Internal Medicine, Division of Human Genetics, Columbus, OH, United States;* [2]*Wexner Medical Center at the Ohio State University, Columbus, OH, United States*

INTRODUCTION

The genetic cardiomyopathies, hypertrophic cardiomyopathy (HCM), dilated cardiomyopathy (DCM), restrictive cardiomyopathy (RCM), or arrhythmogenic cardiomyopathy (ARVC) can be identified in children and may present with heart failure, arrhythmia, or embolus, depending on the contractile or electrophysiological derangements that bring the patient to medical attention. Left ventricular noncompaction (LVNC) can also be identified in concert with any of these phenotypes, as well as in some isolated cases. We refer the reader to specific chapters for the diagnosis, prognosis, and treatment interventions needed for each of these conditions.

A genetic basis may be present in the form of isolated, nonsyndromic disease, or as an inborn error of metabolism, a multisystem syndrome, or neuromuscular disease [1]. Therefore, suspicion of a genetic etiology should be a priority.

Pediatric and early onset left ventricular dilatation accompanied by systolic dysfunction is usually genetic, in contrast to the same phenotype in the older adults among whom coronary artery disease becomes commonplace. Similarly, while adult-onset RCM includes a myriad of causes, e.g., amyloidosis, hypertensive heart disease, and aortic stenosis, pediatric RCM is rare outside of a genetic paradigm. Left ventricular hypertrophy, the hallmark of HCM, can be confounded in adolescents and adults with severe uncontrolled hypertension or as an adaptation to athletic training, and in infants, as the result maternal diabetes exposure [2]. These confounding factors, however, are usually negligible in pediatric HCM cases. ARVC, on the other hand, is considered primarily a genetic condition in both adult and pediatric populations. Preliminary studies in LVNC have identified a genetic overlap with DCM, HCM, and RCM. The approach to a genetic evaluation in these conditions should include a greater degree of sensitivity to detection of multisystem, syndromic disease [3]. An evaluation by a medical geneticist with expertise in dysmorphology, as well as in metabolic screening and interpretation of biochemical findings, is recommended.

Genetics

Most nonsyndromic cardiomyopathies show an autosomal dominant pattern of inheritance. In autosomal dominant inheritance, first-degree relatives of affected individuals have a 50% probability of having the condition, however, reduced penetrance (some family members who carry a pathogenic variant, but escape the condition) and variable expressivity (different degrees of severity among affected individuals) can complicate risk assessment. Locus heterogeneity (many possible genes giving rise to the same condition in different individuals) and allelic heterogeneity (most variants are private to individual families) are also common features of genetic cardiomyopathy. The cardiomyopathies may also be inherited in autosomal recessive (most likely pattern in metabolic disease, with a recurrence risk of 25%), X-linked, and mitochondrial transmission. Regardless of the inheritance pattern, first-degree relatives are at increased risk and thus guidelines recommend periodic cardiovascular screening for them [4].

Genetic Testing

After a thorough clinical evaluation with attention to dysmorphic features, developmental history, and neuromuscular disease, genetic testing (which can identify the cause of familial conditions or those suspected to be heritable) should be considered (Fig. 56.1). In the pediatric population, knowing a specific genetic etiology can provide opportunity for dietary modification (when a metabolic disorder is present) and other forms of clinical intervention to address complications, such as intellectual disability, often present in syndromic disease [3]. Enzyme replacement therapy may also be initiated for patients found to have cardiomyopathy resulting from the biochemical conditions Pompe and Fabry disease. For metabolic

Heart Failure in the Child and Young Adult. http://dx.doi.org/10.1016/B978-0-12-802393-8.00056-9

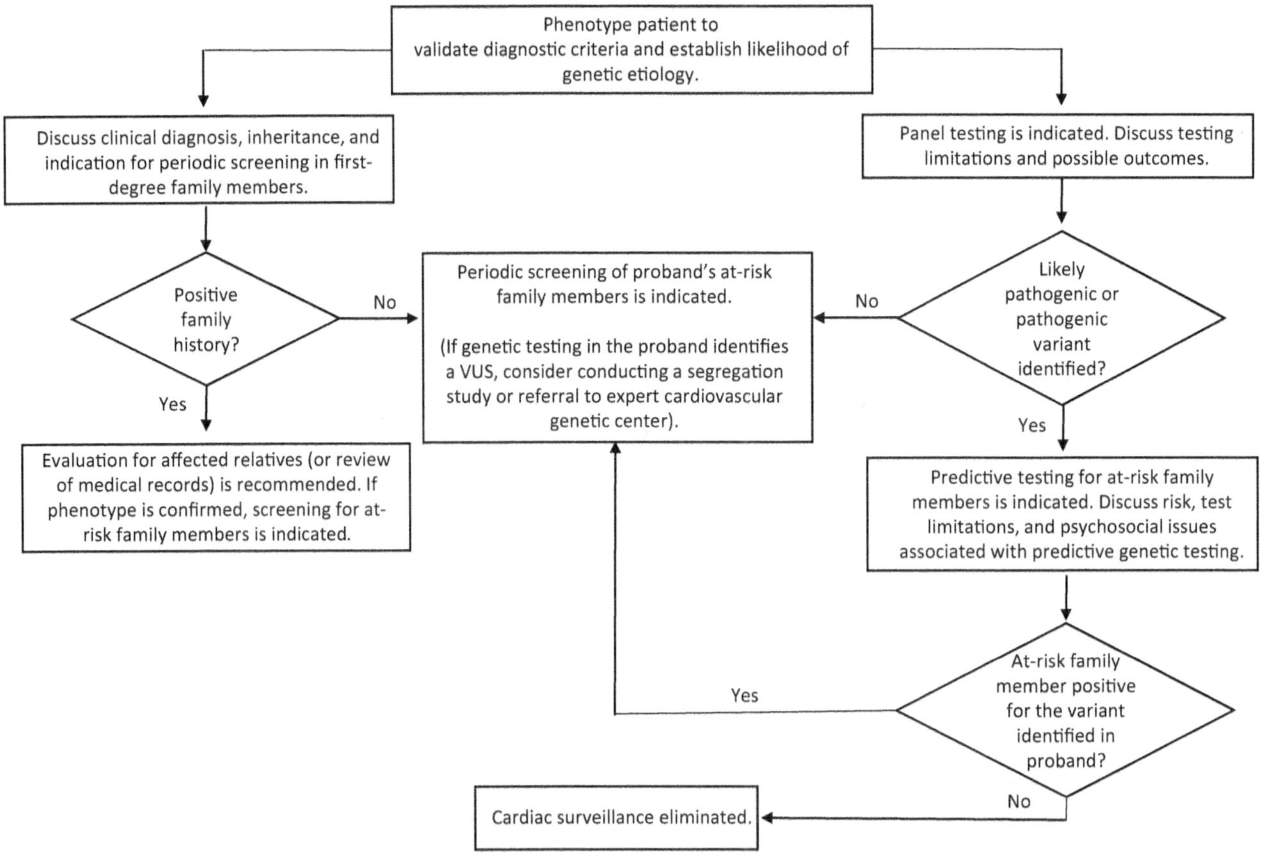

FIGURE 56.1 Flow diagram of genetic testing within the context of a genetic evaluation.

disorders that are diagnosed using biochemical screening, knowledge of the specific molecular variant can help to confirm the diagnosis. Genetic testing can also help to identify who, among all at-risk family members, have inherited the variant(s) for which they are at risk.

While many of the metabolic conditions causing cardiomyopathy are identified by newborn screening [5], next-generation sequencing, which allows testing of a large number of genes at the same time, provides a rapid and effective approach to identify the genetic cause in most other forms of cardiomyopathy. This approach that consists of massive parallel sequencing of DNA fragments makes it possible to assess missense, truncating, and insertion/deletion variants in dozens of genes in a single run. Customized panels can also be built to combine genes associated with a variety of suspected diagnoses. Testing for deletions and duplications, which may rarely be present in genetic cardiomyopathy, is also normally included in the cardiomyopathy panels in the form of multiplex ligation-dependent probe amplification or microarray [3]. Clinical exome sequencing that provides sequencing data from all coding genes may also be considered for mixed or complex phenotypes. A customized panel may also be built on an exome sequencing backbone for future inquiry in genetically inconclusive cases. While next generation sequencing has limitations, such not being able to detect triplet repeat expansions (e.g., involved in Friedrich ataxia), it is of tremendous value to the genetic evaluation of nonsyndromic cardiomyopathy, as it can even identify previously undetected metabolic disease in subclinical cases.

Variant Interpretation

Large reference cohorts, such as the National Heart, Lung, and Blood Institute's Exome Sequencing Project, and the Exome Aggregation Consortium, have brought to light the need for a critical view of the variants identified by genetic testing. This is in large part due to reduced penetrance and the fact that a nonnegligible number of presumably unaffected individuals in these cohorts (who have not been phenotyped to exclude cardiovascular disease) have been found to carry variants in clinically relevant genes. According to the American College of Medical Genetics (ACMG), variants may be classified as pathogenic, likely pathogenic, variant of unknown significance (VUS), likely benign, or benign based on strong, moderate, and supporting criteria [6]. These criteria include, among others, presence of a truncating variant, rare allele frequency, segregation of the variant with disease, de novo origin (when neither unaffected parent carries a variant identified in their affected child), as well as functional data and computational evidence proving a role in disease. These ACMG standards are meant to serve as a baseline guiding variant interpretation. Cardiovascular expertise is therefore key when interpreting variants relevant to cardiomyopathy. For example, the presence of a truncating variant is considered strong criteria for pathogenicity in the baseline standards, however, truncating variants have not been demonstrated to be relevant in MYH7, a gene reported with HCM, DCM, RCM, and LVNC. Similarly, truncating variants in TTN have been reported in from 8% to 20% of DCM; however, truncating variants in this gene are also present in 3% of reference DNA samples. Additional data, including family segregation and titin protein domain location [7], have been applied in an effort to discern the clinical impact of TTN variants. Clinical expertise is also important to assess family history information to select the best testing strategy and to critically evaluate and interpret clinical data related to a variant identified in a patient. Relative to variants causing syndromic disease, sorting variants in isolated, nonsyndromic cardiomyopathy, which is often age-dependent with reduced penetrance, is more difficult. Ultimately, judgment about a variant's role in disease lies with the clinician and may include well-justified factors not documented in sequence interpretation standards.

Genetic Testing Management

Because more than one causative genetic variant may be identified in individuals with cardiomyopathy, it is recommended that genetic testing begins with the most severely affected family member with the earliest age of onset [3]. If a pathogenic variant is identified in the proband, at-risk family members can pursue genetic testing for the variant. Only those testing positive should undergo cardiovascular screening at intervals [4]. The goal of screening for at-risk individuals is to initiate medical therapy at the earliest sign of disease, with the hope to prevent progression to advanced disease. On the other hand, at-risk family members who are found not to carry the disease-causing variant can be discharged from surveillance.

Not all genes causing cardiomyopathy and associated phenotypes have been identified. For isolated cardiomyopathy, the detection rate of genetic testing panels for cardiomyopathy ranges from 40% to 70%. As a consequence, if a pathogenic or likely pathogenic variant is not identified in the proband, a genetic cause cannot be ruled out. Furthermore, VUS, likely benign, and benign results cannot be used for predictive testing in a healthy, at-risk family member. Likely pathogenic variants may be used for predictive testing, as long as the patient undergoing predictive testing understands that there is a small residual risk for disease should they test negative. These individuals should be alert to and report heart disease symptoms immediately. As more genes are discovered or variants get reclassified, new testing options may become available to the family. Notably, at-risk relatives of these individuals remain at risk and periodic screening is indicated.

GENETIC TESTING FOR CARDIOMYOPATHY

Dilated Cardiomyopathy

DCM is the most common cardiomyopathy with an estimated prevalence of >1/500 [8]. Up to 50% of cases are familial and variants in approximately 40 genes of have been identified in approximately 40%, primarily represented in research cohorts by adults. In the pediatric population, DCM is the most common indication for heart transplantation [9,10], and it has been reported in 0.34–3.8 cases per 100,000 per year [11–13]. Fetal and neonatal cases have also been reported. A wide range of causation should be considered in pediatric DCM, including metabolic and syndromic disease, such as Alstrom syndrome [1] and the X-linked disorders Duchenne muscular dystrophy, Barth syndrome, and Danon disease (the latter can represent progression and variability of HCM [3]). Other neuromuscular disorders, including Emery–Dreifuss muscular dystrophy and limb-girdle muscular dystrophy, may be involved. Isolated pediatric DCM can also involve genes normally involved in adult-onset cases. A series of isolated DCM cases in which the proband was of pediatric age [13] identified 15 of 41 pediatric DCM cases with variants in 9 genes. Sarcomeric genes were most commonly represented, with TPM1 and TNNT2 on the lead. The study also found that 35 of the 41 cases had relatives with adult-onset DCM, highlighting the phenotypic variability that can be present within families. Multiple variants were reported in three cases.

Hypertrophic Cardiomyopathy

HCM has an overall prevalence of 1/500, but the incidence in children has been reported to be 4.7 per 1 million children, or 1/200,000 [3,14]. HCM in childhood can be isolated or a feature of a genetic syndrome, including, most commonly, Noonan syndrome, followed by Pompe disease, and Friedrich ataxia [3,14]. A higher rate of heart failure has been reported in HCM caused by metabolic disease [14]. While onset of isolated HCM usually occurs in puberty (with early childhood and late onset cases also reported), most syndromic HCM presents in childhood. Progression to DCM has also been observed in HCM, for example, in cases of Friedrich ataxia [1]. Presentation with DCM has also been observed in carrier mothers of patients with HCM due to Danon disease (caused by LAMP2 variants). Variants in the PRKAG2 gene have been reported with infant-onset HCM and arrhythmia. Genetic testing in isolated HCM patients has identified over 20 genes accounting for 40%–70% of cases with predominant sarcomeric disease [3]. Genetic testing panels include both sarcomeric and some of the syndromic genes, including Noonan syndrome, Fabry, and Danon disease. Compound and digenic variants, which have also been identified in 5% of cases, are associated with early onset, severe disease and the presence of multiple variants [15].

A study that assessed sarcomeric variants as well as variants in LAMP2 and PRKAG2 in 84 pediatric HCM cases (33 familial, 51 nonfamilial) identified variants in 46 (55%) cases [16]. Except for PRKAG2, found in one sporadic case, all other identified variants were sarcomeric. The most represented genes were MYBPC3 and MYH7. These findings support a similar genetic basis between pediatric and HCM not ascertained for pediatric onset.

Restrictive Cardiomyopathy

RCM is a rare cardiomyopathy. Familial disease has been reported in 30% [17]. In children, RCM is rare, accounting for up to 5% of all pediatric cardiomyopathy cases [18,19]. A genetic basis is known, with overlap with DCM and HCM, and may rarely include inborn errors of metabolism [17]. The restrictive physiology characteristic of RCM can be observed in HCM, DCM and LVNC, and RCM families can display a variety of phenotypes in different relatives [17]. It is estimated that one third of patients with pediatric RCM will show a mixed RCM/DCM phenotype while RCM/DCM and RCM/LVNC combinations are less common [3]. It is thus not surprising that variants in HCM and DCM genes have been identified in 30%–50% of RCM.

Arrhythmogenic Right Ventricular Cardiomyopathy

ARVC is predominantly a cardiomyopathy identified in adults with a reported prevalence ranging from 6/10,000 to 1/1000 [20,21], and more recently estimated to be 1/2000 [22]. Onset usually occurs by young adulthood, but childhood onset is rare [1]. Approximately 50% of cases are familial. ARVC mainly results from variants in five desmosomal genes. Rarely, variants in two nondesmosomal genes (TMEM43; a nuclear envelope protein, and RYR2; a calcium channel) are involved. These seven genes account for 40%–50% of cases. Compound and digenic inheritance has been observed in 20%. Finding a pathogenic variant constitutes major diagnostic criteria [23]. Positive predictive genetic testing in an unaffected individual can not only inform need for periodic screening, but it can also inform decision-making regarding exercise restrictions [3].

Left Ventricular Noncompaction

LVNC has an estimated prevalence of 1/7000. Familial disease, found in up to 60% of cases, is more likely when the proband is of pediatric age [3]. The morphological, and, hence, the genetic basis of LVNC, is generally not well understood, but a sarcomeric basis has been reported [24]. It is estimated that a genetic cause can be identified in 20% of cases, and particularly with a phenotypic overlap with DCM and HCM [14]. Variants in TAZ, responsible for Barth syndrome, have been identified. Similarly, LVNC with atrial septal defect has been reported with NKX2-5 [25]. One report suggested an association between Ebstein's anomaly and LVNC with variants in MYH7 [26]. While more research is necessary to confirm these findings, the association with congenital heart defects may be well founded in the setting of LVNC itself being a disorder of cardiac development with relevance to the pediatric population.

GENETIC COUNSELING

Genetic counseling is central to the process of genetic testing. It involves interpretation of family and medical history as well as education of patients and their families about the risk, management, and prevention of disease. The process that relies on patient-centered decision-making also promotes helping individuals to adapt to genetic disease and risk (www.nsgc.org). In the cardiovascular genetics setting, genetic counseling specifically involves a targeted three-generation family history [27] and providing information about screening recommendations while supporting the process of communicating risk to relatives. Cardiovascular genetic counseling also requires expertise in consenting individuals for the possibility of complex results, VUSs, and variant reclassification. Genetic counseling also involves identifying indication for family cosegregation studies once a result is reported by the laboratory. These family studies, which are performed with the goal of strengthening the data associated with a VUS, consist of obtaining extended family history information, medical records, death certificates, as well as cardiovascular and genotyping data from informative relatives.

In families with early onset disease, predictive testing is recommended for at-risk children. In families with aggressive disease, a more frequent screening approach may be considered. Genetic counseling involving predictive testing for minors should explore concerns about negation of autonomy, stigmatization, and adverse family dynamics. In their position statement about genetic testing for minors, the National Society of Genetic Counselors encourages deferring genetic testing for minors when medical management does not immediately impact care (www.nsgc.org). The American Academy of Pediatrics supports this view and adds that predictive genetic testing may be performed for a child in the setting of no clinical impact in the near term, when the uncertainty about the diagnosis interferes with psychosocial well-being and both parent and child are in agreement with testing [28]. The ACMG and Genomics position statement concurs with these views [29]. Clearly, the benefit of early treatment for cardiomyopathy in these cases outweighs any potential risks.

Some patients have raised concerns about genetic information privacy and potential discrimination. For example, testing has been declined based on fear of adverse employment and insurance decisions when genetic testing is likely to identify risk for extracardiac disease in an individual with cardiomyopathy or when an unaffected person is found to carry a predisposing variant. Discussion of the protections provided by the Genetic Information Non-Discrimination Act (GINA), which is meant to protect individuals from discrimination based on family history or genetic testing results, is recommended. The limitations of GINA should also be discussed, including lack of protection against discrimination for individuals seeking life insurance or for those working in companies smaller than 15 employees.

Genetic testing for cardiomyopathy in children and the young has demonstrated clinical utility. Along with genetic counseling, a cardiovascular genetic evaluation is best performed in the setting of a multidisciplinary team represented by cardiology, medical, and molecular genetics. This approach can lead to high-quality patient outcomes.

REFERENCES

[1] S.M. Ware, Evaluation of genetic causes of cardiomyopathy in childhood, Cardiol. Young 25 (Suppl. 2) (August 2015) 43–50 Research Support, Non-U.S. Gov't.

[2] J.P. Moak, J.P. Kaski, Hypertrophic cardiomyopathy in children, Heart 98 (14) (July 2012) 1044–1054 Review.

[3] M. Russell, A. Roberts, D.J. Abrams, A.M. Murphy, J.A. Towbin, W.K. Chung, How to effectively utilize genetic testing in the care of children with cardiomyopathies, Prog. Pediatr. Cardiol. 39 (2015) 3–11.

[4] R.E. Hershberger, J. Lindenfeld, L. Mestroni, C.E. Seidman, M.R. Taylor, J.A. Towbin, Genetic evaluation of cardiomyopathy–a Heart Failure Society of America practice guideline, J. Card. Fail. 15 (2) (March 2009) 83–97 Practice Guideline.

[5] Newborn screening: toward a uniform screening panel and system, Genet. Med. 8 (Suppl. 1) (May 2006) 1S–252S Guideline.

[6] S. Richards, N. Aziz, S. Bale, D. Bick, S. Das, J. Gastier-Foster, et al., Standards and guidelines for the interpretation of sequence variants: a joint consensus recommendation of the American College of Medical Genetics and Genomics and the Association for Molecular Pathology, Genet. Med. 17 (5) (May 2015) 405–424 Research Support, N.I.H., Extramural.

[7] A.M. Roberts, J.S. Ware, D.S. Herman, S. Schafer, J. Baksi, A.G. Bick, et al., Integrated allelic, transcriptional, and phenomic dissection of the cardiac effects of titin truncations in health and disease, Sci. Transl. Med. 7 (270) (January 14, 2015) 270ra6 Research Support, N.I.H., Extramural Research Support, Non-U.S. Gov't.

[8] R.E. Hershberger, D.J. Hedges, A. Morales, Dilated cardiomyopathy: the complexity of a diverse genetic architecture, Nat. Rev. Cardiol. 10 (9) (September 2013) 531–547 Research Support, N.I.H., Extramural Review.

[9] D. Mozaffarian, E.J. Benjamin, A.S. Go, D.K. Arnett, M.J. Blaha, M. Cushman, et al., Heart disease and stroke statistics–2015 update: a report from the American Heart Association, Circulation 131 (4) (January 27, 2015) e29–322.

[10] A. Morales, R.E. Hershberger, The rationale and timing of molecular genetic testing for dilated cardiomyopathy, Can. J. Cardiol. 31 (11) (November 2015) 1309–1312.

[11] A. Arola, E. Jokinen, O. Ruuskanen, M. Saraste, E. Pesonen, A.L. Kuusela, et al., Epidemiology of idiopathic cardiomyopathies in children and adolescents. A nationwide study in Finland, Am. J. Epidemiol. 146 (5) (September 1, 1997) 385–393 Research Support, Non-U.S. Gov't.

[12] J.A. Towbin, A.M. Lowe, S.D. Colan, L.A. Sleeper, E.J. Orav, S. Clunie, et al., Incidence, causes, and outcomes of dilated cardiomyopathy in children, JAMA 296 (15) (October 18, 2006) 1867–1876 Multicenter Study Research Support, N.I.H., Extramural Research Support, Non-U.S. Gov't.

[13] E. Rampersaud, J.D. Siegfried, N. Norton, D. Li, E. Martin, R.E. Hershberger, Rare variant mutations identified in pediatric patients with dilated cardiomyopathy, Prog. Pediatr. Cardiol. 31 (1) (January 1, 2011) 39–47.

[14] S.D. Colan, S.E. Lipshultz, A.M. Lowe, L.A. Sleeper, J. Messere, G.F. Cox, et al., Epidemiology and cause-specific outcome of hypertrophic cardiomyopathy in children: findings from the pediatric cardiomyopathy registry, Circulation 115 (6) (February 13, 2007) 773–781 Research Support, N.I.H., Extramural Research Support, Non-U.S. Gov't.

[15] M. Kelly, C. Semsarian, Multiple mutations in genetic cardiovascular disease: a marker of disease severity? Circ. Cardiovasc. Genet. 2 (2) (April 2009) 182–190 Review.

[16] H. Morita, H.L. Rehm, A. Menesses, B. McDonough, A.E. Roberts, R. Kucherlapati, et al., Shared genetic causes of cardiac hypertrophy in children and adults, N. Engl. J. Med. 358 (18) (May 1, 2008) 1899–1908 Research Support, N.I.H., Extramural Research Support, Non-U.S. Gov't.

[17] J.P. Kaski, P. Syrris, M. Burch, M.T. Tome-Esteban, M. Fenton, M. Christiansen, et al., Idiopathic restrictive cardiomyopathy in children is caused by mutations in cardiac sarcomere protein genes, Heart 94 (11) (November 2008) 1478–1484 Research Support, Non-U.S. Gov't.
[18] A.W. Nugent, P.E. Daubeney, P. Chondros, J.B. Carlin, M. Cheung, L.C. Wilkinson, et al., The epidemiology of childhood cardiomyopathy in Australia, N. Engl. J. Med. 348 (17) (April 24, 2003) 1639–1646 Research Support, Non-U.S. Gov't.
[19] S.W. Denfield, G. Rosenthal, R.J. Gajarski, J.T. Bricker, K.O. Schowengerdt, J.K. Price, et al., Restrictive cardiomyopathies in childhood. Etiologies and natural history, Tex. Heart Inst. J. 24 (1) (1997) 38–44.
[20] A. Rampazzo, A. Nava, G.A. Danieli, G. Buja, L. Daliento, G. Fasoli, et al., The gene for arrhythmogenic right ventricular cardiomyopathy maps to chromosome 14q23-q24, Hum. Mol. Genet. 3 (6) (June 1994) 959–962 Research Support, Non-U.S. Gov't.
[21] S. Peters, M. Trummel, W. Meyners, Prevalence of right ventricular dysplasia-cardiomyopathy in a non-referral hospital, Int. J. Cardiol. 97 (3) (December 2004) 499–501.
[22] J.A. Towbin, Inherited cardiomyopathies, Circ. J. 78 (10) (2014) 2347–2356 Review.
[23] F.I. Marcus, W.J. McKenna, D. Sherrill, C. Basso, B. Bauce, D.A. Bluemke, et al., Diagnosis of arrhythmogenic right ventricular cardiomyopathy/dysplasia: proposed modification of the task force criteria, Circulation 121 (13) (April 6, 2010) 1533–1541 Clinical Trial Research Support, N.I.H., Extramural Research Support, Non-U.S. Gov't.
[24] L.M. Dellefave, P. Pytel, S. Mewborn, B. Mora, D.L. Guris, S. Fedson, et al., Sarcomere mutations in cardiomyopathy with left ventricular hypertrabeculation, Circ. Cardiovasc. Genet. 2 (5) (October 2009) 442–449 Clinical Trial Research Support, Non-U.S. Gov't.
[25] P. Ouyang, E. Saarel, Y. Bai, C. Luo, Q. Lv, Y. Xu, et al., A de novo mutation in NKX2.5 associated with atrial septal defects, ventricular noncompaction, syncope and sudden death, Clin. Chim. Acta 412 (1–2) (January 14, 2011) 170–175 Research Support, N.I.H., Extramural Research Support, Non-U.S. Gov't Research Support, U.S. Gov't, Non-P.H.S.
[26] A.V. Postma, K. van Engelen, J. van de Meerakker, T. Rahman, S. Probst, M.J. Baars, et al., Mutations in the sarcomere gene MYH7 in Ebstein anomaly, Circ. Cardiovasc. Genet. 4 (1) (February 2011) 43–50 Research Support, Non-U.S. Gov't.
[27] A. Morales, J. Cowan, J. Dagua, R.E. Hershberger, Family history: an essential tool for cardiovascular genetic medicine, Congest. Heart Fail. 14 (1) (January–February 2008) 37–45 Review.
[28] Ethical and policy issues in genetic testing and screening of children, Pediatrics 131 (3) (March 2013) 620–622.
[29] L.F. Ross, H.M. Saal, K.L. David, R.R. Anderson, Technical report: ethical and policy issues in genetic testing and screening of children, Genet. Med. 15 (3) (March 2013) 234–245.

Chapter 57

Data Management and Analytics

Anthony C. Chang
Children's Hospital of Orange County, Orange, CA, United States

You can have data without information, but you cannot have information without data.

Daniel Keys Moran, science fiction writer/ computer programmer

BIG DATA: AN INTRODUCTION

We are immersed in a sea of data as a result of a proliferation of Internet-enabled communications: texts in books and publications, sensor data from monitors and self-tracking devices, audiovisual data (recordings, pictures, video clips, etc.), social media postings (Internet, Twitter, blogs, etc.), and even global positioning system (GPS) signals. We, as data agents, are presently creating 2.5 quintillion (2.5 × 1018) bytes of data per day, and incredibly, 90% of all current data that are estimated to be at 2 ZB (or 2 trillion GB) were produced only in the last 2 years with most of this data being unstructured. In short, we are "dying of thirst (for information and knowledge) in an ocean of data" [1].

Big data is a recent data paradigm describing not merely the data being so much more voluminous but also the coupling of this massive amount of data with sophisticated data analytics to acquire new knowledge or insight [2]; this phenomenon has taken place in a myriad of sectors such as business [3], finance [4], sports [5], and even the recent presidential election (in which a data scientist Nate Silver handily proved his data analytical methodology to be superior to opinions of many political pundits in predicting the outcome of the election) [6]. Big data is thus a mainstream data movement and knowledge revolution that emphasizes "insight from data is more reliable than intuition from experts" and is on the descending "peak of inflated expectations" limb of the Gartner's hype cycle for emerging technologies with an estimated 5 years to mainstream maturation and adoption (see Fig. 57.1).

In short, the advent of an unprecedented large amount of data coupled with escalation of computer capability and data analytics lead to this data revolution. In simple layman terms, big data has been cleverly described by Yahoo chief Marissa Mayer as "the planet developing a nervous system" [7]. Big data has recently become such a high priority in the national strategic plan that President Obama approved a $200 million Big Data Research and Development Initiative to glean discoveries from digital data.

Big data has important dimensions that all conveniently start with the letter "v" (see Fig. 57.2): (1) volume—recent data volumes are calculated to be in petabytes (1015) and exabytes (1018) and will be in zettabytes (1021) in the near future (highest unit is the yottabyte which is 1024) (see Fig. 57.3). This data include electronic medical records, home monitoring devices, genomic data, insurance claims, drug information, and imaging data (from echocardiograms, angiograms, and MRI/CT); (2) variety—both structured and unstructured data in numerous forms and combinations need to be considered; and (3) velocity—prior batch delivery, data transfer, and analytics now need to be in fractions of seconds and even in real-time especially with imaging transfer of studies in telemedicine. Additional "v"s include: (4) veracity—the accuracy and trustworthiness of big data and its accompanying analytics; and finally (5) value—ascertainment of just how much this data is worth to the institution and the user.

BIOMEDICAL BIG DATA

Current biomedical big data, amassed by electronic medical records and digital image archiving (about 20 megabytes or MB per image), is reaching a staggering 100–250 EB with an annual growth rate of 1.2–2.4 EB [8]. This biomedical big data, however, remains extremely fragmented and disorganized. Our traditional "top-down" data approach up to now entails either (1) health care databases or registries (that involves manual entry of data with its inherent limitations of accuracy and completeness, followed by data analysis with relatively basic statistical tools) or (2) conventional hypothesis-driven research and randomized-controlled trials that have become prohibitively expensive, limited in scope, and often without definitive answers to the clinical questions posited.

Heart Failure in the Child and Young Adult. http://dx.doi.org/10.1016/B978-0-12-802393-8.00057-0

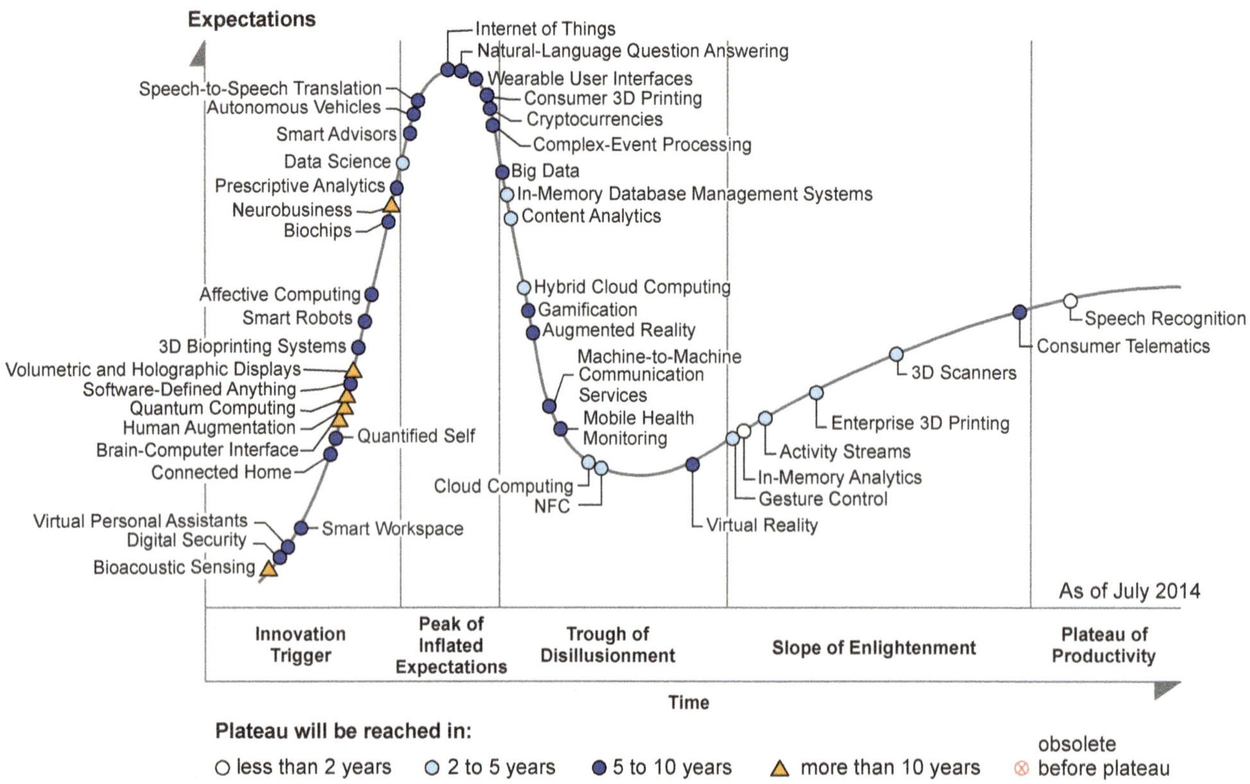

FIGURE 57.1 The hype cycle for emerging technologies, 2014. *(From http://www.mediabuzz.com.sg/asian-emarketing-latest-issue/210-asian-e-marketing/digital-marketing-trends-a-predictions-week-1/2504-gartner-hype-in-2015-around-the-internet-of-things-iot-and-wearables.)*

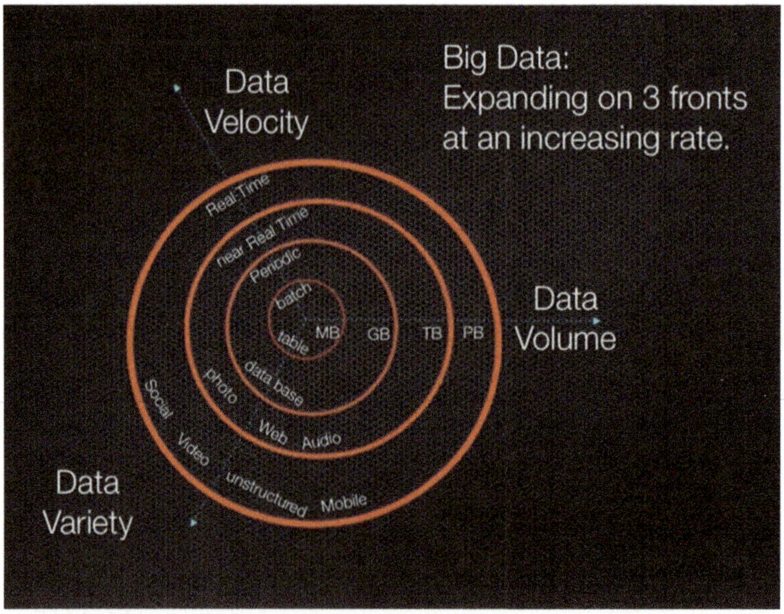

FIGURE 57.2 The "V"s of big data. *(From http://www.datasciencecentral.com/forum/topics/the-3vs-that-define-big-data.)*

Recently, this new big data paradigm has been successfully applied to biomedical science mainly in the form of genomic medicine and its escalating genetic transcript big data [9]. The vast magnitude and rapid acquisition of this genetic big data is absolutely vertiginous, as exemplified by Michael Snyder, a Stanford genetics PhD who has generated 30TB of data of just his own biological data. Despite the daunting challenge, a few have met this challenge and successfully made strides into positive impact on patient care [10,11]. The capstone of this entire data transformation effort in genomic medicine is the ENCyclopedia

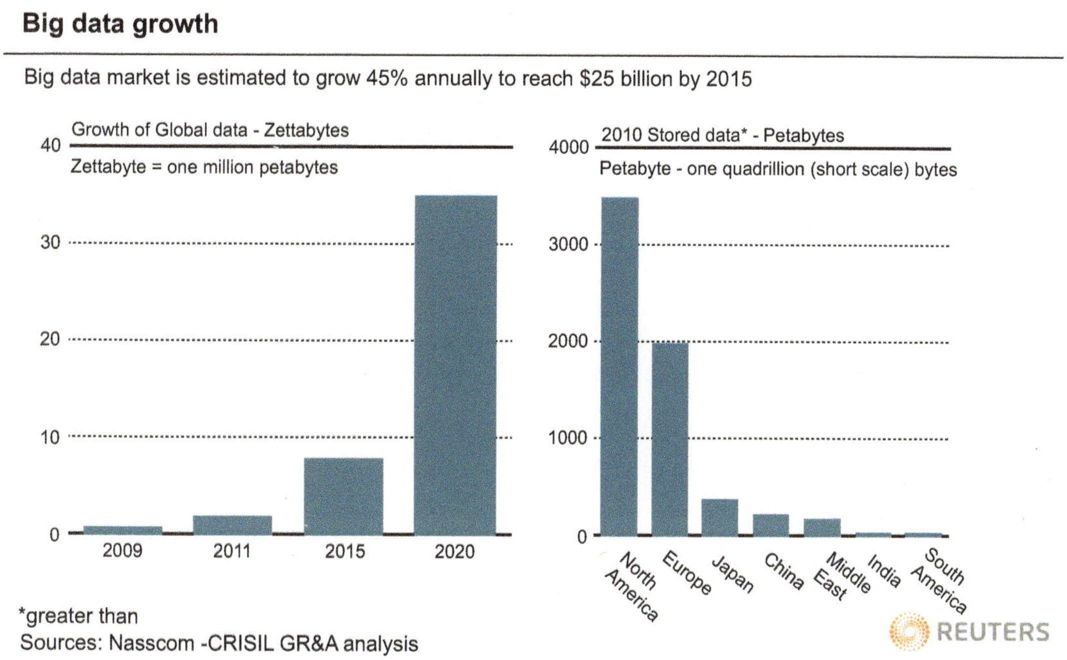

FIGURE 57.3 The worldwide data growth. *(From http://www.theopenstrategist.com/2012/10/big-data-growthchart.html.)*

Of DNA Elements (ENCODE project), an international collaboration of research groups funded by the National Human Genome Research Institute with the aim of delineating the entirety of functional elements encoded in the human genome [12].

DATA MANAGEMENT AND ANALYTICS

The new data paradigm in health care will be a "bottom-up" data management strategy that involves a three-step process after the data is acquired: (1) data extraction with various data warehouses providing data; (2) data transformation with data configured to a uniform format; and (3) data loading with the data entered into an analytical system for final analysis. One example of this data strategy was the tracking of the flu epidemic by Google (called "flu trends") and has been further refined in epidemiological studies using large data sets [13]. The use of big data with real-time collection and analysis is facilitated by the new Hadoop database technology, which minimizes the aforementioned extract–transform–load cycle of data processing [14].

Big data can then strategically utilize methodologies in artificial intelligence to further gain essential information and to even discover new knowledge [15,16]. MIT's Computer Science and Artificial Intelligence Laboratory is leading some of the current efforts to combine big data and artificial intelligence to develop new techniques for big data interpretation that will lead to a genomic data-clinical medicine synergy. The advent of artificial intelligence methodologies such as natural language processing and cognitive computing could enable the medical data manager to not only organize but also mine data from even unstructured electronic medical records automatically (without the tedious and inadequate manual inputting process). In addition, the impressive capability of the computer to perform word-sense disambiguation, or ability to put words into context, was displayed by the IBM computer Watson during its stint on the show Jeopardy! and is presently used effectively for cancer data analytics at Memorial-Sloan-Kettering Cancer Institute.

The perceived value of medical data should not be limited to data analysts and scientists in the IT department of the hospital but be extended to all health care workers to create a data-focused culture. In addition, big data is not merely about mining important information from the medical databases but also demands executing practice changes and transformative innovations. The ultimate data transformation and medical knowledge in the future involves medical databases that will be "living" and "individualized": ongoing clinical research data and analysis with both static and dynamic data (via sensors) from the patient themselves. If embedded with conventional (data mining) [17] or new (machine learning and deep learning) [18] artificial intelligence techniques, these databases will finally enable "intelligence" into health care outcome determinations and decisions.

IMPLEMENTATION OF BIG DATA

Big data is about quality, not quantity, of data. The implementation of big data and analytics could involve a small project in a single hospital sector where data may be easier to be located. In addition, the focus should be on the problem that can be solved by big data, not big data or its analytics itself. The analytic skills even at a basic level should not rest with data analysts but should include everyone. The project should undergo repetitive measurements and analyses to perfect the data analysis strategy. Finally, project execution should have a timeline and progress report throughout the project. Of course all of this data revolution will need adequate storage in the form of cloud computing.

There are some potential limitations of big data in biomedicine. First, there is the "signal-to-noise" problem: true disease data overwhelmed by data that do not truly reflect disease. This could result in over- or underdiagnosis/treatment of the disease. Second, the voluminous data needs to be relatable or at least understandable or visualizable by not just medical caretakers but patients as well. Third, some caretakers may feel intimidated by the decision-making aspects of big data when coupled with artificial intelligence in that intelligent machines may replace certain caretakers. Perhaps the appropriate attitude is to form a human–computer synergy that will surpass the capabilities of either alone, not unlike how the GPS aids the driver (although the autonomous car does come one step closer to replace the driver). There is also some understandable concern that this paradigm shift will depersonalize medicine although the opposite may in fact be true as physicians are liberated from the burden of upkeep and stress of making the appropriate medical decision. There is the potential issue of insufficient data storage capacity even with the cloud, which can be solved by innovative solutions such as using DNA itself as a digital storage medium [19]. Finally, there is the issue of ownership of the data with privacy of information that can lead to identification of patients (especially with a process called triangulation). This problem can be partly mitigated by anonymisation mechanisms.

THE FUTURE: A CLINICAL-DIGITAL CONVERGENCE FOR HEART FAILURE MANAGEMENT

The United States excels in technology and innovation but continually lags far behind other countries in health care data access, transparency, organization, management, and analysis. Our health care organizational and programmatic imperatives in this current era should embrace big data and data analytics/artificial intelligence expertise to harvest meaningful medical data and its hidden information to the fullest extent to improve quality and outcome [20].

In short, big data and strong data governance coupled with data analytics and artificial intelligence will lead to a new paradigm of information and knowledge in heart failure ("medical intelligence"). It therefore behooves us to rethink medical data in traditional forms of tedious databases/registries and even randomized clinical trials to innovate this valuable asset to create a clinical-digital convergence. Big data is therefore not about a collection of technological and analytical tools but rather about a new philosophical transformation in our health care ecosystem in which medical data, artificial intelligence, and personalized health are inextricably intertwined with human intellect and machine intelligence.

The end of theory: The data deluge makes the scientific method obsolete.

Chris Anderson, Wired magazine

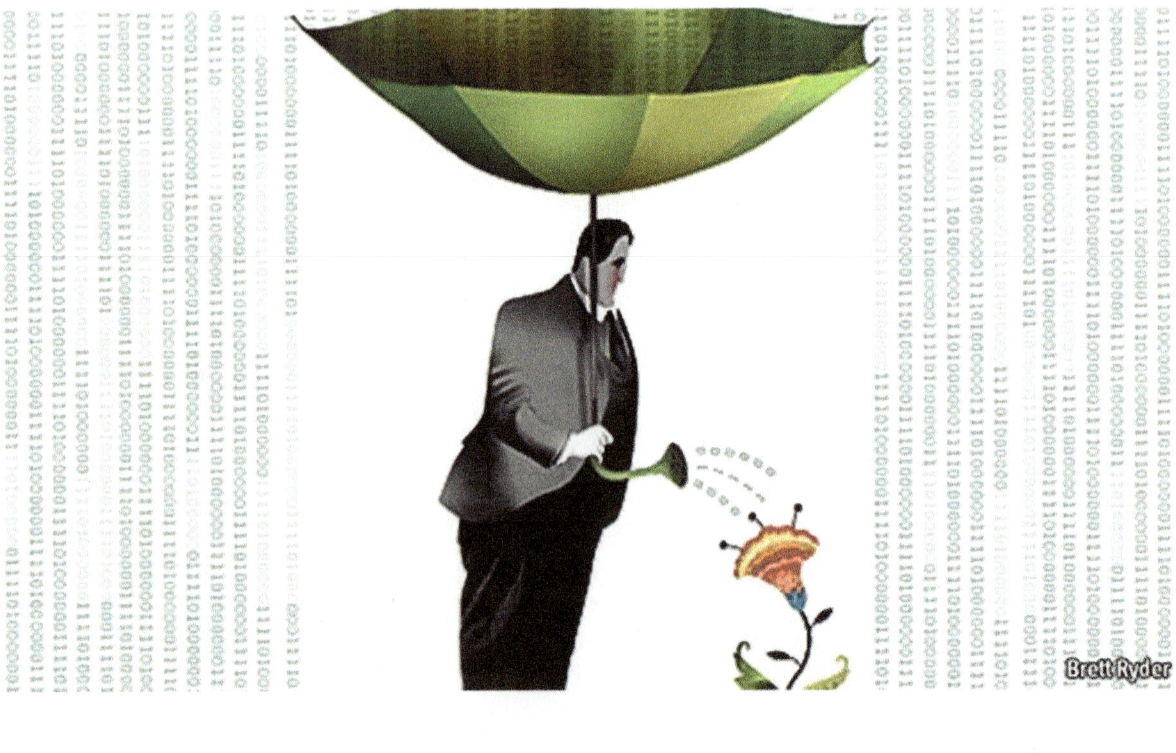

REFERENCES

[1] M. Kohn, Personal Communication (IBM Chief Medical Scientist), February 2013.

[2] A. McAfee, et al., Big data: the management revolution, Harv. Bus. Rev. (October 2012) 60–68.

[3] M. Minelli, et al., Big Data, Big Analytics: Emerging Business Intelligence and Analytic Trends for Today's Businesses, John Wiley and Sons, Inc., Hoboken, New Jersey, 2013.

[4] T. Cosentino, Into the River: How Big Data, the Long Tail, and Situated Cognition are Changing the World of Market Insights Forever, Foundational Insights, LLC, Portland, Oregon, 2011.

[5] The Baseball Prospectus Team of Experts, Baseball Between the Numbers: Why Everything You Know About the Game Is Wrong, Prospetus Entertainment Ventures LLC/Basic Books, New York, NY, 2006.

[6] N. Silver, The Signal and the Noise: Why So Many Predictions Fail But Some Don't, The Penguin Press, New York, NY, 2012.

[7] www.wired.com/wiredscience/2012/10/big-data-is-transforming-healthcare.

[8] G.M.D. Hughes, How Big Is Big Data in Healthcare? From a Shot in the Arm Blog, October 21, 2011.

[9] A. Butte, Personal Communication (Chief, System Medicine at Stanford School of Medicine), February 2013.

[10] E.A. Ashley, et al., Clinical evaluation incorporating a personal genome, Lancet 375 (9725) (2010) 1525–1535.

[11] A. Butte, et al., Computational translating molecular discoveries into tools for medicine: translational bioinformatics articles now featured in JAMIA, J. Am. Med. Inform. Assoc. 18 (4) (2011) 352–353.

[12] The ENCODE Project Consortium, The ENCODE (ENCyclopedia of DNA elements) project, Science 306 (5696) (2004) 636–640.

[13] D.N. Reshef, et al., Detecting novel associations in large data sets, Science 334 (6062) (2011) 1518–1524.

[14] A. Mcafee, What's the big deal about big data? Harv. Bus. Rev. (October 4, 2012) (webinar).

[15] A. Halevy, et al., The Unreasonable Effectiveness of Data, IEEE, March/April, 2009, pp. 8–12.

[16] A.C. Chang, M. Musen, Artificial intelligence in pediatric cardiology: an innovative transformation in patient care, clinical research, and medical education, Congenit. Cardiol. Today 10 (11) (2013) 1–15.

[17] C.W. Hanson, et al., Artificial intelligence applications in the intensive care unit, Crit. Care Med. 29 (2001) 427–435.

[18] R. Hoefen, et al., In silico cardiac risk assessment in patients with long QT syndrome, J. Am. Coll. Cardiol. 60 (2012) 2182–2191.

[19] G.M. Church, et al., Next-generation digital information storage in DNA, Science 337 (6102) (2012) 1628–1631.

[20] J.L. Patel, et al., The coming of age of artificial intelligence in medicine, Artif. Intell. Med. 46 (1) (2009) 5–17.

Chapter 58

Outpatient Monitoring and Self-Care

Jacob Mathew[1], Jennifer Lail[2], Anthony C. Chang[3], John L. Jefferies[2]

[1]*The Royal Children's Hospital, Melbourne, VIC, Australia;* [2]*Cincinnati Children's Hospital Medical Center, Cincinnati, OH, United States;* [3]*Children's Hospital of Orange County, Orange, CA, United States*

This is not the beginning of the end but the end of the beginning…

Winston Churchill (1942)

INTRODUCTION

Heart failure affects approximately 2.4% of American adults, with similar reported prevalence in Northern European populations and is a leading cause of death, disability, and resource usage [1–4]. Much of this resource utilization is attributable to rehospitalization [5]. The burden of heart failure in childhood is less well characterized but increasingly significant [6]. In adult heart failure patients, medical therapy, including ACE inhibitors, angiotensin receptor antagonists, beta-blockers, mineralocorticoid receptor antagonists and, much more recently, the combination of angiotensin receptor blockers with neprilysin antagonists has been shown to reduce mortality [7–15]. In addition, digoxin and ivabradine are known to reduce hospitalization [16,17]. In appropriately selected patients, implantable defibrillators, and cardiac resynchronization therapies are also of potential benefit [18–21]. Though outcomes, as recorded in disease registries and population-based samples, have been improving due to the use of such therapies, they fall short of those achieved in randomized controlled drug trials, even in more recent analyses [22–26]. This outcome gap is likely multifactorial and reflects real-life patients who are older, have more comorbidities, may be less motivated, are less likely to adhere to therapy than those in clinical trials, and who do not benefit from the structured follow-up that occurs in the setting of a research study [27]. Nevertheless, many of these factors are modulated by the mode of health-care delivery, and it is likely that prevailing models of health care have been slow to translate the benefits seen in clinical research to the bedside [28].

Traditional care models have evolved to address acute disease and fall short on many fronts when applied to the care of chronic diseases, such as heart failure. Therapies that have been shown in randomized trials to be of benefit are prescribed less frequently in real-world populations [29]. Even when prescribed, patient adherence is often unacceptably low, while adherence to nonpharmacological aspects of self-care is even lower [30]. Much of this may relate to a failure to adequately engage patients in their care, which may relate to inadequate training of providers in health promotion and motivational interviewing skills, as well as representing a fundamental limitation of care models that center on brief office visits. And, the use of newer therapies may result in increased cost to patients, which results in limited use. The traditional office-visit model of care is simply too unresponsive to adequately address the management of patients whose congestive symptoms may vary daily. At the same time, large gaps in patient education exist, which results in challenges to effective patient self-management [31–34].

As we shall see, successful models for care of chronic disease embrace the patient as a partner in care, with a unique understanding of the impact of chronic disease and their own priorities for care. Skilled providers balance these priorities with an understanding of barriers to effective care, and employ skills such as motivational interviewing, to encourage adoption of and adherence to therapies and lifestyle changes, which are of proven benefit. Such models, therefore, support patient self-care. They exhibit flexibility in provision of care, utilizing multidisciplinary teams, and various modalities of remote care, and increasingly, remote monitoring establishing a dynamic interface between the family and the care team. They utilize comprehensive information systems that allow the integration of multiple sources of information, and coordination of multiple team members, offer decision support, and enable more efficient care for populations as well as patients. However, most of the current strategies in this area have been designed for the care of adults with limited to no data being available in pediatric heart failure.

Heart Failure in the Child and Young Adult. http://dx.doi.org/10.1016/B978-0-12-802393-8.00058-2

In this chapter, we shall review the data supporting some key aspects of successful care models, namely enhancing patient self-care, remote care, and remote monitoring of patients providing information on existing approaches and key differences that should be addressed to deliver optimal care to children and young adults with heart failure.

SELF-CARE MANAGEMENT

Definition and Measurement of Heart Failure Self-Care

A variety of definitions have been applied to self-care, many of which are rather broad. Barlow described self-care as the actions taken by patients "to lead a healthy lifestyle, meet their social, emotional and psychological needs, to care for their long-term condition and to prevent further illness or accidents" [35]. Riegel has emphasized that self-care involves a series of decisions that are made a real-world context, marked by a focus on process rather than outcome, the use of heuristics, strong influence of context and an "availability bias" in deciding what information is applied to a given decision, which they present as an example of naturalistic decision-making, as opposed to the strictly rational view taken by classical decision theory [36]. Riegel further subcategorizes self-care to include "the decision making that underlies the choice of positive health practices (also called 'self-care maintenance') and the behaviors used to manage signs and symptoms of illness and disease (termed 'self-care management')" [37,38]. In the context of heart failure, self-care maintenance behaviors include medication adherence, ensuring attendance at follow-up visits, maintaining a low sodium diet, avoidance of tobacco, moderation of alcohol intake, and receiving influenza vaccination, while self-care management behaviors might include monitoring of weight, recognition of symptoms, reducing fluid intake, and increasing diuretic dose or seeking clinician guidance in response to increase in symptoms or weight.

Specific tools to measure heart failure self-care include the European heart failure self-care behavioral scale (EHFScBS) and self-care of heart failure index (SCHFI) [39–42]. The EHFScBS is a 12-item questionnaire that largely focuses on self-care management, though a refined 9-item version has been described [39,40]. Evaluation in multiple European populations has demonstrated good internal consistency and reasonable retest reliability [40]. Content validity was addressed through involvement of a multinational expert panel throughout an iterative process of refinement and moderate correlation with the Heart Failure Compliance Questionnaire and low correlation with the Minnesota Living with Heart Failure Questionnaire have been presented as evidence of concurrent and discriminative validity, respectively [39,43]. The SCHFI was initially a 15-item instrument with three subscales, evaluating self-care management, self-care maintenance, and self-efficacy. Each subscale is standardized to a score out of 100 [41]. The instrument has undergone revision over time and now includes 22 items [42]. Psychometric testing has confirmed moderate internal consistency, and a number of lines of evidence to support construct and convergent validity [42]. Importantly, the EHFScBS shows moderate correlation with the SCHFI self-care maintenance scale, offering further evidence for concurrent validity of both tools, while the poor correlation between the EHFScBS and SCHFI self-care management and confidence scales, further supports Riegel's assertion that the three subscales measure distinct constructs, and that hence, the scores should be reported separately and not as an aggregate score [42]. Both tools have been validated in diverse populations [44–46]. Despite this, they have not yet found widespread use as clinical tools.

In the pediatric patient, management and measurement of self-care is affected by the child's developmental changes, their dependency on caregivers, the epidemiology and demographics of pediatric heart failure, and the funding mechanisms for their care [47–49]. Caregiver and family dysfunction and social determinant risk factors such as poverty, family conflict, or parental mental health conditions challenge both self-management and adherence in multiple pediatric chronic conditions [50–55]. As the child with chronic illness becomes an adolescent, a gradual evolution of self-efficacy is needed to support condition management and healthy development. Modi et al. have documented decreases in both adherence and self-management skills in the move to adolescence [56].

Predictors of Self-Care and Barriers to Effective Self-Care

In one study, only a third of patients were deemed to be "expert" in self-care [57]. While, as we have noted before, self-care is inevitable, effective self-care is challenged by a number of demographic, medical, psychological and social factors, which interact in a complex interplay to influence self-care in a given patient.

Reported associations between demographic factors and self-care have been somewhat variable. Surprisingly, little data specifically address the impact of age on heart failure self-care, though Artinian found that older patients were more likely to seek attention for changing symptoms, to adhere to prescribed medications and to keep medical appointments, and Chriss found that older patients had better SCHFI scores in a convenience sample of elderly heart failure patients [58–60]. Riegel, however, found that older patients were less likely to recognize heart failure symptoms as such and also found gender to have no consistent impact on self-care in a cross-sectional Australian sample, findings that are consistent with other studies [30,61–63]. Lee et al., however, did report that married women had lower SCHFI confidence and maintenance scores than unmarried women or men and Chriss described higher SCHIFI scores in males [60,64]. In general other factors, notably self-care confidence, better explained self-care in most studies than gender per se [62–64].

Adequate disease-specific knowledge is a necessary, though insufficient, condition for adequate self-care. However, very few patients consider themselves to be knowledgeable in self-care [65,66]. Quality improvement measures such the provision of written instructions to patients on discharge are important step but fail to bridge this knowledge gap [67,68]. Understanding of heart failure symptoms remains poor, and often symptoms are misattributed to old age, or to comorbid conditions [30,32,33,69,70]. When coupled with poor somatic awareness that is prevalent in heart failure populations, this can lead to poor symptom recognition, precluding effective self-care management [71,72]. Knowledge of appropriate heart failure health maintenance behaviors is also often lacking. For example, in many studies, patients prioritized a perceived need to maintain fluid intake to ensure adequate hydration over monitoring of fluid intake and weight [33,34,69]. Even where patients have appropriate recall of specific knowledge (e.g., "I should follow a low sodium diet"), this does not translate into effective decision-making and behavior (e.g., awareness that salt and sodium are synonymous, that the majority of sodium in Western diets is added during manufacture, etc.). Reflecting on this, Riegel et al. have distinguished between heart failure knowledge and the tactical skills required for effective self-care and have suggested that patient education programs need to be more orientated towards the latter [38,73]. Poor general health literacy likely overlaps with poor disease-specific knowledge and has been associated with poorer self-care, and self-efficacy, as well as an increased risk of hospitalization, which was mediated by lower treatment adherence [74,75]. Experience with the disease, however, does seem to be associated with better self-care, as might be expected [45].

Depression and cognitive impairment are frequent comorbidities in adult heart failure populations and may each limit effective self-care maintenance behaviors and self-care management responses to changes in clinical status [76–78]. Depression is associated with decreased dietary and medication adherence, as well as overall self-care [79–81]. However, some have found otherwise and it may be that health management behaviors are affected disproportionately to health maintenance behaviors [82–84]. Similarly, patients with type D personality have been found to present later for medical attention [85]. Cognitive impairment has also been associated with more inconsistent self-care and with poorer self-care management, though not maintenance, which may plausibly reflect the more active processes required to enact self-care management behaviors [86–89]. Similarly, self-care novices were found to have higher daytime sleepiness scores in one study, and sleepiness was found to predict medication nonadherence in another [90,91].

It might be expected that adequate physical capacity is required to implement effective self-care behaviors. However, self-care experts have been found to have higher New York Heart Association (NYHA) classification and lower activity levels, which may reflect increased motivation with increasing disease severity [57,92]. Interestingly, patients with multiple comorbidities tended to exhibit better self-care [69,93].

Social support is an important determinant of self-care. For example, Gallagher and colleagues reported that patient perception of support from their partners predicted EHFScBS score [94]. Those who described high levels of social support were more likely to consult a provider appropriately for weight gain, to adhere to fluid restriction and medications, and to exercise regularly. Riegel reported similar findings in a qualitative study that contrasted self-care experts with novices [90]. Other studies have reported that perceived social support is an important predictor of medication adherence [95]. A systematic metaanalysis performed by DiMatteo reported that various measures of social support were significantly correlated with adherence across 11 reviewed studies [96]. When dimensions of social support were considered individually, functional social support measures, comprised of practical support, emotional support and family cohesiveness, and structural social support measures, comprised of marital status and living arrangements, were each individually associated with adherence using pooled estimates of correlation. However, measures of functional social support, particularly those that measured practical social support, were stronger predictors of adherence than structural measures [96]. Intriguingly, Rohrbaugh found spousal self-confidence to be the strongest assessed predictor of medium term mortality in heart failure, exceeding even patients' own rated self-efficacy [97]. While social support enhances self-care, it remains important to engage the patient as an active contributor to their own care, as those who perceive their role as more passive have been found to have lower SCHFI maintenance and management scores in one study [98].

Data on these topics are lacking in pediatric populations. However, it is reasonable to conclude that children with heart failure must have continuous and reliable access to and funding for care. The March 2014 Standards for Systems of Care for Children and Youth with Special Healthcare Needs identify 10 necessary domains including eligibility for insurance, a medical home with continuity of care and care coordination and geographic and timely access to primary and specialty care, among others [99]. Pediatric cardiomyopathy and resultant heart failure may require travel across state lines for required expertise; even finding pediatric formulations of medications may be a barrier to care, and out-of-pocket costs for families with chronically ill children are higher than acceptable affordability standards [100–102]. These barriers represent proximal impediments to self-care.

For optimal condition management, children with heart failure require regular cardiac surveillance, which is comprised of evaluation and multiple tests and acute care management integrated with their specialty care. The patient/family centered medical home is a standard of care particularly supportive of children with chronic illness, providing a care team of familiar providers, and partnering with the child's family and community [103]. For children with heart failure, school, day care, camp, and recreational activities are critical for growth and development, demanding adaptations to optimize safe participation. An integrated care team, leader and care plan, developed with the family, permits negotiated actions necessary to promote adherence to medications, lifestyle adaptations, and monitoring [104].

Impact of Self-Care on Outcomes in Heart Failure

Multiple lines of observational data support the association of better self-care with improved clinical outcomes in heart failure patients. Firstly, individual components of self-care such as regular weighing, and as noted above, medication adherence, have been shown to predict rates of exacerbation, hospitalization, and mortality [75,105,106]. Other factors such as health literacy, depression, and social support, which are in turn associated with self-care, predict clinical outcomes in adult heart failure patients [75,107]. Lee found that above-average SCHFI self-management scores, though not self-care maintenance or confidence scores, were associated with improved event-free survival in adult heart failure patients, after adjusting for age, gender, diagnosis, ejection fraction, and NYHA class. This largely reflects a reduction in hospitalization in those patients who were more adept at self-care management behaviors [108]. Interestingly, in a retrospective analysis of two previous cross-sectional studies, Lee found that SCHFI self-management scores predicted increased myocardial stress, as measured by NT-proBNP levels, and inflammation as measured by soluble TNF receptor assay, after adjusting for similar covariates [109]. Rathman reported that EHScBS scores (which are higher in patients with poorer self-care) were associated with increased probability of hypervolemic episodes, as determined by thoracic impedance, in elderly heart failure patients [110]. When paired, these findings might suggest that patients with better self-care exhibit improved medication adherence and monitoring behaviors and are therefore less likely to experience hypervolemic episodes, which lead to hospitalization.

Interventional studies of self-management have had more mixed results, particularly with respect to impact on mortality. In a systematic review of 11 randomized studies evaluating disease management programs, most of which were focused on self-care education, McAlister found a reduction in all cause (Relative Risk [RR] 0.73; 95% CI 0.57–0.93) and heart failure hospitalization (RR 0.66; 0.52–0.83) but not mortality [111]. Jovicic and Ditewig reported similar findings in later systematic reviews [112,113].

Medication Adherence

Medication adherence in particular is a key self-care maintenance behavior. It seems self-evident that the therapies found to be of benefit in randomized controlled trials are only likely to be of benefit if patients adhere to them, and indeed this has been shown to be true [106]. While, even in the setting of a research study, adherence is suboptimal, adherence in community samples is substantially poorer [106,114]. Medication adherence is challenged by poor patient understanding of often complicated regimens [32]. Murray reported that poorer health literacy was associated with an increased risk of hospitalization in adult heart failure patients, which was mediated by lower adherence [75]. Patient beliefs about their condition (e.g., consequences of nonadherence, and the perceived impact of illness on daily life) are an important determinant of medication adherence, taking account of which may require a more personalized approach to education [95,115,116].

Similar barriers to medication adherence occur in children, with cost, "forgetting," objections to taste and side effects, and perception of condition remission when symptoms are controlled being cited. Modi described five patterns of adherence with pediatric seizure medications, with lower socioeconomic status being associated with nonadherence. Pediatric medication adherence is complicated by the need for developmentally appropriate formulations of medicine (compounded medications for nonpill swallowers, medication stability in compounding) and delays by required preauthorizations for cardiac medications less used in paediatrics [117]. Additionally, risk-taking behaviors may add to medication nonadherence in adolescent and young adult populations further complicating care delivery.

REMOTE PATIENT MONITORING

Successful self-care of heart failure requires patient education, motivation, and confidence to persist with self-care maintenance and management, the selection of appropriate parameters to monitor for clinical deterioration and the ability for patients to initiate appropriate responses in the event of deterioration. Further for reasons that are described above, some patients and their families are less able to institute effective self-care and may require more frequent monitoring. More frequent clinical contact may address some of these needs, but comes at significant resource cost, and is inconvenient for patients. A range of remote monitoring strategies have been described, which aim to offer a scalable response to this set of needs. By allowing for more frequent monitoring and by reducing barriers to clinician contact they might allow for continued patient education and reinforcement of prior learning, augmented clinical monitoring, and reduce the barriers to an effective response in the face of deterioration. The most studied modalities are structured telephone support (STS) and teleconsultation but advances in technology are offering newer and more scalable possibilities.

Structured Telephone Support

STS refers to scripted and scheduled, rather than solely patient initiated, telephone-based patient evaluation, and decision support. These programs have typically been staffed by specialist nurses under the supervision of a physician. Numerous metaanalyses of randomized STS interventions have been published, which have consistently found a reduction in heart failure hospitalization in middle-aged heart failure patients who received this intervention, over 3–16 months of follow-up [118,119]. In the most recent metaanalysis, which included 25 trials of STS interventions enrolling over 9000 patients, Inglis found that these programs were associated with reduced all-cause mortality (RR 0.87; 0.77–0.98) and heart failure hospitalization (RR 0.85; 0.77–0.93) but not all cause hospitalization [120].

Although no data are available regarding telephone coaching in pediatric heart failure, this approach has been perused in pediatric obesity that revealed a strong interest from parents in such a program [121]. Telephone coaching has also been used to improve self-management behavior in childhood asthma [122].

Noninvasive Remote Monitoring

Telemonitoring refers to the transmission of symptom scores, physiological data including heart rate, blood pressure, oxygen saturation, and weight directly to care providers either via automated electronic means or by web-based or phone-based data entry. Over time these interventions have evolved from automated phone response systems to web, to interactive television-based systems, to mobile phone or PDA-based systems to complex systems, which wirelessly transmit recorded physiological data [120]. Anker has subclassified telemonitoring systems into those which function as nonreactive data collection devices (such as event recorders), those with a delayed analytic and decision-making structure (e.g., only within office hours), those with continuously operating analytic and decision-making infrastructure, and complex systems that integrate invasive and noninvasive data [123]. Metaanalyses have consistently found these interventions to be associated with reduced mortality and heart failure hospitalizations. In the most recent analysis by Inglis, noninvasive telemonitoring reduced all-cause mortality (RR 0.80; 0.68–0.94) in 17 studies with 3740 participants. Heart failure-related hospitalizations were reduced also (RR 0.71; 0.60–0.83) in 8 studies with 2148 subjects [120].

Of note, several interesting prespecified subgroup analyses were performed as part of this metaanalysis. Firstly, the telemonitoring modality was considered. Automated phone response systems were assessed in four studies enrolling 2445 patients, and pooled results suggested no impact on either total mortality (RR 1.01; 0.80–1.28) or on heart failure hospitalization (0.99; 0.86–1.14). In contrast mobile or PDA-based data collection systems were assessed in four studies enrolling 734 patients, and while the effect on total mortality was not significant (RR 0.71; 0.46–1.11), a significant impact on heart failure hospitalization rates was found (RR 0.58; 0.44–0.77). Further, 12 studies that randomized 2885 patients to complex telemonitoring systems that automated data transmission demonstrated significant reductions in total mortality (RR 0.81; 0.68–0.96) and heart failure hospitalization rates (0.78; 0.64–0.94) [120]. This strongly supports the intuitive notion that ease of use and more automated, less patient-dependent systems are more likely to work.

Further subgroup analysis explored the responsiveness of these telemonitoring systems, finding that pooled heart failure hospitalization outcomes from both studies in which the data were acted up on during office hours (RR 0.71; 0.56–0.89) and those that were operational around the clock (RR 0.71; 0.57–0.87) were very similar.

Invasive Remote Monitoring

The clinical variables that are commonly used to assess patient deterioration in clinical studies, such as reported symptoms, heart rate, blood pressure, oxygen saturation, and weight though readily available and useful are imperfect predictive tools heart failure decompensation [124,125]. With increasing utilization of ICD and CRT devices in heart failure patients, the opportunity has arisen to obtain additional invasive physiological data to augment monitoring. These devices have the potential to measure patient activity, heart rate variability (HRV), arrhythmia burden, and thoracic impedance. Alternative strategies have included biomarker-based approaches and those that rely on direct intracardiac or pulmonary pressure measurement.

Biomarker-based monitoring was explored in the HABIT observational study, where patients following a heart failure admission were asked to perform daily weights and finger-prick home-based BNP monitoring daily for 60days. Each natural log increase in BNP was associated with a 1.8-fold increased risk of a composite outcome of death, heart failure admission, or augmentation of diuretic therapy, independently of patient-reported symptoms. This compared to a 3.6-fold increased risk of the outcome on days where weight gain exceeded 5lbs from baseline. When the monitoring period was divided into intervals of continuous trend, positive trending BNP (>1% per day) was associated with an almost 60% increase in risk, while periods of negative trend (<−1% a day) were associated with a 39% decreased risk by comparison to neutral intervals [124].

Adamson investigated HRV as assessed by the standard deviation of 5-min median atrial–atrial intervals in middle-aged heart failure patients with class III to IV systolic heart failure. Reduced HRV (4-week average of <50ms, measured between 5 and 8 weeks after initial hospitalization) was found to predict mortality with a hazard ratio (HR) of 3.2. Further, reductions in HRV occurred a median of 16days and up to 3weeks prior to a heart failure hospitalization. Using an optimal cut-off, 70% of hospitalizations could be predicted by changes in HRV though the false positive rate at this threshold was frequent, at a rate of 2.4 per patient per year. Patient activity and night time heart rate were less useful predictors of clinical events than HRV in this cohort [126].

Measurement of impedance between the generator and typically right ventricular leads of modern pacemaker and defibrillator devices provides a measure of thoracic impedance, which was shown to vary inversely with changes in volume status in the MID-HeFT study [127]. Decreased thoracic impedance is predictive of subsequent decompensation and precedes the latter by an average of 15days [127,128]. In the FAST study, a fluid index derived from impedance measurement by CRT devices was compared to daily weight measurement (for which a change of 3lbs/day, or 5 lbs in 3days was considered significant). Seventy-six percent of heart failure decompensation episodes were marked by fluid indices in excess of a prespecified threshold, while only 23% of these episodes were detected by weight monitoring. Changes in fluid index were more specific predictors of decompensation also, with false positive rate of 1.9 per patient per year, as opposed to 4.3 per patient per year for weight monitoring. Importantly the frequency of successful fluid index recordings was far greater than adherence to weight monitoring (>99% vs. 76%) [129]. In the PARTNERS-HF observational study, Whellan and colleagues explored the predictive value of combinations of device-derived data. On monthly interrogation, two or more of long atrial fibrillation duration, rapid ventricular rate during atrial fibrillation, high fluid index, low patient activity, high night heart rate, low HRV, or device therapy (low CRT pacing or implantable cardioverter–defibrillator shocks), or the presence of a very high fluid index was found to predict heart failure hospitalization (HR 5.5; 3.4–8.8) during the next month. This remained a useful predictor (HR 4.8; 2.9–8.1) after adjustment for age, gender, etiology of heart failure, NYHA class and medical therapy [130]. Contrasting the favorable reports of these earlier observational studies, the SENSE-HF study evaluated the predictive utility of fluid index measurements in a multicentre European observational study. This study found that these measurements had low sensitivity (20.7%) for subsequent heart failure hospitalization and very poor positive predictive value of 4.7%. The discriminatory value did appear to improve over time, perhaps reflecting decreased utility of impedance changes early after implantation. After 6months postimplantation, positive predictive value for worsening heart failure (as opposed to hospitalization) improved to 38.1% [131]. This study raised significant concerns about the false positive rate attributable to this technology, which was finally submitted to randomized trial evaluation with the DOT-HF study. The latter study aimed to determine whether fluid index measurements could reduce a composite endpoint of death and heart failure hospitalization in adult heart failure patients. After recruiting under 15% of the intended number of patients, the trial was terminated due to slow enrollment and anticipated futility. Interim analysis suggested a trend to increased death and hospitalization (HR 1.52; 0.97–2.37) due to increased hospitalization (HR 1.79; 1.08–2.95) in the intervention group, over a mean follow-up of 15months. A threefold increase in outpatient utilization was also noted [132]. These results would seem to confirm the preceding concerns about low specific and sensitivity when these measurements are used in isolation.

Direct pressure measurement approaches have described initially in the multicentre CHRONICLE trial, which enrolled NYHA class III and IV heart failure patients with recent hospitalization, regardless of ejection fraction and on optimal medical therapy. The participants were implanted with continuous pressure monitoring device with subpectoral controller and transvenously placed right ventricular pressure monitor (Chronicle, Medtronic Inc., Minneapolis, MN) and were randomized. Participants were single blinded to their allocation and both groups were asked to transmit data weekly to their clinicians, though only the clinicians of those patients in the treatment group could see and act on the hemodynamic data. A nonsignificant 21% reduction was observed in frequency of heart failure events (urgent care and emergency attendance, or hospitalization). Post hoc analysis suggested a 36% reduced risk of rehospitalization for heart failure [133]. The results were perhaps encouraging though the trial was underpowered, and after the device failed to gain FDA approval, further development has ceased.

The HOMEOSTASIS trial was a small multicentre observational study of class III and IV heart failure patients (independent of left ventricular ejection fraction (LVEF)) who had experienced recent decompensation and underwent twice daily left atrial pressure monitoring using a transvenously implanted (HeartPOD, St Jude Medical Inc., Minneapolis, MN). Clinicians were unblinded to device reported measurements after 3 months. The (uncontrolled) data suggested improvements in mean daily left atrial pressure from 17.6 mmHg (95% CI 15.8–19.4 mmHg) in the first 3 months to 14.8 mmHg (95% CI 13.0–16.6 mmHg; $P = .003$) during pressure-guided therapy. The frequency of elevated readings (≥25 mmHg) was reduced by 67% ($P < .001$). Improvements in NYHA class (−0.7 ± 0.8 units, $P < .001$) and LVEF (7 ± 10%, $P < .001$) was also noted during the latter period [134]. This device and a modification for use with CRT-D devices were employed in the LAPTOP-HF randomized trial [135]. Unfortunately the data safety and monitoring board terminated this trial early on the basis of anticipated futility and a high rate of complications related to transseptal puncture.

The most promising data for invasive pressure monitoring come from the CHAMPION trial, which enrolled class III adult heart failure patients who had previously been hospitalized, independently of ejection fraction and who underwent implantation with a CardioMEMS (CardioMEMS, Atlanta, GA, USA) implantable pulmonary artery pressure monitor. They were then randomized to a control group who transmitted data daily, but whose clinicians were blinded to the hemodynamic data, and an intervention group whose clinicians could amend therapy on the basis of hemodynamic data. The intervention group underwent more changes in drug therapy than the control group and experienced 30% fewer hospitalizations up to 6 months of follow-up. Serious complications arose in 1.4% of participants [136].

Thus far the various invasive and noninvasive remote monitoring parameters that have been reported do suffer from poor sensitivity and specificity when used in isolation. As seen in the DOT-HF impedance monitoring trial, poor positive predictive value is a particular concern because it may result in substantially increased utilization without impacting other outcomes favorably. Nonetheless, it must be noted that the same limitations apply, and predictive value is likely lower still, for the present clinical gold standard of weight monitoring. Further, these technologies generate large amounts of real-time data, which must be analyzed and an effective response initiated. This burden is already substantial in the setting of research trials and the medicolegal implications for harboring and responding to these data are also unclear. One proposal has been to create telemonitoring centers, which operate 24 h a day and provide the first response to telemonitoring data, though it is unclear how such systems should interface with primary care and specialist heart failure teams [123]. It seems likely that increasingly, application of various "big data" or artificial intelligence approaches to data analysis would help to integrate the various types of data generated by remote monitoring and more reliably identify patients at higher risk of decompensation than consideration of individual data points and simple "rules-of-thumb." Such an approach is also more likely to be scalable as these technologies are deployed more widely.

PEDIATRIC CONSIDERATIONS

Pediatric populations present unique challenges to the health system in both outpatient monitoring and self-care in the setting of chronic illness. In the general pediatric population, heart failure from all causes is an uncommon condition; in 2016, Gilboa et al. estimated that 1 million children in the United States were living with congenital heart defects, which may predispose to heart failure, but does not include myocardial dysfunction from other causes [137]. Data on monitoring and self-management are in development for specific populations of pediatric chronic conditions. In juvenile onset diabetes, the validated Problem Recognition in Self-Management tool has shown promise in identifying a specific child's barriers to self-management across six domains [138], including understanding and organizing their care and denial of their disease and consequences, among others. For children with inflammatory bowel disease, routine screening for adherence and self-management, including pill counts and bioassays is recommended [139]. Health system barriers to adherence in pediatric kidney transplant, including legal and insurance have been identified as well [140]. In such high-severity and low-frequency conditions, continuous and reliable access to and funding for care, both pediatric and specialty, and trusted medical and surgical providers must be established by and with families. Ongoing self-care and self-management are complicated by the developmental challenges of the growing child and the child's dependency on their supervising adults and may involve the management of existing medical comorbidities in other organ systems. Finding pediatric formulations of medications are a barrier to care, and out-of-pocket costs for families with chronically ill children are higher than acceptable affordability standards [141]; both are proximal impediments to self-care. Caregiving needs can affect work attendance and job productivity, impacting the family's financial bottom line [142].

Two models of care have been effective in the management of chronic conditions in children: the patient-centered medical home model and the Chronic Care model.

The June 2017 Standards for Systems of Care for Children and Youth with Special Healthcare Needs identify eight necessary domains including eligibility for insurance, a medical home with continuity of care and care coordination and geographic and timely access to primary and specialty care, among others [143]. The medical home model of care for children with chronic conditions has been associated with decreased emergency department visits and hospitalizations [144], decreased time burden for the family in care coordination [145] and notably, decreased unmet specialty care needs [146]. Mosquera et al. using a comprehensive medical home model for high-risk children with chronic illness demonstrated decreased total hospital and clinic costs, with reduced rate and length of inpatient stays [147]. The infant, child, or adolescent with heart disease require ready access to both primary and specialty care for preventive, acute, and chronic care management. Families of children with rare conditions may necessarily seek care and expertise at health centers at distance from their homes and local medical community but require local supports to manage the child's nutrition, learning and development, immunizations, and dental care—all of which can be impacted by and affect their cardiac status. Children, particularly in day care and school settings, have numerous infectious exposures and illnesses, which must be evaluated within the framework of the child's heart failure staging. Accordingly, the patient-centered medical home model of care, endorsed by pediatricians, internists, family physicians, and emergency medicine is particularly valuable to the family and child managing heart failure [148,149]. The medical home model, often implemented in the primary care setting in comanagement with specialty care, offers familiar access into the larger health system, and serves as an organizing force for collaboration between and among families, specialists and the child's larger community. Acute illness management, preventive care, and chronic care management can be accomplished in the medical home in close communication with cardiac specialists, reinforcing the care plan of the cardiologist and supporting the child's participation in school, recreation, and childhood activities. However, while children may have a regular source of care for illness or preventive care, their primary care providers may lack comfort in managing the child's health maintenance in the setting of heart failure, so comanagement with the child's cardiologist is critical [150]. In specific situations of children with high medical complexity, specialty providers may take the lead in management of children, serving as their medical home. Such practices may seek the National Committee on Quality Assurance's certification as a Patient-Centered Specialty Practice [151]. Led by the family, specialists, primary care providers, schools and the child's community must work together to mitigate the psychological impact of the child's illness, which may include anxiety, depression, and altered independence on the child, siblings, and parents [152,153]. Children with chronic illness such as heart failure have a higher risk of emotional problems, complicating their coping with, and self-management of their condition [154]. Families and children may struggle with the possibility of a shortened life span and necessary adaptations for medications, diet and exercise; maintaining friendships, social interests, school attendance, and self-esteem are important challenges. Functional impairments, both behaviorally and emotionally, have been found to be higher in the siblings of children with disabilities [152]. Studies across pediatric chronic illnesses document traumatic stress symptoms in both patient and family, with those children facing potential transplant reporting higher stress [155]. For children and youth with heart failure, school, day care, play, and recreational activities are critical for growth and development, demanding adaptations to optimize safe participation [156]. Caregiver and family dysfunction and social determinant risk factors such as poverty, family conflict, or parental mental health conditions challenge both self-management and adherence in multiple pediatric chronic conditions [56].

There is a growing body of evidence of the efficacy of application of the Chronic Care Model [157] in pediatric chronic illness from Dr. Edward Wagner and the MacColl Institute (Fig. 58.1) [158–161]. Improvement in clinical, functional, and patient-reported outcomes across a diverse array of chronic pediatric conditions through application of the Chronic Care model components [162] has been shown. Highlighting both the prepared, proactive practice team and the informed, empowered patient and family as foundational elements, this model proposes a safe, coordinated health system, designed for cultural competency, both care and decision support and integration of a child's community to optimize their outcomes. As well, clinical information systems and structured self-management are fundamental components of the Chronic Care model. The Chronic Care model acknowledges that systems external to health care, such as community supports, help to address the psychosocial and emotional stressors of chronic illness in childhood.

As the child with chronic illness becomes an adolescent, a gradual evolution of self-efficacy is needed to support condition management and healthy development. Modi et al. have documented decreases in both adherence and self-management skills in the move to adolescence [56]. As early as age 12, condition-specific knowledge, goal-setting, emergency care planning, and accessing the health system are components of the recommended health-care transition to adulthood. There are currently no validated tools that have been developed specifically for pediatric heart failure self-care. This is an area of need that would provide baseline and longitudinal data to inform providers of trends and needs of patients and families.

Adolescents with chronic illness have been shown to have delayed milestones in life skills even as they work on development of autonomy [163]. Support for the ultimate transition to adult care should begin in early adolescence [164], as well as the recommended adolescent screenings for depression, substance use, sexual behaviors, and mood issues [165]. Best practices from the American Heart Association for supporting optimal transition to adulthood for adolescents with

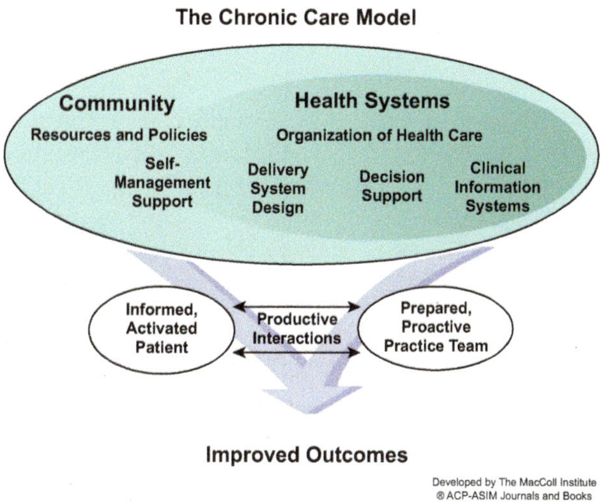

FIGURE 58.1

congenital heart disease have been published [166]. The adolescent's life management capabilities are linked to their condition self-management. Any risk taking behaviors may add to medication nonadherence in adolescent and young adult populations further complicating care delivery. The Maternal and Child Health Bureau and The National Alliance to Advance Adolescent Health created six core elements of health-care transition for young adults, including transition policies, tracking, serial readiness assessments, and a deliberate and informed transfer to the adult care model [167]. Seamless communication between a youth's medical home and cardiologists (adult and pediatric) support a safe and effective transition for the young adult with heart failure.

INTEGRATED DISEASE MANAGEMENT MODELS

It follows from the preceding discussions that successfully addressing the challenges posed by chronic diseases such as heart failure does not occur in the clinician's office but relies on a well-integrated whole system of care. The term "disease management" has been used to describe this shift of attention from discrete episodes of care to a longitudinal continuum of care. The goals of disease management programs include (1) modulation of baseline risk, for example, by enhancing prescription of and adherence to evidence-based therapies, (2) monitoring for and responding promptly to decompensation by enhancing patient self-care management and increasingly, use of remote monitoring technologies. When studied in the context of heart failure, these approaches have overlapped with, and included elements of, self-care education and telecare. Metaanalyses have suggested that these interventions reduce heart failure and all cause hospitalization and total mortality [111]. Interestingly, the benefit appears to be greatest for multidisciplinary models rather than those employing one type of practitioner and for interventions of medium (3–6 months) rather than shorter or longer duration [168].

One well described, and scalable disease management program for chronic diseases, including CHF, is the Veterans' Health Administration's (VHA) care coordination and home telehealth (CCHT) model. This model centers on trained care coordinators, typically with a nursing or social work background who have undergone further training in the VHA's centralized CCHT training program, and who each typically manage a portfolio of 100–150 aging patients. After assessing each patient's disease needs, capacity for self-care management and familiarity with and access to information technology, the care coordinator determines what clinical parameters (e.g., symptom survey, vital signs, weight, blood glucose, etc.) to collect, and the most suitable telemonitoring modality. These data are collected via an integrated health information system. A daily summary of patients in each care coordinator's portfolio is generated, which highlights higher risk patients on the basis of reported symptoms and predefined thresholds for vital signs. Intervention aims to support patient self-management of their condition and videophones and similar devices support teleconsultation on an as-needed basis. The CCHT program, which began in 2003, catered to over 50,000 veterans in 2011. Heart failure patients make up 24% of the total. Compared to the year prior to enrollment, in the 6 months following enrollment, patients experienced a 19% reduction in hospital admission, and a 25% reduction in bed days. These benefits appear to have been realized in both urban and highly rural settings, and across the range of chronic diseases supported (including heart failure) and for patients with multiple morbidities, which is frequently true for heart failure patients [169].

FUTURE DIRECTIONS

Transitional Care at Present

There is a paucity of information on the transitional care of the pediatric patient with heart failure to adulthood. There are, however, many recent reports on children with congenital heart disease and their transition process to adulthood [170–172]. One can gather from these myriad of reports the precise underpinnings of an excellent transition of care from pediatric to adult patient in heart failure and its related issues.

One of the central tenets in transitional self-care in pediatric chronic heart disease management such as heart failure for the older pediatric and adolescent patient is full understanding of the disease pathophysiology as well as therapeutic strategies (such as surgical procedures and medications). Another central tenet is the continual trust and confidence of the patient for the clinician as well as the multidisciplinary health-care system that is rendering the care for the patient. Lastly, successful transitional care for the pediatric heart failure patient will be largely reliant on full 24/7 access to the health-care system for acute and chronic medical and health issues for the patient and family in the current model of population health.

Transitional Care in the Future

A visionary multidisciplinary "intelligent"clinic (or iClinic) for heart failure transitional care of the future (Fig. 58.2) will leverage transitional care principles with current technological advances. The transitional care will focus on: instantaneous biometric measurement so that clinical status and update can be facilitated between clinic visits; intermittent virtual clinical follow-up to increase health-care team patient and family interactions without the necessary burden of travel and waiting; individual therapy to leverage tools that are available for precision medicine that is individualized for that patient in both acute and chronic care; intelligent data-driven medicine that will utilize both state-of-the art evidence-based medicine as well as analytics from wearable devices; and intuitive interactions with educational tools such as virtual avatars and chat-bots that use artificial intelligence-inspired algorithms to enable meaningful interactions between patients and families with the health-care team.

This iClinic will have the following five state-of-the-art technological and clinical capabilities to increase medical intelligence and improve the transitional patient outcome on a long-term basis:

1. Intelligent Sensors: The aforementioned wearable biosensors (for biometric data such as systolic and diastolic blood pressure, heart rate, and oxygen saturation) will be utilized to record and store data (in the electronic health record system) with accompanying data analytics which will be of great value for a myriad of clinical scenarios (such as immediate postdischarge follow-up and heart failure medication initiation and titration) (Fig. 58.3) [173,174]. In the medical Internet of things, biological sensors will enable a continual biomedical data repository for data analytics in chronic diseases such as heart failure [175]. The transitional patient will be empowered with a real-life partnership with the medical team in clinical self-care and management of various situations.

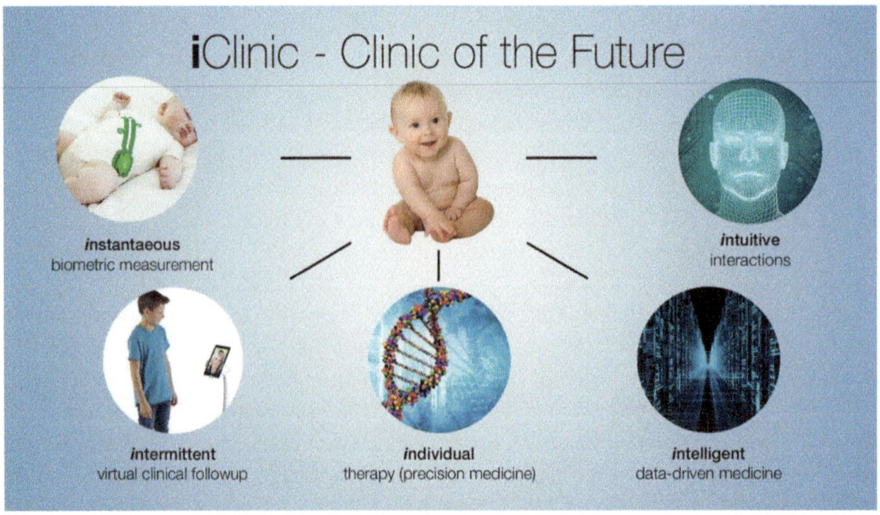

FIGURE 58.2

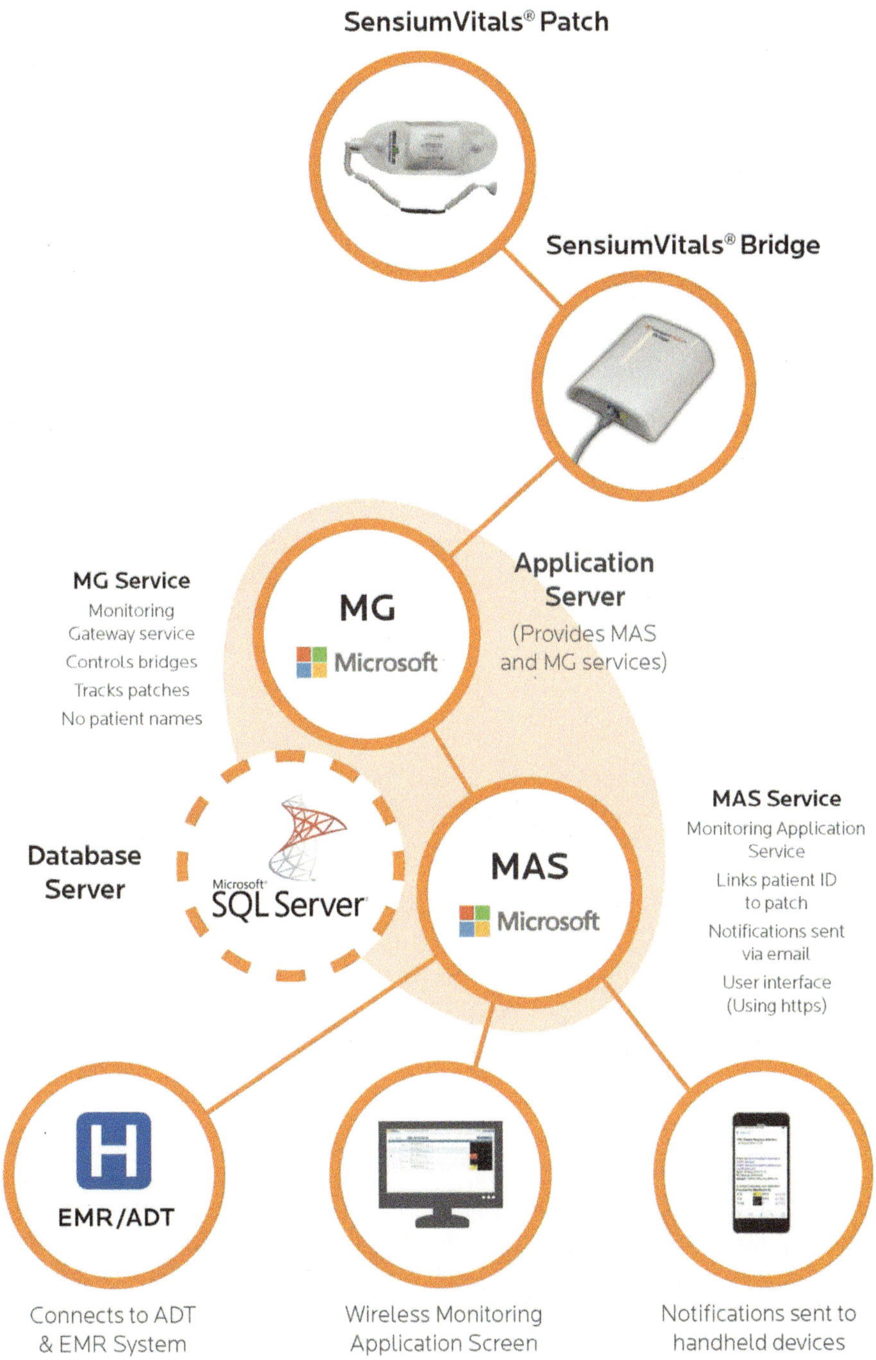

FIGURE 58.3

2. Intelligent Assistant: An artificial intelligence-inspired virtual physician or nurse avatar will be used to function as a health-care assistant to the iClinic families [176]. This capability is a powerful adjunct to telehealth visits as well as wearable technology as the multimedia and empathetic avatars with mapping of physiological signals can add essential patient information to the overall care strategy. While this mode of support is in its infancy, the advent of sophisticated deep learning algorithms will accelerate the capability of such intelligent avatars in the very near future.
3. Intelligent Genomics: Every iClinic transitional patient and immediate family members will have a genomic profile to determine disease genomic subtype for the etiology for heart failure [177]. In addition, these patients will undergo a pharmacogenomic profile to maximize therapeutic benefit while minimizing side effects [178]. The therapy is then individualized since pharmacogenomic testing can identify patients as likely responders or nonresponders as well as

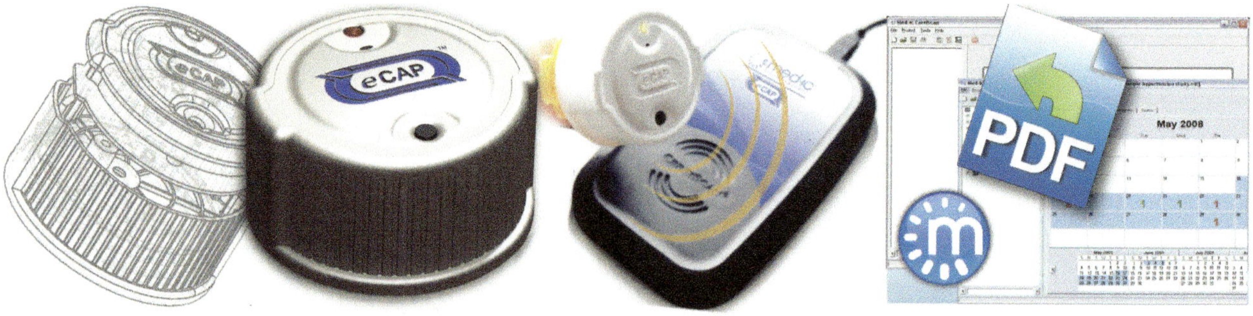

FIGURE 58.4

those who will need a higher or lower dose of the medication(s) [179]. Doses of medications such as beta-blockers, angiotensin-converting enzyme inhibitors, and aldosterone antagonists can be modified on the patient's genetic background. This strategy is particularly relevant to the transitional patients as these patients are usually contemplating their future roles as parents.

4. Intelligent Surveillance: In addition to regular telepresence visits from the medical staff that will increase virtual presence at home, tools such as a medication event monitoring system (eCap) (see Fig. 58.4) will be implemented to increase medication compliance by measuring compliance via an embedded radio-frequency identification (RFID) device without patient input [180]. This smart device can be custom-built with visual or auditory reminders for the transitional patient and family. This type of compliance support is particularly relevant to the transitional patient as compliance in adolescent patients is often suboptimal [181].
5. Intelligent Medicine: The traditional evidence-based medicine in the management of heart failure has served as a basis for therapy for the past few decades [182]. This strategy will need to be replaced with a data-driven and analytics-focused intelligence-based medicine to yield the highest level of intelligent decision-making [183]. Ultimately the clinical decision-making process will be an all-inclusive strategy with comprehensive electronic medical record capture and integration and analysis of clinical, genomic, and molecular information. One such proposal is the BioIntelligence Framework proposed by Farley et al. [184]. In this model, a scalable computational framework leverages a hypergraph-based data model and query language that may be suited for representing complex multilateral, multiscalar, and multidimensional relationships. All of this capability will be particularly useful during transition, as this will be a lifelong clinical strategy based on all of the individual's data.

CONCLUSION

In summary, the optimal care of heart failure patients in the present era is complex, multidisciplinary and multimodal. There are continued learnings from adults with heart failure that can be applied to pediatric patients. However, additional approaches to children and their families will need to be developed that address the unique needs of the pediatric heart failure population.

REFERENCES

[1] V.L. Roger, A.S. Go, D.M. Lloyd-Jones, et al., Heart disease and stroke statistics–2011 update: a report from the American Heart Association, Circulation 123 (2011) e18–e209.

[2] M. Shafazand, M. Schaufelberger, G. Lappas, K. Swedberg, A. Rosengren, Survival trends in men and women with heart failure of ischaemic and non-ischaemic origin: data for the period 1987–2003 from the Swedish Hospital Discharge Registry, Eur. Heart J. 30 (2009) 671–678.

[3] J. Voigt, M. Sasha John, A. Taylor, M. Krucoff, M.R. Reynolds, C. Michael Gibson, A reevaluation of the costs of heart failure and its implications for allocation of health resources in the United States, Clin. Cardiol. 37 (2014) 312–321.

[4] P.A. Heidenreich, N.M. Albert, L.A. Allen, et al., Forecasting the impact of heart failure in the United States: a policy statement from the American Heart Association, Circ. Heart Fail. 6 (2013) 606–619.

[5] A.S. Desai, L.W. Stevenson, Rehospitalization for heart failure: predict or prevent? Circulation 126 (2012) 501–506.

[6] J.W. Rossano, J.J. Kim, J.A. Decker, et al., Prevalence, morbidity, and mortality of heart failure-related hospitalizations in children in the United States: a population-based study, J. Card. Fail. 18 (2012) 459–470.

[7] Effects of enalapril on mortality in severe congestive heart failure. Results of the Cooperative North Scandinavian Enalapril Survival Study (CONSENSUS). The CONSENSUS Trial Study Group, N. Engl. J. Med. 316 (1987) 1429–1435.

[8] Effect of enalapril on mortality and the development of heart failure in asymptomatic patients with reduced left ventricular ejection fractions. The SOLVD Investigators, N. Engl. J. Med. 327 (1992) 685–691.
[9] M.A. Pfeffer, K. Swedberg, C.B. Granger, et al., Effects of candesartan on mortality and morbidity in patients with chronic heart failure: the CHARM-Overall programme, Lancet 362 (2003) 759–766.
[10] Effect of metoprolol CR/XL in chronic heart failure: metoprolol CR/XL randomised intervention trial in congestive heart failure (MERIT-HF), Lancet 353 (1999) 2001–2007.
[11] The cardiac insufficiency Bisoprolol study II (CIBIS-II): a randomised trial, Lancet 353 (1999) 9–13.
[12] M. Packer, M.R. Bristow, J.N. Cohn, et al., The effect of carvedilol on morbidity and mortality in patients with chronic heart failure. U.S. Carvedilol Heart Failure Study Group, N. Engl. J. Med. 334 (1996) 1349–1355.
[13] B. Pitt, F. Zannad, W.J. Remme, et al., The effect of spironolactone on morbidity and mortality in patients with severe heart failure. Randomized Aldactone Evaluation Study Investigators, N. Engl. J. Med. 341 (1999) 709–717.
[14] B. Pitt, W. Remme, F. Zannad, et al., Eplerenone, a selective aldosterone blocker, in patients with left ventricular dysfunction after myocardial infarction, N. Engl. J. Med. 348 (2003) 1309–1321.
[15] J.J. McMurray, M. Packer, A.S. Desai, et al., Angiotensin-neprilysin inhibition versus enalapril in heart failure, N. Engl. J. Med. 371 (2014) 993–1004.
[16] Digitalis Investigation Group, The effect of digoxin on mortality and morbidity in patients with heart failure, N. Engl. J. Med. 336 (1997) 525–533.
[17] K. Swedberg, M. Komajda, M. Bohm, et al., Ivabradine and outcomes in chronic heart failure (SHIFT): a randomised placebo-controlled study, Lancet 376 (2010) 875–885.
[18] A.J. Moss, W. Zareba, W.J. Hall, et al., Prophylactic implantation of a defibrillator in patients with myocardial infarction and reduced ejection fraction, N. Engl. J. Med. 346 (2002) 877–883.
[19] G.H. Bardy, K.L. Lee, D.B. Mark, et al., Amiodarone or an implantable cardioverter-defibrillator for congestive heart failure, N. Engl. J. Med. 352 (2005) 225–237.
[20] M.R. Bristow, L.A. Saxon, J. Boehmer, et al., Cardiac-resynchronization therapy with or without an implantable defibrillator in advanced chronic heart failure, N. Engl. J. Med. 350 (2004) 2140–2150.
[21] J.G. Cleland, J.C. Daubert, E. Erdmann, et al., The effect of cardiac resynchronization on morbidity and mortality in heart failure, N. Engl. J. Med. 352 (2005) 1539–1549.
[22] D. Levy, S. Kenchaiah, M.G. Larson, et al., Long-term trends in the incidence of and survival with heart failure, N. Engl. J. Med. 347 (2002) 1397–1402.
[23] V.L. Roger, S.A. Weston, M.M. Redfield, et al., Trends in heart failure incidence and survival in a community-based population, JAMA 292 (2004) 344–350.
[24] K. MacIntyre, S. Capewell, S. Stewart, et al., Evidence of improving prognosis in heart failure: trends in case fatality in 66 547 patients hospitalized between 1986 and 1995, Circulation 102 (2000) 1126–1131.
[25] S.W. Joffe, K. Webster, D.D. McManus, et al., Improved survival after heart failure: a community-based perspective, J. Am. Heart Assoc. 2 (2013) e000053.
[26] P.S. Jhund, K. Macintyre, C.R. Simpson, et al., Long-term trends in first hospitalization for heart failure and subsequent survival between 1986 and 2003: a population study of 5.1 million people, Circulation 119 (2009) 515–523.
[27] A. Sharma, J.A. Ezekowitz, Similarities and differences in patient characteristics between heart failure registries versus clinical trials, Curr. Heart Fail. Rep. 10 (2013) 373–379.
[28] J.A. Ezekowitz, J. Hu, D. Delgado, et al., Acute heart failure: perspectives from a randomized trial and a simultaneous registry, Circ. Heart Fail. 5 (2012) 735–741.
[29] M. Komajda, P. Lapuerta, N. Hermans, et al., Adherence to guidelines is a predictor of outcome in chronic heart failure: the MAHLER survey, Eur. Heart J. 26 (2005) 1653–1659.
[30] B. Riegel, V.V. Dickson, J. Cameron, et al., Symptom recognition in elders with heart failure, J. Nurs. Scholarsh. 42 (2010) 92–100.
[31] C.M. Cline, A.K. Bjorck-Linne, B.Y. Israelsson, R.B. Willenheimer, L.R. Erhardt, Non-compliance and knowledge of prescribed medication in elderly patients with heart failure, Eur. J. Heart Fail. 1 (1999) 145–149.
[32] A. Rogers, J.M. Addington-Hall, A.S. McCoy, et al., A qualitative study of chronic heart failure patients' understanding of their symptoms and drug therapy, Eur. J. Heart Fail. 4 (2002) 283–287.
[33] C.R. Horowitz, S.B. Rein, H. Leventhal, A story of maladies, misconceptions and mishaps: effective management of heart failure, Soc. Sci. Med. 58 (2004) 631–643.
[34] A. Stromberg, The crucial role of patient education in heart failure, Eur. J. Heart Fail. 7 (2005) 363–369.
[35] J. Barlow, C. Wright, J. Sheasby, A. Turner, J. Hainsworth, Self-management approaches for people with chronic conditions: a review, Patient Educ. Couns. 48 (2002) 177–187.
[36] B. Riegel, V.V. Dickson, A situation-specific theory of heart failure self-care, J. Cardiovasc. Nurs. 23 (2008) 190–196.
[37] K.L. Mickley, P.V. Burkhart, A.N. Sigler, Promoting normal development and self-efficacy in school-age children managing chronic conditions, Nurs. Clin. N. Am. 48 (2013) 319–328.
[38] B. Riegel, C.S. Lee, V.V. Dickson, Medscape, Self care in patients with chronic heart failure, Nat. Rev. Cardiol. 8 (2011) 644–654.
[39] T. Jaarsma, A. Stromberg, J. Martensson, K. Dracup, Development and testing of the European heart failure self-care behaviour scale, Eur. J. Heart Fail. 5 (2003) 363–370.
[40] T. Jaarsma, K.F. Arestedt, J. Martensson, K. Dracup, A. Stromberg, The European heart failure self-care behaviour scale revised into a nine-item scale (EHFScB-9): a reliable and valid international instrument, Eur. J. Heart Fail. 11 (2009) 99–105.

[41] B. Riegel, B. Carlson, D.K. Moser, M. Sebern, F.D. Hicks, V. Roland, Psychometric testing of the self-care of heart failure index, J. Card. Fail. 10 (2004) 350–360.

[42] B. Riegel, C.S. Lee, V.V. Dickson, B. Carlson, An update on the self-care of heart failure index, J. Cardiovasc. Nurs. 24 (2009) 485–497.

[43] C. Shuldham, C. Theaker, T. Jaarsma, M.R. Cowie, Evaluation of the European heart failure self-care behaviour scale in a United Kingdom population, J. Adv. Nurs. 60 (2007) 87–95.

[44] D.S. Yu, D.T. Lee, D.R. Thompson, T. Jaarsma, J. Woo, E.M. Leung, Psychometric properties of the Chinese version of the European heart failure self-care behaviour scale, Int. J. Nurs. Stud. 48 (2011) 458–467.

[45] B. Riegel, A. Driscoll, J. Suwanno, et al., Heart failure self-care in developed and developing countries, J. Card. Fail. 15 (2009) 508–516.

[46] X. Kang, C.R. Dennison Himmelfarb, Z. Li, J. Zhang, R. Lv, J. Guo, Construct validity of the Chinese version of the self-care of heart failure index determined using structural equation modeling, J. Cardiovasc. Nurs. 30 (2015) 222–228.

[47] C. Stille, R.M. Turchi, R. Antonelli, et al., The family-centered medical home: specific considerations for child health research and policy, Acad. Pediatr. 10 (2010) 211–217.

[48] B.H. Fiese, A.J. Sameroff, Family context in pediatric psychology: a transactional perspective, J. Pediatr. Psychol. 14 (1989) 293–314.

[49] C.B. Forrest, L. Simpson, C. Clancy, Child health services research. Challenges and opportunities, JAMA 277 (1997) 1787–1793.

[50] D.A. Ellis, C.L. Podolski, M. Frey, S. Naar-King, B. Wang, K. Moltz, The role of parental monitoring in adolescent health outcomes: impact on regimen adherence in youth with type 1 diabetes, J. Pediatr. Psychol. 32 (2007) 907–917.

[51] B. Reed-Knight, J.D. Lewis, R.L. Blount, Association of disease, adolescent, and family factors with medication adherence in pediatric inflammatory bowel disease, J. Pediatr. Psychol. 36 (2011) 308–317.

[52] T. Wysocki, T.R. Nansel, G.N. Holmbeck, et al., Collaborative involvement of primary and secondary caregivers: associations with youths' diabetes outcomes, J. Pediatr. Psychol. 34 (2009) 869–881.

[53] D. Eckshtain, D.A. Ellis, K. Kolmodin, S. Naar-King, The effects of parental depression and parenting practices on depressive symptoms and metabolic control in urban youth with insulin dependent diabetes, J. Pediatr. Psychol. 35 (2010) 426–435.

[54] A. Hazzard, S.J. Hutchinson, N. Krawiecki, Factors related to adherence to medication regimens in pediatric seizure patients, J. Pediatr. Psychol. 15 (1990) 543–555.

[55] J.K. Orrell-Valente, M.D. Cabana, 'The apple doesn't fall far from the tree': the role of parents in chronic disease self-management, Curr. Opin. Pediatr. 20 (2008) 703–704.

[56] A.C. Modi, A.L. Pai, K.A. Hommel, et al., Pediatric self-management: a framework for research, practice, and policy, Pediatrics 129 (2012) e473–e485.

[57] B. Riegel, C.S. Lee, N. Albert, et al., From novice to expert: confidence and activity status determine heart failure self-care performance, Nurs. Res. 60 (2011) 132–138.

[58] J.E. Zavertnik, Self-care in older adults with heart failure: an integrative review, Clin. Nurse Spec. 28 (2014) 19–32.

[59] N.T. Artinian, M. Magnan, M. Sloan, M.P. Lange, Self-care behaviors among patients with heart failure, Heart Lung 31 (2002) 161–172.

[60] P.M. Chriss, J. Sheposh, B. Carlson, B. Riegel, Predictors of successful heart failure self-care maintenance in the first three months after hospitalization, Heart Lung 33 (2004) 345–353.

[61] B. Riegel, V.V. Dickson, L. Kuhn, K. Page, L. Worrall-Carter, Gender-specific barriers and facilitators to heart failure self-care: a mixed methods study, Int. J. Nurs. Stud. 47 (2010) 888–895.

[62] S. Heo, D.K. Moser, T.A. Lennie, B. Riegel, M.L. Chung, Gender differences in and factors related to self-care behaviors: a cross-sectional, correlational study of patients with heart failure, Int. J. Nurs. Stud. 45 (2008) 1807–1815.

[63] M. Holst, R. Willenheimer, J. Martensson, M. Lindholm, A. Stromberg, Telephone follow-up of self-care behaviour after a single session education of patients with heart failure in primary health care, Eur. J. Cardiovasc. Nurs. 6 (2007) 153–159.

[64] C.S. Lee, B. Riegel, A. Driscoll, et al., Gender differences in heart failure self-care: a multinational cross-sectional study, Int. J. Nurs. Stud. 46 (2009) 1485–1495.

[65] H. Ni, D. Nauman, D. Burgess, K. Wise, K. Crispell, R.E. Hershberger, Factors influencing knowledge of and adherence to self-care among patients with heart failure, Arch. Intern. Med. 159 (1999) 1613–1619.

[66] N.V. Sneed, S.C. Paul, Readiness for behavioral changes in patients with heart failure, Am. J. Crit. Care 12 (2003) 444–453.

[67] G.C. Fonarow, W.T. Abraham, N.M. Albert, et al., Association between performance measures and clinical outcomes for patients hospitalized with heart failure, JAMA 297 (2007) 61–70.

[68] M.E. Patterson, A.F. Hernandez, B.G. Hammill, et al., Process of care performance measures and long-term outcomes in patients hospitalized with heart failure, Med. Care 48 (2010) 210–216.

[69] B. Riegel, B. Carlson, Facilitators and barriers to heart failure self-care, Patient Educ. Couns. 46 (2002) 287–295.

[70] V.V. Dickson, H. Buck, B. Riegel, A qualitative meta-analysis of heart failure self-care practices among individuals with multiple comorbid conditions, J. Card. Fail. 17 (2011) 413–419.

[71] C.Y. Jurgens, Somatic awareness, uncertainty, and delay in care-seeking in acute heart failure, Res. Nurs. Health 29 (2006) 74–86.

[72] B. Carlson, B. Riegel, D.K. Moser, Self-care abilities of patients with heart failure, Heart Lung 30 (2001) 351–359.

[73] V.V. Dickson, B. Riegel, Are we teaching what patients need to know? Building skills in heart failure self-care, Heart Lung 38 (2009) 253–261.

[74] A. Macabasco-O'Connell, D.A. DeWalt, K.A. Broucksou, et al., Relationship between literacy, knowledge, self-care behaviors, and heart failure-related quality of life among patients with heart failure, J. Gen. Intern. Med. 26 (2011) 979–986.

[75] M.D. Murray, W. Tu, J. Wu, D. Morrow, F. Smith, D.C. Brater, Factors associated with exacerbation of heart failure include treatment adherence and health literacy skills, Clin. Pharmacol. Ther. 85 (2009) 651–658.

[76] K.E. Freedland, M.W. Rich, J.A. Skala, R.M. Carney, V.G. Davila-Roman, A.S. Jaffe, Prevalence of depression in hospitalized patients with congestive heart failure, Psychosom. Med. 65 (2003) 119–128.

[77] S.J. Pressler, Cognitive functioning and chronic heart failure: a review of the literature (2002–July 2007), J. Cardiovasc. Nurs. 23 (2008) 239–249.

[78] S.J. Pressler, U. Subramanian, D. Kareken, et al., Cognitive deficits in chronic heart failure, Nurs. Res. 59 (2010) 127–139.

[79] F.S. Luyster, J.W. Hughes, J. Gunstad, Depression and anxiety symptoms are associated with reduced dietary adherence in heart failure patients treated with an implantable cardioverter defibrillator, J. Cardiovasc. Nurs. 24 (2009) 10–17.

[80] M.R. DiMatteo, Variations in patients' adherence to medical recommendations: a quantitative review of 50 years of research, Med. Care 42 (2004) 200–209.

[81] N. Holzapfel, B. Lowe, B. Wild, et al., Self-care and depression in patients with chronic heart failure, Heart Lung 38 (2009) 392–397.

[82] R.A. Hansen, S.B. Dusetzina, L. Song, B.N. Gaynes, W. Tu, M.D. Murray, Depression affects adherence measurement but not the effectiveness of an adherence intervention in heart failure patients, J. Am. Pharm. Assoc. 2009 (49) (2003) 760–768.

[83] D.K. Moser, P.L. Worster, Effect of psychosocial factors on physiologic outcomes in patients with heart failure, J. Cardiovasc. Nurs. 14 (2000) 106–115.

[84] J. Cameron, L. Worrall-Carter, B. Riegel, S.K. Lo, S. Stewart, Testing a model of patient characteristics, psychologic status, and cognitive function as predictors of self-care in persons with chronic heart failure, Heart Lung 38 (2009) 410–418.

[85] A.A. Schiffer, J. Denollet, J.W. Widdershoven, E.H. Hendriks, O.R. Smith, Failure to consult for symptoms of heart failure in patients with a type-D personality, Heart 93 (2007) 814–818.

[86] V.V. Dickson, N. Tkacs, B. Riegel, Cognitive influences on self-care decision making in persons with heart failure, Am. Heart J. 154 (2007) 424–431.

[87] V.V. Dickson, J.A. Deatrick, B. Riegel, A typology of heart failure self-care management in non-elders, Eur. J. Cardiovasc. Nurs. 7 (2008) 171–181.

[88] K. Harkness, G.A. Heckman, N. Akhtar-Danesh, C. Demers, E. Gunn, R.S. McKelvie, Cognitive function and self-care management in older patients with heart failure, Eur. J. Cardiovasc. Nurs. 13 (2014) 277–284.

[89] J. Cameron, L. Worrall-Carter, K. Page, B. Riegel, S.K. Lo, S. Stewart, Does cognitive impairment predict poor self-care in patients with heart failure? Eur. J. Heart Fail. 12 (2010) 508–515.

[90] B. Riegel, V. Vaughan Dickson, L.R. Goldberg, J.A. Deatrick, Factors associated with the development of expertise in heart failure self-care, Nurs. Res. 56 (2007) 235–243.

[91] B. Riegel, S.T. Moelter, S.J. Ratcliffe, et al., Excessive daytime sleepiness is associated with poor medication adherence in adults with heart failure, J. Card. Fail. 17 (2011) 340–348.

[92] J.M. Rockwell, B. Riegel, Predictors of self-care in persons with heart failure, Heart Lung 30 (2001) 18–25.

[93] K.E. Joynt, D.J. Whellan, C.M. O'Connor, Why is depression bad for the failing heart? A review of the mechanistic relationship between depression and heart failure, J. Card. Fail. 10 (2004) 258–271.

[94] R. Gallagher, M.L. Luttik, T. Jaarsma, Social support and self-care in heart failure, J. Cardiovasc. Nurs. 26 (2011) 439–445.

[95] J.R. Wu, D.K. Moser, M.L. Chung, T.A. Lennie, Predictors of medication adherence using a multidimensional adherence model in patients with heart failure, J. Card. Fail. 14 (2008) 603–614.

[96] M.R. DiMatteo, Social support and patient adherence to medical treatment: a meta-analysis, Health Psychol. 23 (2004) 207–218.

[97] M.J. Rohrbaugh, V. Shoham, J.C. Coyne, J.A. Cranford, J.S. Sonnega, J.M. Nicklas, Beyond the "self" in self-efficacy: spouse confidence predicts patient survival following heart failure, J. Fam. Psychol. 18 (2004) 184–193.

[98] V.V.W.-C.L. Dickson, L. Kuhn, B. Riegel, Whose job is it? Gender differences in perceived role in heart failure self-care, J. Nurs. Healthc. Chronic Illn. 3 (2011) 99–108.

[99] V. Hemls, V. Gabor, P. Sloyer, K. VanLandeghem, Developing structure and process standards for systems of care serving children and youth with special health care needs, Washington, DC, in: National Consensus Framework for Systems of Care for Children and Youth with Special Health Care Needs Project, March 14, 2014.

[100] S.L. Porterfield, L. DeRigne, Medical home and out-of-pocket medical costs for children with special health care needs, Pediatrics 128 (2011) 892–900.

[101] K. Kuhlthau, K.S. Hill, R. Yucel, J.M. Perrin, Financial burden for families of children with special health care needs, Matern. Child Health J. 9 (2005) 207–218.

[102] Health Affordable Coverage Hearing. Energy and Commerce Committee, Subcomittee on Health, Energy and Commerce Committee, Washington, DC, 2009.

[103] Council on Children with Disabilities, Medical Home Implementation Project Advisory Committee, Patient- and family-centered care coordination: a framework for integrating care for children and youth across multiple systems, Pediatrics 133 (2014) e1451–e1460.

[104] J.W. McAllister, Achieving a Shared Plan of Care with Children and Youth with Special Health Care Needs: An Implementation Guide, Palo Alto, CA, 2014.

[105] M.H. van der Wal, D.J. van Veldhuisen, N.J. Veeger, F.H. Rutten, T. Jaarsma, Compliance with non-pharmacological recommendations and outcome in heart failure patients, Eur. Heart J. 31 (2010) 1486–1493.

[106] B.B. Granger, K. Swedberg, I. Ekman, et al., Adherence to candesartan and placebo and outcomes in chronic heart failure in the CHARM programme: double-blind, randomised, controlled clinical trial, Lancet 366 (2005) 2005–2011.

[107] T. Rutledge, V.A. Reis, S.E. Linke, B.H. Greenberg, P.J. Mills, Depression in heart failure a meta-analytic review of prevalence, intervention effects, and associations with clinical outcomes, J. Am. Coll. Cardiol. 48 (2006) 1527–1537.

[108] C.S. Lee, D.K. Moser, T.A. Lennie, B. Riegel, Event-free survival in adults with heart failure who engage in self-care management, Heart Lung 40 (2011) 12–20.

[109] C.S. Lee, D.K. Moser, T.A. Lennie, N.C. Tkacs, K.B. Margulies, B. Riegel, Biomarkers of myocardial stress and systemic inflammation in patients who engage in heart failure self-care management, J. Cardiovasc. Nurs. 26 (2011) 321–328.

[110] L.D. Rathman, C.S. Lee, S. Sarkar, R.S. Small, A critical link between heart failure self-care and intrathoracic impedance, J. Cardiovasc. Nurs. 26 (2011) E20–E26.

[111] F.A. McAlister, S. Stewart, S. Ferrua, J.J. McMurray, Multidisciplinary strategies for the management of heart failure patients at high risk for admission: a systematic review of randomized trials, J. Am. Coll. Cardiol. 44 (2004) 810–819.

[112] A. Jovicic, J.M. Holroyd-Leduc, S.E. Straus, Effects of self-management intervention on health outcomes of patients with heart failure: a systematic review of randomized controlled trials, BMC Cardiovasc. Disord. 6 (2006) 43.

[113] J.B. Ditewig, H. Blok, J. Havers, H. van Veenendaal, Effectiveness of self-management interventions on mortality, hospital readmissions, chronic heart failure hospitalization rate and quality of life in patients with chronic heart failure: a systematic review, Patient Educ. Couns. 78 (2010) 297–315.

[114] G.H. Gislason, J.N. Rasmussen, S.Z. Abildstrom, et al., Persistent use of evidence-based pharmacotherapy in heart failure is associated with improved outcomes, Circulation 116 (2007) 737–744.

[115] G.J. Molloy, C. Gao, D.W. Johnston, et al., Adherence to angiotensin-converting-enzyme inhibitors and illness beliefs in older heart failure patients, Eur. J. Heart Fail. 11 (2009) 715–720.

[116] S.J. Bennett, L.M. Hays, J.L. Embree, M. Arnould, Heart Messages: a tailored message intervention for improving heart failure outcomes, J. Cardiovasc. Nurs. 14 (2000) 94–105.

[117] V. Ivanovska, C.M. Rademaker, L. van Dijk, A.K. Mantel-Teeuwisse, Pediatric drug formulations: a review of challenges and progress, Pediatrics 134 (2014) 361–372.

[118] R.A. Clark, S.C. Inglis, F.A. McAlister, J.G. Cleland, S. Stewart, Telemonitoring or structured telephone support programmes for patients with chronic heart failure: systematic review and meta-analysis, BMJ 334 (2007) 942.

[119] S. Inglis, Structured telephone support or telemonitoring programmes for patients with chronic heart failure, J. Evid. Based Med. 3 (2010) 228.

[120] S.C. Inglis, R.A. Clark, R. Dierckx, D. Prieto-Merino, J.G. Cleland, Structured telephone support or non-invasive telemonitoring for patients with heart failure, Cochrane Database Syst. Rev. (2015) CD007228.

[121] R.E. Blaine, L. Pbert, A.C. Geller, E.M. Powers, K. Mitchell, Parent preferences for telephone coaching to prevent and manage childhood obesity, Postgrad. Med. J. 91 (2015) 206–211.

[122] L.M. Swerczek, C. Banister, G.R. Bloomberg, et al., A telephone coaching intervention to improve asthma self-management behaviors, Pediatr. Nurs. 39 (2013) 125–130 45.

[123] S.D. Anker, F. Koehler, W.T. Abraham, Telemedicine and remote management of patients with heart failure, Lancet 378 (2011) 731–739.

[124] A. Maisel, D. Barnard, B. Jaski, et al., Primary results of the HABIT Trial (heart failure assessment with BNP in the home), J. Am. Coll. Cardiol. 61 (2013) 1726–1735.

[125] J. Zhang, K.M. Goode, P.E. Cuddihy, J.G. Cleland, T.-H. Investigators, Predicting hospitalization due to worsening heart failure using daily weight measurement: analysis of the Trans-European Network-Home-Care Management System (TEN-HMS) study, Eur. J. Heart Fail. 11 (2009) 420–427.

[126] P.B. Adamson, A.L. Smith, W.T. Abraham, et al., Continuous autonomic assessment in patients with symptomatic heart failure: prognostic value of heart rate variability measured by an implanted cardiac resynchronization device, Circulation 110 (2004) 2389–2394.

[127] C.M. Yu, L. Wang, E. Chau, et al., Intrathoracic impedance monitoring in patients with heart failure: correlation with fluid status and feasibility of early warning preceding hospitalization, Circulation 112 (2005) 841–848.

[128] R.S. Small, W. Wickemeyer, R. Germany, et al., Changes in intrathoracic impedance are associated with subsequent risk of hospitalizations for acute decompensated heart failure: clinical utility of implanted device monitoring without a patient alert, J. Card. Fail. 15 (2009) 475–481.

[129] W.T. Abraham, S. Compton, G. Haas, et al., Intrathoracic impedance vs daily weight monitoring for predicting worsening heart failure events: results of the Fluid Accumulation Status Trial (FAST), Congest. Heart Fail. 17 (2011) 51–55.

[130] D.J. Whellan, K.T. Ousdigian, S.M. Al-Khatib, et al., Combined heart failure device diagnostics identify patients at higher risk of subsequent heart failure hospitalizations: results from PARTNERS HF (Program to Access and Review Trending Information and Evaluate Correlation to Symptoms in Patients with Heart Failure) study, J. Am. Coll. Cardiol. 55 (2010) 1803–1810.

[131] V.M. Conraads, L. Tavazzi, M. Santini, et al., Sensitivity and positive predictive value of implantable intrathoracic impedance monitoring as a predictor of heart failure hospitalizations: the SENSE-HF trial, Eur. Heart J. 32 (2011) 2266–2273.

[132] D.J. van Veldhuisen, F. Braunschweig, V. Conraads, et al., Intrathoracic impedance monitoring, audible patient alerts, and outcome in patients with heart failure, Circulation 124 (2011) 1719–1726.

[133] R.C. Bourge, W.T. Abraham, P.B. Adamson, et al., Randomized controlled trial of an implantable continuous hemodynamic monitor in patients with advanced heart failure: the COMPASS-HF study, J. Am. Coll. Cardiol. 51 (2008) 1073–1079.

[134] J. Ritzema, R. Troughton, I. Melton, et al., Physician-directed patient self-management of left atrial pressure in advanced chronic heart failure, Circulation 121 (2010) 1086–1095.

[135] M.S. Maurer, P.B. Adamson, M.R. Costanzo, et al., Rationale and design of the Left Atrial Pressure Monitoring to Optimize Heart Failure Therapy Study (LAPTOP-HF), J. Card. Fail. 21 (2015) 479–488.

[136] W.T. Abraham, P.B. Adamson, R.C. Bourge, et al., Wireless pulmonary artery haemodynamic monitoring in chronic heart failure: a randomised controlled trial, Lancet 377 (2011) 658–666.

[137] S.M. Gilboa, O.J. Devine, J.E. Kucik, et al., Congenital heart defects in the United States: estimating the magnitude of the affected population in 2010, Circulation 134 (2016) 101–109.

[138] E.D. Cox, K.A. Fritz, K.W. Hansen, et al., Development and validation of PRISM: a survey tool to identify diabetes self-management barriers, Diabetes Res. Clin. Pract. 104 (2014) 126–135.

[139] K.A. Hommel, R.N. Greenley, M.H. Maddux, W.N. Gray, L.M. Mackner, Self-management in pediatric inflammatory bowel disease: a clinical report of the North American Society for pediatric gastroenterology, hepatology, and nutrition, J. Pediatr. Gastroenterol. Nutr. 57 (2013) 250–257.

[140] E.A. Steinberg, M. Moss, C.L. Buchanan, J. Goebel, Adherence in pediatric kidney transplant recipients: solutions for the system, Pediatr. Nephrol. (2017).

[141] Control NCfHSatCfD. National Survey of Children with Special Health Care Needs, Bureau MaCH, Data Resource Center for Child & Adolescent Health, 2010.

[142] J.M. Perrin, C.F. Fluet, L. Honberg, et al., Benefits for employees with children with special needs: findings from the collaborative employee benefit study, Health Aff. (Millwood) 26 (2007) 1096–1103.

[143] Programs AoMCH, Standards for Systems of Care for CYSHCN, Version 2.0, Association of Maternal & Child Health Programs and the National Academy for State Health Policy, 2017.

[144] J.L. Raphael, W.C. Cooley, A. Vega, et al., Outcomes for children with chronic conditions associated with parent- and provider-reported measures of the medical home, J. Health Care Poor Underserved 26 (2015) 358–376.

[145] J.E. Miller, C.N. Nugent, L.B. Russell, Which components of medical homes reduce the time burden on families of children with special health care needs? Health Serv. Res. 50 (2015) 440–461.

[146] A.A. Boudreau, J.M. Perrin, E. Goodman, D. Kurowski, W.C. Cooley, K. Kuhlthau, Care coordination and unmet specialty care among children with special health care needs, Pediatrics 133 (2014) 1046–1053.

[147] R.A. Mosquera, E.B. Avritscher, C.L. Samuels, et al., Effect of an enhanced medical home on serious illness and cost of care among high-risk children with chronic illness: a randomized clinical trial, JAMA 312 (2014) 2640–2648.

[148] American Academy of Family Physicians AAoP, American College of Physicians, American Osteopathic Association, Joint Principles of the Patient-Centered Medical Home 2007, March 7, 2007.

[149] Physicians ACoE, The Patient-Centered Medical Home Model. Clinical and Practice Management 2015, April 2015.

[150] J. Van Cleave, M.J. Okumura, N. Swigonski, K.G. O'Connor, M. Mann, J.L. Lail, Medical homes for children with special health care needs: primary care or subspecialty service? Acad. Pediatr. 16 (2016) 366–372.

[151] NCQA, 2017. Available from: http://www.ncqa.org/programs/recognition/practices/patient-centered-specialty-practice-pcsp.

[152] A. Goudie, S. Havercamp, B. Jamieson, T. Sahr, Assessing functional impairment in siblings living with children with disability, Pediatrics 132 (2013) e476–e483.

[153] M. Herzer, N. Godiwala, K.A. Hommel, et al., Family functioning in the context of pediatric chronic conditions, J. Dev. Behav. Pediatr. 31 (2010) 26–34.

[154] C. Dell Clark, in: Sickness and in Play: Children Coping with Chronic Illness, 2003.

[155] L.M. Ingerski, K. Shaw, W.N. Gray, D.M. Janicke, A pilot study comparing traumatic stress symptoms by child and parent report across pediatric chronic illness groups, J. Dev. Behav. Pediatr. 31 (2010) 713–719.

[156] S.G. Rice, American Academy of Pediatrics Council on Sports M, Fitness, Medical conditions affecting sports participation, Pediatrics 121 (2008) 841–848.

[157] T. Bodenheimer, E.H. Wagner, K. Grumbach, Improving primary care for patients with chronic illness, JAMA 288 (2002) 1775–1779.

[158] J.S. Adams, E.R. Woods, Redesign of chronic illness care in children and adolescents: evidence for the chronic care model, Curr. Opin. Pediatr. 28 (2016) 428–433.

[159] K. Coleman, B.T. Austin, C. Brach, E.H. Wagner, Evidence on the chronic care model in the new millennium, Health Aff. (Millwood) 28 (2009) 75–85.

[160] The Chronic Care Model. Available from: http://www.improvingchroniccare.org/index.php?p=The_Chronic_Care_Model&s=2.

[161] R. Nuno, K. Coleman, R. Bengoa, R. Sauto, Integrated care for chronic conditions: the contribution of the ICCC Framework, Health Policy 105 (2012) 55–64.

[162] J. Lail, P.J. Schoettker, D.L. White, B. Mehta, U.R. Kotagal, Applying the chronic care model to improve care and outcomes at a Pediatric Medical Center, Jt. Comm. J. Qual. Patient Saf. 43 (2017) 101–112.

[163] H. Stam, E.E. Hartman, J.A. Deurloo, J. Groothoff, M.A. Grootenhuis, Young adult patients with a history of pediatric disease: impact on course of life and transition into adulthood, J. Adolesc. Health 39 (2006) 4–13.

[164] American Academy of Pediatrics, American Academy of Family Physicians, American College of Physicians, Transitions Clinical Report Authoring Group, W.C. Cooley, P.J. Sagerman, Supporting the health care transition from adolescence to adulthood in the medical home, Pediatrics 128 (2011) 182–200.

[165] A. Diaz, H. Fox, M. McManus, K.G. O'Connor, J.D. Klein, Screening Adolescents for High Risk Behaviors: A National Survey, Pediatrics AAo, 2010.

[166] C. Sable, E. Foster, K. Uzark, et al., Best practices in managing transition to adulthood for adolescents with congenital heart disease: the transition process and medical and psychosocial issues: a scientific statement from the American Heart Association, Circulation 123 (2011) 1454–1485.

[167] National Alliance to Advance Adolescent Health CfHCTI. Six Core Elements of Health Care Transition 2.0, 2014.

[168] R. Roccaforte, C. Demers, F. Baldassarre, K.K. Teo, S. Yusuf, Effectiveness of comprehensive disease management programmes in improving clinical outcomes in heart failure patients. A meta-analysis, Eur. J. Heart Fail. 7 (2005) 1133–1144.

[169] A. Darkins, P. Ryan, R. Kobb, et al., Care coordination/home telehealth: the systematic implementation of health informatics, home telehealth, and disease management to support the care of veteran patients with chronic conditions, Telemed. J. E Health 14 (2008) 1118–1126.

[170] I.K. Everitt, J.F. Gerardin, F.H. Rodriguez 3rd, W.M. Book, Improving the quality of transition and transfer of care in young adults with congenital heart disease, Congenit. Heart Dis. 12 (2017) 242–250.

[171] A. Lee, B. Bailey, G. Cullen-Dean, S. Aiello, J. Morin, E. Oechslin, Transition of care in congenital heart disease: ensuring the proper handoff, Curr. Cardiol. Rep. 19 (2017) 55.

[172] J. Nicolarsen, Transition of adolescents and young adults with congenital heart disease: challenges, progress, and future improvements, Pediatr. Ann. 46 (2017) e224–e228.

[173] A.R. Forkan, I. Khalil, A clinical decision-making mechanism for context-aware and patient-specific remote monitoring systems using the correlations of multiple vital signs, Comput. Methods Progr. Biomed. 139 (2017) 1–16.

[174] Sensium, Early Detection of Patient Deterioration, Sensium, 2016.

[175] Z. Yang, Q. Zhou, L. Lei, K. Zheng, W. Xiang, An IoT-cloud based wearable ECG monitoring system for smart healthcare, J. Med. Syst. 40 (2016) 286.

[176] C. Lisetti, F. Nasoz, C. LeRouge, O. Ozyer, K. Alvarez, Developing multimodal intelligent affective interfaces for tele-home health care, Int. J. Hum. Comput. Stud. 59 (2003) 245–255.

[177] K. Dadson, L. Hauck, F. Billia, Molecular mechanisms in cardiomyopathy, Clin. Sci. (Lond.) 131 (2017) 1375–1392.

[178] C. Krittanawong, T. Kitai, Pharmacogenomics of angiotensin-receptor/neprilysin inhibitor and its long-term side effects, Cardiovasc. Ther. (2017).

[179] T.P. Cappola, G.W. Dorn 2nd, Clinical considerations of heritable factors in common heart failure, Circ. Cardiovasc. Genet. 4 (2011) 701–709.

[180] ECAP Smart Bottle Now Available for Liquid Dosing. Information Mediary Corporation (IMC) and Affiliates, 2015, 2017.

[181] V.S. Conn, T.M. Ruppar, M. Enriquez, P. Cooper, Medication adherence interventions that target subjects with adherence problems: systematic review and meta-analysis, Res. Soc. Adm. Pharm. 12 (2016) 218–246.

[182] R. Ghany, L. Tamariz, G. Chen, et al., Screening echocardiograms in a senior focused value based primary care improves systolic heart failure detection and clinical management, Cardiovasc. Diagn. Ther. 7 (2017) 236–243.

[183] B.J. Mortazavi, N.S. Downing, E.M. Bucholz, et al., Analysis of machine learning techniques for heart failure readmissions, Circ. Cardiovasc. Qual. Outcomes 9 (2016) 629–640.

[184] T. Farley, J. Kiefer, P. Lee, et al., The BioIntelligence framework: a new computational platform for biomedical knowledge computing, J. Am. Med. Inform. Assoc. 20 (2013) 128–133.

Chapter 59

Regenerative Medicine/Injured Human Hearts

James T. Willerson
The Texas Heart Institute, Houston, TX, United States

In human development, the fertilized egg gives rise to stem cells, which generate the body's organs and play an important role in forming the appearance, intellect, and uniqueness of each person. Tissues and organs, including the heart, have a rescue system of circulating stem cells and resident stem cells that is intended to repair injuries, such as those caused by heart attacks and strokes. Although this elegant rescue system is critical for sustaining human development and health, the function of stem cells can be limited, and their potential in clinical medicine has not yet been fully explored.

Beyond approximately 2 weeks of life, the mouse heart can no longer regenerate after severe injury [1,2]. This results, at least in part, from the expression of genes in the Hippo pathway, an ancient signaling pathway that controls organ size. The Hippo pathway is a kinase cascade that inhibits the proliferation of developing cardiomyocytes [1]. Dr. James Martin and his team at the Texas Heart Institute have shown that unstressed, Hippo-deficient adult mouse cardiomyocytes reenter the cell cycle and undergo cytokinesis [3]. Hippo deficiency enhances cardiomyocyte regeneration and promotes functional recovery in mice after experimentally induced myocardial infarction (MI) and after postnatal day 8 cardiac apex resection (Fig. 59.1) [4]. In damaged mouse hearts, the proliferation of Hippo mutant cardiomyocytes is elevated, which may explain the heart's inability to regenerate itself after injury beyond 2 weeks of life [2]. In a study by Heallen et al. [3], Hippo signaling was shown to be an endogenous repressor of adult cardiomyocyte renewal and regeneration. Therefore, inhibiting the expression of the Hippo pathway genes in injured human hearts may conceivably have beneficial effects, and studies to evaluate this possibility are being planned.

Clinical studies of stem cell therapy in patients with ischemic cardiomyopathy have shown that human mesenchymal stem cells become increasingly dysfunctional with age [4–6]. At approximately 60 years of age, the ability of human mesenchymal stem cells to replicate is reduced [4,5]. Likewise, the number of stem cells in the bone marrow and circulation is reduced in older individuals [4,6]. The number and effectiveness of bone marrow–derived and circulating stem cells are also reduced in patients with disease and risk factors for cardiovascular disease [7–9]. Therefore, the stem cells in older individuals and patients with severe disease may be unable to repair damage to the hearts, even though the hearts of these individuals are often the ones most in need of repair.

Another potentially important limitation of autologous stem cell therapy is that the composition of the transplanted cell product (i.e., the cellular phenotypes) is often different for each patient because of the inherent heterogeneity of the products isolated from each patient. This probably contributes to the variation observed in the clinical outcomes of stem cell therapy recipients. These are critical issues to consider when designing, implementing, and interpreting the results of any stem cell therapy trial involving patients with cardiovascular disease.

Patients in clinical studies of stem cell therapy are often older, with multiple comorbidities and, frequently, stem cells of reduced potency. However, study findings support that allogeneic mesenchymal cells harvested from the bone marrow or adipose tissue of healthy individuals may be used to treat older patients with ischemic cardiomyopathy and heart failure, thereby improving the mechanical function of the heart and, importantly, reducing the risk of future clinical events [8–10].

RESTORATION OF POTENCY TO AGED MOUSE CELLS IN VITRO AND IN VIVO

The overexpression of myocardin and telomerase has potential as a mechanism for promoting cardiac recovery. Madonna et al. [11] examined this potential by first evaluating the survival, growth, and myogenic differentiation of

Heart Failure in the Child and Young Adult. http://dx.doi.org/10.1016/B978-0-12-802393-8.00059-4

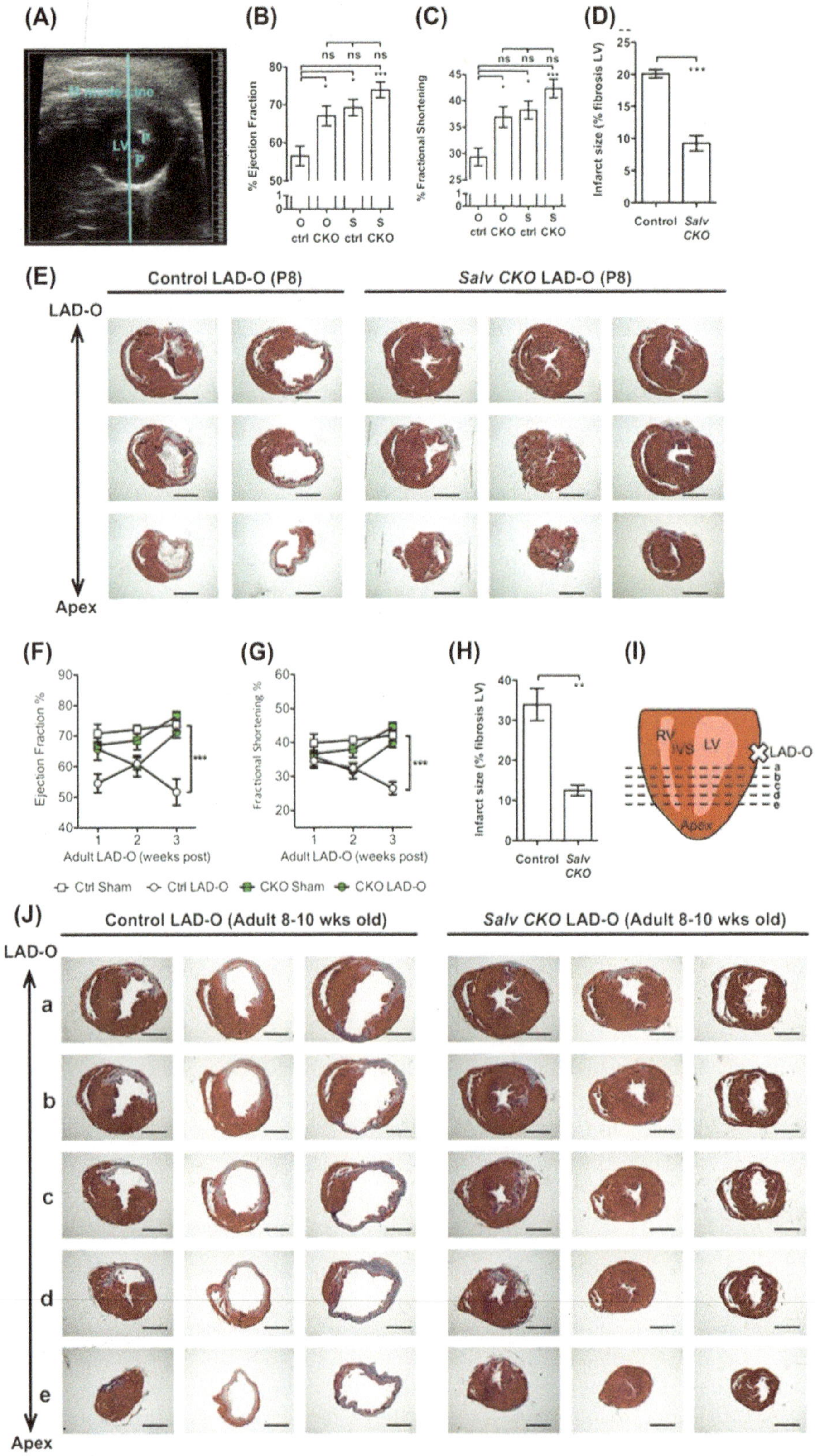

FIGURE 59.1 Cardiac regeneration and functional recovery after myocardial infarction. (A) B-mode echocardiographic image from representative 21-day postocclusion heart. *LV*, left ventricle; *P*, papillary muscle. (B and C) Ejection fraction (B) and fractional shortening (C) percentages of P8 LAD-O hearts. Occluded (O) and sham-operated (S) control (ctrl) and *Salv* CKO (CKO) hearts at 21–32 days postmyocardial infarction (dpmi). Ctrl/O ($n=7$), CKO/O ($n=9$), ctrl/S ($n=6$), CKO/S ($n=9$). Statistical analysis was by one-way ANOVA with the Bonferroni multiple comparison test. (D) Infarct surface area measurements were obtained from multiple specimens, and averages were calculated. Statistical analysis was by unpaired Student *t*-test. Control ($n=6$), *Salv* CKO ($n=8$). (E) Serial transverse sections of 4-week postocclusion hearts. (F and G) Ejection fraction (F) and fractional shortening (G) percentages of adult LAD-O hearts. 1 week: Ctrl Sham ($n=4$), Ctrl LAD-O ($n=6$), CKO Sham ($n=3$), CKO LAD-O ($n=3$); 2 weeks: Ctrl Sham ($n=3$), Ctrl LAD-O ($n=5$), CKO Sham ($n=3$), CKO LAD-O ($n=2$); 3 weeks: Ctrl Sham ($n=7$), Ctrl LAD-O ($n=7$), CKO Sham ($n=3$), CKO LAD-O ($n=5$). (H) Adult LAD-O infarct size 3 weeks postocclusion measured as percentage fibrosis of LV myocardium (total fibrotic area/total myocardial area × 100). Ctrl LAD-O ($n=6$), CKO LAD-O ($n=3$). Statistical analysis was by two-way ANOVA with the Bonferroni multiple comparison test. (I) Illustration of transverse section planes presented in J. Cross indicates plane of occlusion. *IVS*, interventricular septum; *LV*, left ventricle; *RV*, right ventricle. (J) Serial transverse sections of representative 3-week postocclusion adult hearts. All echocardiographic measurements were collected blind from genotype. Scale bars: 1 mm. $*P<.05$, $**P<.01$, $***P<.001$. *From T. Heallen, Y. Morikawa, J. Leach, et al., Hippo signaling impedes adult heart regeneration, Development 140 (2013) 4683–4690. Reproduced with permission.*

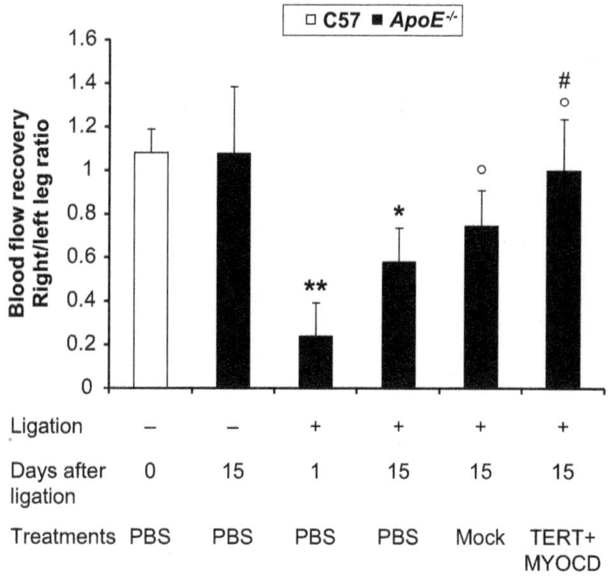

FIGURE 59.2 **Blood flow analysis in *ApoE*$^{-/-}$ mice with hind limb ischemia after the intramuscular injection of adipose tissue–derived mesenchymal stromal cells (AT-MSCs; from 12-month-old green fluorescent protein [GFP]–expressing mice) transduced with or without telomerase reverse transcriptase (TERT) and myocardin (MYOCD).** Hind limb ischemia was induced in 12-month-old *ApoE*$^{-/-}$ mice (ligation; $n=5$). The nonligated contralateral limb was used as a control (no ligation). Nonligated 12-month-old C57/BL6 (C57) mice ($n=3$) were also used as a control. Mice received an injection of phosphate-buffered saline (PBS) or AT-MSCs from 12-month-old mice expressing GFP (GFP+) that were either mock-transduced or transduced with TERT and MYOCD (TERT+MYOCD). Blood flow recovery is expressed as the ratio of the right (ischemic) leg to the left (nonischemic) leg. Graphs represent combined data from three independent experiments ($n=5$ mice per group); results are presented as the mean±SD. **$P<.01$ and *$P<.05$ versus PBS-treated *ApoE*$^{-/-}$ mice without ligation; °$P<.05$ versus PBS-treated *ApoE*$^{-/-}$ mice with ligation; #$P<.05$ versus *ApoE*$^{-/-}$ mice with ligation and treated with mock-transduced AT-MSCs. *From R. Madonna, D.A. Taylor, Y.J. Geng, et al., Transplantation of mesenchymal cells rejuvenated by the overexpression of telomerase and myocardin promotes revascularization and tissue repair in a murine model of hindlimb ischemia, Circ. Res. 113 (2013) 902–914. Reproduced with permission.*

mesenchymal stromal cells (MSCs) isolated from adipose or bone marrow tissues of older mice. Then, they tested the therapeutic efficacy of transplanted MSCs overexpressing myocardin, telomerase, and both together in a mouse model of hind limb ischemia. To this end, they transiently transduced MSCs from the adipose tissue or bone marrow of young (1 mo.) and older (12 mo.) male C57BL/6 apolipoprotein E-null mice with lentiviral vector(s) encoding telomerase, myocardin, or both. The results of flow cytometry and bromodeoxyuridine cell proliferation assays showed that transduction with telomerase and, to a lesser extent, myocardin, increased MSC viability and proliferation. In colony-forming assays, MSCs overexpressing telomerase and myocardin were more clonogenic than were mock-transduced MSCs. Fas-induced apoptosis was inhibited in MSCs overexpressing myocardin and telomerase. The authors showed that MSCs from older mice overexpressing telomerase, myocardin, or both increased myogenic marker expression, blood flow, and arteriogenesis when transplanted into the ischemic hind limb of apolipoprotein E-null mice (Fig. 59.2).

In another study, Mohsin et al. [12] isolated resident cardiac stem cells (CSCs) (c-kit cells) from human heart muscle biopsy samples of patients who had undergone left ventricular assist device implantation. The authors found that the senescence characteristics of the c-kit cells were ameliorated by the genetic modification of stem cells with Pim-1 kinase, which enhances cell proliferation, metabolic activity, differentiation, and prosurvival characteristics by preserving mitochondrial activity and antagonizing intrinsic apoptotic cascades.

These findings offer encouragement with regard to whether reducing senescence in human mesenchymal and c-kit cells might result in enhanced regenerative capacity when these cells are transplanted into injured, failing human hearts.

COMBINED STEM CELL THERAPIES IN ANIMALS WITH EXPERIMENTALLY INDUCED MYOCARDIAL INFARCTION

Williams et al. [13] have shown that combining human MSCs with c-kit myocardial–derived stem cells reduces infarct size more effectively than does either type of stem cell alone in pigs with experimentally induced MI. Immunosuppressed pigs were intramyocardially injected with combined human MSCs and c-kit human CSCs, c-kit CSCs alone, MSCs alone, or placebo in the infarct border zones 14 days after MI. Compared with placebo, each cell treatment reduced the size of the experimentally induced MI ($P < .05$), but the reduction in infarct size was twofold greater with the combination cell therapy than with either therapy alone ($P < .05$). In addition to reducing infarct size, the combination cell therapy significantly improved left ventricle (LV) chamber compliance ($P < .01$) and LV contractility ($P < .05$). The LV ejection fraction was restored to baseline in cell-treated pigs but remained depressed in the placebo-treated group ($P < .05$).

The hypothesis that a combination of human bone-marrow–derived MSCs and cardiac-derived c-kit cells enhances LV contractility and reduces the risk of future clinical adverse events will be tested in patients with ischemic cardiomyopathy in an NHLBI-sponsored clinical trial (the "Concert Trial").

REPEATED INJECTION OF C-KIT STEM CELLS IN A MOUSE MODEL OF MYOCARDIAL INFARCTION

Tokita et al. [14] have recently shown that administering three separate injections of c-kit stem cells several weeks apart improves LV contractility and reduces LV infarct size in mice with experimentally induced MI. These findings suggest that repeated injections of a potent stem cell preparation may have clinical value in enhancing the effectiveness of stem cells and the regenerative potential of the heart. This observation will be evaluated in humans with ischemic cardiomyopathy in the near future.

STEM CELL STUDIES IN PATIENTS WITH CARDIOVASCULAR DISEASE

In the last 15 years, clinical research studies have been conducted in patients with all types of cardiovascular disease: first in patients with MI, ischemic cardiomyopathy, or nonischemic cardiomyopathy, and later in patients with peripheral vascular disease or cerebrovascular disease. To date, the most promising results have been seen in patients with chronic coronary heart disease and significant LV dysfunction (i.e., ischemic cardiomyopathy). Below are three examples of studies that have created considerable optimism about future clinical research in stem cell therapy and the possibility of identifying cell regimens that will benefit humans with cardiovascular disease.

A Phase II Dose-Escalation Study of Allogeneic Mesenchymal Precursor Cells in Patients With Ischemic or Nonischemic Heart Failure

In a phase II dose-escalation study, Perin et al. [8] administered allogeneic mesenchymal precursor cells (MPCs) from a young donor in doses of 25, 75, or 150 million cells to 60 patients with ischemic or nonischemic cardiomyopathy. Each cohort comprised 20 patients: 15 who were injected transendocardially with cells and 5 who were treated with mock procedures. Safety measures for the allogeneic administration of MPCs included antibody testing, and secondary efficacy end points included major adverse cardiac events (MACE: cardiac death, MI, or revascularization), left ventricular imaging, and other clinical-event surrogates. Safety and MACE were evaluated for up to 3 years. No clinically symptomatic immune responses were identified. In a post hoc analysis of heart failure–related MACE, these events were significantly less frequent in the 150m MPC group (0/15) than in the mock-treated group (5/15, 33%), the 25 m cell-treated group (3/15, 20%), or the 75 m cell-treated group (6/15, 40%). In addition, the 150 m cell-treated group had a higher MACE-free survival rate than did all other groups for >3 years ($P = .025$ for the 150 m cell-treated group vs. controls) (Fig. 59.3).

A Study of Cardiac c-kit Stem Cells in Patients With Ischemic Cardiomyopathy Trial

Bolli et al. [15] conducted the Stem Cell Infusion in Patients with Ischemic Cardiomyopathy trial, a phase I randomized open-label trial of c-kit CSCs in patients with postinfarction LV dysfunction (LV ejection fraction ≤40%) who underwent coronary bypass grafting. Autologous CSCs were isolated from the right atrial appendage and reinfused by the intracoronary route at approximately 4 months after surgery. Control patients received no treatment beyond standard medical practice. In Stage A, nine treated and four control patients were consecutively enrolled for the assessment of the short-term safety of the CSCs. In Stage B, patients were randomly assigned to the treatment or control arm in a 2:3 ratio. Primary safety and secondary efficacy end points were evaluated at specific time points after enrollment. In 16 treated patients, no CSC-related adverse events were observed. LV ejection fraction increased from $30 \pm 1.9\%$ before CSC infusion to $38.5 \pm 2.8\%$ at 4 months after infusion ($P = .001$). Regional wall motion score index also improved significantly ($P = .005$), as did NYHA functional class, which decreased from 2.19 ± 0.16 to 1.63 ± 0.16 in the treated patients.

EP activity during culture and tissue development. This work allows for real-time EP evaluation as cellular constructs used in regenerative medicine that are developed and grown in vitro. Response to drug therapies can also be studied in this model, gaining insight to how cultured cells being utilized in the treatment of heart failure may respond to current and investigative drug therapies [10].

STEM CELLS AND NANOTECHNOLOGY

Stem cell used in the field of regenerative medicine is expected to revolutionize the care of patients with heart failure. Nanotechnology is providing additional capabilities into the production, evaluation, and utility of these cells. The production of stem cells for use in treatment of heart failure requires the assurance that pluripotent cells are not included in the culture, as they are at risk for malignant transformation. A labor intense process that involves injection of stem cells into an SCID mouse followed by 3 months of observation and then sacrifice to look for pluripotent cells is currently used and remains insensitive and time-consuming. A novel application of nanotechnology was recently reported by Xu et al. at Emory University. This work utilized gold nanoparticles with an enhanced form of spectroscopy called Raman scattering to identify potential pluripotent cells. Raman scattering of incident light can provide a molecular fingerprint of a molecule. The customized nanoparticles were labeled with antibodies characteristic of pluripotent cells and then incubated with regular myocytes and pluripotent cells (Fig. 60.3). Analysis by Raman spectroscopy yielded a greater than 10,000-fold increase in sensitivity, being able to detect a single abnormal (pluripotent) cell from a million normal myocytes. This represents an application of nanotechnology that will aid in the therapies that can be used for heart disease [11]. The application of stem cells for treatment of heart failure will require extensive physiologic testing. To investigate the electrophysiologic properties of stem cells, Lin and colleagues have developed a vertical nanopillar electrode than can record intracellular action potentials from multiple beating cardiomyocytes [12]. This nanotechnology allows for baseline EP studies, responses to drugs, and evaluates for possible arrhythmias in the stem cell culture prior to use in man (Fig. 60.4). Nanotechnology is also used for the production of unique scaffolds for stem cell growth to be used in regenerative medicine therapies [13–15].

NANOTECHNOLOGY USED IN THE STUDY OF MYOCELLULAR CONTRACTILITY

Actin–myosin interaction and force generation are key to myocardial function and central to the pathophysiology of heart failure. A nano approach to investigation of actin–myosin physiology allows for research to be done at the level of the individual molecule, with the potential to increase the understanding of both normal physiology and the diseased state of the myocardium. Hariadi and colleagues developed a DNA nanoscaffold for studying actin–myosin behavior. Direct visualization of actin filament gliding, recognizing that changes in cross-bridge compliance that influences gliding speed, with myosin ensembles serving as energy reservoirs (Fig. 60.5) [16].

Liu and colleagues evaluated the nanomechanical features of living, single cardiomyocytes, quantitatively measuring torsions, contractions, and calcium intensity using an atomic force cantilever, part of atomic force microscopy [9].

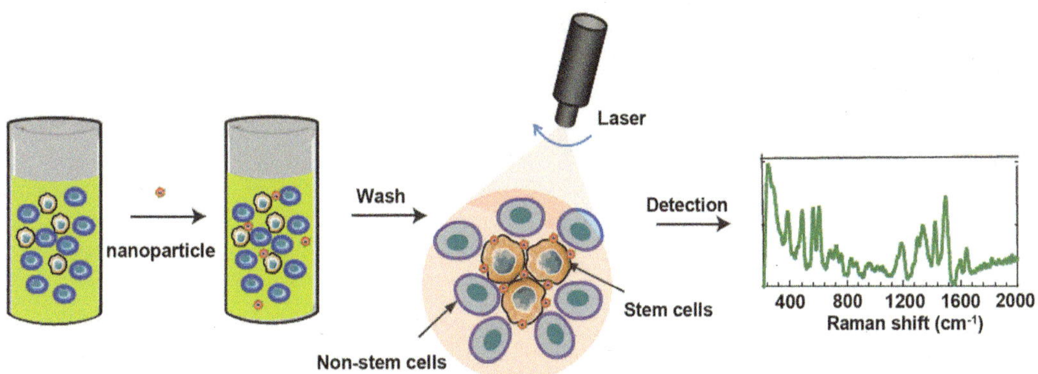

FIGURE 60.3 SERS (surface-enhanced Raman scattering) assay for detection of pluripotent cells: a culture of differentiated cells is incubated with a nanoparticle that will attach to residual pluripotent cells, nanoparticles that do not attach are washed away, and then SERS signals are detected via a laser and the SERS spectra are analyzed to detect pluripotent cells.

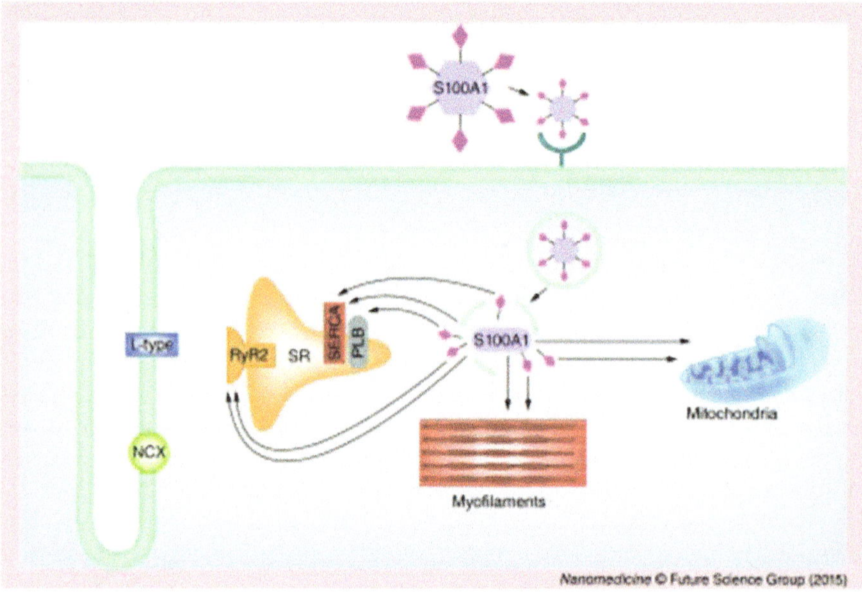

FIGURE 60.4 Diagram of the S100A1 nanoparticle entering a myocyte: the polyketal nanoparticle has been decorated with N-acetyl glucosamine and S100A1 placed as a payload. The nanoparticle is endocytosed into the myocyte and degrades on entry, releasing the payload of S100A1. Physiologic effects are seen on the mitochondria, myofilaments, SERCA, ryanodine receptor2, and phospholamban.

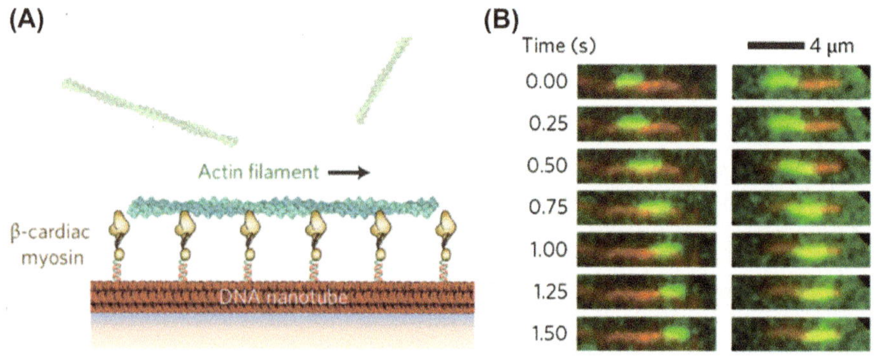

FIGURE 60.5 (A) Schematic of nanotube filament motility assay for actin–myosin model of contraction. (B) Time-lapsed images of actin filaments in green moving along human cardiac myosin labeled nanotubes in red.

The atomic force microscope (Fig. 60.1) was a milestone in nanotechnology development that occurred in the 1980's as the scanning tunneling instrument was also being invented. Drug-induced changes in contractility and force generation at the nanonewton level were determined for the individual myocyte. This type of nano research will allow a greater understanding of force generation within the myocyte, the pathophysiology of heart failure, and can serve as a model for in vitro drug development and testing.

NANOPARTICLES

Nanoparticles can be used for diagnostics and therapeutic applications in heart disease. The opportunity for drug delivery has been well recognized, as nanoparticles can be loaded with therapeutic drugs and delivered to a specific site or organ. An example of this application can be seen when investigators aimed to get a calcium handling molecule (S100A) into myocytes as a potential therapeutic agent. It remained challenging to get this protein across the cell membrane into the myocyte. Wagner and colleagues developed a nanoparticle that can specifically attach to cardiac cells, and then cross the cell membrane, bringing in the payload of S100A [17]. Once inside the cell, the nanoparticle dissolves and releases the payload of S100A. They further went on to identify increased contractility in the rat myocyte following delivery of S100A into the cytoplasm. Nanotechnology will increasingly play a role in drug development and delivery for heart failure therapeutics. New therapeutic agents will be designed and tested using nano techniques to speed development, enhance in vitro testing, and improve the potential for faster development time lines to get drugs from concept to market.

Quantum dots are semiconductor nanoparticles that possess a number of unique optical and electric properties that include size-tunable light emission, narrow emission range, high brightness, and photo stability. They represent a new class of fluorescent labels for molecular imaging and biologic diagnostics, including imaging at the single molecule level. Enhanced cardiac imaging research utilizing QD's is currently underway [18–20].

Other nanotechnogies that will impact heart failure and treatment of cardiac disease include the following:

The use of intracorporeal energy and movement to drive electricity production via nano-based generators, these nano-piezoelectronic devices can be used to generate energy to power cardiac devices [21,22]. Cardiac surgery may benefit from improved wound healing and nano approaches to postoperative bleeding [23,24]. A nano-based ablation utilizing a designed nanoparticle (superparamagnetic nanoparticle that releases a toxic payload when a specific wavelength of laser is delivered) that can destroy cells of interest, while leaving cells a few nanometers away completely intact [25], Fig. 60.6.

CONCLUSION

Nanotechnology, nanoscience, and nanomedicine are interrelated fields of science that focus on the study and manipulation of matter at the molecular and supramolecular level. They represent a new set of research tools and clinical applications that will revolutionize science and medicine. The field of nanoscience is in its infancy despite is having an impact in all areas of scientific endeavor. As we look forward to the next 20 years and beyond for advances in the care of children with heart disease, novel technologies developed through nanomedicine can be expected to change how we care for our patients. These enabling technologies will contribute to our understanding and treatment of heart failure in children and adults for years to come. From a greater understanding of the molecular functioning of the myocyte, to the ability to detect the earliest evidence of rejection of a transplanted heart, to the end of suture material for cardiac surgery, changes will take place at an accelerating rate with application of nanotechnologies. It will be incumbent on the physicians practicing pediatric cardiology/heart failure to help drive this research and ensure that the new technologies are applied.

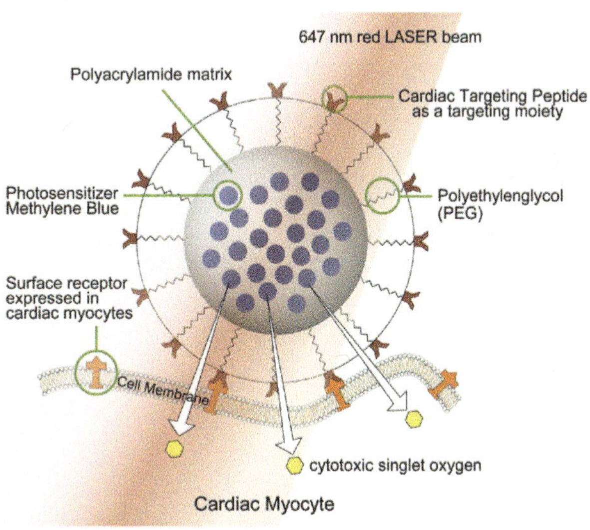

FIGURE 60.6 Schematic of a photodynamic nanoparticle: the nanoparticle attaches in a cell-specific manner to cardiac myocytes. When a 647 nm laser is illuminated on the nanoparticle, the inserted methylene blue is activated and cytotoxic singlet oxygen is released into the attached cardiac myocyte causing cell death.

REFERENCES

[1] Engineering and Science, California Institute of Technology Magazine, February 1960.

[2] N. Taniguchi, On the basic concept of 'nano-technology', in: Proceedings of the International Conference on Production Engineering, Tokyo, 1974, Part II. Japan Society of Precision Engineering, 1974.

[3] Nano.gov.

[4] A. Zhang, Lieber, Nano-bioelectronics, Chem. Rev. 116 (1) (2016) 215–257.

[5] L. Yang, Y. Li, Y. Fang, Nanodevices for cellular interfaces and electrophysiological recording, Adv. Mater. 25 (2013) 3881–3887.

[6] B. Tian, C.M. Lieber, Design, synthesis, and characterization of novel nanowire structures for photovoltaics and intracellular probes, Pure Appl. Chem. 83 (2011) 2153–2169.

[7] T. Cohen-Karni, C.M. Lieber, Nanowire nanoelectronics: building interfaces with tissue and cells at the natural scale of biology, Pure Appl. Chem. 85 (2013) 883–901.

[8] T.W. Barrett, N. Radha Shanmugam, A.P. Selvam, S.C. Kazmierczak, S. Prasad, Novel nanomonitor ultra-sensitive detection of troponin T., Clin. Chim. Acta 10 (442) (2015) 96–101.

[9] Y. Liu, J. Feng, L. Shi, R. Niu, Q. Sun, H. Liu, J. Li, J. Guo, J. Zhu, D. Han, In situ mechanical analysis of cardiomyocytes at nano scales, Nanoscale (4) (2012) 99–102.

[10] X. Dai, W. Zhou, T. Gao, J. Liu, C.M. Lieber, Three-dimensional mapping and regulation of action potential propagation in nanoelectronics-innervated tissues, Nat. Nanotechnol. 11 (2016) 776–782.

[11] J. Han, X. Qian, Q. Wu, R. Jha, J. Dua, Z. Yang, K.O. Maher, S. Nie, C. Xu, Novel surface-enhanced Raman scattering-based assays for ultra-sensitive detection of human pluripotent stem cells, Biomaterials 105 (2016) 66–76.

[12] Z.C. Lin, A.F. McGuire, P.W. Burridge, E. Matsa, H.-Y. Lou, J.C. Wu, B. Cui, Accurate nanoelectrode recording of human pluripotent stem cell-derived cardiomyocytes for assaying drugs and modeling disease, Microsyst. Nanoeng. (2017) 16080.

[13] A. Kumar, A. Patel, L. Duvalsaint, M. Desai, E.D. Marks, Thymosin β4 coated nanofiber scaffolds for the repair of damaged cardiac tissue, J. Nanobiotechnol. 12 (2014) 10.

[14] B. Gorain, M. Tekade, P. Kesharwani, A.K. Iyer, K. Kalia, R.K. Tekade, The use of nanoscaffolds and dendrimers in tissue engineering, Drug Discov. Today 12 (4) (February 2017) 652–664 (Online).

[15] S. Fleischer, M. Shevach, R. Feiner, T. Dvir, Coiled fiber scaffolds embedded with gold nanoparticles improve the performance of engineered cardiac tissues, Nanoscale 6 (2014) 9410–9414.

[16] R.F. Hariadi, R.F. Sommese, A.S. Adhikari, R.E. Taylor, S. Sutton, J.A. Spudich, S. Sivaramakrishnan, Mechanical coordination in motor ensembles revealed using engineered artificial myosin filaments, Nat. Nanotechnol. 10 (2015) 696–700.

[17] J.T. Maxwell, I. Somasuntharam, W.D. Gray, M. Shen, J.M. Singer, B. Wang, T. Saafir, B.H. Crawford, R. Jiang, N. Murthy, M.E. Davis, M.B. Wagner, Bioactive nanoparticles improve calcium handling in failing cardiac myocytes, Nanomedicine 10 (22) (November 2015) 3343–3357.

[18] B.A. Kairdolf, A.M. Smith, T.H. Stokes, M.D. Wang, A.N. Young, S. Nie, Semiconductor quantum dots for bioimaging and biodiagnostic applications, Annu. Rev. Anal. Chem. 6 (2013) 143–162.

[19] R. Bilan, I. Nabiev, A. Sukhanova, Quantum dot-based nanotools for bioimaging, diagnostics, and drug delivery, ChemBioChem 17 (2016) 2103–2114.

[20] J. Liab, J.-J. Zhu, Quantum dots for fluorescent biosensing and bio-imaging applications, Analyst 138 (2013) 2506–2515.

[21] T. Il Lee, S. Lee, E. Lee, S. Sohn, et al., High-power density piezoelectric energy harvesting using radially strained ultrathin trigonal tellurium nanowire assembly, Adv. Mater. (2013) 1–6.

[22] X. Wang, Piezoelectric nanogenerators—harvesting ambient mechanical energy at the nanometer scale, Nano Energy 1 (1) (2012) 13–24.

[23] K.H.L. Kwan, X.L. Liu, M.K.T. To, K.W.K. Yeung, C.M. Ho, K.K.Y. Wong, Modulation of collagen alignment by silver nanoparticles results in better mechanical properties in wound healing, Nanomed. Nanotechnol. Biol. Med. 7 (4) (2011) 497–504.

[24] A. Meddahi-Pellé1, A. Legrand, A. Marcellan, Organ repair, hemostasis, and in vivo bonding of medical devices by aqueous solutions of nanoparticles, Chem. Int. 53 (25) (2014) 6369–6373.

[25] U.M.R. Avula, G. Kim, et al., Cell-specific nanoplatform-enabled photodynamic therapy for cardiac cells, Heart Rhythm 9 (9) (September 2012) 1504–1509.

Chapter 61

Nutritional Assessment and Management in Pediatric Heart Failure

Chitra Ravishankar
Children's Hospital of Philadelphia, Philadelphia, PA, United States

Issues related to nutrition and growth have received considerable attention in children with congenital heart defects (CHD), particularly in those with single ventricle physiology [1,2]. Similarly, there is a growing body of literature on the impact of nutritional status and body habitus on outcomes in children with heart failure. The impact of body habitus on posttransplant survival remains controversial.

ETIOLOGY

The etiology of poor growth in children with heart failure is due to an imbalance between supply (energy intake) and demand (energy consumption). In its most extreme form, it leads to "Cardiac Cachexia." Factors that may contribute to a decrease in energy intake include the following:

- Difficulty in eating due to tachypnea and dyspnea.
- Loss of appetite, early satiety and abdominal discomfort from hepatomegaly, mesenteric ischemia, and ascites.
- Malabsorption from edema of the gastrointestinal tract.
- Gastroesophageal reflux disease.
- Medically imposed fluid restriction.

Consumption of energy may be increased due to the following factors:

- Tachypnea, dyspnea, tachycardia, and diaphoresis.
- Inflammation and catabolism from activation of neuroendocrine system.

ASSESSMENT OF NUTRITIONAL STATUS

Nutritional status is usually assessed in children using anthropometric measurements such as weight, height or length, weight-for-length, and body mass index (BMI). Other measurements such as midarm and calf circumference are rarely used in children with heart failure. There is value in serially monitoring serum albumin and prealbumin levels in children with heart failure especially to assess the effectiveness of nutritional intervention [3,4]. In adults with chronic disease, several screening tools are available to assess nutritional status. One such tool is the Mini Nutritional Assessment (MNA) tool, which has been validated across the world in elderly patients with chronic disease, and has been especially useful in identifying patients at risk for malnutrition [5]. The MNA is an 18 item tool that has four sections: general status, anthropometrics, dietary aspects, and subjective assessment (Fig. 61.1). Anthropometrics include weight, height, BMI, midarm circumference, and midcalf circumference. A score of 24–30 is indicative of a normal nutritional status, 17–23.5 at risk for malnutrition, and <17 is indicative of malnourished status. This tool may have a role in monitoring adolescents in heart failure.

PREVALENCE OF MALNUTRITION AND OVERWEIGHT

In a study of 154 adults with advanced heart failure with a mean ejection fraction of <20% referred for evaluation for placement of a ventricular assist device or heart transplantation, only 10% were classified as normal using the MNA tool [6]. Nearly a quarter of these patients were malnourished and the remainder were in the "at-risk" group. In a retrospective

Heart Failure in the Child and Young Adult. http://dx.doi.org/10.1016/B978-0-12-802393-8.00061-2

Nestlé NutritionInstitute

Mini Nutritional Assessment MNA®

Last name: First name:

Sex: Age: Weight, kg: Height, cm: Date:

Complete the screen by filling in the boxes with the appropriate numbers. Add the numbers for the screen. If score is 11 or less, continue with the assessment to gain a Malnutrition Indicator Score.

Screening

A Has food intake declined over the past 3 months due to loss of appetite, digestive problems, chewing or swallowing difficulties?

0 = severe decrease in food intake
1 = moderate decrease in food intake
2 = no decrease in food intake ☐

B Weight loss during the last 3 months

0 = weight loss greater than 3kg (6.6lbs)
1 = does not know
2 = weight loss between 1 and 3kg (2.2 and 6.6 lbs)
3 = no weight loss ☐

C Mobility

0 = bed or chair bound
1 = able to get out of bed / chair but does not go out
2 = goes out ☐

D Has suffered psychological stress or acute disease in the past 3 months?

0 = yes 2 = no ☐

E Neuropsychological problems

0 = severe dementia or depression
1 = mild dementia
2 = no psychological problems ☐

F Body Mass Index (BMI) (weight in kg) / (height in m²)

0 = BMI less than 19
1 = BMI 19 to less than 21
2 = BMI 21 to less than 23
3 = BMI 23 or greater ☐

Screening score ☐☐
(subtotal max. 14 points)

12-14 points: Normal nutritional status
8-11 points: At risk of malnutrition
0-7 points: Malnourished

For a more in-depth assessment, continue with questions G-R

Assessment

G Lives independently (not in nursing home or hospital)

1 = yes 0 = no ☐

H Takes more than 3 prescription drugs per day

0 = yes 1 = no ☐

I Pressure sores or skin ulcers

0 = yes 1 = no ☐

J How many full meals does the patient eat daily?

0 = 1 meal
1 = 2 meals
2 = 3 meals ☐

K Selected consumption markers for protein intake

- At least one serving of dairy products (milk, cheese, yoghurt) per day yes ☐ no ☐
- Two or more servings of legumes or eggs per week yes ☐ no ☐
- Meat, fish or poultry every day yes ☐ no ☐

0.0 = if 0 or 1 yes
0.5 = if 2 yes
1.0 = if 3 yes ☐.☐

L Consumes two or more servings of fruit or vegetables per day?

0 = no 1 = yes ☐

M How much fluid (water, juice, coffee, tea, milk...) is consumed per day?

0.0 = less than 3 cups
0.5 = 3 to 5 cups
1.0 = more than 5 cups ☐.☐

N Mode of feeding

0 = unable to eat without assistance
1 = self-fed with some difficulty
2 = self-fed without any problem ☐

O Self view of nutritional status

0 = views self as being malnourished
1 = is uncertain of nutritional state
2 = views self as having no nutritional problem ☐

P In comparison with other people of the same age, how does the patient consider his / her health status?

0.0 = not as good
0.5 = does not know
1.0 = as good
2.0 = better ☐.☐

Q Mid-arm circumference (MAC) in cm

0.0 = MAC less than 21
0.5 = MAC 21 to 22
1.0 = MAC 22 or greater ☐.☐

R Calf circumference (CC) in cm

0 = CC less than 31
1 = CC 31 or greater ☐

Assessment (max. 16 points) ☐☐.☐

Screening score ☐☐.☐

Total Assessment (max. 30 points) ☐☐.☐

Malnutrition Indicator Score

24 to 30 points	☐	normal nutritional status
17 to 23.5 points	☐	at risk of malnutrition
Less than 17 points	☐	malnourished

Ref. Vellas B, Villars H, Abellan G, et al. *Overview of MNA®- Its History and Challenges.* J Nut Health Aging 2006; 10: 456-465.
Rubenstein LZ, Harker JO, Salva A, Guigoz Y, Vellas B, Screening for Undernutrition in Geriatric Practice: *Developing the Short-Form Mini Nutritional Assessment (MNA-SF).* J. Geront 2001; 56A: M366-377.
Guigoz Y. The Mini-Nutritional Assessment (MNA®) *Review of the Literature – What does it tell us?* J Nutr Health Aging 2006; 10: 466-487.

For more information: www.mna-elderly.com

FIGURE 61.1 Sample of Mini Nutritional Assessment form. *(Copyright by The American Society for Parenteral and Enteral Nutrition.)*

analysis of 165 children with dilated cardiomyopathy (CM) managed with medical therapy at a single center in Brazil, the mean age at presentation was 2.2±3.2 years, and 80% were in New York Heart Association (NYHA) 3 or 4 [7]. At initial diagnosis, a third of these children were malnourished with a weight-for-age z-score (WAZ) <−2 or below the fifth percentile. During a mean follow-up period of 3.6±4.2 years, WAZ fell below 2 in an additional 27.5%.

In a retrospective analysis of the Organ Procurement and Transplantation Network (OPTN) database of children 2–18 years of age listed for heart transplantation between 1997 and 2011, BMI percentile was calculated at the time of listing [8]. Nutritional groups were classified as follows: BMI 5%–85% normal, <5% underweight, <1% severe wasting, 85%–95% overweight, and >95% obese. The study cohort included 2712 subjects with a median age of 11 years (IQR 6, 11) and a diagnosis of CM in 61% subjects. For the whole group, BMI was normal in 59%, whereas 8% were underweight and 10% were severely malnourished. In a similar analysis of over 4000 children from the United Network of Organ Sharing (UNOS) database listed for heart transplantation between 1995 and 2012, BMI was <5% in 17.4% of subjects [9]. In the underweight group, there was a higher proportion of subjects with a diagnosis of CHD. The proportion of malnutrition decreased over time with 21% being underweight from 1995 to 1999 as opposed to 14% in the most recent era from 2010 to 2012 ($P<.0001$). This may suggest earlier recognition and management of heart failure, including nutritional intervention in the most recent era. In another analysis of the OPTN database of infants less than 2 years of age listed for heart transplantation, 203/1653 (12%) had moderate to severe wasting as defined as weight/height <80% of idealized body weight [10].

DESCRIPTION OF OVERWEIGHT AND OBESITY

As the prevalence of overweight and obesity has increased nationwide, several investigators have studied its prevalence in children listed for heart transplantation and its impact on survival before and after transplantation. Analysis of both the OPTN and United Network of Organ Sharing (UNOS) databases demonstrates a prevalence of obesity (BMI >95%) of 13–14% and overweight (BMI 85%–95%) of 11% at the time of listing among 2- to 18-year-old children listed for heart transplantation [8,9]. Similar to other epidemiologic studies, obesity was more commonly seen among African–American subjects and those of lower socioeconomic status [9]. At the time of listing, 15% of children with CM were obese compared with 9% of those with CHD [8].

IMPACT OF NUTRITIONAL STATUS ON OUTCOMES

In the study from Brazil of 165 children with dilated CM managed medically (without transplantation as a treatment option), WAZ was −0.62±1.43 for survivors during 3 years of follow-up compared with −2.02±1.12 for nonsurvivors ($P<.0001$, Fig. 61.2) [7]. Similarly, malnutrition has been shown to be associated with increase in waitlist mortality in children listed for heart transplantation. Moderate or severe wasting (defined as weight/height <80% idealized body weight) has been independently associated with waitlist mortality in young infants awaiting heart transplantation [10]. Findings were similar in older children between 3 and 18 years of age with higher early waitlist mortality of 16.6% among underweight children (BMI <5%) as opposed to 11.4% among normal weight children [9]. In risk-adjusted multivariable analysis, underweight was independently associated with mortality within 2 months of listing (odds ratio 1.4, 95% CI 0.7–2.2). These findings are consistent with the obesity paradox with obese patients having lower waitlist mortality than undernourished patients

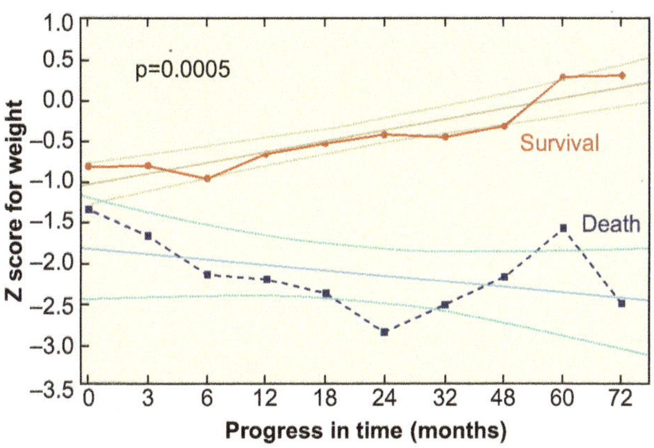

FIGURE 61.2 Impact of weight-for-age z-score on survival in children with dilated cardiomyopathy in Brazil. *(Modified from: V.M. Azevedo, F.M. Albanesi Filho, M.A. Santos, M.B. Castier, B.R. Tura, The impact of malnutrition on idiopathic dilated cardiomyopathy in children. J. Pediatr. (Rio J.) 80 (2004) 211–216.)*

[11–13]. However, the impact of nutrition on outcome does differ by diagnosis. Nutritional status has the biggest impact on children with CM with the highest waitlist mortality among both the severely malnourished (BMI <1%) and obese children [8]. The impact of severe wasting on waitlist mortality for children with CM is not an unexpected finding and is probably reflective of cardiac cachexia in the setting of decompensated heart failure.

There are conflicting data regarding the effect of nutritional status on posttransplant outcomes after heart transplantation in children. In single center studies, both malnutrition (BMI <5%) and obesity (BMI >95%) have been associated with worse survival [14,15]. However, in an analysis of the International Society of Heart and Lung Transplantation database, nutritional status at the time of transplantation was not associated with 1-year or 5-year survival, postoperative length of stay, or adverse events such as infections, stroke, dialysis, or reoperation [16]. Similarly, in the most recent analysis of the UNOS database, BMI did not affect posttransplant mortality in unadjusted analysis. In risk-adjusted multivariable analysis, obesity was associated with borderline higher mortality (odds ratio 1.7, 95% confidence intervals 1–3). Even though immediate postoperative outcomes did not differ across BMI groups, freedom from complications such as diabetes, hypertension, hyperlipidemia, rejection, and renal insufficiency was poorer among the obese children [9].

INTERVENTIONS

Similar to children with CHD and other chronic problems, attention should be paid to nutritional status in children who present with heart failure, with ongoing nutritional surveillance. Many of these children are undernourished at presentation and may require dietary supplementation along with treatment of congestive heart failure. A registered dietician should ideally be part of the multidisciplinary team. Significant feeding issues including vomiting and abdominal pain are quite common with decompensated heart failure, and symptoms may improve with escalation of therapy including initiation of vasoactive medications and/or mechanical ventilation (Fig. 61.3). In the more recent era, feeding intolerance despite escalation

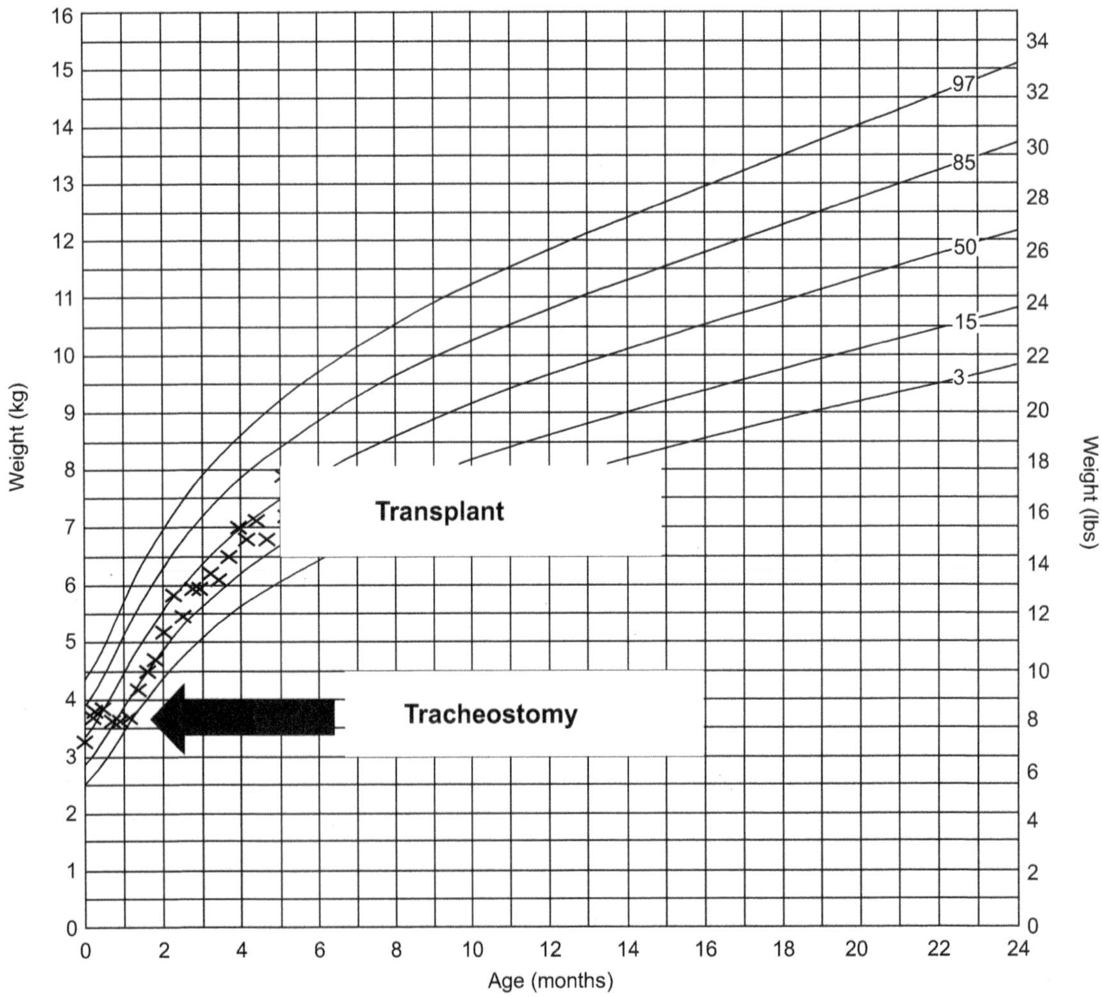

FIGURE 61.3 Impact of tracheostomy on weight in an infant with decompensated heart failure.

of medical therapy may be considered an indication for initiating mechanical circulatory support. Supplementation with nasogastric tube feeds or in the most severe cases nasojejunal feeds should be considered early to provide adequate enteral nutrition. Parenteral nutrition may be required in those with decompensated heart failure with persistent low cardiac output and in the immediate postoperative period after institution of mechanical circulatory support.

Children with heart failure irrespective of nutritional status are often deconditioned. Physical and psychological rehabilitation play an important role especially for children listed for transplantation and those on mechanical circulatory support. For the overweight patients, encouraging healthy dietary habits and physical rehabilitation should be pursued while under medical surveillance before and after transplantation to mitigate the morbidity associated with persistent obesity after transplantation.

CONCLUSION

Undernutrition is associated with worse survival in children with heart failure particularly in children with CM. This underscores the importance of including nutritional surveillance and intervention while managing children with heart failure. Obesity has not been associated with worse early outcome after heart transplantation. Similar to adults, the obesity paradox exists in children, and obesity should not be considered a contraindication to listing for heart transplantation.

REFERENCES

[1] D.T. Hsu, V. Zak, L. Mahony, L.A. Sleeper, A.M. Atz, J.C. Levine, et al., Pediatric heart network investigators. Enalapril in infants with single ventricle: results of a multicenter randomized trial, Circulation 122 (2010) 333–340.

[2] P.T. Burch, E. Gerstenberger, C. Ravishankar, D.A. Hehir, R.R. Davies, S.D. Colan, et al., Pediatric heart network investigators. Longitudinal assessment of growth in hypoplastic left heart syndrome: results from the single ventricle reconstruction trial, J. Am. Heart Assoc. 3 (2014) e000079.

[3] B.R. Don, G. Kaysen, Serum albumin: relationship to inflammation and nutrition, Semin. Dial. 17 (2004) 432–437.

[4] T.B. Horwich, K. Kalantar-Zadeh, R.W. MacLellan, G.C. Fonarow, Albumin levels predict survival in patients with systolic heart failure, Am. Heart J. 155 (2008) 883–889.

[5] J.M. Bauer, M.J. Kaiser, P. Anthony, Y. Guigoz, C.C. Sieber, The mini nutritional assessment–its history, today's practice, and future perspectives, Nutr. Clin. Pract. 23 (2008) 388–396.

[6] A. Aggarwal, A. Kumar, M.P. Gregory, C. Blair, S. Pauwaa, A.J. Tatooles, et al., Nutrition assessment in advanced heart failure patients evaluated for ventricular assist devices or cardiac transplantation, Nutr. Clin. Pract. 28 (2013) 112–119.

[7] V.M. Azevedo, F.M. Albanesi Filho, M.A. Santos, M.B. Castier, B.R. Tura, The impact of malnutrition on idiopathic dilated cardiomyopathy in children, J. Pediatr. (Rio J.) 80 (2004) 211–216.

[8] J. Godown, J.E. Donohue, S. Yu, J.M. Friedland-Little, R.J. Gajarski, K.R. Schumacher, Differential effect of body mass index on pediatric heart transplant outcomes based on diagnosis, Pediatr. Transplant. 18 (2014) 771–776.

[9] R.R. Davies, S. Haldeman, M.A. McCulloch, S.S. Gidding, C. Pizarro, Low body mass index is associated with increased waitlist mortality among children listed for heart transplant, J. Heart Lung Transplant. 34 (2015) 1462–1470.

[10] J. Godown, J.M. Friedland-Little, R.J. Gajarski, S. Yu, J.E. Donohue, K.R. Schumacher, Abnormal nutrition affects waitlist mortality in infants awaiting heart transplant, J. Heart Lung Transplant. 33 (2014) 235–240.

[11] T.B. Horwich, G.C. Fonarow, M.A. Hamilton, W.R. MacLellan, M.A. Woo, et al., The relationship between obesity and mortality in patients with heart failure, J. Am. Coll. Cardiol. 38 (2001) 789–795.

[12] J.P. Curtis, J.G. Selter, Y. Wang, S.S. Rathore, I.S. Jovin, F. Jadbabaie, et al., The obesity paradox: body mass index and outcomes in patients with heart failure, Arch. Intern. Med. 165 (2005) 55–61.

[13] C.J. Lavie, A. Sharma, M.A. Alpert, A. De Schutter, F. Lopez-Jimenez, R.V. Milani, et al., Update on obesity and obesity paradox in heart failure, Prog. Cardiovasc. Dis. 58 (2016) 393–400.

[14] J.W. Rossano, M.A. Grenier, W.J. Dreyer, J.J. Kim, J.F. Price, J.L. Jefferies, et al., Effect of body mass index on outcome in pediatric heart transplant patients, J. Heart Lung Transplant. 26 (2007) 718–723.

[15] B.D. Kaufman, M.L. Nagle, S.R. Levine, N. Vijaynathan, B.D. Hanna, S. Paridon, et al., Too fat or too thin? Body habitus assessment in children listed for heart transplant and impact on outcome, J. Heart Lung Transplant. 27 (2008) 508–513.

[16] B.D. Kaufman, S. Chuai, F. Dobbels, R.E. Shaddy, Wasting or obesity at time of transplant does not predict pediatric heart transplant outcomes: analysis of ISHLT pediatric heart transplant registry, J. Heart Lung Transplant. 28 (2009) 1273–1278.

Index

Note: "Page numbers with "f" and "t" indicate figures and tables".

B

C

D

E

H

I

K

L

M

N

Q

R

S

T

U

V